D1582262

Clinical Radiation Oncology

Clinical Radiation Oncology

Indications, Techniques, and Results

Third Edition

Editor

William Small Jr, MD, FACRO, FACR, FASTRO
Loyola University

Associate Editors

Nancy J. Tarbell, MD, FASTRO
Harvard Medical School

Min Yao MD, PhD
Case Western Reserve University

Section Editors

Jason A. Efstathiou, MD, DPhil
Massachusetts General Hospital

Minesh P. Mehta, MD, FASTRO
University of Maryland School of Medicine

William Small, Jr, MD, FACRO, FACR, FASTRO
Loyola University

Christopher G. Willett, MD, FASTRO
Duke University

Min Yao, MD, PhD
Case Western Reserve University

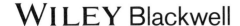

WILEY Blackwell

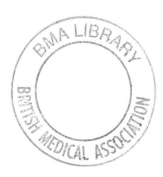

Registered Offices
John Wiley & Sons, Inc., 111 River Street, Hoboken, NJ 07030, USA
John Wiley & Sons Ltd, The Atrium, Southern Gate, Chichester, West Sussex, PO19 8SQ, UK

Editorial Office
9600 Garsington Road, Oxford, OX4 2DQ, UK

For details of our global editorial offices, customer services, and more information about Wiley products visit us at www.wiley.com.

Wiley also publishes its books in a variety of electronic formats and by print-on-demand. Some content that appears in standard print versions of this book may not be available in other formats.

Library of Congress Cataloging-in-Publication Data

Names: Small, William, Jr., editor. | Tarbell, Nancy J., 1951– editor. | Yao, Min (Radiation oncologist), editor.
Title: Clinical radiation oncology : indications, techniques, and results / editor, William Small, Jr. ; associate editors, Nancy J. Tarbell, Min Yao ; section editors, Jason A. Efstathiou, Minesh P. Mehta, William Small, Jr., Christopher G. Willett, Min Yao.
Description: Third edition. | Hoboken, NJ : John Wiley & Sons, Inc., 2017. | Includes bibliographical references and index.
Identifiers: LCCN 2016039773 (print) | LCCN 2016040775 (ebook) | ISBN 9780470905524 (cloth) | ISBN 9781119341215 (pdf) | ISBN 9781119341352 (epub)
Subjects: | MESH: Neoplasms–radiotherapy | Radiation Oncology–methods
Classification: LCC RC271.R3 (print) | LCC RC271.R3 (ebook) | NLM QZ 269 | DDC 616.99/40642–dc23
LC record available at https://lccn.loc.gov/2016039773

Set in 10/12pt WarnockPro by Aptara Inc., New Delhi, India

Printed in the United States of America

10 9 8 7 6 5 4 3 2 1

Contents

Dedication

We dedicate this book in loving memory of Dr C.C. Wang (English pronunciation Wong), a gifted clinician, researcher and an outstanding teacher, mentor, and friend and clearly one of the great figures in the history of our field.

Chiu-Chen, always known as 'C.C.', arrived in the US in 1949 from Canton, China. He was a brilliant and energetic young physician who spent his first year in the US as a medical intern at the University Hospital in Syracuse, NY. He then was admitted to the Department of Radiology at Massachusetts General Hospital (MGH) in 1950, with the encouragement of his older brother, Dr C.A. Wang, an accomplished Professor of Surgery at Harvard and an endocrine surgeon at MGH.

C.C.'s academic career skyrocketed when he reached the MGH and Harvard. Within 20 years, he became Professor of Radiation Oncology at Harvard Medical School and the Clinical Director of the Department under Dr Herman Suit at the MGH. He had a particular interest and expertise in malignancies of the head and neck region and he was world-renowned for his work in this area. Dr Wang was awarded the ASTRO Gold Medal.

He was an inspiration for all of us who knew and worked with him. He changed the treatment of patients with cancer in a profound way. He cured thousands of patients during his career, and I still meet their children and grandchildren who ask me about the legendary Dr Wang. He was always optimistic, telling his patients that 'C.C.' stood for 'cure cancer'. His sense of humor usually led to one of his still-talked-about Chinese aphorisms. For example in identifying the clinical target volume, "…you cannot hit a home run if you do not see the ball", or, on the importance of treating only the tumor, "…you do not burn down a house to kill a mosquito."

In 2005, the C.C. Wang Professorship at Harvard Medical School was established in his honor. I am humbled and grateful to be the first incumbent of the chair named after this very special physician.

C.C. was a devoted husband and father. His daughter, Janice a Harvard Medical School graduate, survives him. C.C. was also an expert gardener. It was a special honor to receive a cantaloupe from his fruit and vegetable garden.

He is still loved and deeply missed by his trainees, his patients, and by all of us who were fortunate to have called 'C.C.' our friend. A day doesn't go by that the Harvard residents don't hear a C.C. story or meet a patient whose life was changed forever by this remarkable human.

With devotion,

Nancy J Tarbell, MD, FASTRO
C.C. Wang Professor of Radiation Oncology
Harvard Medical School

With this Third Edition of *Clinical Radiation Oncology* we hope to continue C.C.'s efforts to provide a comprehensive, clinically relevant and practical guide to radiation oncology. This textbook is the result of our efforts to continue C.C.'s unique ability to bring his clinical talents and superb teaching methods to a new generation of radiation oncologists. We are deeply indebted to C.C., and this book is dedicated to all he has done for his trainees, patients, and the specialty of radiation oncology.

Nancy J Tarbell, MD, FASTRO
Min Yao, MD, PhD
William Small Jr, MD, FACRO, FACR, FASTRO

Preface

Cancer remains a significant cause of morbidity and mortality worldwide: based on GLOBOCAN estimates, about 14.1 million new cancer cases and 8.2 million deaths occurred in 2012, and according to American Cancer Society estimates approximately 1.69 million new cases of cancer will be diagnosed in the United States in 2017, with approximately 601 000 deaths.

It has been nearly 30 years since the first edition of *Clinical Radiation Oncology: Indications, Techniques and Results* was published in 1988, and 17 years since publication of the Second Edition in 2000. Featuring contributions from renowned specialists and prepared by the legendary Dr Chiu-Chen Wang – "… an editor well known for his skilled and no-nonsense methods of dealing with the various types of major organ cancers" – these earlier editions presented clinically relevant information in a user-friendly format.

With this Third Edition, the baton has been passed and I have the onus of the continuation of Dr Wang's legacy. In assuming this responsibility, my colleagues and I have sought to create a text reflective of the changes in the field of clinical radiation oncology, and in so doing, to continue to build on the immeasurable contribution to the medical literature of the textbook's founding editor. The textbook is a strong collaboration of myself, associate editors, section editors, and many outstanding chapter authors.

We have aimed to make the new edition even more useful to our intended readers: students, specialty and subspecialty trainees, practicing clinicians, and academicians. We took as a basic premise that the textbook would continue to be comprehensive, incorporating all of the significant advances made since the last edition, and written by a cast of authors at the forefront of the oncologic field. Therefore, this fully updated and enhanced Third Edition continues to offer a highly practical, application-based review of the biological basis of radiation oncology and the clinical efficacy of radiation therapy.

The chapters discuss disease by anatomic site and cover relevant background information on each tumor, including epidemiology, pathology, diagnostic workup, prognostic factors, treatment techniques, applications of surgery and chemotherapy, end results of treatment, and pertinent clinical trials. The comprehensive and rigorous assessment of each tumor site set forth in this text provides the foundation for the proper application of radiation therapy techniques in the treatment of patients with cancer.

Furthermore, the new edition addresses the latest developments in the field, including intensity-modulated radiation therapy, image-guided radiation therapy, proton beam radiation therapy, and palliative radiotherapy. We have also added chapters on statistics in radiation oncology and quality, which we are confident will provide further insight to our readers. This text is intended as an invaluable reference for radiation oncologists, oncologic surgeons, medical oncologists, oncology nurses, radiation therapists, residents, and students.

I am grateful for the work done by my predecessor as steward of this textbook, and am especially appreciative of the enormous efforts made by the associate editors, Nancy Tarbell and Min Yao. The additional section editors, Minesh Mehta, Jason A. Efstathiou and Chis Willet put together outstanding sections that provide unprecedented comprehensive evaluations of intrathoracic, genitourinary, and gastrointestinal sites. I am deeply indebted to the enormous effort of the chapter authors who provided content that fulfilled the high standards expected. In addition, I want to thank several individuals who worked most closely with this project at Wiley including Claire Brewer, Jon Peacock, James Schultz, Audrey Koh and Claire Bonnett. I want to thank Shalini Sharma, who was critical in the final proofs for the book, and Amy Laleman, my Executive Secretary, whose extraordinary efforts helped get this book completed and state of the art for 2017. A special thanks goes out to Thomas Moore, the original senior editor of this edition, without whose vision and persistence this invaluable resource would not have been possible.

Sincerely,
William Small Jr, MD, FACRO, FACR, FASTRO

Contributors

Kaled M. Alektiar, MD
Department of Radiation Oncology
Memorial Sloan-Kettering Cancer Center
New York, NY, USA

Fiori Alite, MD
Geisinger Medical Center
Department of Radiation Oncology
Danville, PA, USA

Robert J. Amdur, MD
Department of Radiation Oncology
College of Medicine, University of Florida
Gainesville, FL, USA

Jonathan B. Ashman, MD, PhD
Department of Radiation Oncology
Mayo Clinic
Phoenix, AZ, USA

Elizabeth A. Barnes, MD, FRCPC
Department of Radiation Oncology
Odette Cancer Centre
Sunnybrook Health Sciences Centre
University of Toronto
Toronto, Ontario, Canada

Sean Boyer, MS
Northwestern Medicine Chicago Proton
    Center
Warrenville, IL, USA

Kristy K. Brock, PhD
Professor, Department of Imaging Physics
The University of Texas MD Anderson Cancer
    Center
Houston, TX, USA

Timothy A. Chan, MD, PhD
Department of Radiation Oncology
Memorial Sloan Kettering Cancer Center
New York, NY, USA

Allen M. Chen, MD
Joe and Jean Brandmeyer Endowed Chairman and
    Professor
Department of Radiation Oncology
University of Kansas School of Medicine
Associate Director, University of Kansas Cancer Center
Kansas City, Kansas, USA

Changhu Chen, MD
Department of Radiation Oncology
University of Toledo College of Medicine and Life
    Sciences
Toledo, OH, USA

George T.Y. Chen, PhD
Department of Radiation Oncology
Harvard Medical School
Boston, MA, USA

Joanna Y. Tansky, MD, PhD
Department of Radiation Oncology
Massachusetts General Hospital
Boston, MA, USA

Edward Chow, BBS, MSc, PhD, FRCPC
Department of Radiation Oncology
Odette Cancer Center
Sunnybrook Health Sciences Centre
University of Toronto
Toronto, Ontario, Canada

Caitlin Costello, MD
Department of Medicine, Division of Blood and Marrow
    Transplantation
Moores Cancer Center
University of California, San Diego
La Jolla, CA, USA

Brian G. Czito, MD
Department of Radiation Oncology
Duke University
Durham, NC, USA

Roi Dagan, MD, MS
UFHealth Proton Therapy Institute
Department of Radiation Oncology
University of Florida, College of Medicine
Jacksonville, FL, USA

Laura A. Dawson, MD
Radiation Medicine Program
Princess Margaret Hospital
University Health Network;
Department of Radiation Oncology
University of Toronto
Toronto, Ontario, Canada

Phillip M. Devlin, MD, FACR, FASTRO, FFRRCSI(Hon)
Chief, Division of Brachytherapy
Institute Physician, Dana Farber Cancer Institute
Associate Professor of Radiation Oncology
Harvard Medical School
Boston, MA, USA

Jason A. Efstathiou, MD, DPhil
Massachusetts General Hospital
Department of Radiation Oncology
Harvard Medical School
Boston, MA, USA

Patricia Eifel, MD, FASTRO
Professor
Department of Radiation Oncology
The University of Texas MD Anderson Cancer Center
Texas, USA

Avraham Eisbruch, MD
Department of Radiation Oncology
University of Michigan
Ann Arbor, MI, USA

Nicholas Galanopoulos, MD
Mark M. Connolly Center for Cancer and Specialty Care
Presence St. Joseph Hospital
Chicago, IL, USA

Phillip J. Gray, MD
The CHEM Center for Radiation Oncology
Hallmark Health System
Stoneham, MA, USA

Rebecca I. Hartman, MD
Department of Dermatology
Harvard Medical School
Boston, MA, USA

William F. Hartsell, MD
Radiation Oncology Consultants, Ltd
Northwestern Medicine Chicago Proton Center
Warrenville, IL, USA

John P. Hayes, MD
Radiation Oncology
RH Lurie Comprehensive Cancer Center of Northwestern University
Chicago, IL, USA

Draik Hecksel, PhD
Northwestern Medicine Chicago Proton Center
Warrenville, IL, USA

Felix Ho, MD, MPH
SUNY Downstate Medical Center
Brooklyn, NY, USA

Theodore S. Hong, MD
Department of Radiation Oncology
Massachusetts General Hospital
Boston, MA, USA

Boris Hristov, MD
United States Air Force
Radiation Oncology
Dayton, Ohio, USA

Deepak Khuntia, MD
Varian Medical Systems and Precision Cancer Specialists
Palo Alto, CA, USA

Grace J. Kim, MD, PhD
Department of Radiation Oncology
University of Maryland Medical Center
Baltimore, MD, USA

Ann Klopp, MD, PhD
Radiation Oncology
The University of Texas MD Anderson Cancer Center
Houston, TX, USA

Jong H. Kung
Department of Radiation Oncology
Massachusetts General Hospital
Harvard Medical School
Boston, MA, USA

Charles A. Kunos, MD, PhD
Department of Radiation Oncology and Case Comprehensive Cancer Center
University Hospitals Case Medical Center and Case Western Reserve University School of Medicine
Cleveland, OH, USA

Steve Laub, MS
Northwestern Medicine Chicago Proton Center
Warrenville, IL, USA

Pierre Lavertu, MD
Department of Otolaryngology - Head and Neck
    Surgery
University Hospitals Cleveland Medical Center
Case Western Reserve University
Cleveland, OH, USA

Justin W. Lee, MD, FRCPC, MSc
Department of Radiation Oncology
Odette Cancer Center
Sunnybrook Health Sciences Centre
University of Toronto
Toronto, Ontario, Canada

Nancy Lee, MD
Memorial Sloan Kettering Cancer Center
Department of Radiation Oncology
New York, NY, USA

Jay S. Loeffler, MD, FASTRO, FACR
Herman and Joan Suit Professor of Radiation
    Oncology
Professor of Neurosurgery
Harvard Medical School
Chair, Department of Radiation Oncology
Massachusetts General Hospital
Boston, MA, USA

Stephen Lutz, MD
Eastern Woods Radiation Oncology Findlay
Ohio, USA

Shannon M. MacDonald
Department of Radiation Oncology
Massachusetts General Hospital
Harvard Medical School
Boston, MA, USA

Mitchell Machtay, MD
Department of Radiation Oncology
University Hospitals Cleveland Medical Center
Case Western Reserve University
Cleveland, OH, USA

Minesh P. Mehta, MD, FASTRO
Deputy Director, Miami cancer Institute and Chief of
    Radiation Oncology
Baptist health of South Florida
Miami, FL, USA

Loren K. Mell, MD
Department of Radiation Medicine and Applied
    Sciences
University of California, San Diego
La Jolla, CA, USA

James M. Melotek, MD
Department of Radiation and Cellular Oncology
University of Chicago
Chicago, IL, USA

Nasiruddin Mohammed, MD, MBA
Radiation Oncology Consultants, Ltd
Northwestern Medicine Chicago Proton Center
Warrenville, IL, USA

Pranshu Mohindra, MD, MBBS, DABR®
Department of Radiation Oncology
University of Maryland School of Medicine
Baltimore, MD, USA

Monica Morrow, MD
Breast Service, Department of Surgery
Memorial Sloan Kettering Cancer Center
NY, USA

Kent W. Mouw, MD, PhD
Department of Radiation Oncology
Brigham & Women's Hospital
Dana-Farber Cancer Institute
Boston, MA, USA

Caitlin Newhouse, MD
Pediatric Resident, Children's Hospital Los Angeles
Los Angeles, CA, USA

Manisha Palta, MD
Department of Radiation Oncology
Duke University
Durham, NC, USA

Jonathan J. Paly, DO
Department of Radiation Oncology
Fox Chase Cancer Center
Philadelphia, PA, USA

Mark Pankuch, PhD
Northwestern Medicine Chicago
    Proton Center
Warrenville, IL, USA

Simon N. Powell, MD, PhD
Chair, Department of Radiation Oncology
Member, Memorial Sloan Kettering Cancer Center
Molecular Biology Program Member, Sloan Kettering
    Institute
Professor of Molecular Biology, Weill Cornell Graduate
    Medical Sciences
New York, NY, USA

Brent S. Rose, MD
Moores Cancer Center
UC San Diego Health
La Jolla, CA, USA

Parag Sanghvi, MD, MSPH
University of California, San Diego
Center for Advanced Radiotherapy Technologies
Department of Radiation Oncology
La Jolla, CA, USA

Karan Shah, MD, MBA
Department of Radiation Oncology
Midwestern Regional Medical Center
Cancer Treatment Centers of America
Zion, IL, USA

Helen A. Shih, MD, MS, MPH
Massachusetts General Hospital
Department of Radiation Oncology
Francis H. Burr Proton Therapy Center
Boston, MA, USA

William U. Shipley, MD, FACR, FASTRO
Massachusetts General Hospital
Department of Radiation Oncology
Harvard Medical School
Boston, MA, USA

Farzan Siddiqui, MD, PhD
Department of Radiation Oncology
Henry Ford Health System
Detroit, MI, USA

William Small, Jr, MD, FACRO, FACR, FASTRO
Department of Radiation Oncology
Stritch School of Medicine Loyola University Chicago
Cardinal Bernardin Cancer Center
Maguire Center
Maywood, IL, USA

Abhishek A. Solanki, MD, MS
Assistant Professor
Department of Radiation Oncology
Loyola Outpatient Center
Cardinal Bernardin Cancer Center
Stritch School of Medicine Loyola University Chicago
Chicago, IL, USA

Jonathan B. Strauss, MD, MBA
Department of Radiation Oncology
Robert H. Lurie Comprehensive Cancer Center
Northwestern University, Feinberg School of Medicine
Chicago, IL, USA

Mohan Suntharalingam, MD, MBA
Department of Radiation Oncology
University of Maryland Medical Center
Baltimore, MD, USA

Nancy J. Tarbell, MD
C.C. Wang Professor of Radiation Oncology
Harvard Medical School
Boston, MA, USA

Kanokpis Townamchai, MD
Radiation Oncologist
Division of Radiation Oncology
Department of Radiology
Bhumibol Adulyadej Hospital
Bangkok, Thailand

May N. Tsao, MD, FRCPC
Department of Radiation Oncology
Odette Cancer Centre
Sunnybrook Health Sciences Centre
University of Toronto
Toronto, Ontario, Canada

Keith Unger, MD
Department of Radiation Medicine
Georgetown University Hospital
Washington, DC, USA

Tamara Z. Vern-Gross, DO, FAAP
Mayo Clinic-Arizona
Department of Radiation Oncology
Phoenix, AZ, USA

Akila N. Viswanathan, MD, MPH
Professor and Executive Vice Chair
Department of Radiation Oncology and Molecular
   Radiation Sciences
Johns Hopkins Medicine
Baltimore, MD, USA

Angela Wan, MPhil
Department of Radiation Oncology
Odette Cancer Center
Sunnybrook Health Sciences Centre
University of Toronto
Toronto, Ontario, Canada

XiaoShen Wang, MD
Department of Radiation Oncology
Cancer Hospital
Fudan University
Shanghai, China

Randy L. Wei, MD, PhD
Department of Radiation Oncology
University of California, Irvine
Orange, CA, USA

Christopher G. Willett, MD
Department of Radiation Oncology
Duke University, USA

Kathryn Winter, MS
Statistics and Data Management Center
NRG Oncology; RTOG Foundation
American College of Radiology: Center for Research
    and Innovation
Philadelphia, PA, USA

Jennifer Y. Wo, MD
Massachusetts General Hospital
Harvard Medical School
Boston, MA, USA

Charles Woods, MD
Department of Radiation Oncology
University Hospitals Cleveland Medical Center
Case Western Reserve University
Cleveland, OH, USA

Min Yao, MD, PhD
Department of Radiation Oncology
University Hospitals Cleveland Medical Center
Case Western Reserve University
Cleveland, OH, USA

Torunn I. Yock, MD, MCH
Massachusetts General Hospital
Associate Professor, Department of Radiation Oncology
Director, Pediatric Radiation Oncology
Harvard Medical School
Boston, MA, USA

Hannah Yoon, MD
Department of Radiation Oncology
Stony Brook University
Stony Brook, NY, USA

Monique Youl, MBBS, FRANZCR
Department of Radiation Oncology
Peter MacCallum Cancer Centre
Melbourne, Australia

Anthony L. Zietman, MD
Department of Radiation Oncology
Massachusetts General Hospital
Boston, MA, USA

Section 1

Scientific Foundations

Section Editor: William Small Jr.

1

Basic Concepts of Clinical Radiation Oncology

Hannah Yoon, Karan Shah, William Small Jr, Minesh P. Mehta and John P. Hayes

Introduction

Radiation oncology is the practice of utilizing ionizing radiation to treat both malignant and benign diseases. It requires comprehensive medical knowledge coupled with advanced skills in clinical oncology, physics, and radiation biology. In 2017, radiation oncologists are integral team members of modern multidisciplinary care, working in conjunction with specialists in medical oncology, surgical oncology, diagnostic and interventional radiology, pathology, and the entire spectrum of subspecialties involved in oncologic care. The specialty can trace its history back over 100 years, yet as the role it plays continues to change, the primary mission remains the same – to enhance the health of the patient with cancer, and improve the specialty for the benefit of future patients.

To consider the scope of oncology, one can start with an acknowledgement of the extent of the socioeconomic impact. In the United States, deaths from cancer are exceeded only by those resulting from heart disease. In 2017, approximately 1,688,780 new cancer cases will be diagnosed (not including carcinomas in situ or non-melanoma skin cancers), and about 600,920 Americans will die of cancer [1]. It is estimated that 50–60% of patients afflicted with cancer will receive radiation therapy, either for cure or palliation. Radiation oncology is therefore a medical specialty of major importance. Such a specialty demands a working knowledge of the clinical and biologic course, both treated and untreated of various cancers, knowledge of the various stages of the diseases, and knowledge of the efficacy and toxicities of different methods of treatment. It necessitates an understanding of the clinical application of the physical and biologic aspects of ionizing radiation, and an awareness of the significance of rehabilitation and follow-up. The prognosis of patients with malignant diseases depends on many factors, both disease-related (cell type, tumor grade, extent of the primary disease, and presence or absence of regional or distant metastases), and patient-related (comorbidities, performance status, etc.). Consequently, a refined appreciation of palliative care, hospice care, quality of life issues, and end-of-life issues is paramount in this field. Furthermore, since oncology encompasses hundreds of different diseases, with differing natural histories, distinct biologic behaviors, modes of tumor growth and spread, and characteristic responses to radiation therapy, the therapeutic management and results will therefore differ greatly.

Planning and Preparation

The optimal use of radiation therapy requires meticulous planning, preparation, and implementation. First, the goal of treatment needs to be established, be it curative, palliative or to enhance local control in a non-curative patient. For most patients, radiation therapy is a local or local-regional treatment, and therefore, designing treatment starts with the recognition of the known and potential extent of the disease. Hence, the clinician must recognize both the grossly evident disease as well as adjacent areas at risk for harboring subclinical spread, and consider treatment, keeping in mind the normal tissues or organs that will be irradiated.

A thorough history and physical examination, along with a review of diagnostic studies such as laboratory values, plain films, ultrasound, mammograms, CT, MRI, and PET or PET/CT scans, precedes the first planning session. In certain cases of head and neck cancer, gynecologic cancers and genitourinary cancers, an examination under anesthesia may add critical information about the extent of the disease. Except for a few situations in which biopsy is considered impractical or potentially harmful, histologic confirmation of malignancy should be obtained before treatment. This requirement, of course does not extend to the management of benign disease processes with radiotherapy.

Simulation is where the patient is positioned for radiation therapy, a support/immobilization platform often made, and imaging studies obtained that will be used to direct treatment. Most radiation therapy plan calculations today are based on CT data sets that allow three-dimensional (3D) reconstruction of individual patient anatomy. A four-dimensional (4D) CT can also be obtained to account for changes in tumor location during respiration. The definition of both the diseased and normal structures follows, and is primarily an image-based exercise, but incorporates essentially every imaging technique available, and therefore significant familiarity with the specialty of radiology is a key requirement for radiation oncology. Techniques of treatment are then developed and optimized in virtual reality. Today's advanced computer systems enhance the radiation oncologist's ability to compare options, quantify target and normal tissue doses, and create complex distributions of radiation energy that have been customized for each patient. Dose distributions are optimized so as to maximize the dose to the target and minimize the dose to the adjacent normal structures; in modern practice, these dose distributions can be reduced to mathematical representations such as dose–volume histograms, mean doses, maximum doses, and so on, which can be correlated with predicted toxicities, allowing, effectively for 'multicriteria' optimization, to generate the best possible treatment plan for a patient. In parlance that the patient can understand, treatment is designed to "hit what we want to hit, and miss what we don't want to hit."

With few exceptions, most external beam radiation therapy is given with megavoltage linear accelerators with energies ranging from 4 to 25 MV. Superficial areas such as the skin may be treated with low-energy x-rays (e.g. 50–100 kV) or electron beam therapy. The basic physical properties of radiation are reviewed in Chapter 3.

Radiation doses are quantified in units called Gray (Gy), that represent the energy absorbed within the tissue. Prescribed doses are based on accepted standards of normal tissue tolerances, which were historically developed from observation and, more recently, from quantifiable dose–response analyses.

Radiation Therapy in the Clinic

Radiation therapy is used as primary, curative treatment, as palliative treatment, and as adjunctive therapy (most commonly to surgery), yet often in combination with chemotherapy, targeted molecular therapies, and now also immune-modulating therapies. Additionally, it can be combined with either tumor-radiosensitizing drugs,

or normal tissue-protecting radioprotectors, or physical methods which enhance the effectiveness of radiation therapy, ranging from tissue displacement devices to local and regional hyperthermia, and potentially to alternating electrical field antimitotic therapy. Palliative treatment may be given with the hope of relieving symptoms and/or prolonging survival. Palliative doses of radiation may be more limited, and risks therefore minimized. In less-common cases, radiation can be administered for benign diseases, such as heterotopic ossification, keloids and pterygium. Radiation therapy with curative intent may require doses that carry significant risks of permanent morbidity. These treatments may be prolonged and taxing due to acute toxicities, both local and systemic. As with any cancer therapy the goals of treatment – be they curative or palliative – need to be weighed against potential side effects and risks.

The effects of a given dose of radiation on malignant tissue varies with multiple factors, including the total dose administered, the time over which it is given, and the amount that is administered during each treatment (called the fraction, hence, fractionation). Tumor responses to any given dose sequence vary, although generalization based on previous study helps determine expectations. Some cancers, such as lymphomas and germ cell tumors, are considered radioresponsive as doses ranging from 24 to 45 Gy given with standard daily fractionation of 1.8–2.0 Gy result in high rates of local control; in fact, in some modern regimens doses as low as 4 Gy are employed in certain situations. Most other cell types require higher doses, on the order of 60–70 Gy or beyond, to obtain reasonable rates of local or local-regional control. Some cell types (e.g., renal cell carcinoma) are notoriously capricious in their response, while others (e.g., melanoma, glioblastoma, pancreatic carcinoma, and anaplastic thyroid cancer) often require prohibitive doses to try to eradicate gross, or even microscopic, disease.

Other than cell type, the primary determinant of the likelihood of eradicating disease at a given site is the volume of disease, sometimes called the *tumor burden*. Although a dose of 60–70 Gy may lead to the sterilization of a 1 cm squamous cell carcinoma on 90% of occasions, the same tumor is much less likely to be eradicated if it is 3–4 cm, and will recur in most instances if it is 5–6 cm or larger and treated with standard fractionation external beam therapy alone. Recognizing this, alternative paradigms of treatment have been developed. Examples used at specific disease sites are reviewed in later chapters.

The *therapeutic index* or *window* is the balance of risk and reward that accompanies all treatment decisions in oncology, as there is no condition, nor any treatment, without risk. Outcomes are never guaranteed. Simply put, the ideal treatment separates the likelihood of benefit as far as possible from the probability of damage or dysfunction. Although theoretically logical and definable, this combination is notoriously difficult to define, and achieve.

Combining Radiation Therapy with Surgery

Surgery and radiation therapy may be competitive or complementary in the treatment of localized or locally and regionally limited malignancies. Each has its merits, indications and limitations, all of which are site- and diagnosis-specific. Radiation therapy can offer the advantage of controlling disease *in situ*, thus avoiding removal of useful, even critical organs, thereby preserving the function of these vital organs. Examples of organ-sparing treatment that preserve function in a high proportion of patients include the treatment of cancer of the larynx and anal canal cancers. In early-stage lung cancer, treatment with stereotactic body radiotherapy can obviate the need for a lobectomy (especially in patients with significant cardiopulmonary compromise), preventing morbidity from invasive surgery. Surgery may provide an expeditious alternative without functional or cosmetic compromise, and can provide treatment for lesions that are notoriously difficult to eradicate with acceptable doses of radiotherapy. Rather than considering these alternatives in a hierarchical way, each can be supported based on its applicability in a given clinical setting.

In the management of locally advanced carcinomas, the failure of surgery to cure the disease may be due to its inability to remove unrecognized microscopic tumor (subclinical disease) at the periphery of resection, thus resulting in a marginal recurrence. Tumor seeding in the wound and metastases via lymphatic or hematogenous routes are additional means to account for therapeutic failures of surgery. In contrast, radiation therapy may be unable to sterilize bulky tumors because of the volume of malignant cells, or because of relatively radioresistant cells (e.g., hypoxic cells) that may comprise a component of large tumors. Tumor cells that are well-oxygenated, well-nourished, and therefore more radiosensitive, may be more common at the periphery of the cancer. Radiation therapy failures are thus often central rather than marginal. Distant failures, be they from lymphatic or hematogenous spread, are also the bane of both surgery and radiotherapy.

Thus, it can easily be seen how the spatial strengths of radiation therapy and surgery can be complementary.

Preoperative Radiation Therapy

The aims of preoperative radiation therapy are to eradicate subclinical disease around the primary site and in the lymph nodes, or to convert technically inoperable tumors into operable ones. Preoperative treatment has been found to decrease the risk of iatrogenic scar implants as well as marginal and regional (nodal) recurrences,

and in some cases, the incidences of distant metastases [2].

The disadvantages of preoperative radiation include: (i) the full extent of the primary tumor or regional spread may never be known due to the response to treatment; (ii) the risk of postoperative complications such as wound healing may be increased; (iii) the delay until surgery may create a great deal of anxiety; and (iv) if there is significant radioresistance the opportunity for surgical cure may be lost.

The doses employed in preoperative radiation therapy are usually moderate, on the order of 45–50 Gy over five weeks [3–5]. Surgery is usually performed one to two months later to allow healing of any inflamed tissue, facilitating visualization and resection. Examples of this approach include the treatment of head and neck cancers, rectal tumors, and soft-tissue sarcomas. Lower doses (e.g., 25 Gy in five fractions) followed by immediate surgery have been used in the treatment of rectal cancer, and more recently in mesothelioma, with similar success [6–8]. Some protocols have used preoperative treatment to gauge responsiveness of the disease, avoiding surgery when possible, often with the advantage of potential organ preservation [9, 10].

Postoperative Radiation Therapy

Postoperative radiation therapy is used in an effort to eradicate residual disease at the periphery of the surgical bed, in the unresected regional lymphatics, and to prevent recurrence in the scar [11, 12]. Time is required for adequate healing before postoperative radiation therapy can begin, usually at least three to four weeks. Doses are commonly 50–66 Gy for completely resected tumors, while subtotal resection requires higher doses that are often equivalent to those used for inoperable situations. Although exceptions include primary CNS malignancies, planned subtotal resection must be used selectively as the benefit of postoperative radiation therapy in these cases may be marginal.

The question of whether to use preoperative versus postoperative radiation therapy is unresolved in many cases. Each method has its advantages and disadvantages, proponents and opponents. The decision should be driven by evidence-based data whenever possible, individualizing for each patient and, very importantly, should include consideration of the experience of the treating clinicians.

Combining Radiation Therapy with Chemotherapy

Commonly used chemotherapeutic agents that exert cytotoxic or cytostatic effects on neoplastic cells include vinca alkaloids, alkylating agents, antimetabolites, epipodophyllotoxins, platinoids, and taxanes. Many of these drugs cause damage during specific phases of the cell cycle, while other agents such as platinum and alkylators are non-cell cycle-specific. Multi-agent chemotherapy regimens with different mechanisms of action may help overcome drug resistance through either additive or synergistic outcome.

Chemotherapy alone is rarely efficacious in tumor eradiation or cure. However, the combination of chemotherapy with radiation in clinical trials for many sites of cancer has demonstrated improved local control, decreased distant metastases, and improved overall survival. At the present time, chemotherapeutic agents such as cisplatin, 5-florouracil, gemcitabine, temozolomide, paclitaxel and docetaxel are often combined with radiation to treat head and neck, lung, CNS, breast, gastrointestinal, gynecological, and genitourinary cancers.

The interaction of radiotherapy and chemotherapy may be additive or synergistic, and various mechanisms of interaction have been theorized. Spatial cooperation is a condition in which various agents may be used to target tissue in spatially different areas (local versus distant), or within the same tumor mass but in areas with different environmental factors. Independent cell kill explains how two therapies at full dose can produce a greater tumor response than with either agent alone. A third theory – debulking – explains that radiotherapy can more effectively kill cells after chemotherapy is employed to shrink the tumor beforehand, as there are fewer tumor cells remaining. Finally, enhanced tumor response explains how chemotherapy can inhibit radiation-induced DNA damage repair, and also kill cells that are resistant to one modality of treatment [13]. Optimally, the combined treatment should be lethal to tumor cells but nontoxic to normal tissue.

Biologically, oxygen plays an important role in modulating the radiation response via reactions downstream of toxic free radical production, and this interaction is the mechanism of action of several radiosensitizing chemotherapeutic agents. Tirapazamine functions specifically on radiation-resistant hypoxic tumor cells, by converting itself into a highly reactive free radical under hypoxic conditions. Mitomycin functions in a similar fashion to damage hypoxic cells.

Combining Radiation Therapy with Biologic Agents

Molecular targeted agents have more recently been employed to further modulate response to radiation, while causing less normal tissue toxicity when compared to more traditional chemotherapeutic agents. Biologic agents targeting the EGFR, VEGFR, integrin, and mTOR pathways are being used concurrently with radiation therapy. For instance, EGFR-inhibitors, such as erlotinib and cetuximab, are often included in combined modality treatment for lung and head and neck cancers, while trastuzumab, which inhibits the ErbB-2 receptor, is routinely used to treat Her2/Neu-positive breast cancers.

Molecular agents may enhance radiation sensitivity and cell killing by improving tumor oxygenation, inhibiting angiogenesis, promoting cell arrest, and activating apoptosis [14]. Similarly, there is a strong preclinical rationale for combining radiotherapy with anti-angiogenic therapies. Emerging preclinical data and some early clinical results have provided insights into how immune checkpoint inhibitors could potentially be combined with radiation, with the latter effectively acting as a 'stimulatory vaccine,' a relatively novel role for radiotherapy [15–17].

Combining Radiation Therapy with Hormonal Agents

The use of hormonal agents either as monotherapy or part of multimodality regimen has implications for the treatment of breast, prostate, uterine, thyroid, and carcinoid tumors. These agents can directly bind to a hormone receptor, thereby either inhibiting (antagonizing) or enhancing (agonizing) the effects of the specific hormone. Alternatively, these molecules can exert their actions by binding to a receptor upstream or downstream in the hormonal pathway.

The use of hormonal agents is widely prevalent in the treatment of prostate cancer. In 1941, Huggins and Hodges first showed that bilateral orchiectomy results in a significant decrease in circulating testosterone levels within hours after the procedure, and thereby represented an effective, fast therapy to treat prostate cancer. In later years, the use of androgen deprivation therapy (ADT) – either as luteinizing hormone-releasing agonists or antagonists – has replaced surgical interventions and other pharmacotherapy agents, such as diethylstilbestrol, cyproterone acetate, and ketoconazole. Luteinizing hormone-releasing hormone (LHRH) agents can effectively reduce circulating testosterone levels by 90% [18].

The use of ADT in combination with radiation therapy for prostate cancer has shown to improve treatment-related outcomes, including local control, disease-free survival, time to the development of metastases, biochemical control, and overall survival in multiple Phase III randomized trials [19]. Furthermore, several investigators have proposed radiobiology synergism between ADT and radiation therapy, including enhanced apoptosis, decreased tumor hypoxia, and prostate volume reduction (improving radiation therapy delivery and reducing adverse effects) [20–22].

Radiosensitivity and Tumor Control Probability

Clinically, 'radiosensitivity' is often used interchangeably with 'radioresponsiveness.' In radiation biology, the former term refers to the innate sensitivity of the cells to radiation. As shown in the dose–response cell survival

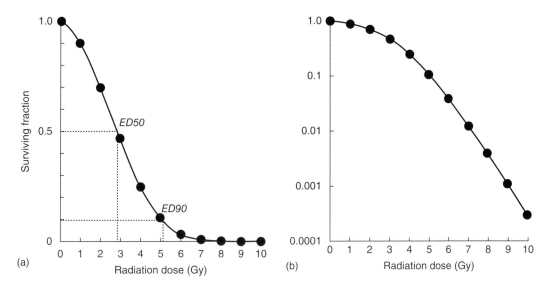

Figure 1.1 A typical cell survival curve. *Source:* Horsman 2002 [23]. Reproduced with permission of Taylor and Francis.

curves in Figure 1.1, the radiosensitivity for various normal and malignant mammalian cell lines is related to the slope of the curve that shows increasing cell death with increasing dose [24].

Factors influencing radiosensitivity include the ability to repair damage that does not immediately cause cell death (sublethal damage repair), the cell's location in the cell cycle (most sensitive in G_2 and M, least in G_1), the degree of oxygenation or relative hypoxia, the dose rate, fractionation, total dose, and the quality of radiation.

Fractionation and Fraction Size

The effects of a single dose of radiation energy on mammalian cells are more pronounced than those produced by the same amount of energy delivered in divided doses. Because of this, a higher total dose is necessary to obtain the same amount of cell kill whenever an identical amount of radiation is given in multiple smaller doses. Therefore, *fractionation* – or the breaking up of the total dose into multiple smaller doses – may seem counterproductive when considering the goal of tumor eradication. However, tumors and normal tissues are intimate, and what might be desirable for the tumor can be hazardous for the normal tissues.

The benefit of fractionation is based on the fact that normal tissues can accept a certain amount of radiation energy, and avoid death, if the damage they incur is reparable. As the cell has avoided death the damage is called *sublethal*, and the corrective process is termed *sublethal damage repair*.

Most commonly in the clinic, treatment is given once a day, five days a week. This allows for the repair of sublethal damage by normal tissue, as this process normally requires less than 24 h, and some may be completed in as little as 4–6 h [25, 26]. Malignant cells are frequently

much less efficient or incapable of similar sublethal damage repair. Standard fractionation external beam radiation therapy schedules try to take advantage of this difference. As such, a course of treatment may require higher total doses over five to eight weeks than would be necessary if given in smaller amounts over two or three weeks.

Fractionation also allows for changes in the tumor environment that may improve the effectiveness of subsequent treatments. An example of this is the death of well-oxygenated cells causing a reduction in tumor size, leading to a better oxygenation of previously hypoxic cells, which thereby increases their radiosensitivity. Another example is *redistribution*, during which the cell progresses from a radioresistant phase of the cell cycle to a more radiosensitive phase, such as M phase.

Conventional radiation therapy is generally given with one fraction per day, five days per week. The total dose prescribed is dependent on a number of factors, including the presence of gross versus microscopic disease, whether it is being given in a preoperative or postoperative setting (postoperative situations generally require a greater dose), and the nature of the surrounding normal tissues. Such programs were derived from empiric observations in the clinic, yet may not be the actual best treatment course for many human cancers. Altered fractionation schedules vary the dose and frequency of administration to try to take advantage of additional factors beyond sublethal damage repair, and have become part of the normal lexicon of radiation oncology.

Linear Energy Transfer (LET) and Relative Biologic Effectiveness (RBE)

In trying to understand why one type of radiation energy is more effective in causing cell death than another, characteristics of energy, mass, and charge need to be considered. In simple terms, the greater the mass of a particle, the more damage it is likely to inflict along its path. Charged particles are more likely to interact over a short distance than are uncharged particles, while the energy of the radiation (expressed in electron volts) affects the location where these interactions will occur. Energy is deposited in the cell along that path of the particle, and their subsequent effects will be produced at that point or within a very short distance. Therefore, mass, charge, and energy combine to express the quality of any given type of radiation energy used in the clinic. The resulting concept is referred to as the linear energy transfer (LET).

LET is designated as the average energy deposited in each unit of length; it is measured in electron volts per micrometer ($eV\ \mu m^{-1}$) or kilo-electron volts per micrometer ($keV\ \mu m^{-1}$). Protons, fast neutrons and other forms of particulate radiation have dense ionization (energy deposition) along their paths, and therefore high LET. Photons and megavoltage electrons (which, although charged, have a relatively small mass) have more sparse ionization, and therefore a low LET.

Biologic damage to cells is related to LET. In general, high-LET radiation is more likely to produce substantial damage in a given volume of living matter, regardless of other factors. This is true for both normal and malignant cells. Because high-LET energy can cause such severe effects, there is little chance for the repair of sublethal damage, and therefore the benefits of fractionation are minimized. Again, damage to malignant and normal tissue may be similar, so the benefits of high-LET radiation can only be accrued if there is spatial separation of the targeted tumor and nearby critical normal structures.

Relative biologic effectiveness is a term used to describe comparisons of radiation quality against a benchmark of 200 kV x-rays as the standard. For cobalt-60 x-rays and low-megavoltage photons, the RBE approaches one, whereas higher-LET radiation has RBEs up to 3.5. Although extremely high-LET radiation deposits large amounts of energy in a given space, its RBE reaches a ceiling after maximum lethality has been reached.

The RBE of electrons, which are charged but consist of low mass, is similar to that of low-LET photons, typically 0.85 to 0.9.

Oxygen Enhancement Ratio

In most biologic systems under both normal and malignant conditions, the effects of radiation are greater when the cells are well oxygenated. Poorly oxygenated cells (i.e., hypoxic cells) comprise 10–20% of tumor cells [23]. It has been shown that regions more than 150–180 μm distant from functional capillaries often contain hypoxic cells [27]. These cells are viable and can proliferate, yet may be relatively resistant to the effects of radiation due to the lack of oxygen. The difference in radiosensitivity under oxygenated conditions is in the neighborhood of two- to threefold; this is known as the *oxygen enhancement ratio* (OER).

In order for oxygen to be a radiation sensitizer, it must be present in the cells during irradiation. The mechanism of oxygen enhancement is believed to be through radiation-induced free radicals that initiate a chain of events that begin with DNA damage and finally results in biologic damage. High-LET radiation operates in a more direct manner, so the OER is either low or non-existent for these types of radiation.

Clinical situations where hypoxic cells are likely to exist, such as bulky tumors or anemia, have been associated with poorer outcomes with standard treatment [28]. However, attempts to overcome cellular hypoxia – including transfusions, hyperbaric oxygen, and hypoxic cell radiosensitizers – have been disappointing for the most part.

Radiocurable Tumors

Clinically, 'radioresponsiveness' is judged by the extent of regression of the gross tumor before surgery, or the extent of residual disease found during pathologic analysis. The sensitivity of various cancers is determined by many factors, including cell type and the growth kinetics of the individual cancer. The kinetics of growth include the rate of proliferation and cell loss from factors such as apoptosis, and adequate vascular and connective tissue support. Human tumors are extremely complex, and the aggregate of cell growth and tumor represents an enormous biologic disorder; consequently, there is a wide range of factors that affect a given tumor's response. In spite of this tremendous variability, some types of cancer respond to radiation therapy more consistently than others (as noted above), and are commonly cured with tolerable doses associated with limited long-term sequelae. That is, radiocurability means that the tumor–normal tissue relationship is such that a dose of radiation energy can be delivered to eradicate the growth without leading to organ dysfunction. In these cases, the therapeutic window is open; in other words, there is a good separation between the likelihood of tumor sterilization and the risk of damage. Importantly, radiocurable tumors may be innately sensitive, or they may have normal sensitivity but be limited in extent (i.e., early stage), and therefore in a radiocurable state.

Examples of radiocurable tumors include:

1. Non-melanoma skin cancers (basal and squamous cell carcinomas).
2. Epithelial cancers of the head and neck.
3. Carcinoma of the uterine cervix.
4. Carcinoma of the prostate.
5. Hodgkin's and non-Hodgkin's lymphomas.

6. Seminoma of the testicle and dysgerminoma of the ovary.
7. Medulloblastoma, pineal germinoma, and ependymoma.
8. Retinoblastoma.
9. Choroidal melanoma (treated by proton beam therapy or plaque brachytherapy).

Technological Advances in Radiotherapy

During the past 25 years, the field of radiation oncology has undergone significant changes due to advancements in technology and a better understanding of how radiobiological principles can be utilized. Altered fractionation – that is, changing the dose of radiation per treatment – and the frequency of the treatments, including multiple doses of radiation per day, has become a commonplace regimen. Combining chemotherapy with radiation therapy, either sequentially or concurrently, has also become a standard approach for numerous disease sites. A brief review of some of the technical advancements in radiation therapy is provided in the following sections.

Intensity-Modulated Radiation Therapy (IMRT)

Classically, when external beam radiation therapy was utilized, the radiation therapy technique was determined by first considering the tumor location and the surrounding normal structures, and then selecting the direction, energy, and number of beams to be used so as to provide optimal coverage of the target with the least exposure of the adjacent normal structures. The distribution of radiation with this approach is manipulated by changing the field size or weighting, adding blocking to protect normal structures, and adding other devices such as wedges that act as tissue compensators to redistribute the energy. This is known as *forward treatment planning*.

More recently, using advances in computer technology and equipment engineering, a different paradigm has been developed termed *inverse treatment planning*. Here, the radiation oncologist designs treatment by first establishing the dose parameters for the target tissues as well as the normal organs. Priority or rank is given to each contoured object. A computer program is allowed to proffer solutions for how the radiation therapy can be given to meet the desired goals. Multiple possibilities are considered and numerous iterations are evaluated. This assessment is optimized by the use of dose–volume histogram analysis, a technique whereby the critical normal tissue doses are quantified. Only after finding an acceptable distribution of the radiation is a technique chosen.

The delivery of IMRT is achieved either via a step-and-shoot (static) or a sliding window technique (dynamic IMRT). In the static method, the beam is off while the multileaf collimator (MLC) adjusts their proper shape, whereas in the latter method the beam is continuously modulated by moving the MLC. IMRT plans are highly conformal with the optimal sparing of organs at risk, especially with coverage of concave-shaped targets. However, IMRT plans tend to have higher overall monitor units (MUs) and increase low-dose radiation to the surrounding tissues.

An extension of IMRT is that of volumetric modulated arc therapy (VMAT), which combines gantry rotation, dynamic MLC movement, and changes in dose rate to create highly conformal radiation dose distributions. VMAT plans can use a single 360° arc or multiple arcs for treatment delivery, or a helical, CT-like delivery approach. The major advantage of VMAT over traditional IMRT is the reduction in treatment delivery time with a possible decrease in integral dose; for highly complex targets, it is also more likely to produce greater tumor dose conformality [29].

Image-Guided Radiotherapy (IGRT)

Moving from the planning phase to treatment requires an exact implementation of the chosen technique of treatment. This may be achieved in several ways after first confirming that the patient's position is correct within the support platform that has been created during simulation. The direct observation of superficial tumors with a clinical set-up of the overlying field may be used in cases of cutaneous or superficial malignancies, although most patients receive radiation therapy for more deep-seated locations. Plain film images of each field or beam have been used for decades. Here again, with advances in technology, there has been a fusion of diagnostic imaging into therapy such that treatment may be directed based on CT scans obtained with the patient in the treatment position. The radiation oncologist might utilize megavoltage or cone beam CT scans to directly visualize the target, making adjustments based on the immediate location of the target, while adjacent normal tissues can be seen and taken into consideration. Surrogates such as fiducial markers that are placed in or near the tumor may be used to assess the focus of the radiation therapy. Other systems include (but are certainly not limited to) ultrasound-guided imaging, 3D optical surface monitoring, infra-red or optical marker tracking, and radiofrequency-beacon-guided modalities. Image-guided radiotherapy (IGRT) is thus the use of real-time imaging for treatment localization during radiotherapy.

The information gathered from IGRT can be used to modify treatment plans. During a typical six-week treatment course, changes in tumor volume, patient anatomy and patient positioning can significantly affect the location and volumes of both the target and organs at risk.

Hence, image-guidance can help identify these interfraction patient variations, which may lead to re-planning, re-simulation, or both. This process, termed *adaptive radiotherapy*, refers to adjusting the radiation delivery based on anatomic changes. Adaptive radiotherapy can be combined with functional imaging, such as ^{18}F-FDG-PET, to differentially boost residual tumor or radioresistant intratumor regions. This latter technique is termed *dose-painting*. IGRT combined with adaptive radiotherapy allows for dose escalation to the target, while sparing organs at risk [30–32].

Stereotactic Radiosurgery (SRS)/Stereotactic Body Radiation Therapy (SBRT)

In 1951, Lars Leskell, a Swedish neurosurgeon, first introduced the concept of delivering high doses of radiation to treat brain lesions. SRS delivers a large dose per fraction (usually single or three to five fractions) to treat focal brain lesion(s), while minimizing toxicity to the surrounding normal tissues due to a sharp dose gradient. More recently, stereotactic body radiation therapy (SBRT), an extension of SRS to treat extracranial metastasis, has been made possible by the advances in real-time image guidance. SBRT can be used to treat focal lesions in the lung, spine, liver, pancreas, kidney, and prostate [33, 34].

Particle Beam Radiotherapy

Although radiation therapy most commonly utilizes uncharged packets of energy called *photons*, it may also be given with charged particles such as electrons or protons, or uncharged particles such as neutrons. These particles have different advantages in their physical qualities, and thus their distribution within tissues as well as their biologic effectiveness also differ.

In *proton therapy*, the main advantage is spatial distribution, which potentially can deliver high doses to areas that would otherwise need a more conservative approach. This is most evident when considering tumors in close proximity to dose-limiting tissues such as the eye, brain, and spinal cord. With protons, there is also minimal exit dose beyond the target area. Carbon ions may provide a similar dose gradient with increased biologic effectiveness. Importantly, expertise in these forms of radiation is needed as increased conformality carries the risk of missing the intended target. That is, the avoidance of normal structures carries an increased risk of inadequate coverage of the malignancy. Another axiom: "Don't miss what you want to miss if you don't hit what you need to hit."

Neutrons can be helpful in treating slower-growing tumors. They do not carry a spatial advantage as other particles may, but their radiobiologic effectiveness is greater and this can be advantageous when treating relatively unresponsive ('radioresistant') tumors. The lack of spatial advantage leads to a limited clinical potential due to difficulties in delivering adequate doses to the tumor without taking potentially prohibitive risks to adjacent structures. One approach to addressing this problem has been the use of boron-neutron capture therapy (BNCT). For this, a boron-containing compound is preferentially concentrated in the tumor, which is subsequently irradiated with neutrons. The interaction of the neutrons with the boron leads to a release of alpha particles (heavy, positively charged particles) and lithium nuclei. Both of these have very short ranges and so can interact preferentially with the immediately adjacent cells, causing significant damage to the tumor. This type of treatment has been used in malignant brain tumors [35].

Brachytherapy

Brachytherapy or 'short-distance' therapy is defined as the placement of sealed radioactive sources near the tumor. Historically, radium was used but now sources that are safer and have more practical characteristics, such as iodine, palladium, iridium and cesium, are used. Brachytherapy occurs in three forms: (i) in the first type, molds or plaques are placed on the skin or mucosa of a superficial lesion; for example, eye plaques have been used to treat retinoblastoma, ocular melanoma, and pterygium; (ii) in interstitial implants, catheters containing radioactive sources or seeds are placed within soft tissue; prostate interstitial implants can be an elegant and highly effective example of this; and (iii) in intracavitary implants, radioactive sources are placed in a body cavity; for instance, vaginal brachytherapy is often used in the adjuvant treatment of endometrial cancer.

Brachytherapy implants can utilize either temporary or permanent implantation of the source of radioactivity. Temporary implants, either low-dose rate or high-dose rate, typically utilize afterloading systems whereby the radioactive material is loaded into a previously placed holding device that was designed specifically for the purpose. Examples of this include treatment for endometrial and cervical carcinomas. In each case the devices are inserted into and secured in the endometrial cavity and/or vagina with the radioactive sources added later. This enables the clinician to minimize personal exposure to radioactivity.

In permanent implants, radioactive sources are placed into tissue and their activity allowed to progressively decay while in the body. Once the compound's energy has dissipated, the inert source remains.

Intraoperative Radiotherapy

Despite intraoperative radiotherapy (IORT) technology having been in existence for the past three decades, the technique has gained increasing popularity during recent years. This is partly due to the success of the TARGIT-A trial, a multi-international, randomized, prospective Phase III non-inferiority trial, in which early-stage breast cancer patients were randomized to whole-breast radiotherapy versus targeted IORT to the tumor bed, using low-energy x-rays (kV range) [36].

IORT is delivered to the surgical bed after removal of the tumor (primary or recurrent setting) under anesthesia. The theoretical advantage of IORT is a higher therapeutic ratio by maximally sparing/shielding normal tissues and delivering a large single-fraction dose to the tumor bed to improve local control. IORT can be used as monotherapy, but is more often used in combination with external-beam RT (± chemotherapy). Currently, intraoperative machines using electrons, low-kV photons and ^{192}Ir high-dose rates exist in the marketplace [37].

Unsealed Sources

Unsealed radioisotopes have been used for the treatment of malignancies for many decades. In this type of treatment the radiopharmaceutical is delivered either alone or in conjugated form, orally or parenterally, to the patient. Examples include phosphorus-32, iodine-131, yttrium-90, strontium-89, and samarium-153, all of which decay by high-energy beta-particle emission. While the very first radiopharmaceuticals typically had intrinsic tendencies to accumulate in a target organ or site, they were of limited potential use due to their hematopoietic toxicity. More recently, a new wave of research has led to the development of biologic molecular targeted radiopharmaceuticals that optimize the delivery of cytotoxic agents to specific body cell types, by manipulation of the immune system.

Radioimmunotherapy is commonly used to treat non-Hodgkin's lymphoma that has proved refractory to other treatments. Two compounds have recently been approved by the Food and Drugs Administration (FDA) which consist of murine monoclonal anti-CD20 antibodies attached to radioactive isotopes; these are yttrium-90 ibritumomab tiuxetan (Zevalin®) and iodine-131 tositumomab (Bexxar®). Prior to treatment, the patient must undergo an hematopoietic work-up to ensure that he/she will tolerate treatment without significant toxicity, and also to determine the appropriate dosage. Patients can be discharged shortly after both types of therapy [38–41].

Radiopharmaceuticals have also been shown in multiple studies to significantly palliate pain caused by bone metastases, albeit without improving survival. They are most often given as second-line therapies for patients who have failed other local palliative treatments. Contraindications to treatment include poor hematopoietic reserve, impending pathologic fracture, spinal cord

or nerve root compression, significant extra-osseous extension of disease, extensive bony destruction, and poor uptake of lesions on bone scan. Strontium-89 (Metastron™) is indicated in metastatic prostate cancer, while samarium-153 (Quadramet®) has been shown to accumulate preferentially in osteoblastic lesions rather than in normal bone. After injection, all bodily fluids should be monitored. Radium-223 has recently been shown to palliate symptoms and prolong survival in metastatic prostate cancer [42].

The thyroid gland's innate ability to absorb and sequester iodine can be utilized to deliver radioactive iodine-131 for certain disorders. Radioactive iodine treatment may be indicated for benign disorders such as hyperthyroidism and toxic nodular goiter, or as adjuvant therapy to ablate residual thyroid tissue after thyroidectomy for differentiated thyroid carcinoma. Indications for adjuvant treatment include high-risk features such as large tumor size, multifocal disease, thyroid capsule, vascular, or soft tissue invasion. The standard postoperative activity delivered two to six months after thyroidectomy is 30–100 mCi. Iodine-131 is also given for recurrent or metastatic thyroid carcinoma, and an activity of 150–250 mCi is indicated.

Phosphorus-32 can be delivered as radioimmunotherapy in two distinct forms. In its soluble state, it accumulates in bone marrow, spleen and liver, and is hence useful to treat hematopoietic disorders such as polycythemia vera and thrombocytosis. In its colloid state, phosphorus-32 accumulates in intracavitary surfaces and is useful to treat malignant ascites, pleural effusions, and ovarian and endometrial carcinoma [43–46].

Hyperthermia

The addition of heat to radiotherapy can enhance the cell-killing potential of a given dose of energy. The mechanism of action is multifactorial and includes, but is not limited to, the inactivation of proteins that may be involved in DNA repair necessary for cell survival. Hyperthermia is also complementary to radiotherapy in that the S phase of the cell cycle, typically a relatively radioresistant time, is sensitive to hyperthermia. In addition, hypoxic cells (which are relatively radioresistant) are nevertheless heat-sensitive due to the acidic pH of nutrient-deprived cells at the border of viability. It is not known if the combination of heat and radiation has a synergistic or additive effect. Regardless, this therapeutic combination may be a useful option for superficial tumors such as locally recurrent breast cancer. Historically, technologic limitations made heating deep-seated tumors difficult [47]. However, a Dutch randomized trial comparing radiotherapy with or without deep hyperthermia showed dramatic improvements in complete response rates with the latter, associated with a survival benefit. Newer-generation deep hyperthermia devices are coupled with *in vivo* magnetic resonance imaging (MRI) to provide precise thermometry, and this combination is beginning to generate renewed interest [48].

Radiation Complications

The deposition of radiation energy into tissues leads to both immediate effects and potentially delayed reactions. The former is referred to as the *acute reaction*, while the latter is best described as *chronic toxicity*. It is important to understand that acute effects – that is, temporary side effects – are different from permanent changes. The latter are what most would call damage, and these are the true risks of treatment, more accurately described as treatment complications.

Acute toxicities are expressed as a function of the tissues or organs exposed, the total dose, and the time over which it is given. These side effects are *probable*, normally temporary, and are the result of both cell depletion in normal tissues and inflammatory reaction. Healing occurs when the injured tissue repopulates the lost cells, and the body's defense reaction resolves. The time course over which this occurs is usually weeks to months for both the development of the reaction as well as the recovery.

The late toxicity of radiation therapy results from damage primarily to the vasculoconnective tissues and slowly proliferating parenchymal cells, leading to an increase in cell loss, that results in fibrotic replacement-associated tissue dysfunction. Examples include subcutaneous fibrosis and osteoradionecrosis, among others.

The probability of a long-term complication such as these is most commonly associated with larger fraction sizes and/or higher total doses. Looking again at the idea of therapeutic window, as seen in Figure 1.2, expresses this idea graphically [49].

Trying to increase the probability of tumor control from 90% to 95% by increasing the total dose from point A to point B will lead to a proportionately greater increase in the risk of late damage. In practice, the data – and therefore the position of the two curves – is never so

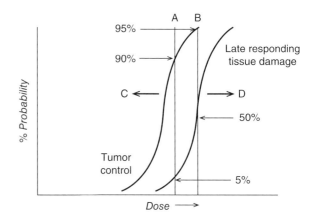

Figure 1.2 The therapeutic window. *Source:* Hall and Giaccia 2012 [49]. Reproduced with permission of Wolters Kluwer Health.

clearly defined. Just as importantly, individual patient responses are never obliged to follow previous patterns, so there is always a risk of damage in any situation. This concept should never be forgotten.

Radiation oncologists must counsel patients regarding the risks of treatment, acknowledging that subcutaneous fibrosis, chronic enteritis or proctitis, and transverse myelitis result in substantially different quality of life repercussions. In the case of palliation, there is usually minimal tolerance for risk, while in curative treatment it is reasonable to accept a finitely low level of risk, especially when options for management of the complication are available. The difficult decisions arise when palliative treatments have a significant risk of organ damage due to previous therapy or pre-existing comorbidities, or when even high-dose radiation therapy is unlikely to provide much chance of cure. Although a clinician's experience can be invaluable, there is no substitute for communicating the realities of the situation to the patient and their loved ones, and cooperatively reaching an agreement on how best to proceed. As much as the field of radiation oncology relies on quantifiable measurements of physics and statistics, it is the clinical art of implementation that brings the value to the patient.

References

1 Siegel, R., Miller, K., Jemal, A. (2017) Cancer Statistics 2017. *CA Cancer J. Clin.*, **67**, 7–30.

2 O'Sullivan, B., Davis, A.M., Turcotte, R., *et al.* (2002) Preoperative versus postoperative radiotherapy in soft-tissue sarcoma of the limbs: a randomized trial. *Lancet*, **359**, 2235–2241.

3 Pollack, A., Zagars, G.K., Goswitz, M.S., *et al.* (1998) Preoperative versus postoperative radiotherapy in the treatment of soft tissue sarcomas: a matter of

presentation. *Int. J. Radiat. Oncol. Biol. Phys.*, **42**, 563–572.

4 Sauer, R., Becker, H., Hohenberger, W., *et al.* (2004) Preoperative versus postoperative chemoradiotherapy for rectal cancer. *N. Engl. J. Med.*, **351**, 1731–1740.

5 Cole, C.J., Pollack, A., Gunar, K., *et al.* (1995) Local control of muscle-invasive bladder cancer: Preoperative radiotherapy and cystectomy versus cystectomy alone. *Int. J. Radiat. Oncol. Biol. Phys.*, **32** (2), 331–340.

6 Kapiteijn, E., Marijnen, C.A.M., Nagtegaal, I.D., *et al.* (2001) Preoperative radiotherapy combined with total mesorectal excision for resectable rectal cancer. *N. Engl. J. Med.*, **345**, 638–646.

7 Pahlman, L., Glimelius, B., *et al.* (1997) Improved survival with preoperative radiotherapy in resectable rectal cancer: Swedish Rectal Cancer Trial. *N. Engl. J. Med.*, **336**, 980–987.

8 Rosenzweig, K.E. (2013) Current readings: improvement in intensity-modulated radiation therapy for malignant pleural mesothelioma. *Semin. Thorac. Cardiovasc. Surg.*, **25** (3), 245–250.

9 Mendenhall, W., Amdur, R., Morris, C., Hinerman, R. (2001) T1-T2N0 squamous cell carcinoma of the glottis larynx treated with radiation therapy. *J. Clin. Oncol.*, **19**, 4029–4036.

10 Tester, W., Caplan, R., Heaney, J., *et al.* (1996) Neoadjuvant combined modality program with selective organ preservation for invasive bladder cancer: results of Radiation Therapy Oncology Group phase II trial 8802. *J. Clin. Oncol.*, **14**, 119–126.

11 Looser, K.J., Shah, J.P., Strong, E.W. (1978) The significance of 'positive' margins in surgically resected epidermoid carcinomas. *Head Neck Surg.*, **1**, 107–111.

12 Johnson, J.T., Barnes, E.L., Myers, E.N., Schramm, L., Borochovitz, D., Sigler, B.A. (1981) The extracapsular spread of tumors in cervical node metastasis. *Arch. Otolaryngol.*, **107**, 725–729.

13 Wood, C.G., Hahn, S.M. (2009) Combined modality, in *Handbook of Radiation Oncology: Basic Principles and Clinical Protocols*, 1st edition (eds B.G. Haffty, L.D. Wilson), Jones and Bartlett, Sudbury, MA, pp. 89–110.

14 Scaringi, C., Enrici, R.M., Minniti, G. (2013) Combining molecular targeted agents with radiation therapy for malignant gliomas. *OncoTargets Ther.*, **6**, 1079–1095.

15 Xuan, Z.X., Li, L.N., Zhang, Q., *et al.* (2014) Fully human VEGFR2 monoclonal antibody BC001 attenuates tumor angiogenesis and inhibits tumor growth. *Int. J. Oncol.*, **45** (6), 2411–2420.

16 Liu, Y., Zhang, L., Liu, Y., *et al.* (2015) DNA-PKcs deficiency inhibits glioblastoma cell-derived angiogenesis after ionizing radiation. *J. Cell Physiol.*, **230** (5), 1094–1103.

17 Pilones, K.A., Vanpouille-Box, C., Demaria, S. (2015) Combination of radiotherapy and immune checkpoint inhibitors. *Semin. Radiat. Oncol.*, **25** (1), 28–33.

18 Gomelia, L., Singh, J., Costas, L., Edouard, T. (2010) Hormone therapy in the management of prostate cancer: evidence-based approaches. *Ther. Adv. Urol.*, **2** (4), 171–181.

19 Wang, T., Languino, L., Lian, J., Stein, G., Blute, M., FitzGerald, T. (2011) Molecular targets for radiation oncology in prostate cancer. *Front. Oncol.*, **1** (17), 1–11.

20 Joon, D.L., Hasegawa, M., Sikes, C., *et al.* (1997) Supra-additive apoptotic response of R3327-G rat prostate tumors to androgen ablation and radiation. *Int. J. Radiat. Oncol. Biol. Phys.*, **38** (5), 1071–1077.

21 Al-Ubaidi, F., Schultz, N., Egevad, L., Granfors, T., Helleday, T. (2012) Castration therapy of prostate cancer results in downregulation of HIF-1α levels. *Int. J. Radiat. Oncol. Biol. Phys.*, **82** (3), 1243–1248.

22 Langenhuijsen, J.F., Van Lin, E.N., Hoffmann, A.L. *et al.* (2011) Neoadjuvant androgen deprivation for prostate volume reduction: the optimal duration in prostate cancer radiotherapy. *Urol. Oncol.*, **29** (1), 52–57.

23 Horsman, M.R., Overgaard, J. (2002) Overcoming tumour radioresistance resulting from hypoxia, in *Basic Clinical Radiobiology*, 3rd edn (ed. G.G. Steel), Arnold, London, pp. 169–181.

24 Casarett, A.P. (1968) Radiation effects on microorganisms and independent cell systems, in *Radiation Biology*, 1st edn (ed. A.P. Casarett), Prentice-Hall, Englewood Cliffs, CA, pp. 136–158.

25 Puck, T.T., Marcus, P.I. (1956) Actions of x-rays on mammalian cells. *J. Exp. Med.*, **103**, 653–666.

26 Elkind, M.M., Sutton, G., Moses, W.B., *et al.* (1967) Sub-lethal and lethal radiation damage. *Nature*, **214**, 1088–1092.

27 Thomlinson, R.H., Gray, L.H. (1955) The histological structure of some human lung cancers and the possible implications for radiotherapy. *Br. J. Cancer*, **9**, 539–549.

28 Harrison, L.B., Chadha, M., Hill, R.J., Hu, K., Shasha, D. (2002) Impact of tumor hypoxia and anemia on radiation therapy outcomes. *Oncologist*, **7**, 492–508.

29 Teoh, M., Clark, C.H., Wood, K., Whitaker, S., Nisbet, A. (2011) Volumetric modulated arc therapy: a review of current literature and clinical use in practice. *Br. J. Radiol.*, **84**, 967–996.

30 Castadot, P., Lee, J., Geets, X., Grégoire, V. (2010) Adaptive radiotherapy of head and neck cancer. *Semin. Radiat. Oncol.*, **20**, 84–93.

31 Duprez, F., De Neve, W., De Gersem, W., Coghe, M., Madani, I. (2011) Adaptive dose painting by numbers for head-and-neck. *Int. J. Radiat. Oncol. Biol. Phys.*, **80** (4), 1045–1055.

32 Grégoire, V., Jeraj, R., Lee, J.A., O'Sullivan, B. (2012) Radiotherapy for head and neck tumors in 2012 and beyond: conformal, tailored, and adaptive? *Lancet Oncol.*, **13**, 292–300.

33 Suh, J. (2010) Stereotactic radiosurgery for the management of brain metastases. *N. Engl. J. Med.*, **362**, 1119–1127.

34 Chang, B., Timmerman, R. (2007) Stereotactic body radiation therapy: A comprehensive review. *Am. J. Clin. Oncol.*, **30**, 637–644.

35 Diaz, A.Z. (2003) Assessment of the results from the phase I/II boron neutron capture therapy trials at the

Brookhaven National Laboratory from a clinician's point of view. *J. Neurooncol.*, **62**, 101–109.

36 Vaidya, J.S., Wenz, F., Bulsara, M., *et al.* (2014) Risk-adapted targeted intraoperative radiotherapy versus whole-breast radiotherapy for breast cancer: 5-year results for local control and overall survival from the TARGIT-A randomised trial. *Lancet*, **383** (9917), 603–613.

37 Willett, C., Czito, B., Tyler, D. (2007) Intraoperative radiation therapy. *J. Clin. Oncol.*, **25** (8), 971–977.

38 Pohlman, B., Sweetenham, J., Macklis, R.M. (2006) Review of clinical radioimmunotherapy. *Expert Rev. Anticancer Ther.*, **6**, 445–462.

39 Kassis, A.I., Adelstein, S.J. (2005) Radiobiologic principles in radionuclide therapy. *J. Nucl. Med.*, **46**, S4–S12.

40 McLaughlin, P., Grillo-Lopez, A.J., Link, B.K., *et al.* (1998) Rituximab chimeric anti-CD20 monoclonal antibody therapy for relapsed indolent lymphoma: Half of patients respond to a four-dose treatment program. *J. Clin. Oncol.*, **16**, 2825–2833.

41 Hernandez, M.C., Knox, S.J. (2004) The radiobiology of radioimmunotherapy: Targeting CD20 B-cell antigen in non-Hodgkin's lymphoma. *Int. J. Radiat. Oncol. Biol. Phys.*, **59**, 1274–1287.

42 Brady, D., Parker, C.C., O'Sullivan, J.M. (2013) Bone-targeting radiopharmaceuticals including radium-223. *Cancer J.*, **19** (1), 71–78.

43 U.S. Nuclear Regulatory Commission: Part 35-medical use of byproduct material. http://www.nrc.gov/reading-rm/doc-collections/cfr/part035/.

44 Perez, C., Brady, L., Halperin, E., *et al.* (eds) (2013) *Principles and Practice of Radiation Oncology*, 6th edn. Lippincott Williams and Wilkins, Philadelphia, PA.

45 Serafini, A.N. (2001) Therapy of metastatic bone pain. *J. Nucl. Med.*, **42**, 895–906.

46 Bauman, G.G., Charette, M., Reid, R., *et al.* (2005) Radiopharmaceuticals for the palliation of painful bone metastases – a systematic review. *Radiother. Oncol.*, **75**, 258–270.

47 Leibel, S.A., Phillips, T.L. (eds) (2010) *Textbook of Radiation Oncology*, 3rd edn. Saunders, Philadelphia, PA.

48 Van der Zee, J., Gonzalez, D.G., van Rhoon, G.C., *et al.* (2010) Comparison of radiotherapy alone with radiotherapy plus hyperthermia in locally advanced pelvic tumours: A prospective, randomised, multicenter trial. *Lancet*, **355**, 1119–1125.

49 Hall, E.J., Giaccia, A.J. (2012) *Radiobiology for Radiologists*, 7th edn. Lippincott Williams and Wilkins, Philadelphia, PA.

2

Radiation Biology for Radiation Oncologists

Timothy A. Chan, Boris Hristov and Simon N. Powell

During the past 15 years, the molecular mechanisms of how exposure to ionizing radiation affects molecules, proteins, cells, organisms – and ultimately humans – have been intensively investigated. The effect of radiation exposure is to generate many forms of cellular stress, including direct effects on cell membranes, oxidative stress, and DNA damage. DNA damage is thought to be the major determinant of cell death, although the full spectrum of effects on cells contributes to the overall complex radiation response.

DNA Damage, DNA Repair, and Cell Survival

DNA Damage After Irradiation

Initial DNA damage refers to the measured DNA damage in the cell after rapid biochemical modification has occurred but before biological processing (i.e., via enzymatic reactions with relatively long half-lives) has taken place. This is the DNA damage that is present after irradiation, prior to the onset of DNA repair. In practical terms, this is the measured DNA damage when cells are irradiated on ice, preventing active repair. A variety of types of DNA damage have been described; the main types are summarized in Table 2.1. High-LET radiations, such as heavy charged particles, are more likely to cause breakage of both strands of DNA due to a higher probability of clustered ionizations, leading to double-strand breaks (DSB) (Figure 2.1). Low-LET radiations such as photons can also cause DSBs but produce less per unit dose relative to single-strand breaks and other lesions, due to sparse ionizations. A significant proportion of the damage from photons results from indirect effects and free radical-associated damage, which are amenable to free

radical scavenging. Typically, 1 Gy of photon irradiation will generate 40 DSBs and up to 2000 nucleotide base lesions, many of the latter resulting from free radical-dependent damage.

Many techniques are available to measure DNA damage (Figure 2.2). The measurement of single- or double-strand breaks is based on DNA fragmentation in alkaline (denaturing) or neutral conditions, respectively. DNA fragments can be separated according to size by a variety of means, including velocity sedimentation, filter elution, or pulsed-field gel electrophoresis (PFGE). An adaptation of a DNA fragmentation assay that is commonly used is the single-cell gel electrophoresis or 'comet' assay [1]. In this assay, cells are embedded in agarose on a microscope slide and lysed with detergent and high salt to form nucleoids containing supercoiled loops of DNA linked to the nuclear matrix. Subsequently electrophoresis results in structures resembling comets, with the tail of the comet running in front of the head, due to DNA fragmentation. The comet assay allows an assessment of DNA fragmentation in the context of chromatin, since the protein is retained in this method (in contrast to PFGE). The intensity of the comet tail relative to the head reflects the number of DNA breaks. The relative intensities of fluorescence are recorded using imaging software, and computerized analysis can be used to calculate the extent of DNA damage.

DNA protein crosslinks are quantified by the reduction in strand breaks detected when no protein digestion is allowed in the preparation of the test DNA. Base damage can be measured by a variety of chemical methods, and these have been used to characterize more than 20 different radiation products of thymine. Specific antibodies have been made to recognize certain types of base lesions. In addition, high-performance liquid chromatography (HPLC) is commonly used to separate and

Clinical Radiation Oncology: Indications, Techniques, and Results, Third Edition. Edited by William Small Jr.
© 2017 John Wiley & Sons, Inc. Published 2017 by John Wiley & Sons, Inc.

Table 2.1 Major types of DNA damage after ionizing radiation.

	Damage type	No./Gy/cell
	base damage	>1000
	single-strand break (SSB)	500–1000
	double-strand break (DSB)	~40
	sugar damage, DNA-DNA and DNA-protein cross links	*various*

characterize different base adducts that form following exposure to genotoxins. Lastly, fluorescence *in-situ* hybridization (FISH) is increasingly used to directly visualize chromosomal breaks after DNA damage.

Of the radiation-induced lesions listed in Table 2.1, DSBs are most closely associated with cell lethality. While the number of DSBs correlates closely with the extent of lethality, it is important to note that this association does not exclude the possibility that some other lesion produced in proportion to DSBs also plays a critical role. The ratio of DSBs to single-strand breaks (SSBs) can vary by altering the agents to which cells are exposed. For example, if hydrogen peroxide is present, the DSB:SSB ratio is reduced and this causes less cell lethality per measured lesion. In contrast, when irradiation is performed in the presence of bleomycin, the ratio is increased and more cell deaths per lesion results. Between DSBs and SSBs, the absolute number of DSBs correlates most well with cell survival probability, irrespective of the agent used to cause those breaks. Hence, it is concluded that the DSB is the biologically important lesion. But, could two independently produced SSBs combine to form a DSB?

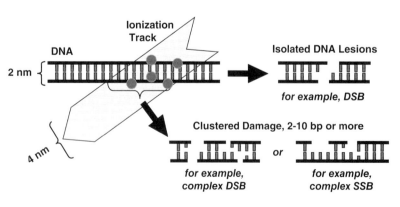

Figure 2.1 Ionizing radiation induces sparse and clustered lesions in DNA, including oxidized purines and pyrimidines, abasic (AP) sites and SSB. As LET increases, the proportion of clustered lesions increases. Clustered lesions are more likely to result in a DSB. (Adapted from Ref. [1a].

- **Sucrose gradients**
- **Filter elution** } alkaline for SSB
- **Gel electrophoresis** } neutral for DSB
- **Nucleoid sedimentation**
- **Comet assay**
- **Foci of** *γ***H2AX**

Figure 2.2 Assays for measuring DNA damage from ionizing radiation. Sucrose gradients, filter elution and pulsed-field gel electrophoresis are used to measure DNA fragmentation, so that alkaline or neutral conditions determine single- or double-stranded measures. Nucleoid and comet assays retain protein with DNA, and reflect chromatin damage. *γ*-H2AX reflects DNA damage indirectly via histone post-translational modifications.

For radiation doses within the clinically used range, the answer is yes, but only with an extremely low probability. However, when two SSBs are on opposite strands within three nucleotides, conversion to a DSB is likely. The majority of DSBs are produced from a single clustered ionization at clinically relevant doses of radiation, whereas interaction of two independent events becomes more likely at higher doses.

Although the majority of DNA DSBs (i.e., DNA fragments) are rejoined, the fidelity or accuracy of the repair process is less than perfect in many instances (Figure 2.3) [1a]. The consequence is that although the DSB is rejoined, it may not correct the function of a critical gene in the vicinity of the lesion. In addition, the repair process may also induce more significant deletions and rearrangements. The balance of high-fidelity repair and misrepair can be altered under certain conditions, such as stem cells that attach a priority on error-free repair, whereas terminally differentiated cells are content to repair broken chromosomes with errors.

Residual DNA lesions can remain because of either saturation of DNA repair processes leading to a failure to rejoin in the available time, or misrepair of the broken ends. Specific subsets of DSBs, either by nature or position, may have a higher probability of repair failure. One

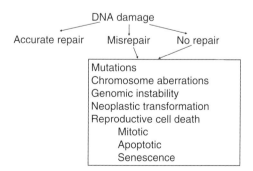

Figure 2.3 DNA damage can be linked to biological effects that lead to a number of physiologic results.

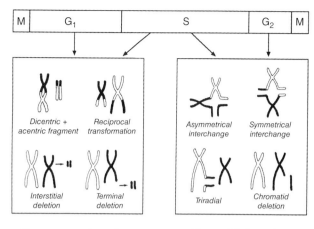

Chromosome aberrations   Chromatid aberrations

Figure 2.4 Ionization radiation-induced chromosomal aberrations depend on the cell cycle. Chromosomal aberrations arising in G_1 produce effects on both chromatids, whereas aberrations produced in S and G_2 produce breaks in chromatids which produce radial chromosomes.

possibility is that the ability to repair a DNA DSB may be influenced by the presence of other minor types of DNA damage in the immediate vicinity (i.e., within 10 base pairs or one helical turn of the site of cleavage). Such effects produce what is called a locally multiply damaged site (LMDS) [2]. At these sites, a cluster of ionizations has caused a group of lesions to form close together, which can result in a greater probability of loss of genetic material and cell death.

At the level of chromosomes, DNA damage from irradiation can manifest as different types of aberrations (Figure 2.4). These aberrations can be visualized when cells are in metaphase. The two primary classes of aberrations are chromosomal aberrations and chromatid aberrations.

Chromosomal aberrations result if a cell is irradiated early in interphase (G_1), before chromosomal material has been duplicated. In this situation, the radiation-induced DSB affects the duplex of a single chromosome. Subsequently, during DNA synthesis, this strand of chromatin is copied and the break is replicated. This leads to a chromosome aberration that is visible at the next mitosis, because there is an identical break in the corresponding points of a pair of chromatids. Two types of chromosomal aberrations that are lethal to the cell are the ring and the dicentric chromosome, as neither chromosome is capable of completing cell division. These chromosomal aberrations are produced by abnormal end-joining, either intra- or inter-chromosomally.

If the DNA break occurs later in interphase (G_2) after DNA synthesis has occurred (when chromosomes exist as two strands of chromatin), then the defects produced are called *chromatid aberrations*. In this case, a break occurs in a single chromatid arm after DNA replication and leaves the opposite arm of the same chromosome undamaged. The chromosomal break is revealed at the next cell cycle in the daughter cell. Another common type of chromatid aberration is that produced by an exchange event, which result in abnormal junctions between chromatids. Radial chromosomes can be produced by this mechanism. A consequence of abnormal exchange events is also the anaphase bridge seen at mitosis, which presumably leads to cell death. In summary, the consequence of DNA damage and subsequent repair is the major determinant of cell survival or cell death after exposure to ionizing radiation. Cell death pathways will be discussed later in the chapter.

Immediate Biochemical Modification of Radiation-Induced Damage

Once ionized biological target molecules are formed after exposure to ionizing radiation, either by direct action at the DNA or indirectly from the interaction of DNA with OH• radicals produced by the incident ionizing radiation, rapid biochemical reactions can process the ionized species to determine the biologically relevant effects that result. For example, one direct effect of ionization is a loss of hydrogen atoms from DNA, which can be rapidly reversed by hydrogen donor molecules such as those containing sulfhydryl groups (-SH). In order to act upon DNA, these molecules need access to damaged sites and necessarily are either small or already present adjacent to DNA. Reduced glutathione (GSH; the most abundant sulfhydryl hydrogen donor molecule) (Figure 2.5) and cysteamine are potent modifiers of DNA damage. Sulfhydryl compounds are efficient radioprotectors against sparsely ionizing x- or gamma-rays. The mechanisms most implicated in sulfhydryl-mediated cytoprotection include: (i) scavenging free-radicals and thus protecting against oxygen-based free-radical generation by radiation or chemotherapy; and (ii) hydrogen atom donation to promote direct chemical repair at sites of DNA damage or DNA-radical formation.

In some cases, a direct correlation between sulfhydryl levels and radiosensitivity is observed, but this relationship is by no means universal [3]. Artificial manipulation of thiol levels has a clear effect on measurable initial DNA damage – that is, the damage that can be measured in cells after energy deposition and immediate modification. For example, when the intracellular GSH content is reduced using buthionine sulphoximine or diethyl maleate, sensitivity to DNA damage is significantly increased [4].

Another mechanism of 'immediate' biological modification of DNA damage is rapid enzymatic metabolism of the products of water hydrolysis. Hydrogen peroxide

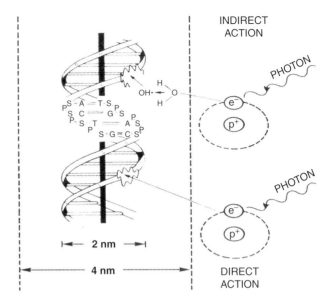

Figure 2.5 Ionizations that occur in water and free radical interactions within 2 nm can lead to radical formation in DNA. However, indirect action can also be quenched by glutathione (GSH) and other thiol-containing free radical scavengers. Adapted from Ref. [1a].

is generated from hydroxyl radicals, and is converted to water and oxygen by the enzyme catalase, or to water and dehydrogenated cosubstrates by peroxidases. Superoxide radicals are catalyzed by the enzyme superoxide dismutase. Thus, levels of these enzymes can affect the amount of DNA damage sustained after exposure to ionizing radiation.

A third mechanism that can affect how much damage is sustained is the conformation or compactness of the exposed DNA, but evidence for this is conflicting. Cells grown as multicellular spheroids can be more radioresistant than the same cells grown in monolayer culture. The ability of DNA to unwind is greater in monolayer-cultured cells. The decreased sensitivity may be explained by tighter packing of chromatin in the cells of the spheroids, which results in less residual DNA damage. However, the mechanism of observing less residual damage is not clearly ascribed to either less initial damage or improved DNA repair. Direct measurements of radiosensitivity correlated with the state of chromatin seem to support this hypothesis. In an interesting series of experiments, Rajab *et al.* directly measured both the radiosensitivity and chromatin compaction patterns in a series of human bladder cell lines. It was found that radiosensitive lines typically possessed more relaxed chromatin, whereas radioresistant lines exhibited condensed chromatin [5]. The impact of chromatin on DNA repair has been recognized as a major regulator during recent years [6, 7].

DNA Damage Sensing and DNA Repair

The repair of DNA DSBs is a complex biological process that is carried out by one of two pathways of DNA repair, namely non-homologous end-joining (NHEJ) or homologous recombination (HR). NHEJ is intrinsically error-prone, in which the cells modify the broken ends of DNA before they are ligated. It can occur at any point in the cell cycle, as well as in non-cycling cells. In contrast, HR faithfully repairs DSBs through the use of homologous DNA sequences, primarily the sister chromatids, which are present in the late S and G_2 phases of the cell cycle. The process of HR is also used by cells to repair other types of DNA damage, including stalled replication forks, inter-strand DNA crosslinks, sites of meiotic DSBs, and abortive topoisomerase II lesions. Although the predominant method of repairing DNA DSBs caused by ionizing radiation is by NHEJ, based on genetic determinants of radiosensitivity, there is a growing view that DSBs in cancer cells may be frequently repaired by HR [8].

Over the past several years, many molecular components of the DNA damage response have been elucidated (Figure 2.6). Sensors of DNA DSBs are recruited to the site of damage, which activate a variety of cellular signaling pathways, including repair, checkpoints, senescence or cell death. The question of which protein is the 'first responder' has been debated for many years, but both the Ku heterodimer (Ku70/Ku80) and the Mre11 complex are capable of binding rapidly to DNA DSBs. Whether there are chromatin changes that actually signal the presence of the double-strand break is also questioned, but not clearly demonstrated. Poly ADP-ribose polymerase (PARP) activation remains a possible mechanism for DNA damage recognition.

Once DNA DSB binding proteins are located at the break, the signaling cascade is activated. Ataxia telangiectasia mutated (ATM) activation that is dependent on DNA DSBs (as opposed to ATM activation by other means) is linked to Mre11 complex binding [9,10], which then initiates a local cascade of phosphorylations at and around the break site [11]. Ku heterodimer binding recruits the DNA-dependent protein kinase catalytic subunit (DNA-PKcs), which also results in local phosphorylation of itself, of Ku, and other local targets. In the setting of a stalled replication fork, the combination of RPA binding to single-stranded DNA and Ataxia telangiectasis-related (ATR) interacting protein (ATRIP) binding, there is activation of ATR, the third member of the DNA damage-dependent protein kinases. These protein kinases are responsible for all aspects of the DNA damage response, including cell cycle checkpoint activation, recruitment of downstream DNA repair proteins, and the activation of cell death or cell senescence depending on the cell context.

The choice of DNA DSB repair pathway, once the DSB is recognized, remains an interesting question that is not fully understood. When a cell is non-cycling, the HR pathway is inactive, since the production of Rad51 and other key HR proteins is dependent on entering the cell cycle. For many cells in the human body, NHEJ is clearly the predominant and important pathway of repair (Figure 2.7). After the Ku heterodimer has recruited DNA-PKcs, auto-phosphorylation and phosphorylation of Ku follow, which results in release of the catalytic

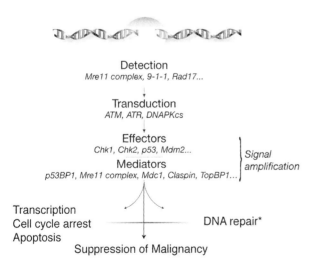

Detection
Mre11 complex, 9-1-1, Rad17...

Transduction
ATM, ATR, DNAPKcs

Effectors
Chk1, Chk2, p53, Mdm2...

Mediators
p53BP1, Mre11 complex, Mdc1, Claspin, TopBP1...

} *Signal amplification*

Transcription
Cell cycle arrest
Apoptosis

DNA repair*

Suppression of Malignancy

* incl. programmed gene rearrangement

Figure 2.6 Sensing DNA damage. Proteins that bind directly to DNA strand breaks recruit additional proteins that activate a cascade of signaling. The product of DNA damage signaling is not only DNA repair, but also cell cycle arrest, cell death and suppression of malignant transformation.

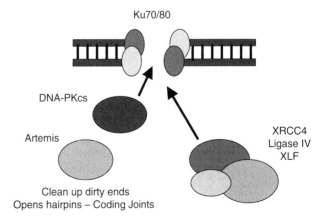

Ku70/80

DNA-PKcs

Artemis

XRCC4
Ligase IV
XLF

Clean up dirty ends
Opens hairpins – Coding Joints

Figure 2.7 Non-homologous end-joining. Ku proteins bind directly to DNA strand breaks and additional proteins are recruited, such as DNA-PKcs that phosphorylate the Ku heterodimer. The resultant translocation of the Ku heterodimer allows recruitment of the ligase complex.

subunit and the translocation of the Ku heterodimer from the blunt ends of DSB. By a mechanism that is not fully understood, the XRCC4/XLF/Ligase IV complex is formed, which functions as a ligase by using the space vacated by the Ku heterodimer. Occasionally, the ends of the DSB need end modification, such as when the end is a closed hairpin, which requires the recruitment of a specific endonuclease (Artemis in this case) to nick the hairpin and create a near-blunt DSB. Additional clipping of covalently bound DNA ends, such as topoisomerase intermediates, can be achieved using the tyrosyl-DNA phosphodiesterase 1 (TDP1). Relatively blunt ends, without chemical modifications of the nucleotides, are critical for the completion of NHEJ.

The interesting question becomes how is HR recruited for DSB repair? There is evidence that one of the key initiators of HR is the CtIP protein, which is activated by cyclin-dependent kinases to initiate DNA 5′-end resection [12]. In addition, the Mre11 complex recruits CtIP, which is then additionally dependent on BRCA1 to complete the resection process [13]. The process of HR repair requires the generation of a 3′-single-stranded DNA (ssDNA) by 5′ to 3′ resection at the site of the DSB, which is bound by replication protein A (RPA). The transition from RPA binding to the formation of RAD51 filaments, which is an essential step before strand exchange can occur, is a complex process controlled by many proteins (Figure 2.8). One of the key players in this transition is the BRCA2 protein, which appears to replace RPA on ssDNA and promotes the formation of Rad51 multimeric filaments on ssDNA. Once the Rad51 filament is formed, the process of invasion of an intact DNA duplex and the search for homology can be initiated. Strand invasion leads to the displacement on one strand of the intact DNA duplex and the formation of a 'D-loop,' which is the simplest form of HR and can act directly as the template for repairing the DSB. DNA can then be synthesized using the homologous template from the D-loop, but how the D-loop is disengaged is less clearly understood. The

front edge of the D-loop creates a structure, which is similar to a replication fork, but the resolution of this structure to allow re-ligation of the two original duplexes is a mechanism that still needs to be elucidated. The ligation step to join the free DNA strands probably involves DNA ligase I (replication-like), but the use of DNA ligase III (SSB repair, the final step in base-excision repair) has not been excluded.

Overall, the effectiveness of the different pathways of DNA DSB repair is the major determinant of a cell surviving exposure to ionizing radiation. Failure to survive is brought about by having too much residual DNA damage to survive cell division, mostly at the first cell division, but occasionally at the second, third or later cell divisions, if the DNA damage cannot be repaired adequately. The mode of cell death can also be variable, and is determined by the 'programming' of the cell: apoptosis, senescence, autophagy, necrosis and post-mitotic loss of genome integrity are all examples of how a cell can prevent further cell division cycles.

Modes of Cell Death Following DNA Damage

Radiation exposure can kill cells if the exposed cells fail to adequately repair the damaged DNA. A large volume of work performed during the past few decades has unveiled detailed information about the different modes of cell death that can occur following DNA damage (Figure 2.9). Much of the information about how cells die following radiation exposure comes from experiments performed on cultured cells. Following irradiation, most cells in culture undergo *mitotic death*, or cell death that occurs during attempted cell division. Mitotic death does not necessarily occur at the first post-irradiation mitosis. Cells may undergo one, two, or more mitoses before the damaged chromosomes cause the affected cell to die during

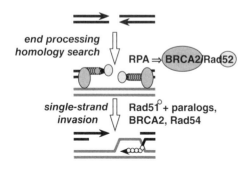

Figure 2.8 Homologous recombination. Resection of the 5′-end of DSB reveals a 3′ tail, which is coated with RPA. HR mediator proteins facilitate the formation of RAD51 filaments, which initiates the strand exchange reactions of the repair pathway.

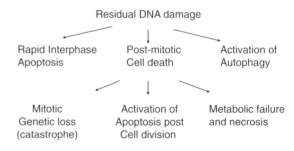

Figure 2.9 Unrepaired DNA damage can trigger cell death. Most cell death occurs following one or more transitions through mitosis, either by excessive genetic loss, or delayed activation of apoptosis. Metabolic failure and necrosis can also occur. Rapid cell death can be triggered by interphase activation of apoptosis, which is p53-dependent. Autophagy, which is initially a pro-survival pathway, can be converted to a death pathway when the extent of the auto-phagocytic process is too large.

attempted division [14]. Death results because the chromosome and chromatid aberrations that go unrepaired ultimately cause mitosis to fail or render the daughter cells incapable of subsequent cell division. Time-lapse microscopy of cells treated with radiation has confirmed that this process of mitotic death is a dominant cause of cell death and loss of reproductive integrity. At the molecular level, mitotic death results if DNA damage is severe enough so that DNA damage repair mechanisms are unable to repair enough of the damage so that reproductive integrity is preserved. This can happen either because the DNA damage itself is too severe or if, during tumorigenesis, tumor suppressors required for cell cycle arrest or checkpoint activation are inactivated, resulting in an inability to properly repair damage prior to progression through the cell cycle [15–18].

Following irradiation, not all cells undergo mitotic death. Some cells, especially those of the hematopoietic lineage, undergo programmed cell death, or *apoptosis*. The latter is an essential process during normal development to eliminate cells during ontogeny or to remove damaged cells. Apoptosis is an active, scheduled process that requires the expenditure of energy, and is characterized by a well-defined sequence of morphologic events. First, cells condense and compartmentalize to form many membrane-enclosed bodies. These bodies are then either shed (i.e., colonic epithelial cells) or phagocytized and destroyed by neighboring cells. Within apoptotic cells, chromatin condensation and DNA fragmentation occurs, giving rise to characteristic DNA laddering [19, 20].

At the molecular level, apoptosis is activated and carried out by a well-orchestrated cascade of events. Apoptosis can be triggered by a diverse range of extracellular or intracellular stimuli. Pro-apoptotic signals may include toxic insults such as radiation, chemotherapy, or secreted proteins such as Fas ligand (FasL) or tumor necrosis factor (TNF) [21–23]. These signals ultimately converge upon and activate a series of cysteine aspartate proteases, called *caspases*, which act in a proteolytic cascade that is required for programmed cell death. Caspases are normally synthesized as inactive precursors, and become activated by internal cleavage during apoptosis. Activated caspases, which are abundant in apoptotic cells, are potent activators of themselves as well as downstream caspases. Typically, upon activation, caspace-8 cleaves BH3-only molecules such as Bid, which translocates to the mitochondrial membrane, where these proteins release cytochrome c. The latter activates caspase-9, and along with apoptotic protease-activating factor 1 (Apaf-1), forms a large complex called the *apoptosome* [24]. The apoptosome then activates the effector caspases such as caspase-3, -6, and -7, which carry out the downstream events of apoptosis [25]. Interestingly, recent studies examining the molecular details of apoptosis

and mitotic death have shown that the molecular underpinnings of the two may overlap to some extent. For example, during mitotic death, effector caspases can become activated, which helps to promote cellular degradation [26, 27].

In contrast to apoptosis, *necrosis* is an unscheduled mode of cell death. Necrosis can result from severe damage to tissues and cells caused by hypoxia, trauma, toxins, or a variety of other damaging exposures. During necrotic death, the mitochondrial and cellular membranes become damaged, and this results in a shutdown of the osmotic pump, leading to cellular swelling. As necrosis progresses, cytoplasmic organelles swell and nuclear chromatin clumps into chaotic masses. Ultimately, the plasma and nuclear membranes completely disintegrate and organelles are extruded into the extracellular space. Necrotic death can attract the cells of the immune system and result in inflammation. Necrotic death can be seen following exposure to radiation, especially at high doses.

In conclusion, the cellular response to radiation exposure is a complex interplay of radiation-induced DNA damage, the damaged cell's attempt to repair DNA and other types of damage, and the dynamic balance between cell cycle arrest and death. The ultimate fate of the exposed cell depends on the extent of DNA damage and the physiologic environment of the affected cell.

Biological Factors that Influence Radiation Response

While the cellular response to radiation is influenced by intrinsic factors, such as the ability to repair DNA, a number of other biological factors can help determine radiation response. These factors include specific elements of the tumor microenvironment, oxygen tension, the nutritional state of the tumor, and other variables. Combined, these factors impart a powerful influence on radiation sensitivity and resistance.

The Oxygen Effect and the Significance of Hypoxia

One of the most important modifiers of radiation sensitivity of cells is molecular oxygen. In general, under physiological conditions, the presence of oxygen is sensitizing to radiation-induced damage. When a cell is exposed to radiation, free radicals form and react with organic molecules such as DNA, making the organic molecule itself highly reactive. O_2 acts at the level of free radicals. Free radical-dependent DNA damage caused by radiation can be repaired by the cell unless O_2 reacts with the site first. If O_2 reacts with the site, the damage can be 'fixed' and remain unrepaired. Furthermore, O_2 can combine with hydroxyl radicals (OH•) generated from the interaction of radiation with water to form H_2O_2, which is highly reactive and can cause damage to DNA and other organic molecules in the cell. These effects occur within 5 ms of exposure to molecular oxygen. The oxygen enhancement ratio (OER), defined as the ratio of radiation dose in anoxic versus oxic conditions to produce equal effect, is used to quantify the extent of oxygen-dependent radiosensitization. OER is given by the following equation:

$$OER = \frac{\text{Dose of radiation without oxygen to give a biological effect}}{\text{Dose of radiation with oxygen to obtain the same effect}}$$

Under physiological conditions, the OER is in the range of 2.5 to 3.0 [28]. This range is applicable for low-linear energy transfer (LET) photons, electrons, or protons, but is diminished in the setting of high-LET modalities. The OER is approximately 1.7–1.8 at LET values of about 100 keV μm^{-1} [29, 30]. The degree to which the OER is reduced is a reflection of the greater biological effectiveness of high-LET radiation.

This sensitizing effect of oxygen is of particular interest to the radiation oncologist because oxygen is maximally sensitizing at physiological concentrations. The pO_2 in normal tissues is in the range of 15 to 100 mmHg, and the pO_2 of venous blood is 40 mmHg [31]. Accordingly, if the oxygen in the target tissue is below a specific threshold concentration, radiation resistance occurs. Resistance to radiation due to hypoxia begins to appear when the pO_2 falls below approximately 20–30 mmHg. As the oxygen tension increases, the irradiated cells or tissues become progressively more sensitive to radiation until, in the presence of 100% oxygen, it is about threefold as sensitive compared to complete anoxia. An O_2 concentration of 0.5% will shift the survival curve half-way towards the fully aerated condition. Increasing the oxygen concentration past this point to 30 mmHg rapidly increases radiosensitivity to an OER of about 3. Further increases in oxygen tension to an atmosphere of pure oxygen have little additional effect. Therefore, only small amounts of oxygen are necessary to produce the very significant radiosensitization due to the oxygen effect.

Extensive data are available relating to the relationship between oxygen tension and radiation sensitivity. One classic study details a series of cell survival curves for Chinese hamster ovary (CHO) cells, equilibrated with variable oxygen tensions form 0.0001% to 100% oxygen. Data from this study are shown in Figure 2.10 [32]. For the CHO cells irradiated under hypoxic and full media conditions, oxygen was dose-modifying. When the results were modeled using the multitarget model (requiring a dose threshold to initiate cell killing, with an extrapolation number of *n*, and a slope of the logarithm

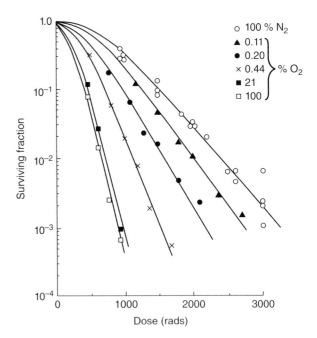

Figure 2.10 Cell survival curves for CHO cells equilibrated with oxygen at various pressures. *Source:* Ling 1981 [32]. Reproduced with permission of Radiation Research Society.

of survival against dose represented by D_0 – the dose to reduce survival to 1/e or ∼0.37) D_0 was seen to be dependent on pO_2 but *n* was independent. In these experiments, *n* was constant at 7 for all conditions at irradiation. The importance of hypoxic cells to radiation therapy is, of course, dependent on the extent to which hypoxic tumor cells *in vivo* exhibit radiation resistance. To assess the sensitivity of hypoxic tumor cells *in vivo* requires an understanding of the role of severity of the hypoxia, the duration of the hypoxia, and the levels of other metabolites on the radiation sensitivity of hypoxic cells.

There is evidence for some cell lines that *n* approaches 1.0 under conditions of extreme hypoxia [33]. This is important because the smaller shoulder on the survival curve for hypoxic cells means that OER decreases progressively with a reduction in dose or dose per fraction. The smaller *n* for hypoxic CHO cells, in the study conducted by Palcic *et al.*, was associated with a decrease in OER from 2.0 to 1.6 as the dose was decreased from 2.0 to 0.3 Gy; at 10 Gy, the OER was 2.7. Taylor and Brown [34] reported that for 20 doses of 1.7 Gy to contact-inhibited C3H-10T1/2 cells, the OER was 1.34, but for the same cell system the OER for single-dose irradiation at a dose of 5 Gy was 3.0. This low OER for multiple small fractions was attributed to a reduced repair of sublethal damage by the hypoxic cells. Others have also observed low OER values for radiation administered in small doses [35]. Therefore, tumor cells under extremely hypoxic conditions may be particularly resistant to radiation delivery using standard fractions compared with larger fractions.

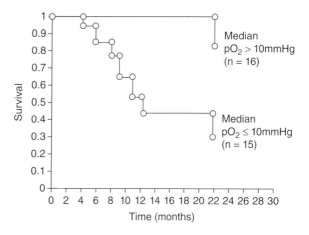

Figure 2.11 Recurrence-free survival in patients with advanced cervical carcinoma treated by a combination of external beam radiation therapy and brachytherapy. The patients were stratified on the basis of pretreatment oxygen probe measurements as indicated on the graph. *Source:* Hockel *et al.* 1993 [41]. Reproduced with permission of Elsevier.

By the early half of the twentieth century, radiotherapists began to realize that oxygen tension influences the sensitivity of tumors to radiation. In 1955, a report by Thomlinson and Gray greatly stimulated interest in the effects of oxygen on tumor radiation response [36]. These authors noted that the distance between capillaries and microscopically demonstrated necrosis in human lung cancer corresponded to the predicted diffusion length of oxygen. Specifically, they examined large numbers of bronchial carcinoma specimens and observed that the tumor cells grew in distinct cords. Each cord was made up of a rim of viable tumor cells, was surrounded by stroma containing blood vessels, and contained necrotic tissue in the middle. The apparent conclusion was that the tumor cells could proliferate and grow only if the cells were close enough to an oxygen supply from the stroma. Using assumed values for capillary pO_2, length, blood flow rate, oxygen diffusion coefficient in tumor cells, and O_2 consumption for tumor and stromal cells, Thomlinson and Gray calculated the distance to which oxygen could diffuse in respiring tissues and deduced a distance of about 150 μm. This value was approximately the width of the viable part of the tumor cords, and from this observation it was concluded that oxygen depletion was the likely cause of necrosis in the tumors. Accordingly, these findings implied that there are hypoxic but viable cells adjacent to the necrotic areas. Hence, the tumor would be comprised of viable cells that are aerobic as well as hypoxic, resulting in heterogeneity of radiosensitivity as a consequence of differences in cellular pO_2. With the advent of modern approaches to measure oxygen tension in tissues (Eppendorf probe, etc.), the presence of hypoxia in tumors has been validated [37–39]. With more refined values for oxygen diffusion coefficients and consumption values, an improved estimate of the distance oxygen can diffuse in respiring tissues is approximately 70 μm.

Powers and Tolmach were the first to demonstrate the presence of aerobic and hypoxic cells in a rodent tumor using an analysis of cell-survival curve profiles [40]. These initial experiments showed that the survival curves of the tumors were biphasic, indicating distinct subsets of tumor cells with differing radiosensitivity. This study was the first to show unequivocally that a solid tumor could contain cells sufficiently hypoxic to be protected from cell killing by x-rays, but could still retain clonogenicity and the capability to seed tumor regrowth. Of course, tumor cells are not simply aerobic or anaerobic; rather, there exists a gradient of oxygen from the capillary to the necrotic zone. Accordingly, a gradient of radiosensitivity is present over a region of varying pO_2. For convenience, the hypoxic fraction is spoken of as the fraction of cells that respond, as would hypoxic cells. The proportion of cells in solid tumors that are hypoxic in a radiobiologic sense varies from zero to about half. Accordingly, these hypoxic cells would be radiation-resistant relative to the cells of normal tissue (aerobic). The presence of hypoxia in tumors has been shown to be associated with increased local failures following treatment with conventional radiation treatment. Hockel *et al.* showed that survival was worse in patients with advanced cervical cancer treated with radiotherapy for which tumor pO_2 levels were less than or equal to 10 mmHg [41]. The results from this study are shown in Figure 2.11.

Knowledge of the shape of the survival curve at low doses is important in applying the findings of radiation biology to radiation therapy, where small doses per fraction are still largely employed. Furthermore, the laboratory systems need to be pertinent to the application in mind. In the Thomlinson–Gray model, hypoxia develops gradually as the cells are displaced away from the capillaries. This results not only in low pO_2 values but also in reduced levels of important metabolites (glucose, glutamine, adenosine-5′-triphosphate, etc.) and an increase in catabolites (e.g., lactate, CO_2). Hence, such chronically hypoxic tissues may be characterized not only by hypoxia but also by low levels of nutrients, low pH, and so on. These conditions may also affect the response of the tumor cells to genotoxic stress. Interestingly, evidence suggests that hypoxia may result in clonal selection of cells deficient in the tumor suppressor p53 [42,43]. Hypoxia leads to the activation of p53 in intact cells and triggers programmed cell death. Tumor cells deficient in p53 function do not exhibit this response; rather, they survive to proliferate and dominate the surviving population.

Hypoxia is a potent stress signal for both normal and tumor cells. Extensive studies examining the effect of hypoxia on cells have indicated that hypoxia leads to profound changes in the patterns of gene expression [44].

The transcriptional changes – and correspondingly the biological responses to hypoxia – have been shown to be due in large part to the actions of hypoxia-inducible factor 1 (HIF-1), a transcription factor complex that is activated by low oxygen tension [45, 46]. HIF-1, which is a heterodimer composed of the HIF-1α and -1β, is an integral component of the cellular response to changes in the amount of environmental oxygen. HIF-1 has been shown to play an extremely important role in the oncogenic process and to strongly influence the pathobiology of tumor cells [47]. Interestingly, hypoxia-induced gene expression signatures correlate with a poor prognosis in a number of human cancers [44, 48].

There is accumulating evidence that prolonged exposure to low oxygen tension under conditions of general metabolic deprivation induces less radiation resistance than acute hypoxia with normal metabolite availability, namely, a smaller D_0 and a lesser repair of radiation damage. Spiro *et al.* [49] reported that hypoxic V79 cells were unable to repair sublethal damage if maintained at 10^{-5} ppm oxygen in a simple balanced salt solution (e.g., no glucose). If the glucose were present, repair was about half that seen if normal culture conditions were present (aerobic, full media). Gupta *et al.* [50] found that Ehrlich ascites and P388 tumor cells had OERs of 1.22 and 1.17, respectively, if maintained at 0.1% oxygen during and following irradiation. The respective values were 2.51 and 2.87, however, for cells incubated in oxygen after irradiation. In studies on a C3H mouse mammary carcinoma system, repair of sublethal damage was reduced in the chronically hypoxic cells [51, 52].

In tumors, the oxygen environment can be extremely heterogeneous. It is now well established that this heterogeneity is due in large part to the fact that the tumor vasculature is abnormal and chaotic. Tumor vessels are dilated, saccular, tortuous, and irregular in their spatial distribution, causing blood flow through tumor capillaries to be intermittent [53, 54]. For variable time periods, flow through a particular tumor capillary may be markedly reduced or even stopped [52, 55]. Thus, the pO_2 of tumor cells adjacent to such a capillary would be reduced to virtually zero and the cells would be acutely hypoxic. Such cells exhibit full hypoxic resistance, namely maximum D_0 and n. If acutely hypoxic cells occur in human tumors, they might constitute a more serious problem for the success of radiotherapy than the chronically hypoxic cells of the Thomlinson–Gray model.

During the course of fractionated irradiation of a tumor, there is often an improvement in the tissue pO_2 (reoxygenation) [56]. This process occurs as a consequence of tumor regression with reduction of intercapillary distances, a decrease in the number of metabolically active (and hence oxygen-consuming) cells, and a decreased intratumoral pressure. All of these changes promote improved blood flow.

Radiation Sensitivity, the Cell Cycle, and Checkpoints

The replication cycle for somatic cells was described as four stages by Howard and Pelc at the Hammersmith Hospital (London) in 1952 [57]. From studies of the incorporation of ^{32}P into the nuclei of growing root tips of the broad bean *Vicia faba*, the four stages of the cell cycle were deduced: M phase (mitosis, during which chromosomes are segregated and cell division occurs); S phase (during which DNA replication occurs); and two gap phases: G_1 phase (the period between M and S); and G_2 phase (the period between S and M). The cell cycle is illustrated in Figure 2.12. The length of the cell cycle (the interval of time between the end of one mitosis to the end of the next) exhibits wide variation. For mammalian cells, there is a relatively narrow distribution of times for S, G_2, and M phases, but G_1 exhibits wide variation. Furthermore, there is a G_0 (or quiescent) phase of cells of many different tissue types. These G_0 cells are not in an active cell cycle, but are brought back into active proliferation by homeostatic control mechanisms. G_0 cells are in most cases subpopulations of G_1 cells; they re-enter the cell cycle after an appropriate signal at a point within G_1, and shortly after they enter S phase. Tissues with prominent G_0 populations include liver, periosteum, and skin, as shown by the rapid increase in proportion of S-phase cells following damage to those organs or tissues.

During the decades following the initial identification of the stages of the cell cycle, knowledge of the molecular mechanisms underlying cell cycle control increased exponentially. The sequence of discoveries that led to the current understanding of the molecular basis of cell cycle control is a remarkable story of the convergence of two different disciplines, biochemistry and genetics.

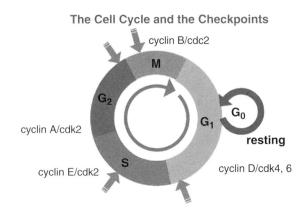

Figure 2.12 The stages of the cell cycle for somatic cells. For mammalian cells, there is not much variation in the duration of S, G_2, and M phases of the cycle. In contrast, G_1 may be be extremely varied. The cyclin and cyclin-dependent kinases associated with each phase of the cell cycle are shown. The red arrows indicate the locations along the cycle at which primary cell cycle checkpoints act.

Masui [58] and Smith and Pardee [59] independently discovered a substance in frog eggs called maturation-promoting factor (MPF), which controls when mitosis begins. The same factor was active in a wide range of cells, from yeast to mammalian cells. The injection of a crude extract of MPF could trigger mitosis even when protein synthesis was inhibited. At approximately the same time, Hartwell [60] identified mutant yeast strains that were arrested at specific points in the cell cycle. Paul Nurse, working with fission yeast (*Schizosaccharomyces pombe*), found that the *cdc2* gene was required for entry into mitosis [61]. At the time, the relationship between the *cdc2* gene and the biochemical factor MPF was unknown.

In 1988, MPF was purified and found to consist of two protein molecules, one of which was encoded by the *cdc2* gene. The cdc2 protein was found to be present in constant amounts throughout the cell cycle. The second protein component of MPF was found to be a cyclin. Originally discovered in 1971, it was observed that this protein abruptly disappeared after mitosis, only to accumulate during interphase [62]. Failure to synthesize cyclin led to a block of entry into mitosis, while failure to degrade cyclin resulted in a corresponding inability to exit from mitosis, also resulting in a cell cycle block [63]. The combination of cyclin and cdc2, which encodes a kinase, was confirmed to be MPF. These studies were the first to identify the fundamental molecular components of the cell cycle machinery, the cyclin and the cyclin-dependent kinase (cdk). Subsequent studies showed that a whole series of different cyclin–cdk complexes function in different phases of the cell cycle. Moreover, it was discovered that a number of other proteins are important in activating and inactivating the cyclin–cdk complex to regulate the cell cycle. The disruption of many of these proteins occurs in human cancers and underlies the disruption of cell cycle regulation seen in tumor cells.

Following the initial discoveries described above, models of cell cycle control have blossomed into increasing complexity. Since the discovery of the *cdc2* gene, an entire family of genes encoding related cyclin-dependent kinases was soon identified. Monoclonal antibodies and cloning of the different genes have allowed the distinction of a family of cdc2-like proteins. Similarly, many cyclins have also been discovered and distinct complexes identified. Cdc2 (also called cdk1) associates with cyclin B. Cdk2, a 33 kDa kinase, associates with the G_1/S cyclins (E and A), while Cdk3 rescues cdc2 mutants but it is not abundant in cells. Cdk4 and cdk6 associate with D-type cyclins, and when combined, function to phosphorylate the retinoblastoma protein pRb. Cdk4 does not complement the cdc2 mutants of yeast. Based on the results of these experiments, it quickly became apparent that the different cyclin–cdk complexes had different functions.

Subsequently, studies showed that the different cyclin–cdk complexes were operative during different phases of the cell cycle: cyclin D–cdk4 and –cdk6 during G_1; cyclin E–cdk2 during the transition from G_1 to S phase; cyclin A–cdk2 during S phase; and cyclin B–cdc2 during mitosis (see Figure 2.12).

The concept of cell cycle checkpoints was derived from experiments seeking to identify genes responsible for controlling entry into mitosis. Initial experiments showed that ionizing radiation leads to an accumulation of cells predominantly in G_1 and G_2. There is also a direct inhibition of replicon initiation and elongation, resulting in a transient arrest in S phase. The *rad9* mutant of *Saccharomyces cerevisiae* shows a lack of G_2 arrest and a corresponding increase in radiation sensitivity, but if time for repair is given artificially (by chemical blockade), the *rad9* yeast are no longer radiosensitive [64, 65]. The process of establishing a cell cycle progression blockade in response to genotoxic agents was termed a 'checkpoint' [64]. During the last decade, significant progress has been made in understanding the relationship between DNA damage and cell cycle progression. DNA constitutes a uniquely important molecule in the cell, and there is virtually no redundancy for many segments of the genome. Hence, damage to essential portions of the DNA molecule (i.e., essential genes) that are not repaired could be fatal to the cell. Furthermore, attempting cell division in the presence of unrepaired DNA can lead to mitotic cell death or the passing on of incomplete genetic material to the daughter cells. To ensure that damaged DNA is repaired prior to cell division, cells utilize checkpoints to control progression through the cell cycle until replication is safe to resume.

In mammalian cells, the molecular mechanisms underlying cell cycle checkpoints involve a large number of gene products. DNA-damaging agents such as ultraviolet radiation or ionizing radiation can activate the ataxia telangiectasia and Rad3-related (ATR) and ataxia telangiectasia-mutated (ATM) kinases, respectively. These kinases can phosphorylate and activate the p53 tumor suppressor gene. The p53 gene product is a transcription factor which, when activated, enhances transcription of the *CDKN1A* gene, which encodes p21. The latter binds to and inhibits cdk2, cdk4, and cdk6 with the appropriate cyclin complexes (D and E), and thereby blocks progression through G_1 and S phases [66, 67]. In some cells, p53 activation can trigger apoptosis. P53 can also activate transcription of the 14-3-3σ protein, which helps enforce the G_2 checkpoint block [15, 68]. In addition, activation of the ATM kinase can, in turn, activate the CHK1 and CHK2 kinases. These kinases inactivate CDC25C, a phosphatase required for progression into mitosis, which ultimately leads to a block at G_2/M [69, 70]. The important elements of key checkpoints in mammalian cells are summarized in Figure 2.13.

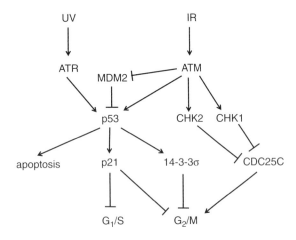

Figure 2.13 Summary of the mammalian G_1/S and G_2/M checkpoints. UV, ultraviolet radiation; IR, ionizing radiation.

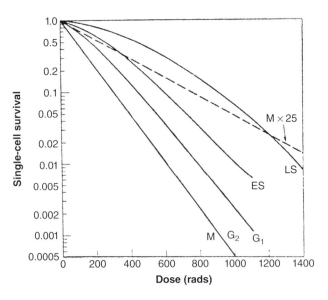

Figure 2.14 Cell survival curves for Chinese hamster cells irradiated (single dose) in the M, G_1, early S, and late S phases of the cell cycle. *Source:* Sinclair 1968 [79]. Reproduced with permission of Radiation Research Society.

The *p53* gene plays an exceptionally important role in the normal functioning of cell cycle checkpoints and warrants further discussion. The gene is located in chromosome 17 and produces a 53 kDa protein containing 393 amino acids. *P53* is mutated in approximately 50% of all human cancers, and is among the most frequently inactivated tumor suppressors [71]. Wild-type p53 protein forms tetramers for which the central core region is the location of its site-specific binding to double-stranded DNA. The majority of mutations found in cancer occur in this part of the gene. After DNA damage occurs, p53 is phosphorylated and stabilized, and translocates to the nucleus. There, p53 binds to transcriptional coactivators such as p300/CBP and activates gene transcription. As explained above, p53 can activate p21 transcription and establish the G_1/S cell cycle block. In the absence of p53, cells have defective G_1 checkpoints. Similarly, in the absence of p21, p53 is no longer able to arrest the cell cycle at the G_1 phase in response to DNA damage, demonstrating that p21 is the crucial p53-dependent effector of G_1 arrest [67,72]. P53 also activates the transcription of GADD45, which is involved in cell differentiation. In addition to activating cell cycle checkpoints, p53 is also able to trigger apoptosis [73,74] by activating the transcription of pro-apoptotic proteins such as PUMA and BAX [75,76].

Terasima and Tolmach were the first to demonstrate that radiation sensitivity varies with the cell's position in the cell cycle [77,78], results that were confirmed by others in many different types of cells [79]. Cell-survival curves for synchronized Chinese hamster cells irradiated in the M, G_1, early S, or late S phases of the cell cycle are shown in Figure 2.14. Cells in mitosis (M phase) show the greatest sensitivity to radiation. The survival curve for M-phase cells was exponential, with little or no shoulder, whereas cells in late S phase had a very broad shoulder and a less steep straight-line segment. Cells in G_1

and early S phase were intermediate. More recent studies have shown that these cells are also quite radiosensitive at the G_1/S transition, but less so than M-phase cells.

The effect of a single dose of radiation on a population of asynchronously dividing cells will depend on the distribution of cells according to age in the cell replication cycle (age–density distribution) and the variation in sensitivity with cell age (age–response function). For fractionated radiation, the surviving cells after a first dose of radiation will predominantly be the cells that were in a relatively radioresistant phase of the cell cycle at irradiation. Following irradiation, the surviving and relatively resistant cells progress into more sensitive phases. There is a delay in progression of the cells through the cell cycle (arrest). The delay is dependent on cell type, dose, and cell age at irradiation. The delay is maximum for cells in G_2. The result is a rapid decline in the mitotic index, essentially to zero, as cells accumulate in G_2 but cannot enter M. After a period of time, the surviving cells begin to progress through the cell cycle and the mitotic index returns to higher levels. Thus, radiation treatment kills the more sensitive cells and results in partial synchrony, such that most of the surviving cells are in a relatively resistant phase. Because of the broad distribution of cell cycle times, the partial synchrony is rapidly dampened and then lost. However, even the partial synchrony may be of consequence in the setting of highly fractionated irradiation, such as is used in clinical treatment. Proliferation of surviving clonogens during each inter-treatment period increases the number of cells that must be inactivated to achieve a specific response. Clonogen proliferation for a particular cell population between treatments will be a function of time between fractions and dose per fraction. Accordingly, the optimal fractionation pattern will be dependent on the differential proliferation kinetics of the cells of the tumor and the critical normal tissues.

For tumor tissues, three main parameters of cell proliferation kinetics are important to understand about the biology of tumor growth: mean cell cycle time (T_c); growth fraction (GF); and cell loss factor (Φ). These variables can be used to model the growth rate of tumors. Growth fraction is calculated from the following:

$$Growth\ fraction = \frac{Number\ of\ proliferating\ cells}{Number\ of\ proliferating\ cells + Number\ of\ quiescent\ cells}$$

The kinetics of proliferation are assayed by labeling cells in S phase by a pulse or continuous exposure to [^{3}H]-TdR or BrdUrd, and then determining the proportion of cells in S during the exposure to the label [80]. From such data, the GF, T_c, and Φ can be derived. In tumor tissue, only a proportion of the cells are in active cell cycle, and therefore the GF is usually <1.0. The influence of GF on tumor growth rate is illustrated by the following example. If a cell population has 1×10^6 cells and the GF = 0.6, after one cell cycle, there would be $(0.6 \times 10^6) \times 2 + 0.4 \times 10^6 = 1.6 \times 10^6$ cells, assuming no cell loss. The potential doubling time (T_{pot}) is the doubling time for a cell population with GF less than 1.0 and no cell loss. $T_c = T_{pot}$ when GF = 1. If there were a constant proportion of the progeny of each cell cycle remaining in the growth fraction, T_{pot} is calculated as follows:

$$T_{pot} = \frac{ln2(Tc)}{\ln(1 + GF)}$$

In the example with GF = 0.6, $T_{pot} = 1.47 \times T_c$. The Φ is the fractional loss in the expected increment in cell number after one cell cycle period. For example, if there were 10^6 cells and all were in cell cycle (GF = 1.0), after one cell cycle, 2×10^6 cells would be expected; that is, the increase should be 1×10^6. If the observed total number of cells after one cell cycle were 1.1×10^6, the increment would have been 0.1×10^6 instead of 1.0×10^6. Hence, 0.9×10^6, or 90% of expected increment, would have been lost. Here, Φ is defined as 0.9. The tumor doubling time, T_D, is related to T_c by the following formula:

$$T_D = \frac{T_{pot}}{1 - \phi}$$

Thus, for $\Phi = 0.9$ and GF = 0.6, $T_D = 14.7 \times T_c$.

T_{vol} is the actual observed volume doubling time measured for a tumor during growth. In actual tumors, T_{vol}

Table 2.2 Examples of tumor kinetic parameters in various tumor types.

	T(pot) (days)	T(vol) (days)	Growth Fraction (%)	Cell Loss (%)
Embryonic tumors	2-4	27	90	93
Lymphomas	1.1	2.8	95	70
Sarcomas	23	44	15	40
Colorectal adenomas	3-4	95	35	96
Breast cancers	10	90	25	90

and not T_{pot} is measured since most tumors have significant cell loss. These two variables are related to Φ according to the following formula:

$$\phi = 1 - \frac{T_{pot}}{T_{vol}}$$

In small tumors, where nearly all cells may be dividing and loss is low, there is a good correlation between T_{pot} and T_{vol}. However, in large tumors, T_{vol} is usually much larger than T_{pot} because only a small fraction of cells in the tumor are actively dividing. In human tumors, the observed volume doubling time is usually much longer than the measured cell cycle time. In fact, the difference may be quite large. T_D may be many months but T_c is usually a few days. This discrepancy is due primarily to a large Φ and to a lesser extent a small GF. For example, Φ may commonly exceed 0.9 and indeed even be close to 1.0. Some typical examples of parameters for tumor kinetics described above are listed in Table 2.2. During tumor growth, there is a progressive broadening of distribution of T_c, an increase in Φ, and a decrease in GF. This results in progressively slower growth of the tumor with increasing tumor age.

In summary, the biological factors that influence how a tumor responds to radiation involve many types of physiological processes. Oxygen levels, molecular signaling underlying cell cycle checkpoints, DNA damage repair activity, and the balance between cell death and repair all influence the ultimate response of a tumor to radiation treatment.

Physical Parameters Affecting Radiation Response

The biological effect that results following exposure to radiation is in large part determined by a number of important physical parameters of the radiation itself. Knowledge of these parameters and the effects they have is critical for a complete understanding of the effects of radiation on tissues.

Dose Rate

The rate of irradiation is an important determinant of response to x- or γ-rays. As the dose rate is lowered and the exposure time is increased, the biological effect of a given dose of radiation is typically reduced. This has long been recognized because clinical observations showed that tissues tolerate 50–70 Gy given in 5–10 days by low-dose-rate continuous irradiation (via radium brachytherapy, for example), whereas with high-dose-rate external beam irradiation, the time required to administer comparable doses and have tolerable reactions was 6–7 weeks. Hall showed that in HeLa cells the D_0 increased by a factor of 2 as the dose rate decreased from 1.0 Gy min^{-1} to 0.01 Gy min^{-1}; n decreased to 1.0 with a decrease in dose rate to 0.1 Gy min^{-1} [81]. Survival curves for V79 cells in plateau phase that were irradiated at 1.43 Gy min^{-1} and at 1.54 and 0.55 Gy h^{-1} are shown in Figure 2.15 [82]. The survival curves at high dose rate had D_0 and n values of 2.7 Gy and 5.0, while at low dose rates the D_0 and n values were 5.6 Gy and 2.0. The slope of the low-dose-rate curve approximates that of the slope of the initial part of the high-dose-rate curve and reflects cell inactivation by single-hit events (e.g., the α component of the LQ model). The extrapolation number approaches but does not reach 1 at the low dose rates in V79 cells [82].

The reduced effect of radiation at lower dose rates is explained by the presence of repair of radiation damage that occurs during the period of irradiation. The magnitude of the dose-rate effect correlates with the extent of sublethal damage repair observed with split-dose radiation studies. The dose-rate effect caused by sublethal damage repair is most dramatic between the range of 0.01 and 1 Gy min^{-1}. Response to radiation is modified only slightly as dose rates extend outside of this range. Only small dose-rate effects occur outside this range because the dose rate was adequate to block cell proliferation, with the consequent accumulation of cells in G_2, a relatively radiosensitive phase [83].

At very low dose rates an inverse dose rate can occur, in which decreasing the dose rate results in a paradoxical increase in cell killing. This is illustrated by experiments conducted by Mitchell *et al.* using HeLa cells and shown in Figure 2.16 [84]. Decreasing the dose rate for HeLa cells from 1.54 to 0.37 Gy h^{-1} increases the efficiency of cell killing. Interestingly, at this low dose rate, killing is nearly as effective as an acute treatment. The mechanism is that, at about 0.3 Gy h^{-1}, cells tend to progress through the cell cycle and become arrested in the G_2 phase, which is a radiosensitive part of the cycle. In contrast, at higher dose rates, cells tend to be arrested in the phase of the cycle they were in at the start of the irradiation. Below a threshold of dose level, cells can continue to cycle up to a certain point, during irradiation. The OER is reduced at low dose rates and constitutes a potential advantage of

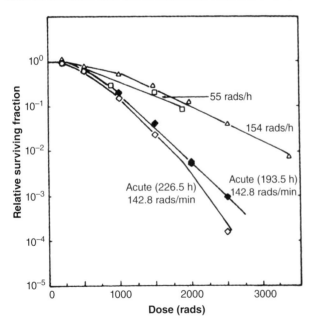

Figure 2.15 Cell survival curves for plateau phase V79 cells irradiated at 143 rads min^{-1}, 154 rads h^{-1}, and 55 rads h^{-1}. For acute exposures, the treatments were performed at 193.5 and 226.5 h into the experiment. *Source:* Mitchell 1979 [82]. Reproduced with permission of Radiation Research Society.

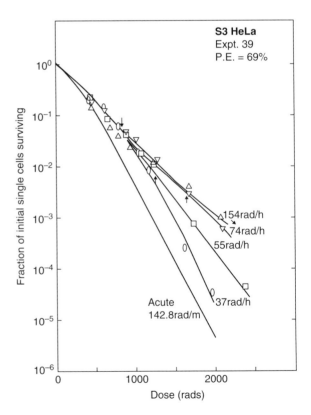

Figure 2.16 Example of the inverse dose-rate effect. A range of dose rates can be found for HeLa cells such that lower dose rates leads to more cell killing. *Source:* Mitchell 1979 [84]. Reproduced with permission of Radiation Research Society

Figure 2.17 Dependence of LET on radiation particle type and energy. For each type of radiation, the energy is noted along the top of the plot and the corresponding LET is noted along the bottom.

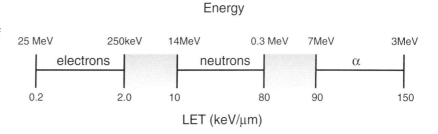

low-dose-rate radiation in treating hypoxic tumors [85]. Although redistribution of cells to radiosensitive phases underlies part of the mechanism of the inverse dose-rate effect, the full complexity for low-dose-rate effects is not completely understood. The mechanisms are likely to encompass a complex interplay of the effect of repair, cell cycle arrest and recovery, and re-oxygenation.

Linear Energy Transfer and Relative Biological Effectiveness

When radiation passes through biological matter, the ionizations and excitations that occur are not distributed randomly but are localized along the pathways of individual charged particles. The pattern in which energy is deposited from these charged particles depends largely on the type of radiation used. For instance, when photons strike molecules in the tissue they produce fast electrons, particles carrying unit electric charge but having a small mass. Alpha particles, on the other hand, carry two electric charges on a particle that is four times as massive as a proton. The charge-to-mass ratio for alpha particles, as a result, differs from that for electrons by a factor of approximately 8000. Because of differences such as these, the spatial distribution of the ionizing events produced by different types of particles differs immensely. The ionization density of low-LET photons results in ionizations being more separated in space and sparsely ionizing. In contrast, the ionization density of large charged particles, such as alpha particles, produces a dense column of ionizations.

LET is a parameter of beam quality and refers to the transfer of energy of the irradiated material per unit path length of a particle or photon. The unit used for LET is kiloelectron volt per micrometer (keV μm^{-1}) of unit density material. For ^{60}Co radiation, the average LET is about 0.6 keV per micrometer of path. This means that along the photon path there is, on average, a transfer of 0.6 keV to the irradiated material in each micrometer of photon path length. For fast neutrons, LET is much higher, typically 5–10 keV μm^{-1}. At the upper end of the LET range, heavy particle radiations have an LET of up to 100 to 1000 keV μm^{-1}. As LET increases, there is a decrease in the distance between ionizing events. For ^{60}Co and fast neutron radiation, there are approximately 17 and

150–200 ion pairs produced per micrometer, respectively. The average energy for production of an ion pair is 34 eV. In general, for each type of radiation LET decreases as the energy of the particle increases. As such, the ranges of LET for various radiation types are highly dependent on particle type and energy; this is illustrated in Figure 2.17 and Table 2.3. There is significant variation in the density of ionization events along the photon or particle path with LET; this is illustrated in Figure 2.18a for electrons and neutrons in a Wilson cloud chamber [86].

Ionizations produced by radiation are not randomly distributed throughout the irradiated material. Rather, they typically occur along the paths of photons or particles. Along such paths, they are not distributed randomly but occur in clusters. Furthermore, the ionizations along a path are produced at virtually the same instant. Accordingly, for high-LET radiation there are likely to be ionizations at nearly the same site in space and at the same time, with resultant massive damage locally. Such concentrated damage is likely to be more difficult to repair, although whether there are types of damage that are irreparable is not clear. Sublethal damage repair and potentially lethal damage repair are sharply reduced or absent following fast neutron irradiation or irradiation with higher-LET particles [87, 88]. OER and cell cycle effects are also decreased with high-LET radiations. The OER for low-LET photons is about 3 and approaches 1 at LET values greater than 200 keV μm^{-1}. For fast neutron radiation, OER is 1.5–2.0. In addition, cell cycle-dependent radiation sensitivity (age–response function) decreases in the setting of high-LET radiation [89]. Likewise, the effectiveness of radiation response modifiers (e.g., radiation sensitizers and radiation protectors) is

Table 2.3 Examples of linear energy transfer values.

Radiation	Linear energy transfer, keV μm^{-1}
Cobalt 60 γ-rays	0.2
250 kV x-rays	2.0
10 MeV protons	4.7
150 MeV protons	0.5
2.5 MeV α-particles	166
2 GeV Fe ions	1000

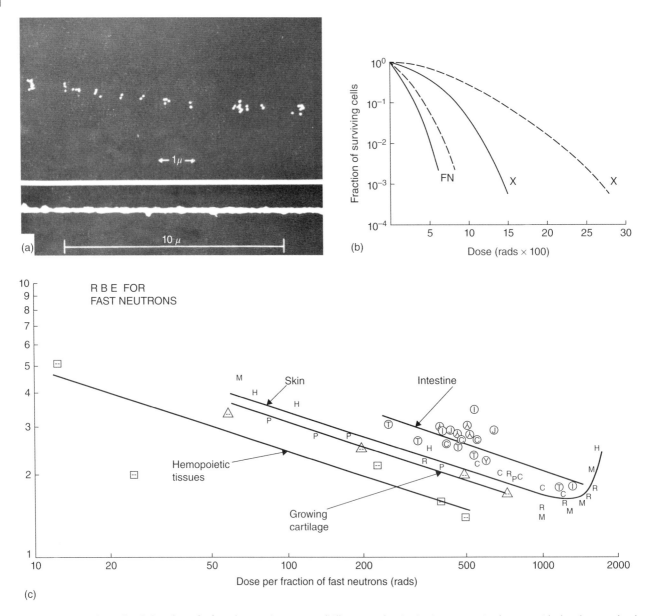

Figure 2.18 (a) Wilson cloud chamber of a fast electron (upper panel) illustrates that ionization occurs in clusters, with the clusters clearly separated. In contrast, fast neutrons (lower panel) show the ionizations to be a continuous track. *Source:* Bacq 1961 [86]. Reproduced with permission of Elsevier. (b) Cell survival curves for rat rhabdomyosarcoma R1 cells subjected to 300 keV(p) x-ray or 15 MeV fast neutron (FN) irradiation under aerobic (solid line) or hypoxic (dashed line) conditions. (c) Relative biological effectiveness (RBE) as a function of neutron dose for various tissues. *Source:* Field 1974 [91]. Reproduced with permission of Elsevier.

diminished or absent in the setting of high-LET radiation. Cell-survival curves are shown in Figure 2.18b for cells irradiated *in vitro* by 300 kV_p x-rays and 15 MeV neutrons [90].

Equal doses of different types of radiation (i.e., different LETs) do not produce equal biological effects. The relative biological effectiveness (RBE) of a radiation is described in terms of the ratio of doses to produce a defined level of damage or cell-surviving fraction for a beam of interest to that for a conventional beam, usually 250 kV_p (kilovolt peak) or ^{60}Co photons. Thus, RBE is defined as:

$$RBE = \frac{\textit{Dose of standard radiation } (250\,kV_p\textit{ x-rays}) \textit{ to produce a biological effect}}{\textit{Dose of test radiation to produce the same biological effect}}$$

The RBE is influenced by a number of factors. Different target tissues can have different RBEs from the same radiation treatment because of differences in microenvironment and inherent differences in cellular repair capacities

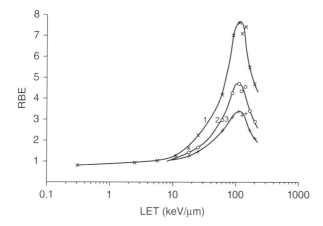

Figure 2.19 Relationship between linear energy transfer (LET) and relative biological effectiveness. Data from human cells are shown. The RBE rises to a maximum at an LET of about 100 keV mm^{-1} and subsequently falls for higher LET values. Curves 1, 2 and 3 refer to cell survival levels of 0.8, 0.1, and 0.01, respectively, illustrating that the absolute value of the RBE is not unique but rather depends on the level of biological damage and dose level.

(killing curve shoulder and D_0). RBE is also dependent on dose, decreasing with increasing dose. This dependence of RBE on dose or dose per fraction is shown in Figure 2.18C [91]. Furthermore, because the quality of radiation affects recovery and cellular repair, spreading the treatment over longer periods of time (increasing fractions or lowering the dose rate) will increase the RBE. Lastly, RBE is also known to depend on LET, increasing with rising LET. The relationship between LET and RBE is shown in Figure 2.19. As LET increases, RBE increases slowly at first and then more rapidly as the LET increases beyond 10 keV μm^{-1}. RBE reaches a maximum at about 100 keV μm^{-1}, beyond which the RBE begins to fall. The RBE reaches a maximum value because this peak LET is the most biologically effective due to it being the point at which there is a coincidence between the diameter of the DNA helix and the average separation of ionization events from the radiation.

Tumor and Tissue Responses to Ionizing Radiation

Most effects of radiation on tissues result from the depletion of a cell population by cell killing, with the overall tissue response depending primarily on the inherent cellular radiosensitivity, the overall proportion of cells that survive, the ability of the surviving cells to proliferate and repopulate the damaged tissue, and the rate at which dead cells are removed from the affected tissue. How radiation affects the delicate balance between cell birth and cell death in a given tissue ultimately determines that tissue's response to ionizing radiation.

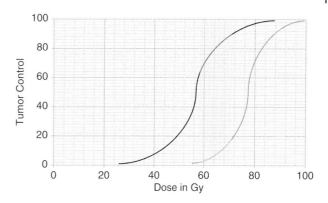

Figure 2.20 Dose–response curve for tumor (black curve) and for normal tissue damage (gray curve). The therapeutic window is depicted by the shaded gray area.

Dose–Response Curves and the Therapeutic Window

When radiation therapy is contemplated as part of a treatment strategy, it is important to consider the dose–response curves for the tumor and the surrounding normal tissues in an attempt to optimize tumor cell kill while minimizing collateral damage to essential normal tissues. As illustrated in Figure 2.20, under ideal circumstances the dose–response curve for the tumor is well to the left of that for normal tissues, with an optimum dose range (also known as the 'therapeutic window') that allows for tumor control with minimal normal tissue damage. In radiobiology, this ratio of tumor response to normal tissue damage is defined in terms of the therapeutic ratio or index. In most cases, however – and especially with radioresistant tumors – there is an approximation or an overlap of the two curves, at which point higher doses are required to achieve tumor control and the incidence of normal tissue complications starts to rise. The aim of novel strategies in radiation oncology, be they in the form of radiosensitizing agents, normal tissue radioprotectors, or state-of-the-art modalities that increase targeting precision (e.g., stereotactic radiation, proton therapy), is precisely this: to widen the therapeutic range or window in an attempt to optimize tumor control while minimizing complications.

Tumor Cell Radiation Sensitivity

In-vitro studies of tumor cell lines derived from human tumors have yielded important findings over the years. These experiments, in which cell culture lines are exposed to varying doses of radiation, have shown that after exposure some lines lose their capacity to divide and cannot form colonies, some continue to divide but more slowly, while others degenerate and die. The remaining cells that are not affected by the radiation represent the surviving fraction (SF). Indeed, SF2 is a commonly used

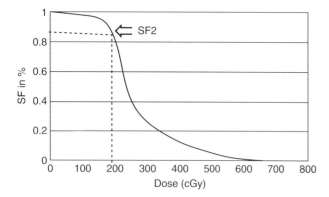

Figure 2.21 Sigmoid cell survival curve showing the relation between radiation dose and the SF. The SF2 is the survival fraction after 2 Gy of exposure (arrow).

marker of cell sensitivity and is defined as the surviving fraction after 2 Gy of ionizing radiation (Figure 2.21).

Two important and interrelated factors affecting the tumor-control probability are the cellular type of the tumor and the intrinsic tumor radiosensitivity. Comparing the SF after the same exposure dose (e.g., SF2) between different tumor types can offer some insight into the differential tumor line responses to ionizing radiation and the inherent differences in radiosensitivity between tumor types. For example, the classic experiments by Deacon *et al.* (Figure 2.22) showed not only a broad distribution but also some substantial overlap of SF2 ranges for the various tumor groups [92]. As a result, the relatively sensitive tumor types (e.g., lymphoma) overlap the values for traditionally radioresistant tumors, such as melanoma. Even though these and other *in-vitro* studies have clearly shown a wide variability in radiation response between different tumor types, there is also variability that can be noted for individual

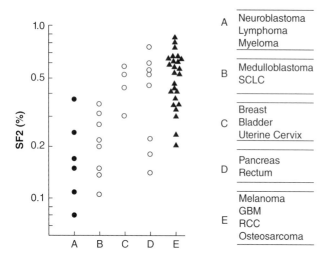

Figure 2.22 SF at 2 Gy for various tumor cell types. *Source:* Deacon, Peckham, and Steel 1984 [92]. Reproduced with permission of Elsevier.

Table 2.4 Surviving fractions (SF) after treatment of a model cell population with one or with 30 equal doses.

SF	
After One Dose	**After 30 Equal Doses**
0.8	1.2×10^{-3}
0.6	2.2×10^{-7}
0.4	1.2×10^{-12}
0.2	1.1×10^{-21}

tumor types. For example, the SF2 for melanoma and some other tumors extends from less than 0.2 to 0.9 (Figure 2.22). Other studies also support a similar broad and overlapping distribution in SF2 values for different tumor types [93, 94]. These other studies are particularly notable in that their data are derived from cell lines studied in a single laboratory and that some of them measured cell proliferation, rather than colony formation, as their endpoint.

The importance of relatively small differences in survival fraction becomes even more pronounced after repeated doses of radiation, as evident from Table 2.4. For example, while a tumor with a SF2 of 0.8 would have a SF of 1.2×10^{-3} after 30 treatments, a cell line with a SF2 of 0.4 would have an exponentially lower SF of 1.2×10^{-12} after repeat exposures to irradiation. One problem, however, is that this model assumes that the SF is constant for all 30 treatments, which is not necessarily the case *in vivo*. This and other issues, such as inconsistencies in accurately measuring SF2 values and the occasional lack of clear correlation between *in vitro* SF2 values and tumor control rates in patients, clearly demonstrate that living tumors in a host can respond very differently to radiation and are subject to significantly more variables that may affect their radiosensitivity than isolated tumor cells cultured in a controlled environment. For example, it is now known that a patient's normal tissue radiosensitivity clearly affects the radiosensitivity of that patient's tumor. Ataxia telangiectasia (A-T) patients have been reported to show significant responses to irradiation after only a third of the dose that would be normally required for patients without this host mutation. This is clear evidence that the radiation sensitivity of tumor clonogens closely tracks that of the normal tissues.

In addition to inherent host factors, however, it has recently become clear that the path to cancer progression that a tissue takes (the tumor genesis sequence) can also have an important effect on that tumor's inherent response to radiation. For example, there is an association between human papillomavirus (HPV)-16 (plus other oncogenic HPV viruses) and oropharyngeal carcinoma, particularly tonsillar carcinoma. It is now the

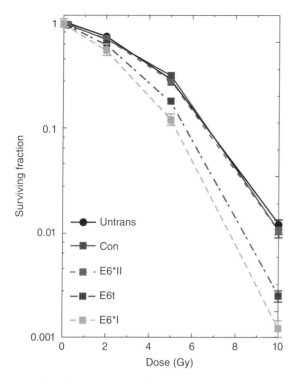

Figure 2.23 Radiosensitization of oropharyngeal squamous cell carcinoma (OSCC) cells by E6 isoforms (dotted) lines.

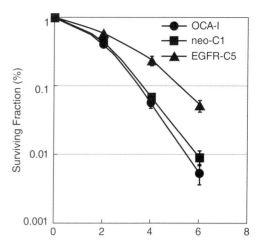

Figure 2.24 Survival fractions are plotted against single doses of 2, 4, or 6 Gy. Expression of EGFR after transfection of a human EGFR cDNA fragment (clone 5 or triangles) clearly increases the survival fraction at the same exposure, whereas transfection with a control vector (clone-1 or squares) shows survival similar to that of the parental ovarian carcinoma line (OCA-1).

consensus opinion that this subtype of carcinomas occurs more often in younger patients who do not have the typical risk profile of smoking or alcohol abuse, and that the disease in these individuals tends to respond better to therapy, including radiation [95]. Even though the exact mechanism for this enhanced radiosensitivity of HPV-positive tumors remains to be fully elucidated, a few investigators have noted some important correlations. For example, the downregulation of SMG-1 due to promoter hypermethylation correlates with improved survival in HPV-positive tumors [96]. Others have postulated that certain HPV proteins confer an enhanced radiosensitivity to HPV-positive tumors. For example, Pang *et al.* showed that overexpression of the oncoprotein E6∗I significantly sensitized tumor cells to radiation, resulting in an approximately eightfold lower surviving cell fraction at 10 Gy (Figure 2.23) [97]. The complex interplay between virus and host – whatever the precise mechanism may prove to be ultimately – appears to profoundly affect the tumor's radiosensitivity and overall response to therapy.

HPV is just one example of how additional and hitherto unknown intrinsic tumor factors, rather than simply the tumor's basic histologic type, can affect that tumor's radiosensitivity. For instance, some cancer cells exhibit a phenotype characterized by the upregulation of epidermal growth factor receptor (EGFR) and one of its ligands, transforming growth factor α. Some of the first

evidence that EGFR expression might affect intrinsic cellular radiation sensitivity emerged from studies of a murine model by Akimoto and colleagues [98]. In another seminal study, the same group demonstrated a causal relationship between cellular EGFR expression and relative radiation resistance [99]. The investigators' findings showed that the transfection of human EGFR expression vectors into a low-EGFR-expressing murine ovarian carcinoma cell line (OCA-1) resulted in an EGFR level-dependent increase in resistance to ionizing radiation (Figure 2.24). There is reason to believe that the poor survival of patients with EGFR-overexpressing head and neck tumors is mostly due to failure of locoregional tumor control as opposed to distant metastasis. These observations suggest that EGFR plays an important role in tumor-cell repopulation, which is a significant contributor to treatment failure in patients with head and neck malignancies treated with radiotherapy. Even though all of the mechanisms for EGFR-dependent radioresistance have not been fully delineated, it is now thought that EGFR affects the DNA repair process and that its inhibition governs radiosensitivity by affecting certain downstream DNA repair genes/proteins. A greater understanding of these pathways is already translating into more effective therapies for patients, and may one day lead to a de-escalation of the radiation doses required for optimal tumor control.

The response of a solid tumor *in vivo* to local radiation is clearly not simply the response of a pure colony of tumor cells. Rather, the response reflects both the direct ability of radiation to kill tumor cells, and to an undefined extent the indirect effect of the radiation on the stromal and capillary environment around the tumor. In other words, radiation may also have a profound effect on the tumor's milieu, thereby indirectly and additionally affecting the its survival chances after exposure. For example, the control of tumor angiogenesis has recently become an area of intense study. Even though *in-vitro* studies have shown that radiation killing of endothelial cells makes at most a minor impact on tumor control probability by radiation, it is also clear that some cells will be inactivated because of metabolic inadequacies as a result of vascular compromise (e.g., severe hypoxia, hypoglycemia), and that this effect may have been underestimated for tumors *in vivo*. For example, recent studies have demonstrated that single large doses of radiation (8–20 Gy) may primarily target tumor endothelial cells, leading to secondary tumor clonogenic cell death [100]. These studies suggest that blood vessels play an important role in radiation response. This may be of particular importance in the future, particularly with the advent of new technologies that allow radiation oncologists to deliver higher (ablative) doses of radiotherapy with greater accuracy and precision. As a result, various strategies have been proposed to more effectively combine radiation with vascular targeting agents, and certain antiangiogenic drugs have actually been demonstrated to enhance radiation therapy by targeting endothelial cells (described in more detail in later sections). Briefly, when combined with radiation, these agents are believed to cause even more localized vascular destruction and to accelerate the tumor's clonogenic cell death. Interestingly, a comparison of different sequencing strategies of radiation therapy and antiangiogenic therapy in a mouse lung carcinoma model showed that the concurrent administration of radiation and angiostatin was more effective than was radiation therapy followed by angiostatin [101]. However, a more recent study of another agent (the vascular endothelial growth factor receptor antagonist PTK787) in a human squamous cell carcinoma mouse model showed that the compound enhanced the radiation response, but only when it was administered after radiation therapy [102].

Dose–Response Curves for Tumors Irradiated *In Situ*

Following irradiation, tumors exhibit a retarded growth rate. The tumor growth curve may show flattening or may exhibit temporary regression followed by regrowth. Also, there may be complete regression followed by regrowth. The most desired response is, of course, complete and permanent regression. The two endpoints that have been used extensively in experimental radiation therapy have been tumor-growth delay (TGD) and tumor control probability (TCP). 'Tumor control' means complete and permanent regression or absence of growth for the period of observation. Thus, even though regression may be incomplete, tumor control would be scored provided there was no growth during the study period.

One example of progressively longer delays in tumor growth with increasing radiation dose is shown in Figure 2.25a for the benzpyrene-induced fibrosarcoma line RIB5 in rats. There is clearly an increase in the delay of tumor growth with radiation dose, and the slope of the regrowth curve becomes progressively less steep [103]. Alternatively, Figure 2.25b shows TGD as a function of radiation dose for the same tumor under conditions of clamp hypoxia, air (0.2 atm O_2), or hyperbaric oxygen. What is notable is that the TGD curve for air closely follows that for hyperbaric oxygen in the low dose range, indicating that the response to lower doses is predominantly determined by the aerobic cells of the tumor. At higher doses, the curve follows that for irradiation under clamp hypoxia, implying that at higher doses the response is largely influenced by the hypoxic cells [104]. From the ratio of doses to achieve a specified TGD, an enhancement ratio (ER) can be calculated to estimate the magnitude of the effect of an oxygenated environment on the irradiated tissues. It is obvious from the shapes of the different curves that this ER is dose-dependent.

Unfortunately, an accurate analysis of TGD curves is complicated by the effects of radiation on the stroma as well as on the tumor cells. In other words, TGD is not simply a function of the fraction of tumor cells surviving at each dose level. This is largely because, with increasing radiation doses, there are progressively longer mean cell cycle times, increasing probabilities of unsuccessful cell division, and changes in the normal tissue environment (e.g., capillary network) that prevent it from keeping pace with tumor expansion and supporting tumor growth. This effect on the irradiated stroma is called the tumor-bed effect (TBE) and is most easily demonstrated experimentally by observing the time for a tumor to grow to a specified size following transplantation of tumor cells into normal or irradiated tissue. For example, 50 days post-transplantation into unirradiated tissue, the TD_{50} (number of tumor cells required to produce a tumor in 50% of inoculations) for the mammary carcinoma MCaIV was 2×10^4 [105]. In contrast, there were virtually no tumors when the tumor cells were inoculated into legs previously irradiated to 35 Gy. However, between 200 and 250 days after irradiating the tumor bed site, the TD_{50} values were comparable for transplantation into normal or irradiated legs. This TBE is not, however, observed for all tumor systems. For example, Milas *et al.* reported that sarcomas exhibit little or no such effect [106]. The main point is that the irradiation of normal tissue retards the growth of some transplanted tumors, but does not appreciably affect transplantability in normal and irradiated tissue. Thus, TBE cannot be considered to be a significant component of the response to radiation

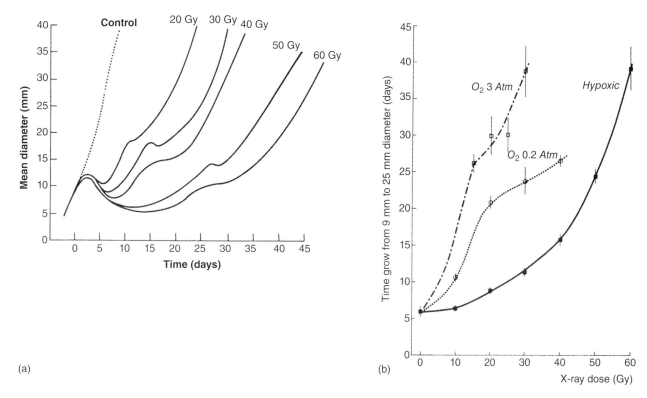

(a)

(b)

Figure 2.25 (a) Tumor growth curves for the benzpyrene-induced fibrosarcoma RIB5 of the rat following single radiation doses given to air-breathing animals with no restriction in blood flow to the tumor. *Source:* Thomlinson 1961 [103]. Reproduced with permission of Camelot Press. (b) Tumor growth delay versus radiation dose after irradiation of RIB5 under air, hyperbaric oxygen, and clamp hypoxia conditions. *Source:* Thomlinson 1967 [104]. Reproduced with permission of Camelot Press.

that ultimately contributes to tumor control. However, TBE may nonetheless complicate the use of TGD as an endpoint, and in such studies the potential role of the TBE should be taken into account.

Tumor-Control Assays

Tumor control is the endpoint of most obvious relevance to clinical radiation therapy. The TCD_{50} is the dose at which 50% of the tumors are controlled for the time specified. The dose–response curve for a model tumor is defined by three important factors: (i) clonogens; (ii) clonogens that die only as a result of direct radiation exposure; and (iii) tumor recurrence if one or more clonogens survive treatment. As a result, TCP is a reflection of the probability that all clonogens are inactivated, whereas TCD_{50} means that in half of the irradiated tumors no clonogens survive and that in the other half one or more cells survive. The relationship between TCP, SF, and clonogen number (M) can be defined by the following equations:

$$TCP = \exp\{-(SF \times M)\}$$
$$\ln TCP = SF \times M$$

The lnTCP represents the average number of surviving cells per tumor; as a result, at the TCP_{50}, the average number of cells surviving per tumor would be 0.693.

At TCD_{50} and TCD_{37} dose levels, the average numbers of cells surviving among tumors that recur are 1.39 and 1.58, respectively. What these values imply is that there is an extremely small number of cells that survive radiation treatment in tumors that recur. For example, even after treatments yielding a TCP of only 0.1, more than 90% of all recurrences seem to develop from one to four surviving cells. Perhaps this lends some credence to the recently proposed cancer stem cell (CSC) theory, which postulates that there is a subgroup of CSCs within most tumors that persist as a distinct population and cause relapse and metastasis by giving rise to new tumors. This theory suggests that conventional therapies (perhaps including radiation) kill differentiated or differentiating cells, which form the bulk of the tumor, but are unable to target CSCs, which form only a very small proportion of the tumor. As a result, a population of CSCs, which gave rise to it, could conceivably remain unaffected and cause a relapse of the disease at a later time.

A competing but related concept is the theory of *tumor hierarchy*. This concept claims that a tumor is a heterogeneous population of mutant cells, all of which share some mutations but vary in specific phenotype. In this model, the tumor is made up of several types of stem cell lines, some optimal to their specific environment and several less successful ones. These secondary lines can

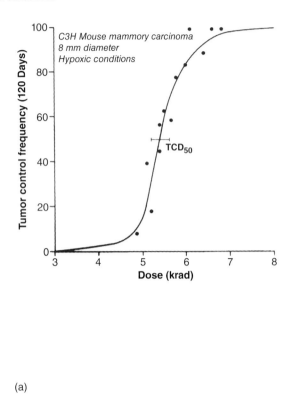

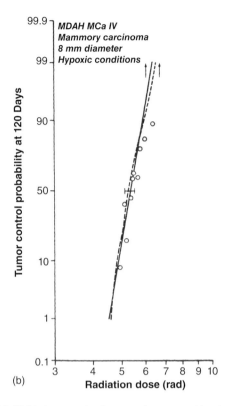

(a)

(b)

Figure 2.26 (a) Dose–response curves for local control at 120 days, of an 8 mm MCaIV third-generation isotransplant treated by single-dose 250 kV(p) x-radiation under clamp hypoxia. *Source:* Suit 1973 [108]. Reproduced with permission of Elsevier. Data plotted on a standard linear grid. (b) Same data plotted on a logit of tumor control versus log dose: solid line, logit regression line through the data points; dashed line, that predicted by the multitarget model. *Source:* Suit 1973 [108]. Reproduced with permission of Elsevier.

ultimately become more successful in some environments, allowing the tumor to adapt to its environment, including the methods by which it can be treated [107]. The result of this rapid tumor evolution and adaptation is that the targeting strategy for different subtypes of cells within the tumor may vary considerably, making it difficult for conventional therapies to target all the repopulating cells within the tumor.

The TCD_{50} and the slope of the TCP curve can be defined from dose–response assays for tumor control. In experiments of this type, animals with tumors of uniform size are subdivided into groups and the tumors are irradiated locally with escalating doses. Tumor diameters are then measured at appropriate frequencies following treatment so as to permit the construction of tumor growth curves. The period of observation permits at least 90% of the regrowths to be scored, and animals are also scored for deaths. At completion, the tumor control results are plotted and a regression line is fitted to allow computation of the TCD_{50} and the slope of the curve at the TCD_{50}. As an example, Figure 2.26 shows the dose–response curve for control at 120 days of 8 mm MCaIV isotransplants subjected to single-dose radiation under clamp hypoxia [108]. The dose–response curve, as plotted on a linear–linear grid is S-shaped, being quite steep

in the TCP range of 5% and 40%, and less steep in the range above 60%. Figure 2.26b shows the same data plotted on a logarithmic grid, yielding a nearly straight line. This line characterizes the relationship between single radiation exposures and tumor control probability and can be approximated by the following equation:

$$TCD_p = D_0[\ln M + \ln n - \ln(-\ln P)]$$

According to this relationship, the TCD_{50} for tumors comprising a particular cell population (uniform D_0, n) will increase with $D_0[\ln M]$. For tumors of a particular clonogen number (M), D_0, and n, TCDp increases with $(D_0)[-\ln(-\ln P)]$, where P represents the proportion of tumors in which all tumor cells are killed. Thus, the dose increment required to raise TCP from 0.1 to 0.9 would be $3.08 \times D_0$. The clinical implication of these observations is that the last few fractions of a conventional course of fractionated radiotherapy are critical to achieve the desired tumor control.

The relationship between radiation dose and tumor control probability for fractionated irradiation is somewhat more complex and will be addressed only briefly. Data from a typical experiment using mammary carcinoma cell lines is presented in Figure 2.27. Tumors were grown by transplanting cells into the external portion

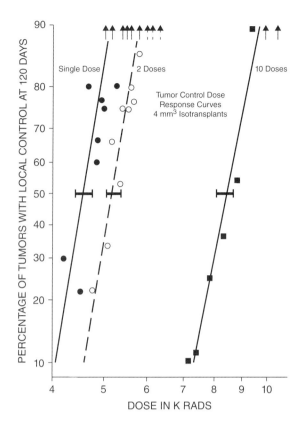

TCD$_{50}$ AT 120; DAYS, FOR X-IRRADIATION GIVEN IN ONE, TWO, OR TEN FRACTIONS TO 4-MM^3 ISOTRANSPLANTS OF THE C$_3$H MOUSE MAMMARY CARCINAOMA UNDER CONDITIONS OF LOCAL TISSUE HYPOXIA AT THE TIME OF EACH TREATMENT

Number of fractions	Interval between fractions	TCD$_{50}$ at 120 days with 95% Confidence Limits
1	—	4420...4575...4740
2	6 hours	5030...5190...5350
2	24 hours	4950...5110...5280
10	24 hours	8040...8400...8780

Figure 2.27 Tumor control results and fitted log lines for three dose fractionation schemes.

of the mouse ear, and radiation was performed when the tumors reached a size of 4 mm^3. Uniform hypoxia was achieved before the treatments by clamping the base of the ear for at least a minute. Single-dose, two-dose, and ten-dose experiments were performed, with a 24-h interval between fractions [109]. As evident from the figure, the TCD$_{50}$ increased from 45.75 Gy for the single treatment to 51.1 Gy for two fractions, and to 84 Gy if the radiation was delivered in ten equal sessions. These data indicate that there must be extensive repair of damage (sublethal damage repair) that takes place during a protracted multifraction regimen. Clearly, this important phenomenon must be taken into account by the clinician in the radiation planning process.

Slope of Dose–Response Curve and Heterogeneity in Treated Tumors

The slope of the dose–response curve is also affected by the heterogeneity in size of the tumors included in the dose–response assays, as seen in Figure 2.28. In this experiment, MCaIV tumors were treated under aerobic conditions with two equal doses of radiation. The tumors ranged in size from 4 to 12 mm diameter. The solid line is the resultant and relatively flat curve if all the independently determined dose–response curves for the 4–5, 8,

and 12 mm tumors were combined. Tumor heterogeneity clearly results in an overall flattening of the curve.

Tumor Volume and TCD$_{50}$

It is well known in clinical radiation oncology that tumor size or tumor volume at irradiation is an important determinant of the likelihood of success following a particular total dose and fractionation schedule. This has also been observed for tumors in experimental animal models. As stated earlier, the TCD$_{50}$ values for a series of transplanted mammary carcinomas subjected to single-dose radiation under clamp hypoxia have been shown to increase with tumor volume [110, 111]. In another study of MCaIV tumors, radiation was administered under aerobic conditions to microcolonies and to tumors of 0.6 and 250 mm^3. The observed TCD$_{50}$ values were 15.2, 22, and 54.3 Gy, respectively [112]. The extremely steep increase in the TCD$_{50}$ between 0.6 and 250 mm^3 tumor volumes strongly suggests that the tumor growth was accompanied by a deterioration of metabolic conditions in the tumor: in other words, a significant fraction of tumor clonogens became hypoxic as the tumors increased in size. These data conform to the expectation of increasing TCD$_{50}$ with tumor volume due to increasing number

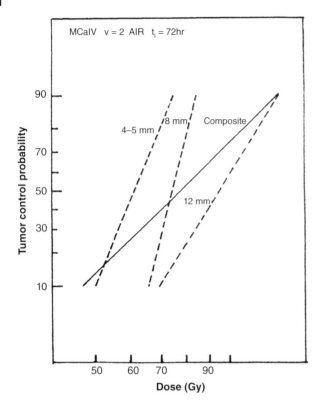

Figure 2.28 Dose–response curves for local control of MCaIV treated under air by two equal doses of ^{137}Cs radiation separated by 72 h; the tumors were 4–5, 8, or 12 mm in diameter. The solid line is the calculated dose–response curve if all data from the three assays were pooled.

of clonogens and the appearance of relatively radiation-resistant foci of cells as tumors achieve larger sizes.

Recurrent Tumors

As described earlier, cells that survive large radiation doses have heritable changes, including increased radiation sensitivity. Experiments have been performed to assess the radiation response of tumors derived from failures after high doses. For example, a CH3 mouse mammary carcinoma that had recurred following a single radiation dose (the TCD$_{95}$) was transplanted into fresh isologous recipients. This tumor grew slowly: the volume doubling time was 17 days, compared with 3–4 days for the untreated tumor growing in the untreated tissue. The TCD$_{50}$ at 240 days was 59.9 Gy for the control tumor but 51.3 Gy for the recurrent tumor growing in unirradiated tissue. The difference between these two TCD$_{50}$ values, which were measured concurrently, was significant at p <0.01 [111]. The treatments were performed under conditions of clamp hypoxia to obviate concerns regarding the status of oxygenation in the primary and the recurrent tumors. Ando *et al.* reported similar findings in their study of a recurrent fibrosarcoma [113]. A

recurrent tumor may be comprised of cells of greater sensitivity than the original tumor, but this does not mean that the gross response would be greater for the recurrent tumor than for the primary. The recurrent tumor would be growing in an irradiated tumor bed with attendant vascular system inadequacies and probably a higher proportion of hypoxic cells.

Historically in the clinic, recurrent lesions have not been typically subjected to full dose levels because of the limited tolerance of the normal tissues. However, the infrequency of good clinical results in the treatments of local failures cannot be taken as proof of an increased inherent radiation resistance of the tumor cells. The induction of radiation resistance before undertaking re-irradiation is extremely uncommon, and this contrasts markedly with the rapid appearance of drug-resistant mutants in tumor cell populations exposed to chemotherapy. Interestingly, with the advent of novel technologies and more sophisticated radiation delivery systems, high-dose radiation can be now be directed with extreme precision with concurrent improvements being noted for patients retreated for recurrences. For example, some authors have recently reported on re-irradiation alone with more modern techniques. A total of 34 patients with recurrent head and neck tumors were treated with a second course of high-dose radiotherapy. Patients were selected for re-irradiation in case of inoperable and/or unresectable tumors, and doses of up to 60 Gy with conventional fractionation were achieved using these new technologies. In this study, reasonable locoregional control rates could be achieved with re-irradiation [114].

Immune Reaction and Tumor Response

The potential of an immune reaction to cause partial or complete response of a tumor has been studied comprehensively in experimental animal tumor systems. These have been based primarily on tumors induced by chemicals or viruses (e.g., SV40). The immunogenicity of these tumors is demonstrated by the effect of specific immunization against a particular tumor on the TD$_{50}$ and TCD$_{50}$. The first demonstration of an immune reaction by an inbred mouse against an isogenic tumor was reported by Foley for fibrosarcoma [115]. It was found that if a mouse had been exposed to the tumor antigen by transplantation of the tumor, followed by excision of the transplanted tumor at an appropriate size, the animal was able to reject subsequent tumor challenge. In another experiment, when the TD$_{50}$ assay was used with iso-transplantation of the fibrosarcoma, FSaI, the TD$_{50}$ was significantly increased by previous immunization and significantly decreased by whole-body irradiation before transplantation. Similarly, the TCD$_{50}$ values were 34.8, 25.9, and 43.1 Gy for control mice, and for mice that had been immunized or given 4 Gy whole-body irradiation prior to transplantation, respectively [116]. Interestingly, immune checkpoint blockade therapy can increase the rate by which radiation causes an *abscopal effect*, a phenomenon in which local radiation treatment of a tumor results in the shrinkage of other tumors outside the radiation field due to immune system activation. In fact, radiation can result in the expansion of T-cell diversity within irradiated tumors.

Normal Tissue Response

As a result of studies vigorously supported by the US Atomic Energy Commission and the Department of Defense during the early years of the era of nuclear weapons, extensive data are now available on the effects of ionizing radiation on diverse normal tissues, organs, and organisms. Such studies generated a vast array of dose–response assays for death after irradiation for a wide variety of species. Those studies were based primarily on conventional photons at conventional dose rates, which were complemented by comprehensive determinations of life shortening and causes of death versus dose for different species. Since then, intensive studies have been conducted in experimental animals of the response of normal tissues to localized irradiation. The effort has been directed at evaluating the response of tissues to radiation under conditions similar to those employed in clinical radiation therapy. These studies have been performed principally on mice, rats, and miniature pigs. For many tissues, ingenious experimental strategies have permitted the derivation of values for the parameters of survival curves including D_0, n, and α/β ratios (see Table 2.5). An observation by Withers that has been of importance to clinical radiation therapy was that the total dose to produce a specified level of damage was much more dependent on dose per fraction in late-responding than in acute-responding tissues [117]. This is clearly demonstrated in Figure 2.29, in which the dose is plotted to produce the defined effect versus dose per fraction. The slopes of the curves are steeper for late-responding tissues (e.g., spinal cord, kidney, lung) than for the acutely responding tissues (e.g., skin, testis, jejunal crypt cells). A comprehensive review by Williams *et al.* showed that the α/β ratios for tumors are comparable to those for acutely responding normal tissues [118]. Thus, the α/β ratio is high (>5) for acutely responding tissues and tumors, and low (<5) for most late-responding normal tissues. The major implication for radiation therapy is that smaller doses per fraction (<3 Gy) should be used where late-responding normal tissues are to receive the full dose in a radical course of treatment. In other words, when the dose-limiting toxicity is the late-responding normal tissue, the optimum therapeutic ratio is obtained by the use of small doses per fraction.

Table 2.5 Values of α/β ratios for various normal tissues determined from multifraction experiments on animals.

Effects	α/β (Gy)
ACUTE	
Skin desquamation	
Mouse	8–14
Rat	9–10
Pig	8–11
Human	9–11
Jejunal clones	6–11
Colon clones	8–9
Colon weight loss	12–13
Testis clones	9–13
Mouse tail necrosis	7–26
Mouse LD$_{50}$ (30 days)	
LATE	
Rat spinal cord	
Cervical	1.0–2.7
Lumbar	2.3–4.9
Kidney	
Rabbit	1.7–2
Pig	1.7–2
Mouse	1.0–3.5
Lung, mouse	2.0–6.3
Bladder, mouse	3.5–7
Pig skin, late contraction	2.0–5

Source: Adapted from Fowler [134].

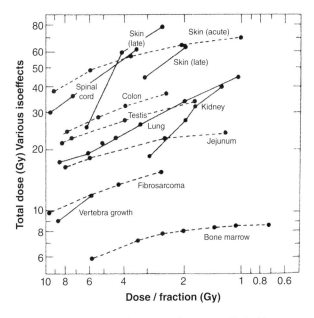

Figure 2.29 Plots of total dose to produce a specified effect versus dose per fraction for various late- and acutely responding (solid and dashed lines, respectively) tissues. *Source:* Withers 1985 [117]. Reproduced with permission of John Wiley & Sons.

However, it is now known that there is a much more sophisticated interplay and co-dependence between early- and late-responding tissues than previously thought or evident from past *in-vitro* studies. For example, the term 'consequential late effect' was recently coined to describe a non-healing acute response that can directly progress into a late effect [119]. This concept has particular relevance in cases where more aggressive radiotherapy protocols result in additional acute toxicity (i.e., an increase in the severity and duration). In such cases, intensive fractionation protocols are thought to deplete the stem cell population below levels needed for eventual tissue restoration. Organ systems in which a barrier against mechanical and/or chemical stress is established by the acutely responding tissue are at a particular risk from this phenomenon. As a result, the subsequent damage is often attributable to an acutely responding overlying epithelial tissue (e.g., fibrosis of skin as a result of desquamation and acute ulceration). Therefore, rather than thinking of early- and late-responding tissues as independent entities, the radiation oncologist should consider them as two potentially linked and interconnected entities along the broader toxicity spectrum.

The radiation biology of each of the various important normal tissues, including the various tissue classification schemes, cannot be reviewed comprehensively here and are beyond the scope of this introductory chapter. However, details relevant to each site and tumor type are included in chapters covering specific entities. To summarize, the response of normal tissues to a course of radiation depends on the number of stem cells, the total dose, the number of fractions, the time between fractions, the dose per fraction, the inherent cellular radiation sensitivity, the micrometabolic milieu of the cells of the constituent tissues, the tumor cell proliferative activity and cell divisions during treatment, the cellular age redistribution during treatment, and the capacity and the kinetics of repair after radiation damage.

Attempts to Reduce the Impact of Hypoxic Cells on Tumor Resistance

Soluble oxygen in tissues increases the stability and toxicity of free radicals, thereby increasing the deleterious effects of radiation on the affected tissues. In order for oxygen to act as a sensitizer, however, it must be present during the radiation exposure, or at least during the lifetime of the free radicals that are involved in the indirect action of radiation, which is a fleeting 10^{-5} s. This radiosensitizing effect of oxygen can be quantified as the OER and was defined earlier in this chapter. The effect of oxygen on the cell-survival curve is illustrated in Figure 2.30. When an animal tumor that is made up

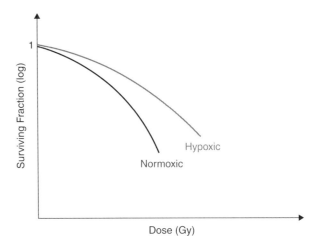

Figure 2.30 The effect of oxygen on the surviving fraction after radiation. Note that the OER (effect of oxygen) is generally greater at higher doses.

of a mixture of aerated and hypoxic cells is irradiated, the aerated cells are killed preferentially because of their greater sensitivity, and the survivors contain a preponderance of hypoxic cells. However, this situation is not static, and over time the proportion of hypoxic cells tends to return to the pre-irradiation level. In virtually all solid tumor systems of experimental animals, reoxygenation during the course of fractionated irradiation results in a decrease in the proportion of cells that are hypoxic. Despite this reoxygenation phenomenon, the available evidence indicates that some hypoxic cells can persist and are the major determinants of the dose required for tumor inactivation. Much preclinical laboratory and clinical research in radiation oncology has been directed towards reducing the number and/or the importance of hypoxic cells in tumors and towards improving the efficacy of radiation therapy. These various approaches have included: (i) dose fractionation; (ii) blood transfusion; (iii) respiration of oxygen at higher concentrations than air or even at high pressures (hyperbaric oxygen); (iv) the use of chemical sensitizers of hypoxic cells; (v) suppression of the consumption of O_2; (vi) increase of tumor blood flow; (vii) decrease of blood viscosity; (viii) changing erythrocyte rigidity; (ix) high-LET radiation; and (x) hyperthermia [120, 121]. For instance, fractionation of the total dose allows for reoxygenation of previously hypoxic regions between fractions, thereby minimizing the overall effect of hypoxia during treatment. The magnitude of the benefit achieved through any of these various approaches may be described in terms of the therapeutic gain factor, which is defined as the ER of the tumor, divided by the ER of the normal tissue.

It was suspected for a long time that previously untreated rodent and human tumors harbored hypoxic regions within them. As a result of meticulous

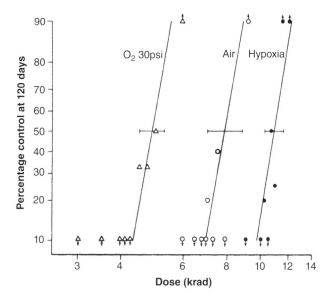

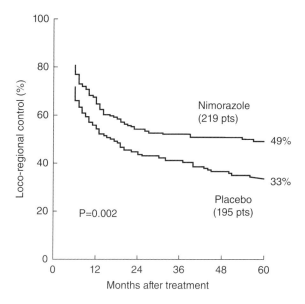

Figure 2.31 Dose–response curves for local control of 8 mm MCaIV isotransplants treated by five equal doses (one day between treatments) given under air, clamp hypoxia, or hyperbaric (O23ATA) conditions. *Source:* Suit 1974 [124]. Reproduced with permission of Radiation Research Society.

Figure 2.32 Actuarial locoregional tumor control in patients randomized to receive nimorazole or placebo in conjunction with conventional radiotherapy for carcinoma of the pharynx and supraglottic larynx.

studies employing ultraviolet cryophotometric methods to determine the oxyhemoglobin-deoxyhemoglobin ratio of individual erythrocytes in the capillaries of frozen histologic sections, there is now unambiguous evidence of the presence of hypoxic cells in several untreated solid tumor lines [122]. For example, Moulder and Rockwell reported that of 42 tumor types surveyed, 37 contained hypoxic cells, with the hypoxic fractions ranging from 0% to 50% (average approximately 15%) [123]. In some experiments, attempts were made to reduce this hypoxic fraction by improving the tumor tissue PO_2 using hyperbaric oxygen [122]. As an example, Figure 2.31 shows the effect of clamp hypoxia versus hyperbaric oxygen on the dose–response curve for an 8 mm MCaIV tumor that was treated with five equal fractions of radiation [124]. The three dose–response curves are steep, parallel, and widely separated. The TCD_{50} enhancement ratio for the hypoxic versus hyperbaric set-up was 2.3. Hyperbaric oxygen also achieved a large reduction in TCD_{50} over that for air conditions, with an ER of 1.75.

Hyperbaric oxygen has increased the response to fractionated radiation of virtually every solid tumor of rodents tested, prompting clinical trials using several of these approaches. The largest multicenter trials of hyperbaric oxygen were performed by the Medical Research Council in the United Kingdom and showed significant benefits in local control and survival for patients with carcinoma of the uterine cervix and advanced head and neck cancer [125]. Hyperbaric oxygen treatment has fallen into disuse, however, partly because of its cumbersome nature and partly because drugs were thought to be able to

achieve the same outcomes by other means. Using a different approach, Bush *et al.* demonstrated a gain in survival of anemic (hemoglobin $10–12$ g dl^{-1}) patients with stage III carcinoma of the uterine cervix by transfusing and maintaining hemoglobin levels at 12 g dl^{-1} or more [126,]. Alternatively, in the seminal Danish head and neck trials conducted by Overgaard *et al.*, a gain in local control was observed with the use of nimorazole, a radiation sensitizer of hypoxic cells (Figure 2.32) [127].

Many trials of other radiation sensitizers and modifiers, however, have yielded equivocal results. In 1996, Overgaard and Horsman published the results of a meta-analysis of 10 602 patients treated in 82 randomized clinical trials involving various oxygen sensitizers, reporting that these various antihypoxic cell treatments improved local tumor control by only 4.6% and the overall survival rate by 2.8% [128]. Because of the modest benefit in many trials and the cumbersome nature of these interventions, currently neither radiation sensitizers nor hyperbaric oxygen are in routine clinical use today. Perhaps with the recent popularization of hypofractionated and stereotactic radiation methods, where the effect of tumor oxygenation is more pronounced, some of these techniques will be revisited.

Dose Fractionation and Tissue Response

Biological Significance of Dose Fractionation

Clinical research in radiation therapy continues to study dose-fractionation and its effects on tissue responses to irradiation. The standard dose fractionation of conventional treatments employed in 2015 in the United States for definitive treatment of patients with solid tumors remains 1.8 to 2.0 Gy per fraction. Usually, five fractions are given per week. The total dose of radiation given depends on the type of tumor being treated and tolerance of the surrounding normal tissues. Typical doses given for the eradication of solid tumors range from 60 to 75 Gy. In the adjuvant or neoadjuvant setting (i.e., when radiation is given in conjunction with surgery), the total radiation dose is often reduced. However, during the past 20 years, there has been an increasing trend towards altered fractionation schemes or single-dose delivery. Planning new fractionation schemes is based on the biological and radiobiological characteristics of the cells of the tumor and the critical normal tissues. These characteristics include repair capacity, cellular sensitivity, and proliferative kinetics, but also include the more complex aspects of the vascular and tumor bed effects of radiation, which can modify the response of the tumor cells.

The improving metabolic status of tumor cells, which may occur as fractionated treatment progresses, may cause cells to enter into active cell cycle and hence to increase cell number between fractions. This phenomenon is termed *proliferative response* or *accelerated repopulation*. The effect of this process is to increase the tumor-control dose. In any given tumor, a significant proportion of the tumor cells are in a prolonged G_1 phase as a result of metabolic insufficiency and, as this is alleviated, the cells resume proliferation. The result is a reduction in mean cell cycle time and cell loss factor along with a higher growth fraction. Consequently, there is an acceleration of clonogen population growth. These observations support the idea that, in the treatment of those tumors capable of showing accelerated repopulation and increased growth fraction, a shortened overall treatment time would be of greater effectiveness than a pure increase in total dose. Clinical studies have supported this theory. For head and neck cancer, accelerated repopulation during protracted overall treatment times leads to a well-documented loss of tumor-control probability [129]. It is estimated that 1–2% of tumor control is forfeited for each day of delay during delivery of the radiation regimen in head and neck cancer patients [130]. The prolongation of treatment time also results in decreased tumor control in other disease sites [131]. For example, Chen *et al.* observed that the prolongation of treatment time during radiotherapy for cervical cancer resulted in a decrease of pelvic control by 0.67% per day of delay [132, 133].

As a general rule, for relatively faster-growing tumors such as squamous cell carcinomas of the head and neck, accelerated fractionation (i.e., reduction in the overall treatment time) helps to offset the increased proliferation during treatment [134]. However, acceleration cannot be achieved simply by giving a larger fraction size per day. This would result in a greater risk of complications in late-responding tissues, as explained earlier. Therefore, acceleration is achieved by delivering two smaller fractions of treatment per day, making the total dose per day higher. This approach commonly adopts 1.5–1.6 Gy twice a day, reaching doses of 55–60 Gy in 3.5–4 weeks, before acute toxicities necessitate a gap in therapy [135, 136]. Even with a short break in therapy, the overall treatment time for the delivery of doses in the range of 70 Gy can be 5.5–6 weeks. A randomized trial of accelerated fractionation was undertaken in a study conducted by the European Organization for Research on the Treatment of Cancer (EORTC) for head and neck cancer [137]. Actuarial survival at five years was 13% better in the accelerated arm compared with the standard arm, a significant improvement in survival. Subgroup analysis suggested that the greatest benefit was seen in the tumors with fast proliferation kinetics (short T_{pot}) [138]. Similarly, in a randomized trial performed by Turrisi *et al.*, patients with small cell lung cancer were randomized to 45 Gy given by 1.8 Gy fractions once a day or 1.5 Gy fractions given twice a day (accelerated fractionation). Median survival was better in the patients that were treated twice a day (23 months versus 19 months, p = 0.04) [139].

One way to try to improve the acute tolerance of accelerated fractionation is to use a concomitant boost. This refers to the treatment of the large field (covering tumor and regional nodes) once a day and a smaller cone down field (tumor volume only) once a day, resulting in the tumor being treated twice daily and the regional nodes daily. This may be suitable if the regional nodes are being treated electively, but less appropriate if there is a large amount of detectable disease in the nodes. During the past ten years, the use of concomitant boost has gained increasing acceptance in the treatment of head and neck squamous cell carcinomas. In the Radiation Therapy Oncology Group (RTOG) 90-03 study, Fu *et al.* randomized patients to one of four treatment arms: (i) conventional radiotherapy (70 Gy in 2-Gy daily fractions); (ii) hyperfractionated radiotherapy (81.6 Gy in two 1.2-Gy fractions per day); (iii) concomitant boost (72 Gy by 1.8 Gy per day and then for the last 12 fractions, a second 1.5-Gy fraction to the primary tumor); and (iv) split course hyperfractionated accelerated radiation therapy (67.2 Gy by 1.6-Gy fractions given twice a day with a two-week break after 38.4 Gy) [140]. The concomitant boost regimen (and the hyperfractionated regimen) resulted in improved two-year local control. Concomitant boost has also been shown to improve local control in the setting of definitive chemoradiation for head and neck tumors [141].

An alternative manipulation of the fractionation schedule is to increase the total radiation dose, and achieve this by giving small doses per fraction; this is known as hyperfractionation. The rate of delivery of treatment is usually around 2 Gy per day, 1 Gy twice a day or 1.2 Gy twice a day being the most commonly used schemes. A randomized trial in the treatment of bladder cancer showed an improvement in outcome with 84 Gy, 1.2 Gy twice a day over 7 weeks, compared with 64 Gy, 2 Gy daily [142].

For both types of twice-a-day therapy, the time interval between treatment fractions is usually set at least 4 h and preferably more than 6 h. The optimum inter-treatment interval remains uncertain. The recovery of tumor cells in cell culture in split-dose experiments appears to be about 6 h. For late-responding tissues (e.g., spinal cord, neural tissue), a period of 6–12 h may be essential to realize the full benefit of hyperfractionation. Since clinical therapy is designed to limit potential side effects to the spinal cord to an extremely low frequency, it will be difficult to distinguish between an inter-treatment interval of 6 and 12 h, for example. Animal data may help bring some insight, but characteristics for the tolerance of rodent spinal cord may not answer such a subtle question due to interspecies differences. Data from murine models seem to demonstrate that sublethal repair continues in the mouse beyond 8 h [143]. Tolerance studies on the spinal cord using monkey and swine models, as well as newer computation-based models, have provided important additional data to understanding fractionation dependence [144–146].

The strategies of acceleration and hyperfractionation may be combined. A rigorous test of this general strategy was conducted by Dische and Saunders in the United Kingdom on patients with cancer of the lung and cancer of the head and neck [147–150]. The investigators employed 1.4 Gy initially, and then 1.5 Gy, three times a day with 6 h between fractions, in 36 fractions over a 12-day period. Treatment continued over the weekend. The total dose was 50.4 Gy, escalating to 54 Gy in 12 days. This regimen is termed continuous hyperfractionated accelerated radiation therapy (CHART). Because the preliminary data gave encouraging results, the United Kingdom Medical Research Council sponsored randomized trials [151, 152] which initially showed promising results, but further follow-up suggested significant late toxicity that required some degree of caution as to its widespread use [151, 153]. Unfortunately, CHART is labor-intensive and, from a logistics perspective, it is not clear whether it adds any worthwhile benefit in the setting of modern concurrent chemoradiation regimens. As such, this strategy has not been widely adopted in current practice.

Taken to its logical conclusion, the ultimate evaluation of the efficacy of hyperfractionation is to use low-dose-rate continuous radiation therapy. Pierquin *et al.* [154] investigated this approach using 8–10 Gy per day at 1 Gy h^{-1} for total treatment times of several weeks.

Results from clinical trials of low-dose-rate therapy versus conventional fractionated treatment for head and neck cancer and breast cancer have indicated promising results for the low-dose-rate therapy approach. In addition, results using low-dose-rate brachytherapy from a variety of disease sites (e.g., cervical cancer, sarcoma, prostate cancer) indicate favorable results using this approach.

Models of Fractionation Dependence

Radiobiological characterization of tissues for assessing fractionation dependence is typically done in terms of the α/β ratio. The ratio is used in conjunction with the linear quadratic model to calculate effective biological doses. The reason for the increasing use of the α/β ratio is its simplicity for calculating fraction size dependence and for equating different doses per fraction (d) and total dose (D). For a single acute dose D, the biological effect is given by:

$$E = \alpha D + \beta D^2$$

For n well-separated fractions of dose d, the biological effect is given by:

$$E = n(\alpha d + \beta d^2)$$

This equation may be rewritten as:

$$E = (nd)(\alpha + \beta d)$$
$$= (\alpha)(nd)(1 + d/(\alpha/\beta))$$

Because nd equals the total dose, D,

$$E = \alpha(\text{total dose})(\text{relative effectiveness})$$

where $(1 + d/(\alpha/\beta))$ is called the relative effectiveness. This equation can again be converted to the following form:

$$\frac{E}{\alpha} = (\text{total dose})(\text{relative effectiveness})$$
$$= nd(1 + (d/(\alpha/\beta)))$$

Here, E/α is called the biologically effective dose (BED) and is typically the quantity used to compare different fractionation regimens. This equation can be used to convert between biologically equivalent regimens of fractionated radiation. For example, to calculate the late effects of a 2 Gy per fraction regimen of 30 fractions (assuming $\alpha/\beta = 3$):

$$BED_{\text{late}} = 30 \times 2 \text{ Gy} \left(1 + \frac{2}{3}\right) = 100.2 \text{ Gy}$$

What total dose must be used to obtain the same late effects with 1.4 Gy per fraction with 2 Gy per fraction? This is calculated as follows:

$$30 \times 2 \text{ Gy}(1 + 2/3) = n(1.4 \text{ Gy})(1 + 1.4/3)$$
$$100.2 = 2.05n$$

$$n = 48.8$$

$$48.8 \text{ fractions } (1.4 \text{ Gy}) = 68.43 \text{ Gy}$$

Below is a simplified version of this equation for comparing two different fractionation schemes, where the aim is to compare 5 Gy per fraction with 2 Gy per fraction for a site with an α/β of 3 Gy.

$$\frac{nd5}{nd2} = \frac{\dfrac{\alpha}{\beta} + d2}{\dfrac{\alpha}{\beta} + d5}$$

If the total dose in 2 Gy per fraction is 72 Gy (36 fractions), then the total dose in 5 Gy per fraction would need to be reduced by 5/8 (of 72 Gy), which is 45 Gy (nine fractions).

Use of this modeling approach must be made with explicit recognition that there is no consideration for the time factor. This is an important consideration for treatment protracted over more than four to five weeks, because there may be a proliferative response in the acutely responding tissues (malignant and normal). Corrections for the general equations above have been developed and can be used when allowances for tumor proliferation need to be made.

There are methods that assess different overall treatment times and different number of fractions, for example, nominal standard dose and time dose fractionation models [155, 156]. The models employ exponents of dose per fraction and time appropriate to the normal tissue of concern. The models must be used only as guidelines, not rules, for changes in dose per fraction within a relatively small range. This point needs to be emphasized because there have been untoward reactions when major extrapolations or extensions from conventional treatments have been based on these formulas. The exact values of the exponents in the model are not necessarily constant. Certainly, for acutely responding tissues, the exponent for the time factor is approximately 0.11 for the overall time of treatment, which can make a significant difference to the calculated equivalent dose. For late-responding tissues, the exponent for time is reduced, since the overall treatment time is less significant than dose per fraction.

In summary, the effect of radiation on biologic tissues depends not only on the total dose of radiation given but on how that treatment is divided and applied over time.

Combination of Radiation and Chemotherapeutic Agents: Cytotoxics, Sensitizers, and Protectors

The primary goal of combining chemotherapy with radiation is to improve the therapeutic ratio or to enhance the tumoricidal effect while minimizing the toxicity of the treatment to critical normal tissues. The mechanism of action of chemotherapeutic agents and the manner in which the cellular response to radiation is modified by chemotherapy is governed in large part by five overarching principles:

1. The pharmacokinetics of the drug or the time course of drug concentrations in the various tissues of the body.
2. The cell cycle dependence of the drug: some drugs affect cells at specific phases of the cell cycle (e.g., vincristine in G_2/M, etoposide in S/G_2, etc.), whereas others affect cells at all stages of the cell cycle (e.g., alkylating agents).
3. The mechanism of action in terms of direct cytotoxicity or sensitization of radiation effect.
4. The timing and magnitude of the drug-induced proliferative response.
5. The dose–response relationship.

The chemotherapy agent may act as a cytotoxic agent and/or to modify the response to radiation. The major classes of chemotherapeutic agents and the mechanisms by which they are thought to mediate radiosensitization are listed in Table 2.6.

Sensitization refers to an enhanced response where the chemical agent is not cytotoxic at the dose levels employed. This is illustrated in Figure 2.33, which

Table 2.6 Chemotherapeutic drugs classes and mechanisms of radiosensitization.

Chemotherapy Class	Sensitization Mechanism
Antimetabolites	Nucleotide pool perturbation
	Lowering apoptotic threshold
	Tumor cell reoxygenation
	Cell cycle redistribution
Taxanes	Cellular arrest in the G_2M phase
	Reoxygenation of tumor cells
	Induction of apoptosis
Topoisomerase I inhibitors	Inhibition of repair of radiation-induced DNA strand breaks
	Redistribution into G_2 phase of the cell cycle
	Conversion of radiation-induced single-strand breaks into double-strand breaks
Hypoxic cell cytotoxins	Complementary cytotoxicity with radiation on normoxic and hypoxic tumor cells
Platinum-based	Inhibition of DNA synthesis
	Inhibition of repair of radiation-induced DNA damage
	Inhibition of transcription elongation by DNA interstrand cross-links

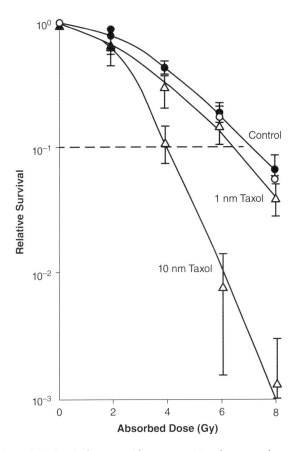

Figure 2.33 Survival curves with concurrent taxol expressed relative to unirradiated controls.

shows the survival curves for astrocytoma cells treated with radiation and taxol [157]. In this report on the radioenhancing effect of taxanes, the radiosensitivity was increased by approximately a factor of 1.8 and radiosensitization was achieved only when the cells were in phase G_2 or M at the time of irradiation, a result subsequently confirmed in other *in-vitro* and *in-vivo* studies [158].

Sensitizing agents such as taxol appear to reduce D_0 on the cell-survival curve, but do not affect n. Chemotherapy-enhancing or cytotoxic agents, on the other hand, reduce D_0 and/or n. The radiosensitizing effect (ER) for a particular drug-radiation treatment can be easily quantified from most survival curves by obtaining the ratio of radiation doses to produce a specified effect for radiation alone to radiation plus the drug in question.

The observed ER also depends on other factors, including the timing of the radiation in relation to administration of the drug, the drug and radiation doses, the drug pharmacokinetics, the kinetics of tissue repair, and the oxygenation status of the tissues. For example, bleomycin exhibits increased cell kill in an oxygenated state, whereas mitomycin is activated and at its most effective under hypoxic conditions. There can also be major

cytotoxicity in the recovering tissues, even if the drug is administered some time after the irradiation. This has been shown to be particularly true for drugs such as doxorubicin, docetaxel, and gemcitabine, and is seen occasionally clinically when normal tissues (e.g., the skin) are affected in the so-called 'recall' phenomenon. Along the same lines, the term 'spatial cooperation' was coined to describe the effective treatment at a different site (radiation for the primary site and chemotherapy for distant foci of disease). In many cases, however, chemotherapeutic agents, in addition to enhancing the tumoricidal effect of radiation locally, are also sufficiently potent to eliminate micrometastatic foci at distant anatomic sites.

Early trials of combined chemoradiation for solid tumors yielded limited evidence of clinical benefit. However, important gains have recently been realized by combining chemotherapy and radiation in the treatment of patients with a variety of tumors, from Ewing's sarcoma and Wilms' tumor in the pediatric population, to locally advanced head and neck cancer, rectal, and breast cancer in the adult population. Indeed, with modern advances in chemotherapy sequencing and targeted drug design, the need for radiation therapy has gradually decreased for certain tumor types (e.g., Hodgkin lymphoma). As a result of mounting evidence in favor of a survival benefit with chemoradiation, combined modality therapy has now become standard for many cancers, often in lieu of surgery. Important studies of this combined approach in both nasopharyngeal and laryngeal carcinoma have led to a paradigm shift over the past two decades, with definitive chemoradiation being now the preferred approach to upfront surgical resection [133, 134, 159, 160]. For example, the Intergroup 0099 randomized trial comparing cisplatin-based chemoradiation to radiation alone for locally advanced nasopharyngeal carcinoma demonstrated an impressive 30% improvement in overall survival at three years with the addition of chemotherapy [159]. Two important randomized trials – one from Europe and another from the United States – have also confirmed the superiority of combined chemoradiation in the adjuvant setting for select patients with head and neck cancer undergoing upfront surgery [161, 162]. In breast cancer, especially for locally advanced and/or node-positive disease, the best treatment results after surgery are now obtained through the judicious sequencing of chemotherapy with radiation. With the recent explosion in the fields of rational drug and design and targeted therapy, continued advancement of the present knowledge on the complex interactions between drugs and radiation will continue to be instrumental in helping to predict favorable and unfavorable combinations.

In summary, there are important rationales for combining chemotherapy with radiation, including better cell cycle optimization of tumor kill, arrest of tumors in a more radiosensitive phase of the cell cycle, inhibition of repair after radiation damage, improved efficacy against radioresistant hypoxic tumor clones, reduced proliferation between radiation fractions, and tumor mass reduction as a result of improved oxygenation. Precisely because of these multiple beneficial advantages and interactions, combined-modality treatment using chemotherapy and radiation is a mainstay of oncologic care.

Radiation Protectors

Considerable research has been devoted to the design and identification of agents that can protect normal tissues against the effects of ionizing radiation. The goal is to preferentially concentrate these drugs in normal tissues, but not in tumor tissues. The principal and most fruitful approaches to date have been directed toward drugs that inactivate radiation-induced radicals. As mentioned earlier, sulfhydryl-containing compounds, such as cysteine, were among the first compounds to be shown as effective in this capacity [163].

Unfortunately, these early compounds were highly toxic in humans at the doses that were protective against radiation. During the early years of the nuclear arms race, the possibility of a compound that would protect against whole-body irradiation was of great interest to the military. As a result, the Walter Reed Army Hospital synthesized several thousand compounds that were similar in structure to cysteine with the aim of finding one that was less toxic. Ultimately, by covering the sulfhydryl group with a phosphate, scientists were able to develop compounds that were similarly radioprotective but significantly better tolerated. One such compound, WR-2721 (amifostine), was found to confer a significant protective effect on a variety of normal tissues, including bone marrow, jejunal crypt cells, intestine, lung, testis, spinal cord, and hair follicles. Later, as this drug became available to clinicians, the question arose as to whether the drug protects tumor cells from cytotoxicity as well. Even though protection has not been observed for large rodent tumors, Milas *et al*. reported that WR-2721 did protect CH3 mouse fibrosarcoma micrometastases in the lungs [164]. Similar to experiments in animals, clinical studies with WR-2721 have shown protection of the skin, mucous membranes, bladder, and pelvic structures against late, moderate, and severe reactions [165]. In addition, the RTOG conducted a Phase III randomized clinical trial in which amifostine was found to reduce xerostomia (dry mouth) without affecting tumor control in patients with head and neck cancer given radiation therapy [166]. Despite these promising studies, the use of radioprotectants such as amifostine has not gained widespread acceptance. Toxicity trials of amifostine conducted in humans in the United States have shown that the main dose-limiting toxicity is hypotension; this and other adverse effects (sneezing, somnolence) have also tended to limit the amount of drug given to less than the dose needed to achieve maximum protection. Finally, recent advances in precision radiotherapy (e.g., intensity-modulated radiation therapy, stereotactic radiation) and the concomitant shrinkage of treatment volumes have led to a gradual reduction in damage to surrounding normal tissues (e.g., the parotid glands in head and neck malignancies), thus further obviating the need for potentially toxic radioprotectors.

Rationale for the Combination of Surgery and Radiotherapy

The three most important and somewhat interrelated goals of combining surgery and radiation are to: (i) reduce the extent of surgery and the dose of radiation needed; (ii) maintain or improve tumor-control probability compared with radical surgery or radical irradiation alone; and (iii) achieve a superior cosmetic and functional result without compromising cure. Conservative surgery removes the grossly evident lesion, whereas radical surgery typically includes all of the tissues suspected of involvement by subclinical disease. If surgery alone was to be performed, in order to achieve adequate locoregional control the margins around the radiographically evident mass must be enlarged substantially enough to include all the microscopic extensions of disease. This resection of additional tissue likely to be involved by subclinical disease would, however, result in greater functional and/or cosmetic compromise. In contrast, the reverse holds true for radiation. Radical or high-dose radiation is required to eradicate all cells in the primary tumor mass, whereas radiation at moderate dose levels is typically adequate to inactivate microscopic extension of disease into the surrounding normal tissues. Therefore, combining moderate dose radiation and conservative surgery can produce a result similar to that achieved by extending the surgical procedure from simple excision to radical resection. This is perhaps best illustrated by the modern approach of performing the less-invasive lumpectomy (in lieu of radical mastectomy) for patients with early-stage breast cancer, followed by moderate doses of whole-breast irradiation to eradicate any residual microscopic disease. Multiple randomized control trials (e.g., National Surgical Adjuvant Breast and Bowel Project B-06, Milan trials) have demonstrated the non-inferiority of this approach vis-à-vis radical surgery, both in terms of locoregional control and overall survival, with the added advantage of organ preservation and improved cosmesis for patients undergoing combined modality therapy [167, 168]. Combining radiation and surgery on a planned basis has also been very successful for many other anatomic sites, including gynecological malignancies, bladder cancer, rectal cancer, primary brain tumors, and sarcoma.

Naturally, the exact strategy for combining radiation and surgery depends on the local circumstances for the individual anatomic site. As such, radiation may be given before, after, or during the surgical procedure. For example, preoperative radiation has the following advantages and may, therefore, be occasionally preferred for certain tumor types:

1. A closer coordination of overall therapy planning between surgeons and the radiation oncologist.
2. Radiation given preoperatively includes only tissues known or suspected of involvement based on clinical examination and imaging, whereas postoperative radiation must encompass not only the tumor bed but all tissues handled during the surgical procedure; the consequence is that postoperative radiation will in most instances require larger treatment fields with potential increases in toxicity.
3. Some tumors may regress substantially before surgery, allowing for a more conservative and often less morbid surgical resection.
4. The probability of tumor seeding as a result of surgical manipulation is decreased as typical preoperative doses (on the order of 50 Gy) are sufficient to inactivate virtually all microscopic extensions of disease.
5. There is no delay in the start of radiation; for example, postoperatively, problems with wound healing may

delay the start of radiation, allowing residual tumor cells to grow and repopulate the tumor bed.

6. Preoperative radiation allows for the targeting of tumors with an intact vasculature; postoperatively, the vasculature of the tumor site may be compromised, leading to hypoxic conditions that render the tumoricidal properties of radiation less effective.

The principal disadvantage of giving radiation preoperatively is that there may be increased difficulty in achieving primary wound healing after surgery. In addition, an advantage of radiation given postoperatively is that the entire surgical specimen is available for analysis and for determination of the histologic grade and pattern of microscopic extension.

Multiple experiments have been performed to evaluate the effectiveness of preoperative radiation combined with conservative or radical surgery versus amputation in mice bearing isotransplants of various tumor types. Dose–response curves for single-dose irradiation of 8 mm fibrosarcoma (FSaII) isotransplants treated by radiation alone or with radiation followed by local excision, or en bloc excision, are shown in Figure 2.34a [169]. On the one hand, there is a clear and significant shift of the dose–response curve to the left when radiation is combined with surgery. The shift of the dose–response curve by going from conservative to radical resection is, on the other hand, quite minimal. Figure 2.34b shows the extent of leg shortening versus tumor control probability for radiation alone or in combination with resection. In this experiment there was a small but clear benefit

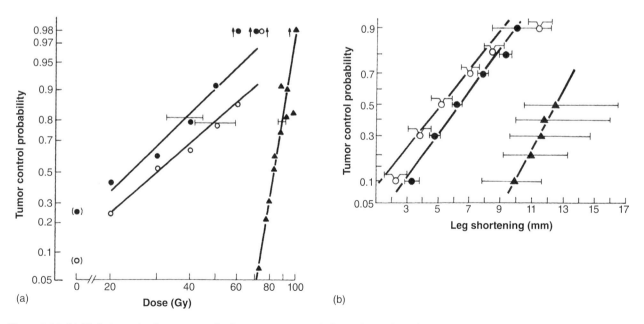

Figure 2.34 (a) FSaII, 8 mm in diameter, single dose. Tumor control–dose relationship after preoperative radiation or radiation alone as treatment of 8 mm tumor. Solid circles, en bloc resection four days after radiation; open circles, local resection four days after radiation; open circle with parenthesis, local resection alone; solid triangles, radiation alone. The 95% confidence limit is shown at 80% tumor control level. (b) Tumor control versus leg shortening for 8 mm tumors, with three different treatment options as shown in (a).

for radiation combined with local rather than extensive surgery. Even though such experiments hardly represent a perfect model for clinical studies, they do indicate that combined-modality treatment results in a major reduction in the dose required to achieve a given tumor control probability with a concomitant reduction in treatment-related toxicity.

New Approaches to Optimize Radiation Therapy

The past few decades have brought about an explosion in understanding the biological mechanisms that drive tumor initiation and progression. Rapid advances in molecular biology and cancer genetics have enabled the elucidation of key pathways that drive tumor-cell survival and growth [170]. This increased understanding has paved the way for exploration of novel approaches to enhance the therapeutic ratio of ionizing radiation as a cancer treatment.

Inhibition of Kinase-Dependent Signaling Pathways to Enhance Radiotherapy

It is now widely accepted that an aberrant activation of kinases is a common event in human cancers. Abnormal kinase activation has been found to occur in, and help promote the growth of, many types of human malignancies. These include lung cancer, leukemias, thyroid cancer, head and neck cancer, breast cancers, gliomas, melanomas, and others [171–175]. One example of a particularly important kinase in solid tumors is the EGFR, a member of the ERB family of receptor tyrosine kinases. EFGR was touched on above as a factor that influenced sensitivity to radiation. EGFR is mutated, amplified, or aberrantly activated in a number of different types of cancers, including non-small-cell lung cancer, glioblastomas, and head and neck squamous cell carcinomas. EGFR activation leads to activation of the phosphatidylinositol 3-kinase (PI3K), RAS/MEK, and signal transducer and activator of transcription 3 (STAT3) signaling pathways, which ultimately leads to increased tumor cell growth. Many cancers are effectively 'addicted' to EGFR signaling, as the inhibition of EGFR often leads to decreased growth or cell death in tumors with activating EGFR mutations [176]. Because of the dependence of tumor growth on activated EGFR signaling, much effort has been dedicated to developing agents that can target EGFR for use as targeted anticancer agents. These agents include the small-molecule inhibitors gefitinib and erlotinib, and monoclonal antibodies against EGFR, such as cetuximab. Erlotinib has been used to treat EGFR mutant non-small-cell lung cancer successfully, although

an eventual development of resistance and tumor recurrence nearly always occurs when it is used as a single agent [177, 178].

The combination of EGFR inhibitors and radiation has shown promise as a means to increase tumor control above and beyond the level obtained with radiotherapy alone. In preclinical models, it has been shown that the hyperactivity of EGFR can increase the radioresistance of tumor cells [99]. Accordingly, in both *in-vitro* and *in-vivo* model systems, the treatment of cancer cells with a combination of EGFR inhibitors and radiation has resulted in marked radiosensitization and enhanced cell killing [179]. Chinnaiyan *et al.* showed that, when given concomitantly with radiation, erlotinib causes striking radiosensitization. An examination of the genetic programs that were altered showed that erlotinib enhanced the response to radiation at multiple levels, by modulating processes such as cell cycle progression, apoptosis, and DNA repair [180]. The robust synergy seen between EGFR inhibitors and radiation in preclinical studies spawned a number of clinical trials to test the efficacy of the combination for the treatment of cancers. In one noteworthy trial, Bonner *et al.* randomized 211 patients with clinically advanced squamous cell carcinoma of the head and neck to receive either radiotherapy alone or concomitant radiotherapy with cetuximab. With a median follow-up of 54 months, the median duration of locoregional control was 24.4 months among patients treated with cetuximab and radiation, and 14.9 months among those receiving radiotherapy alone (p = 0.005). The median duration of overall survival was 49 months in the combined treatment arm, and 29.3 months among those treated with radiation alone (p = 0.03) (Figure 2.35). It was concluded that concomitant cetuximab and radiation improved both locoregional control and reduced mortality in the test population [181]. Currently, a number of other ongoing trials are being conducted to study many different disease types, testing the efficacy of EGFR inhibitors in combination with radiotherapy. These trials will determine the general clinical usefulness of combining anti-EGFR agents with radiation.

Aside from EGFR, a number of kinases have been shown as promising targets for combining targeted agents with radiotherapy. Most of these are still in the preclinical stages of development or in early Phase I clinical study. PIK3CA is a lipid kinase that is very frequently mutated and activated in a number of human cancers [182]. The mutation of PIK3CA and other PI3Ks results in the aberrant activation of AKT and the mTOR pathway, which promotes cell growth. PIK3CA is one of the most frequently mutated genes across all human cancers. A number of novel PI3K inhibitors have been developed as potential anticancer agents. Interestingly, Gupta *et al.* showed that the combination of inhibitors of PI3K with radiation results in significantly enhanced

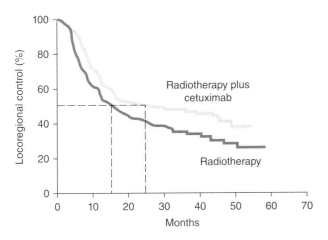
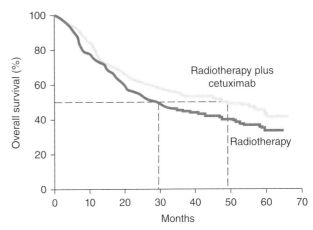

Figure 2.35 Addition of EGFR inhibition to radiation therapy results in significant improvements in locoregional control and overall survival rates for patients with locally advanced head and neck cancer.

radiosensitivity [183]. Similarly, Fokas *et al.* found that dual PI3K/mTOR inhibitors enhanced the radiation-induced cell killing in both tumor and endothelial cells [184]. Ongoing studies will determine the clinical utility of combining PI3K inhibitors with radiation therapy.

Modulation of Apoptosis to Increase Tumor Cell Kill or Protect Normal Tissues

As summarized earlier in the chapter, the tumor suppressor p53 is critically important in both G_1 arrest and apoptosis induction in response to DNA damage [71]. The ultimate importance of apoptosis to radiation-induced loss of clonogenicity remains to be fully clarified. Based on the initial observations that cells without wild-type p53 function did not undergo G_1 arrest [185], it was expected that cells with mutant or no p53 would be radiation-sensitive because they would replicate prior to repairing their DNA [186]. Although a few reports have shown increased radiation sensitivity in association with loss of wild-type p53 function, most have shown no difference or increased radiation resistance with the loss of wild-type p53 [187]. The increased resistance observed is predominantly due to the lack of radiation-induced apoptosis. This conclusion stems from studies on cells of hematopoietic origin [73, 188], or transformed fibroblasts [189]. Interestingly, human uroepithelial cells that are immortalized by the E6 protein of human papillomavirus have low or no detectable p53 and do not exhibit radiation-induced apoptosis, whereas their E7-immortalized counterparts, with wild-type p53, do undergo apoptosis when exposed to ionizing radiation [190]. The latter study was particularly intriguing because the authors reported that the normal E6 and E7-immortalized cells had similar survivals, based on trypan blue exclusion assays, despite the differences in apoptosis levels. This suggested that the presence of functional

p53 protein may change the mode of cell death, but not the ultimate amount of cell death after irradiation. This possibility raises problems about the validity of the endpoint when only apoptosis after exposure to radiation is assessed, and not clonogenic survival.

The clinical relevance of apoptosis following radiation treatment is still not clear. Initially, studies using murine tumor systems showed that increased pretreatment apoptosis levels correlated with a greater radiation-induced apoptosis, longer tumor growth delays, and lower TCD_{50} values. Additional studies were undertaken to determine whether the pretreatment apoptosis index predicts for the response of patients' tumors to radiotherapy. Thus far, the data indicate that this relationship is highly tumor-type and context-specific, but that in general the propensity to undergo apoptosis does *not* predict for clinical outcome following radiation treatment. For example, two reports – one examining cervical cancer and one transitional cell carcinoma of the bladder – concluded that the higher the pretreatment apoptosis level in biopsy samples, the better the response to radiotherapy [191,192]. In contrast, other reports have concluded that patients whose biopsy samples showed pre-therapy apoptosis levels above the median had worse survival rates than those with apoptosis indices below the median [193]. Because of the conflicting data and the lack of consensus, apoptotic potential is currently not used as a predictive marker for radiation response.

The variable relationship between apoptosis and radiotherapy is likely due in part to the different mechanisms of cell death induced by radiation in the specific cell type irradiated. While hematopoietic cells are known to be primed to undergo apoptosis and do so following radiation therapy, cells of other types – such as epithelial or glial cells – do not necessarily undergo classic apoptosis following irradiation. As noted above, irradiated epithelial cells more routinely undergo post-mitotic death

[15]. At the molecular level, the distinction between mitosis-triggered cell death (sometimes referred to as 'mitotic catastrophe') and apoptosis is not always clear. In some cells, genotoxic agent-induced mitotic catastrophe proceeds via a caspase-dependent mechanism, while in other cells mitotic catastrophe occurs in a caspase-independent manner [27, 194]. In other types of cells, a mixture of these two types of events can occur. Because of these overlapping molecular mechanisms, the propensity of non-hematopoietic cells to undergo programmed cell death is not a strong predictor of their response to radiotherapy.

When considering the relevance of apoptosis to radiation therapy for cancer, many questions remain. Do some tumor types that were thought not to undergo apoptosis after irradiation in fact die by that mode, but after longer times? Do proliferating cells that undergo late apoptosis divide one or more times between the radiation exposure and manifestation of apoptosis? Are these cells responding to a persistent lesion that remains in the cells through one or more cell cycles, or to a lesion created by replication of damaged DNA, or both? Are proliferating cells more susceptible to radiation-induced apoptosis than quiescent cells, or vice versa?

An example of the potential significance of these questions is highlighted in clinical studies undertaken by RTOG. In a randomized prospective trial (RTOG 86-10), the results showed an increased control of advanced prostate cancer and improved disease-specific mortality in patients treated with combined androgen deprivation and ionizing radiation [195]. Similar results were obtained from a European randomized trial also testing the efficacy of the addition of androgen deprivation to definitive radiotherapy for advanced prostate cancer [196, 197]. It is well documented that androgen deprivation causes apoptosis in normal prostate tissue, and prostate tumor cells have been shown to undergo apoptosis after radiation exposure [198–200]. Examination of the tissues from RTOG 86-10 for levels of BCL2 and BAX – two critical determinants of apoptosis – showed no relationship with clinical outcomes [201]. Interestingly, survivin, a member of the inhibitor of apoptosis family, does correlate with clinical outcome and prostate cancer-specific survival [202]. However, survivin regulates not only apoptosis but also cytoskeletal dynamics and the mitotic checkpoint, suggesting that the determinants of clinical response to radiation and androgen deprivation are likely to involve a number of biological processes aside from programmed cell death.

Although the propensity to undergo classic apoptosis across different tumor types may not necessarily be a good predictor of response to radiotherapy, direct manipulation of the apoptotic machinery – at least in certain tumor cells – has been shown capable of modulating the response to radiation. Studies have been conducted in attempts to increase radiation-induced apoptosis in tumors by using small molecules. For example, Moretti *et al.* have shown that a pan-BCL2 inhibitor leads to significant radiosensitization of non-small-cell lung cancer cells [203]. Hormonal manipulations may be useful in a proportion of tumors, or perhaps in a subset of cells within individual tumors. In addition, manipulation of apoptosis in normal tissues, in concert with radiation therapy, might have therapeutic benefit by protecting normal tissue from injury, but obtaining additional biological information about radiation-induced apoptosis will be important in the design of new regimens.

This paradigm has been explored by Fuks and others, who have shown that basic fibroblast growth factor (bFGF) can protect the lung against radiation-induced injury mediated via apoptosis [204]. As noted above, another approach used in the clinic is to administer a protective agent such as amifostine, an organic thiophosphate prodrug that is converted *in vivo* into WR-1065, a cytoprotective thiol [166, 205]. Amifostine is thought to help protect against radiation damage, in part by preventing apoptosis and other forms of DNA damage-induced cell death [206]. Understanding the mechanism of radiation-induced apoptosis will become increasingly important. Studies investigating the intricacies of these mechanisms demonstrate that processes outside of the classic caspase-mediated events are important. For example, membrane signaling via ceramide and sphingomyelinase have been reported to play key roles [207, 208]. The relative role of the ceramide pathway in regulating radiation-induced apoptosis is both dependent on the dose of radiation and on the cell type in question [209]. An additional variable is whether the irradiated cell is treated *in vivo* or *in vitro*. The results of studies published to date suggest that cells irradiated *in vivo* undergo apoptosis much more rapidly than cells irradiated *in vitro*. This difference is due to the influence of environmental factors such as cytokines, hormones, and lower oxygen levels in the tumor microenvironment.

Angiogenesis as a Target for Cancer Therapy

Tumors have long been known to contain large numbers of blood vessels. Indeed, tumor hypervascularity was initially thought to be a result of inflammatory vasodilation of pre-existing host vessels, a response to tumor metabolite and necrotic tumor products that was of no benefit to the tumor. Subsequently, it has become accepted that tumor growth and metastasis depends on angiogenesis and that chemical signals from tumor cells, such as vascular endothelial growth factor (VEGF) [210, 211] can shift resting endothelial cells into a phase of rapid growth. The production of VEGF by tumor cells can initiate and promote the growth of capillaries in tumors. Although, initially these ideas were not widely accepted, a clear

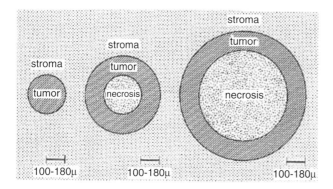

Figure 2.36 Extent of necrosis rises with increasing tumor size. Thomlinson and Gray saw that no necrosis occurred in small tumor cords with a radius of less than about 160 mm. As the tumor size increased, the necrotic volume increased. *Source:* Thomlinson and Gray 1955 [36]. Reproduced with permission of Nature Publishing Group.

concept of the role of angiogenesis in cancer and other diseases such as macular degeneration has now emerged [212, 213].

Most tumors in humans persist *in situ* for months to years without neovascularization. Subgroups of cells in the tumor can become 'vascularized' when genetic switches promoting an angiogenic phenotype are turned on. In the prevascular phase, the tumor is rarely larger than 2–3 mm in diameter and may contain about a million or so cells. Such asymptomatic lesions are usually clinically undetectable, although some are directly visible on the skin, surface of the cervix, or on the bladder. Cells in the prevascular tumors or dormant micrometastases may replicate as rapidly as cells in expanding, vascularized tumors, but without the growth of new vessels, the rate of proliferation of these cells reaches an equilibrium with their rate of death. Without tumor neovascularization, the poorly vascularized cells in the mass die and become necrotic (Figure 2.36) [36]. This is because the distance to which sufficient levels of oxygen and nutrients can diffuse is limited, and because of increased interstitial pressure in the middle of the tumor.

The switch to the neoangiogenic phenotype involves a change in the local equilibrium between positive and negative regulators of the growth of microvessels. Tumor cells may overexpress one or more of the positive regulators of angiogenesis, may mobilize an angiogenic protein from the extracellular matrix, may recruit host cells such as macrophages (which produce their own angiogenic proteins), or may engage in a combination of these processes. In addition to VEGF, a number of common pro-angiogenic proteins found in tumors, are produced either by tumor cells themselves, the tumor stroma, or via recruited cells in the tumor microenvironment. Members of the FGF family are strongly implicated in tumor angiogenesis. The FGF family includes at least 22 known

members, of which acidic FGF (aFGF) and basic FGF (bFGF) are the best studied [214]. Basic FGF was the first angiogenic protein to be isolated and purified from a tumor (in 1982), followed shortly by aFGF [215, 216]. Acidic and basic FGFs stimulate endothelial cell mitosis and migration, and are very potent angiogenic proteins *in vivo*. Elevated levels of FGF are produced by many different types of tumor [217]. Angiopoietins are another type of secreted factor that are pro-angiogenic. Angiopoietin-1, the prototypic angiopoietin, promotes vascular growth in tumors, much like VEGF. Angiopoietin-1 is a 70-kDa ligand that binds to a specific tyrosine kinase expressed only on endothelial cells, called Tie2 (or Tek), and in contrast to VEGF it is not a direct endothelial mitogen. Rather, it induces endothelial cells to recruit pericytes and smooth muscle cells to become incorporated into vessel walls, promoting vascular maturation and expansion. The angiogenic activities of factors such as these can be synergistic, especially VEGF and bFGF.

The upregulation of an angiogenic factor is not sufficient by itself for a tumor to become angiogenic. Certain negative regulators or inhibitors of vessel growth must be downregulated as well. These endogenous inhibitors normally defend the vascular endothelium from mitogenic stimuli. These proteins include endostatin, tumstatin, and thrombospondin-1. Significant effort has gone into attempting to devise ways to use these molecules in anticancer therapy, with mixed responses to date. Indeed, more than a trillion endothelial cells line the inside of blood vessels and cover an area of approximately $1000\,m^2$ in a typical 70 kg adult human. The turnover time of these normally quiescent cells can exceed 1000 days. During angiogenesis, however, capillary endothelial cells can proliferate as rapidly as bone marrow cells, with a mean turnover time of about five days. The foundations of this drastic difference are based on the relative activities of endogenous pro-angiogenic and anti-angiogenic factors. In tumors, this angiogenic switch is disrupted, resulting in an environment that favors capillary construction.

It is now well accepted that neovascularization plays a critical role in tumor progression. New tumor vessel development permits tumors to grow and metastasize, and the conversion of angiogenic switch to being pro-neovascular often heralds the onset of clinical symptoms. Most tumors become symptomatic and clinically detectable only after neovascularization has occurred. It should be noted, however, that the change to an angiogenic phenotype does not always result in a rapidly proliferating tumor. For example, in metastases, angiogenesis may be suppressed by local inhibitors. The successful remodeling of the distant site into a hospitable metastatic niche often entails changing the microenvironment to enable neovascularization [218]. Furthermore, angiogenesis in distant metastases may be suppressed by circulating inhibitors from the primary tumor and may become apparent only after the removal of the primary tumor. In addition, there are circulating bone marrow-derived monocytes which have the potential to colonize a metastatic niche or a treated tumor bed. The relative importance of circulating factors to promote vascular growth, relative to local factors, remains to be determined and may depend on the tumor type.

A variety a new agents to target tumor angiogenesis have been developed over the past decade. Perhaps the most widely used to date is bevacizumab, a humanized monoclonal antibody that inhibits VEGF-A. Bevacizumab was the first clinically available angiogenesis inhibitor in the United States. It is approved for use in certain metastatic cancers, such as colon and lung carcinoma, and for use in patients with glioblastoma multiforme [219, 220]. The compound binds to and blocks VEGF which, as described above, is needed for the formation and maintenance of tumor vasculature. Infusion of bevacizumab decreases tumor perfusion, tumor vascular volume, microvascular density, interstitial fluid pressure, and the number of viable, circulating endothelial cells [221]. Paradoxically, neovascularization gradually reduces a tumor's accessibility to chemotherapeutic drugs and the amount of oxygen carried to the tumor by the blood. Tumors do not outgrow their blood supply but instead compress it. By the time they are clinically detectable, increased interstitial pressure from leaky vessels in the tumor and the relative absence of intratumor lymphatics, cause vascular compression and eventually central necrosis. Anti-VEGF therapy results in the destruction of immature nonfunctional vessels in tumors, leading to a vascular 'normalization' and a better blood flow provided by remnant mature vessels; this increases exposure of the tumor cells to molecules carried in the bloodstream, including chemotherapeutic drugs and oxygen [221]. In addition to bevacizumab, there are a variety of other anti-angiogenic compounds in clinical use or at various stages of development. Noteworthy are the kinase inhibitors sunitinib and sorafenib,

both of which are inhibitors of VEGF receptor kinase activity. Their mechanisms of action involve blocking tumor angiogenesis by preventing VEGF receptor signaling [222]. Currently, sunitinib and sorafenib are approved for use in the treatment of kidney cancer.

To date, a marked interest has been expressed in combining inhibitors of angiogenesis with radiotherapy to achieve better tumor control, and until now bevacizumab has received the most attention in this regard. The blockage of angiogenesis during radiotherapy by bevacizumab has significantly improved the efficacy of irradiation in experimental model systems [223]. It is hypothesized that the vascular 'normalization' that is brought about by bevacizumab improves the efficacy of radiation by reducing tumor hypoxia [221]. A number of early-stage clinical trials have suggested that such combination therapies result in improved clinical outcomes, although definitive Phase III trials are still ongoing. Data from several tumor types demonstrate potentially improved outcomes with the combination of bevacizumab and radiation. These include locally advanced rectal cancer [224], glioblastoma [225, 226], head and neck cancers [227] and a number of other malignancies. Initial evidence has shown that the combination of anti-angiogenic compounds and radiation can achieve higher frequencies of complete clinical regression, at least for some cancers. More widespread clinical use of such combination strategies awaits the results of definitive randomized trials and long-term outcome data.

Summary

The complexities of the response of cells, tissues and whole organisms to ionizing radiation are manifest. Which of these responses offer the best opportunities for improved effect of radiation against the cancer or for reduced effect on normal tissues remains the key challenge of radiation biology.

References

1 Singh, N.P., McCoy, M.T., Tice, R.R., Schneider, E.L. (1988) A simple technique for quantitation of low levels of DNA damage in individual cells. *Exp. Cell Res.*, **175** (1), 184–191.

1a Hall, E.J. (2000) Radiobiology for the Radiologist, 5th edition. Lippincott, Williams and Wilkins.

2 Ward, J.F. (1985) Biochemistry of DNA lesions. *Radiat. Res. Suppl.*, **8**, S103–S111.

3 Bristow, R.G., Hardy, P.A., Hill, R.P. (1990) Comparison between in vitro radiosensitivity and in vivo radioresponse of murine tumor cell lines. I:

Parameters of in vitro radiosensitivity and endogenous cellular glutathione levels. *Int. J. Radiat. Oncol. Biol. Phys.*, **18** (1), 133–145.

4 Vos, O., van der Schans, G.P., Roos-Verheij, W.S. (1986) Reduction of intracellular glutathione content and radiosensitivity. *Int. J. Radiat. Biol. Relat. Stud. Phys. Chem. Med.*, **50** (1), 155–165.

5 Rajab, N.F., McKenna, D.J., Diamond, J., Williamson, K., *et al.* (2006) Prediction of radiosensitivity in human bladder cell lines using nuclear chromatin phenotype. *Cytometry A*, **69** (10), 1077–1085.

6 Ball, A.R., Jr, Yokomori, K. (2011) Damage site chromatin: open or closed? *Curr. Opinion Cell Biol.*, **23** (3), 277–283.

7 Miller, K.M., Jackson, S.P. (2012) Histone marks: repairing DNA breaks within the context of chromatin. *Biochem. Soc. Trans.*, **40** (2), 370–376.

8 Powell, S.N., Kachnic, L.A. (2008) Therapeutic exploitation of tumor cell defects in homologous recombination. *Anti-cancer Agents Med. Chem.*, **8** (4), 448–460.

9 Lee, J.H., Paull, T.T. (2005) ATM activation by DNA double-strand breaks through the Mre11-Rad50-Nbs1 complex. *Science*, **308** (5721), 551–554.

10 Lee, J.H., Paull, T.T. (2004) Direct activation of the ATM protein kinase by the Mre11/Rad50/Nbs1 complex. *Science*, **304** (5667), 93–96.

11 Bakkenist, C.J., Kastan, M.B. (2003) DNA damage activates ATM through intermolecular autophosphorylation and dimer dissociation. *Nature*, **421** (6922), 499–506.

12 Sartori, A.A., Lukas, C., Coates, J., Mistrik, M., *et al.* (2007) Human CtIP promotes DNA end resection. *Nature*, **450** (7169), 509–514.

13 Yun, M.H., Hiom, K. (2009) CtIP-BRCA1 modulates the choice of DNA double-strand-break repair pathway throughout the cell cycle. *Nature*, **459** (7245), 460–463.

14 Terasima, T., Ohara, H. (1968) Chromosome aberration and mitotic death in x-irradiated HeLa cells. *Mutat. Res.*, **5** (1), 195–197.

15 Chan, T.A., Hermeking, H., Lengauer, C., Kinzler, K.W., Vogelstein, B. (1999) 14-3-3Sigma is required to prevent mitotic catastrophe after DNA damage. *Nature*, **401** (6753), 616–620.

16 Fragkos, M., Beard, P. (2011) Mitotic catastrophe occurs in the absence of apoptosis in p53-null cells with a defective G1 checkpoint. *PLoS ONE*, **6** (8), e22946.

17 Galluzzi, L., Vitale, I., Abrams, J.M., Alnemri, E.S., *et al.* (2011) Molecular definitions of cell death subroutines: recommendations of the Nomenclature Committee on Cell Death 2012. *Cell Death Differ.*, **19** (1), 107–120.

18 Mir, S.E., De Witt Hamer, P.C., Krawczyk, P.M., Balaj, L., *et al.* (2010) In silico analysis of kinase expression identifies WEE1 as a gatekeeper against mitotic catastrophe in glioblastoma. *Cancer Cell*, **18** (3), 244–257.

19 Nagata, S. (2000) Apoptotic DNA fragmentation. *Exp. Cell Res.*, **256** (1), 12–18.

20 Nagata, S. (2002) Breakdown of chromosomal DNA. *Cornea*, **21** (2 Suppl.1), S2–S6.

21 Itoh, N., Yonehara, S., Ishii, A., Yonehara, M., *et al.* (1991) The polypeptide encoded by the cDNA for human cell surface antigen Fas can mediate apoptosis. *Cell*, **66** (2), 233–243.

22 Wong, G.H., Goeddel, D.V. (1994) Fas antigen and p55 TNF receptor signal apoptosis through distinct pathways. *J. Immunol.*, **152** (4), 1751–1755.

23 Wajant, H. (2002) The Fas signaling pathway: more than a paradigm. *Science*, **296** (5573), 1635–1636.

24 Li, P., Nijhawan, D., Budihardjo, I., Srinivasula, S.M., *et al.* (1997) Cytochrome c and dATP-dependent formation of Apaf-1/caspase-9 complex initiates an apoptotic protease cascade. *Cell*, **91** (4), 479–489.

25 Danial, N.N., Korsmeyer, S.J. (2004) Cell death: critical control points. *Cell*, **116** (2), 205–219.

26 Chan, Y.W., Chen, Y., Poon, R.Y. (2009) Generation of an indestructible cyclin B1 by caspase-6-dependent cleavage during mitotic catastrophe. *Oncogene*, **28** (2), 170–183.

27 Mansilla, S., Priebe, W., Portugal, J. (2006) Mitotic catastrophe results in cell death by caspase-dependent and caspase-independent mechanisms. *Cell Cycle*, **5** (1), 53–60.

28 Gray, L.H., Conger, A.D., Ebert, M., Hornsey, S., Scott, O.C. (1953) The concentration of oxygen dissolved in tissues at the time of irradiation as a factor in radiotherapy. *Br. J. Radiol.*, **26** (312), 638–648.

29 Frankenberg-Schwager, M., Frankenberg, D., Harbich, R., Beckonert, S. (1994) Evidence against the 'oxygen-in-the-track' hypothesis as an explanation for the radiobiological low oxygen enhancement ratio at high linear energy transfer radiation. *Radiat. Environ. Biophys.*, **33** (1), 1–8.

30 Wenzl, T., Wilkens, J.J. (2011) Modelling of the oxygen enhancement ratio for ion beam radiation therapy. *Phys. Med. Biol.*, **56** (11), 3251–3268.

31 Guyton, A.C. (1976) *Textbook of Medical Physiology*, p. 545.

32 Ling, C.C., Michaels, H.B., Gerweck, L.E., Epp, E.R., Peterson, E.C. (1981) Oxygen sensitization of mammalian cells under different irradiation conditions. *Radiat. Res.*, **86** (2), 325–340.

33 Revesz, L., Palcic, B. (1985) Radiation dose dependence of the sensitization by oxygen and oxygen mimic sensitizers. *Acta Radiol. Oncol.*, **24** (3), 209–217.

34 Taylor, Y.C., Brown, J.M. (1987) Radiosensitization in multifraction schedules. I. Evidence for an extremely low oxygen enhancement ratio. *Radiat. Res.*, **112** (1), 124–133.

35 Dasu, A., Denekamp, J. (1998) New insights into factors influencing the clinically relevant oxygen enhancement ratio. *Radiother. Oncol.*, **46** (3), 269–277.

36 Thomlinson, R.H., Gray, L.H. (1955) The histological structure of some human lung cancers and the

possible implications for radiotherapy. *Br. J. Cancer*, **9** (4), 539–549.

37 Brizel, D.M., Rosner, G.L., Harrelson, J., Prosnitz, L.R., Dewhirst, M.W. (1994) Pretreatment oxygenation profiles of human soft tissue sarcomas. *Int. J. Radiat. Oncol. Biol. Phys.*, **30** (3), 635–642.

38 Movsas, B., Chapman, J.D., Horwitz, E.M., Pinover, W.H., *et al.* (1999) Hypoxic regions exist in human prostate carcinoma. *Urology*, **53** (1), 11–18.

39 Movsas, B., Chapman, J.D., Hanlon, A.L., Horwitz, E.M., *et al.* (2001) Hypoxia in human prostate carcinoma: an Eppendorf PO_2 study. *Am. J. Clin. Oncol.*, **24** (5), 458–461.

40 Powers, W.E., Tolmach, L.J. (1963) A multicomponent x-ray survival curve for mouse lymphosarcoma cells irradiated in vivo. *Nature*, **197**, 710–711.

41 Hockel, M., Knoop, C., Schlenger, K., Vorndran, B., *et al.* Intratumoral pO_2 predicts survival in advanced cancer of the uterine cervix. *Radiother. Oncol.*, **26** (1), 45–50.

42 Graeber, T.G., Peterson, J.F., Tsai, M., Monica, K., Fornace, A.J., Jr, Giaccia, A.J. (1994) Hypoxia induces accumulation of p53 protein, but activation of a G1-phase checkpoint by low-oxygen conditions is independent of p53 status. *Mol. Cell. Biol.*, **14** (9), 6264–6277.

43 Graeber, T.G., Osmanian, C., Jacks, T., Housman, D.E., *et al.* (196) Hypoxia-mediated selection of cells with diminished apoptotic potential in solid tumours. *Nature*, **379** (6560), 88–91.

44 Chi, J.T., Wang, Z., Nuyten, D.S., Rodriguez, E.H., *et al.* (2006) Gene expression programs in response to hypoxia: cell type specificity and prognostic significance in human cancers. *PLoS Med.*, **3** (3), e47.

45 Wang, G.L., Semenza, G.L. (1993) General involvement of hypoxia-inducible factor 1 in transcriptional response to hypoxia. *Proc. Natl Acad. Sci. USA*, **90** (9), 4304–4308.

46 Wang, G.L., Semenza, G.L. (1993) Characterization of hypoxia-inducible factor 1 and regulation of DNA binding activity by hypoxia. *J. Biol. Chem.*, **268** (29), 21513–21518.

47 Semenza, G.L. (2011) Oxygen sensing, homeostasis, and disease. *N. Engl. J. Med.*, **365** (6), 537–547.

48 van Malenstein, H., Gevaert, O., Libbrecht, L., Daemen, A., *et al.* (2010) A seven-gene set associated with chronic hypoxia of prognostic importance in hepatocellular carcinoma. *Clin. Cancer Res.*, **16** (16), 4278–4288.

49 Spiro, I.J., Kennedy, K.A., Stickler, R., Ling, C.C. (1985) Cellular and molecular repair of X-ray-induced damage: dependence on oxygen tension and nutritional status. *Radiat. Res.*, **101** (1), 144–155.

50 Gupta, V., Rangala, N.S., Belli, J.A. (1986) Enhancement of radiation sensitivity by postradiation hypoxia. *Radiat. Res.*, **106** (1), 132–136.

51 Suit, H., Urano, M. (1969) Repair of sublethal radiation injury in hypoxic cells of a C3H mouse mammary carcinoma. *Radiat. Res.*, **37** (2), 423–434.

52 Brown, J.M. (1979) Evidence for acutely hypoxic cells in mouse tumours, and a possible mechanism of reoxygenation. *Br. J. Radiol.*, **52** (620), 650–656.

53 Jain, R.K. (1988) Determinants of tumor blood flow: a review. *Cancer Res.*, **48** (10), 2641–2658.

54 Chang, Y.S., di Tomaso, E., McDonald, D.M., Jones, R., Jain, R.K., Munn, L.L. (2000) Mosaic blood vessels in tumors: frequency of cancer cells in contact with flowing blood. *Proc. Natl Acad. Sci. USA*, **97** (26), 14608–14613.

55 Jain, R.K. (1998) Integrative pathophysiology of solid tumors: role in detection and treatment. *Cancer J. Sci. Am.*, **4** (Suppl. 1), S48–S57.

56 van Putten, L.M. (1968) Tumour reoxygenation during fractionated radiotherapy; studies with a transplantable mouse osteosarcoma. *Eur. J. Cancer*, **4** (2), 172–182.

57 Howard, A., Pelc, S.R. (1952) Synthesis of deoxyribonucleic acid in normal and irradiated cells in its relationship to chromosome breakage. *Heredity*, **6**, 216.

58 Masui, Y. (1996) A quest for cytoplasmic factors that control the cell cycle. *Prog. Cell Cycle Res.*, **2**, 1–13.

59 Smith, H.S., Pardee, A.B. (1970) Accumulation of a protein required for division during the cell cycle of *Escherichia coli. J. Bacteriol.*, **101** (3), 901–909.

60 Hartwell, L.H. (1974) *Saccharomyces cerevisiae* cell cycle. *Bacteriol. Rev.*, **38** (2), 164–198.

61 Nurse, P. (1975) Genetic control of cell size at cell division in yeast. *Nature*, **256** (5518), 547–551.

62 Evans, T., Rosenthal, E.T., Youngblom, J., Distel, D., Hunt, T. (1983) Cyclin: a protein specified by maternal mRNA in sea urchin eggs that is destroyed at each cleavage division. *Cell*, **33** (2), 389–396.

63 Murray, A.W., Solomon, M.J., Kirschner, M.W. (1989) The role of cyclin synthesis and degradation in the control of maturation promoting factor activity. *Nature*, **339** (6222), 280–286.

64 Weinert, T.A., Hartwell, L.H. (1988) The RAD9 gene controls the cell cycle response to DNA damage in *Saccharomyces cerevisiae. Science*, **241** (4863), 317–322.

65 Weinert, T., Hartwell, L. (1989) Control of G2 delay by the rad9 gene of *Saccharomyces cerevisiae. J. Cell Sci. Suppl.*, **12**, 145–148.

66 Xiong, Y., Hannon, G.J., Zhang, H., Casso, D., Kobayashi, R., Beach, D. (1993) p21 is a universal inhibitor of cyclin kinases. *Nature*, **366** (6456), 701–704.

67 el-Deiry, W.S., Tokino, T., Velculescu, V.E., Levy, D.B., *et al.* (1993) WAF1, a potential mediator of p53 tumor suppression. *Cell*, **75** (4), 817–825.

68 Hermeking, H., Lengauer, C., Polyak, K., He, T.C., *et al.* (1997) 14-3-3 sigma is a p53-regulated inhibitor of G2/M progression. *Mol. Cell*, **1** (1), 3–11.

69 Peng, C.Y., Graves, P.R., Thoma, R.S., Wu, Z., *et al.* (1997) Mitotic and G2 checkpoint control: regulation of 14-3-3 protein binding by phosphorylation of Cdc25C on serine-216. *Science*, **277** (5331), 1501–1505.

70 Graves, P.R., Lovly, C.M., Uy, G.L., Piwnica-Worms, H. (2001) Localization of human Cdc25C is regulated both by nuclear export and 14-3-3 protein binding. *Oncogene*, **20** (15), 1839–1851.

71 Vogelstein, B., Kinzler, K.W. (1992) p53 function and dysfunction. *Cell*, **70** (4), 523–526.

72 Waldman, T., Kinzler, K.W., Vogelstein, B. (1995) p21 is necessary for the p53-mediated G1 arrest in human cancer cells. *Cancer Res.*, **55** (22), 5187–5190.

73 Lowe, S.W., Schmitt, E.M., Smith, S.W., Osborne, B.A., Jacks, T. (1993) p53 is required for radiation-induced apoptosis in mouse thymocytes. *Nature*, **362** (6423), 847–879.

74 Symonds, H., Krall, L., Remington, L., Saenz-Robles, M., *et al.* (1994) p53-dependent apoptosis suppresses tumor growth and progression in vivo. *Cell*, **78** (4), 703–711.

75 Miyashita, T., Reed, J.C. (1995) Tumor suppressor p53 is a direct transcriptional activator of the human bax gene. *Cell*, **80** (2), 293–299.

76 Yu, J., Wang, Z., Kinzler, K.W., Vogelstein, B., Zhang, L. (2003) PUMA mediates the apoptotic response to p53 in colorectal cancer cells. *Proc. Natl Acad. Sci. USA*, **100** (4), 1931–1936.

77 Terasima, T., Tolmach, L.J. (1963) Variations in several responses of HeLa cells to x-irradiation during the division cycle. *Biophys. J.*, **3**, 11–33.

78 Terasima, T., Tolmach, L.J. (1961) Changes in x-ray sensitivity of HeLa cells during the division cycle. *Nature*, **190**, 1210–1211.

79 Sinclair, W.K. (1968) Cyclic x-ray responses in mammalian cells in vitro. *Radiat. Res.*, **33** (3), 620–643.

80 Gray, J.W., Dolbeare, F., Pallavicini, M.G., Beisker, W., Waldman, F. (1986) Cell cycle analysis using flow cytometry. *Int. J. Radiat. Biol. Relat. Stud. Phys. Chem. Med.*, **49** (2), 237–255.

81 Hall, E.J. (1972) Radiation dose-rate: a factor of importance in radiobiology and radiotherapy. *Br. J. Radiol.*, **45** (530), 81–97.

82 Mitchell, J.B., Bedford, J.S., Bailey, S.M. (1979) Dose-rate effects in plateau-phase cultures of S3 HeLa and V79 cells. *Radiat. Res.*, **79** (3), 552–567.

83 Mitchell, J.B., Bedford, J.S., Bailey, S.M. (1979) Dose-rate effects in mammalian cells in culture III. Comparison of cell killing and cell proliferation during continuous irradiation for six different cell lines. *Radiat. Res.*, **79** (3), 537–551.

84 Mitchell, J.B., Bedord, J.S., Bailey, S.M. (1979) Dose-rate effects on the cell cycle and survival of S3 HeLa and V79 cells. *Radiat. Res.*, **79** (3), 520–536.

85 Steel, G.G. (1991) The ESTRO Breur lecture. Cellular sensitivity to low dose-rate irradiation focuses the problem of tumour radioresistance. *Radiother. Oncol.*, **20** (2), 71–83.

86 Bacq, Z., Alexander, P. (1961) *Fundamentals of Radiobiology*, 2nd edition. Pergamon Press, New York.

87 Urano, M., Nesumi, N., Ando, K., Koike, S., Ohnuma, N. (1976) Repair of potentially lethal radiation damage in acute and chronically hypoxic tumor cells in vivo. *Radiology*, **118** (2), 447–451.

88 Shipley, W.U., Stanley, J.A., Courtenay, V.D., Field, S.B. (1975) Repair of radiation damage in Lewis lung carcinoma cells following in situ treatment with fast neutrons and gamma-rays. *Cancer Res.*, **35** (4), 932–938.

89 Raju, M.R., Bain, E., Carpenter, S.G., Jett, J., *et al.* (1980) Effects of argon ions on synchronized Chinese hamster cells. *Radiat. Res.*, **84** (1), 152–157.

90 Barendsen, G.W. (1968) Res tumours and normal different linear energy, in *Current Research*, vol. **4** (ed. A. Howard), Amsterdam, p. 283.

91 Field, S.B., Hornsey, S. (1974) Tissue, in *High LET Radiotherapy* (eds G.W. Barendsen *et al.*), Oxford, pp. 181–186.

92 Deacon, J., Peckham, M.J., Steel, G.G. (1984) The radioresponsiveness of human tumours and the initial slope of the cell survival curve. *Radiother. Oncol.*, **2** (4), 317–323.

93 Rofstad, E.K., Wahl, A., Brustad, T. (1987) Radiation sensitivity in vitro of cells isolated from human tumor surgical specimens. *Cancer Res.*, **47** (1), 106–110.

94 Brock, W.A., Baker, F.L., Peters, L.J. (1989) Radiosensitivity of human head and neck squamous cell carcinomas in primary culture and its potential as a predictive assay of tumor radiocurability. *Int. J. Radiat. Biol.*, **56** (5), 751–760.

95 Ringstrom, E., Peters, E., Hasegawa, M., Posner, M., Liu, M., Kelsey, K.T. (2002) Human papillomavirus type 16 and squamous cell carcinoma of the head and neck. *Clin. Cancer Res.*, **8** (10), 3187–3192.

96 Gubanova, E., Brown, B., Ivanov, S.V., Helleday, T., *et al.* (2012) Downregulation of SMG-1 in HPV-positive head and neck squamous cell carcinoma due to promoter hypermethylation correlates with improved survival. *Clin. Cancer Res.*, **18** (5), 1257–1267.

97 Pang, E., Delic, N.C., Hong, A., Zhang, M., Rose, B.R., Lyons, J.G. (2011) Radiosensitization of oropharyngeal squamous cell carcinoma cells by human papillomavirus 16 oncoprotein E6 *I. *Int. J. Radiat, Oncol. Biol. Phys.*, **79** (3), 860–865.

98 Akimoto, T., Hunter, N.R., Buchmiller, L., Mason, K., Ang, K.K., Milas, L. (1999) Inverse relationship between epidermal growth factor receptor expression and radiocurability of murine carcinomas. *Clin. Cancer Res.*, **5** (10), 2884–2890.

99 Liang, K., Ang, K.K., Milas, L., Hunter, N., Fan, Z. (2003) The epidermal growth factor receptor mediates radioresistance. *Int. J. Radiat. Oncol. Biol. Phys.*, **57** (1), 246–254.

100 El Kaffas, A., Tran, W., Czarnota, G.J. (2012) Vascular strategies for enhancing tumour response to radiation therapy. *Technol. Cancer Res. Treat.*, **11** (5), 421–432.

101 Gorski, D.H., Mauceri, H.J., Salloum, R.M., Gately, S., *et al.* (1998) Potentiation of the antitumor effect of ionizing radiation by brief concomitant exposures to angiostatin. *Cancer Res.*, **58** (24), 5686–5689.

102 Zips, D., Krause, M., Hessel, F., Westphal, J., *et al.* (2003) Experimental study on different combination schedules of VEGF-receptor inhibitor PTK787/ZK222584 and fractionated irradiation. *Anticancer Res.*, **23** (5A), 3869–3876.

103 Thomlinson, R.H. (1961) The oxygen effect in mammals. *Brookhaven Symp. Biol.*, **14**, 204–219.

104 Thomlinson, R.H. (1967) *Oxygen therapy - Biological considerations.* Camelot Press, London.

105 Urano, M., Suit, H.D. (1971) Experimental evaluation of tumor bed effect for C3H mouse mammary carcinoma and for C3H mouse fibrosarcoma. *Radiat Res.*, **45** (1), 41–49.

106 Milas, L., Ito, H., Hunter, N., Jones, S., Peters, L.J. (1986) Retardation of tumor growth in mice caused by radiation-induced injury of tumor bed stroma: dependency on tumor type. *Cancer Res.*, **46** (2), 723–727.

107 Clarke, M.F., Dick, J.E., Dirks, P.B., Eaves, C.J., *et al.* (2006) Cancer stem cells – perspectives on current status and future directions: AACR Workshop on cancer stem cells. *Cancer Res.*, **66** (19), 9339–9444.

108 Suit, H.D. (1973) Radiation biology: A basis for radiotherapy, in *Textbook of Radiotherapy*, pp. 75–121.

109 Suit, H., Wette, R. (1966) Radiation dose fractionation and tumor control probability. *Radiat Res.*, **29** (2), 267–281.

110 Suit, H.D., Shalek, R.J. (1963) Response of spontaneous mammary carcinoma of the C3H mouse to x irradiation given under conditions of local tissue anoxia. *J. Natl Cancer Inst.*, **31**, 497–509.

111 Suit, H.D. (1966) Response to x-irradiation of a tumour recurring after a TCD95 radiation dose. *Nature*, **211** (5052), 996–997.

112 Suit, H.D., Maeda, M. (1967) Hyperbaric oxygen and radiobiology of a C3H mouse mammary carcinoma. *J. Natl Cancer Inst.*, **39** (4), 639–652.

113 Ando, K., Koike, S., Ikehira, H., Hayata, I., Shikita, M., Yasukawa, M. (1985) Increased radiosensitivity of a recurrent murine fibrosarcoma following radiotherapy. *Jpn. J. Cancer Res.*, **76** (2), 99–103.

114 Langendijk, J.A., Kasperts, N., Leemans, C.R., Doornaert, P., Slotman, B.J. (2006) A phase II study of primary reirradiation in squamous cell carcinoma of head and neck. *Radiother. Oncol.*, **78** (3), 306–312.

115 Foley, E.J. (1953) Antigenic properties of methylcholanthrene-induced tumors in mice of the strain of origin. *Cancer Res.*, **13** (12), 835–837.

116 Suit, H.D., Kastelan, A. (1970) Immunologic status of host and response of a methylcholanthrene-induced sarcoma to local x-irradiation. *Cancer*, **26** (1), 232–238.

117 Withers, H.R. (1985) Biologic basis for altered fractionation schemes. *Cancer*, **55** (9 Suppl.), 2086–2095.

118 Williams, M.V., Denekamp, J., Fowler, J.F. (1985) A review of alpha/beta ratios for experimental tumors: implications for clinical studies of altered fractionation. *Int. J. Radiat. Oncol. Biol. Phys.*, **11** (1), 87–96.

119 Dorr, W., Hendry, J.H. (2001) Consequential late effects in normal tissues. *Radiother. Oncol.*, **61** (3), 223–231.

120 Suit, H.D. (1984) Modification of radiation response. *Int. J. Radiat. Oncol. Biol. Phys.*, **10** (1), 101–108.

121 Fowler, J.F. (1983) The second Klaas Breur memorial lecture. La Ronde – radiation sciences and medical radiology. *Radiother. Oncol.*, **1** (1), 1–22.

122 Mueller-Klieser, W., Vaupel, P., Manz, R. (1983) Tumour oxygenation under normobaric and hyperbaric conditions. *Br. J. Radiol.*, **56** (668), 559–564.

123 Moulder, J.E., Rockwell, S. (1984) Hypoxic fractions of solid tumors: experimental techniques, methods of analysis, and a survey of existing data. *Int. J. Radiat. Oncol. Biol. Phys.*, **10** (5), 695–712.

124 Howes, A.E., Suit, H.D. (1974) The effect of time between fractions on the response of tumors to irradiation. *Radiat. Res.*, **57** (2), 342–348.

125 Henk, J.M. (1986) Late results of a trial of hyperbaric oxygen and radiotherapy in head and neck cancer: a rationale for hypoxic cell sensitizers? *Int. J. Radiat. Oncol. Biol. Phys.*, **12** (8), 1339–1341.

126 Bush, R.S., Jenkin, R.D., Allt, W.E., Beale, F.A., Bean, H., Dembo, A.J., Pringle, J.F. (1978) Definitive

evidence for hypoxic cells influencing cure in cancer therapy. *Br. J. Cancer Suppl.*, **3**, 302–306.

127 Overgaard, J., Hansen, H.S., Overgaard, M., Bastholt, L., *et al.* (1998) A randomized double-blind phase III study of nimorazole as a hypoxic radiosensitizer of primary radiotherapy in supraglottic larynx and pharynx carcinoma. Results of the Danish Head and Neck Cancer Study (DAHANCA) Protocol 5-85. *Radiother. Oncol.*, **46** (2), 135–146.

128 Overgaard, J., Horsman, M.R. (1996) Modification of hypoxia-induced radioresistance in tumors by the use of oxygen and sensitizers. *Semin. Radiat. Oncol.*, **6** (1), 10–21.

129 Slevin, N.J., Hendry, J.H., Roberts, S.A., Agren-Cronqvist, A. (1992) The effect of increasing the treatment time beyond three weeks on the control of T2 and T3 laryngeal cancer using radiotherapy. *Radiother. Oncol.*, **24** (4), 215–220.

130 Dale, R.G., Hendry, J.H., Jones, B., Robertson, A.G., Deehan, C., Sinclair, J.A. (2002) Practical methods for compensating for missed treatment days in radiotherapy, with particular reference to head and neck schedules. *Clin. Oncol. (R. Coll. Radiol.)*, **14** (5), 382–393.

131 Bese, N.S., Hendry, J., Jeremic, B. (2007) Effects of prolongation of overall treatment time due to unplanned interruptions during radiotherapy of different tumor sites and practical methods for compensation. *Int. J. Radiat. Oncol. Biol. Phys.*, **68** (3), 654–661.

132 Chen, S.W., Liang, J.A., Yang, S.N., Ko, H.L., Lin, F.J. (2003) The adverse effect of treatment prolongation in cervical cancer by high-dose-rate intracavitary brachytherapy. *Radiother. Oncol.*, **67** (1), 69–76.

133 Perez, C.A., Grigsby, P.W., Castro-Vita, H., Lockett, M.A. (1995) Carcinoma of the uterine cervix. I. Impact of prolongation of overall treatment time and timing of brachytherapy on outcome of radiation therapy. *Int. J. Radiat. Oncol. Biol. Phys.*, **32** (5), 1275–1288.

134 Fowler, J.F. (1984) Fractionated radiation therapy after Strandqvist. *Acta Radiol. Oncol.*, **23** (4), 209–216.

135 Wang, C.C. (1988) Local control of oropharyngeal carcinoma after two accelerated hyperfractionation radiation therapy schemes. *Int. J. Radiat. Oncol. Biol. Phys.*, **14** (6), 1143–1146.

136 Garden, A.S., Morrison, W.H., Ang, K.K., Peters, L.J. (1995) Hyperfractionated radiation in the treatment of squamous cell carcinomas of the head and neck: a comparison of two fractionation schedules. *Int. J. Radiat. Oncol. Biol. Phys.*, **31** (3), 493–502.

137 Horiot, J.C., Bontemps, P., van den Bogaert, W., Le Fur, R., *et al.* (1997) Accelerated fractionation (AF) compared to conventional fractionation (CF) improves loco-regional control in the radiotherapy of advanced head and neck cancers: results of the EORTC 22851 randomized trial. *Radiother. Oncol.*, **44** (2), 111–121.

138 Begg, A.C., Hofland, I., Moonen, L., Bartelink, H., *et al.* (1990) The predictive value of cell kinetic measurements in a European trial of accelerated fractionation in advanced head and neck tumors: an interim report. *Int. J. Radiat. Oncol. Biol. Phys.*, **19** (6), 1449–1453.

139 Turrisi, A.T., 3rd, Kim, K., Blum, R., Sause, W.T., *et al.* (1999) Twice-daily compared with once-daily thoracic radiotherapy in limited small-cell lung cancer treated concurrently with cisplatin and etoposide. *N. Engl. J. Med.*, **340** (4), 265–271.

140 Fu, K.K., Pajak, T.F., Trotti, A., Jones, C.U., *et al.* (2000) A Radiation Therapy Oncology Group (RTOG) phase III randomized study to compare hyperfractionation and two variants of accelerated fractionation to standard fractionation radiotherapy for head and neck squamous cell carcinomas: first report of RTOG 9003. *Int. J. Radiat. Oncol. Biol. Phys.*, **48** (1), 7–16.

141 Semrau, R., Mueller, R.P., Stuetzer, H., Staar, S., *et al.* (2006) Efficacy of intensified hyperfractionated and accelerated radiotherapy and concurrent chemotherapy with carboplatin and 5-fluorouracil: updated results of a randomized multicentric trial in advanced head-and-neck cancer. *Int. J. Radiat. Oncol. Biol. Phys.*, **64** (5), 1308–1316.

142 Littbrand, B., Edsmyr, F., Revesz, L. (1975) A low dose-fractionation scheme for the radiotherapy of carcinoma of the bladder. Experimental background and preliminary results. *Bull. Cancer*, **62** (3), 241–248.

143 Lavey, R.S., Johnstone, A.K., Taylor, J.M., McBride, W.H. (1992) The effect of hyperfractionation on spinal cord response to radiation. *Int. J. Radiat. Oncol. Biol. Phys.*, **24** (4), 681–686.

144 Ang, K.K., Price, R.E., Stephens, L.C., Jiang, G.L., Feng, Y., Schultheiss, T.E., Peters, L.J. (1993) The tolerance of primate spinal cord to re-irradiation. *Int. J. Radiat. Oncol. Biol. Phys.*, **25** (3), 459–464.

145 Levin-Plotnik, D., Niemierko, A., Akselrod, S. (2000) Effect of incomplete repair on normal tissue complication probability in the spinal cord. *Int. J. Radiat. Oncol. Biol. Phys.*, **46** (3), 631–638.

146 Medin, P.M., Foster, R.D., van der Kogel, A.J., Sayre, J.W., McBride, W.H., Solberg, T.D. (2012) Spinal cord tolerance to reirradiation with single-fraction radiosurgery: a Swine model. *Int. J. Radiat. Oncol. Biol. Phys.*, **83** (3), 1031–1037.

147 Dische, S., Saunders, M.I. (1989) Continuous, hyperfractionated, accelerated radiotherapy (CHART): an interim report upon late morbidity. *Radiother. Oncol.*, **16** (1), 65–72.

148 Dische, S., Saunders, M.I. (1989) Continuous, hyperfractionated, accelerated radiotherapy (CHART). *Br. J. Cancer*, **59** (3), 325–326.

149 Saunders, M.I., Dische, S. (1990) Continuous, hyperfractionated, accelerated radiotherapy (CHART) in non-small cell carcinoma of the bronchus. *Int. J. Radiat. Oncol. Biol. Phys.*, **19** (5), 1211–1215.

150 Saunders, M.I., Dische, S., Barrett, A., Parmar, M.K., Harvey, A., Gibson, D. (1996) Randomised multicentre trials of CHART vs conventional radiotherapy in head and neck and non-small-cell lung cancer: an interim report. CHART Steering Committee. *Br. J. Cancer*, **73** (12), 1455–1462.

151 Saunders, M., Dische, S., Barrett, A., Harvey, A., Gibson, D., Parmar, M. (1997) Continuous hyperfractionated accelerated radiotherapy (CHART) versus conventional radiotherapy in non-small-cell lung cancer: a randomised multicentre trial. CHART Steering Committee. *Lancet*, **350** (9072), 161–165.

152 Dische, S., Saunders, M., Barrett, A., Harvey, A., Gibson, D., Parmar, M. (1997) A randomised multicentre trial of CHART versus conventional radiotherapy in head and neck cancer. *Radiother. Oncol.*, **44** (2), 123–136.

153 Saunders, M., Dische, S., Barrett, A., Harvey, A., Griffiths, G., Palmar, M. (1999) Continuous, hyperfractionated, accelerated radiotherapy (CHART) versus conventional radiotherapy in non-small cell lung cancer: mature data from the randomised multicentre trial. CHART Steering committee. *Radiother. Oncol.*, **52** (2), 137–148.

154 Pierquin, B., Calitchi, E., Mazeron, J.J., Le Bourgeois, J.P., Leung, S. (1987) Update on low dose rate irradiation for cancers of the oropharynx – May 1986. *Int. J. Radiat. Oncol. Biol. Phys.*, **13** (2), 259–261.

155 Ellis, F. (1971) Nominal standard dose and the ret. *Br. J. Radiol.*, **44** (518), 101–108.

156 Ulmer, W. (1985) On the problem of time, dose and fractionation (TDF) in the linear-quadratic model. *Strahlentherapie*, **161** (3), 177–185.

157 Tishler, R.B., Geard, C.R., Hall, E.J., Schiff, P.B. (1992) Taxol sensitizes human astrocytoma cells to radiation. *Cancer Res.*, **52** (12), 3495–3497.

158 Milas, L., Milas, M.M., Mason, K.A. (1999) Combination of taxanes with radiation: preclinical studies. *Semin. Radiat. Oncol.*, **9** (2 Suppl.1), 12–26.

159 Al-Sarraf, M., LeBlanc, M., Giri, P.G., Fu, K.K., *et al.* (1998) Chemoradiotherapy versus radiotherapy in patients with advanced nasopharyngeal cancer: phase III randomized Intergroup study 0099. *J. Clin. Oncol.*, **16** (4), 1310–1317.

160 Forastiere, A.A., Goepfert, H., Maor, M., Pajak, T.F., *et al.* (2003) Concurrent chemotherapy and radiotherapy for organ preservation in advanced laryngeal cancer. *N. Engl. J. Med.*, **349** (22), 2091–2098.

161 Bernier, J., Domenge, C., Ozsahin, M., Matuszewska, K., *et al.* (2004) Postoperative irradiation with or without concomitant chemotherapy for locally advanced head and neck cancer. *N. Engl. J. Med.*, **350** (19), 1945–1952.

162 Cooper, J.S., Pajak, T.F., Forastiere, A.A., Jacobs, J., *et al.* (2004) Postoperative concurrent radiotherapy and chemotherapy for high-risk squamous-cell carcinoma of the head and neck. *N. Engl. J. Med.*, **350** (19), 1937–1944.

163 Patt, H.M., Tyree, E.B., Straube, R.L., Smith, D.E. (1949) Cysteine protection against X irradiation. *Science*, **110** (2852), 213–214.

164 Milas, L., Hunter, N., Reid, B.O., Thames, H.D., Jr. (1982) Protective effects of S-2-(3-aminopropylamino)ethylphosphorothioic acid against radiation damage of normal tissues and a fibrosarcoma in mice. *Cancer Res.*, **42** (5), 1888–1897.

165 Kligerman, M.M., Liu, T., Liu, Y., Scheffler, B., He, S., Zhang, Z. (1992) Interim analysis of a randomized trial of radiation therapy of rectal cancer with/without WR-2721. *Int. J. Radiat. Oncol. Biol. Phys.*, **22** (4), 799–802.

166 Brizel, D.M., Wasserman, T.H., Henke, M., Strnad, V., *et al.* (2000) Phase III randomized trial of amifostine as a radioprotector in head and neck cancer. *J. Clin. Oncol.*, **18** (19), 3339–3345.

167 Fisher, B., Anderson, S., Bryant, J., Margolese, R.G., *et al.* (2002) Twenty-year follow-up of a randomized trial comparing total mastectomy, lumpectomy, and lumpectomy plus irradiation for the treatment of invasive breast cancer. *N. Engl. J. Med.*, **347** (16), 1233–1241.

168 Veronesi, U., Cascinelli, N., Mariani, L., Greco, M., *et al.* (2002) Twenty-year follow-up of a randomized study comparing breast-conserving surgery with radical mastectomy for early breast cancer. *N. Engl. J. Med.*, **347** (16), 1227–1232.

169 Todoroki, T., Suit, H.D. (1986) Effect of fractionated irradiation prior to conservative and radical surgery on therapeutic gain in a spontaneous fibrosarcoma of the C3H mouse. *J. Surg. Oncol.*, **31** (4), 279–286.

170 Hanahan, D., Weinberg, R.A. (2011) Hallmarks of cancer: the next generation. *Cell*, **144** (5), 646–674.

171 Parsons, D.W., Jones, S., Zhang, X., Lin, J.C., *et al.* (2008) An integrated genomic analysis of human glioblastoma multiforme. *Science*, **321** (5897), 1807–1812.

172 Ding, L., Getz, G., Wheeler, D.A., Mardis, E.R., *et al.* (2008) Somatic mutations affect key pathways in lung adenocarcinoma. *Nature*, **455** (7216), 1069–1075.

173 Davies, H., Bignell, G.R., Cox, C., Stephens, P., *et al.* (2002) Mutations of the BRAF gene in human cancer. *Nature*, **417** (6892), 949–954.

174 Kimura, E.T., Nikiforova, M.N., Zhu, Z., Knauf, J.A., Nikiforov, Y.E., Fagin, J.A. (2003) High prevalence of BRAF mutations in thyroid cancer: genetic evidence for constitutive activation of the RET/PTC-RAS-BRAF signaling pathway in papillary thyroid carcinoma. *Cancer Res.*, **63** (7), 1454–1457.

175 Irish, J.C., Bernstein, A. (1993) Oncogenes in head and neck cancer. *Laryngoscope*, **103** (1 Pt 1), 42–52.

176 Mendelsohn, J., Baselga, J. (2000) The EGF receptor family as targets for cancer therapy. *Oncogene*, **19** (56), 6550–6565.

177 Tsao, M.S., Sakurada, A., Cutz, J.C., Zhu, C.Q., *et al.* (2005) Erlotinib in lung cancer – molecular and clinical predictors of outcome. *N. Engl. J. Med.*, **353** (2), 133–144.

178 Kobayashi, S., Boggon, T.J., Dayaram, T., Janne, P.A., *et al.* (2005) EGFR mutation and resistance of non-small-cell lung cancer to gefitinib. *N. Engl. J. Med.*, **352** (8), 786–792.

179 Sartor, C.I. (2004) Mechanisms of disease: Radiosensitization by epidermal growth factor receptor inhibitors. *Nat. Clin. Pract. Oncol.*, **1** (2), 80–87.

180 Chinnaiyan, P., Huang, S., Vallabhaneni, G., Armstrong, E., *et al.* (2005) Mechanisms of enhanced radiation response following epidermal growth factor receptor signaling inhibition by erlotinib (Tarceva). *Cancer Res.*, **65** (8), 3328–3335.

181 Bonner, J.A., Harari, P.M., Giralt, J., Azarnia, N., *et al.* (2006) Radiotherapy plus cetuximab for squamous-cell carcinoma of the head and neck. *N. Engl. J. Med.*, **354** (6), 567–578.

182 Samuels, Y., Wang, Z., Bardelli, A., Silliman, N., *et al.* (2004) High frequency of mutations of the PIK3CA gene in human cancers. *Science*, **304** (5670), 554.

183 Gupta, A.K., Cerniglia, G.J., Mick, R., Ahmed, M.S., *et al.* (2003) Radiation sensitization of human cancer cells in vivo by inhibiting the activity of PI3K using LY294002. *Int. J. Radiat. Oncol. Biol. Phys.*, **56** (3), 846–853.

184 Fokas, E., Yoshimura, M., Prevo, R., Higgins, G., *et al.* (2012) NVP-BEZ235 and NVP-BGT226, dual phosphatidylinositol 3-kinase/mammalian target of rapamycin inhibitors, enhance tumor and endothelial cell radiosensitivity. *Radiat. Oncol.*, **7**, 48.

185 Kastan, M.B., Onyekwere, O., Sidransky, D., Vogelstein, B., Craig, R.W. (1991) Participation of p53 protein in the cellular response to DNA damage. *Cancer Res.*, **51** (23 Pt 1), 6304–6311.

186 Lane, D.P. (1992) Cancer. p53, guardian of the genome. *Nature*, **358** (6381), 15–16.

187 Bristow, R.G., Benchimol, S., Hill, R.P. (1996) The p53 gene as a modifier of intrinsic radiosensitivity: implications for radiotherapy. *Radiother. Oncol.*, **40** (3), 197–223.

188 Clarke, A.R., Purdie, C.A., Harrison, D.J., Morris, R.G., *et al.* (1993) Thymocyte apoptosis induced by p53-dependent and independent pathways. *Nature*, **362** (6423), 849–852.

189 Lowe, S.W., Bodis, S., McClatchey, A., Remington, L., *et al.* (1994) p53 status and the efficacy of cancer therapy in vivo. *Science*, **266** (5186), 807–810.

190 Puthenveettil, J.A., Frederickson, S.M., Reznikoff, C.A. (1996) Apoptosis in human papillomavirus16 E7-, but not E6-immortalized human uroepithelial cells. *Oncogene*, **13** (6), 1123–1131.

191 Wheeler, J.A., Stephens, L.C., Tornos, C., Eifel, P.J., Ang, K.K., Milas, L., Allen, P.K., Meyn, R.E., Jr. (1995) ASTRO Research Fellowship: apoptosis as a predictor of tumor response to radiation in stage IB cervical carcinoma. *Int. J. Radiat. Oncol. Biol. Phys.*, **32** (5), 1487–1493.

192 Chyle, V., Pollack, A., Czerniak, B., Stephens, L.C., Zagars, G.K., Terry, N.H., Meyn, R.E. (1996) Apoptosis and downstaging after preoperative radiotherapy for muscle-invasive bladder cancer. *Int. J. Radiat. Oncol. Biol. Phys.*, **35** (2), 281–287.

193 Levine, E.L., Renehan, A., Gossiel, R., Davidson, S.E., *et al.* (1995) Apoptosis, intrinsic radiosensitivity and prediction of radiotherapy response in cervical carcinoma. *Radiother. Oncol.*, **37** (1), 1–9.

194 Kroemer, G., Galluzzi, L., Vandenabeele, P., Abrams, J., *et al.* (2009) Classification of cell death: recommendations of the Nomenclature Committee on Cell Death 2009. *Cell Death Differ.*, **16** (1), 3–11.

195 Roach, M., 3rd, Bae, K., Speight, J., Wolkov, H.B., *et al.* (2008) Short-term neoadjuvant androgen deprivation therapy and external-beam radiotherapy for locally advanced prostate cancer: long-term results of RTOG 8610. *J. Clin. Oncol.*, **26** (4), 585–591.

196 Bolla, M., Collette, L., Blank, L., Warde, P., *et al.* (2002) Long-term results with immediate androgen suppression and external irradiation in patients with locally advanced prostate cancer (an EORTC study): a phase III randomised trial. *Lancet*, **360** (9327), 103–106.

197 Bolla, M., Gonzalez, D., Warde, P., Dubois, J.B., *et al.* (1997) Improved survival in patients with locally advanced prostate cancer treated with radiotherapy and goserelin. *N. Engl. J. Med.*, **337** (5), 295–300.

198 Colombel, M., Olsson, C.A., Ng, P.Y., Buttyan, R. (1992) Hormone-regulated apoptosis results from reentry of differentiated prostate cells onto a defective cell cycle. *Cancer Res.*, **52** (16), 4313–4319.

199 Berges, R.R., Furuya, Y., Remington, L., English, H.F., Jacks, T., Isaacs, J.T. (1993) Cell proliferation, DNA

repair, and p53 function are not required for programmed death of prostatic glandular cells induced by androgen ablation. *Proc. Natl Acad. Sci. USA*, **90** (19), 8910–8914.

200 Algan, O., Stobbe, C.C., Helt, A.M., Hanks, G.E., Chapman, J.D. (1996) Radiation inactivation of human prostate cancer cells: the role of apoptosis. *Radiat Res.*, **146** (3), 267–275.

201 Khor, L.Y., Desilvio, M., Li, R., McDonnell, T.J., *et al.* (2006) Bcl-2 and bax expression and prostate cancer outcome in men treated with radiotherapy in Radiation Therapy Oncology Group protocol 86-10. *Int. J. Radiat. Oncol. Biol. Phys.*, **66** (1), 25–30.

202 Zhang, M., Ho, A., Hammond, E.H., Suzuki, Y., *et al.* (2009) Prognostic value of survivin in locally advanced prostate cancer: study based on RTOG 8610. *Int. J. Radiat. Oncol. Biol. Phys.*, **73** (4), 1033–1042.

203 Moretti, L., Li, B., Kim, K.W., Chen, H., Lu, B. (2010) AT-101, a pan-Bcl-2 inhibitor, leads to radiosensitization of non-small cell lung cancer. *J. Thorac. Oncol.*, **5** (5), 680–687.

204 Fuks, Z., Alfieri, A., Haimovitz-Friedman, A., Seddon, A., Cordon-Cardo, C. (1995) Intravenous basic fibroblast growth factor protects the lung but not mediastinal organs against radiation-induced apoptosis in vivo. *Cancer J. Sci. Am.*, **1** (1), 62–72.

205 Anne, P.R., Machtay, M., Rosenthal, D.I., Brizel, D.M., *et al.* (2007) A Phase II trial of subcutaneous amifostine and radiation therapy in patients with head-and-neck cancer. *Int. J. Radiat. Oncol. Biol. Phys.*, **67** (2), 445–452.

206 Belkacemi, Y., Rat, P., Piel, G., Christen, M.O., Touboul, E., Warnet, J.M. (2001) Lens epithelial cell protection by aminothiol WR-1065 and anetholedithiolethione from ionizing radiation. *Int. J. Cancer, 96 Suppl.*, 15–26.

207 Haimovitz-Friedman, A., Kan, C.C., Ehleiter, D., Persaud, R.S., McLoughlin, M., Fuks, Z., Kolesnick, R.N. (1994) Ionizing radiation acts on cellular membranes to generate ceramide and initiate apoptosis. *J. Exp. Med.*, **180** (2), 525–535.

208 Santana, P., Pena, L.A., Haimovitz-Friedman, A., Martin, S., *et al.* (1996) Acid sphingomyelinase-deficient human lymphoblasts and mice are defective in radiation-induced apoptosis. *Cell*, **86** (2), 189–199.

209 Garcia-Barros, M., Paris, F., Cordon-Cardo, C., Lyden, D., *et al.* (2003) Tumor response to radiotherapy regulated by endothelial cell apoptosis. *Science*, **300** (5622), 1155–1159.

210 Shweiki, D., Itin, A., Soffer, D., Keshet, E. (1992) Vascular endothelial growth factor induced by hypoxia may mediate hypoxia-initiated angiogenesis. *Nature*, **359** (6398), 843–845.

211 Kim, K.J., Li, B., Winer, J., Armanini, M., Gillett, N., Phillips, H.S., Ferrara, N. (1993) Inhibition of vascular endothelial growth factor-induced angiogenesis suppresses tumour growth in vivo. *Nature*, **362** (6423), 841–844.

212 Folkman, J. (1997) Angiogenesis and angiogenesis inhibition: an overview. *EXS*, **79**, 1–8.

213 Folkman, J. (2002) Role of angiogenesis in tumor growth and metastasis. *Semin. Oncol.*, **29** (6 Suppl. 16), 15–18.

214 Ornitz, D.M., Itoh, N. (2001) Fibroblast growth factors. *Genome Biol.*, **2** (3), REVIEWS3005.

215 Shing, Y., Folkman, J., Sullivan, R., Butterfield, C., Murray, J., Klagsbrun, M. (1984) Heparin affinity: purification of a tumor-derived capillary endothelial cell growth factor. *Science*, **223** (4642), 1296–1299.

216 Friesel, R.E., Maciag, T. (1995) Molecular mechanisms of angiogenesis: fibroblast growth factor signal transduction. *FASEB J.*, **9** (10), 919–925.

217 Nguyen, M., Watanabe, H., Budson, A.E., Richie, J.P., Hayes, D.F., Folkman, J. (1994) Elevated levels of an angiogenic peptide, basic fibroblast growth factor, in the urine of patients with a wide spectrum of cancers. *J. Natl Cancer Inst.*, **86** (5), 356–361.

218 Duda, D.G., Jain, R.K. (2010) Premetastatic lung 'niche': is vascular endothelial growth factor receptor 1 activation required? *Cancer Res.*, **70** (14), 5670–5673.

219 Kabbinavar, F., Hurwitz, H.I., Fehrenbacher, L., Meropol, N.J., *et al.* (2003) Phase II, randomized trial comparing bevacizumab plus fluorouracil (FU)/leucovorin (LV) with FU/LV alone in patients with metastatic colorectal cancer. *J. Clin. Oncol.*, **21** (1), 60–65.

220 Hurwitz, H.I., Fehrenbacher, L., Hainsworth, J.D., Heim, W., *et al.* (2005) Bevacizumab in combination with fluorouracil and leucovorin: an active regimen for first-line metastatic colorectal cancer. *J. Clin. Oncol.*, **23** (15), 3502–3508.

221 Willett, C.G., Boucher, Y., di Tomaso, E., Duda, D.G., *et al.* (2004) Direct evidence that the VEGF-specific antibody bevacizumab has antivascular effects in human rectal cancer. *Nat. Med.*, **10** (2), 145–147.

222 Rini, B.I. (2007) Vascular endothelial growth factor-targeted therapy in renal cell carcinoma: current status and future directions. *Clin. Cancer Res.*, **13** (4), 1098–1106.

223 Gorski, D.H., Beckett, M.A., Jaskowiak, N.T., Calvin, D.P., *et al.* (1999) Blockage of the vascular endothelial growth factor stress response increases the antitumor effects of ionizing radiation. *Cancer Res.*, **59** (14), 3374–3378.

224 Koukourakis, M.I., Giatromanolaki, A., Sheldon, H., Buffa, F.M., *et al.* (2009) Phase I/II trial of bevacizumab and radiotherapy for locally advanced inoperable colorectal cancer: vasculature-independent

radiosensitizing effect of bevacizumab. *Clin. Cancer Res.*, **15** (22), 7069–7076.

225 Lai, A., Tran, A., Nghiemphu, P.L., Pope, W.B., *et al.* (2011) Phase II study of bevacizumab plus temozolomide during and after radiation therapy for patients with newly diagnosed glioblastoma multiforme. *J. Clin. Oncol.*, **29** (2), 142–148.

226 Vredenburgh, J.J., Desjardins, A., Reardon, D.A., Peters, K.B., *et al.* (2011) The addition of bevacizumab to standard radiation therapy and temozolomide followed by bevacizumab, temozolomide, and irinotecan for newly diagnosed glioblastoma. *Clin. Cancer Res.*, **17** (12), 4119–4124.

227 Fury, M.G., Lee, N.Y., Sherman, E., Lisa, D., *et al.* (2012) A phase 2 study of bevacizumab with cisplatin plus intensity-modulated radiation therapy for stage III/IVB head and neck squamous cell cancer. *Cancer*, **118** (20), 5008–5014.

3

Treatment Planning

George T.Y. Chen and Jong H. Kung

Introduction

The goal of radiation treatment planning is to design an optimized and deliverable radiation distribution resulting in a tumoricidal dose to the target, while sparing adjacent normal tissues. Treatment planning is a computational simulation exercise, where a personalized model of the patient's anatomy is constructed, and beams are configured to irradiate the target. A radiation transport calculation is performed, resulting in a volumetric dose distribution. Dose is ideally calculated within the patient to an accuracy of 5% or better, based on the radiobiological concept that a steep dose–response curve exists, and a greater uncertainty could result in the suboptimal probability of local tumor control.

Current treatment planning concepts and technology are discussed in this chapter, specifically describing key elements of the process, including imaging in treatment planning and fundamentals of dose computation. Discussions are included on the sources of uncertainty associated with treatment planning. Example treatment plans provide a concrete context for explaining the information provided by treatment planning.

Imaging

Imaging for Treatment Planning

Imaging has many roles in radiation oncology. It is used to localize the extent of disease, to design radiation portals, to provide quantitative data for dose calculations, and to guide treatment delivery and monitor therapy response.

Computed Tomography

Computed tomography (CT) is the most commonly used imaging modality for radiation treatment planning. A CT scan provides a quantitative map of the body's organ shape and location, and the relative linear attenuation coefficient in the transverse imaging plane. Briefly, a fan beam of x-rays rotates around the patient, and the transmitted radiation at each angle is measured. From these projections, image reconstruction algorithms generate an image matrix, typically 1024×1024 pixels, with a slice thickness of a few millimeters. Each image pixel is a measure of μ_x, the linear attenuation coefficient (relative to water μ_w) at diagnostic x-ray energies. Pixel values are quantified in Hounsfield units (HU):

$$HU = 1000(\mu_x - \mu_w)/\mu_w$$

The linear attenuation coefficient is a function of the electron density and atomic number of the tissue and the x-ray beam energy. The assignment of a specific HU value to a pixel does not uniquely characterize the tissue. Voxels of the same HU can consist of either a tissue of higher Z and unit density, or a water equivalent Z with a higher physical density. Accurately estimating the electron density of a voxel is important in radiation transport calculations. Fortunately, tissues (in different patients) have similar physical and chemical properties [1], and therefore similar atomic numbers, allowing approximations to be made to estimate tissue electron density. If tissue characterization is essential for special radiation transport calculations, methods to unfold the relative components of atomic composition and electron density may

Clinical Radiation Oncology: Indications, Techniques, and Results, Third Edition. Edited by William Small Jr.
© 2017 John Wiley & Sons, Inc. Published 2017 by John Wiley & Sons, Inc.

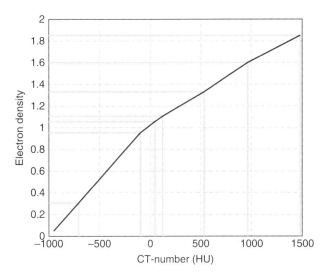

Figure 3.1 CT WEL calibration curve maps a CT voxel to a water equivalent pathlength.

be achieved with dual-energy scanning (scans at two different diagnostic energies), although most radiotherapy planning scans are performed at a single x-ray tube potential.

In a planning scan (~120 kVP), the HUs associated with specific tissues and materials are: air, −1000 HU; fat, −100 HU; water; 0 HU; muscle, ~40 HU; liver, ~80 HU and bone variable, up to 1000 HU. The HU-values of different tissues at diagnostic energies can be approximately mapped to electron density values that are used for dose calculations [2]. A typical calibration curve to convert HU to relative electron density (relative to water) is shown in Figure 3.1. Other implementations have a smooth or piecewise continuous mapping rather than the discontinuity. Fat has a disproportionately high electron density relative to other tissues due to the abundance of hydrogen.

This calibration curve has two segments. Below ~50 HU, tissues have atomic numbers near water; tissues can be considered to be mixtures of water and air, which have similar *Z*. Above ~100 HU, tissues have increasing amounts of high-*Z* elements (e.g., calcium), which disproportionally attenuates photons at diagnostic energies but does not significantly affect megavoltage photon attenuation. This results in a decreased slope of the curve. Treatment planning systems use these graphs to map HU to voxel electron densities relative to water.

Contrast media are frequently used to improve visualization of tumor and organs at risk. Because of the high *Z* of contrast materials, areas of contrast uptake may require image editing to reset HU for specialized treatment planning (e.g., proton beam planning) so as not to be interpreted as high-electron density materials present during treatment.

Practical Aspects of CT Image Acquisition

To acquire a scan that is most representative of anatomy in the treatment position, the patient is scanned as treated. Multidetector CT (MDCT) simulators have a wide bore (80 cm) that accommodates most treatment-positioning accessories (e.g., breast board, body immobilization cradles). MDCT scanning is three- to fivefold faster than a single-slice scanner, depending on the number of detector rings (between four and 64) and the slice thickness. High-speed scanning can capture a bolus of intravenous contrast before dissipation and potentially reduce motion artifacts.

The scan field of view is selected to include the external skin contour, which is required for dose calculations. Longitudinal scan limits are chosen to capture the tumor extent and the complete volume of organs at risk (to accurately calculate dose to the entire organ at risk). A three-dimensional (3D) planning study may contain about 200 or more slices.

CT acquisition modes include step-and-shoot as well as helical mode. In step-and-shoot, a scan is acquired in the axial plane while the patient couch is at rest; the x-ray source is gated off after image acquisition, and the couch is advanced to the next longitudinal position. The next slice of data is then taken, and the sequence is repeated. In helical mode, the couch is continuously advanced while the x-ray tube continuously rotates, leading to faster volumetric scan acquisitions. The tube rotation time is ~0.5 s. CT simulators are typically diagnostic quality, having the same spatial and temporal resolution.

Artifacts

Imaging artifacts degrade CT information content. Commonly observed artifacts include:

- *Streak artifacts*: Beam hardening causes streaks when the x-ray beam crosses particularly opaque regions, for example in the posterior fossa of the brain, bony pelvis, or when metallic clips (Figure 3.2a) [3] or dental fillings are present. Physiologic motion can also cause streak artifacts (e.g., gas bubble movement during abdominal scanning). These artifacts distort the HU values within the streaks and therefore introduce errors in the calculation of radiographic path length. Such perturbations can affect an intensity-modulated fluence calculation or the calculated penetration of a charged particle beam.
- *Partial volume sampling*: this artifact occurs when an anatomical feature (e.g., bone) partially intersects the scan plane, resulting in inaccuracies in HU assignment. The selection of slice thickness influences the detectability of small lesions. Thin slices mitigate the effects of partial volume sampling errors.

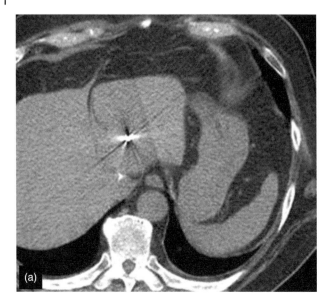
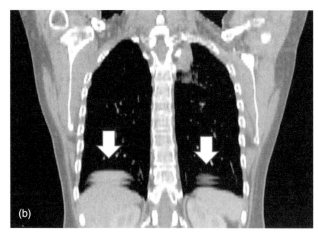

Figure 3.2 (a) Streak artifact from metallic clip. (b) Temporal artifact at lung/diaphragm interface (arrows) observed in a helical scan of a patient breathing lightly.

- *Motion artifacts*: When the scanner rotation period is comparable to the periodicity of organ motion, interference can occur. This may result in imaging artifacts that severely distort the shape and volume of structures of interest (e.g., target or organ at risk). Respiratory motion artifacts during CT scans have been noted for some time [4,5]. A common artifact in the CT scan of a patient breathing lightly during helical scanning is the presence of discontinuities at the diaphragm/lung interface. Figure 3.2b shows an example of such an artifact, where the diaphragm/lung interface is unrealistically jagged due to motion.

These temporal aliasing artifacts have been studied in phantom and simulation experiments to elucidate both their source and magnitude [6]. In Figure 3.3, the first column is a photograph of test objects embedded in a foam block, scanned on a moving stage to simulate periodic respiratory motion. Surface rendering of the phantom in a static state shows life-like realism, as seen in the second column. When the phantom is set into respiration-like craniocaudal motion and scans are acquired in the conventional helical scan mode, the resulting images of the spherical objects are significantly distorted, as shown in the next three columns. The specific distortion is dependent on the relative phases of organ and scanner motion. Motion artifacts spurred the development of algorithms that image object motion as a function of time, or four-dimensional (4D) imaging.

One approach to minimizing motion artifacts is to scan (and treat) by suspending respiratory motion. Breath-hold scanning and treatment have been reported [7]. This requires patient compliance and lengthens the treatment room time. Deep inspiration breath-hold (DIBH) CT scanning and treatment has also been applied to displace organs at risk. In the treatment of the left breast [8], DIBH external beam treatment can reduce the dose to the heart.

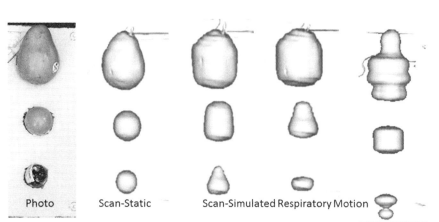

Figure 3.3 Left to right: Column 1 shows photographs of phantom objects. Column 2 shows surface rendering of scan with no motion. Columns 3 to 5 show scans during 1 cm amplitude sinusoidal S/I motion with varying phases.

Photo   Scan-Static   Scan-Simulated Respiratory Motion

4D CT Scanning

The goal of 4D CT scanning is to capture the shape and trajectory of moving organs during respiration. The term 4D CT is used interchangeably with respiratory correlated CT (RCCT), to mean scanning during respiration. Symantically, serial CT studies conducted over the course of therapy are also '4D.'

Proof of principle of 4D CT was demonstrated on single-slice scanners [9–11]. RCCT uses either a surrogate signal, such as the position of the abdominal surface, the volume of air measured by spirometry, or internal anatomy, to provide a signal needed to re-sort the approximately 1500 slices of reconstructed image data to coherent spatiotemporal CT data sets at specific instances of the respiratory phase. The scan times for a 4D CT scan with multidetector scanners are of the order of a few minutes, and this results in about 10 CT volumes, each with a temporal spacing of approximately one-tenth of the respiratory period (ca. 0.4 s). Details of the 4D CT acquisition methods are described elsewhere [12]. The dose administered during a 4D CT scan is approximately fivefold that of a conventional treatment planning scan, but this may be reduced by altering the radiographic technique without any significant reduction of motion information or image quality [13].

4D CT provides an imaging technique that quantifies and characterizes tumor and normal tissue shape and motion as a function of time. This enables radiation planning to design an aperture that adequately covers the target (assuming respiration during treatment is reproducible to that during CT simulation). The 4D CT data can also be used to decide if a motion mitigation strategy is needed (e.g., gating).

Images of a moving ball from a helical scan, as well as a 4D scan, are shown in Figure 3.4. The amplitude of sinusoidal motion is 1 cm in the S/I direction, simulating

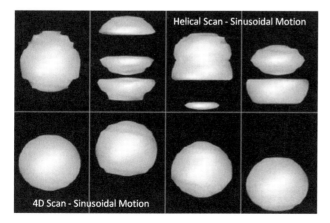

Figure 3.4 Upper row: Sphere imaged during sinusoidal motion scanned helically. Lower row: 4D scan showing the trajectory of the sphere.

breathing motion. The helical scan shows severe artifacts, while the 4D scan shows the ball's trajectory.

Limitations of 4D CT

While 4D CT allows for the visualization of anatomical displacement and deformation as the result of respiratory motion, 4D acquisition can still have residual artifacts. Phase-based 4D CT reconstruction, which is the predominant method used in commercially available 4D CT systems, models the patient's respiration as cyclical, assigning a physiological phase ($0-2\pi$) to fixed points (inhale $\rightarrow$ exhale $\rightarrow$ inhale) during a single period of the respiratory cycle. Images reconstructed at common phase points are used to form a single static CT reflecting a fixed phase point in the patient's respiratory cycle. Amplitude variations during different breathing cycles of a 4D scan result in residual geometric errors. Implicit in applying and utilizing 4D CT for treatment planning is the assumption that the patient will breath as he/she breathes during CT simulation. Serial 4D CT (acquired on different days) could be used to justify this assumption.

A 4D scan is suitable for assessing organ motion at the ~1 s time scale, but does not have adequate temporal resolution to study motion associated with the heart. Ultrafast scanners, initially designed for cardiac imaging, have been used to study the motion of structures in the radiation field near the heart [14]. Gated cardiac scans now provide insight into cardiac motion, but are typically acquired during breath-hold, which reduces its usefulness for therapy planning.

Magnetic Resonance Imaging

Magnetic resonance imaging provides information complementary to CT for target delineation, particularly for treatment sites involving the central nervous system (CNS). A few radiation oncology departments have installed MRI scanners dedicated to radiotherapy imaging. MRI is used generally used in conjunction with CT scans.

The primary advantage of MRI imaging over CT imaging is superior soft-tissue discrimination. In general, MRI is more sensitive than CT in detecting soft-tissue abnormalities. One area where MRI was used early on was for brain tumors, where the CT image is degraded by beam-hardening artifacts. Radiation oncologists frequently contour targets or suspected brain targets on both CT and MRI and combine them [15, 16]. In the abdomen and pelvis, multiplanar imaging and improved contrast enable a more accurate delineation of the extent of the malignancy. Limitations of MRI in treatment planning include susceptibility to geometric distortions (from magnetic field inhomogeneities) and the lack of electron density information in scans. These limitations are mitigated by combining CT and MRI.

In parallel with the use of MRI in external beam treatment planning, it has also been explored in brachytherapy. Its superior soft-tissue visualization provides insight into tumor localization and normal structures in adaptive conformal brachytherapy of gynecological cancers, such as cervix cancer. Over the past decade, guidelines have been published standardizing imaging techniques, terminology, and dose specification [17, 18]. Today, both MRI and CT routinely provide images used in image-guided brachytherapy.

Functional MRI

Functional MRI (fMRI) reveals physiologic and neurologic activity in contrast to structural information [19]. fMRI techniques can detect changes in blood flow associated with activation of specific regions of the brain (BOLD technique). When a task is performed (e.g., tapping a finger), oxygen demands in the region of the motor cortex increase, resulting in a net increase in oxyhemoglobin due to overcompensation. Increased blood flow results in perturbations in the MRI signal which can be superimposed on an anatomical MRI image. The geometric localization of functional regions could in principle be useful in avoiding such areas in treatment planning. Functional imaging of the brain is feasible at magnetic field strengths of clinically available scanners (1.5 T) and is capable of mapping the human visual system during visual stimulation [20], language processing areas, and sensory and motor cortex [21].

MR Spectroscopy (MRS)

The dominant MR signals result from ^{1}H nuclei of water, which is abundant in the body. Because of its abundance, the hydrogen signal tends to overpower signals from other nuclei. Suppression of water signals permits the measurement and analysis of other compounds. MRS was initially limited to small regions of interest but has evolved to imaging multiple voxels. Water-suppressed ^{1}H spectroscopy techniques are commercially available. For each voxel, the MR spectrum reveals the chemical composition. Differences in metabolite concentrations – either observed by peak heights, peak ratios of different peaks, or the integral of the spectrum – can be used to characterize the tissue. Applications of MRS imaging in radiation therapy include the characterization of prostate tumors [22].

Diffusion-Weighted Imaging (DWI) of the Brain

Specialized imaging techniques such as DWI-MRI provide data on the anisotropic flow of water along white matter tracts of the brain. These data have potential use in estimating clinical target volumes in treatment of high-grade gliomas [23], but the procedure is still under investigation and is not the standard of care.

MR Dynamic Studies

Specialized imaging sequences can provide information on organ motion. An advantage of MRI over CT is that no ionizing dose is present in this imaging modality. Cine MRI can be used to study organ motion [24, 25]. When acquired every few seconds over ~30 minutes, physiologic motion in the bowel, and bladder filling can be visualized and quantified, providing organ motion data over a time period comparable to a therapeutic treatment. Development of a MRI image guided treatment system is being researched. Various approaches to hardware for MRI guided treatment machines have been reported, with the anticipation that clinical studies with these devices will be forthcoming [26, 27]

Emission Tomography

Biological imaging provides information on the biochemical activity of tumors. Positron emission tomography (PET)-based imaging of tumor hypoxia, degree of cell proliferation, angiogenesis, apoptosis and response to therapy are under investigation. Nuclear imaging by emission tomography is of increasing importance in oncologic imaging, and therefore of use to radiation oncology.

Tomographic imaging based on the detection of γ-rays emitted from administered radionuclides includes single-photon emission computed tomography (SPECT) and PET. Coincidence detection technology to identify back-to-back photon events during positron annihilation was developed at MIT/MGH [28]. This technology was then applied to generate projections resulting in the generation of the first PET (tomographic) images by the Washington University group [29]. The positron radionuclides administered are conjugated with biomolecules chosen to bind to selected tissue, producing images that measure biochemical distribution. In SPECT imaging, γ-emitting isotopes are used, while for PET positron emitters are chosen. Positrons annihilate nearby electrons with emission of opposed γ-rays. PET and SPECT scanners use scintillation detector rings to capture the gamma ray geometry. Volumetric data sets are acquired at several couch positions, requiring about 20 min at each position.

Since the anatomical information from CT and MRI is complementary to the biochemical/biological information from emission tomography, it is logical to combine the information from these modalities. The PET CT scanner is a union of a conventional multislice CT scanner with a PET scanner [30, 31]. By mechanical integration of these imaging devices, many image registration issues are resolved, although data acquisition times for the modalities are very different (CT <1 min; PET ~20 min). This significant difference can result in ambiguities in distributions that arise from different organ positions due to motion during scans.

Image Processing

Image processing (IP) is applied to the acquired image data sets to synthesize images that have specific functions in radiation treatment planning. Selected IP tasks include image registration, segmentation or contouring, generation of beam's-eye view images, and volume visualization. The objective of these image processing procedures is to distill the gigabytes of image data acquired to the most essential elements for accurate treatment and assessment.

Image Registration

The use of multiple modality imaging studies typically requires that the images be analyzed in a common coordinate system. For example, the extent of a tumor might be visible on MRI, but must be accurately mapped into the coordinate system of a CT image for treatment planning. The enabling technology for mapping information between different image data is known as image registration. Ideally, image registration defines a one-to-one mapping between the coordinates of a points in one space with a corresponding point in the second space. Image registration has additional uses in radiation planning, mapping organs from one respiratory phase to another, alignment of planning and treatment images, and combining dose distribution from serial studies.

Reviews of medical image registration have been published [32, 33]. Registration can be performed manually, semi-automatically, or fully automatically. Manual registration is common for routine clinical use, especially when performing rigid translational or rigid translational or rotational matching. The operator visually inspects and adjusts the match using interactive tools, such as a custom viewport where the operator can slide the images back and forth, or a landmark selection tool to define matching points. Semi-automatic tools allow for a limited degree of feedback from the user, such as a starting

guess or an incomplete set of matching points. Fully automatic methods generate a transformation matrix without operator feedback, but still requires inspection of the final alignment to validate its correctness.

Besides commercial software, there are a number of open source implementations of image registration algorithms. General-purpose registration software are included in the Insight Toolkit [http://www.itk.org], or 3D Slicer [http://slicer.org]. Other free software for registration include Plastimatch [34] or DIRART [35]

Deformable Image Registration (DIR)

Soft tissues can deform due to physiologic processes, or through patient positioning variations. Deformation may be large, for example in the increase in lung volume expansion during respiration. It is useful to find the geometric transformation that permits one-to-one mapping of tissue voxels in the presence of deformation [36]. This is done through the process of deformable image registration. At the current time, the validated accuracy of deformable image registration is approximately 2–3 mm, compared to the 'gold standard' of human identification of homologous points in a structure (e.g., bifurcation of a specific airway branch at multiple phases of a 4D lung scan).

Examples are provided here of the application of deformable registration relevant to radiation therapy planning. In Figure 3.5(a) the inhale volumetric CT was registered to the exhale scan using deformable image registration (DIR) (Plastimatch). This open-access software performs the deformable registration of the two data sets over the entire volume, and then applies the transformation to map all voxels from inhale to exhale. No segmentation of any structures is required for the deformable registration, and the computation takes a few minutes.

The result of the deformable registration is shown in Figure 3.5(b). Again, this is a composite image, mapping the (red) exhale data set with the transformed (green)

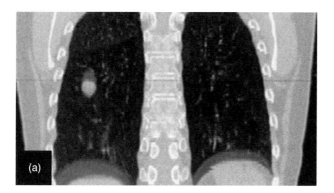 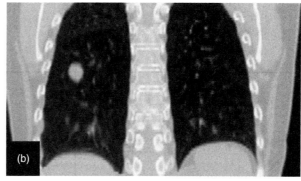

Figure 3.5 (a) Image at inhale and exhale showing different positions of the tumor and diaphragm. (b) After deformable image registration, the organs are aligned in 3D. Note after optimized DIR alignment, the vessels and airways show residual differences. For a color version of this figure, see the color plate section.

Table 3.1 Target and normal organ volume nomenclature.

Abbreviation	Description	Definition
GTV	Gross Tumor Volume	Visible tumor volume
CTV	Clinical Target Volume	Region of subclinical disease
ITV	Internal Target Volume	CTV plus motion margin
PTV	Planning Target Volume	ITV plus setup margin
PRV	Planning Organ at Risk	OAR with margin

inhale scan. With the exception of a few vessels/airways in the lower right lung, the registration is clinically useable. The estimated accuracy of the transformation is about 2–3 mm [37].

One application of DIR is *dose mapping.* Consider 10 phases of 4D CT; the patient is irradiated during respiration; the dose distribution can be calculated for each phase. To sum the dose over breathing, DIR would be used to map the individual dose distributions back to a reference phase. Dose–volume histograms (DVHs) computed on this summed distribution would then be more accurate in assessing normal tissue complication probability (NTCP). Pilot studies have shown that the mean dose to normal liver could be underestimated by ~1–2 Gy when a static 3D plan is compared to a 4D dose distribution.

Image Segmentation

After image acquisition, volumes of interest (target, organs at risk, and landmarks) must be identified and contoured. Contouring the target is a manual process, and the contouring of many normal organs and planning structures can be semi-automated (e.g., skin, spinal canal, bones). These semi-automatic methods generally depend on a high contrast boundary, and commonly use threshold edge detection algorithms.

Standard nomenclature is recommended to identify a variety of targets and organs at risk. The terminology and definitions associated with volumes of interest has evolved over time [38]. The terminology commonly used is defined in Table 3.1. Target volume delineation is subjective, and there are uncertainties introduced by inter-observer and modality specific [39, 40].

Another application of deformable registration is the propagation of contours of organs from one respiratory phase to another, an example of which is shown in Figure 3.6. In this case, the liver was segmented by the radiation oncologist on the T30 (mid-respiration). To study organ deformation and perform 4D dose calculations, it is necessary to contour the liver on all 10 phases. This is a tedious and inefficient task. Image registration may be used to propagate contours. During the process of deformable registration, the vector mapping of each voxel from one phase to all other phases is calculated.

This transformation is then be applied to the voxels that define the liver contour, to map the liver outline to other respiratory phases. There are small discrepancies (as seen in Figure 3.6), but most contours are acceptable. Editing can be done to correct the propagated contours as needed. A full set of 3D contours at each phase permits the calculation and quantitative assessment of organ trajectories [41].

Uncertainties in Target Delineation

Defining the extent of the target volume in an accurate, consistent, and efficient manner is clearly important. It must be recognized that these targets are drawn at an instant in time (on CT simulation scan). With positional uncertainties due to physiologic processes [42] (e.g., breathing, variable bladder filling), the location, size, and shape of the drawn structures may vary for a number of treatment sites.

Beam's-Eye View and Digitally Reconstructed Radiographs

Beam's-eye views (BEVs) [43] and digitally reconstructed radiographs (DRRs) are processed images that provide guidance on radiation portal design and placement for treatment. The two components, BEV and DRR are

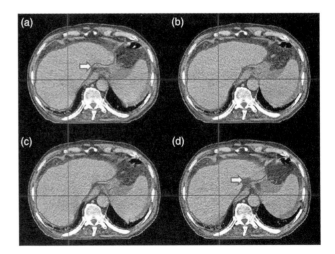

Figure 3.6 (a–d) Propagation of liver contour from manually contoured phase (panel b) to other phases. The arrows indicate imperfect registration at areas of high curvature. For a color version of this figure, see the color plate section.

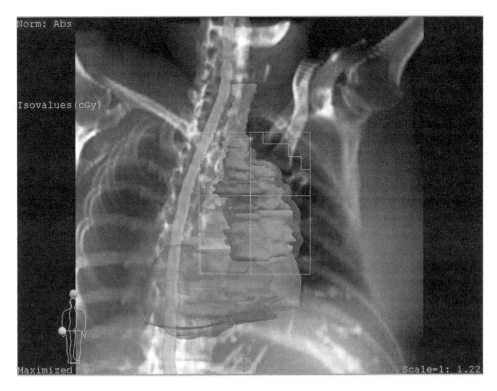

Figure 3.7 Beam's-eye view from a commercial treatment planning system. This right anterior oblique view shows separation of various CTVs of target (purple, red) and spinal cord (green). The lower heart is shown in gold. For a color version of this figure, see the color plate section.

complementary. The target and adjacent organs at risk are segmented on the volumetric CT scan, and represented as a ring stack of contours, extrema outlines, or as a surface. The DRR component generates a projection image principally of the bony and low-density anatomy (airways, lung) which provide an patient anatomical coordinate system. The DRR is generated by 3D ray tracing from the radiation source through the volume of CT data, projecting the final image onto a plane [43]. The DRR is the reference image against which the image guidance radiograph is compared to make final adjustments in patient position. The two components are typically fused into one image on the treatment planning workstation display. A planning BEV DRR oblique field for a lung tumor is shown in Figure 3.7

Since the viewpoint is from the radiation source, the BEV image accurately portrays the projection of the radiation field as it passes through both target and normal organs. The 3D target projected onto a 2D plane defines the aperture shape, and interactively varying the beam angle permits the choice of a portal entry to avoid or minimize the irradiation of critical structures while encompassing the target.

Volume Visualization

An alternative to ring-stack contour display of structures over DRRs is volume visualization, as initially described in computer science literature [44]. In volume rendering, the opacity and hue of a voxel of a 3D image data set is set by the operator to be a function of its CT number. Such displays provide an intuitive representation of anatomy not unlike a 'surgeon's eye view.' Volume-rendered displays have been used in treatment planning for radiotherapy, although to a somewhat limited extent. 3D volume-rendering laboratories are now commonly found in radiology departments, and are used in the simulation of operative procedures, often by neurosurgeons.

An advantage of volumetric visualization in radiotherapy planning is that this technique can display anatomic structures not normally segmented. Nerves, vessels, and lymph nodes are difficult to identify and laborious to segment on axial cuts. Yet, these structures may be seen directly in a volumetric rendering from a selected BEV. An example of volume rendering of a lung tumor is shown in Figure 3.8. Visualization of these structures may help in aperture design of the clinical target volume and anatomy to be excluded from radiation portals.

The challenge in volume visualization is that so much anatomy, including overlying tissues, is visualized, and some organs or structures are not relevant to the planning task. Methods to display only the relevant anatomy from a given beam perspective are yet to be developed. Interactive tools capable of selectively dissolving tissues obscuring the volume of interest must be incorporated into these techniques to reveal the interior volumes of interest.

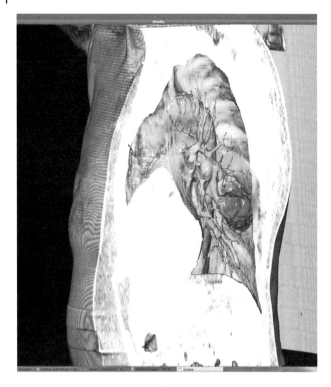

Figure 3.8 Volume rendering of a lung tumor. A cut plane is advanced from patient's left. The tumor, vessels and airways are visualized without image segmentation. The colors encode radiological pathlength variations from the skin surface to structures. For a color version of this figure, see the color plate section.

Dose Calculations

Dose (energy absorbed per unit mass) is a surrogate for biological effect. It is not possible to measure dose in the patient throughout the entire irradiated volume. Hence, reliance is placed on dose calculations to estimate doses to the target and normal tissues. Radiobiological considerations show that both dose and volume to a structure (target or OAR) influence the biological/therapeutic outcome (tumor control/normal tissue complication or damage). Thus, in dose calculations, a 3D assessment of dose to target and normal tissues is needed. The dose in each voxel irradiated is calculated, after which the dose to an organ is computed, summarizing the dosimetry in a cumulative dose–volume histogram [45]. Models have been devised to use the dose distribution to estimate the tumor control probability [46] and the normal tissue complication probability [47, 48]. Awaiting further validation, such estimates of probabilities are most often used to compare the relative merit of rival treatment plans.

Single-Field Dosimetry

Features of a single megavoltage field are depicted in Figure 3.9, which shows a 6 MV radiation field incident on a water phantom. The color wash represents a 2D dose distribution through the central axis; dose values are seen at the left margin. Several features of the dose distribution are worthy of comment. First, the dose at point P is the sum of two components: (i) the primary beam, which does not interact until reaching the point of interest; and (ii) scattered radiation, which is represented schematically as radiation that undergoes scatter at point S, and finds its way to point P. It should also be noted that there is a low dose component near the surface which appears unusually wide (arrow a). This superficial radiation region is due to electron contamination of the photon beam as well as scattered photons from the collimator.

The reduction in dose as a function of depth is due to two factors: (i) the radiation field is exponentially attenuated as it traverses matter; and (ii) the intensity of the radiation decreases as it diverges from the point source (inverse square law). Note the bowed shape of low isodose lines (~3–5%). This is attributed to an increased dose from scattered radiation initially, but the narrowing as a function of depth is due to less scatter as the beam is attenuated.

The central axis dose distribution is shown in Figure 3.9(b). As the photon beam enters the medium, interactions between photons and matter result in electrons set in motion in the beam direction. Dose in the buildup region (the first few millimeters) rapidly increases, as electronic equilibrium is established. The dose peaks at D_{max}, and as photons are removed from the beam, the dose falls exponentially. Higher-energy photon beams have a deeper D_{max}, resulting in more sparing of tissues between beam entrance and D_{max}.

Figure 3.9(c) shows a transverse dose profile at several depths (normalized at the central axis). The transverse radiation field is flat in the central portions of the field (created by field flatteners in the linac head), and the penumbra is relatively sharp. At deeper depths, the penumbra (the distance for the dose to fall from 80% to 20% of the central axis value) enlarges. Sharper penumbras spare organs at risk that are lateral to the beam edge.

Dose computation algorithms have evolved to calculate dose at a point. Simple algorithms compute the attenuation of photons and estimate the scattered radiation from tabular data. More sophisticated algorithms sum the contributions of multiple pencil beams [49]. Monte Carlo dose calculations apply the physics of the interactions of individual photons with matter. Several million photon histories can be statistically summed to estimate the resulting dose distribution. With faster treatment planning computers and parallel computation techniques, Monte Carlo dose calculations are becoming sufficiently fast to be considered for routine treatment planning. This approach is the most accurate method of estimating the dose in a patient.

Figure 3.9 (a) Single-field dosimetry schematically indicating dose at point P is sum of primary dose from radiation source, and secondary scattered dose from point S. (b) Depth dose along the central axis. (c) Transverse profile at different depths show that the penumbra increases with depth. For a color version of this figure, see the color plate section.

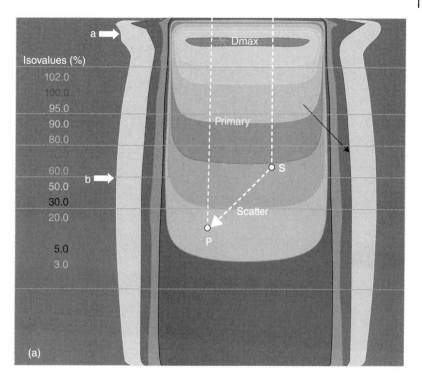

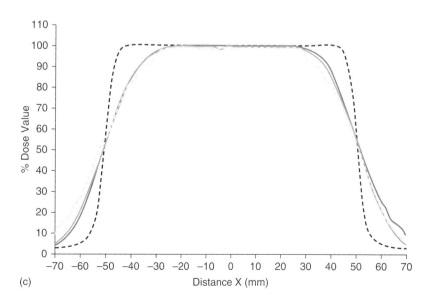

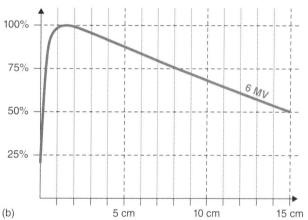

Multifield Plans-3D Conformal and IMRT Dose Distributions

In 3D conformal radiotherapy, the apertures are designed to geometrically conform to the target shape from each beam's viewpoint. A 3D CT scan is used to localize the target relative to adjacent critical structures. A beam fluence illuminates the apertures, producing a convex dose distribution. Beam's-eye view is generally used to geometrically exclude distal critical structures.

With intensity-modulated radiotherapy (IMRT), the radiation fluence over the aperture is modulated. Beamlets of varying intensity are applied often in a grid-like pattern. The specific intensity of a beamlets is determined through a process of inverse treatment planning (optimization). The mathematical optimization process uses input that describe the target geometry in 3D, the desired dose and dose uniformity within the target, and dose volume limits to adjacent organs at risk. Using multiple intensity-modulated beams from user-selected directions, the resulting summation dose distribution ideally irradiates the target and maximally spares the OARs. An important feature of IMRT is its ability to produce concave indentations in the resulting dose distribution. Such a capability can be useful in, for example, in the irradiation of a head and neck tumors, where IMRT can be used to spare the parotid glands and spinal cord. Images of the relative fluence in an IMRT portal for the irradiation of a prostate are shown in Figure 3.10

Several techniques can be used to deliver IMRT, and these depend on the specific beam delivery capabilities of the equipment. Descriptions of some of the most common IMRT delivery techniques are:

- Step-and-shoot IMRT [50]: In this approach, typically five to nine beam directions are used. At each beam angle, a computer-controlled multileaf collimator (MLC) is used to deliver an intensity-modulated segment of treatment. The leaves of the MLC are moved into position in the radiation beam is turned on. After the appropriate number of monitor units are delivered, the beam is turned off, the MLC leaves are set to the next position, and the irradiation is turned on again. In this process, the desired intensity-modulated radiation beam is built up from a series of static complements. Because the radiation is given in small segments, with much of the field blocked, a large number of monitor units are used. This prolongs the treatment session.

- Sliding Window IMRT [51]: Fixed gantry angles are again used, but rather than pausing the irradiation during MLC motion, the leaves move at specified velocities during 'beam on.'

- Volumetric Intensity Arc Therapy (VMAT/Rapid Arc) [52,53]: Volumetric-modulated arc therapy (VMAT) is another approach to IMRT delivery. VMAT involves controlled rotational arc therapy where the MLC leaves are computer-controlled during rotation to deliver an intensity-modulated arc. The dose rate, gantry speed and other parameters are computer-controlled during beam delivery. The superposition of multiple arcs can lead to highly conformal resultant dose distributions. Generally, this technique requires fewer MU for irradiation, resulting in faster treatment delivery times and improved treatment room utilization than step-and-shoot IMRT. Treatment times may be reduced by as much as a factor of 3.

Treatment Planning Case Examples

Three examples are provided to illustrate the features of imaging, image processing, dose computation, and interpretation.

Prostate

A patient with Stage 1 carcinoma of the prostate is treated with two courses of radiation to a total dose of 79 Gy. The first course includes irradiation of the prostate and seminal vesicles to 45 Gy in 1.8-Gy per fraction. Geometric margins of 1.0 cm are applied to encompass the target along the anterior and lateral axes. A 0.5-cm margin is used along the posterior GTV border to spare the anterior rectal wall. A conedown to the prostate gland itself, with a 0.5 cm isotropic margin was then delivered for an additional 34 Gy at 2 Gy per fraction.

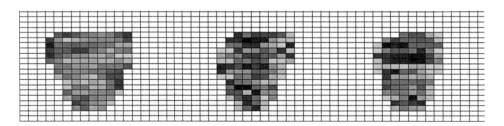

Figure 3.10 Multiple intensity modulated fields at different gantry angles ultimately yield an intensity-modulated composite distribution, which can have concave properties that spare critical structures. Darker pixels indicate greater radiation fluence.

Table 3.2 Prostate planning instructions.

Target prescription:
45 Gy to prostate + svs34 Gy to prostate boost
Dose constraints to OARs
Bladder v80 <15%, v75 <25%
Rectum v75 <15%, v70 <25%
Hips D_{max} <45 Gy

In addition to contouring the prostate and seminal vesicles, OARs are outlined, including the femoral heads, bladder, and rectum. An additional OAR volume often computed is 'non-target tissue,' which includes all tissues within the dose calculation matrix minus target volume(s).

IMRT planning includes upfront stipulation of dose–volume histogram constraints. Boundary conditions include that the hotspot be less than 115% and that there be no hotspot at or near the anterior rectal wall. The 95% isodose line ideally conforms to the PTV boundary. The specific constraints in this prostate plan were communicated as planning instructions shown in Table 3.2

The commercial planning system used in this example documents statistics of the dose distribution in Table 3.3. The output provides a summary of the statistics of the treatment plan, including the goal, what percentage of the structure is below the goal, statistics of the minimum, maximum and mean dose delivered to a structure, the dose standard deviation, and the structure volume. These statistics are viewed by the radiation oncologist to determine if the plan is satisfactory. If not, he/she may ask the treatment planner to tune the plan. By adjusting importance factors in plan input, and possibly adding avoidance structures (outlines of regions where hotspots must not occur), some flexibility is available in adjusting the plan.

Prostate Dose Distributions

The isodose distributions in orthogonal planes are shown in Figure 3.11(a). Normal structures are shown as solid color-coded regions, while the prostate is shown in red, the rectum in brown, and the femoral heads in light blue. The (yellow) bladder is not visible in the displayed axial plane, but is prominent in the coronal and sagittal cuts. Color-coded isodose lines indicate the dose levels in percentage of the maximum dose of ~86 Gy. The 90% isodose is seen to enclose the prostate gland, and is slightly indented along the posterior margin to spare the anterior rectal wall.

Cumulative DVHs are shown in Figure 3.11(b). Target DVHs are ideally step function-shaped. Ideally, 100% of the target is irradiated to the prescribed dose, and no part of the target receives greater than the prescribed dose. However, this rarely occurs. The high dose tail of a target DVH is due to the presence of hot spots within the target. These hotspots should be less than 115% of the prescribed dose. The soft shoulder below the prescribed dose of the target DVH also indicates that parts of the target are slightly underdosed. The underlying reason for the underdose is generally a dose constraint on an OAR that is very close to the high dose gradient. Information within DVHs may be reduced further to summarize dose distribution characteristics to a single number (e.g., conformity index [54]) or to estimate the probability of tumor control or of normal tissue complication (NTCP) [46].

Comparison of the DVHs with the planning goals show that the dose objectives were reached to the satisfaction of the radiation oncologist by the proposed plan. Specifically, dose to the femoral heads is less than the maximum allowed by planning instructions (32 Gy versus 45 Gy). The bladder and rectal DVHs of the plan satisfy the dose volume criteria stated in Table 3.2. The CTV target (CTV as well as CTV plus 0.5 cm margin) satisfy the goals within acceptable variations.

Table 3.3 Prostate dosimetry after planning to various targets and organs at risk.

Desired Target Dose:
Delivered Dose:
Deliver 79.00 Gy at 91.3% of maximum.
(minimum dose to Prostate - target (PTV), 74.45 Gy, is 86.0% of maximum
(maximum dose is 86.57 Gy at the 100.0% isodose line)

	Goal (Gy)	Below (%)	Goal (cc)	Min (Gy)	Max (Gy)	Mean (Gy)	S.D. (Gy)	Vol. (cc)
Prostate - target				78.34	86.13	82.39	1.29	43.18
Seminal Vesicles - target				64.06	85.70	80.41	3.76	7.91
	Limit (Gy)	Above (%)	Limit (cc)	Min (Gy)	Max (Gy)	Mean (Gy)	S.D. (Gy)	Vol. (cc)
Non-target Tissue				0.00	86.57	4.61	10.40	32651.22
Tissue				0.00	86.57	4.73	10.83	32702.31
Femoral Head RT				2.16	36.79	15.55	8.44	115.45
Femoral Head LT				2.16	36.36	15.03	8.68	123.20
Rectum				2.60	80.94	34.94	28.89	68.22
Sim Bladder Bat				3.03	85.27	26.00	26.23	155.15

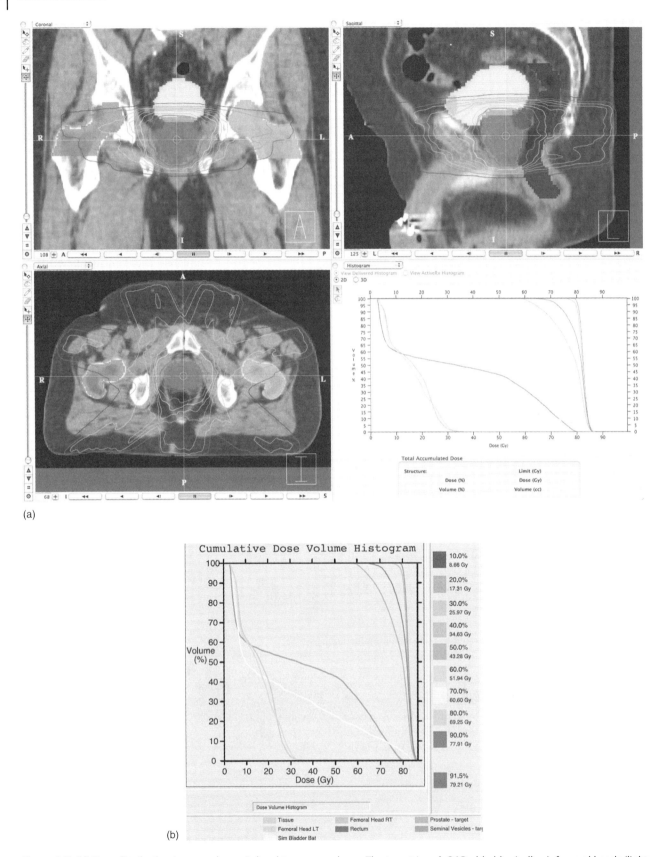

Figure 3.11 (a) Dose distribution in coronal, saggital and transverse planes. The target is red; OARs: bladder (yellow); femoral heads (light and dark blue). (b) Expanded view of the prostate plan cumulative DVH. For a color version of this figure, see the color plate section.

Table 3.4 List of segmented structures in a lung treatment plan.

Contour Information		
Contour description	Electron Density	Volume (cc)
patient	1.00	40378.46
Tumor	1.00(forced)	– – –
GTV 1		– – –
GTV 2		– – –
CTV 1		– – –
CTV 2		– – –
CTV 3		– – –
Atria	1.00	297.97
BoostPTV	1.00	267.67
BoostPTV+1	1.00	617.98
Carina	1.00	2.83
Esophagus	1.00	51.29
ITVp	1.00	11.24
ITVp Rescan	1.00	11.24
Left Lung	1.00	1196.25
Right Lung	1.00	1455.49
Spinal Cord	1.00	33.87
Spinal Cord+0.5	1.00	151.57
Ventricles	1.00	480.89
iTV-Nl	1.00	110.62
iTV-Nl Rescan	1.00	77.66
iTV-N2	1.00	56.83
iTV-N2 Rescan	1.00	55.86

Lung

The next example case involves the treatment of a Stage 3a small-cell lung cancer in a 57-year-old woman. Lung cases are dosimetrically more complex because of the presence of a significant density inhomogeneity (lung density 0.3 g ml^{-1}) and the consideration of tumor motion. This example has the added complexity of a planned re-scan to define conedown targets. The use of an IMRT technique also requires extended MLC leaf travel; mechanical limits of leaf travel separately required that the fields are decomposed into two parts. While the plan may be complex, attention is focused on the core aspects of this lung treatment plan to illustrate key considerations in planning.

4D CT is used in treatment planning of moving tumors. The patient was immobilized in a personalized body cast, used for both CT scanning and treatment. The 4D CT scan generates 10 phases. Multiple structures were contoured, as listed in Table 3.4. The primary tumor was observed to move laterally by ~3 mm, superiorly to inferiorly by 6 mm and anteriorly-posteriorly by 3 mm. Appropriate margins were applied to account for motion (defining the ITVs).

There are several approaches to constructing the geometric envelop that encompasses the target during respiratory motion. In this case, a maximum intensity projection (MIP) is used to bound the primary target. A MIP of a lung tumor is computed by projecting all ten phases of the axial slice onto a blank CT matrix and assigning the maximum HU as the pixel value. Given the HU difference between tumor (~0 HU) and lung parynchema (~-700 HU), the resulting image is an outline of the voxels swept out by the moving tumor in the axial plane, forming the ITV. ITVs for various subtargets are segmented by the physician. These include an ITV that defines the primary tumor, and an ITV of nodal groups N1 and N2. DVHs for each of these separate targets are computed for the treatment plan.

Alternative approaches to maximum intensity projection definition of the ITV exist. One approach is to outline the target in all 10 phases (by deformable registration) and then form the union volume. Another approach is to visually observe the motion of the tumor in a movie loop, and artistically draw the contour that encloses the target motion, in arbitrary planes. Both approaches have been experimented with at the present authors' institution for research purposes.

The target volumes were re-assessed after 36 Gy by a second 4D CT scan, and targets were redefined. The PTV was reduced by more than 100 ml in the conedown. Target volume reduction is a clinical decision by the radiation oncologist. While a GTV can grossly shrink during treatment, there can still be questions about the extent of microscopic disease which cannot be seen by CT.

Multiple OARs were contoured and included the spinal cord (with an expansion of 5 mm), esophagus, heart-ventricles, heart-atria, right and left lungs (separately), and a union of the right and left lungs, or total lung. The structure labeled '5-7-6-8' in the DVHs is the Boolean union of right lung minus volumes of the ITVs of the primary and nodal volumes. Thus, it represents the normal lung tissue in the right lung. Volume '4+5-7-6-5' represents the normal right lung tissue and normal left lung tissue minus targets. Cumulative DVHs for structures of interest are shown in Figure 3.12 (b and c).

The dose calculation algorithm was superposition convolution. Inhomogeneity corrections were based on the HU pixel values from the CT scan. This algorithm sums the contribution of pencil beam kernels, providing a more accurate dose distribution. Constraints were provided to the inverse planning system, and are shown in Table 3.5. An IMRT treatment plan was designed and DVHs of volumes of interest were computed.

While the ITV target includes the effects of tumor motion, the dose calculation is fundamentally 3D; no explicit motion captured in the 4D CT is incorporated into the dose calculations. The dose calculation is performed in the average CT (a numerical average of all 10 phases). 4D treatment planning, the explicit calculation of dose at each temporal phase, and combined by

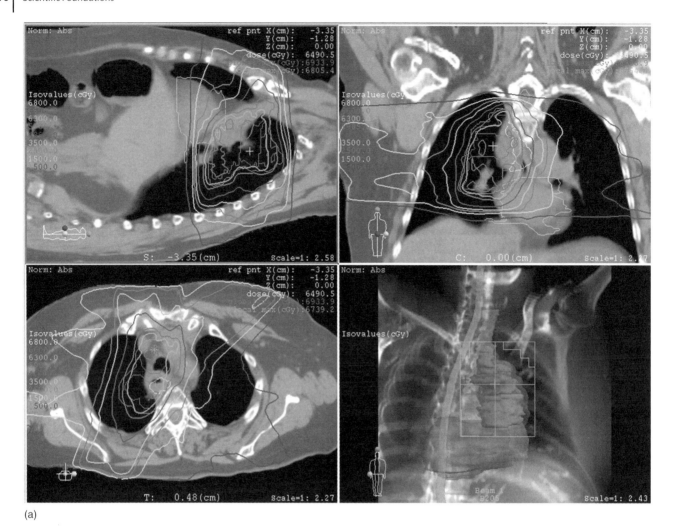

(a)

Figure 3.12 (a) Lung dose distributions in saggital, coronal and axial plane. A BEV view from the right anterior oblique field is also included. (b, c) Dose–volume histograms for lung example case (composite plan). The cumulative DVHs are color-coded to match the structure label in the legend (upper left-hand corner). For a color version of this figure, see the color plate section.

deformable image registration, is not routinely (commercially) available.

A composite treatment plan was then calculated by adding the dose distributions from the initial course and the conedown. This image-processing technique in principle provides a mapping of one CT scan to another, taking into account the deformation or shrinkage of organs. In this particular instance, the transformation was a simpler rigid translation, because the immobilization body cast used in scanning and treatment provided good relocalization of the patient. The desired and achieved dose to target, as determined from treatment planning, is shown in Table 3.6

A comparison of dosimetry goals and what the plan computed is shown in Table 3.6. Goals were generally achieved, the target was irradiated to 63 Gy, and the hotspot was less than 15% of the prescription. The dose

to the spinal column was less than the value not to be exceeded.

While this is a state-of-the-art assessment of the dose expected to be delivered by this plan, there are limitations to the accuracy of the computed DVHs. The actual patient geometry varies during respiration, but this is not explicitly taken into account. There may be organ deformations from day to day, and inaccuracies in set-up. While these geometric variations are largely mitigated by a body cradle, they are not totally eliminated. The difference between 4D CT planned dose distributions and approximate 3D calculations are currently being investigated. Margins provide some assurance that the target is irradiated as intended, but dose to normal tissue that moves in and out of the field during respiration is not as accurately calculated. Depending on the motion, modality (e.g., proton therapy) and other variables, the

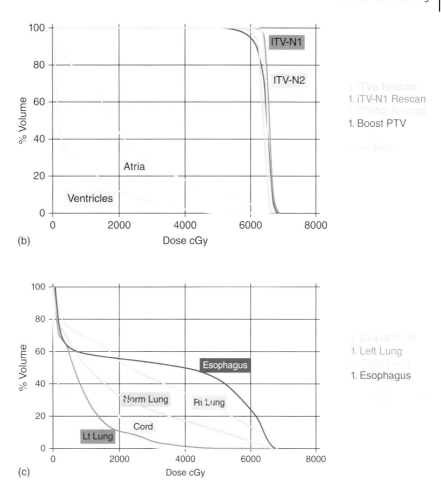

Figure 3.12 (*Continued*)

differences between normal tissue DVHs calculated in 3D and 4D could be substantial.

Head and Neck

The final example case involves the treatment of a head and neck tumor. The patient was scanned in helical mode with head immobilization (litecast). Multiple targets were defined, including a primary GTV and two CTV volumes, 1 and 2 respectively. Normal tissues segmented included brainstem, right and left parotid glands, spinal cord, oral cavity, mandible, larynx, skin contour, and esophageal constrictors. Segmenting structures can require several hours. PET and MRI may be used as additional aids in contouring. Dose volume limits were specified for some critical segmented structures for the inverse planning process (as in the prescription; see Table 3.7).

Using IMRT, distinct targets are irradiated simultaneously to different dose levels, which is a form of dose painting. The dose goal to the GTV is 70 Gy in 2.0-Gy fractions. The prescribed dose to CTV1 is 64 Gy, in 1.83 Gy/fx and CTV2 is to be irradiated to 60 Gy at 1.71 Gy/fx. The dose is to be delivered over 35 fractions.

The dose was delivered by a seven-field 6 MV IMRT plan. The linear accelerator has limitations in MLC carriage travel, and thus some beam portals are delivered in two parts. The CTV dose statistics are shown in Table 3.8

The isodose distribution is shown in Figure 3.13(a), where structures are shown in solid colors. The blue structure is the mandible, while the red and gold solid regions are CTV1 and CTV2 targets, respectively. The yellow structure is the primary target. Other structures are color-coded in the legend in the left panel. Isodose colors identify dose levels.

The DVHs for this case are shown in Figure 3.13(b). The plan was accepted and delivered.

Summary

Treatment planning continues to evolve as dose algorithm accuracy and interactivity improve. Increases in computer power should enable the generation of 4D dose distributions which, with deformable image registration, will provide a more accurate assessment of cumulative organ dose in the presence of respiratory motion and anatomic change (e.g., tumor shrinkage). Yet,

Table 3.5 Constraints in lung plan.

IMRT• PHYSICIAN'S INSTRUCTIONS
TARGET VOLUMES AND MARGINS:

GTV specifications	Sup/inf margins		Radial margins	
	CTV (mm)	PTV (mm)	CTV (mm)	PTV (mm)
ITV-p+N1+N2:63Gy/35Fx	5 mm	5 mm	5 mm	5 mm

Margins to be generated by Physics(all other margins already drawn by MD on workstation):
All CTVs and PTVs.
Special comments:
Please print carina on DRRs. Do not expand CTV and PTV into the heart or spinal column.
TREATMENT PLAN:
Total Dose - *please conform 95% isodose line to PTV,MD will pick isodose line (95-100%) for prescription*:
V-Sim date: 2012
Start date: 2012
Field and isocenter suggestions:
Cone-down: **Repeat CT-Sim needed?**
Yes. 4D CT at 36 Gy is planned   Yes.
DVH restraints (lungs, spinal cord, et cetera):
Lung DVH: V5<65%, V10<55%, V20<33%, V30<25%, V40<20%, V50<15%, V60<12%, V65<5%, V70 = 0%
Esophagus DVH: V20<50%, V30<40%, V40<30%, V50<20%, V60<10%, V65<0%, V70 = 0%
Ventricle-Heart DVH: V20<30%, V30<25%, V40<15%, V50<1%, V60 = 0%
Atrium-Heart DVH: V20<50%, V30<40%, V40<25%, V50<20%, V60<10%, V65 = 0%.
Spinal Cord: maximum dose <45 Gy

Tumor Motion (mm)	**X (mm)**	**Y (SI) (mm)**	**Z (mm)**
ITVp	3	6	3

Table 3.6 Comparison of goal and achieved dose to structures – lung.

Structure	Prescription	Constraint	Plan Dose	Plan Mean Dose	Comment
ITVp-rescan	63 Gy		67 Gy	63.9 Gy	
ITV-N1		Max dose 66.75 Gy	69.3 Gy	65.9 Gy	99% of volume receives 63 Gy
ITV-N2		Max dose 66.75 Gy	68 Gy	65.3 Gy	99% of volume receives 63 Gy
Atria		Max dose 63 Gy	68.6 Gy	22.5 Gy	3% of atria receive 63 Gy
Right Lung		Max dose 65 Gy	~65 Gy		Constraint satisfied
Total Lung		V20 <40%	~33%		Constraint satisfied
Spinal Cord		Max dose 42 Gy	32.6 Gy		Constraint satisfied

Table 3.7 Prescription for head and neck cancer case.

GTV (primary and LN) 70 Gy in 35 fx (2.0 Gy per fx)
CTV1 (high-risk) 64 Gy in 35 fx (1.82 Gy per fx)
CTV2 (low-risk) 60 Gy in 35 fx (1.71 Gy per fx)
PTV: add 0.5 cm to CTV1 and CTV2. No expansion of GTV
Avoidance:
Spinal cord (requires a 7 mm PTR expansion) <46 Gy and PTR <56 Gy.
Parotid glands mean dose 26 Gy or less (but not to compromise CTV1 coverage)
Larynx <50 Gy
Oral cavity <50 Gy
Brainstem <54 Gy
Mandible <70 Gy (but not to compromise CTV1 coverage)
Esophageal constrictors <54 Gy
PTV coverage: No more than 20% of PTV may receive >110% of prescribed dose.
No more than 3% of PTV may receive <95% of prescription dose. No more than 1 ml
of tissue outside the PTV may receive >110% of prescription dose.

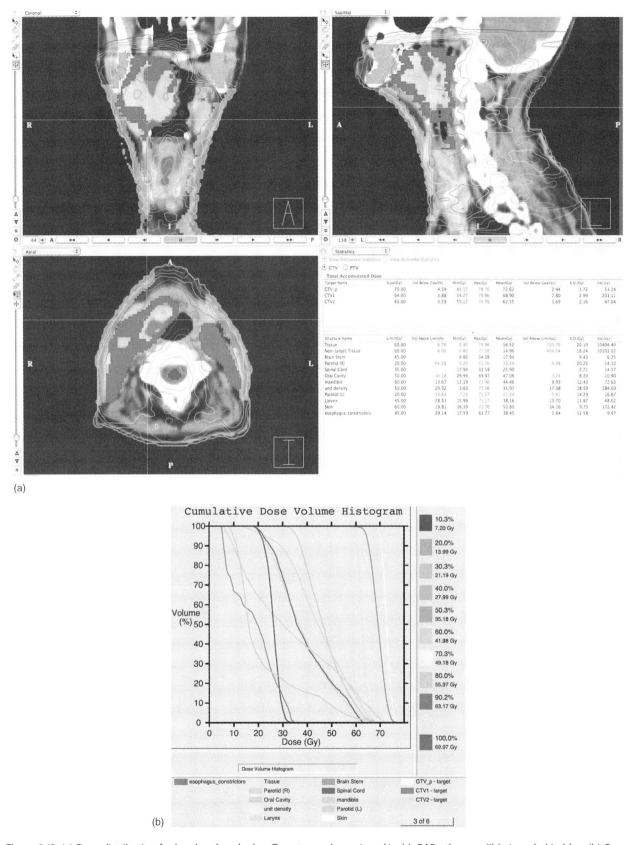

Figure 3.13 (a) Dose distribution for head and neck plan. Targets are shown in red/gold. OARs, the mandible is coded in blue. (b) Corresponding cumulative DVHs for targets and multiple OARs. For a color version of this figure, see the color plate section.

Table 3.8 Dose statistics for composite head and neck plan.

Desired Target Dose:

    Deliver 35 fractions over 35 days(inclusive)

        Goal dose to GTV_p - target   70.00 Gy, 2.00 Gy per fraction

        Goal dose to CTV1 - target   64.00 Gy, 1.83 Gy per fraction

        Goal dose to CTV2 - target   80.00 Gy, 1.71 Gy per fraction

Delivered Dose:

    Deliver 70.00 Gy at 87.5% of maximum, 2.00 Gy per fraction

    (minimum dose to GTV_p - target (PTV), 65.17 Gy, is 81.5% of maximum)

    (maximum dose is 79.96 Gy at the 114.2% isodose line)

	Goal (Gy)	Below (%)	Goal (cc)	Min (Gy)	Max (Gy)	Mean (Gy)	S.D. (Gy)	Vol. (cc)
GTV_p-target	70.00	4.59	2.44	*65.17*	**78.76**	72.62	1.72	53.24
CTV1- target	64.00	3.88	7.80	*54.77*	**79.96**	68.90	2.99	201.11
CTV2- target	60.00	3.59	1.69	*55.17*	**74.76**	62.55	2.16	47.04
	Limit (Gy)	Above (%)	Limit (CC)	Min (Gy)	Max (Gy)	Mean (Gy)	S.D. (Gy)	Vol. (cc)
Non-target Tissue	60.00	**4.00**	404.54	**0.40**	77.56	14.96	18.24	10103.02
Tissue	60.00	**6.76**	703.76	**0.40**	79.96	16.52	20.10	10404.40
Brain Stem	45.00	0.00	0.00	4.80	34.38	17.94	9.43	6.25
Parotid (R)	20.00	**64.38**	9.08	**5.20**	72.76	**33.59**	20.25	14.10
Spinal Cord	35.00	0.00	0.00	17.99	33.58	25.90	2.71	14.57
Oral Cavity	50.00	**34.28**	3.74	29.99	69.97	47.06	8.20	10.90
mandible	60.00	13.67	9.93	13.19	**71.96**	44.46	12.43	72.63
unit density	50.00	20.32	37.38	3.60	**77.56**	31.97	18.59	184.00
Parotid (L)	20.00	**33.64**	5.61	**7.20**	**71.17**	**22.24**	14.29	16.67
Larynx	45.00	28.53	13.70	15.99	**71.17**	38.16	11.87	48.02
Sldn	60.00	19.81	34.16	16.39	**72.76**	50.80	9.73	172.42
esophagus_constrictors	45.00	29.14	2.64	17.59	62.77	38.45	11.58	9.07

there are still additional challenges; advances in imaging may provide more specific information on tumor characteristics and geometric extent; advanced scientific visualization may be able to more efficiently and effectively present the gigabytes of information to the planning team. An improved understanding of the relationship between physical dose and the biological effect – specifically tumor control probability and normal tissue complication probability – will be valuable if capable of being personalized to the individual patient.

Acknowledgements

The authors wish to thank their clinical colleagues, radiation oncologists, medical physicists and dosimetrists in the preparation of this chapter. Particular thanks go to Drs Annie Chan, Noah Choi, and Anthony Zietman for the case example plans and Drs. John Wolfgang and Gregory Sharp for technical assistance on volume rendering and deformable image registration.

References

1 ICRP (1975) ICRP Publication 23: Report of the Task Group on Reference Man: Anatomical, Physiological and Metabolic Characteristics. *Ann. ICRP*, **4** (3–4).

2 Schneider, W., Bortfeld, T., Schlegel, W. (2000) Correlation between CT numbers and tissue parameters needed for Monte Carlo simulations of clinical dose distributions. *Phys. Med. Biol.*, **45** (2), 459–478.

3 Gould, R.G. (1991) CT overview and basics, in *Specifications, Acceptance Testing, and Quality Control of Diagnostic X-Ray Imaging Equipment* (eds J.A. Siebert, G.T. Barnes, and R.G. Gould), American

Association of Physicists in Medicine, Summer School. American Institute of Physics, Woodbury, NY, pp. 801–831.

4 Balter, J.M., Ten Haken, R.K., Lawrence, T.S., Lam, K.L., Robertson, J.M. (1996) Uncertainties in CT-based radiation therapy treatment planning associated with patient breathing. *Int. J. Radiat. Oncol. Biol. Phys.*, **36** (1), 167–174.

5 Balter, J.M., McGinn, C.J., Lawrence, T.S., Ten Haken, R.K. (1998) Improvement of CT-based treatment-planning models of abdominal targets using static exhale imaging. *Int. J. Radiat. Oncol. Biol. Phys.*, **41** (4), 939–943.

6 Chen, G.T., Kung, J.H., Beaudette, K.P. (2004) Artifacts in computed tomography scanning of moving objects. *Semin. Radiat. Oncol.*, **14** (1), 19–26.

7 Wong, J.W., Sharpe, M.B., Jaffray, D.A., Kini, V.R., *et al.* (1999) The use of active breathing control (ABC) to reduce margin for breathing motion. *Int. J. Radiat. Oncol. Biol. Phys.*, **44** (4), 911–919.

8 Rosenzweig, K.E., Hanley, J., Mah, D., Mageras, G., *et al.* (2000) The deep inspiration breath-hold technique in the treatment of inoperable non-small-cell lung cancer. *Int. J. Radiat. Oncol. Biol. Phys.*, **48** (1), 81–87.

9 Ford, E.C., Mageras, G.S., Yorke, E., Ling, C.C. (2003) Respiration-correlated spiral CT: a method of measuring respiratory-induced anatomic motion for radiation treatment planning. *Med. Phys.*, **30** (1), 88–97.

10 Low, D.A., Nystrom, M., Kalinin, E., Parikh, P., *et al.* (2003) A method for the reconstruction of four-dimensional synchronized CT scans acquired during free breathing. *Med. Phys.*, **30** (6), 1254–1263.

11 Keall, P.J., Starkschall, G., Shukla, H., Forster, K.M., *et al.* (2004) Acquiring 4D thoracic CT scans using a multislice helical method. *Phys. Med. Biol.*, **49** (10), 2053–2067.

12 Pan, T., Lee, T.Y., Rietzel, E., Chen, G.T. (2004) 4D-CT imaging of a volume influenced by respiratory motion on multi-slice CT. *Med. Phys.*, **31** (2), 333–340.

13 Wang, J., Li, T., Liang, Z., Xing, L. (2008) Dose reduction for kilovotage cone-beam computed tomography in radiation therapy. *Phys. Med. Biol.*, **53** (11), 2897–2909.

14 Ross, C.S., Hussy, D.H., Pennington, E.C. (1990) Analysis of movement in intrathoracic neoplasm using ultrafast computerized tomography. *Int. J. Radiat. Oncol. Biol. Phys.*, **18**, 671–677.

15 Nelson, S.J. (2003) Multivoxel magnetic resonance spectroscopy of brain tumors. *Mol. Cancer Ther.*, **2** (5), 497–507.

16 Thornton, A.F., Sandler, H.M., Ten Haken, R.K., *et al.* (1992) The clinical utility of MRI in 3-dimentional treatment planning of brain neoplasms. *Int. J. Radiat. Oncol. Biol. Phys.*, **24**, 767–775.

17 Small, W., Beriwal, S., Demanes, D.J., Dusenbery, K.E., *et al.* (2012) American Brachytherapy Society consensus guidelines for adjuvant vaginal cuff brachytherapy after hysterectomy. *Brachytherapy*, **11** (1), 58–67.

18 Nag, S., Cardenes, H., Chang, S., Das, I.J., *et al.* (2004) Proposed guidelines for image-based intracavitary brachytherapy for cervical carcinoma: report from Image-Guided Brachytherapy Working Group. *Int. J. Radiat. Oncol. Biol. Phys.*, **60** (4), 1160–1172.

19 Orrison, W.W., Lewine, J.D., Sanders, J.A, Hartshorne, M.F. (1995) *Functional Brain Imaging. Year Book.* Mosby, Chicago.

20 Nakajima, T., Fujita, M., Watanabe, H., *et al.* (1994) Functional mapping of the human visual system with near-infrared spectroscopy and BOLD functional MRI. *Society of Magnetic Resonance Medicine*, San Francisco.

21 Cao, Y., Towel, V., Levin, D., Balter, J. (1993) Functional mapping of human motor cortical activation with conventional MR imaging at 1.5 T. *J. Magn. Reson. Imag.*, **3**, 869–871.

22 Kurhanewicz, J., Thomas, A., Jajodia, P., Weiner, M.W., *et al.* (1991) 31P spectroscopy of the human prostate gland in vivo using a transrectal probe. *Magn. Reson. Med.*, **22** (2), 404–413.

23 Berberat, J., McNamara, J., Remonda, L., Bodis, S., Rogers, S. (2014) Diffusion tensor imaging for target volume definition in glioblastoma multiforme. *Strahlenther. Onkol.*, **190** (10), 939–943.

24 Ghilezan, M.J., Jaffray, D.A., Siewerdsen, J.H., van Herk, M., *et al.* (2005) Prostate gland motion assessed with cine-magnetic resonance imaging (cine-MRI). *Int. J. Radiat. Oncol. Biol. Phys.*, **62** (2), 406–417.

25 Feng, M., Balter, J.M., Normolle, D., Adusumilli, S., *et al.* (2009) Characterization of pancreatic tumor motion using cine MRI: surrogates for tumor position should be used with caution. *Int. J. Radiat. Oncol. Biol. Phys.*, **74** (3), 884–891.

26 Mutic, S., Dempsey, J.F. (2014) The ViewRay system: magnetic resonance-guided and controlled radiotherapy. *Semin. Radiat. Oncol.*, **24** (3), 196–199.

27 Lagendijk, J.J.W., Raaymakers, B.W., Raaijmakers, A.J.E., Overweg, J., *et al.* (2008) MRI/linac integration. *Radiother. Oncol.*, **86** (1), 25–29.

28 The Beginning of Positron Emission Tomography (PET) (1953) HistoryofInformation.com [Internet]. [cited 2015 Dec 15]. Available from: http://www.historyofinformation.com/expanded.php?id = 2043

29 Ter-Pogossian, M.M., Phelps, M.E., Hoffman, E.J., Mullani, N.A. (1975) A Positron-Emission Transaxial Tomograph for Nuclear Imaging (PETT). *Radiology*, **114** (1), 89–98.

30 Townsend, D.W. (2001) A combined PET/CT scanner: the choices. *J. Nucl. Med.*, **42** (3), 533–534.

31 Townsend, D. (2008) Combined positron emission tomography-computed tomography: the historical perspective. *Semin. Ultrasound CT MR*, **29** (4), 232–235.

32 Maurer, C.R., Fitzpatrick, J.M. (1993) A review of medical image registration, in *Interactive Image Guided Neurosurgery* (ed. R.J. Macinuas). AAN, Park Ridge, IL, pp. 17–44.

33 Pluim, J.P.W., Maintz, J.B.A., Viergever, M.A. (2003) Mutual information based registration of medical images: a survey. *IEEE Trans. Med. Imaging*, **22** (8), 968–1003.

34 Sharp, G. Plastimatch [Internet]. Available from: http://plastimatch.org.

35 Matlab. DIRART [Internet]. Available from: code.google.coom/p/DIRART.

36 Glocker, B., Sotiras, A., Komodakis, N., Paragios, N. (2011) Deformable medical image registration: setting the state of the art with discrete methods. *Annu. Rev. Biomed. Eng.*, **13**, 219–244.

37 Sharp, G.C., Peroni, M., Li, R., Shackleford, J., Kandasamy, N. (2010) Evaluation of plastimatch B-Spline registration on the EMPIRE10 data set, in *Medical Image Analysis for the Clinic: A Grand Challenge* (in conjunction with MICCAI'10) (MICCAI, Beijing, China), pp. 99–108. Available at http://empire10.isi.uu.nl/staticpdf/article_mgh.pdf.

38 Berthelsen, A.K., Dobbs, J., Kjellén, E., Landberg, T., *et al.* (2007) What's new in target volume definition for radiologists in ICRU Report 71? How can the ICRU volume definitions be integrated in clinical practice? *Cancer Imaging*, 7, 104–116.

39 Gao, Z., Wilkins, D., Eapen, L., Morash, C., Wassef, Y., Gerig, L. (2007) A study of prostate delineation referenced against a gold standard created from the visible human data. *Radiother. Oncol.*, **85** (2), 239–246.

40 Rasch, C., Barillot, I., Remeijer, P., Touw, A., van Herk, M., Lebesque, J.V. (1999) Definition of the prostate in CT and MRI: a multi-observer study. *Int. J. Radiat. Oncol. Biol. Phys.*, **43** (1), 57–66.

41 Hallman, J.L., Mori, S., Sharp, G.C., Lu, H.-M., Hong, T.S., Chen, G.T.Y. (2012) A four-dimensional computed tomography analysis of multiorgan abdominal motion. *Int. J. Radiat. Oncol. Biol. Phys.*, **83** (1), 435–441.

42 Langen, K.M., Jones, D.T. (2001) Organ motion and its management. *Int. J. Radiat. Oncol. Biol. Phys.*, **50** (1), 265–278.

43 Goitein, M., Abrams, M., Rowell, D., *et al.* (1983) Multidimensional treatment planning: 2. Beam's eye view, back projection, and projection through CT sections. *Int. J. Radiat. Oncol. Biol. Phys.*, **9**, 789–797.

44 Drebin, R., Carpenter, L., Hanrahan, P. (1988) Volume Rendering. *Comput. Graph.*, **22**, 65–74.

45 Lyman, J.T. (1985) Complication probability as assessed from dose-volume histograms. *Radiat. Res.*, **104** (2s), S13–S19.

46 Niemierko, A., Goitein, M. (1993) Implementation of a model for estimating tumor-control probability. *Radiother. Oncol.*, **29** (2), 140–147.

47 Kutcher, G.J., Burman, C. (1989) Calculation of complication probability factors for non-uniform normal tissue irradiation: the effective volume method. *Int. J. Radiat. Oncol. Biol. Phys.*, **16** (6), 1623–1630.

48 Marks, L.B., Yorke, E.D., Jackson, A., Ten Haken, R.K., *et al.* (2010) Use of normal tissue complication probability models in the clinic. *Int. J. Radiat. Oncol. Biol. Phys.*, **76** (3 Suppl.), S10–S19.

49 Ahnesjo, A., Aspradakis, M.M. (1999) Dose calculations for external photon beams in radiotherapy. *Phys. Med. Biol.*, **44** (11), R99–R155.

50 Bortfeld, T., Boyer, A.L., Schlegel, W., Kahler, D.L., Waldron, T.J. (1994) Realization and verification of three-dimensional conformal radiotherapy with modulated fields. *Int. J. Radiat. Oncol. Biol. Phys.*, **30** (4), 899–908.

51 Williams, P.C. (2003) IMRT: delivery techniques and quality assurance. *Br. J. Radiol.*, **76** (911), 766–776.

52 Yu, C.X. (1995) Intensity-modulated arc therapy with dynamic multileaf collimation: an alternative to tomotherapy. *Phys. Med. Biol.*, **40** (9), 1435–1449.

53 Otto, K. (2008) Volumetric modulated arc therapy: IMRT in a single gantry arc. *Med. Phys.*, **35** (1), 310–317.

54 Feuvret, L., Noël, G., Mazeron, J.-J., Bey, P. (2006) Conformity index: A review. *Int. J. Radiat. Oncol. Biol. Phys.*, **64** (2), 333–342.

4

Image-Guided Radiation Therapy

Monique Youl, Kristy K. Brock and Laura A. Dawson

Introduction

The primary goal of image-guided radiation therapy (IGRT) is to minimize the difference between the actual delivered dose and the dose that was originally planned to be delivered. Over the past decade, advances in IGRT have paralleled advances in radiation planning, and the combination of advanced technologies has resulted in the development of high-precision radiation therapy techniques allowing novel tumor sites to be treated to doses that would not have previously been possible [1]. The spectrum of imaging modalities available for IGRT ranges from two-dimensional imaging, such as electronic portal images, to three-dimensional volumetric imaging such as cone beam computed tomography (CBCT) and magnetic resonance (MR) imaging, and includes near-real and real-time tracking solutions [2–4].

Rationale and Benefits of IGRT

Traditionally, skin marks alone were used to align patients for radiation therapy. Skin marks or tattoos are marked on the patient during the planning session when the treatment region is defined. The skin marks are used at the start of each radiation session, in conjunction with room-mounted lasers, to reproduce the position of the patient at the planning session. The radiation treatment is then expected to be delivered to the original planned treatment volume. During radiation treatment, however, the internal anatomy – including the tumor – can change in position, shape and/or size, relative to adjacent anatomy, including skin and bones. Hence, skin marks are often poor surrogates for the internal tumor position. Whilst skin marks are still used to initially help set the patient up in the same position each day,

IGRT is now widely utilized as the primary tool to position patients, with increased accuracy compared to skin marks.

Internal changes of the planned treatment volume may be due to direct changes in the tumor itself or they can result from changes in neighboring normal tissues. They can be classified as either *inter-fractional*, occurring between fractions, or *intra-fractional*, occurring during the delivery of a specific radiotherapy fraction. At present, most clinical use of IGRT is predominantly geared to correct for inter-fractional changes, for example with imaging and repositioning immediately prior to each fraction. Intra-fractional changes, for example due to peristalsis or respiration, are often smaller in magnitude and have smaller dosimetric consequences than inter-fractional changes [5]. Non-IGRT techniques can also minimize the magnitude of some intra-fractional uncertainties. For example, breath-hold techniques (e.g., active breathing control), respiratory gating, abdominal compression and tumor tracking technology can reduce the amplitude of breathing motion, and an anti-gas preparation can minimize intra-fractional moving gas. In addition to causing organ motion, both breathing motion and moving gas can cause artifacts in images acquired for IGRT. Changes in the target volume position can be classified as a random or systematic uncertainty. As illustrated in Figure 4.1 [6], the systematic component of a set-up error is a positional deviation, relative to the planned position, that occurs in the same direction with each fraction during a course of radiation therapy. The random component, in comparison, can vary in its direction for any given fraction, but overall the mean offset compared to the planned position from random uncertainty is close to zero [7]. It is important to note that both random and systematic errors can result from the same source [6]. For example, both patient set-up errors and

Clinical Radiation Oncology: Indications, Techniques, and Results, Third Edition. Edited by William Small Jr.
© 2017 John Wiley & Sons, Inc. Published 2017 by John Wiley & Sons, Inc.

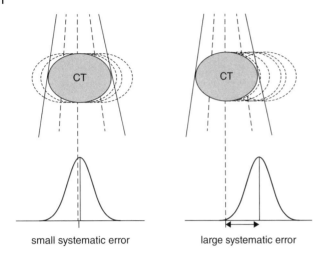

small systematic error   large systematic error

Figure 4.1 Systematic and random errors. The dotted line circles depict daily tumor positions. The frequency of the tumor positions are indicated by the distribution curves in the lower two panels. The dark gray circles indicate where the tumor was at the time of the planning CT. *Source:* Stroom and Heijmen 2002 [6]. Reproduced with permission of Elsevier.

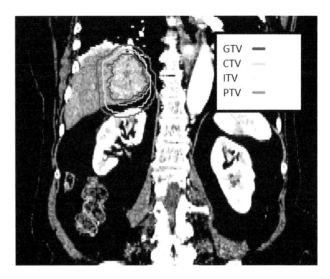

Figure 4.2 The gross tumor volume (GTV), clinical target volume (CTV) and internal target volume (ITV) to account for asymmetrical motion due to respiration (with the patient set-up in exhale breath-hold), and the planned target volume (PTV). For a color version of this figure, see the color plate section.

changes in the target position/shape can result in either a systematic or a random error. However, a target delineation error – that is, an error in defining the clinical target volume (CTV) on the planning CT – would only lead to a systematic error as the error will be present for all treatment fractions [5].

Systematic errors have a larger negative impact on radiation therapy delivery compared to random error, as they may lead to a shift in the dose distribution compared to what was planned, and can, in turn, cause a geometric miss in (part of) the target volume. By comparison, random errors tend to blur the dose distribution, with less effect on the minimum dose to the target volume. Of note, as a treatment course becomes more hypofractionated, random errors can have a larger negative impact.

Changes in tumor position need to be accounted for at the time of radiation therapy planning. The simplest method to account for such uncertainties is by irradiating a volume larger than the tumor itself, for example the planned target volume (PTV) (Figure 4.2). The PTV includes the gross tumor volume (GTV) which is the tumor visible on the planning imaging and sometimes on clinical examination, with a margin for microscopic spread (the CTV) and a margin to account for uncertainties in tumor position. This margin for uncertainty (specifically the PTV margin) takes into account a set-up margin and the internal margin [18, 19].

The *set-up margin* is designed to account for uncertainties in patient positioning and alignment of therapeutic beams during treatment planning and through all treatment sessions [18, 19]. It accounts for a range of uncertainties, including day-to-day changes in patient positioning during a course of radiation therapy, differences

between the set-up at the planning CT versus the linear accelerator, equipment uncertainties (e.g., sagging of the gantry), and dosimetric uncertainties.

The *internal margin* is defined as a margin to account for physiological variations in size, shape, and position of the CTV relative to anatomical reference points (Table 4.1) [18, 19]. For example, it helps to account for changes in tumor position due to changes in organ filling or respiration. The CTV plus the internal margin is designated the internal target volume (ITV) which, in addition to the set-up margin, is considered when defining the PTV. The PTV is a geometric concept designed to ensure that the prescribed dose will be delivered to the CTV, in the presence of expected uncertainties. A planning organ at risk (OAR) volume (PRV) is a normal organ with a margin to account for set-up uncertainty and physiological changes, and is analogous to the PTV margin for the tumor. At radiation therapy planning, the goal is that the PTV is covered by the prescription isodose, while the normal organ dose limits should be applied to the PRV around that normal tissue or OAR.

The ICRU Reports 62 and 83 [19, 20] caution that adding the internal margin and the set-up margin linearly can result in unacceptably large PTVs. Rather, it is recommended that sources of uncertainty be added quadratically [20]. Numerous 'margin recipes' have been published for this purpose. For example, van Herk *et al.* [21] proposed the following simplified PTV margin: $2.5\Sigma + 0.7\sigma$, where Σ is the standard deviation of the systematic uncertainties and σ is the standard deviations of random uncertainties. While the specifics of margin recipes are beyond the scope of this chapter, it should be

Table 4.1 Example of changes in the internal treatment volume.

Normal tissue-related	Examples
Organ volume changes	Prostate cancer Inter-fractional: bladder or bowel distension position variable Intra-fractional [8,9]: peristalsis of bowel
Weight loss or gain	Head and neck cancer Weight loss leading to loose-fitting immobilization mask and increased variability in position (inter- and intra-fractional)
Respiration	Lung, liver and upper abdominal tumors [9–13] Intra-fractional: with respiration, lung and liver tumors can move by up to 20 mm and 30 mm, respectively Inter-fractional: average position of organs relative to bones varies day-to-day

Tumor-related	Examples
Progression	Head and neck and lung cancers. Inter-fractional: tumor growth may lead to extension beyond the planned target volume and/or change in tumor position (e.g., due to tumor-related atelectasis)
Tumor response	Head and neck, cervix and lung cancers [14–17] Inter-fractional: ~70% reduction in tumor volume, during a course of radiation therapy, has been documented, which may lead to increased doses to normal tissues Changes in tumor volume may be asymmetrical and unpredictable (e.g., tumor growth followed by regression) [15]

noted that the previous equation reflects that systematic errors have a larger negative impact than random uncertainties, which is a characteristic of all margin recipes. Quantifying the uncertainties and applying such formulae may not be clinically possible in some situations, and in these cases the treatment team will determine a PTV margin utilizing their knowledge of possible uncertainties and their potential impact on the treatment and outcomes. More quantitative measurements of set-up error and motion can then occur based on the imaging obtained for IGRT in these patients, so that subsequent patients can have evidence-based PTVs.

IGRT improves the likelihood that radiation therapy is delivered to the target volumes as planned, through increased accuracy and precision of tumor localization. This improvement due to IGRT also allows for a reduction in the PTV margin. The reduced PTV further lowers normal tissue toxicity, which in turn provides the opportunity for safe dose escalation, which in some tumor sites (e.g., prostate, liver and lung cancer [22–27]) can even further improve local control and, potentially, survival.

IGRT has a role to play in ensuring the accurate delivery of radiotherapy in any clinical situation. However, in certain clinical situations, IGRT becomes crucial and often a necessity if treatment is to be delivered safely. IGRT becomes vital when tumors are directly adjacent to critical normal tissues, as an expansion of the PTV in this circumstance is undesirable and often impossible if tumoricidal doses are to be delivered safely. Highly conformal treatment techniques, including intensity-modulated radiotherapy (IMRT), are required in the

clinical circumstances where the tumor and critical normal tissues are intimately related; for example, a nasopharyngeal carcinoma is usually in close proximity to the brainstem and cranial nerves. Conformal plans with their inherent steep dose gradient outside the PTV are vulnerable to geographic misses, if systematic geometric uncertainties were to occur. That is, a small internal movement of the target volume could result in the delivery of a higher dose to the adjacent critical structures and under-dosage of the tumor. IGRT minimizes this risk. IGRT also facilitates hypofractionated courses of radiotherapy, including stereotactic body radiotherapy (SBRT), due to the confidence that the high dose per fraction is being delivered to the PTV and not inadvertently to surrounding normal tissues. SBRT plans are highly conformal, and additionally each fraction delivers a large dose (generally >6–10 Gy). Therefore, whilst with conventional radiotherapy any single daily error is small in the scheme of the whole course of treatment, with SBRT – where each fraction represents 20% or more of the total treatment dose – the error is magnified. Hypofractionation can improve resource utilization, leading to cost savings as well as enhancing patient convenience [28]. The higher biological dose delivered via SBRT has led to even further improvements in patient outcomes. An example of this is lung SBRT for Stage 1 non-small-cell lung cancer, where values of ~90% two-year local control and ~65% (up to 90% in some studies) two-year overall survival rates are superior to those achievable with a conventional fractionated course, and rival the results of surgical series [29–31].

SBRT can also provide new treatment opportunities for patients who were previously without feasible options. Examples of this include the use of SBRT to a spine metastasis to safely re-irradiate within the tolerance of the spinal cord, as well as SBRT for liver metastases or hepatocellular carcinoma that were not suitable for surgery and where conventional non-IGRT radiation therapy to a meaningful dose would have resulted in an unacceptable risk of radiation-induced liver damage. The potential for serious toxicity to occur with such examples of SBRT is far higher than with conventional fractionated radiation therapy. Thus, IGRT is crucial as it ensures there is less chance of a systematic geometric error and allows for a smaller PTV margin, a reduced volume or normal tissues irradiated, and less risk of toxicity.

In summary, IGRT allows for a lowered normal tissue toxicity, an improved local control (and potentially survival) and also facilitates dose escalation, hypofractionation and highly conformal radiation therapy treatments.

Process of IGRT

Image Registration

Once an image has been obtained at the treatment unit (i.e., the verification image), it must be registered to the corresponding image from the radiation therapy planning session and fused to it for visualization. Image registration is the mathematical description of the transformation that would align the images, whereas fusion is the visualization of the registered images (Figure 4.3). Since the primary structure for alignment (e.g., the tumor or a critical normal tissue) is not always directly visible on imaging, the clinician and treatment team must determine which anatomic structure set should be used as a surrogate for the tumor or critical normal tissue (e.g., vertebral body for spinal cord or whole liver for liver cancer) for image registration. Registration may occur in either two or three dimensions, and may be automated or manual. A bone match, for which there are many commercially available automated tools, is often the first step taken, and this can determine if there is a rotation in the overall patient position. Whether further adjustments are required depends on the modality of imaging used and the clinical scenario. For example, if the patient is being treated for a liver metastasis with SBRT then bony anatomy is a poor surrogate for the liver tumor. Baseline shifts in the liver tumor position relative to the bones often occur on a day-to-day basis. While the liver metastasis itself is not usually visible on CBCT, the liver may be used as a surrogate to further refine the registration and aid in positioning. A 'clip box,' which designates a region for the automated registration to focus, around a soft-tissue region of interest (ROI) may be used. In this example the ROI would be the liver, excluding the chest wall

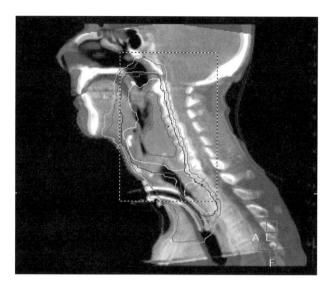

Figure 4.3 Overlay of planning CT scan and verification cone beam CT acquired during a course of radiation therapy for a posterior pharyngeal wall cancer. The gray color represents excellent alignment, whereas purple (reference CT) and green (CBCT) represents regions not well aligned due to deformation. Image registration was focused on the primary tumor and the cervical spine vertebral bodies adjacent to the tumor, as shown within a 'clipbox' (dotted line box). This region was registered to the planning CT dataset. For a color version of this figure, see the color plate section.

and spine. The anatomy within the clip box is then used to drive the registration to match the verification image acquired at the treatment unit to the liver from the planning CT image. As many tumors are often not well visualized, the insertion of radiopaque fiducial markers around the target volumes may be helpful. Manual adjustments to refine the registration may also be performed. These may be required because despite advanced automated registration algorithms, organ rotation and deformation may occur, in which case the match of anatomy near the tumor or critical normal tissue should be the priority. Visualization of the fused images is therefore always required for clinical interpretation.

Off-Line, On-Line, and Real-Time Corrections

Once imaging and image registration has been performed, the offset of the tumor position (or nearby surrogates) is calculated. That is, the position at the treatment unit, relative to the patient and tumor, is compared with its location on the planning CT and a decision is then made regarding how to act on this information. This process of determining a positional offset requires the IGRT technology to be calibrated relative to the isocenter of the linear accelerator (LINAC) (e.g., the relationship of the isocenter of a kilovoltage imaging system relative to the megavoltage(MV) treatment isocenter must be known).

An '*on-line*' *correction* is where the patient's position is corrected (e.g., via couch movements) prior to the delivery of that treatment fraction, based on the pretreatment image. An on-line shift is made when the error in the treatment volume position is greater than a predetermined tolerance. These tolerances will vary depending on the clinical situation, the institution, and the anatomic site. For example, if a tolerance for a palliative case is 5 mm, and the offset position is more than 5 mm, then the patient's position will be corrected. In contrast, a radical head and neck case being treated with IMRT may have a tolerance of 0 mm. That is, an on-line shift is always required unless the image registration results in a perfect match (<1 mm offset). Another predetermined tolerance should be defined to determine if and when a verification image should be performed after a patient has been repositioned. For example, if this tolerance is 10 mm, when the shift is greater than 10 mm a verification image will be performed prior to treatment. On-line corrections help to decrease both random and systematic errors. An '*off-line*' *correction* refers to obtaining images before each treatment without immediate intervention. The images are reviewed at regular intervals away from the treatment unit, while the patient is not on the treatment couch. The trend in offsets are evaluated, and if there is a systematic error beyond a specified tolerance level, a decision can be made to include a set adjustment of the treatment couch for all subsequent fractions to correct for this systematic error. For example, if a patient is consistently shown to be setting up 3.0 mm superior than desired, the radiation oncologist may direct the radiation therapists to set-up the patient 3.0 mm inferior to the previous set-up position for all remaining fractions. Off-line corrections help to decrease systematic errors. In practice, both on-line and off-line corrections may be made during the course of a patient's treatment. *Real-time imaging* is currently less widely used and refers to imaging that occurs whilst the radiation treatment is being delivered. Technological advances are still being made in this area, and current examples include real-time fluoroscopy and near-real-time imaging (where a 2-D x-ray image is acquired immediately before or between radiation delivery). While patient repositioning, via couch movements, is the most common intervention triggered as a result of IGRT, other possible outcomes include re-planning the treatment or stopping the treatment altogether (e.g., if the tumor spreads to regions not treatable with radiation therapy). Re-planning the treatment could occur for a variety of reasons. Tumor progression outside the PTV noticed on CBCTs acquired early during a course of therapy may trigger re-planning with a larger GTV, CTV, and PTV margin. Re-planning may also be performed if the tumor volume or its surrogates are noted to be less reproducible in position than expected, or normal tissue changes are predicted to increase the doses delivered exceeding OAR tolerance levels. In such situations, a new plan may be developed with more generous PTV margins or PRV margins. Tools that may help in visualizing changes in anatomy and organ deformation include overlying normal tissue contours and isodose lines from the planning CT to the daily treatment verification image (e.g., the CBCT). This can help to highlight whether sensitive normal tissues have moved, and where they currently lie in relation to a dose region. For example, the close proximity of small bowel or stomach to an inappropriately high isodose line may indicate that the OARs have moved towards the high-dose region. The use of isodose overlay can be complementary to anatomic information by highlighting changes in anatomy in regions where doses close to or beyond an OAR limit are expected. In the previous example of the stomach moving towards the high-dose region, the patient may be given instructions about bowel preparation prior to subsequent treatments (e.g., a gastrointestinal gas minimization regimen) with the goal of reducing the volume of the stomach and increasing the distance from the stomach and the target volume (Figure 4.4). However, it should be noted that isodose line overlay is only an approximation of how the dose will be delivered, as changes in organ position and deformation between planning and the treatment image will impact the true dose deposition.

Imaging Modalities Employed for IGRT

Two-Dimensional (2-D) Planar Imaging

Megavoltage (MV) 2-D Portal Imaging

This is 2-D radiographic imaging produced using the megavoltage treatment beam, and was one of the first uses of imaging for positioning the patient prior to radiotherapy delivery. Film was used initially, but this has now been widely replaced by electronic portal imaging (EPI). Most often, orthogonal (e.g., anterior-posterior (AP) and lateral) beams are used to position the patient. This relies on the stereoscopic principle that two planar images at different angles can identify the position of a 3-D object.

The disadvantages of MV imaging for IGRT include the extra radiation dose received by the patient, which is more than with kV imaging. MV images also have much less soft-tissue delineation than kilovoltage (kV) imaging due to Compton scattering, versus the photoelectric effect that is dominant with KV imaging. As soft-tissue densities are not usually identified, fiducial markers inserted into or around the target volume have been used in conjunction with MV imaging to allow 'soft-tissue' positioning, for example in for prostate cancer [32].

When fiducial markers are not in use, bony landmarks on the MV portal image are often used for alignment, with comparison to a digitally reconstructed radiograph

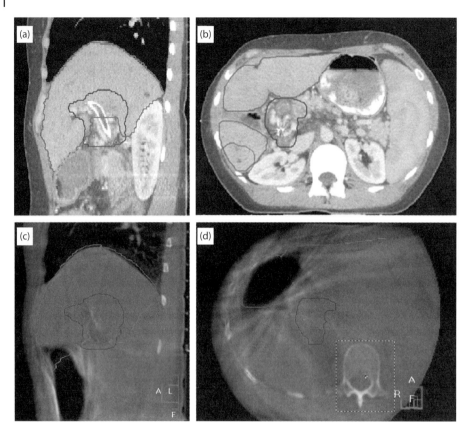

Figure 4.4 Stereotactic body radiotherapy, 33 Gy in six fractions, to treat a cholangiocarcinoma. (a,b) Images from the planning CT. The PTVs (primary tumor PTV = dark blue, liver metastasis PTV = light blue) and the liver (pink) are overlaid on the planning CT and the CBCT. (c,d) On day 1 of treatment, the CBCT showed an increase in gastric gas that resulted in deformation of the liver, as well as bringing the stomach in close proximity to the PTV of the primary tumor. Radiation was not delivered on this day and an anti-gas preparation was recommended for subsequent treatments. For a color version of this figure, see the color plate section.

(DRR) from the CT planning scan. In addition to orthogonal positioning imaging, actual beam's-eye view MV images can also be obtained during treatment delivery. These are less useful if there is no anatomy of contrast in the beam's-eye view, but if some anatomy can be visualized (e.g., the diaphragm for an upper-abdominal target) this can provide reassurance that the treatment is being delivered as planned. IMRT techniques, with their variable apertures and modulation of the treatment beam, makes verification of the treatment volume with the treatment beam itself practically not useful.

Kilovoltage (kV) 2-D Imaging

kV imaging systems are either attached to the LINAC gantry (which can also allow for 3-D Cone beam CT as the gantry rotates) or are room-mounted. kV imaging has the advantage of delivering a lower dose of radiation than MV imaging, and produces images with higher soft-tissue contrast. As the imaging is no longer performed with the treatment beam (as in MV imaging), commissioning and quality assurance (QA) must be performed to ensure that the kV imaging isocenter corresponds with the MV treatment isocenter. A potential disadvantage is that kV images are more sensitive to artifact from metallic implantations within the patient, such as hip prostheses or dental fillings. This can be important in certain clinical situations, for example,

treating a spinal tumor where there is orthopedic spinal stabilization apparatus *in-situ*. The metallic artifact occurs for both 2-D kV imaging and also 3-D KV imaging (e.g., Cone beam CT) and MV imaging results in superior soft-tissue imaging in these cases [33]. Similar to MV imaging, orthogonal kV x-rays can be utilized for positioning, when they are compared with DRRs prior to therapy. In addition, kV images may be obtained in near-real-time to facilitate intra-fraction positioning or tumor tracking. An example of how room-mounted orthogonal kV x-rays can be employed for IGRT includes the Cyberknife (Accuray, Sunnyvale, CA, USA). The Cyberknife (Figure 4.5) is a frameless robotic radiosurgery system that consists of a compact 6 MV LINAC attached to a robotic arm. Orthogonal x-rays are acquired to determine the 3-D position of a tumor surrogate (bony landmark or fiducial marker) immediately prior to each radiation beam being delivered [4]. The robotic arm moves the LINAC (rather than the patient being repositioned) to compensate for any misalignment of the target. However, patient repositioning with couch translations are used when larger corrections are necessary. The process of image acquisition, target localization and positional corrections may be repeated, approximately, every 30–60 s during treatment delivery, producing near-real-time tracking of the target. This highlights one advantage of 2-D kV imaging, in that it can be

Figure 4.5 Cyberknife. Image provided courtesy of Accuray, Sunnyvale, CA, USA.

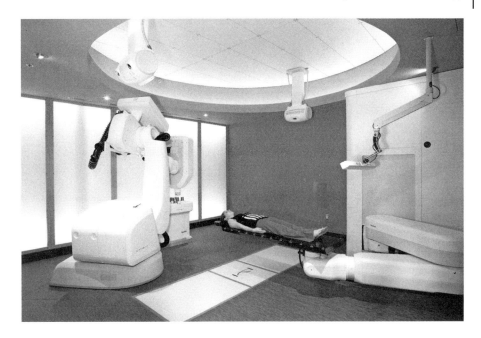

obtained almost instantaneously. By comparison, a 3-D CBCT generally takes 30–180 s for image acquisition and volumetric reconstruction.

Similar to the Cyberknife, the Novalis ExacTrac IGRT system (BrainLAB, Germany) also uses a pair of 2-D kV X-rays, but in this case a non-orthogonal pair is utilized. Two x-ray tubes are set in the floor of the treatment room and two x-ray silicon detectors are attached to the ceiling (Figure 4.6). The x-ray beam axes overlap with the LINAC's isocenter. Projections from the two x-ray tubes in oblique directions are automatically registered via bony anatomy or fiducials to a DRR taken from the

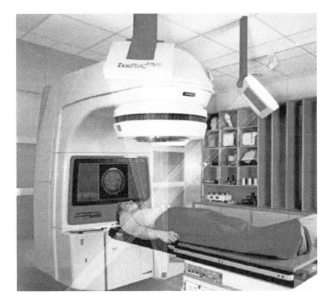

Figure 4.6 The ExacTrac IGRT system (Novalis, BrainLAB, Germany). *Source:* Jin 2008 [74]. Reproduced with permission of Elsevier.

planning CT. A positional offset and rotational error is then calculated. The robotics in the treatment couch, which includes an ability to correct for up to 3–4° of rotation, then repositions the patient in six directions using an infrared-based positioning system. The overall spatial accuracy has been noted to be in the range of 0.7 mm [34, 35]. This system allows for frameless central nervous system radiosurgery, and is also in use for prostate and lung cancer treatments with implanted fiducial markers. In addition to the 2-D kV X-rays used to position the patient, the ExacTrac also has a real-time infrared monitoring system. This consists of body markers, which are attached to the patient and an infrared camera which tracks the patient's position during treatment. Whilst the precise delivery of radiation therapy is achieved using technology as described above, one disadvantage of all planar imaging systems is that soft-tissue targets and normal tissues are usually not well visualized. Thus, if unexpected changes in normal tissues occur it is possible that higher doses than intended may be delivered to the normal tissue, even if fiducial markers are used for positioning.

Fluoroscopy

Fluoroscopy is another capability of some 2-D kV x-ray imaging systems. Imaging may be used to assess organ motion prior to (or during) treatment delivery. Fluoroscopy may be used alone but is also often used as a complementary technique to 2-D static or 3-D imaging. It allows for the quantification of motion due to respiration, reproducibility of breath-hold and potentially may be used for real-time imaging and tracking of the tumor via implanted fiducials. The Department of Radiation

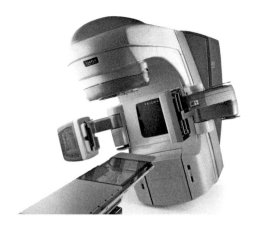

Figure 4.7 Varian cone beam CT. Image provided courtesy of Varian Medical Systems, Inc., Palo Alto, CA, USA.

Medicine in Sapporo, Japan, developed an elegant fluoroscopic real-time tumor tracking system (Mitsubishi Electronics Co. Ltd, Tokyo, Japan). Four sets of fluoroscopy systems are utilized so that there may always be two real-time fluoroscopic images that are not blocked by the LINAC gantry during therapy. Using two fluoroscopic images, the 3-D position of the implanted fiducial, in relation to the isocenter of the LINAC, is determined. A gating control unit results in the LINAC being triggered to irradiate only when the fiducial is within a set volume relative to the LINAC's isocenter [36–39].

Three-Dimensional (3-D) Volumetric CT Imaging

Cone Beam CT (CBCT)

When a kV imaging system is attached to the LINAC's gantry, a cone beam CT image can be obtained by a partial or full rotation of the gantry around the patient. A kV x-ray generator is typically mounted 90° from the treatment head with a flat-panel detector mounted orthogonal to it (Figures 4.7 and 4.8). A single rotation takes approximately 60 s or more, and obtains hundreds of 2-D KV images that are tomographically reconstructed to form a 3-D image. One disadvantage of CBCT is the longer acquisition and reconstruction time when compared with planar imaging. This can lead to the introduction of artifacts due to the anatomy moving during the acquisition (e.g., organs moving secondary to respiration or moving gas in the digestive tract). Metal implants (e.g., implanted fiducials, dental implants, or prosthetic hips) can also cause image artifacts. The advantages of CBCT are that soft-tissue anatomy can be directly visualized, so that deformations and changes in normal tissues and target volumes can be measured and accounted for. Soft-tissue imaging is a necessity for adaptive planning and dose re-calculation.

Breath-hold CBCT is available commercially for patients who are simulated and treated in breath-hold. Furthermore, there is the potential to obtain a respiratory sorted (or 4D) CBCT. Analogous to a 4DCT performed during treatment planning, 4D CBCT has the potential to allow for quantification of the amplitude of breathing motion, and more accurate patient positioning (since breathing motion introduces artifacts in 3-D CBCT). The respiration sorting for 4D CBCT is typically performed using internal anatomy (i.e., the diaphragm interface) compared to 4DCT, where external surrogates are typically used [40].

Some MV cone beam CT scanners are available commercially which use the treatment beam (6 MV) to produce a cone beam CT; an example is the Siemens

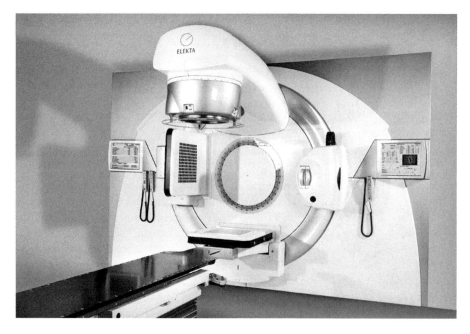

Figure 4.8 Elekta cone beam CT. Image provided courtesy of Elekta AB, Stockholm, Sweden.

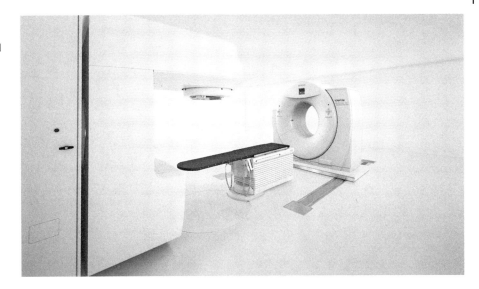

Figure 4.9 Siemens CTVision 'CT-on-Rails.' Image provided courtesy of Siemens Canada Limited on behalf of Siemens AG. All rights reserved 2012.

MVision Megavoltage Cone Beam (Siemens AG, Erlangen, Germany). Utilizing the treatment beam for IGRT has the advantage of there being only one isocenter. The potential disadvantages of MV cone beam CT imaging is the inferior soft-tissue contrast compared with kV cone beam CT for most anatomical sites, and a higher delivered dose to the patient compared with kV CBCT.

In-Room CT

This refers to a CT scanner being positioned within the treatment room allowing a diagnostic-quality CT scan to be performed prior to treatment. An example is the Siemens CTVision System, 'CT-on-Rails' (Siemens AG, Erlangen, Germany) (Figure 4.9), where theCT scanner slides on rails in the treatment room floor. The treatment couch is rotated towards the CT scanner, which is then moved towards the patient and the CT scan is acquired. The main advantage of in-room CT imaging is the superior soft-tissue contrast provided by a diagnostic-quality scan which, can be further enhanced by intravenous or oral contrast if desired. The CT image acquired can also be used directly for re-planning should this be required. It also allows for a direct CT-to-CT image registration. A potential disadvantage is that that the imaging is not performed in the exact treatment position, as the treatment couch must be rotated between the CT scanner and the linear accelerator.

Helical MV CT imaging

A TomoTherapy unit (Accuray, TomoTherapy, Madison, WI, USA) obtains a helical 6 MV CT scan prior to treatment, while the patient is in the treatment position (Figure 4.10). It has a 6 MV source and x-ray detector mounted on a ring gantry, similar to a diagnostic kV CT machine. The ring gantry continuously rotates as the treatment couch moves through its bore. The MV CT

scan is then registered to the planning kV CT scan. In this system, the imaging device and the treatment device are the same, ensuring exact correspondence of the imaging and treatment isocenters. A potential disadvantage is a reduction in the tissue contrast and increase in dose to the patient compared to kV CBCT images.

Transabdominal Ultrasound

Transabdominal ultrasound imaging has been successfully used as an IGRT modality in prostate cancer and upper gastrointestinal cancers [41–43]. The technique is inexpensive, relative to other image guidance equipment, does not expose the patient to any further radiation, and is portable. Potential disadvantages include inter-technician variability [44], the possibility of anatomical displacement of the tumor due to pressure from the ultrasound probe during imaging [45–47], and the interferences of bone and air cavities with the ultrasound signal [48].

In-Room Magnetic Resonance Imaging

In-room MRI is a new development in IGRT. An MR-guided cobalt machine is currently available (ViewRay, Oakwood Village, OH, USA), which integrates a 0.35 T MRI with a cobalt source treatment unit. MRI-guided LINACs are also being investigated commercially (e.g., Elekta plans to introduce MRI-guided radiation system in 2017), and in the research setting. In-room MRI is also being investigated (similar to the 'CT on Rails') where the MRI scanner is on rails adjacent to a standard linear accelerator [49, 50]. Potential advantages of in-room MRI are the superior soft-tissue contrast obtained from an MR compared to CT imaging modalities, the direct tumor visualization, which may aid in measuring tumor

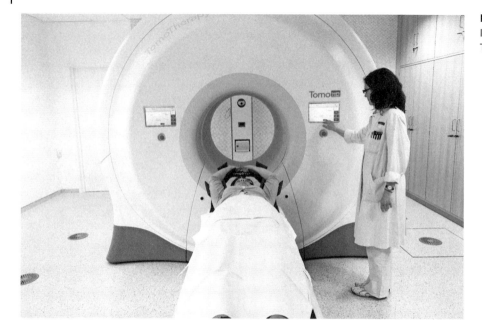

Figure 4.10 A TomoTherapy unit. Image provided courtesy of Accuray, TomoTherapy, Madison, WI, USA.

regression or progression during a course of therapy, and the possibility of measuring organ function using MR immediately pre- or post-radiotherapy. It also enables the possibility of near-real-time soft-tissue imaging during irradiation, and should detect changes in the tumor and other soft tissues during a course of radiation, making it an elegant platform upon which decisions can be made about re-planning (i.e., adaptive radiation therapy). Potential disadvantages include accounting for the influence of the magnetic field on the deposited dose [51].

Complementary Techniques and Non-Imaging Based Localization of the Tumor During Radiotherapy Delivery

Implantable Fiducials

Implantable fiducials are commonly used in combination with 2-D imaging (and less commonly 3-D imaging) to improve the localization of tumors. The most common fiducial in use is gold seed markers, which are inserted into the prostate prior to a course of external beam radiotherapy (EBRT) for prostate cancer. However, other radiographic implantable markers have also been used for lung [11,52], pancreatic [53], esophageal/gastric [54], and liver cancers [55]. Vascular clips from previous surgery in the region can also be exploited as a fiducial marker. With the fiducials in place, the patient can be imaged daily prior to treatment and the radiotherapy field matched to the location of the fiducials.

The disadvantage of this approach is that the insertion procedure is invasive and complications can occur, such as prostatitis with the gold seed markers for prostate cancer [56–60] and pneumothorax for lung fiducials [52]. The issue of fiducial migration has been raised, although it may be more likely in lung and liver cancers [3], as intraprostatic fiducials have been shown to be stable by multiple authors [61, 62]. The measurement of intermarker distance (when more than one fiducial is inserted) is a well-documented method for detecting fiducial migration, which may occur in a minority of patients [61]. In prostate cancer, the use of two or more fiducial markers is recommended as it is has been shown to be more accurate than a single fiducial, which may not represent the position of the entire prostate gland due to organ deformation. However a single fiducial has still been noted to result in more accurate and reproducible set-up compared to using bone alignment alone [63].

Electromagnetic System

The Calypso 4D Localization System (Varian, Calypso Medical Technologies, Seattle, WA, USA) have designed an implantable radiofrequency transponder which allows for real-time localization and continuous monitoring of the tumor position during treatment. The transponders, which are the size of a grain of rice, have been approved by the FDA for implantation within soft tissue throughout the body (with the exception of lung). To date, most experience has been in the treatment of prostate cancer.

This Calypso 'GPS body' transponder is inserted under ultrasound guidance into the patient's prostate prior to commencing a course of radiotherapy. An electromagnetic energy source positioned in the treatment room excites the implanted transponder to release radiofrequency waves, which are then detected by infrared cameras within the treatment room that are calibrated with the LINAC's isocenter. The ability to perform continuous tracking during the delivery of radiotherapy allows for the continuous evaluation of intra-fraction movement in addition to measuring and correcting for the inter-fraction movement at set-up [64,65].

Optical Tracking Equipment

A camera is used, with an inherent coordinate system (which is calibrated with the LINAC's isocenter) to detect light reflected or emitted from markers placed on the patient, or the surface of the patient. The wavelengths of these photons range in the electromagnetic spectrum from ultraviolet through to visible light and infrared light. Optical tracking may be used to facilitate the initial patient positioning, as well as to continuously monitor a patient during radiation therapy, so as to provide real-time feedback on the patient's position. This can allow the detection of intra-fractional movement and treatment gating when an optically tracked tool is placed on a region of interest, such as the chest for respiratory gating. The limitation of optical tracking equipment is that it uses an external surrogate, rather than the treatment volume itself, to determine positional offset. A clear advantage is that it does not require the patient to be exposed to any further radiation. It also has high spatial resolution; to within a fraction of a millimeter [66]. Current examples of optical tracking equipment includes real-time 3-D surface-image-guided beam set up for breast cancer treatment [67], and the ExacTrac system (Novalis, BrainLAB, Germany) which, as previously described, incorporates optical guidance with a dual x-ray system.

Potential Disadvantages and Limitations of IGRT

While the benefits of IGRT appear to be substantial, there are some disadvantages and limitations. One limitation is that while there are a number of different technologies available for IGRT, not one technology is ideal for all potential clinical scenarios [1]. There are also no prospective randomized trials investigating IGRT. With the apparent advantages of IGRT and its role as an advanced quality assurance tool, it has rapidly become the new standard of care, despite the lack of Phase III evidence. Given this, future randomized trials are unlikely to be performed as they would be unlikely to pass ethical standards to meet accrual goals [68]. A common concern regarding IGRT is that the increased dose received by patients from the various methods employed could lead to an increased risk of neo-carcinogenesis [69, 70]. The dose from kV imaging is lower than that from MV portal imaging [71]; however, all kV- or MV- based imaging techniques deposit dose, and the long-term impact of the cumulative low doses from imaging during a long course

of treatment may not be inconsequential (although estimated risks are very low). Discussions regarding extra dose from new treatment techniques with higher integral doses, such as IMRT, have highlighted this issue [72]. However, an alternative view is that IGRT allows for smaller PTV margins, which reduces the volume of tissue receiving an inappropriately high dose and should thus ultimately reduce second cancer risk. Regardless, the principle of ALARA (as low as reasonable achievable) should be applied in all cases of IGRT.

Other disadvantages are an increase in treatment time [68] due to IGRT that may lead to decreased patient convenience and impact on radiotherapy resources. The financial expense of these technical advancements is also a trade-off against the potential benefits. There is also a change in roles with the introduction of IGRT, with a higher burden on radiation therapists to interpret and make decisions based on the imaging. While this can be overcome with education and protocols to aid decisions, there is still the issue of the time required to implement these processes and deal with the outcomes, which could include re-planning. The clinicians and medical physicists also require further training on how to safely implement, interpret and maintain an IGRT program, given that at the time of their original training many of the IGRT processes now available did not exist. The introduction of IGRT has also heightened the need for inter-profession communication. For example, the clinician may need to be available to give guidance when images obtained prior to treatment are required to be analyzed without delay, as the patient is still on the treatment couch awaiting treatment. The extra time required at the treatment unit in addition to time spent training, writing and implementing protocols, and contouring normal structures on the planning CT (to aid with patient alignment) is an extra workload placed on the radiation team. Perhaps the largest potential pitfall of IGRT is not acknowledging and accounting for all uncertainties, both related and unrelated to positioning. This can lead to the use of inappropriately small PTV margins, which may in turn lead to tumor miss and under-dosage. An institution must have a good understanding of the precision of its own IGRT system before modifying PTV margins. Sources of uncertainties in the IGRT process that need to be considered include image-acquisition uncertainties, image-registration uncertainties, inter-observer variations, and uncertainties in making corrections [73]. Other important sources of uncertainty that need to be considered in the PTV margins include target contouring variability [28].

Image-acquisition uncertainties include imaging artifacts (e.g., moving gas) and low image resolution. IGRT imaging is not designed to be of diagnostic quality, but if the image quality is too poor to serve its role for detecting set-up errors then an uncertainty will be introduced. Image-registration uncertainties can stem from image-acquisition issues, in that the software may not be able to produce an accurate registration due to the poor image quality. Organ deformation and the rotation of internal organs, relative to the vertebral bodies, may also limit the ability of the registration process. When the registration process does not result in the best alignment of the treatment volume, manual adjustments are required, and this then introduces the possibility for inter-observer variations. The ability to accurately identify the treatment volume and align it with the planning image can be difficult for the treatment team due to many of the same factors, such as deformation, organ rotation, and poor image quality. If the treatment volume is not able to be identified, then surrogates are used, but this also introduces another source for uncertainty, as there is always the potential that the surrogate does not accurately represent the true treatment volume [73]. The movement of organs at risk in relation to the target poses yet another challenge for the treatment team, and may result in the best possible registration not being implemented due to concern about critical organs. Uncertainties in correcting positional offsets also exist. Treatment couches can correct for translational shifts, but specialized couches that correct for both translational and rotational shifts ('tilt and roll couches') are not yet widely available. The current specialized couches that do also correct for rotational shifts are limited regarding the maximal degree of correctable rotation [74,75]. In the absence of a rotational couch, a 'best fit' translation must be determined to best account for the translation and rotation using only translation. Limitations will be associated with this approximation, dependent on the degree of rotation.

Image acquisition, registration and analysis can take time to complete. Any couch shifts will only correct for the positional offset error that was determined at the time the image was acquired. It will not correct for any changes that may have taken place between image acquisition and the correction. A confirmatory image may help reduce this uncertainty and may be performed if a particularly long time has been spent analyzing the fusion image or if a large correction was made. Therefore, while one of the goals of IGRT is to minimize set-up errors, the uncertainty associated with a treatment delivery cannot be reduced to zero. The amount a PTV margin can be reduced is dependent on the ability of the IGRT system to reduce set-up errors, and also on other factors such as whether intra-fractional changes are being monitored and corrected for. In addition, treatment planning uncertainties also need to be considered when designing margins. For example, uncertainty in contouring may be the largest potential uncertainty in the process, and this needs to be considered in PTV margins [28].

Future Potentials of IGRT

Implementation of Dose Painting

This new notion aims to provide a heterogeneous delivery of radiation within the tumor volume. The aim would be to deliver a higher dose to a radioresistant region (e.g., a hypoxic region) that could be defined by functional imaging such as PET and functional MRI. Investigations have been conducted in this area regarding head and neck malignancies as well as prostate cancer. IMRT techniques are used in this situation to deliver a non-uniform dose distribution to the tumor volume. As previously described, a steep dose gradient makes a treatment vulnerable to geometrical miss, and therefore IGRT will be a necessity in the further development and clinical validation of such techniques.

Determining More Accurate Normal Tissue Complication Probabilities

IGRT use in clinical trials is expected to lead to improved uniformity of dose delivery, to both normal tissues and tumor, in a population of patients due to the improved accuracy of delivery. As this will lead to less heterogeneity in the doses delivered to tumors and normal tissues across the patient population studies, it is envisioned that this will help to determine the appropriate dose threshold between normal tissue complication probability (NTCP) and tumor control [28].

Adaptive IGRT

Various forms of adaptive radiotherapy exist. In general, this refers to changing the radiation treatment plan to account for changes in internal anatomy that may lead to a change in the intended dose to the tumor or normal tissues (e.g., tumor regression or normal tissues changes such as weight loss). One example of a type of clinical application of adaptive therapy is the TROG 10.01 BOLART study (closed to accrual, follow-up continuing) [76]. This feasibility study is assessing the use of three different treatment plans for radical chemoradiotherapy for bladder urothelial cancer. The choice of which treatment plan to use on any day is dependent on whether the bladder is assessed as being small, medium, or large (on cone beam CT) on the day of treatment. The implementation of adaptive IGRT can be on-line or off-line. In an on-line approach the plan or treatment is modified at the treatment unit, in real time (e.g., 'on the fly' treatment planning). In an off-line approach, the anatomical or functional changes are quantified and a new treatment plan is developed and implemented at a subsequent treatment fraction.

Adaptive IGRT has many potential uses, one being the situation of tumor response. As noted above, tumor shrinkage has been documented in head and neck, cervix and lung tumors [14–17]. While this is obviously the aim of the radiotherapy, it does lead to the potential for sensitive normal tissues to move into a high-dose region; for example, in head and neck tumors, parotid migration into the high-dose volume has been documented [15]. Situations such as this have sparked interest in adaptive radiotherapy, where the treatment plan can be modified to account for such changes, to potentially exploit or improve the therapeutic ratio by re-planning and adapting to change [77,78]. Caution should be used when clinically implementing adaptive therapy and reducing volumes irradiated, as macroscopic tumor shrinkage does not necessarily mean that the underlying microscopic tumor may be safely treated to lower doses. The present authors recommend that adaptive therapy, using a 'shrinking volume', should be investigated in clinical trials, due to the potential for under-dosing of microscopic tumor. Further research in this intriguing area is therefore required to ensure there is no detriment in local control rates. Technological advances are also required before adaptive radiotherapy can be used routinely in the clinic (e.g., in deformable image registration, dose recalculation and accumulation, and rapid planning and QA).

Conclusion

While IGRT has been present for more than a decade, it is now a rapidly expanding area of radiotherapy development. It has allowed an improved awareness of the magnitude of change that occurs in tumors and normal tissues during a course of radiotherapy. IGRT acts to minimize the difference between the planned dose and the actual delivered dose. It has the potential to lower normal tissue toxicity, improve local control (and potentially survival), and has paved the way for safe dose escalation, hypofractionation and highly conformal treatments. Finally, it has enabled the development of new treatments including frameless CNS radiosurgery and SBRT, and is essential to future clinical applications of adaptive radiotherapy and dose painting.

References

1 Dawson, L.A., Jaffray, D.A. (2007) Advances in Image-Guided Radiation Therapy. *Am. J. Clin. Oncol.*, **25**, 938–946.

2 Shirato, H., Shimizu, S., Kitamura, K., *et al.* (2007) Organ motion in image-guided radiotherapy: lessons from real-time tumor-tracking radiotherapy. *Int. J. Clin. Oncol.*, **12**, 8–16.

3 Shirato, H., Harada, T., Harabayashi, T., *et al.* (2003) Feasibility of insertion/implantation of 2.0-mm-diameter gold internal fiducial markers for precise setup and real-time tumor tracking in radiotherapy. *Int. J. Radiat. Oncol. Biol. Phys.*, **56**, 240–247.

4 Saw, C.B., Chen, H., Wagner, H. (2008) Implementation of fiducial-based image registration in the Cyberknife robotic system. *Med. Dosim.*, **33**, 156–160.

5 Van Herk, M. (2004) Errors and margins in radiotherapy. *Semin. Radiat. Oncol.*, **14**, 52–64.

6 Stroom, J.C., Heijmen, B.J. (2002) Geometrical uncertainties, radiotherapy planning margins, and the ICRU-62 report. *Radiat. Oncol.*, **64**, 75–83.

7 Li, C.P., Chao, Y., Chi, K.H., *et al.* (2003) Concurrent chemoradiotherapy treatment of locally advanced pancreatic cancer: gemcitabine versus 5-fluorouracil, a randomized controlled study. *Int. J. Radiat. Oncol. Biol. Phys.*, **57**, 98–104.

8 Ghilezan, M.J., Jaffray, D.A., Siewerdsen, J.H., *et al.* (2005) Prostate gland motion assessed with cine-magnetic resonance imaging (cine-MRI). *Int. J. Radiat. Oncol. Biol. Phys.*, **62**, 406–417.

9 Langen, K.M., Jones, D.T. (2001) Organ motion and its management. *Int. J. Radiat. Oncol. Biol. Phys.*, **50**, 265–278.

10 Shirato, H., Seppenwoolde, Y., Kitamura, K., *et al.* (2004) Intrafractional tumour motion: lung and liver. *Semin. Radiat. Oncol.*, **14** (1), 10–18.

11 Seppenwoolde, Y., Shirato, H., Kitamura, K., *et al.* (2002) Precise and real-time measurement of 3D tumor motion in lung due to breathing and heartbeat, measured during radiotherapy. *Int. J. Radiat. Oncol. Biol. Phys.*, **51**(3), 822–834.

12 Suramo, I., Paivansalo, M., Myllyla, V. (1984) Cranio-caudal movements of the liver, pancreas, and kidneys in respiration. *Acta Radiol. Diagn.*, **25** (2), 129–131.

13 Brock, K.K., Dawson, L.A. (2010) Adaptive management of liver cancer radiotherapy. *Semin. Radiat. Oncol.*, **20**, 107–115.

14 Hatano, K., Sekiya, Y., Araki, H., *et al.* (1999) Evaluation of the therapeutic effect of radiotherapy on cervical cancer using magnetic resonance imaging. *Int. J. Radiat. Oncol. Biol. Phys.*, **45**, 639–644.

15 Barker, J.L., Garden, A.S., Ang, K.K., *et al.* (2004) Quantification of volumetric and geometric changes occurring during fractionated radiotherapy for head-and-neck cancer using an integrated CT/linear

accelerator system. *Int. J. Radiat. Oncol. Biol. Phys.*, **59**, 960–970.

16 Britton, K.R., Starkschall, G., Tucker, S.L., *et al.* (2007) Assessment of gross tumor volume regression and motion changes during radiotherapy for non-small-cell lung cancer as measured in four-dimensional computed tomography. *Int. J. Radiat. Oncol. Biol. Phys.*, **68**, 1036–1046.

17 Van De Bunt, L., Van Der Heide, U.A., Ketelaars, M., *et al.* (2006) Conventional, Conformal, and Intensity-modulated radiation therapy treatment planning of external beam radiotherapy for cervical cancer: the impact of tumor regression. *Int. J. Radiat. Oncol. Biol. Phys.* **64**, 189–196.

18 ICRU R, 50 (1993) Prescribing, Recording and Reporting Photon Beam Therapy. International Commission on Radiation Units and Measurements, pp. 3–16.

19 ICRU R, 62 (1999) Prescribing, Recording and Reporting Photon Beam Therapy. International Commission on Radiation Units and Measurements, pp. 3–20.

20 ICRU R, 83 (2010) Prescribing, Recording, and Reporting Intensity-Modulated Photon-Beam Therapy (IMRT) - Definition of Volumes, vol. 10, pp. 41–53.

21 Van Herk, M., Remeijer, P., Rasch, C., *et al.* (2000) The probability of correct target dosage: Dose-population histograms for delivering treatment margins in radiotherapy. *Int. J. Radiat. Oncol. Biol. Phys.*, **47**, 1121–1135.

22 Perez, C.A., Stanley, K., Rubin, P., Kramer, S., *et al.* (1980) A prospective randomized study of various irradiation doses and fractionation schedules in the treatment of inoperable non-oat-cell carcinoma of the lung. Preliminary report by the radiation therapy oncology group. *Cancer*, **45**, 2744–2753.

23 Perez, C.A., Pajak, T.F., Rubin, P., Simpson, J.R., *et al.* (1987) Long-term observations of the patterns of failure in patients with unresectable non-oat cell carcinoma of the lung treated with definitive radiotherapy. Report by the Radiation Therapy Oncology Group. *Cancer*, **59**, 1874–1881.

24 Dearnaley, D.P., Sydes, M.R., Graham, J.D., *et al.* (2007) Escalated-dose versus standard-dose conformal radiotherapy in prostate cancer: first results from the MRC RT01 randomised controlled trial. *Lancet Oncol.*, **8**, 475–487.

25 Kuban, D.A., Tucker, S.L., Dong, L., *et al.* (2008) Long-term results of the M.D. Anderson randomized dose-escalation trial for prostate cancer. *Int. J. Radiat. Oncol. Biol. Phys.*, **70**, 67–74.

26 Peeters, S.T., Heemsbergen, W.D., Koper, P.C., *et al.* (2006) Dose-response in radiotherapy for localized prostate cancer: results of the Dutch multicenter randomized phase III trial comparing 68Gy of radiotherapy with 78Gy. *J. Clin. Oncol.*, **24**, 1990–1996.

27 Park, C.H., Seong, J., Han, K.H., *et al.* (2002) Dose-response relationship in local radiotherapy for hepatocellular carcinoma. *Int. J. Radiat. Oncol. Biol. Phys.*, **54**, 150–155.

28 Kim, J., Meyer, J.L., Dawson, L.A. (2011) IGRT and the new practice of radiotherapy. *Front. Radiat. Ther. Oncol.*, **43**, 196–216.

29 Timmerman, R., Papiez, L., McGarry, R., Likes, L., *et al.* (2003) Extracranial stereotactic radioablation: results of a phase I study in medically inoperable stage I non-small cell lung cancer. *Chest*, **124**, 1946–1955.

30 Onishi, H., Nagata, Y., Shirato, H., Gomi, K., *et al.* (2004) Stereotactic hypofractionated high-dose irradiation for stage I nonsmall cell lung carcinoma: clinical outcomes in 245 subjects in a Japanese multiinstitutional study. *Cancer*, **101**, 1623–1631.

31 Chi, A., Liao, Z., Nguyen, N.P. (2010) Systematic review of the patterns of failure following stereotactic body radiation therapy in early-stage non-small-cell lung cancer: clinical implications. *Radiother. Oncol.*, **94**, 1–11.

32 Langen, K.M., Zhang, Y., Andrews, R.D., *et al.* (2005) Initial experience with megavoltage (MV) CT guidance for daily prostate alignments. *Int. J. Radiat. Oncol. Biol. Phys.*, **62**, 1517–1524.

33 Tome, W.A., Jaradat, H.A., Nelson, I.A., *et al.* (2007) Helical tomotherapy: Image guidance and adaptive dose guidance. *Front. Radiat. Ther. Oncol.*, **40**, 162–178.

34 Takakura, T., Mizowaki, T., Nakata, M., *et al.* (2010) The geometric accuracy of frameless stereotactic radiosurgery using a 6D robotic couch system. *Phys. Med. Biol.*, **55**, 1–10.

35 Ackerly, T., Lancaster, C.M., Geso, M., *et al.* (2011) Clinical accuracy of ExacTrac intracranial frameless stereotactic system. *Med. Phys.*, **38**, 5040–5048.

36 Shirato, H., Shimizu, S., Kitamura, K., *et al.* (2000) Four-dimensional treatment planning and fluoroscopic real-time tumor tracking radiotherapy for moving tumor. *Int. J. Radiat. Oncol. Biol. Phys.*, **48**, 435–442.

37 Shimizu, S., Shirato, H., Kitamura, K., *et al.* (2000) Use of an implanted marker and real-time imaging for the positioning of prostate and bladder cancers. *Int. J. Radiat. Oncol. Biol. Phys.*, **48**, 1591–1597.

38 Shirato, H., Shimizu, S., Shimizu, T., *et al.* (1999) Real-time tumour-tracking radiotherapy. *Lancet*, **353**, 1331–1332.

39 Shirato, H., Shimizu, S., Kunieda, T., *et al.* (2000) Physical aspects of a real-time tumor tracking system for gated radiotherapy. *Int. J. Radiat. Oncol. Biol. Phys.*, **48**, 1187–1195.

40 Sonke, J.J., Zijp, L., Remeijer, P., *et al.* (2005) Respiratory correlated cone beam CT. *Med. Phys.*, **32**, 1176–1186.

41 Fuss, M., Salter, B.J., Cavanaugh, S.X., *et al.* (2004) Daily ultrasound-based image-guided targeting for radiotherapy of upper abdominal malignancies. *Int. J. Radiat. Oncol. Biol. Phys.*, **59**, 1245–1256.

42 Lattanzi, J., McNeeley, S., Pinover, W., *et al.* (1999) A comparison of daily CT localization to a daily ultrasound-based system in prostate cancer. *Int. J. Radiat. Oncol. Biol. Phys.*, **43**, 719–725.

43 Morr, J., DiPetrillo, T., Tsai, J.S., *et al.* (2002) Implementation and utility of a daily ultrasound-based localization system with intensity-modulated radiotherapy for prostate cancer. *Int. J. Radiat. Oncol. Biol. Phys.*, **53**, 1124–1129.

44 Langen, K.M., Pouliot, J., Anezinos, C., *et al.* (2003) Evaluation of ultrasound-based prostate localization for image-guided radiotherapy. *Int. J. Radiat. Oncol. Biol. Phys.*, **57**, 635–644.

45 Artignan, X., Smitsmans, M.H., Lebesque, J.V., *et al.* (2004) Online ultrasound image guidance for radiotherapy of prostate cancer: Impact of image acquisition on prostate displacement. *Int. J. Radiat. Oncol. Biol. Phys.*, **59**, 595–601.

46 Serago, C.F., Chungbin, S.J., Buskirk, S.J., *et al.* (2002) Initial experience with ultrasound localization for positioning prostate cancer patients for external beam radiotherapy. *Int. J. Radiat. Oncol. Biol. Phys.*, **53**, 1130–1138.

47 McGahan, J.P., Ryu, J., Fogata, M. (2004) Ultrasound probe pressure as a source of error in prostate localization for external beam radiotherapy. *Int. J. Radiat. Oncol. Biol. Phys.*, **60**, 788–793.

48 Dawson, L.A., Sharpe, M.B. (2006) Image-guided radiotherapy: rationale, benefits, and limitations. *Lancet Oncol.*, **7** (10), 848–858.

49 Crijns, S.P., Kok, J.G., Lagendijk, J.J., *et al.* (2011) Towards MRI-guided linear accelerator control: gating on an MRI accelerator. *Phys. Med. Biol.*, **56**, 4815–4825.

50 Kron, T., Eyles, D., Schreiner, J. (2006) Magnetic resonance imaging for adaptive cobalt tomotherapy: A proposal. *Med. Phys.*, **31**, 242–254.

51 Raaymakers, B.W., Raaijmakers, A.J., Kotte, A.N., *et al.* (2004) Integrating a MRI scanner with a 6MV radiotherapy accelerator: Dose deposition in a transverse magnetic field. *Phys. Med. Biol.*, **49**, 4109–4118.

52 Kupelian, P.A., Forbes, A., Willoughby, T.R., *et al.* (2007) Implantation and stability of metallic fiducials within pulmonary lesions. *Int. J. Radiat. Oncol. Biol. Phys.*, **69**, 777–785.

53 Park, W.G., Yan, B.M., Schellenberg, D., *et al.* (2010) EUS-guided gold fiducial insertion for image-guided radiation therapy of pancreatic cancer: 50 successful cases without fluoroscopy. *Gastrointest. Endosc.*, **71**, 513–518.

54 Chandran, S., Vaughan, R., Jacob, A., Hamilton, C., *et al.* (2016) A novel endoscopic marker for radiological localization and image-guided radiotherapy in esophageal and gastric cancers (with video). *Gastrointest. Endosc.*, **83** (2), 309–317.

55 Balter, J.M., Dawson, L.A., Kazanjian, S., McGinn, C., *et al.* (2001) Determination of ventilatory liver movement via radiographic evaluation of diaphragm position. *Int. J. Radiat. Oncol. Biol. Phys.*, **51** (1), 267–270.

56 Fonteyne, V., Ost, P., Villeirs, G., Oosterlinck, W., *et al.* (2012) Improving positioning in high-dose radiotherapy for prostate cancer: Safety and visibility of frequently used gold fiducial markers. *Int. J. Radiat. Oncol. Biol. Phys.*, **83** (1), 46–52.

57 Henry, A.M., Wilkinson, C., Wylie, J.P., *et al.* (2004) Trans-perineal implantation of radio-opaque treatment verification markers into the prostate: An assessment of procedure related morbidity, patient acceptability and accuracy. *Radiother. Oncol.*, **73**, 57–59.

58 Igdem, S., Akpinar, H., Alco, G., *et al.* (2009) Implantation of fiducial markers for image guidance in prostate radiotherapy: Patient-reported toxicity. *Br. J. Radiol.*, **82**, 941–945.

59 Langenhuijsen, J.F., Van Lin, E.N., Kiemeney, L.A., *et al.* (2007) Ultrasound-guided transrectal implantation of gold markers for prostate localization during external beam radiotherapy: complication rate and risk factors. *Int. J. Radiat. Oncol. Biol. Phys.*, **69**, 671–676.

60 Mosman, M.R., Van Der Heide, U.A., Kotte, A.N., *et al.* (2010) Long-term experience with transrectal and transperineal implantations of fiducial gold markers in the prostate for position verification in external beam radiotherapy; feasibility, toxicity and quality of life. *Radiother. Oncol.*, **96**, 38–42.

61 Kupelian, P.A., Willoughby, T.R., Meeks, S.L., *et al.* (2005) Intraprostatic fiducials for localization of the prostate gland: Monitoring inter-marker distances during radiation therapy to test for marker stability. *Int. J. Radiat. Oncol. Biol. Phys.*, **62**, 1291–1296.

62 Pouliot, J., Aubin, M., Langen, K.M., *et al.* (2003) (Non)-migration of radiopaque markers used for on-line localization of the prostate with an electronic portal imaging device. *Int. J. Radiat. Oncol. Biol. Phys.*, **56**, 862–866.

63 Kudchadker, R.J., Lee, A.K., Yu, Z.H., *et al.* (2009) Effectiveness of using fewer implanted fiducial markers for prostate target alignment. *Int. J. Radiat. Oncol. Biol. Phys.*, **74**, 1283–1289.

64 Willoughby, T.R., Kupelian, P.A., Pouliot, J., *et al.* (2006) Target localization and real-time tracking using the Calypso 4D localization system in patients with localized prostate cancer. *Int. J. Radiat. Oncol. Biol. Phys.*, **65**, 528–534.

65 Kupelian, P.A., Willoughby, T.R., Mahadevan, A., *et al.* (2007) Multi-institutional clinical experience with the Calypso system in localization and continuous, real-time monitoring of the prostate gland during external radiotherapy. *Int. J. Radiat. Oncol. Biol. Phys.*, **67**, 1088–1098.

66 Meeks, S.L., Tome, W.A., Willoughby, T.R., *et al.* (2005) Optically guided patient positioning techniques. *Semin. Radiat. Oncol.*, **15**, 192–201.

67 Djajaputra, D., Shidong, L. (2005) Real-time 3D surface-image-guided beam setup in radiotherapy of breast cancer. *Med. Phys.*, **32**, 65–75.

68 Bujold, A., Tim, C., Jaffray, D., *et al.* (2012) Image-guided radiotherapy: has it influenced patient outcomes? *Semin. Radiat. Oncol.*, **22**, 50–61.

69 Islam, M.K., Purdie, T.G., Norrlinger, B.D., *et al.* (2006) Patient dose from kilovoltage cone beam computed tomography imaging in radiation therapy. *Med. Phys.*, **33**, 1573–1582.

70 Ding, G.X., Coffey, C.W. (2009) Radiation dose from kilovoltage cone beam computed tomography in an image-guided radiotherapy procedure. *Int. J. Radiat. Oncol. Biol. Phys.*, **73**, 610–617.

71 Walter, C., Boda-Heggemann, J., Wertz, H., *et al.* (2007) Phantom and in-vivo measurements of dose exposure by image-guided radiotherapy (IGRT): MV portal images vs. kV portal images vs. cone-beam CT. *Radiat. Oncol.*, **85**, 418–423.

72 Hall, E.J. (2006) Intensity-modulated radiation therapy, protons, and the risk of second cancers. *Int. J. Radiat. Oncol. Biol. Phys.*, **65**, 1–7.

73 Palta, J.R., Mackie, T.R. (eds) (2011) *Uncertainties in External Beam Radiation Therapy. AAPM Medical Physics.* Monograph No.35. Proceedings of the 2011 AAPM Summer School. Medical Physics Publishing, Madison, WI.

74 Jin, J., Yin, F., Tenn, S., *et al.* (2008) Use of the BrainLAB ExacTrac X-Ray 6D system in image-guided radiotherapy. *Med. Dosim.*, **33**, 124–134.

75 Ma, J., Chang, Z., Wang, Z., *et al.* (2009) ExacTrac x-ray 6 degree-of-freedom image-guidance for intracranial non-invasive stereotactic radiotherapy: Comparison with kilo-voltage cone-beam CT. *Radiat. Oncol.*, **93**, 602–608.

76 Trans Tasman Radiation Oncology Group, TROG, Cancer Research program. Available at: Trog.com.au.

77 Ramsey, C.R., Langen, K.M., Kupelian, P.A., *et al.* (2006) A technique for adaptive image-guided helical tomotherapy for lung cancer. *Int. J. Radiat. Oncol. Biol. Phys.*, **64**, 1237–1244.

78 Mohan, R., Zhang, X., Wang, H., *et al.* (2005) Use of deformed intensity distributions for on-line modification of image-guided IMRT to account for interfractional anatomic changes. *Int. J. Radiat. Oncol. Biol. Phys.*, **61**, 1258–1266.

5

A Guide to Understanding Statistics in Radiation Oncology

Kathryn Winter

Introduction

"The purpose of a clinical trial is to provide valid and convincing evidence about the effects of medical therapy" [1]. This important clinical trial work requires the collaboration of many individuals, starting with the principal investigator and the study statistician. "No amount of analysis can salvage a poorly designed study" [2]. Additionally, a well-designed study with an incorrect analysis is not useful and could potentially be harmful. Both, the design and the corresponding analyses of a clinical trial are based on statistical methodology that has been developed over time, originally created mainly for testing drugs, but extrapolated and revised as needed over time for all cancer-treatment modalities, including radiation therapy. The aim of this chapter is not to turn radiation oncologists into statisticians, as that takes formal education and training. No offense intended, but just because doctors have easier access to statistical analysis software than a statistician has to the proton machine does not mean that radiation oncologists without formal statistical education should be doing their own statistics any more than a statistician should be treating cancer patients with radiation therapy, in the event that they ever had access to the treatment machines. While the 'damages' that could be caused by this role reversal are very different, in the statistician's world, an incorrect design or analysis leading to erroneous conclusions that are interpreted as fact, which could lead to other incorrect research or patients receiving or missing out on treatments that are less than ideal or potentially beneficial respectively, could rank as a serious adverse event (SAE) if there were a common toxicity criteria adverse event (CTCAE) equivalent scale for grading the statistical AEs from non-statisticians behaving as one. So, what is the aim of this chapter? It is to provide a base of statistical knowledge for clinical trials that will aid radiation oncologists in their collaborations with statisticians for clinical trial research endeavors and when reading the clinical trials literature.

Consider the following multiple choice question. "When should the radiation oncologist involve the statistician in their project?: (a) Never; (b) 18 h before the ASTRO abstract deadline; (c) After the radiation oncologist has an Excel spreadsheet with some data; or (d) from the beginning of a trial idea through the publication of the trial. If you as the reader chose any answer except for (d), please read this chapter carefully and multiple times. Even those that know that the correct answer is (d) will benefit from reading this chapter, as it will aid in the many discussions they will have with statisticians as they conduct clinical trials.

Terminology and Definitions

It is always good to start with some terminology and definitions. The *null hypothesis*, often denoted H_0, is the starting point and the hypothesis that will be tested against. Usually, the H_0 is one of no difference between treatment arms. The *alternative hypothesis*, often denoted H_A, is the hypothesis that the investigator is hoping to validate, generally that there is a difference between the treatment arms or even more specifically that the new treatment (experimental) is better than the standard treatment (control). Once these hypotheses are determined, statistical tests are formulated such that if the data observed in the trial are not consistent with H_0 then it can be concluded that the data are supportive of H_A. As it is not realistic to include all patients with a particular disease, say primary hepatocellular carcinoma (HCC), to evaluate a potential treatment, *hypothesis testing* provides a systematic and formal way to help investigators come to a conclusion about a *population* (all HCC patients) by studying a *sample* (a group of patients

Clinical Radiation Oncology: Indications, Techniques, and Results, Third Edition. Edited by William Small Jr.
© 2017 John Wiley & Sons, Inc. Published 2017 by John Wiley & Sons, Inc.

with HCC that participate in a given clinical trial). For example, sorafenib is a current standard of care for treating HCC. An investigator has a hypothesis that treating patients first with stereotactic radiation body therapy (SBRT) followed by the standard sorafenib regimen will improve overall survival (OS) for HCC patients. The null hypothesis is that the OS is the same for patients treated with sorafenib and patients treated with SBRT followed by sorafenib. The alternative hypothesis is that the OS is improved for patients treated with SBRT followed by sorafenib, as compared to patients treated with sorafenib alone. A trial can be designed to accrue a sample of HCC patients who are randomized to the two treatments, data collected, and then an analysis to answer the question posed in the hypotheses. This specific question is currently being addressed in the NRG Oncology RTOG 1112 trial. For any hypothesis test, there is an underlying truth, which if were known would negate the need to conduct the clinical trial and put a lot of statisticians out of work. The reality is that that underlying truth is not known, which is why clinical trials are conducted.

Type I and Type II Errors

Given the underlying truth, it is possible that the results of a clinical trial may not reflect that truth and result in errors, called *Type I and Type II errors*. A *type I error*, denoted by α, is a false positive rejecting the H_0 when it is true, meaning that the results of the trial concluded that there is a difference in the treatment arms, when the underlying truth is that the treatment arms are the same. A *type II error*, denoted by β, is a false negative rejecting the H_A when it is true, meaning that the results of the trial did not conclude that there is a difference in the treatment arms, when the underlying truth is that the treatment arms are different.

Decision based on data	Truth	
	H_0 True	H_0 False (H_A True)
Reject H_0	False Positive: Type I Error (α)	Correct Action (Power)
Fail to Reject H_0	Correct Action	False Negative: Type II Error (β)

It is important to note that the two decisions based on the data in the table above are 'Reject H_0' and 'Fail to Reject H_0.' It is not a semantics choice that the bottom row is not labeled 'Accept H_0.' Although investigators say it and this statistician has heard it on multiple occasions,

'accepting H_0' is not a correct statistical decision for a hypothesis test. This is due to the fact that the data in a trial, gathered from a sample of the population of interest, either provides sufficient evidence that is not consistent with the H_0, in which case the H_0 can be rejected, or the data does not provide sufficient evidence that is not consistent with the H_0, in which case the H_0 cannot be rejected. The best analogy is the current legal system. When the jury foreperson reads the verdict, they either state that the defendant is guilty (sufficient evidence to support) or not guilty (not sufficient evidence to support). Although the defendant is assumed to be innocent, as the H_0 is assumed to be true, he/she is never pronounced to be innocent. One might say, if there is the chance for error, why not make both errors as small as possible? Unfortunately, all other parameters held constant, α and β are inversely proportional to each other, so as the type II error is decreased, the type I error increases. As a general rule for prospectively designed clinical trials, the type II error should be ≤ 0.20, while the type I error should be ≤ 0.05 for Phase III trials and anywhere from 0.05 up to 0.20 in Phase II trials. The exact error values that are used for a given trial are determined on a trial-by-trial basis as part of the sample size determination discussed later in this chapter.

Statistical Power

Another important definition is *statistical power*, which is related to the type II error. If in a given clinical trial the underlying truth is that the H_A is true, there are two outcomes – either the data supports that and a correct decision is made, or the data do not support that and a type II error is made. Under the laws of probability, when adding up all of the probabilities of a given scenario they have to sum to 1. In this case, there are only two things that can happen which means that (type II error + correct decision) have to equal 1, or conversely (1 – type II error) equals the probability of a correct decision. While the probability of a correct decision does not have a special name when the H_0 is true, it does when H_A is true – it is called *statistical power*. This is the probability of concluding the H_A is true when it really is. When designing and interpreting clinical trials, it is more common to refer to the statistical power than to the type II error, although knowing one always allows the other to be calculated. Prospectively designed clinical trials should have a minimum of 80% statistical power or correspondingly a type II error or no more than 0.20. When reading the results of a prospectively designed clinical trial, the statistical power for the primary hypothesis is typically reported. However, it is important to know – or at least be aware of the impact of – the statistical power for retrospective analyses as well, especially when 'negative' results are reported. If a retrospective analysis reports a negative association, but does not give any information about the statistical power that was available to detect the hypothesized difference, caution should be taken in interpreting the results. Consider an example retrospective analysis with a null hypothesis of no association between pelvic radiation and second primaries, and an alternative hypothesis that there is such an association. If the results of that analysis report that there is no statistical association between pelvic radiation and the appearance of second primaries, it is difficult to interpret that result without information about how much statistical power there actually was to detect the hypothesized association. If there was at least 80% statistical power, the reader can feel confident in the results. However, if there was only 26% statistical power, then the probability of being able to detect the hypothesized association between pelvic radiation and second primaries (if it really exists) is only 26%, so the 'negative' results would not be surprising, but they also cannot be interpreted as truly conclusive negative results. For time-to-event endpoints, this power is driven by the number of events of interest – second primaries in this example – and not the number of patients (as discussed later in the chapter). Basically, sufficient statistical power provides reliable results, while insufficient power does not, but that cannot be determined if the statistical power is not reported. The take-away message here is to be cognizant of this issue when reading and interpreting reported negative results.

p-Values

It is time now to talk about *p-values* which, while important, are not the end-all-be-all of a clinical trial and, unlike the cheese, should never stand alone. What is a p-value? The answer is not 'a number that needs to be <0.05 so the trial can be published in a good journal.' A p-value is simply the probability of obtaining a result from the data (which comes from a sample) that is equal to or more extreme than the observed result, *given that the H_0 is true*. Generally a small p-value indicates that the observed results are not likely to have occurred if the H_0 is true, so either the H_0 is not true or a type I error has occurred. In hypothesis testing a significance level, also denoted α, is set a priori and then the p-value from the data is compared such that if the data p-value $\leq \alpha$, reject H_0. A widely held perception is that when comparing any two p-values, a smaller p-value indicates greater evidence for the experiment treatment, such as $p = 0.04$ versus $p = 0.0001$. That perception would be INCORRECT! A p-value only indicates how likely the result would be if the H_0 is true, it gives absolutely no information about the magnitude of the observed difference or about the number of patients from which the data came. Consider the example table below which shows the results of four trials that all had 40% two-year OS for the

control arm and 42% two-year OS for the experimental arm.

Trial	p-value	No. of patients in trial
A	0.77	200
B	0.39	2000
C	0.16	5000
D	0.004	20 000

As evidenced by the table above, any difference – however small – can be shown to be statistically significant with enough patients. This is why statisticians design clinical trials with the appropriate number of patients (to achieve the required number of events for time-to-event trials; as discussed later) to answer the hypothesis of interest. This also illustrates why the p-value should never be reported alone. In a time-to-event scenario comparing two treatments, it should always be accompanied by the effect size (hazard ratio) and estimates at meaningful time points (e.g., two- and/or five-year OS), both of which should also include relevant confidence intervals.

One-Sided and Two-Sided Hypothesis Tests

Hypothesis tests can be either one-sided or two-sided. If an investigator is interested in testing two treatments A and B to determine if there is a difference between them in either direction, then a *two-sided* hypothesis test is appropriate. Using OS as an example there are three possible outcomes:

- OS is significantly different between treatments A and B, with treatment A having better OS than treatment B.
- OS is significantly different between treatments A and B, with treatment B having better OS than treatment A.
- OS is not significantly different between treatments A and B.

Note that the wording of that last bullet, as discussed earlier, is that the treatments are 'not significantly different,' as opposed to stating that the treatments are the same. Now, when an investigator is testing an experimental treatment (A) and is interested only in determining if it is better than the control arm treatment (B), then a *one-sided* hypothesis test is appropriate and would have the following two possible outcomes:

- OS for the experimental treatment A is significantly better than OS for treatment B.
- OS for the experimental treatment A is *not* significantly better than OS for treatment B.

Even if the treatment curves are completely separated in the opposite direction than was hypothesized, the only definitive statistical conclusion that can be made is that treatment A is not significantly better than treatment B. An example of this is the RTOG 0617 non-small-cell lung cancer trial [3]. It was hypothesized that a higher radiotherapy dose regimen would result in an increase in OS as compared to the standard radiotherapy dose, and the trial was designed as a one-sided test in that direction. Unfortunately, the results were completely opposite to what was hypothesized, with a clear separation of the survival curves. Given that, the trial conclusion, relative to the one-sided hypothesis, was that the higher radiotherapy dose regimen did not result in a statistically significant increase in OS.

When a two-sided test is designed, the type I error (α) is equally divided between the two possible scenarios of a statistically significant difference, such that a test with an overall α of 0.05 really provides 0.025 in the direction of treatment A being better than B, and 0.025 in the direction of treatment B being better than A, since in reality, if the data shows a difference in the treatments it can only be in one direction. In a one-sided test, the entire α goes to the one scenario of a statistically significant difference in the hypothesized direction. For a one-sided trial testing treatment A being better than B, using an overall α of 0.05, the 0.05 false positive rate is all in that one direction. Due to that, a one-sided test of the same overall significance level as a two-sided test has a higher false-positive rate, for the selected direction [4]. Given that, one-sided tests for definitive Phase III trials frequently use an alpha of 0.025 (half of a two-sided 0.05 test), though it is not uncommon to see a one-sided test with an α of 0.05, especially in trials of more rare tumors, as the α-level plays a key role in the sample size that is required. For example, the NRG/RTOG 1112 liver trial uses a one-sided test with an α of 0.05 (the full design of the trial is described later in the chapter). When the results of that study are reported, the possible conclusions will be 'Liver cancer patients treated with SBRT + sorafenib have a statistically significant increase in overall survival compared to patients treated with sorafenib alone,' or 'It cannot be concluded that liver cancer patients treated with SBRT + sorafenib have a statistically significant increase in overall survival compared to patients treated with sorafenib alone.' If positive, the conclusion can only go in one direction. NRG/RTOG 1010, a trimodality esophageal trial examining the addition of trastuzumab to chemoradiation for HER2-positive patients, with a disease-free survival (DFS) primary end-point, was designed with a two-sided hypothesis and an overall α-level of 0.05. As a side note, with all other parameters being held constant, the sample size required for this trial would be exactly the same as if the trial had been designed as a one-sided test with an overall α-level of 0.025. When this trial is analyzed,

the possible conclusions will be 'There is a statistically significant difference in DFS between patients treated with chemoradiation with or without trastuzumab (more specifically, depending on the direct of the difference: There is a statistically significant improvement in DFS for patient treated with chemoradiation and trastuzumab,' or 'There is a statistically significant decrease in DFS for patient treated with chemoradiation and trastuzumab) or 'It cannot be concluded that there is a statistically significant difference in DFS between patients treated with chemoradiation with or without trastuzumab.' If this trial is positive (meaning a statistically significant difference, it can go in one of two directions, hence the two-sided hypothesis and test.

Hazard Ratios

What is a *hazard ratio* (HR)? A hazard is an event of interest occurring (e.g., death for OS). A hazard rate is the probability of failure for a given end-point at any given point in time, and is usually denoted by λ. The HR is the ratio of two hazard rates and is used to measure a treatment effect where the question is to what extent can an experimental treatment lengthen the time to the event of interest. If HR = 1, this means that the two treatments have the same hazard rates and therefore there is no treatment effect. For two treatments A and B, it does not matter which way the hazard rates are divided, λ_A/λ_B or λ_B/λ_A, but knowing which way the division was done is needed for the interpretation. A HR >1 means an increased risk for the treatment on top, while a HR <1 means a decreased risk for the treatment on top. For example, the following two HRs, for an OS end-point, are the same, but the way they are reported is generally based on whether the HR is > or <1. A HR = 2.0 for (λ_A/λ_B) is reported as patients on Arm A are twice as likely to experience the event (death), while a HR = 0.5 for (λ_B/λ_A) is reported as a 50% reduction in experiencing the event (death) for patients on Arm B. Hazard ratios are an important statistic for reporting efficacy results, but equally important are the confidence intervals (CIs) for the reported effect size. For example, a HR of 0.53 may look very promising in and of itself, but would be interpreted very differently with a 95% CI of (0.40, 0.71) than with a CI of (0.26, 2.85). In the first CI the results indicate 95% confidence that the HR is below 1, whereas the second CI indicates 95% confidence that the HR is between two values that include 1, so it cannot be concluded that there is a treatment effect.

Data Monitoring Committee

In brief, a Data Monitoring Committee (DMC; also referred to as a Data and Safety Monitoring Board or Committee) provides oversight for a clinical trial and makes recommendations to the organization that is leading the trial. For cancer clinical trials, a DMC consists of members with the appropriate scientific/disease expertise and should always include a statistician. The DMC generally reviews the accrual, relative to projected targets, and adverse events on a regular basis (e.g., twice a year, as is done by the NRG Oncology DMC), as well as reviewing any protocol-specified interim analyses (e.g., primary end-point, early safety analyses, etc.) either at the regularly scheduled meetings or in between as needed.

Determining a Sample Size for a Clinical Trial

How many patients are needed for a clinical trial? Investigators are often overheard saying things like, "I have an idea for a clinical trial. Fifty patients should be enough to do it, right?" or "I did a quick calculation and this trial is going to need 120 patients, right?" Determining a sample size is not done by picking a number out of thin air, nor – contrary to popular belief – do statisticians have a key board with magic keys like the one below:

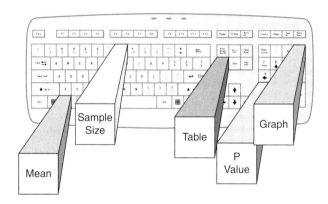

Determining the sample size for a clinical trial is a collaborative process that absolutely requires input from the radiation oncologist, or other researchers, but should be done by the statistician. The following are the main pieces of information that a statistician needs to determine a sample size: primary endpoint; control arm data; effect size of interest; accrual rate; one- or two-sided test; and Type I and II error rates.

Clinical trials are designed based on the primary endpoint, so that needs to be determined first. Some examples based on trial phase would be: Phase I trial – specific adverse events of interest to determine the maximum tolerated dose; Phase II trial – disease-free survival, complete response, and so on; Phase III – OS, disease-free survival, and so on. Defining the endpoint is very important. Some are straightforward; for example it is universal

that failure for OS is death due to any cause. Distant metastases, in the non-metastatic disease setting, is also rather straightforward with failure being the appearance of any distant metastasis. Some people use disease-free survival (DFS) and progression-free survival (PFS) interchangeably, but there is a difference. As a general rule, in the DFS setting it is expected that the treatment will eradicate the disease, whereas in the PFS setting the expectation is that the treatment will keep the disease from getting worse and it is a bonus if it actually gets better. There are some specific challenges in radiotherapy-focused trials with respect to endpoints, given that the clinical trial world has a heavy bent towards drugs and radiotherapy is obviously anatomically targeted, while drugs are systemically targeted. A particular radiotherapy regimen may be very effective for addressing local-regional disease, but that may get lost in a trial with an OS endpoint if there are systemic issues. The radiotherapy effect needs to be over and above and/or synergistic with other treatments. Thinking about this is important when determining the best primary endpoint for a trial and what secondary endpoints are important to include.

Once the primary endpoint is finalized, the effect size needs to be determined for efficacy endpoints and for a Phase I trial, the upper limit for the percentage of dose-limiting toxicities (DLTs). The remainder of the present discussion will focus on determining sample sizes for efficacy endpoints. In order to determine effect size, the investigator needs to provide information about the control arm, generally the current standard of care, and then information about how much they think the experimental treatment will improve the endpoint of interest. For example, it may be that the control arm has a median OS of 23 months and the investigator thinks that the experimental treatment will increase the median OS to 31 months, or the standard of care has a five-year OS of 28% and the investigator thinks that the experimental treatment will increase that to 42.5%. It is important to remember that the difference to be detected and the required sample size are inversely proportional, which means that the smaller the difference the larger the required sample size. When a statistician is working on a sample size, they do not just calculate a single number and say "…here it is." They generally calculate potential sample sizes under several scenarios determined by varying parameters such as the effect size, error and accrual rates, and length of follow-up, among others. The different scenarios are then discussed with the trial's principal investigator. Ideally, a trial should be designed to test the smallest clinically meaningful difference with acceptable error rates; however, due to resource limitations, sometimes that required sample size is not feasible. In those cases, it becomes a balancing act between a feasible sample size and a realistic effect size. It does not make any sense, nor is it really ethical, to conduct a trial that is looking for such a large difference that no one believes would ever occur just to get to a sample that can meet funding constraints. Consider a scenario where the control arm median OS is 23 months. The table below shows potential sample sizes when looking for an increase in median OS, using a two-sided alpha of 0.05 and 85% power.

Increase in Median OS to	Hazard Ratio	Required Evaluable Sample Size
37	0.62	256
34.5	0.67	321
33	0.70	381
31	0.74	513

In the discussions between the investigator and statistician, it may be concluded that accruing 513 patients really is not feasible and perhaps an increase in median OS from 23 to 37 months is overly optimistic. That would eliminate the top and bottom row options, and then further discussions would determine if the trial would use a sample size of 321 or 381.

Types of Trial

Phase I Trials

The purpose of a Phase I trial is to determine the maximum tolerated dose of the regimen of interest that will move forward through the clinical trial system in the hopes of eventually becoming a new standard of care and improving the lives of cancer patients. The most important point about a Phase I trial is the correct and specific definition of what will count as a dose-limiting toxicity (DLT). Broader is not better in this situation, because at the time of the analysis of a given Phase I dose regimen the radiation oncologist cannot tell the statistician "Oh, when the DLT was defined as all grade 3 and higher AEs, we didn't mean grade 3 fatigue or heme toxicity that was expected from the concurrent chemo and resolved, etc." The DLTs defined at the time the study is activated are those that need to be used for the analysis. The DLTs will vary from disease site to disease site, and even within a disease site. For example, here is a list of the AEs that defined the DLT for evaluating SBRT in a Phase I trial for patients with liver metastases:

- Grade 4 or 5 hepatic.
- Grade 4 or 5 gastrointestinal.
- Grade 4 or 5 thrombocytopenia.

- Radiation-induced liver disease (RILD) requiring treatment (including diuretics). RILD will be defined using the following adverse events:
  - Grade 3 or higher alkaline phosphatase (ALP) in the presence of ascites occurring in the absence of disease progression.
  - Grade 4 hepatic liver enzyme elevations persisting for ≥5 days.
- Any adverse event requiring interruption of therapy by ≥2 weeks (14 calendar days). This does not include patient desire to discontinue therapy. It does include failure for thrombocytopenia to improve to a level of 80 requiring interruption of therapy.
- Any grade 5 treatment-related adverse event.

If a Phase I trial were being conducted in early-stage prostate cancer, lower grades would be included because there is a tradeoff between the extent of the AEs that are willing to be accepted for a potentially life-prolonging treatment given the current standard of care and outcomes. In the drug research world, it is standard to use a 3+3 design where three patients are entered, receive the drug, and then evaluated for DLTs. If none is observed, the trial continues to the next dose level. If two or more DLTs are observed, then the dose is determined to be too toxic. If one DLT is observed, then three more patients are entered and treated. If no DLTs are observed in these three cases then the trial continues to the next dose level, otherwise the dose level is determined to be too toxic. This approach works well for drug development because generally the DLTs for these trials are those that will happen quickly. In the radiation therapy setting, the DLTs of interest are often those that happen later, and the amount of follow-up required makes the 3+3 approach logistically challenging for completing a Phase I trial in a timely fashion. An alternative approach is to use a time-to-event continual reassessment method (TITE-CRM). The CRM uses a more mathematical formula based on dose–response modeling to assign the dose to the next patient entered, based on any DLTs experienced by patients already entered. The primary objective is to estimate the target dose corresponding to the target rate, which is the acceptable probability of DLT. This approach minimizes patients being treated at much lower, potentially ineffective doses, and allows more patients to be treated at the dose that will eventually be determined to be the maximally tolerated dose (MTD). The TITE-CRM is a refinement of the CRM design, which provides the advantage of continued accrual, unlike in the 3+3 design [5–9]. Under this methodology, the starting dose can be much closer to the expected MTD and then escalated and de-escalated based on the data collected over time. The NRG/RTOG 0813 trial for non-small-cell lung cancer was the first national multi-institutional trial to implement this method. A common question asked by investigators at the end of a Phase I trial is, "Hey, can we compare the OS between the dose arms?" The short answer if NO! The more detailed answer is that Phase I trials are not intended – and therefore not designed – to statistically estimate and/or answer questions about the efficacy of a regimen; that is why there are Phase II and Phase III clinical trials. If a Phase I trial ends up with three dose levels, each with six patients, there is no appropriate statistical test to compare the OS between those arms. The TITE-CRM methodology does allow for some efficacy estimation of the final dose chosen, but that is built in prospectively within the trial design and such a trial would actually be considered a Phase I/II trial.

Phase II Trials

Phase II trials take a regimen that has Phase I level safety data and further evaluates it for efficacy, as well as providing more information about the AE profile, generally with the plan to move promising regimens forward to a definitive Phase III trial. For a long time, it was very common to design single-arm Phase II trials, the results of which would be compared to historical control data. While information can be gained from such trials, these results can often be biased due to the differences in the patients treated with the new regimen, as compared to those on which the historical control data is based. This can be due to a variety of reasons including – but not limited to – shifts in patient staging over time, different distributions of factors not known to be associated with the outcome of interest, improved support care, and so forth. Do not be fooled by the word 'randomization' in the trial title. This type of trial design is just a more efficient way of conducting a single-arm Phase II trial when there are multiple experimental treatments to be evaluated, and is subject to the same biases as a single-arm Phase II trial. More recently, there has been a move towards randomized Phase II trials with a current control arm treated with the standard of care to help account for these biases, often referred to as a randomized Phase II screening trial. There are some disadvantages to this trial design as more patients are needed, but the advantages of being able to assess a new regimen relative to contemporary patients being treated with the standard of care and better determine which regimens should be considered for definitive Phase III trials, which are very resource intensive, outweigh those [10]. Just to alleviate any confusion, a trial that randomizes patients to multiple experimental arms and compares each back to historical controls, and may even have some 'statistical selection' to choose between the arms if more than one meets the historical control comparison criteria, is not the same as a randomized Phase II screening trial that contains a current control

arm. That does not mean that single-arm Phase II trials should never be conducted. There are some patient populations where there is no well-established standard of care, and unfortunately the survival has not shifted over long periods of time. Pilot information from trials in these populations is very useful in helping to appropriately design the randomized Phase II screening trials.

Randomized Phase II trials are designed to determine if there is a sufficient signal for the experimental treatment to warrant a Phase III trial. The key word here is 'signal.' By design, a Phase II-R trial has a smaller sample size than a Phase III trial because the Type I error (false-positive rate) used is higher, usually 0.10–0.20, as opposed to the Type I error in a Phase III trial, which is usually ≤ 0.05. This is the reason why the results of a Phase II-R trial are used for signal purposes only and the definitive results are provided by a Phase III trial. Because Phase II-R trials are looking for a signal, they are generally powered at 85%, 90%, or sometimes even 95%, to help safeguard against a Type II error of missing that signal if it truly exists. While Phase II-R trials play a very important role, they are not meant to be conducted in place of a Phase III trial. That said, there are circumstances in rare tumor populations where an appropriately designed Phase III trial would never be able to be completed. It is possible in that setting that a well-designed Phase II-R trial with a Type I error on the lower end of the scale and a large observed effect may change clinical practice, but that is certainly the exception. No matter the setting, a Phase II-R trial should never ever be referred to as a 'mini Phase III trial.'

Phase III Trials

Phase III trials are large, multicenter, randomized, multiarm comparative trials of efficacy with the goal of changing current clinical practice. These trials are also able to support other important endpoints such as correlative science and quality of life/patient reported outcomes (QoL/PRO) and are conducted in order to make a definitive decision about a whether or not a treatment should become the new standard of care. Randomized Phase III trials are considered the 'gold standard.' Randomized trials help to minimize patient selection bias by physicians, and the randomization also helps to balance for known and unknown prognostic factors [11]. There are three main types of Phase III trials: superiority; non-inferiority; and equivalence.

Superiority trials are the most common and aim to show that a new treatment is better than an existing treatment. Non-inferiority trials are used to test a new treatment that has one or more benefits such as fewer side effects, shorter treatment time, less costly, more accessible, and so on, with the goal of showing that these benefits exist for the new treatment at a low cost relative to the loss of effectiveness compared to the current standard of care. By design, there is going to be a little give on the efficacy side (i.e., an acceptable amount of potential reduction in efficacy), so non-inferiority trials in cancer are generally conducted in populations with very high survival/low local failure rates. For example, the NRG Oncology trial RTOG 1005 is a Phase III non-inferiority trial for early-stage breast cancer designed to determine if hypofractionated whole-breast radiation (WBRT) with a concurrent boost is non-inferior to standard fractionation WBRT with a sequential boost with respective to local failure. Another non-inferiority example is NRG Oncology trial RTOG 1016, which is a Phase III trial in HPV-associated oropharynx cancer patients looking to replace the chemotherapy in the standard chemoradiation regimen with something less toxic. The trial is specifically designed to determine if accelerated IMRT + cetuximab is non-inferior to the standard chemoradiation regimen, with respect to OS. The null hypothesis in non-inferiority trials is that the experimental treatment is significantly worse than the standard treatment, by a specified amount, and the alternative is that it is not. The determination of the size of that 'specified amount' – often referred to as the non-inferiority margin – is a critical part of designing a non-inferiority trial. There is no 'gold standard' for what this margin should be, but it must defined a priori as part of the trial design and should be less than what would be considered a clinically meaningful decrease in efficacy. This margin is often chosen relative to an effect size and it is common to choose a fraction ($\leq 1/2$) of the effect size of the standard intervention [12]. Investigators often use the words non-inferiority and equivalence interchangeably, but they are not the same. While a non-inferiority trial is designed to show that the experimental treatment is no worse than the standard treatment by a specified amount, an equivalency trial is designed to determine that the difference between the experimental and standard treatments, in either direction, is no bigger than the specified amount. With respect to sample size, keeping in mind the relationship between effect size and sample size, the number of patients needed for a non-inferiority trial are generally larger than for a superiority trial, and larger yet for an equivalency trial, with the exact numbers obviously driven by the relevant parameters for a given trial.

For any randomized trial, the point at which a patient should be randomized needs to be considered. Ideally, the randomization should occur at the point at which the treatments differ. In Figure 5.1(a) the patients are randomized at the beginning of treatment to receive either 64.8 Gy or 50.4 Gy, but that is not the point at which the treatments differ. Figure 5.1(b) shows all patients receiving 50.4 Gy and then being randomized to receive another 14.4 Gy, or not. That is the purest randomization

as it helps to reduce any bias that could arise from an imbalance in patients dropping out prior to the point the treatments differ. However, a randomization such as that in Figure 5.1(b) may have challenges due to the treatment versus no treatment scenario after randomization, especially if patients are not even approached to participate in the trial until that point. A patient may be more willing to participate in a trial such as that in Figure 5.1(a) and have no problem being randomized to 50.4 Gy, since they fully know which treatment they will be receiving, rather than the situation in Figure 5.1(b) where they will not know until after they have completed the 50.4 Gy, at which point they may not want to be randomized to 'no treatment,' even though a randomization to no treatment in this scenario is still 50.4 Gy. Yet another scenario exists which sometimes is needed for logistical purposes and may aid in addressing the patient's perspective. Figure 5.1(c) shows a different trial where patients receive three cycles of chemotherapy, are re-staged, and if there is no progression they are then randomized to either one more cycle of chemotherapy followed by SBRT, or one more cycle of chemotherapy. Having some amount of time prior to the SBRT was necessary due to prospective radiotherapy quality assurance reviews that were required for patients randomized to the SBRT arm. This does not fully address the patient's issue of wanting to know their complete planned treatment at the time of study entry, but knowing that they will receive some treatment after being randomized can be very helpful. From the statistical perspective, although this last scenario is not as pure as randomizing after the fourth chemotherapy cycle, performing the randomization after three cycles and restaging versus randomizing at the point of study entry helps to significantly reduce potential biases.

Randomization Ratio

The most common allocation of experimental to control is 1:1, and this results in the smallest sample size. Sometimes more patients are allocated to the experimental arm, e.g. two or three patients on the experimental arm for every one patient on the control arm, denoted as 2:1 or 3:1. A common reason for doing this is if there are concerns about accrual in the setting where there is a 50:50 chance of receiving the experimental treatment. This appears to be more of an issue in a setting where the randomization is a treatment versus no treatment scenario, such as radiotherapy versus no radiotherapy. It's also been used in order to get more information quickly on the toxicity profile for the experimental treatment. From a statistical design perspective, keeping all other parameters constant, a 2:1 allocation requires a larger sample size than 1:1 in order to have a similar study duration, approximately 12% larger. This is due to the fact that the sample size is driven by the number of events needed

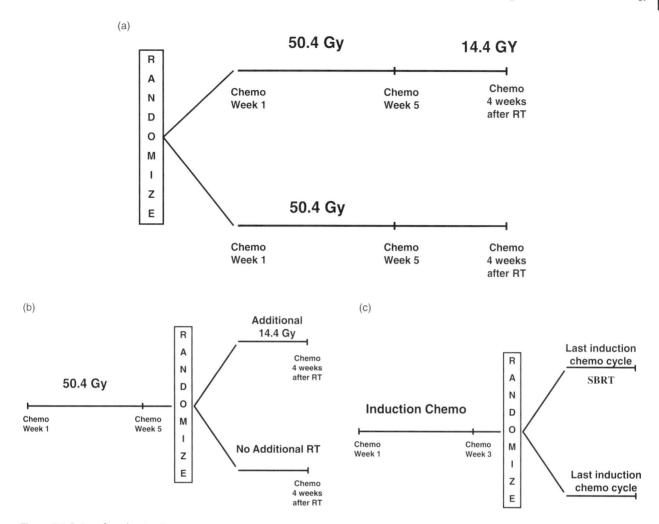

Figure 5.1 Point of randomization.

to detect the hypothesized effect size. Under the alternative hypothesis that the experimental treatment will have a better outcome, there will be more events (e.g., deaths for an OS endpoint) on the control arm. Consider a 600-patient trial that requires 326 events. In a 1:1 randomization, half of the patients (i.e., 300) will be on the control arm and the other 300 on the experimental arm. In a 2:1 randomization, 200 patients will be on the control arm and 400 on the experimental arm. While both scenarios have 600 patients, under the alternative hypothesis the second scenario will have fewer events because more of the patients are on the experimental arm. In order to have a trial with a similar study duration as the 1:1 setting, the sample size will need to be increased in order to reach the required 326 events. Another option that can potentially be used is to keep the same sample size, but extend the follow-up time to reach the required number of events.

Stratification Factors

While randomization helps with balancing factors between the treatment arms, stratification will ensure balance for factors known to be associated with the primary outcome. Using gender as an example in a two-arm randomized trial, there is a common misconception that stratifying by gender will result in 50% males and 50% females on each treatment arm. Wrong! The distribution of the levels of a given stratification factor will not be known until the trial has finished accruing. What stratification does is provide balance between the treatment arms with respect to the levels of the factor. Using the gender example again, if the overall distribution of males and females is ~25% and 75%, then stratifying by gender provides that each treatment arm will have ~25% males and 75% females. For example: Arm A has 25% males and 75% females; Arm B has 24% males and 76% females. There is no hard and fast rule for how much stratification is too much, but over-stratification can reduce precision. A rough rule of thumb used by some is to have 20–60 patients per stratification cell. To determine the number of stratification cells, multiply the number of levels for each factor. For example, if a trial is stratifying by gender (male versus female), histology (adenocarcinoma versus squamous), and T-stage (T1 versus T2 versus T3/T4), then there are $2 \times 2 \times 3 = 12$ stratification cells. The cells would be male/adenocarcinoma/T1, male/adenocarcinoma/T2, and so forth. All of that said, significant thought should be given to which variables are included for stratification. If a tumor marker is going to be used for stratification, there are logistical issues that need to be considered. Will the marker determination be done centrally or at each treating institution? If done centrally, how is that built into the trial design? One approach is to enter the patients onto the trial and start a common treatment while the marker is being centrally assessed, so that the results will be available for stratification at the time of randomization following the common treatment completion. This was done in the NRG Oncology/RTOG 0825 GBM trial. In a scenario where patients will not be randomized or any treatment started until the marker assessment is completed, it is important to be able to get the marker assessment done in a very timely fashion. In the postoperative H&N trial, NRG Oncology/RTOG 0920, patients were entered so that specimens could be submitted for epidermal growth factor receptor (EGFR) assessment for all patients and human papilloma virus (HPV) for oropharyngeal patients. These centrally determined results are available within two weeks of study entry so that they can then be used for stratification purposes at the time the patient is randomized.

Study Duration

For time-to-event endpoint trials, study duration is the time interval between starting accrual and the definitive treatment analysis, which is generally driven by reaching the required number of primary endpoint events. Increasing the total sample size shortens the study duration as there are more patients for which the primary endpoint can occur. Conversely, decreasing the sample size lengthens the study duration. In a prospective clinical trial, the time to reach the required number of primary endpoint events is projected based on the assumed null and hypothesized alternative hypotheses. While the actual time to reach the required number of events may be slightly shorter or longer than projected, unless otherwise released by the study's data monitoring committee, the primary endpoint analysis will not occur until the required number of events is reached.

Interim Analyses

As part of the trial design, it must be determined if any interim analyses will be included. If a treatment really is extremely effective (efficacy) or will never be positive (futile), it is better to know sooner rather than later; however it is also important – even more so on the futility side – not to write off a treatment erroneously based on results with very little information on the primary endpoint. Phase III trials often include interim analyses for both efficacy and futility. There are several methods that can be used for both, and various philosophies on how conservative or liberal a rule should be used. It is not a one-size fits all, but rather needs to be determined on a study-by-study basis. Generally, the threshold for determining efficacy at an interim analysis is very high at the initial of multiple looks, as things could change as the data matures. One method is the Lan–DeMets alpha-spending function [13]. For example, if a trial is designed with two interim analyses and a final analysis (total three snap-shots) with an overall Type I error of $\alpha = 0.05$, the thresholds for crossing the efficacy boundary at the two interim looks could be p-values <0.001 and <0.012, respectively. Because some alpha has been spent for those looks, the final analysis would be made at an α of 0.046 so as to preserve the overall α of 0.05. Interim futility analyses are based on the idea that, employing the current data, even if the trial were to complete to the final planned analysis, it is very unlikely that the results will show the hypothesized difference. In a Phase III trial, if a decision is taken to stop accrual to a trial early and/or report the trial results prior to the final planned analysis, it is with the understanding that these results are determined to be definitive. With that in mind, it should not be surprising that as a general rule for randomized Phase II trials only futility analyses are included. Phase II-R trials are designed to detect a signal for efficacy with α levels of 0.10–0.20, so looking to stop early for definitive efficacy results is not applicable. On the other hand, since the goal of the Phase II-R trial is to have sufficient signal to warrant a Phase III trial, if it can be determined part way through the trial that no such signal will ever be seen, it makes sense to determine futility and direct resources towards other potential treatments. The number and the timing of interim analyses are done on a trial-by-trial basis and the results are reported to the data monitoring committee (DMC) responsible for the trial. The DMC reviews the results and makes recommendations regarding early stopping of accrual and/or early reporting or continuation of the trial to the next planned interim analysis.

Based on all of the parameters discussed, two sample size examples are now provided: one for a Phase II-R screening trial, and one for a Phase III trial.

Phase II-R Trial Example (Figure 5.2)

For each comparison: chemotherapy versus radiotherapy regimen:

- Primary endpoint: Overall survival (OS)
- Control arm 2-year OS rate = 10%
- Experimental arm 2-year OS rate = 22.5%
- 12.5% absolute improvement in OS with new Rx (HR = 0.65)

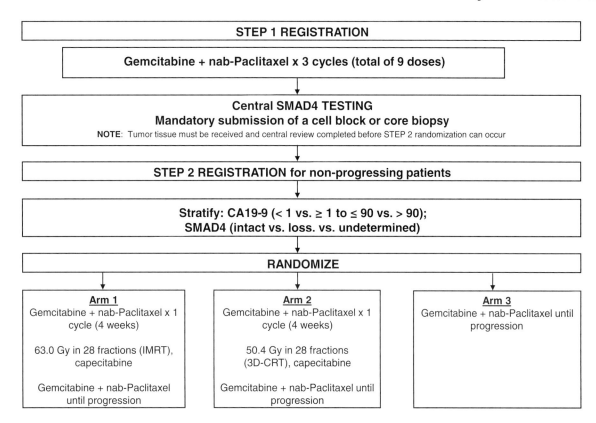

Figure 5.2 NRG Oncology/RTOG 1201 schema.

- Power = 90%; 1-sided Type I error of 0.10
- Allow for 10% ineligible/lost
- n = 96 per arm
- Total of 288 randomized
- If the resulting p-value for overall survival is ≤0.10 for a given radiotherapy regimen, the result will be interpreted as an indication to test that regimen in a definitive Phase III trial
- Phase II-R results are NOT definitive – looking for a signal.

Phase III Trial Example (Figure 5.3)

- Primary endpoint: overall survival
- Control arm: median survival = 10.5 months
- Experimental arm: median survival = 14.5 months
- HR = 0.72 (28% reduction in the hazard rate of death)
- 85% Power; 1-sided Type I error of 0.05
- Five years accrual and one-year follow-up
- Two interim analyses
- 13% adjustment for ineligible/lost cases
- 320 evaluable patients
- Targeted sample size = 368
- If the resulting p-value for overall survival is ≤0.05, the result will be that SBRT significantly improved overall survival
- **Results ARE definitive.**

Given the discussions above about the various parameters that play a role in determining a sample size, the table below further shows examples of how parameter changes impact sample size calculations:

Parameters	O	P	S	H	F
Two-sided significance level (α)	0.05		0.01		
Statistical power ($1-\beta$)	80%	90%			
Control arm yearly hazard rate (based on two-year survival of 36%)	0.511				
Hazard ratio (based on inc. in 2-year survival to 50%)	0.68			0.80	
Accrual years	4				
Follow-up years	2				5
Total sample size	266	356	396	776	222
No. of primary endpoint events	209	281	312	632	209

Columns: O: original parameters; P: increasing power; S: decreasing significance level; H: higher hazard ratio (i.e. closer to 1); F: longer follow-up time

For example, increasing the statistical power from 80% to 90% increases the required number of events and hence the sample size, keeping all other parameters constant, whereas increasing the follow-up years does not impact the required number of events but does decrease the required sample size.

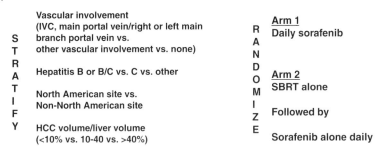

Figure 5.3 NRG Oncology/RTOG 1112 schema.

Analyses

Protocol interim and final analyses of the primary endpoint and of secondary endpoints are made at the times specified in the protocol, which are generally event- or time-driven. Interim analyses are reported to the DMC responsible for the trial, and unless a boundary is crossed and the trial results are released early by the DMC, the study investigator does not see the results of interim analyses. When an analysis report is provided to the investigator, it includes information on accrual, patient and tumor characteristics, treatment delivery, adverse events, and the protocol endpoint-specific analyses, along with the statistical interpretations of the results. Which endpoints are included, and when they are reported, is determined by the protocol-specified timing of the trial's endpoints. For example, if the primary endpoint is complete response (CR) at three months post radiotherapy completion and there are secondary endpoints for overall survival and local failure after patients have been followed for three years, the intimal analysis report would include the CR endpoint, but not the OS and local failure endpoints. After the analysis report is sent to the investigator, there is continued collaboration with the statistician in order to present and publish the results. It bears repeating that the timing of the analyses of protocol endpoints is driven by the statistical design. This timing should be specified in the protocol, and while one should never say never, this timing is almost never the day after the protocol has completed its accrual. While this is stated a bit tongue in cheek, it is more common than one might think for an investigator to contact the trial statistician right after accrual has completed to ask "Can we analyze the trial now?" Do not be that investigator. That said, checking in with your statistician when the study closes to accrual, and routinely while the trial is in follow-up for an analysis that is depending on a certain number of primary endpoint events occurring, to discuss when the analysis will happen is completely reasonable.

Interpreting p-Values

While the official statistical conclusion of a hypothesis test is based on the p-value, please remember (as mentioned previously in this chapter) that the p-value alone does tell the whole story for the analysis. That message understood, for a result to be statistically significant, the p-value from the test based on the collected data must be less than or equal to the a priori-specified alpha level, with the key term there being a priori. It is completely inappropriate and downright wrong to bump up the a priori alpha level because the resulting p-value was a little higher than the original alpha, and equally as wrong to collect the data, do the hypothesis test and then choose an alpha level. The p-value from a test can be either one-sided or two2-sided. Whether a one-sided or two-sided p-value is reported should be based on and consistent with whether the hypothesis test was designed as a one-sided or two-sided test. By default, statistical software packages report a two-sided p-value, which is divided in half to obtain the one-sided p-value. Consider a trial designed with a two-sided hypothesis test for an OS endpoint with an overall α of 0.05. If the results of the trial produce a two-sided p-value of 0.036, then statistical significance has been met. If the results produce a two-sided p-value of 0.062, then statistical significance has not been met. There is no such thing as 'almost statistically significant.' Much like a woman either is or is not pregnant, hypothesis test results either are or are not statistically significant. However, let us revisit the important fact that the p-value alone does not tell the whole story. From the non-statistically significant example above, a p-value of 0.062 or 0.29 or 0.75 would all result in statistical significance not being met; however, the additional important information would be very different. Let us assume that the trial was designed to detect and absolute difference in two-year OS of at least 12%. The observed absolute differences for p-values of 0.062, 0.29, and 0.75 could hypothetically be 10%, 6%, and 2%, with the actual values less important than the understanding that a p-value result closer to the designed α will have an OS difference closer to the hypothesized difference. It may be that 10% is a clinically meaningful difference in OS for this patient population, but resources did not allow for a trial large enough to be designed to detect a 10% difference. The take-away message for a trial as a whole with such a result would be very different from a trial with an absolute difference in OS of 2%, which for the given population is not clinically meaningful and would never change the standard of care. All of that being said, it is important to note that the p-value of 0.062 example does not guarantee that if the trial had been designed to detect a 10% difference in OS it would have produced a statistically significant result, but further hammers home the point that the p-value alone does not provide the whole story for an analysis. Consider the following example for a one-sided hypothesis test. If the trial was designed with a one-sided α of 0.025 and the data produces a two-sided p-value of 0.04, the corresponding one-sided p-value would be 0.02, which is ≤ 0.025 and therefore statistical significance can be concluded. It is important to be aware of what p-values are being reported and how the trial was designed. This is especially true in the setting of journals that require all reported p-values to be two-sided. From a statistically purist perspective, this can be extremely frustrating, but not so much as to not publish in such journals. For these journals, in the one-sided example above, the actual one-sided design would be described, but the two-sided p-value of 0.04 would be reported. The manuscript would also state the corresponding two-sided α level, in this case $2 \times 0.025 = 0.05$, that would be used for comparison of the required two-sided p-values that would be reported.

Survival Analyses

The most common approach for analyzing survival data is to use the Kaplan-Meier approach [14] to estimate survival, and the log-rank test [15] to compare survival between treatments. This approach starts with all patients surviving (100% survival) and decreases as failures occur (graphically, the curves go from the top left down to the right over time). This is a good way to present survival data for endpoints where eventually, if followed long enough, the survival would reach 0%. This applies to OS and any endpoint where death due to any cause is a failure, as eventually everyone dies. There are other endpoints that require a different approach due to events that occur prior to the event of interest, called *competing risk events*. If a patient dies before experiencing a local failure, there is no way to know whether or not he/she would have experienced a local failure if they had continued living. These endpoints can also be thought of in terms of not having a guaranteed occurrence with enough follow-up, such as local failure. While death – along with taxes – is inevitable, patients can be cured and there is no inevitability to local failure. For endpoints with competing risks, the cumulative incidence methodology [16] is used to account for patients who experience the competing risk before the event of interest, instead of treating them the same as patients that have not experienced the event of interest or a competing risk event, as would be done with the Kaplan-Meier method, in order to estimate the failure. Gray's test [17] is then used to compare the failure between treatments. This approach starts with no patients having failed (0% failure) and increases as failures occur (graphically, the curves go from the bottom left up to the right over time). When reporting results at a given time point for an endpoint with competing risks, it is most appropriate to report as a percentage failure, instead of subtracting that percentage from 100% and reporting the percentage control. This can best be exemplified by the following sentence: The two-year overall survival was 50% and the two-year local control was 95%. How in the world can there be 95% local control at two years when only half of the patients are even alive at two years? The appropriate way to report this is: The two-year overall survival was 50% and the two-year local failure 5%. Understandably investigators – at least the glass-half-full type – prefer to report on 'control' rather than 'failure,' but hopefully the example shown here helps to explain why that is not appropriate numerically and will facilitate your understanding.

Subgroup Analyses

A subgroup analysis, in the context of treatment clinical trials, is looking at the treatment effect in a subset of patients based on a particular characteristic (e.g., tumor stage, gender, race, etc.). Why are subgroup analyses done? Appropriate subgroup analyses are performed because there is patient heterogeneity and there are scientific reasons to suggest that treatment effects may be different in different subgroups. Subgroup analyses should not be done because the overall clinical trial result was negative and the investigator wants to analyze every possible subgroup in order to find a positive p-value. Good subgroup analyses are defined a priori – that is, before the study results are collected, are based on characteristics known at randomization and with a specified hypothesis. There are two basic approaches to analyzing differences by subgroup: (i) modeling interaction effects (i.e., using a treatment by t-stage variable); and (ii) doing separate analyses within subgroups (i.e., comparing treatments within the T1/T2 patients and separately within the T3/T4 patients). One of the biggest problems with subgroup analyses is a lack of statistical power. By definition, a given subgroup will have fewer events than the overall trial, and since the statistical power to detect the hypothesized difference is driven by number of events, there will be less statistical power within the subgroup to detect the same alternative hypothesis that was used to design the overall trial. However, if the treatment effect within a subgroup is larger than the hypothesized effect for the overall study, there may be sufficient statistical power to detect it. One might say "Why not power the trial for an interaction effect or for a given subgroup?" Sometimes that is done, but that may overpower (i.e., require significantly more patients/resources) the overall trial. If the trial is powered for an interaction effect, the approximate required increase in the sample size is fourfold. That should only be done if the interaction is of primary interest. The original NRG/RTOG 9704 adjuvant pancreas trial allowed head, body, and tail pancreas cancers and was designed to detect an increase in OS, with a projected monthly accrual of 5. Once the accrual was ramped up, and very importantly before any interim analysis looks at the data, the actual monthly accrual was much higher than projected, over 10 patients per month. There was a definite interest in an a priori-defined subgroup of head of the pancreas patients, but under the original accrual projections this was not able to be included. Given the increased accrual, the trial was amended to increase the sample size to include a specific analysis of treatment effect for the head of the pancreas patients at 80% statistical power, and the overall trial power increased to 85%. Given that the subgroup of head of the pancreas was defined a priori and sufficiently powered, results of that subgroup from this Phase III trial are considered definitive. Subgroup analyses that are not defined a priori and/or not sufficiently powered are exploratory, not definitive. While not definitive, they may still be hypothesis-generating. This is a very important point, especially when subgroup analyses are reported as being negative, without any information as to the statistical power for the hypothesized difference. Another important issue in subgroup analyses is multiple testing. Remember that for any hypothesis test there is always a false positive rate (α). Within a dataset, when there are many tests being done, the probability of finding at least one statistically significant result increases with multiple testing, as shown in the table below:

No. of tests	1	2	3	5	10	20
Probability*	0.05	0.10	0.14	0.23	0.40	0.64

*Probability of at least one statistical significant result at $\alpha = 0.05$, given no true differences.

Investigators have jokingly said "…this is great – if I do enough tests I can get a significant result." That clearly is not the take-home message here. There are many ways to adjust for the issue of multiple comparisons [18]. One way is to take the overall α and divide it by the number of tests being done (Bonferroni) so that if there are 10 multiple tests, instead of comparing to an α of 0.05, each test result would be compared to an α of 0.005. Another approach is to set a stricter level than 0.05, such as 0.01. The important point is that the approach for multiple testing needs to be set prior to doing the multiple testing.

While the ideal is a priori, sufficiently powered subgroup analyses, that is not always possible, so it is important to be complete with the reporting of any subgroup analysis. The number of subgroup analyses done (not just the number reported), whether or not they were planned a priori, and the rationale for the chosen subgroups, should all be included. As is true for most analyses, go beyond the p-value! The number of patients, number of events, effect sizes (e.g., hazard ratios), appropriate point estimates (e.g., two-year OS) and all corresponding confidence intervals should be reported. Although this may sound heretical to some investigators, it is often appropriate to report all of the above information without formal statistical testing – meaning no p-values, which are often misinterpreted in subgroup analyses. When reporting subgroups (a priori or not) as part of an overall prospective clinical trial, they should not be in place of the primary endpoint of the study.

Non-Positive Trials

Figure 5.4 Panel 1 shows data from a positive trial where the blue survival curve represents the increase in OS as hypothesized in the trial design, and the log-rank analysis met the criteria for being statistically significant (i.e., the p-value was less than or equal to the a prior set α-level). Panel 2 shows a non-positive trial with the survival curves on top of each other at the level of the hypothesized control arm. Panel 3 shows a clear separation in the survival curves, but unfortunately in the opposite direction than was hypothesized. When results such as this occur, the first question the investigator usually asks the statistician is "Did you code the treatment arms correctly?" Interestingly enough, when there is clear separation in the treatment arms in the hypothesized direction, the investigator never asks the statisticians about correct coding. In all honesty, when a statistician sees a result in a completely opposite direction, they themselves are double- and triple-checking their coding. Results like this do occur, and when they do additional analyses are generally performed to try and explain the results. Finally, Panel 4 shows a clear separation of the

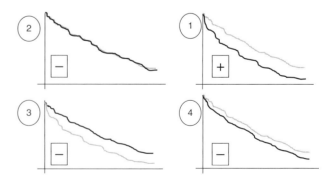

Figure 5.4 Types of non-positive trials.

survival curves in the hypothesized direction, but not to the extent that was hypothesized, and therefore the log-rank analysis did not meet the criteria for being statistically significant (i.e., the p-value was greater than the a priori set α-level). Does a statistically non-significant result imply that the difference observed is not clinically meaningful? Not necessarily, which is why it is important to look beyond the p-value at the reported effect size and corresponding confidence intervals. As discussed earlier in the chapter, although the ideal clinical trial is designed for the smallest clinically meaningful difference, that is not always feasible. Although a negative result per the protocol design, these results may still be clinically meaningful and should be discussed further. There are various reasons why a Phase III trial ends up with non-positive results. It may be that there really is no clinical benefit to the treatment. Perhaps the early phase clinical evidence that led to the Phase III trial was biased in an unknown way, or those results fell into the false-positive category. Another possibility is that the endpoints used for early phase trials were not predictive of the endpoint used in the definitive Phase III trial (e.g., CR and OS). Of course, there is always the possibility of a false-negative result. Using Phase III trials as the setting, many people examine the results of a Phase III trial and when they see what is in Panel 1, there is much of celebration and a plan for a sub-

mission to the *New England Journal of Medicine*. Unfortunately, too many people, when they do not see what is in Panel 1, they say 'bummer, negative trial' and more often than they should (which is really never) make much less of an effort to publish the results. While this example is in terms of a Phase III trial, the importance of publishing 'non-positive' results of trials that are well designed and executed is true across the board. NCI's National Clinical Trials Network (NCTN) Groups, who conduct well-designed and executed trials, have an outstanding track record of making sure all trial results are submitted for publication.

Conclusion

In summary, the statistician plays an integral role as a co-investigator from the beginning of a clinical trial idea, through study design, data collection, analyses, and the interpretation and publication of the results. Neither the statistician nor the principal investigator is in it or can truly do it alone, it needs to be a true collaboration and communication is key. The statistical topics discussed in this chapter provide a sound foundation for a radiation oncologist, or any investigator, in understanding the various statistical aspects of a clinical trial.

References

1 Piantadosi, S. (1988) Principles of clinical trial design. *Semin. Oncol.*, **15**, 423–433.

2 Leventhal, B.G. (1988) An overview of clinical trials in oncology. *Semin. Oncol.*, **15**, 412–422.

3 Bradley, J.D., Paulus, R., Komaki, R., Masters, G., *et al.* (2015) Standard-dose versus high-dose conformal radiotherapy with concurrent and consolidation carboplatin plus paclitaxel with or without cetuximab for patients with stage IIIA or IIIB non-small-cell lung cancer (RTOG 0617): a randomised, two-by-two factorial phase 3 study. *Lancet Oncol.*, **16** (2), 187–199.

4 Ellenberg, S. (1989) Biostatistics in clinical trials: Part 2 Determining sample sizes for clinical trials. *Oncology*, **3**, 39–46.

5 O'Quigley, J., Pepe, M., Fisher, L. (1990) Continual reassessment method: a practical design for Phase I clinical trials in cancer. *Biometrics*, **46**, 33–48.

6 Piantadosi, S., Fisher, J., Grossman, S. (1998) Practical implementation of a modified continual reassessment method for dose-finding trials. *Cancer Chemother. Pharmacol.*, **41**, 429–436.

7 O'Quigley, J. (1990) Another look at two Phase I clinical trial designs. *Stat. Med.*, **18**, 2638–2690.

8 Cheung, K., Chappell, R. (2000) Sequential designs for phase I clinical trials with late-onset toxicities. *Biometrics*, **56**, 1177–1182.

9 Normolle, D., Lawrence, T. (2006) Designing dose escalation trials with late onset toxicities using the time-to-event continual reassessment method. *J. Clin. Oncol.*, **24**, 4426–4433.

10 Rubinstein, L.V., Korn, E.L., Freidlin, B., *et al.* (2005) Design issues of randomized phase II trials and a proposal for phase II screening trials. *J. Clin. Oncol.*, **23** (28), 7199–7206.

11 Lachin, J.M. (1988) Statistical properties of randomization in clinical trials. *Control. Clin. Trials*, **9**, 289–311.

12 Temple, R., Ellenberg, S.S. (2000) Placebo-controlled trials and active control trials in the evaluation of new treatments. Part 1: Ethical and scientific issues. *Ann. Intern. Med.*, **133**, 455–463.

13 Lan, K., DeMets, E. (1983) Discrete sequential boundaries for clinical trials. *Biometrika*, **70**, 659–663.

14 Kaplan, E.L., Meier, P. (1958) Nonparametric estimation from incomplete observations. *J. Stat. Assoc.*, **53**, 457–481.

15 Mantel, N. (1966) Evaluation of survival data and two new rank order statistics arising in its consideration. *Cancer Chemother. Rep.*, **50**, 163–170.

16 Kalbfleish, J.D., Prentice, R.L. (1980) *The Statistical Analysis of Failure Time Data*. John Wiley & Sons, New York.

17 Gray, R.J. (1988) A class of K-sample tests for comparing the cumulative incidence of a competing risk. *Ann. Stat.*, **16**, 1141–1154.

18 Green, S., Benedetti, J., Crowley, C. (2012) *Clinical Trials in Oncology*, 3rd edition. Chapman & Hall/CRC.

6

Use of Protons for Radiation Therapy

Mark Pankuch, Nasiruddin Mohammed, Draik Hecksel, Steve Laub, Sean Boyer and William F. Hartsell

Introduction

The goal of any radiation therapy treatment is to deliver the prescribed dose to the target area while minimizing dose to all surrounding healthy tissues. In the past several years, there have been many advances in which x-ray therapy can be delivered, including three-dimensional (3D) conformal methods, intensity-modulated radiation therapy (IMRT), and **volumetric-modulated arc therapy** (VMAT). Each of these advanced techniques improves some component of the treatment plan, but all are limited by the physical properties of the incident photon beam. High-energy photon fields are bound by the laws of physics which require an initial build-up of dose in the first several millimeters, followed by an exponential deposition of photon dose as the beam progresses deeper in the patient, then eventually exiting through the patient. The initial build-up and subsequent deposition of dose beyond the target of an x-ray field results in unwanted dose to non-target structures. Often, it is this unwanted dose to critical structures that generates the dose limitations to the target and therefore decreases the therapeutic ratio.

In 1946, Robert R. Wilson published the first work that suggested that the unique properties of heavy charged particles (a mass much larger than an electron) could present a radiobiological advantage over standard photon therapy [1]. Heavy charged particles deliver a low entrance dose, and then at a depth determined by the incident particle's energy deposit a highly concentrated dose, and stop with no further dose released to tissues downstream. This property can be exploited to reduce integral dose to the patient and potentially increase the therapeutic ratio.

The concentrated dose at the end of a particle path is a consequence of a dramatic change in the rate of energy transfer from the particle to the media. The loss of energy per unit path length of the particle is characterized by the linear energy transfer (LET) of the particle and may be very different when compared to photons. Local LET values may result in different radiobiological consequences to both target and healthy tissue presenting another potential benefit and/or drawback of particle therapy [2].

Heavy charged particles used for therapy have included several different large ions such as helium, neon, argon, carbon, negative pi measons (pions) and, most commonly, a single hydrogen ion, a proton [2]. The aim of this chapter is to describe the use of protons in the clinical environment as these treatments are by far the most common forms of particle therapy currently being offered.

The Desire for Better Radiation Therapy

The goal of a curative radiotherapy treatment is to deliver a dose to the tumor that is high enough to establish local control and prevent metastatic spread while avoiding toxicities, both acute and long-term to all nearby structures. Very often, unacceptable dose to nearby structures is the limiting constraint to the total dose delivered to the target. New techniques in photon-based radiotherapy such as 3D conformal and IMRT have allowed more conformity of the high prescription dose to targets. These methods also enable good control of the placement of the mid- and low-dose spillover, which are characteristic of all photon beams. Unfortunately, for the planner, low- and mid-dose spillover regions must be delivered somewhere, and spillover locations with their associated dose levels are prioritized based on reported toxicity information [3]. This leaves the radiation oncologist with a struggle to negotiate between potential local tumor control and normal tissue damage. The unique properties of protons, with their very different dose distributions,

Clinical Radiation Oncology: Indications, Techniques, and Results, Third Edition. Edited by William Small Jr.
© 2017 John Wiley & Sons, Inc. Published 2017 by John Wiley & Sons, Inc.

can be used in some cases to not only reduce dose the healthy tissues but also to eliminate all dose to an organ at risk. This provides the radiation oncologist with a very different options and priorities in the plan optimization process.

Local Tumor Control

Rates of local failure for malignant tumors vary widely from about 10% to 90%, and will depend on several factors including tumor size, tumor pathology, and tumor location [4–8]. For patients that present with local tumor progression after a completing a course of radiation therapy, cure rates of less than 30% are found in cases where salvage surgery is even possible [9]. If a local failure does occur, the patient's long-term prognosis and quality of life are generally very poor [10–12]. These poor outcomes emphasize the importance of delivering an effective and accurate therapeutic dose to the target when a curative intent is the main goal for treatment.

The shape of a typical tumor control probability (TCP) curve indicates that there is an increasing probability of tumor control as the treatment doses are increased. The incremental increase in TCP is not linear as the dose increases. There is an increase in the incremental TCP per unit dose up to a maximum value at the mid-portion of the curve. The incremental increase in TCP per unit dose then begins to decrease above the mid portion of the curve until some point where any amount of additional dose will show no benefit to control probability. The shape of the TCP curve identifies that, in some cases, even small amounts of additional dose may results in large increases in tumor control. The magnitude of the benefit in increasing dose depends where each patient's prescribed dose falls on their specific tumor's control probability. If the distinctive properties of particle therapy can be used to enable the radiation oncologist to increase the treatment doses – either through a higher relative biological effectiveness or by diminishing dose escalation limitations resulting from normal tissue complications – an increased control rate for patient treated with protons can be expected.

Normal Tissue Damage

The modern clinical environment using photons for treatment have set dosing protocols to ensure that a significant amount of normal tissue damage is not typically observed in everyday practice. Photon doses are prescribed to ensure acceptable morbidity rates of 5% or less for most curative treatments. In some cases, the dose limits are set using these expected toxicity levels with an acceptance of the resulting TCP at this dose. TCP is therefore constrained by the normal tissue's limiting dose.

Emami *et al.* reported tolerance doses to several healthy organs based on the relative volume of the organ irradiated [13]. More recently the QUANTEC report [3] provided a more detailed, model-based collection of dose–response and dose–volume relationships specific to several organ-specific locations. These reports are currently used as the 'gold standards' to predict normal tissue complications.

According to these dose–response reports, the incidence and severity of treatment-related morbidity is a function the volume of critical organ included in the irradiated volume, the dose delivered to that organ, and the functional capacity of the organ. An obvious conclusion can therefore be made that reducing the dose to uninvolved functional tissues will decrease the potential for morbidity. Particle beams reduce the amount of integral dose as compared to photon beams. Exploiting this benefit in an effort to decrease integral dose to healthy tissues is one of the main driving motivations for particle therapy.

Improvements in Dose Distributions

It is most likely that there will be limitations to the magnitude of improved tumor control that can be expected if higher dose protocols are achievable by using the new technical advances in radiation therapy. Using new technology with improved dose control can enable the radiation oncologist to decrease dose to organs at risk. In addition, the radiation oncologist can consider increasing target doses up to the limits of prior equivalent doses to the organs at risk. This ability will create the need to validate new dosing protocols that may be very specific to the treatment delivery technology.

The ability to treat the target to the planned doses has improved remarkably during the past two decades. Advanced imaging techniques, specifically computed tomography (CT), positron emission tomography (PET) and magnetic resonance imaging (MRI) can provide accurate 3D models of the patient for better calculations and improved organ and target delineation. Four-dimensional (4D) CT scanning has been clinically adopted in many departments to provide additional information of the internal motion of organs and target volumes throughout the respiratory cycle. This 4D information can be correlated in the treatment delivery process with methods such as beam gating to spare more healthy tissues. Image guidance in the treatment position has improved the alignment of the treatment beam with the patient's target on a day-to-day basis. With better knowledge of tumor position, margins that are added to account for set-up errors can be reduced, sparing more healthy tissues. Notably with particle therapy, the clinical adaption of proton tomography or proton radiography with Monte Carlo calculation methods may soon improve dose calculation reliability [14–18].

Each of these advancements has improved the overall quality of the treatment for the patients. Large improvements have been realized and quickly implemented into the clinical environment. Additional incremental improvements when using photons may be reaching a technological limit. The exploitation of alternative dose-delivery methods, including the special dose-delivery properties of particle therapy, is one potential method to continue these positive trends.

History of Proton Beam Therapy

Some 70 years ago, Robert Wilson suggested that protons offered several advantages for use in clinical radiotherapy because of their physical characteristics [1]. Comparative dose distributions for protons, photons and electrons were presented in 1972 by Koehler and Preston [19], while potential advantages of protons for para-aortic irradiation were proposed in 1974 by Archambauu *et al.* [20]. Clinical studies were first reported from the University of California at San Francisco (UCSF) and the Lawrence Berkely Laboratory (LBL) in 1955 [21,22], from the University of Uppsala, Sweden, in 1957 [23], from the Massachusetts General Hospital and the Harvard Cyclotron laboratory in 1961 [24–26], and from the Physics Research Institute at Dubna, Russia, in 1964 and the Institute for Experimental and Theoretical Physics (ITEP) in Moscow in 1969 [27]. The treatments applied during the 1950s at Uppsala resulted in the creation of techniques such as beam scanning for the production of large treatment fields, and range modulation for the creation of the Bragg peak which were first implemented at the University of Uppsala [28,29]. The Harvard Cyclotron Laboratory demonstrated the first use of passive scattering for lateral beam spreading and rotating modulator wheels for range modulation [28]. Proton therapy started in Japan in 1979 at the National Institute for Radiological Science at Chiba, and by 1980 this group had developed a pencil beam scanning (PBS) system [28]. The Particle Radiation Medical Science Center in Tsukuba was the first center to use a vertical treatment beam and multileaf collimator in 1983 [28,30]. The first hospital-based proton therapy center was established at Loma Linda University Medical Center in California, and the first patient was treated there in 1990 [28]. The Loma Linda facility was built around a dedicated synchrotron that provided protons to four treatment rooms, including three gantries, and a research room.

Through the 2000s there was a large increase in the number of proton therapy centers in operation. In 2004, there were four centers in operation in the United States, but by the end of 2010 there were 10 proton therapy centers treating patients [31]. Currently there are 16 proton therapy treatment centers in operation in the United States, and an additional 33 treatment centers worldwide. As of December 2014, over 118 000 patients had been treated using proton therapy, and over 137 000 if including patients treated with other heavy particles besides protons [32]. Proton therapy centers treat a wide range of sites including pediatrics, breast, lung, head and neck, central nervous system, lymphoma, sarcoma, liver and eye [33].

Charged Particle Beam Therapy – Better Dose Distributions

Charged Particles Versus X-Ray

Charged particle beams such as protons and heavier ions provide a dosimetric advantage over megavoltage x-rays due to their energy deposition characteristics. The following discussion relates specifically to proton beams, but is generally applicable to heavier ions. Protons have a low ionization density at the surface of tissue, but this slowly increases as the proton reaches the end of its finite penetration depth. Near the end of the proton's path, the ionization density increases sharply over a narrow region, resulting in a Bragg peak [19]. The penetration depth can be calculated based on the initial energy of the incident proton and the stopping power of the medium. For treatment purposes, the maximum proton energy is selected so that a portion of the delivered protons reach their maximum penetration depth at the distal end of the target volume relative to the beam direction. The proton beam avoids depositing energy in tissue beyond the intended volume. This is a very different dose-deposition behavior when compared to x-rays that undergo an exponential decrease in intensity through tissue. One unavoidable characteristic of an exponential decrease in dose is the unwanted exit radiation dose to healthy tissue beyond the radiation target volume. Additionally, in x-ray fields tissues proximal to the target along the photon beam direction will receive an increasing dose as the distance increases from the target. An example of the depth dose curves for a megavoltage x-ray beam, a single energy proton beam and a modulated proton beam are shown in Figure 6.1.

Spread-Out Bragg Peak and Dose Uniformity

A mono-energetic proton beam is of limited clinical value owing to the narrow region of high dose in the Bragg peak. By summing a distribution of decreasing proton energies, a uniform region of dose can be produced at the depth of interest within the patient. This is commonly known as a spread out Bragg peak (SOBP).

Depth Dose Curves for Different Treatment Modalities

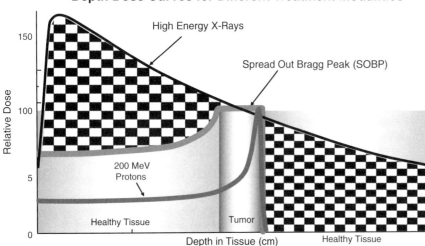

Figure 6.1 Depth dose curves for protons and photons. A single Bragg peak (red line) does not cover the target area, so several peaks are integrated together to form the spread-out Bragg peak (blue line). The checkered areas define where dose is deposited with photons, but is not delivered with protons. For a color version of this figure, see the color plate section.

In order to create a uniform 3D dose distribution, the proton beam extracted from the accelerator must be spread in two directions, both laterally and in depth. Passive scattering systems use combinations of scattering foils to create the lateral distribution and rotating modulator wheels or ridge filters to create the distribution in depth [34, 35]. Uniform scanning systems use magnets to spread the beam laterally, and similar range-shifting hardware to create the distribution in depth [36]. Both scattering and uniform scanning systems use a compensator at the end of the treatment nozzle to further shape the distal end of the treatment field to account for variances in desired proton path length, and to modify proton energy to account for inhomogeneities along the beam path. Compensators are used to improve conformity to the distal shape of the target. Scattering and uniform scanning systems also use brass apertures to shape the proton field around the target volume laterally (see Figure 6.2) [35]. The use of multileaf collimators (MLCs) has been introduced into proton therapy and has been used clinically [37–39].

Another delivery method used to shape the beam both laterally and in depth is known as pencil beam scanning (PBS). In PBS, the range is modulated upstream of the treatment nozzle, and scanning magnets place the proton beam at individual spot locations throughout the treatment volume. [40–42]. A full 3D volume is treated using a pattern of spots at various proton energies corresponding to the depths required to cover the target volume. The ability to weight individual spots within the treatment volume allows for more complex dose distribution for a single treatment field, especially when combined with multiple intensity modulated proton fields. The differences in dose distributions of a proton field treating a simple sphere using an open SOBP, an SOBP with a compensator, and a PBS field is demonstrated in Figure 6.3.

The use of any proton-delivery method allows for the creation of elegant dose distributions that may be relatively simple when compared to equivalent x-ray dose distributions that require using multiple treatment angles, field sizes, beam energies, intensities, and modifiers. When compared to x-rays, protons provide a lower

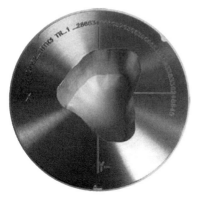

Brass Aperture

(a)

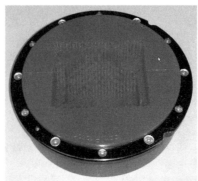

Machinist Wax Compensator

(b)

Figure 6.2 A patient-specific aperture and compensator. (a) Apertures define the field shape in the direction lateral to the beam direction. Compensators are used to shape the distal edge to the apertures and compensator, and are unique to every patient and every field.

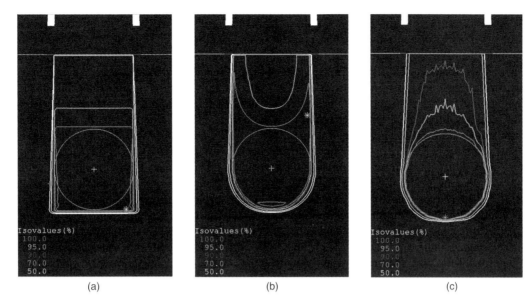

Figure 6.3 A sphere is treated with a single proton field from the top. (a) An uncompensated SOBP. (b) A SOBP with a range compensator providing improved distal conformality. Distal dose is displaced from the distal side to the proximal end when using the compensator. (c) A PBS beam; PBS allows for both distal and proximal shaping of the dose. For a color version of this figure, see the color plate section.

dose proximal to the target volume, a uniform dose distribution across the target volume, and no exit dose. These characteristics give protons their advantage during treatment planning.

Relative Biologic Effectiveness (RBE) and Linear Energy Transfer (LET)

Both proton and photons are classified as low-LET radiation. Except for in the most distal region of the Bragg peak, particles lose relatively low amounts of their total energy via ionization, excitation and nuclear interactions as they progress along the beam's path. The rate of energy loss is ~35 keV μm^{-1} in the entrance region [2]. Near the end of a proton beam's range, a rapid loss of energy occurs, associated with production of a limited zone of high-LET radiation (dense ionization). This results in the characteristic Bragg peak of the proton beam shown in Figure 6.1. In an SOBP, the LET of many distal peaks will be distributed across the entire SOBP and will increase up to a maximum at the distal edge. The higher average LET increases the biological effectiveness of the proton beam. A summary of both *in vitro* and *in vivo* data examining proton RBE can be found in ICRU report 78 [2]. The experimental data have shown that the average RBE for protons in a laboratory setting is 1.1. There are no proton RBE values based on clinical experience, so experimental data has been applied and is in the process of validation in the clinical setting. At the present time, clinical experience has not shown that a generic proton RBE value is significantly different than 1.1. It is therefore recommended by ICRU report 78 that a proton dose be reported as $D_{(RBE)}$, which is equal to the physical proton dose multiplied by the constant RBE factor of 1.1 which is independent of depth, LET, and target cell type.

It should also be noted that experimental and theoretical data show that there is potential of an additional increase in RBE on the declining edge of the SOBP where the average LET is the greatest. The higher RBE in this region results in an effective increase of the range of the RBE weighted absorbed dose by 1–2 mm, depending on the energy of distal layer of the SOBP [2]. This effect is not accounted for when using the generic RBE value of 1.1. It is necessary to consider this potential 'distal edge effect' during treatment planning if the distal edges of many fields overlap. or if a distal edge is near a critical structure.

Treatment Planning Considerations with Protons

Treatment Planning in Proton Therapy

Treatment planning for proton radiation therapy has many similarities to traditional x-ray radiation therapy. A 3D model of the patient is obtained via CT-based, volumetric imaging of the patient in the treatment position. The images of the treatment planning CT can be registered with complementary diagnostic imaging modalities, such as PET and MRI to assist the radiation oncologist in defining target regions and organs at risk (OARs). Based on the specifications of the delivery system, the treatment planner will choose treatment angles, beam energies and field weights with careful consideration of the position of the targets relative to the OARs. Additional margins are required to account for systematic and random errors that may be present in the patient set-up procedure, internal motion within the patient during treatment, and the accuracy limitations of the delivery system. The patient then is treated with a dose in accordance with the written directive. The following sections will illuminate some of the major differences between proton and x-ray radiation treatments with respect to treatment planning.

Computed Tomography (CT) and the Volumetric Model of the Patient

The volumetric model obtained of the patient in the treatment position has several purposes. The model is used to define targets and OARs. In addition, the 3D map of the CT's Hounsfield Units (HU) is converted and used by the treatment planning system to calculate the expected dose distribution. Photon treatment planning systems often use a look-up table to convert the HU into a physical density or electron density relative to water. For proton planning, the relative stopping power is needed. The conversion of x-ray HU to proton relative stopping power (RSP) is not direct, and stoichiometric methods [43] have been described to approximate this conversion. Because the RSP conversion is an approximation, a thorough evaluation of the uncertainty in this method is necessary and must be accounted for in the planning process. These additional distal and proximal margins, often referred to as range uncertainties, are unique to protons and must be accounted for to avoid the unacceptable potential of underdosing the targets and/or overdosing of OARs [14–16]. A consensus on the magnitude of range uncertainties is still under investigation and has been assigned to a Task Group 202 within the American Association of Medical Physicists. In general, these uncertainties are 2.5–4% of the proton's incident range plus 1–3 mm.

Any degradations of the image quality of a patient's model CT must also be carefully reviewed to accurately calculate the expected dose and range in the patient. Any image artifacts resulting from high-density material need to be properly defined and forced to the appropriate density. Images where the patient's external contour is not included in the reconstruction algorithm can lead to incorrect derivation of HU and therefore incorrect RSP values. Any implanted devices, such as a silicone prosthesis, should be independently verified to minimize potential calculation errors [43]. Typical planning processes avoid treating with a proton beam directly through high-density materials whenever possible.

Care is taken in the simulation process to produce an environment that will assist in reproducibly positioning the patient throughout the entire treatment course. Additional care in the case of protons is needed to mitigate any potential perturbations of the proton beam generated by changes in path length of the proton beam within the set-up immobilization devices. Smooth, rounded shapes of uniform thickness without discrete edges within the beam path are preferred in the case of protons, and can be more easily modeled within the planning system. Treatment couches of known relative stopping power with of uniform thicknesses are used with treatment plans developed to avoid any beam from entering through treatment couch edges.

Target Definitions

The delineation of anatomy in photon therapy and in proton therapy is identical. For appropriate comparisons between photon and proton treatments, it is essential that OARs, gross target volume (GTV) and clinical target volume (CTV) are defined by the same guidelines. In the treatment planning process, additional volumes are often derived by adding geometric margins to account for various alignment uncertainties that cannot be avoided during the actual treatment process. Volumetric expansions to the GTV and CTV to account for internal motion by using and internal target volume (ITV) can be added to avoid a geometric miss of a moving target. Planning target volume (PTV) expansions are added to account for the day-to-day geometric variations in the patient's set-up. Both of these expansions used in photon therapy still apply in the case of protons to avoid a geometric miss of the target in the directions lateral to the proton treatment beam. However, in the direction parallel to the proton beam, distal and proximal margins are needed to account for the range uncertainty discussed above, in addition to any potential range changes which resulted from a set-up uncertainty. The latter effect can be easily accounted for when using aperture/compensator based delivery in a method known as 'smearing' of the compensator, and is discussed below. The addition of range uncertainties is slightly more complex due to the fact that these margins must be added in terms of water equivalent path lengths of the proton beam and are not just geometric expansions. The distal range uncertainty across a given proton field therefore can vary, depending on the RSP of the tissues downstream of the target and the direction of the incident beam. This is demonstrated for a lung patient in Figure 6.4. The standard PTV expansion concept is a not valid representation for appropriate margins of a proton beam, and alternative methods that are specific to the treatment delivery method are used [45–47].

Treatment Delivery Techniques

In all proton-delivery systems, the protons are accelerated to the required energy and then are spread across the target. For treatment planning purposes, delivery systems can be broken down into two types: (i) those that use apertures and compensators (single scattered,

Figure 6.4 A GTV (red) and CTV (blue) are defined. The PTV (yellow) is generated by expanding the CTV by 0.5 cm. The physical expansion of 0.5 cm can be used to avoid geometric misses of the target. When addressing range uncertainty, expansions are dependent on the water equivalent thicknesses (WET), which can be very different depending on the beam angle. In panel (a), the physical distance of 0.5 mm is only 0.12 cm of WET due to the low density of the lung tissues. In panel (b) the WET is 0.57 cm, and is greater than the physical expansion of 0.5 cm due to the higher-density bone. For a color version of this figure, see the color plate section.

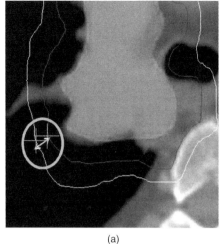
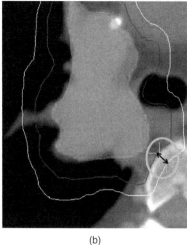

(a) (b)

double scattered, and uniform scanning); and (ii) those that use PBS.

Aperture/Compensator-Based Planning Methods

Aperture and compensator-based planning uses forward-planning methods, analogous to 3D conformal radiation therapy (3DCRT). With the aid of the treatment planning system, the planner designs beam portal openings and compensator thickness in an effort to conform the dose to the target and minimize dose to nearby OARs. The aperture is used to conform the dose in the direction lateral to the beam direction, and is essentially a silhouette of the target projection. The compensator is used to conform the high-dose regions to the distal end of the target in the direction parallel to the treatment beam.

The aperture used in proton treatments are analogous to the high-density blocks used in 3DCRT planning and the MLCs used more commonly today in photon therapy. The lateral edges of the proton treatment portal are defined by the aperture, and an appropriate aperture thickness is needed to ensure all incident protons are completely stopped within the aperture. Apertures are often made of high-density materials such as brass or lead alloys (see Figure 6.2a). Depending on the size of the portal, some apertures can be large and must be made thick to stop high-energy protons. In these cases, duplicate apertures can be manufactured and used collectively to limit the weight of any individual device.

In aperture- and compensator-based delivery, the projected proton source is large due to the scattering of the proton beam [2]. Much like Co-60 teletherapy of the past, this large source size increases the geomantic penumbra of the field and undesirably blurs the field edges, giving additional unwanted dose to the patient. To mitigate this effect, the apertures are brought as close to the patient as possible by using a retractable snout that holds the

apertures and compensators in place during treatment. The air gap, or the distance between the patient and the distal edge of the snout, is often less than 10 cm.

A compensator (see Figure 6.2b) – also called a 'bolus' at some proton centers – is placed after the aperture and is used to modify the range of the incident protons across a specific field. Compensators are designed to create distal conformity to the target's shape. They are manufactured using low-atomic number materials such as Lucite or machinist's wax to minimize proton scattering while degrading the proton's energy. Compensator are often plunge-milled using modern CNC (computerized numerical control) milling machinery. It should be noted that every patient and every field will require a unique set of apertures and compensators for each field. Any changes in target or the patient that may require adaptive planning most often require complete remanufacturing of these devices.

The compensator is designed by the treatment planning system with specific considerations of the discrete path lengths of protons originating at the surface of the patient and tracked to distal edge of the target. Along each ray, the path length of the proton beam is calculated and any difference from the deepest depth is added to the compensator. This additional compensator material pulls the range back where it is needed and produces the desired distal conformity.

Another benefit of the physical compensator is that fact that uncertainties in the range due to patient set-up error can be included in the compensator design. This process is known 'compensator smearing.' As each individual ray is calculated during planning, adjacent rays can be evaluated for the effects of potential patient misalignment. Including any potential effects of patient misalignment by adding smearing will decrease the conformity to the distal end of the target, but will ensure that the appropriate range is available to treat the deepest edge of the target.

Pencil Beam Scanning

Treatment planning for PBS delivery uses inverse-planning, which is analogous to IMRT. In inverse planning, a set of desired dosing goals are prioritized and evaluated using iterative methods to improve the plan. The optimizer varies spot position, beam energy and spot weights in an effort to minimize the cost function defined by the dosing goals. PBS plans may use several thousand spots to reach the desired target coverage with the lowest OAR doses. There have been several studies demonstrating that inverse-planning with PBS delivery can provide better target coverage along with OAR sparing when compared to photon IMRT and aperture/compensator-based proton therapy [48,49].

As in aperture/compensator-based planning, PBS allows lateral and distal conformity to the target regions. The scanning system controls the positions of each spot, eliminating the need for both an apertures and compensators. An additional advantage that PBS offers is the added ability for proximal conformity that is not available when using aperture/compensator-based methods (see Figure 6.3c). With the control of spot intensity, spatially variable dosing is also possible with PBS methods including such techniques as integrated simultaneous boost.

There are two planning techniques that can be used when optimizing more than one PBS treatment field on an individual target. These include single-field uniform dose (SFUD) optimization and multifield optimized (MFO). SFUD requires that each single beam delivers a uniform dose over the entire target region on its own. SFUD-optimized fields will not rely on other beams to for target coverage. In SFUD, the dose is very uniform within the target area and there are no high gradients of dose within the target regions. This makes SFUD-optimized plans less sensitive to misalignments, but may limit how well a target can be covered and how effectively the OARs can be spared. MFO optimization methods allow the dose of one field to supplement the dose of the other fields. Each field can rely on the dose delivered by other beams to give proper target coverage. Because individual beams from an MFO plan are not constrained to fully cover the target, this optimization method can create greater flexibility in dose-sparing. A disadvantage when using MFO is that internal motion, set-up errors and range uncertainty can produce very large dose deviations. Figure 6.5 shows the SFUD and MFO concept on an 'L'-shaped target near an OAR.

Internal motion, set-up errors and range uncertainty may create the condition that the dose delivered to the patient will not match that represented in the original treatment plan. Potential deviations must be evaluated during the planning process to determine whether these uncertainties are adequately considered – a process called 'robustness evaluation' [50]. A plan with good robustness will deliver the prescribed target dose even in the presence of specific uncertainties and maintain appropriate dose levels to OARs. Robust evaluation includes the re-calculations of planned spot patterns with misalignments of the treatment fields. To simulate range uncertainty, errors are introduced to the HU conversion process and planned spot patterns are recalculated; the resulting distribution is then evaluated. Coverage of the CTV in all of these potential scenarios must be evaluated and declared to be appropriate before determining if the plan can be safely delivered to the patient. This is an additional step in the plan evaluation process that is very unique to PBS planning. Newer treatment planning systems are able to include robustness directly into the optimization process. By including robustness at the time of optimization, individual spots that are more dependent on patient set-up errors or range uncertainty will be preferentially penalized and decreased in overall weight. This process may decrease target coverage and increase OAR doses, but will aid in generating a plan that that will have a greater probability of delivering the dose distribution presented in the nominal plan. At the present time, there are no unified procedures and no universally accepted criteria for robustness,

Clinical Results from Proton Therapy

The longest historical clinical experience with fractionated proton beam therapy has been in patients with uveal melanomas, skull base chordomas and chondrosarcomas, and prostate cancer. With the more recent growth in accessibility to particle beams, there has been an expansion in efforts to delineate other treatment sites that may benefit from the unique properties of protons. The subsections that follow discuss clinical indications, planning considerations, and current treatment protocols for patients with the historical sites of ocular neoplasms, skull-based targets and prostate cancer, along with more recently investigated sites actively being treated, including pediatric malignancies, lung, and breast.

Ocular Neoplasms

Choroidal melanomas occur in approximately 2000 to 2500 people annually in the United States. Until the past two decades the standard treatment for these tumors was enucleation. While enucleation remains an appropriate option for treatment, either plaque brachytherapy or proton beam therapy are good alternative treatments which provide similar long-term survival and disease-free survival outcomes, with preservation of the eye in many patients and also preservation of eyesight in a proportion of cases.

The COMS (Collaborative Ocular Melanoma Study) prospective trial of enucleation versus plaque

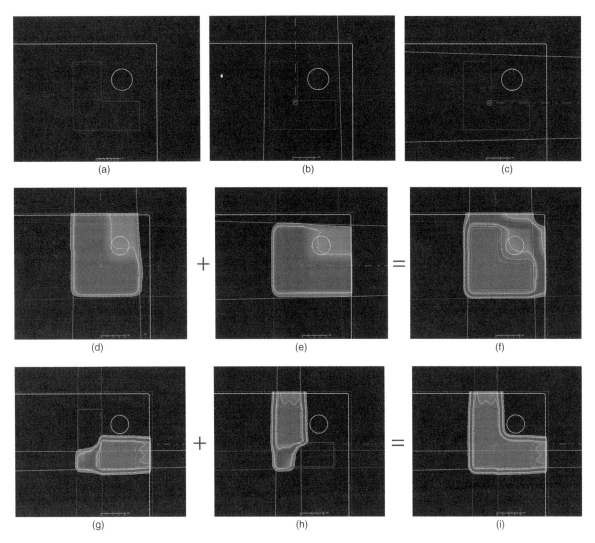

Figure 6.5 (a) A target (blue) is surrounding an OAR (yellow). (b) The target is treated with an anterior beam. (c) The target is treated with a lateral beam. (d–f) Single-field uniform dose (SFUD) optimized. Each proton field delivers a uniform dose to the target. SFUD plans are less sensitive to uncertainties. (g–i) Multi-field-optimized (MFO). Each individual field is optimized with dosimetric information of other fields. MFO allows for better sparing of OARs but is more sensitive to set-up and range uncertainties. For a color version of this figure, see the color plate section.

brachytherapy evaluated 1317 patients with localized choroidal tumors less than 16 mm in basal diameter and less than 10 mm in apical height. [51]. Patients were randomly assigned to enucleation or plaque brachytherapy. There was no difference in survival and disease-free survival between the two treatments at a median of 12 years' follow-up. The ten-year rates of death from metastatic melanoma were 17% following enucleation, and 18% with brachytherapy. The primary predictors of time to death were older age and larger tumor size. A prospective randomized trial from the University of California at San Francisco and the Lawrence Berkley National Laboratory evaluated plaque brachytherapy versus particle therapy in patients with localized ocular melanomas [52]. A total of 184 patients was randomly

assigned to plaque brachytherapy ($n = 98$) or treatment with helium particles ($n = 86$). At a median follow-up of greater than 12 years, there was no difference in survival between the two groups. However, the local control for patients treated with particles was 100% and 98% at 5 and 12 years, versus 84% and 79% for the patients treated with plaques (p-0.0006). The enucleation rate was significantly lower in the particle-treated patients (17% after particles versus 37% after plaques at 12 years), and treatment with particles was a significant predictor of long-term disease-free survival.

Wang *et al.* [53] performed a meta-analysis evaluating particle therapy versus brachytherapy, utilizing 27 studies with a total of 8809 ocular melanoma patients. Patients treated with particle therapy had a significantly lower risk of local recurrence than those with brachytherapy, although there were no significant differences in mortality or enucleation rates. There was also a lower risk of retinopathy or cataract formation rates with charged particle therapy compared to plaque brachytherapy.

Multiple institutions have lengthy experiences of using protons for the treatment of large numbers of patients with uveal melanomas. The group from Massachusetts General began treating patients at the Harvard cyclotron in 1975 [54], and reported their experience with more than 3000 patients in 2005, most of whom were treated with 70 Gy RBE in five fractions. The all-cause mortality rates were 49.0%, 58.6%, and 66.8% at 15, 20, and 25 years; melanoma-related mortality rates at those same intervals were 24.6%, 25.8%, and 26.4%. Younger patients (aged ≤60 years) with smaller tumors (≤11 mm) had a significantly lower melanoma-related mortality rate of 8.6% compared to older patients with larger tumors (40.1%).

The Paul Scherrer Institute (PSI) in Switzerland has used protons for the treatment of ocular melanomas since 1984 [55]. A total of 2645 patients was treated between 1984 and 1999 at PSI, and the overall eye-retention rates at 5, 10, and 15 years were 88.9%, 86.2%, and 83.7%. Using a continuous quality improvement program, the five-year eye-retention rates for patients treated more recently had improved to 100%, 99.7%, and 89.5%, for small, medium, and large tumors. Patients more likely to require eventual enucleation included those with larger tumor size (primarily apical height), proximity to optic disc, male gender, and retinal detachment at the time of treatment.

A large number of ocular melanoma patients have been treated at the Curie Institute proton center in Orsay [56]. Dendale *et al.* reported outcomes in 1406 patients treated between 1991 and 2001 with 60 Gy RBE in four fractions. The five-year survival and metastasis-free survivals were 79% and 80.6%, with a five-year local control rate of 96%. Only 7.7% of patients required enucleation at five years for recurrence or complications. As with other large series, the most important prognostic factors for survival and tumor control were large tumor size, older age, male gender, and tumors close to the optic nerve.

The optimal total dose and fractionation scheme with protons is not clear. There does appear to be universal agreement on the use of a hypofractionated treatment schedule, with doses of 10–15 Gy RBE per treatment for four to five treatments. Gragoudas *et al.* reported on a double-blind, randomized prospective trial from Massachusetts General and the Harvard Cyclotron, conducted between 1989 and 1994 [57]. Patients in this trial had tumors up to 5 mm in apical height and up to 15 mm in basal dimension. These were centrally located tumors, within 6 mm of the macula or optic disc. The patients were assigned to either 70 Gy RBE in five treatments (standard arm) or 50 Gy RBE in five treatments. There

was no difference in tumor regrowth, rate of metastases, visual acuity or maculopathy at five years after treatment. The lower dose group had a better retention of visual fields, and a non-significantly lower risk of papillopathy.

The process of care involves close collaboration by the ophthalmology and radiation oncology teams. The initial evaluation is performed by a retinal specialist. Although biopsy may be performed, the diagnosis is typically made based on clinical examination. The ophthalmologic examination includes fundoscopic images which are used to map the position of the tumor, while ultrasound images of the eye are performed to evaluate the dimensions of the tumor. The patient undergoes evaluation by the radiation oncologist and typically also a medical oncologist. A metastatic work-up is performed, primarily evaluating potential systemic disease. Special attention is directed to the liver and lungs. This had been done in the past using chest x-radiography and liver function blood tests, but currently is more commonly done using contrast-enhanced CT scans of the chest and abdomen, or CT/PET scans. The patient then undergoes a surgical procedure for placement of radio-opaque markers, such as tantalum clips. These clips are discs which are 2.5 mm in diameter, with holes in the center which allow for suturing to the sclera. Three to five clips are used to demarcate the tumor borders and as fiducials during treatment. Trans-illumination of the eye during this procedure is often used to help delineate the extent of the tumor. The patients then undergoes simulation, which is often performed in the seated position. A thermoplastic mask (or similar device, often including a dental mold) is used for immobilization, and the patients are instructed to gaze at a specific marker during the treatment. The gaze position depends on the location of the tumor in the eye. Metallic lid retractors may be used to more widely open the eyelids during treatment. Treatment is given over a period of four to ten days, with common fractionation schemes including 70 Gy RBE in five fractions, 60 Gy RBE in four fractions, 56 Gy RBE in four fractions, and 50 Gy RBE in five fractions.

Complications of treatment include rubeosis iridis, neovascular glaucoma, cataract formation, maculopathy, and optic neuropathy. There are certain cases in which protons would typically not be used as the primary treatment. These include patients with no vision in the eye, patients with very large tumors, or those with significant extrascleral extension of tumor. In such patients enucleation would be the preferred treatment.

In summary, proton beam therapy is an effective method for treating ocular melanoma, with obvious advantages over enucleation for most patients. Protons also have advantages over plaque brachytherapy in some patients. Only a single surgical procedure is required for protons (for the placement of high-density clips), whereas two procedures are required for plaques (placement and removal of the plaque). Placement of the plaque in certain tumor locations requires the cutting of an extra-ocular muscle, which may result in a risk of diplopia after the procedure when the muscle is reattached. There are also radiation safety issues for patients receiving plaque brachytherapy; in some cases this may mean an inpatient hospital stay of four to seven days. In addition, protons may be used to treat some patients with tumors which are not good candidates for brachytherapy treatment; these include tumors near the optic disc and/or tumors with an apical height >10 mm. Protons are at least as effective as plaque brachytherapy in terms of tumor control, and there is some evidence that the risk of complications leading to enucleation may also be lower with protons.

Skull-Base Chordomas and Chondrosarcomas

One of the primary indications for proton treatment historically has been skull-based tumors, primarily chordoma and chondrosarcoma. Both of these tumors are relatively slow growing, but very difficult to control. This is a difficult area to approach surgically, and requires significant expertise. For sarcomas, a wide local resection is typically recommended, but is very difficult to achieve in this area. There is a high risk of significant complications with extensive surgery. The adjacent normal structures are often critical for normal functioning, including the brainstem (and basilar artery), optic chiasm, internal carotid arteries, cranial nerves, temporal lobes and other neurologic structures. Postoperative treatment is needed for almost all (if not all) of these patients. Despite the need for postoperative treatment, a maximal safe resection is indicated [58]. This will likely require the expertise of an experienced skull-base surgeon (or team of surgeons). It may also require two or more procedures, because both an anterior approach (trans-nasal/trans-sphenoidal) and a posterolateral approach may be needed for maximal debulking of the tumor.

Risk factors include age (children tend to have poorer outcomes); there may also be some difference in outcome based on gender, but this is not as clear (males have fared better in the Harvard series, but in other series males had poorer outcomes). The outcomes with chondrosarcoma tend to be better than those with chordoma.

Radiation therapy techniques have included standard radiation therapy, stereotactic radiosurgery, fractionated stereotactic radiotherapy, or particle therapy. There are multiple issues to consider for the treatment technique to be utilized. The treatment of somewhat larger volumes are needed; for example, chordomas may recur along the surgical pathway, have a tendency to involve the inferior aspect of the clivus, and may track along the longus colli muscles. Postoperative treatment may need to include all of those volumes. This is more difficult with focal treatments such as stereotactic radiosurgery or fractionated stereotactic radiotherapy. The doses required for local control are also quite high. This can be difficult with standard fractionated radiation therapy techniques, and it is for these reasons that proton/particle treatment of clival tumors is the standard method for postoperative treatment of these lesions [58].

The definition of tumor control is also important. If local control is defined as 'tumor control within the treated area,' this may exclude failures adjacent to the original primary tumor, but in areas which should have been targeted initially. The definition of local control should include those areas adjacent to the primary tumor which are known sites of potential recurrence (prepontine cistern, sphenoid sinus in patients who have endoscopic resection, and the longus colli muscles in those same patients).

Using this definition, the highest rates of long-term local control have been achieved with particle therapy, primarily with proton beam therapy. Munzenrider and Liebsch reported their experience with 290 patients with skull-base chordomas treated at the Harvard Cyclotron [59]. These authors achieved a five-year local control rate of 73%, with an 8% incidence of grade 3 toxicity (primarily temporal lobe injury). Hug *et al.* reported the experience from Loma Linda [60], where the local control rate was 92% for patients with chondrosarcoma and 74% for those with chordoma, despite 91% of patients having residual gross tumor postoperatively, including 59% with brainstem involvement. Symptomatic grade ≥3 toxicities occurred in 5% of patients. Ares *et al.* reported their experience with proton therapy for skull-base tumors, treated at the Paul Scherrer Institute in Switzerland [61]. In this case, the five-year local control for patients with chordomas was 81%, and for chondrosarcomas was 94%. The median dose for the chordoma patients was 73.5 Gy RBE, and 68.4 Gy RBE for the chondrosarcoma patients. No patients experienced brainstem toxicity, but one patient developed a grade 4 unilateral optic neuropathy.

The importance of long-term follow-up of these patients is also important. These tumors may recur at extended periods of time following treatment, and there are multiple toxicities which may become apparent with long-term follow-up. For patients treated with protons, the incidence of brainstem injury has been low, despite very high doses of treatment given to the brainstem surface (up to 64 Gy RBE). In part, this was because of the treatment techniques, which limit the brainstem core to <53 Gy RBE. Neurocognitive testing was performed prospectively in 17 patients who received high-dose therapy for chordomas or chondrosarcomas. There was no significant decline in neurocognitive functioning at four years, other than a mild decline in psychomotor (processing) speed [62]. Endocrine dysfunction is also quite common, because of the high dose to the pituitary gland [63]. This will include the majority of patients by the 10-year follow-up.

Pediatrics

Combined modality therapy has led to a significant improvement in the outcomes for many pediatric cancers. Radiation therapy is a major component of treatment for many central nervous system tumors (these comprise the largest group of solid tumors in children), and is frequently used for the treatment of sarcoma. The use of radiation therapy is associated with better outcomes in many pediatric cancers, but is also associated with significant long-term side effects, including the risk of secondary cancers. These side effects may become apparent decades after the treatment. The side effects are also related to the volume of and dose to the normal tissues which are included in the treatment. Clearly, a reduction in the volume of tissue treated will mean fewer long-term side effects for these patients. A major benefit of proton beam therapy is a reduction of the integral dose given during treatment, because of distal tissue-sparing as there is no exit dose. The use of PBS may also afford proximal tissue-sparing.

Dosimetric evaluations have shown the benefit of protons for many tumor types in children, including medulloblastoma, craniopharyngioma, retinoblastoma, parameningeal rhabdomyosarcoma, and pelvic sarcomas [64–67]. A useful example of the potential benefits of proton beam therapy in children is medulloblastoma. Treatment of the craniospinal axis with photons is typically performed with a posterior beam, whereby the exit of the beam provides dose to the lungs, esophagus, heart, pancreas, small bowel (and potentially to the ovaries in girls). Although these are relatively low doses, they may be associated with long-term side effects. In contrast, treatment with protons gives no significant exit dose to the heart, small bowel, ovaries or pancreas, and a much lower dose to the lungs and esophagus. Treatment of the posterior fossa boost with protons allows for better sparing of the cochlea, pituitary gland, hippocampus, and supratentorial brain [68].

The planning techniques for protons include several considerations which are of much less concern with photons. Altered growth dynamics is a concern for treatment of the spinal axis in pre-pubertal children. The specific concern is that the treatment of a portion of the vertebral body may lead to uneven growth, potentially causing musculoskeletal issues including kyphosis or scoliosis. In treatment of the spinal axis with photons, this is usually not a major concern. There is an exit dose through the entire vertebral body, which gives significant dose from the posterior elements all the way to the anterior portion of the vertebral body. For protons, the dosimetric

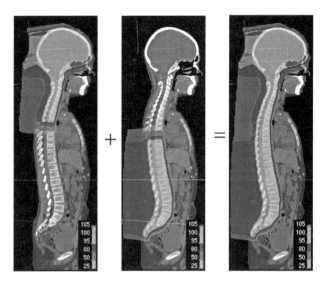

Figure 6.6 A typical CSI dose distribution using PBS delivery. The entire cranial and spinal axis for most children can be treated with two fields. Smooth intensity gradients are planned into the matchline regions to minimize sensitivities to misalignment. For a color version of this figure, see the color plate section.

issues are considerably different. If the spinal canal is set as the target, the dose fall-off will be rapid within the vertebral body. The dose to the posterior aspect of the vertebral body will be close to 100% of the prescription dose, while the dose to the anterior aspect may be nearly 0%. This differential has the potential to cause significant skeletal growth issues. For that reason, the entire vertebral body is typically included in the PTV for children who are still skeletally immature. Figure 6.6 shows a typical craniospinal irradiation (CSI) dose distribution using PBS delivery. With pencil beam, the entire cranial and spinal axis can be treated with two fields for most children. Smooth intensity gradients are intentionally planned into the match lines to minimize any potential of high dose overlap.

A second planning consideration involves the end of proton range. As the protons slow, the linear energy transfer increases, and thus the radiobiologic effectiveness increases. Because there are fewer protons (and fewer interactions) just beyond the Bragg peak, the total dose in this area is lower than within the Bragg peak, but the RBE may be higher. In the central nervous system, this seems to be of more importance than in most other sites in the body. For that reason, the recommendations for treatment near critical normal structures in the brain is to avoid overlap of the distal ends of the treatment fields, and to use at least three beams whenever possible (to minimize the potential RBE effects). This is especially a concern near the brainstem, as brainstem toxicity has been noted in some patients treated with protons. In a series from the University of Florida Proton Therapy Institute, the incidence of grade ≥3 brainstem toxicity was 2.1% [69]. This was associated with young patients (aged <5 years), with a larger volume of brainstem treated, and with aggressive surgical resection. The authors' recommendation was to consider more conservative brainstem dosimetric guidelines, especially in younger children who have undergone aggressive surgery. The MRI changes seen after proton beam therapy may be more common than with IMRT. Many of these changes resolve without treatment, but some require treatment with steroids, bevacizumab, or hyperbaric oxygen [70].

Clinical outcomes with proton beam therapy in children have shown promising results for multiple tumor types. The dosimetric results show a clear benefit for protons in many disease sites with sarcoma. A review of the clinical data has shown that the outcomes with regards to tumor control are equivalent or superior to standard radiation therapy techniques, with an apparent reduction in toxicity [71]. The tumor types for which there are data showing these excellent outcomes include rhabdomyosarcoma, soft tissue sarcomas, osteosarcoma, Ewing sarcoma, chordoma, and chondrosarcoma.

Second malignant neoplasms are a potential risk of radiation therapy, especially in children. Because of the lower integral dose with protons, the risk of secondary cancers should be reduced for proton therapy compared to standard radiation therapy techniques. A cohort series of patients treated in Boston evaluated over 500 patients treated with protons, matched to a group of patients treated with photons from the SEER database [72]. There were fewer second malignancies in the proton-treated patients (5.2%) compared to the photon group (7.5%), with an adjusted hazard ratio of 0.52 (95% confidence interval 0.32-0.85). Patients with retinoblastoma have a very high risk of secondary cancers, especially after treatment with radiation therapy. An evaluation of retinoblastoma patients treated from the same institution showed the 10-year risk of second malignancies to be much higher after photon irradiation (14%) compared to protons (0%) [73].

Lung

Lung cancer is the most common cause of cancer death in the US for both men and women. Systemic therapies (especially targeted treatments) and surgical techniques have made significant advances over the past two decades, but local control of the lung cancer remains a significant problem. In addition, patients with lung cancer often have significant co-morbidities from the heart or lungs, and treatment may negatively impact those organs.

Stereotactic body radiation therapy (SBRT) has become the standard of care for patients with inoperable Stage I non-small-cell lung cancer. SBRT allows for a much larger biologically effective dose to the tumor, while in most cases limiting doses to normal lung and mediastinal tissues. Protons have been used for the treatment of early-stage lung cancers, using SBRT or similar hypofractionated techniques. The outcomes are good for Stage I tumors, with local controls rates of 82–97% [74–76]. There may be a dosimetric advantage for protons in some patients with Stage I lung cancer, especially in tumors adjacent to the mediastinal structures. However, photon-based SBRT is very effective for most Stage I non-small-cell lung cancers. The primary advantage for protons may be in larger tumors; the tumor size limit for most SBRT photon series has typically been 5 cm, and there is a decreasing dosimetric advantage for photon-based-SBRT in tumors greater than that size. However, treatment with protons may still retain a significant dosimetric advantage over standard techniques. Bush *et al.* performed a dose escalation study of hypofractionated proton treatment in 111 patients with T1 and T2 non-small-cell lung cancer. The majority of patients ($n = 64$) had T2 primary tumors (>5 cm) and received 70 Gy in 10 fractions. The four-year local control rate was 74% and the overall survival was 54% [75].

For patients with Stage III non-small-cell lung cancer, the standard treatment is combined chemotherapy and radiation therapy. The RTOG 0617 trial tested the hypothesis that a higher dose of radiation therapy (74 Gy in 37 treatments) would improve outcomes compared to the standard dose (60 Gy in 30 treatments) [77]. However, the reported outcomes showed the opposite results: median survival was 28.7 months in the 60-Gy arm compared to 20.3 months in the 74-Gy arm. On multivariate analysis, heart V(5 Gy) and V(30 Gy) were associated with an increased risk of death. It is not clear if this is the primary reason for the differences in outcomes between the lower dose and higher dose radiation therapy treatments. Protons allow for significant sparing of the heart compared with IMRT, and should allow dose escalation [78].

Sejpal *et al.* evaluated three consecutive treatment techniques in patients with locally advanced non-small-cell lung cancer [79]. Patients were treated at the same institution by the same physicians, initially utilizing 3D conformal techniques, followed by IMRT and then protons. Patients treated with 3D or IMRT received 63 Gy, while those with protons received 74 Gy. Despite the higher doses, patients treated with protons had significantly lower rates of grade ≥3 esophagitis (5%, compared to 18% for 3D and 44% for IMRT) and pneumonitis (2%, compared to 30% for 3D and 9% for IMRT).

The current NRG/RTOG 1308 trial is evaluating patients with locally advanced non-small-cell lung cancer, attempting to determine whether treatment with protons will improve outcome [80]. All patients receive platinum-based doublet chemotherapy concurrently with radiation (either carboplatin/paclitaxel or cisplatin/etopsoide). The randomization is between protons and photons, with a target total dose of 70 Gy in 35 treatments. However, the treatment plan must be delivered without exceeding dose–volume tolerance limits for all critical structures; if these cannot be met, the total doses is lowered until those constraints can be met (with a minimum of 60 Gy in 30 fractions). This study will help to determine whether normal tissue toxicity can be reduced with protons for lung cancer.

A clear understanding of potential effects of respiratory motion to the planned dose distribution of lung targets is essential. Knowledge of the time structure of the proton delivery system in coordination with the patient's respiratory cycle is necessary to anticipate interplay effects [81,82]. Interplay effects tend to be greater when treating with PBS delivery, and can be mitigated through gantry angle-specific robustness predictions [83], gating [82], and repainting [84]. When planning, appropriate distal and proximal margins are required that account for the low water equivalent thickness of lung tissues. Figure 6.7 shows a treatment plan for a squamous cell carcinoma in the right hilar region. The posterior angles can be used very efficiently to keep the spinal cord below tolerance dose while sparing much of the heart and lung.

Lymphoma

The management of both Hodgkin's and non-Hodgkin's lymphoma and the improvements in outcomes over the past few decades represent some of the greatest successes in oncology. With the introduction of multimodality therapy, a malignancy that was uniformly fatal prior to the 1950s now carries an excellent cure rate with many long-term survivors. Many of these survivors live to experience late treatment-related side effects which can include cardiovascular disease and secondary malignancies. Thus, the focus of treatment moving forward is to maintain the excellent cure rates while further reducing treatment-related morbidity and mortality.

While radiotherapy was the primary modality for curative treatment several decades ago, the use of multi-agent chemotherapy has resulted in a cure for some patients without radiation. Studies have shown, however, that chemotherapy alone results in its own toxicity and may not be as effective in bulky areas.

More recent trials have focused on de-intensifying radiotherapy rather than eliminating radiotherapy all together. The German Hodgkin's Study Group HD10 trial established the new standard of care for limited-stage favorable Hodgkin's lymphoma as two cycles of ABVD (doxorubicin, bleomycin, vinblastine, dacarbazine) followed by 20 Gy of involved field radiation [85]. Adaptive radiotherapy based on PET response to chemotherapy is also an area of active study [86]. Radiation fields have gradually become more limited, evolving from subtotal nodal irradiation, to involved field irradiation, to involved site radiation [87, 88]. The smaller fields, lower doses, improved treatment setup, and image guidance have undoubtedly improved long-term toxicity [89]. Proton therapy provides further improvement

Organs often exposed to the toxicity of radiation are the heart, lungs, and breasts. The combined toxicity of doxorubicin and heart exposure with radiation is of particular concern. Two large retrospective studies have found that Hodgkin's lymphoma survivors were more likely to have late cardiac toxicities, and that this excess risk was associated with radiation exposure of the heart, anthracycline or vincristine exposure, radiation doses >30 Gy, minimal cardiac blocking, and young age at exposure [90]. Secondary cancers are also an obvious concern and reduced doses/field sizes are desirable.

The unique dosimetric advantages of proton therapy are beneficial for the above concerns [91]. The ability to spare organs with any form of radiotherapy will ultimately depend on the location of the pre-chemotherapy disease. That said, the physical properties of protons and photons are different, with protons providing certain clinical advantages over x-rays. The reduced dose to neighboring critical structures, the elimination of exit dose, and lower integral dose results in less acute and late treatment-related side effects.

Figure 6.8 shows a PBS plan of a 40-year-old female with Hodgkin's lymphoma. The proton beam is incident, *en face* to the chest in an anterior superior oblique angles. Protons were considered in this patient to minimize dose to the heart, lungs, and breast. The couch kick and anterior incidence gantry angle was chosen specifically to minimize breast dose. PBS allows for greater proximal dosing control of the proton dose, and can be used to decrease breast dose even further along the beam's path. The effects of respiratory motion on the pencil beam pattern should be carefully monitored throughout the respiratory cycle as part of the robustness evaluation. Based on patient-specific target location and priorities of the organs at risk, the posterior beam can be considered to lower breast dose to nearly zero at the cost of a potentially higher dose to the lung, spinal cord, and heart.

Breast

Several studies have demonstrated clear survival benefits of irradiation of breast cancer for locoregional control in early-stage and locally advanced breast cancer patients [92,93]. Unfortunately, increased mortality, in the form of increased treatment-related cardiovascular toxicity has been reported [94–96]. Postmastectomy radiation therapy has been shown to increase the risk for ipsilateral lung carcinoma between 10–20 years after radiation

Figure 6.7 The dose distribution for a squamous cell carcinoma of the right hilum. Posterior oblique angles are used to keep the spinal cord below tolerance while sparing much of the heart and lungs. For a color version of this figure, see the color plate section.

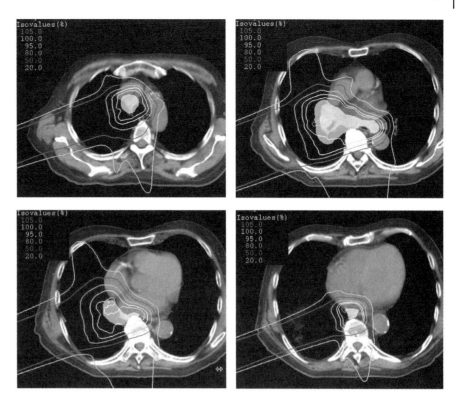

exposure [97]. For more advanced stages, in which inclusion of the internal mammary nodes is required, increased doses to the heart, coronary arteries, and lung have been observed [98].

The reports of increased toxicities have prompted the development of various treatment techniques to reduce heart and lung dose as low as possible while ensuring appropriate target coverage. Techniques such as deep

Figure 6.8 A PBS dose distribution for a 40-year-old female with Hodgkin's lymphoma. Protons were considered in this patient to minimize dose to the heart, lungs, and breast. For a color version of this figure, see the color plate section.

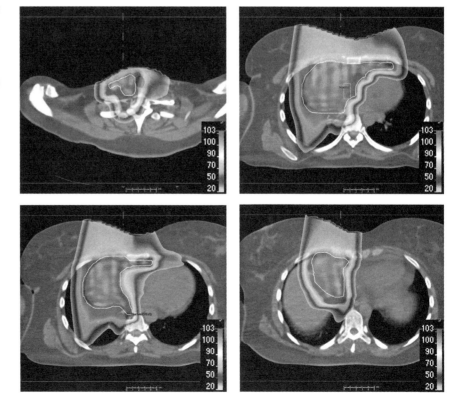

inspiration breath-hold [99] and field gating can be used to trigger treatment when the heart is physically displaced from the treatment areas. Methods such as IMRT and VMAT can be used to increase the conformity of the high-dose areas around the target at the cost of increased low-dose scatter and integral dose [100].

In an attempt to quantify clinically relevant improvements that protons might offer for localized and locoregional breast cancer, Ares *et al.* [101] performed dosimetric comparisons using intensity-modulated proton therapy (IMPT) protons, IMRT, and 3D conformal radiotherapy. The same patients were evaluated with increasing complexity of targets from breast or chest wall only, to breast/chest wall plus supraclavicular and axilla and finally breast/chest wall, supraclavicular, axilla and internal mammary chain (IMC). Results showed that IMPT proton plans could offer improved target coverage with reduced doses to OARs in cases when regional lymphatics were treated. The benefits of IMPT protons were greatest for the most complex cases where IMCs were included. Other dosimetric evaluations of plans that included the internal mammary chain irradiation compared the use of protons to deep photon tangents and photon/electron combined plans [102], and VMAT [98]. Fagundes *et al.* [98] quantified increased dose in photon plans when the IMC were added to the irradiated volume, and showed that the addition of IMC in protons plan did not significantly increase heart nor ipsilateral lung dose.

Proton treatment plans of the breast/chestwall and regional lymphatics make use of a single or multiple, nearly *en-face* fields rather than tangent type fields that are most often used in photon treatments. The proton beams are positioned so that the distal edge of the deepest proton layers are stopped in the intercostal spaces of the chest wall, before the lung and heart. Figure 6.9 shows single-field, IMPT left-sided breast dose distribution. The entire treatment volume, including the IMC, axilla and supraclavicular areas are all encompassed within one field. With this arrangement, typical breathing motion is mostly in the direction parallel to the proton's incidence. This parallel type motion of the breast will cause slight displacement of the breast but will not cause thickness changes to the target tissues, making these plans less sensitive to respiratory motion. Thickness changes within the breast due to on-treatment swelling or seroma resolution can create significant path length differences that will require adaptive planning methods.

Many patients present for radiotherapy with tissue expanders or breast prosthesis. Careful attention to these implants is necessary to ensure that the planning system will properly account for these implanted materials. It has been reported [103] that considerable errors in the dose distribution calculation can occur if uncorrected HU conversions are used by the planning system.

A pragmatic Phase III randomized trial, RTOG 3510, has recently been funded through the Patient Centered Outcome Research Institute (PCORI). This study will randomize non-metastatic patients receiving comprehensive nodal irradiation either to photon/electron or to protons. The study is a radiotherapy comparative effectiveness consortium trial (RADCOMP) with a

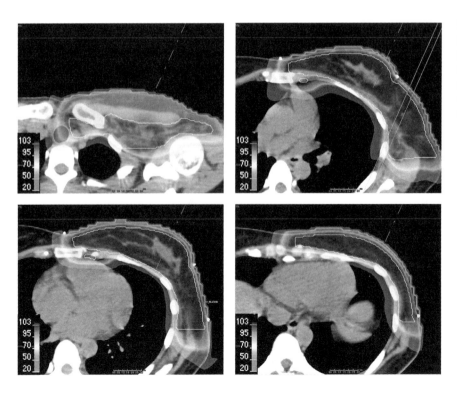

Figure 6.9 A PBS dose distribution for a left-sided breast with comprehensive nodal irradiation, including the internal mammary chain. This plan makes use of a single, *en-face* PBS field. For a color version of this figure, see the color plate section.

primary endpoint to evaluate cardiovascular morbidity and mortality. The study is designed to enroll approximately 1700 patients with long-term follow-up.

Prostate

Proton therapy has been used for the treatment of prostate cancer for more than 30 years. The initial techniques used protons as a boost dose, following x-ray treatment to the whole pelvis. The imaging modalities and limitations of the early proton systems required techniques which are not commonly used today. A randomized prospective trial from 1981 to 1992 at the Harvard cyclotron utilized an *en face* perineal boost to the prostate, for patients with Stage C (locally advanced – T3 or T4, N0) prostate cancer [104]. The patients all received 50.4 Gy in 28 fractions to the pelvis, followed by a boost of either 17 Gy in eight fractions with lateral fields using x-rays, or 25.2 Gy RBE in 12 fractions using the perineal proton field. This was in the pre-prostate-specific antigen (PSA) era, and patients were classified by standard grading (well, moderately or poorly differentiated); none of the patients received hormonal therapy. The patients treated with protons had a trend towards improved local control (77% at 8 years, compared to 60% with x-rays, p = 0.089); those with poorly differentiated tumors had significantly better local control (64% at 8 years versus 19% with x-rays, p = 0.0014). There was no improvement in overall survival, and there were significantly more complications in the patients who were treated with protons, primarily grade 2 rectal bleeding [105].

Treatment using more modern techniques began at Loma Linda during the early 1990s. At that time, standard treatment for prostate cancer with x-rays utilized a four-field box treatment to larger field to 45–50 Gy, followed by boost to a total of 65–70 Gy, typically using 10–18 MV photons. At Loma Linda, treatment with protons was initially used for the boost portion of the treatment. Patients were treated with a rectal balloon, which affords better stabilization of the pelvic anatomy

during treatment. Their five-year results for more than 900 patients treated between 1991 and 1996 showed very promising results, with a five-year bNED (biologic no evidence of disease) survival of 82%, with no grade 3–4 toxicity, and low levels of grade 2 rectal (3.5%) and bladder (5.4%) toxicities [106].

The Proton Radiation Oncology Group (PROG) conducted a prospective randomized dose escalation trial in which patients all received 50.4 Gy in 28 fractions to a larger field covering the prostate and seminal vesicles using a four-field x-ray technique [107]. The patients were randomly assigned to receive a boost to the prostate using protons with a dose of either 19.8 Gy RBE in 11 fractions or 28.8 Gy RBE in 16 fractions. The 10-year results from the PROG 95-09 trial showed significantly better outcomes in the higher-dose arm, with lower rates of local failure and biochemical failure. This was a similar finding to multiple other concurrent prospective randomized dose escalation trials using x-rays alone. The differences between these studies were primarily in the side-effect profiles. In nearly all of the x-ray studies there was a significantly higher risk of grade 3 gastrointestinal or genitourinary complications in patients who received the higher doses. In contrast, there was no difference in grade 3 gastrointestinal or genitourinary toxicity between the high- and low-dose patients on PROG 9509 (Table 6.1). The rates of complications in the high-dose arm were lower in the PROG 9509 study than in the x-ray-only studies. As noted in Table 6.1, the planning and treatment process for most of these studies utilized 3D conformal radiation therapy techniques.

Single-institution studies have confirmed the low incidence of significant long-term toxicities with proton treatment for prostate cancer. Pugh *et al.* evaluated 291 consecutive patients treated at MD Anderson Cancer Center with protons for low- or intermediate-risk prostate cancer [108]. Their two-year rate of grade 2 genitourinary toxicity was 13.4%, with no grade ≥3 toxicity. The two-year gastrointestinal grade 2 toxicity rate was 9.6%, with only one patient experiencing a grade 3 toxicity. Mendenhall *et al.* reported the University of Florida

Table 6.1 Summary of reported outcomes and toxicity for external beam treatment of prostate cancer.

Trial/Reference	Boost modality	Planning technique	High-dose arm	Five-year bNED	GU toxicity Grade 2	Grade 3
MD Anderson [114]	X-rays	2D/3D	78.0 Gy	78%	28%	10%
CKVO96-10 [115]	X-rays	3D	78.0 Gy	64%	32%	5%
MRC RT01 [116]	X-rays	3D	74.0 Gy	71%	33%	10%
GETUG [117]	X-rays	3D/IMRT	80.0 Gy	77%	27%	6%
PROG 95-09 [107]	Protons	3D	79.2 Gy	92%	17%	1%

bNED, biologic no evidence of disease; GU, genitourinary.

Proton Therapy Institute five-year results on 211 patients with low- ($n = 89$), intermediate- ($n = 82$) or high-risk ($n = 40$) prostate cancer [109]. The five-year bNED rates were 99% for the low- and intermediate-risk patients, and 76% for the high-risk group. The rate of toxicity was quite low: using the CTCAE version 4 criteria, the five-year rate of grade 3 gastrointestinal toxicity was 0.5% and the genitourinary toxicity was 1.0%.

While there is evidence that protons are safe and effective for the treatment of prostate cancer, there is still uncertainty as to whether protons are superior to – or equivalent to – IMRT. A current randomized prospective trial is evaluating protons versus IMRT for low- and intermediate-risk prostate cancer. The PARTIQoL study is designed to detect differences in quality of life parameters, with a primary endpoint of bowel function at 24 months following treatment [110].

One potential advantage of protons is the possibility of altered dose delivery, either with escalation or hypofractionation. It is unlikely that dose escalation will be of benefit in patients with Stage I (low-risk) disease, since the outcomes are so good already. Coen *et al.* reported a dose escalation study on 85 men with localized prostate cancer, evaluating 82 Gy RBE in 41 fractions [111]. Most of the patients in the study had T1c disease (76%), with PSA levels <10 (87%) and a Gleason score of 6 (60%). The late grade 3 toxicity rate was 6.1%. The image guidance used at that time was ultrasound localization of the prostate without a rectal balloon, or rectal balloon plus orthogonal radiographs (without fiducial markers). In contrast, a prospective study of hypofractionation for patients with low-risk prostate cancer has shown no evidence of increased toxicity for a very short course of therapy; patients in that study were treated utilizing both fiducial markers and rectal balloons. Patients on the Proton Collaborative Group PCG GU002 study were randomly assigned to either 79.2 Gy RBE in 44 fractions or 38 Gy RBE in five fractions [112]. There have been no grade 3 toxicities reported thus far in either arm.

There are new techniques for proton beam treatment of prostate cancer which may further improve outcomes. The standard treatment now utilizes image guidance, typically with interstitial fiducial markers [113]. This allows for smaller treatment margins, especially posteriorly towards the rectum. PBS techniques are being used with increasing frequency, providing the opportunity for not only distal beam shaping but also better proximal conformity. This will reduce the integral dose, and may improve treatment for patients with more difficult anatomy (e.g., better bladder-sparing in patients with a large median lobe of the prostate). The use of a spacer between the rectum and prostate may allow for even further reductions in the rectal wall doses [113]. Although this can be used with any radiation therapy technique (IMRT, brachytherapy, or protons), the use of a hydrogel

space may allow treatment with protons in which there is minimal rectal dose. This will be especially useful for treatment with hypofractionation, in which rectal toxicity has been the primary dose-limiting structure.

Head and Neck Cancers

Treatment of head and neck cancers is difficult and may be especially problematic. These patients frequently have significant comorbidities, often require combined modality therapy, and have difficulties with nutrition and hydration during the course of therapy that are directly related to the tumor and its treatment. In addition, there are multiple organs at risk within or adjacent to the treatment volume, which may permanently impact on quality of life following treatment. IMRT has allowed for improvements in quality of life by sparing some of these organs (e.g., salivary glands), but does so by spreading low doses over large volumes of the oral cavity and posterior fossa. A Dutch research group has evaluated normal tissue complication probabilities for multiple normal tissues within the head and neck, and developed a model which can be prospectively applied to individual treatment plans. This model has been used to predict whether there would be benefits from changes in treatment techniques [118]. Proton beam therapy may provide a dosimetric advantage over IMRT in certain areas of the head and neck, primarily in the paranasal sinuses, nasal cavity, nasopharynx, and oropharynx [119]. However, there is increasing evidence that these dosimetric advantages translate also into clinical improvements.

Acute tolerance of treatment appears to be better with IMPT compared to IMRT for nasopharynx, paranasal sinus, and oropharyngeal cancers. McDonald *et al.* performed a cohort comparison of patients with nasopharyngeal and paranasal sinus cancers, and found a significantly lower risk of opioid dependence or need for G-tube placement in patients who received protons compared to IMRT [120]. Sio *et al.* evaluated a cohort comparison of patients with oropharyngeal cancers, and found that symptoms in the subacute recovery phase were significantly better with protons compared to IMRT; this same group had previously noted a decrease in the need for G-tubes with protons (20%) compared to IMRT (48%) [121].

Patel *et al.* performed a meta-analysis of treatment for paranasal sinus cancers, and included a total of 41 studies in the analysis. Patients who were treated with protons had significantly better disease-free survival compared to photon therapy, both at five years and at longest follow-up. The overall survival at five years was significantly higher for patients treated with particle therapy compared to photons [122].

Even for patients receiving only ipsilateral treatment, there is a significant advantage of proton therapy for acute toxicities. Romesser *et al.* compared consecutive cohorts of patients with salivary and mucosal head and neck malignancies treated to the tumor and ipsilateral cervical nodes [123]. Those patients treated with protons had significantly lower risks of grade ≤2 dysguesia (5.6% versus 65.2%, P <0.001), mucositis (16.7% versus 52.2%, P = 0.019), and nausea (11.1% versus 56.5%, P = 0.003), compared to the cohort treated with IMRT.

Careful treatment planning is required for patients who receive proton beam therapy for head and neck cancers. Frequently, there may be high-density metal in the oral cavity (e.g., dental amalgam fillings) which may cause significant difficulties both with visualization of the target volume and normal tissues, as well as with uncertainties in the treatment range [124]. Similarly, variations in densities within the sinuses may cause changes to the potential path length of the protons during the course of treatment [125]. Weight loss is common amongst patients being treated for head and neck cancers, and volumetric re-imaging during treatment may be needed to determine if plan adaptations are required.

There is an ongoing prospective randomized study which will help to clarify the differences in outcomes between IMRT and IMPT in head and neck cancers. Patients with Stage III or IV oropharyngeal cancers are randomly assigned to either IMPT or IMRT, both given to a total of 70 Gy in 33 fractions, with concomitant chemotherapy. The primary endpoint of the study is a comparison of the rates and severity of late grade 3–5 toxicity between IMRT and IMPT following the treatment of oropharyngeal tumors [126].

The Value of Proton Therapy: Clinical Trials

The James M. Slater Proton Treatment and Research Center at Loma Linda University Medical Center, which opened in 1990 [31], was the first hospital-based cancer treatment center in the US, and for the next decade it would remain the only one [31,127]. Research institutions that possessed cyclotrons, such as the Harvard Cyclotron Laboratory and Crocker Nuclear Laboratory, treated some cancers [128,129], but proton therapy was largely unknown as a treatment for cancer for many years. Among the many factors that contributed to the obscurity of proton therapy were limited access and limited clinical knowledge. From 2001 to 2015, the number of dedicated medical proton facilities grew from three to 17 [31]. The rise in the number of medical proton centers increased access dramatically, which in turn necessitated and facilitated an increase in clinical knowledge. As protons become a more viable and mainstream treatment option, it is the proton community's responsibility to use this increase in clinical knowledge to develop new

treatment techniques that take full advantage of the benefits that protons can provide.

As protons are a relatively new form of treatment, there are many opportunities for clinical research. Currently, most non-protocol proton treatments and fractionation schemes are based on data gathered from standard photon treatments. It is important that proton-specific research be conducted to discover how to fully utilize the advantages that protons can offer, rather than continue to treat patients according to photon-specific data, with its inherent limitations. Clinical trials are a time-tested method of conducting this research.

Several institutions sponsor clinical trials involving proton therapy. The Proton Collaborative Group (PCG), formed in 2009, is currently the only collaborative group in the world dedicated exclusively to proton therapy research [130]. The PCG is an independent, not-for-profit organization comprised of several proton therapy centers throughout the US. PCG-sponsored protocol categories include breast, CNS, pediatrics, prostate, and lung, as well as others. Other research organizations sponsor clinical trials that include proton therapy. The Radiation Therapy Oncology Group (RTOG) is an NCI-funded clinical cooperative group that has been conducting clinical oncology research since 1968 [131]. The RTOG has now become part of NRG Oncology, a National Cancer Institute sponsored non-profit research organization developed to conduct multi-institutional Phase II and Phase III clinical trials, as well as Phase I and translational biological studies ([32]. NRG Oncology sponsors proton-related clinical trials, some of which originated in the RTOG. In addition to dedicated research organizations, virtually every open proton center participates in proton-related clinical trials [133–136].

New Proton Therapy Centers

Between 1990 and 2015, the number of proton centers treating cancer patients in the US grew from one to 17, with the majority of new centers having been built after 2005. All proton centers operating in the US are listed in Table 6.2 [31]. Not included in this list is the Indiana University Health Proton Therapy Center (originally the Midwest Proton Radiotherapy Institute), which opened in 2004 and closed in 2014 [137]. Proton centers in the US currently under construction are listed in Table 6.3

As can be seen from the information in Tables 6.2 and 6.3, most PTCs have multiple treatment rooms. Multiple rooms require a large support system and infrastructure to house them, which translates to large dedicated centers and multimillion dollar price tags. While the number of proton centers has grown in recent years, a continuing

Table 6.2 Proton centers operating in the US, as of December 2016. Details include the location, number of treatment rooms, and the year of first treatment.

Proton Therapy Center	State	Rooms	Year opened
J. Slater PTC, Loma Linda	CA	4	1990
UCSF, San Francisco/UC Davis	CA	1	1994
MGH Francis H. Burr PTC, Boston	MA	3	2001
MD Anderson Cancer Center, Houston	TX	4	2006
University of Florida PTI, Jacksonville	FL	4	2006
ProCure PTC, Oklahoma City	OK	4	2009
Roberts PTC, University of Pennsylvania, Philadelphia	PA	5	2010
Chicago Proton Center, Warrenville	IL	4	2010
Hampton University PTI, Hampton	VA	5	2010
ProCure ProtonTherapy Center, Somerset	NJ	4	2012
SCCA ProCure Proton Therapy Center, Seattle	WA	4	2013
S. Lee Kling PTC, Barnes Jewish Hospital, St. Louis	MO	1	2013
Provision Center for Proton Therapy, Knoxville	TN	3	2014
Scripps Proton Therapy Center, San Diego	CA	5	2014
Willis Knighton Proton Therapy Cancer Center, Shreveport	LA	1	2014
Ackerman Cancer Center, Jacksonville	FL	1	2015
RobertWood Johnson, New Brunswick	NJ	1	2015
Mayo Clinic Proton Beam Therapy Center, Rochester	MN	4	2015
Texas Center for Proton Therapy, Irving	TX	3	2015
St Jude Red Frog Events PTC, Memphis	TN	3	2016
Maryland Proton Treatment Center, Baltimore	MD	5	2016
Mayo Clinic Proton Beam Therapy Center, Phoenix	AZ	4	2016
MD Anderson, Orlando	FL	1	2016
UH Seidman Cancer Center, Cleveland	OH	1	2016
Cincinnati Children's Proton Therapy Center, Cincinnati	OH	3	2016

PTC = Proton Therapy Center; PTI = Proton Therapy Institute.

challenge to increasing treatment access is the cost associated with building these large, multi-room centers. Until recently, the multi-room 'mega' center was the only option that made economic and logistical sense. However, a new generation of proton-producing accelerators has recently been introduced commercially from multiple vendors that allow for more compact treatment hardware. These accelerators are designed to be 'one-room solutions,' or proton therapy rooms without the need for an entire building dedicated to the treatment. This design may be the future of proton therapy. These one-room cyclotrons are generally cheaper than the models used in multi-room centers, and can be added to existing clinics rather than requiring all-new construction. These two factors greatly reduce the cost of implementing a proton therapy program and can make protons a more realistic option for a greater number of oncology centers. This reduction in cost could eventually result in reduced cost of the treatment itself, which would further patients' access to protons.

Table 6.3 Proton therapy centers under construction in the US, as of December 2016. Details include the number of treatment rooms and the anticipated year of first treatment.

Proton Therapy Center	State	Treatment rooms	Year of planned opening
Oklahoma University, Oklahoma City	OK	1	2017
McLaren Proton Therapy Center, Flint	MI	3	2017
Emory Proton Therapy Center, Atlanta	GA	5	2017
Massachusetts General Hospital, Boston	MA	1	2017
Lombardi Comprehensive CC, Georgetown Univ., Washington	DC	1	2017

CC = Cancer Center.

References

1 Wilson, R.R. (1946) Radiological Use of Fast Protons. *Radiology*, **47**, 487–491.

2 *Journal of the ICRU*, Vol. 7, No. 2 (2007), Report 78.

3 Bentzen, S.M., *et al.* (2010) Quantitative Analyses of Normal Tissue Effects in the Clinic (QUANTEC): An Introduction to the Scientific Issues. *Int. J. Radiat. Oncol. Biol. Phys.*, **76** (3, Suppl.), S3–S9.

4 Cancer Treatment Symposia (1983) Proceedings of The Workshop on Patterns of Failure after Cancer Treatment, Vol. 2.

5 DeVita, V.T., Lawrence, T.S., Rosenberg, S.A., DePinho, R.A. (eds) (2011) *Cancer: Principles & Practice of Oncology*, 9th edition., Lippincott Williams & Wilkins, Philadelphia.

6 Fletcher, G.H. (1980) *Textbook of Radiotherapy*, 3rd edition. Lea & Febiger, Philadelphia.

7 Halperin, E.C., Brady, L.W. (eds) (2013) *Perez and Brady's Principles and Practice of Radiation Oncology*, 6th edition. Lippincott Williams and Wilkins, Philadelphia.

8 Wang, C.C. (2000) *Clinical Radiation Oncology: Indications. Techniques and Results*, 2nd edition. Wiley Liss, New York.

9 Suit, H.D. (1982) Potential for improving survival rates for the cancer patient by increasing the efficacy of treatment of the primary lesion [American Society of Therapeutic Radiology, Presidential address, October 1981]. *Cancer*, **50**, 1227–1234.

10 Fuks, Z., Leibel, S.A., Wallner, K.E., *et al.* (1991) The effect of local control on metastatic dissemination in carcinoma of the prostate: Long-term results in patient treated with I implantation. *Int. J. Radiat. Oncol. Biol. Phys.*, **21**, 537–547.

11 Leibel, S.A., Scott, C.B., Mohiuddin, M., *et al.* (1991) The effect of local-regional control on distant metastatic dissemination in carcinoma of the head and neck: Results of an analysis from the RTOG head and neck database. *Int. J. Radiat. Oncol. Biol. Phys.*, **21**, 549–555.

12 Suit, H.D. (1992) Local control and patient survival. *Int. J. Radiat. Oncol. Biol. Phys.*, **23**, 653–660.

13 Emami, B., Lyman, J., Brown, A., *et al.* (1991) Tolerance of normal tissue to therapeutic irradiation. *Int. J. Radiat. Oncol. Biol. Phys.*, **21**, 109–122.

14 Paganetti, H. (2012) Range uncertainties in proton therapy and the role of Monte Carlo simulations. *Phys. Med. Biol.*, **57** (11), R99–R117

15 Moyers, M.F., Sardesai, M., Sun, S., Miller, D.W. (2010) Ion stopping powers and CT numbers. *Med. Dosim.*, **35** (3), 179–194.

16 Yang, M., Zhu, X.R., Park, P.C., Titt, U., *et al.* (2012) Comprehensive analysis of proton range uncertainties related to patient stopping-power-ratio estimation using the stoichiometric calibration. *Phys. Med. Biol.*, **57** (13), 4095–4115.

17 Plautz, T., Bashkirov, V., Feng, V., Hurley, F., *et al.* (2014) A 200 MeV proton radiography studies with a hand phantom using a prototype proton CT scanner. *IEEE Trans. Med. Imaging*, **33** (4), 875–881

18 Poludniowski, G., Allinson, N.M., Evans, P.M. (2015) Proton radiography and tomography with application to proton therapy. *Br. J. Radiol.*, **88** (1053), 20150134.

19 Koehler, A.M., Preston, W.M. (1972) Protons in radiation therapy. Comparative dose distributions for protons, photons and electrons. *Radiology*, **104**, 191–195.

20 Archambeau, J.O., Bennett, G.W., Chen, S.T. (1974) Potential of proton beams for nodal irradiation. *Acta Radiol. Ther. Phys. Biol.*, **13**, 393–401.

21 Raju, M.R. (1980) *Heavy Particle Radiotherapy*. Academic Press, New York.

22 Tobias, C.A., Lawrence, J.H., Born, J.L., McCombs, R.K., *et al.* (1958) Pituitary irradiation with high energy proton beams: A preliminary report. *Cancer Res.*, **18**, 121–134.

23 Graffmau, S., Jung, B. (1970) Clinical trials in radiotherapy and the merits of high energy protons and electrons. *Acta Radiol. Ther. Phys. Biol.*, **9**, 1–23.

24 Kjellberg, R.N., Shintaml, A., Frantz, A.G., *et al.* (1968) Proton bean therapy in acromegaly. *N. Engl. J. Med.*, **278**, 689–695.

25 Kjellberg, R.N., Kliman, B. (1974) Bragg peak proton treatment for pituitary related conditions. *Proc. R. Soc. Med.*, **67**, 32–33.

26 Kjellberg, R.N., Kliman, B. (1979) Lifetime effectiveness – A system of therapy for pituitary adenomas, emphasizing proton hypophysectomy, in *Recent Advances in Diagnosis and Treatments in Pituitary Tumors* (ed. J.A. Linfoot). Raven Press, New York, pp. 269–288.

27 Chllvilo, I.V., Goldin, L.L., Khoroshkoy, V.S., *et al.* (1984) lTEP synchrotron proton beam in radiotherapy. *Int. J. Radiat. Oncol. Biol. Phys.*, **10**, 185–195.

28 Miller, D.W. (1995) A review of proton beam radiation therapy. *Med. Phys.*, **22**, 1943–1954.

29 Larsson, B., Larsson, B., Leksell, L., Rexed, B., Sourander, P., Mair, W., Andersson, B. (1958) The high-energy proton beam as a neurosurgical tool. *Nature*, **182**, 1222–1223.

30 Matsuda, T., Inamura, K. (1981) Computer controlled multi-leaf conformation radiotherapy (in Japanese). *Nippon Acta Radiol.*, **41**, 965–974.

31 http://www.ptcog.ch/index.php/facilities-in-operation.

32 http://www.ptcog.ch/archive/patient_statistics/ijpt-15-00013.pdf.

33 http://www.ptcog.ch/index.php/clinical-protocols.

34 Koehler, A.M., Schneider, R.J., Sisterson, J.M. (1975) Range modulators for protons and heavy ions. *Nucl. Instrum. Methods*, **131**, 437–440.

35 Koehler, A.M., Schneider, R.J., Sisterson, J.M. (1977) Flattening of proton dose distributions for large-field radiotherapy. *Med. Phys.*, **4**, 297–301.

36 Farr, J.B., Mascia, A.E., Hsi, W.C., Allgower, C.E., *et al.* (2008) Clinical characterization of a proton beam continuous uniform scanning system with dose layer stacking. *Med. Phys.*, **35**, 4945–4954.

37 Bues, M., Newhauser, W.D., Titt, U., Smith, A.R. (2005) Therapeutic step and shoot proton beam spot-scanning with a multi-leaf collimator: A Monte Carlo study. *Radiat. Prot. Dosim.*, **115**, 164–169.

38 Gottschalk, B. (2011) Multileaf collimators, air gap, lateral penumbra, and range compensation in proton radiotherapy. *Med. Phys.*, **38** (11), 10.1118/1.3653297.

39 Daartz, J., Bangert, M., Bussiere, M.R., Engelsman, M., Kooy H.M. (2009) Characterization of a mini-multileaf collimator in a proton beamline. *Med. Phys.*, **36**, 1886–1894.

40 Bacher, R., Bladdmann, H., Boehringer, T., Coray, A., *et al.* (1989) Development and first results of discrete dynamic spot scanning with protons. Proc. Int. Heavy Particle Therapy Workshop (PTCOG/EORTC/ ECNE)U, PSI Report No. 69 Paul Scherrer Institute, Villigen, Switzerland, pp. 9–12.

41 Pedroni, E., Enge, H. (1995) Beam optics design of compact gantry for proton therapy. *Med. Biol. Eng. Comput.*, **33** (3), 271–277.

42 Pedroni, E., Bacher, R., Blattmann, H., Böhringer, T., *et al.* (1995) The 200-MeV proton therapy project at the Paul Scherrer Institute: conceptual design and practical realization. *Med. Phys.*, **22** (1), 37–53.

43 Schneider, U., Pedroni, E., Lomax, A. (1996) The calibration of CT Hounsfield units for radiotherapy treatment planning. *Phys. Med. Biol.*, **41**, 111.

44 Moyers, M.F., Mah, D., Boyer, S.P., Chang, C., Pankuch, M. (2014) Use of proton beams with breast prostheses and tissue expanders. *Med. Dosim.*, **39** (1), 98–101.

45 Moyers, M.F., Miller, D.W., Bush, D.A., Slater, J.D. (2001) Methodologies and tools for proton beam design for lung tumors. *Int. J. Radiat. Oncol. Biol. Phys.*, **49** (5), 1429–1438.

46 Moyers, M.F., Miller, D.W. (2003) Range, range modulation, and field radius requirements for proton therapy of prostate cancer. *Technol. Cancer Res. Treat.*, **2** (5), 445–447.

47 Depauw, N., Batin, E., Daartz, J., Rosenfeld, A., *et al.* (2015) A novel approach to postmastectomy radiation therapy using scanned proton beams. *Int. J. Radiat. Oncol. Biol. Phys.*, **91** (2), 427–434.

48 Zhao, J., Hu, W., Cai, G., Wang, J., Xie, J., Peng, J., Zhang, Z. (2016) Dosimetric comparisons of VMAT, IMRT and 3DCRT for locally advanced rectal cancer with simultaneous integrated boost. *Oncotarget*, 7, 6345–6351.

49 Chen, G.P., Liu, F., White, J., Vicini, F.A., *et al.* (2015) A planning comparison of 7 irradiation options allowed in RTOG 1005 for early-stage breast cancer. *Med. Dosim.*, **40** (1), 21–25.

50 Lomax, A.J. (2008) Intensity modulated proton therapy and its sensitivity to treatment uncertainties 2: the potential effects of inter-fraction and inter-field motions. *Phys. Med. Biol.*, **53** (4), 1043–1056

51 Collaborative Ocular Melanoma Study Group (2006) The COMS randomized trial of iodine 125 brachytherapy for choroidal melanoma: V. Twelve-year mortality rates and prognostic factors: COMS report No. 28. *Arch. Ophthalmol.*, **124**, 1684–1693.

52 Mishra, K.K., Quivey, J.M., Daftari, I.K., *et al.* (2015) Long-term results of the UCSF-LBNL randomized trial: Charged particle with helium ion versus iodine-125 plaque therapy for choroidal and ciliary body melanoma. *Int. J. Radiat. Oncol. Biol. Phys.*, **92**, 376–383.

53 Wang, Z., Nabhan, M., Schild, S.E., *et al.* (2013) Charged particle radiation therapy for uveal melanoma: a systematic review and meta-analysis. *Int. J. Radiat. Oncol. Biol. Phys.*, **86**, 18–26.

54 Lane, A.M., Kim, I.K., Gragoudas, E.S. (2015) Long-term risk of melanoma-related mortality for patients with uveal melanoma treated with proton beam therapy. *JAMA Ophthalmol.*, **133**, 792–796.

55 Egger, E., Zografos, L., Schalenbourg, A., *et al.* (2003) Eye retention after proton beam radiotherapy for uveal melanoma. *Int. J. Radiat. Oncol. Biol. Phys.*, **55**, 867–880.

56 Dendale, R., Lumbroso-Le Rouic, L., Noel, G., *et al.* (2006) Proton beam radiotherapy for uveal melanoma: results of Curie Institut-Orsay proton therapy center (ICPO). *Int. J. Radiat. Oncol. Biol. Phys.*, **65**, 780–787.

57 Gragoudas, E.S., Lane, A.M., Regan, S., *et al.* (2000) A randomized controlled trial of varying radiation doses in the treatment of choroidal melanoma. *Arch. Ophthalmol.*, **118**, 773–778

58 Campbell, R.G., Prevedello, D.M., Ditzel Filho, L., Otto, B.A., Carrau, R.L. (2015) Contemporary management of clival chordomas. *Curr. Opin. Otolaryngol. Head Neck Surg.*, **23**, 153–161.

59 Munzenrider, J.E., Liebsch, N.J. (1999) Proton therapy for tumors of the skull base. *Strahlenther. Onkol.*, **175** (Suppl. 2), 57–63.

60 Hug, E.B., Loredo, L.N., Slater, J.D., *et al.* (1999) Proton radiation therapy for chordomas and chondrosarcomas of the skull base. *J. Neurosurg.*, **91**, 432–439.

61 Ares, C., Hug, E.B., Lomax, A.J., *et al.* (2009) Effectiveness and safety of spot scanning proton radiation therapy for chordomas and chondrosarcomas of the skull base: first long-term report. *Int. J. Radiat. Oncol. Biol. Phys.*, **75**, 1111–1118.

62 Glosser, G., McManus, P., Munzenrider, J., *et al.* (1997) Neuropsychological function in adults after high dose fractionated radiation therapy of skull base tumors. *Int. J. Radiat. Oncol. Biol. Phys.*, **38**, 231–239.

63 Pai, H.H., Thornton, A., Katznelson, L., *et al.* (2001) Hypothalamic/pituitary function following high-dose conformal radiotherapy to the base of skull: demonstration of a dose-effect relationship using dose-volume histogram analysis. *Int. J. Radiat. Oncol. Biol. Phys.*, **49**, 1079–1092.

64 Lee, C.T., Bilton, S.D., Famiglietti, R.M., Riley, B.A., *et al.* (2005) Treatment planning with protons for pediatric retinoblastoma, medulloblastoma and pelvic sarcoma: how do protons compare with other techniques? *Int. J. Radiat. Oncol. Biol. Phys.*, **63**, 362–372.

65 St Clair, W.H., Adams, J.A., Bues, M., Fullerton, B.C., *et al.* (2004) Advantage of protons compared to conventional x-ray or IMRT in the treatment of a pediatric patient with medulloblastoma. *Int. J. Radiat. Oncol. Biol. Phys.*, **58**, 727–734.

66 Kozak, K.A., Adams, J., Krejcarek, S.J., Tarbell, N.J., Yock, T.I. (2009) A dosimetric comparison of proton and intensity modulated photon radiotherapy for pediatric parameningeal rhabdomyosarcomas. *Int. J. Radiat. Oncol. Biol. Phys.*, **74**, 179–186.

67 Yeung, D.A., McKenzie, C., Indelicato, D. (2013) A dosimetric comparison of intensity modulated proton therapy optimization techniques for pediatric craniopharyngiomas. *Pediatr. Blood Cancer*, **61**, 89–94.

68 Yuh, G.E., Loredo, L.N., Yonemoto, L.T., Bush, D.A., *et al.* (2004) Reducing toxicity from craniospinal irradiation, using proton beams to treat medulloblastoma in young children. *Cancer J.*, **10**, 386–390.

69 Indelicato, D.J., Flampouri, S, Rotondo, R.L., *et al.* (2014) Incidence and dosimetric parameters of pediatric brainstem toxicity following proton therapy. *Acta Oncol.*, **53**, 1298–1304.

70 Gunther, J.R., Sato, M., Chintagumpala, M., *et al.* (2015) Imaging changes in pediatric intracranial ependymoma patients treated with proton beam radiation therapy compared to intensity modulated radiation therapy. *Int. J. Radiat. Oncol. Biol. Phys.*, **93**, 54–63.

71 Ladra, M.M., Yock, T.I. (2014) Proton radiotherapy for pediatric sarcoma. *Cancer*, **6**, 112–127.

72 Chung, C.S., Yock, T.I. (2013) Incidence of second malignancies in patients treated with proton versus photon irradiation. *Int. J. Radiat. Oncol. Biol. Phys.*, **87**, 46–52.

73 Sethi, R.V., Shih, H.A., Yeap, B.Y., Mouw, K.W., *et al.* (2014) Second nonocular tumors among survivors of retinoblastoma treated with contemporary photon and proton radiotherapy. *Cancer*, **120**, 126–133.

74 Nakayama, H., Sugahara, S., Tokita, M., Satoh, H., *et al.* (2010) Proton beam therapy for patients with medically inoperable stage I non-small-cell lung cancer at the University of Tsukuba. *Int. J. Radiat. Oncol. Biol. Phys.*, **78** (2), 467–471.

75 Bush, D.A., Cheek, G., Zaheer, S., Wallen, J., *et al.* (2013) High-dose hypofractionated proton beam radiation therapy is safe and effective for central and peripheral early stage non-small cell lung cancer: results of a 12-year experience at Loma Linda University Medical Center. *Int. J. Radiat. Oncol. Biol. Phys.*, **86** (5), 964–968.

76 Kanemoto, A., Okumura, T., Ishikawa, H., Mizumoto, M., *et al.* (2014) Outcomes and prognostic factors for recurrence after high-dose proton beam therapy for centrally and peripherally located stage I non-small-cell lung cancer. *Clin. Lung Cancer*, **15** (2), e7–e12.

77 Bradley, J.D., Paulus, R., Komaki, R., *et al.* (2015) Standard-dose versus high-dose conformal radiotherapy with concurrent and consolidation carboplatin plus paclitaxel with or without cetuximab for patients with Stage IIA or IIIB non-small-cell lung cancer (RTOG 0617): a randomized, two-by-two factorial phase 3 study. *Lancet Oncol.*, **16**, 187–199.

78 Zhang, X., Li, Y., Pan, X., *et al.* (2010) Intensity modulated proton therapy reduces the dose to normal tissue compared with intensity modulated radiation therapy or passive scattering proton therapy and enables individualized radical radiotherapy for extensive stage IIIB non-small-cell lung cancer: a virtual clinical study. *Int. J. Radiat. Oncol. Biol. Phys.*, **77**, 357–366.

79 Sejpal, S., Komaki, R., Tsao, A., *et al.* (2011) Early findings on toxicity of proton beam therapy with concurrent chemotherapy for nonsmall cell lung cancer. *Cancer*, **117**, 3004–3013.

80 Comparing photon therapy to proton therapy to treat patients with lung cancer. https://clinicaltrials.gov/ct2/show/NCT01993810.

81 Li, Y., Kardar, L., Li, X., Li, H., *et al.* (2014) On the interplay effects with proton scanning beams in stage III lung cancer. *Med. Phys.*, **41**, 021721.

82 Seco, J., Sharp, G., Wu, Z., Gierga, D., Buettner, F., Paganetti, H. (2008) Dosimetric impact of motion in free-breathing and gated lung radiotherapy: A 4D Monte Carlo study of intrafraction and interfraction effects. *Med. Phys.*, **35**, 356.

83 Chang, J., Li, H., Zhu, X.R., Liao, Z., *et al.* (2014) Clinical implementation of intensity modulated proton therapy for thoracic malignancies. *Int. J. Radiat. Oncol. Biol. Phys.*, **90** (4), 809–818.

84 Bernatowicz, K., Lomax, A., Knopf, A. (2013) Comparative study of layered and volumetric rescanning for different scanning speeds of proton patients. *Phys. Med. Biol.*, **58** (22), 7905–7920.

85 Engert, A., Plutschow, A., Eich, H.T., *et al.* (2010) Reduced treatment intensity in patients with early-stage Hodgkin's lymphoma. *N. Engl. J. Med.*, **363** (7), 640–652.

86 Raemaekers, J.M., Andre, M.P., Federico, M., *et al.* (2014) Omitting radiotherapy in early positron emission tomography-negative stage I/II Hodgkin lymphoma is associated with an increased risk of early relapse: clinical results of the preplanned interim analysis of the randomized EORTC/LYSA/FIL H10 trial. *J. Clin. Oncol.*, **32** (12), 1188–1194.

87 Illidge, T., Specht, L., Yahalom, J., *et al.* (2014) Modern radiation therapy for nodal non-Hodgkin lymphoma-target definition and dose guidelines from the International Lymphoma Radiation Oncology Group. *Int. J. Radiat. Oncol. Biol. Phys.*, **89** (1), 49–58.

88 Specht, L., Yahalom, J., Illidge, T., *et al.* (2014) Modern radiation therapy for Hodgkin lymphoma: field and dose guide- lines from the International Lymphoma Radiation Oncology Group (ILROG). *Int. J. Radiat. Oncol. Biol. Phys.*, **89** (4), 854–862.

89 Hoppe, R.T. (2013) Evolution of the techniques of radiation therapy in the management of lymphoma. *Int. J. Clin. Oncol.*, **18** (3), 359–363.

90 Hancock, S.L., Tucker, M.A., Hoppe, R.T. (1993) Factors affecting late mortality from heart disease after treatment of Hodgkin's disease. *JAMA*, **270** (16), 1949–1955.

91 Chung, C.S., Yock, T.I., Nelson, K., Xu, Y., Keating, N.L., Tarbell, N.J. (2013) Incidence of second malignancies among patients treated with proton versus photon radiation. *Int. J. Radiat. Oncol. Biol. Phys.*, **87** (1), 46–52.

92 Clarke, M., Collins, R., Darby, S., *et al.* (2005) Effects of radiotherapy and of differences in the extent of surgery for early breast cancer on local recurrence and 15-year survival: An overview of the randomized trials. *Lancet*, **366**, 2087–2106.

93 Ragaz, J., Olivotto, I.A., Spinelli, J.J., Phillips, N., *et al.* (2005) Locoregional radiation therapy in patients with high-risk breast cancer receiving adjuvant chemotherapy: 20-year results of the British Columbia randomized trial. *J. Natl Cancer Inst.*, **97**, 116–126.

94 Marks, L.B., Yu, X., Prosnitz, R.G., Zhou, S.M., *et al.* (2005) The incidence and functional consequences of RT-associated cardiac perfusion defects. *Int. J. Radiat. Oncol. Biol. Phys.*, **63**, 214–223.

95 Hojris, I., Overgaard, M., Christensen, J.J., Overgaard, J. (1999) Morbidity and mortality of ischaemic heart disease in high-risk breast-cancer patients after adjuvant postmastectomy systemic treatment with or without radiotherapy: analysis of DBCG 82b and 82c randomised trials. Radiotherapy Committee of the Danish Breast Cancer Cooperative Group. *Lancet*, **354**, 1425–1430.

96 Early Breast Cancer Trialists' Collaborative Group. (2000) Favourable and unfavourable effects on long-term survival of radiotherapy for early breast cancer: an overview of the randomised trials. *Lancet*, **355**, 1757–1770.

97 Zablotska, L., Neugut, A. (2003) Lung carcinoma after radiation therapy in women treated with lumpectomy or mastectomy for primary breast carcinoma. *Cancer*, **97**, 1404–1411.

98 Fagundes, M., Hug, E.B., Pankuch, M., Fang, C., *et al.* (2015) Proton therapy for local-regionally advanced breast cancer maximizes cardiac sparing. *Int. J. Particle Ther.*, **1** (4), 827–844.

99 Smyth, L.M., Knight, K.A., Aarons, Y.K., Wasiak, J. (2015) The cardiac dose-sparing benefits of deep inspiration breath-hold in left breast irradiation: a systematic review. *J. Med. Radiat. Sci.*, **62** (1), 66–73.

100 Zhao, H., He, M., Cheng, G., Han, D., *et al.* (2015) A comparative dosimetric study of left sided breast cancer after breast-conserving surgery treated with VMAT and IMRT. *Radiat. Oncol.*, **10**, 231.

101 Ares, C., Khan, S., Macartain, A.M., *et al.* (2010) Postoperative proton radiotherapy for localized and locoregional breast cancer: potential for clinically relevant improvements? *Int. J. Radiat. Oncol. Biol. Phys.*, **76** (3), 685–697.

102 MacDonald, S.M., Jimenez, R., Paetzold, P., Adams, J., *et al.* (2013) Proton radiotherapy for chest wall and regional lymphatic radiation; dose comparisons and treatment delivery. *Radiat. Oncol.*, **8**, 71.

103 Moyers, M.F., Mah, D., Boyer, S.P., Chang, C., Pankuch, M. (2014) Use of proton beams with breast prostheses and tissue expanders. *Med. Dosim.*, **39** (1), 98-101.

104 Shipley, W.U., Verhey, L.J., Munzenrider, J.E. (1995) Advanced prostate cancer; the results of a randomized comparative trial of high dose irradiation boosting with conformal protons compared with conventional dose irradiation using photons alone. *Int. J. Radiat. Oncol. Biol. Phys.*, **32**, 3–12.

105 Benk, V.A., Adams, J.A., Shipley, W.U., *et al.* (1993) Late rectal bleeding following combined x-ray and proton high dose irradiation for patients with Stages T3-T4 prostate carcinoma. *Int. J. Radiat. Oncol. Biol. Phys.*, **26**, 551–557.

106 Schulte, R.W., Slater, J.D., Rossi, C.J., Jr, Slater, J.M. (2000) Value and perspectives of proton radiation therapy for limited stage prostate cancer. *Strahlenther. Onkol.*, **176**, 3–8.

107 Zietman, A.L., Bae, K., Slater, J.D., *et al.* (2010) Randomized trial comparing conventional-dose with high-dose conformal radiation therapy in early-stage adenocarcinoma of the prostate: long-term results from Proton Radiation Oncology Group/American College of Radiology 95-09. *J. Clin. Oncol.*, **28**, 1106–1111.

108 Pugh, T.J., Munsell, M.F., Choi, S.T., *et al.* (2013) Quality of life and toxicity from passively scattered and spot-scanning proton beam therapy for localized prostate cancer. *Int. J. Radiat. Oncol. Biol. Phys.*, **87**, 946–953.

109 Mendenhall, N.P., Hoppe, B.S., Nichols, R.C., *et al.* (2014) Five-year outcomes from 3 prospective trials of image-guided proton therapy for prostate cancer. *Int. J. Radiat. Oncol. Biol. Phys.*, **88**, 596–602.

110 Efstathiou, J. (2012) Proton Therapy vs. IMRT for Low or Intermediate Risk Prostate Cancer (PARTIQoL). Available at: https://clinicaltrials.gov/ct2/show/NCT01617161.

111 Coen, J.J., Bae, K., Zietman, A.L., *et al.* (2011) Acute and late toxicity after dose escalation to 82 GyE using conformal proton radiation for localized prostate cancer: initial report of American College of Radiology Phase II study 03-12. *Int. J. Radiat. Oncol. Biol. Phys.*, **81**, 1005–1009.

112 Vargas, C.E., Hartsell, W.F., Dunn, M., Keole, S.R., *et al.* (2015) Hypofractionated Versus Standard Fractionated Proton-beam Therapy for Low-risk Prostate Cancer: Interim Results of a Randomized Trial PCG GU 002. *Am. J. Clin. Oncol.* [Epub ahead of print].

113 Ng, M., Brown, E., Williams, A., Chao, M, *et al.* (2014) Fiducial markers and spacers in prostate radiotherapy: Current applications. *Br. J. Urol. Int.*, **113** (Suppl. 2), 13–20.

114 Kuban, D.A., Tucker, S.L., Dong, L., *et al.* (2008) Long-term results of the M. D. Anderson randomized dose escalation trial for prostate cancer. *Int. J. Radiat. Oncol. Biol. Phys.*, **70**, 67–74.

115 Peeters, S.T., Heemsbergen, W.D., Koper, P.C., *et al.* (2006) Dose-response in radiotherapy for localized prostate cancer: results of the Dutch multicenter randomized phase III trial comparing 68 Gy of radiotherapy with 78 Gy. *J. Clin. Oncol.*, **24**, 1990–1996.

116 Dearnaley, D.P., Sydes, M.R., Graham, J.D., *et al.* (2007) Escalated dose versus standard-dose conformal radiotherapy in prostate cancer: first results from the MRC RT01 randomised controlled trial. *Lancet Oncol.*, **8**, 475–487.

117 Beckendorf, V., Guerif, S., Le Prise, E., Cosset J.M., *et al.* (2011) 70 Gy versus 80 Gy in localized prostate cancer: 5-year results of GETUG 06 randomized trial. *Int. J. Radiat. Oncol. Biol. Phys.*, **80**, 1056–1063.

118 Widder, J., van der Schaaf, A., Lambin, P., Marijnen, C.A., *et al.* (2015) The quest for evidence for proton therapy: model-based approach and precision medicine. *Int. J. Radiat. Oncol. Biol. Phys.*, **95**, 30–36 [E-pub ahead of print].

119 van de Water, T.A., Bijl, H.P., Schilstra, C., Pijls-Johannesma, M., Langendijk, J.A. (2011) The potential benefit of radiotherapy with protons in head and neck cancer with respect to normal tissue sparing: a systematic review of the literature. *Oncologist*, **16**, 366–377.

120 McDonald, M.W., Liu, Y., Moore, M.G., Johnstone, P.A. (2016) Acute toxicity in comprehensive head and neck radiation for nasopharynx and paranasal sinus cancers: cohort comparison of 3D conformal proton therapy and intensity modulated radiation therapy. *Radiat. Oncol.*, **11**, 32.

121 Sio, T.T., Lin, H.K., Shi, Q., Gunn, G.B., *et al.* (2016) Intensity-modulated proton therapy (IMPT) versus intensity-modulated photon radiotherapy (IMRT) for oropharyngeal cancer: first comparative results of patient-reported outcomes. *Int. J. Radiat. Oncol. Biol. Phys.*, **95** 1107-1014.

122 Patel, S.H., Wang, Z., Wong, W.W., Murad, M.H., *et al.* (2014) Charged particle therapy versus photon therapy for paranasal sinus and nasal cavity malignant diseases: a systematic review and meta-analysis. *Lancet Oncol.*, **15**, 1027–1038.

123 Romesser, P.B., Cahlon, O., Scher, E., Zhou, Y., *et al.* (2016) Proton beam radiation therapy results in significantly reduced toxicity compared with intensity-modulated radiation therapy for head and neck tumors that require ipsilateral radiation. *Radiother. Oncol.*, **118** 286-292.

124 Richard, P. Sandison, G., Dang, Q., Johnson, B., Wong, T., *et al.* (2015) Dental amalgam artifact: Adverse impact on tumor visualization and proton beam treatment planning in oral and oropharyngeal cancers. *Pract. Radiat. Oncol.*, **5**, e583–e588.

125 Fukumitsu, N., Ishikawa, H., Ohnishi, K., Terunuma, T., *et al.* (2014) Dose distribution resulting from changes in aeration of nasal cavity or paranasal sinus cancer in the proton therapy. *Radiother. Oncol.*, **113**, 72–76.

126 http://www.cancer.gov/about-cancer/treatment/clinical-trials/search/view?cdrid = 751031&version =

HealthProfessional#link/StudyIdInfo_
CDR0000751031.

127 http://www.proton-therapy.org/UShospitals_
191A.pdf.

128 http://cerncourier.com/cws/article/cern/27943.

129 http://cyclotron.crocker.ucdavis.edu/.

130 http://www.pcgresearch.org/.

131 https://www.rtog.org/.

132 https://www.nrgoncology.org/.

133 https://protons.com/proton-treatments/clinical-
trials.

134 http://www.massgeneral.org/radiationoncology/
research/.

135 http://www.mdanderson.org/patient-and-cancer-
information/proton-therapy-center/clinical-trials/
index.html.

136 http://cancer.northwestern.edu/clinicaltrials/
DS206_All.

137 http://iuhealth.org/proton-therapy-center//how-
proton-therapy-works/index.html.

7

Principles of Palliative Radiation Therapy

Randy L. Wei, Bo A. Wan, Edward Chow and Stephen Lutz

The History of End-of-Life Care

Early Hospice and Palliative Medicine

The term hospice is derived from the Latin word *hospes,* which refers to either a traveler or a traveler's host. The first hospice-like facilities originated in the 11th century and provided care for injured or dying Crusaders [1]. Religious institutions became the main providers for terminal care from the 11th to the 19th centuries, and that assistance was most commonly provided to travelers, the poor, and those with no family support group [2]. The early 20th century saw a shift towards hospice facilities dedicated to patients with a single diagnosis such as cancer or tuberculosis [3]. The number of hospice programs in the United States has increased from a single facility in 1974 to over 5000 in 2010 [4]. Recent studies have shown that admission to hospice or a palliative care consult at the time of a life-threatening diagnosis can improve quality of life, and in some cases even increase life expectancy [5,6]. Hospice is therefore a subset of the larger approach to symptom management offered by palliative care, which is defined by the World Health Organization as "…an approach that improves the quality of life of patients and their families facing the problems associated with life-threatening illness, through the prevention and relief of suffering by means of early identification and impeccable assessment and treatment of pain and other problems, physical, psychosocial and spiritual" [7]. The rise of the modern hospice and palliative care movement within the past hundred years has coincided with the use of radiotherapy for the palliation of symptoms due to locally advanced or metastatic neoplasm [8].

Origins of Palliative Radiotherapy

Radiotherapy was first used to control symptoms of cancer shortly after Roentgen discovered the x-ray in 1895 [9]. The lack of depth of penetration of comparatively low-energy radiation machines limited the use of this treatment to disease present on superficial structures for several decades. Technological advances in linear accelerators over the past 50 years have allowed the use of radiotherapy for symptom relief that is safe, effective, time-efficient, and not limited by anatomic site or tumor histology. Radiotherapy may provide relief from tumors causing symptoms in the central nervous system, aerodigestive tract, genitourinary system, skeletal system, and integument (Table 7.1).

While much of the early use of radiotherapy was delivered with a small number of large doses, or even a single treatment, the discovery that normal tissue may heal itself with multiple doses led to 'standard' fractionation between 1.8 Gy and 2.0 Gy per day [10]. However, for patients with a limited life expectancy and difficulties with transportation, a shorter, hypofractionated course is less cumbersome for both the patient and caregiver. Thus, the majority of palliative radiotherapy is given with fractionation schema ranging from a single 8 Gy fraction to 30 Gy in 10 fractions. The recent discovery of methods for providing highly conformal therapy, such as intensity-modulated radiation therapy (IMRT) and stereotactic body radiation therapy (SBRT), has added both an opportunity for improved outcomes as well as an increased complexity of care for patients receiving palliative care.

Table 7.1 Clinical circumstances where palliative radiotherapy may be worthwhile.

Anatomic site	Palliative circumstance	Common EBRT fractionation scheme(s) (total Gy/# of fractions)
Skeleton	1. Painful bone metastases 2. Spinal cord compression 3. Status post vertebral body decompression 4. Status post fixation of long bone	1. 30/10, 24/6, 20/5, 8/1 2. 40/20, 30/10, 16/2, 8/1 3. 30/10, 20/5 4. 30/10, 20/5
Brain	1. Neurologic dysfunction, headaches, seizure 2. Status post resection of metastasis	1. 30/10, 20/5 2. 30/10, 20/5
Lung	1. Cough, shortness of breath, hemoptysis, chest pain, post-obstructive pneumonia, superior vena cava syndrome	1. 60/30, 50/20, 45/25, 30/10, 20/5, 17/2, 8–10/1
Esophagus	1. Dysphagia, pain	1. 50/25, 45/25, 30/10, 20/5
Head and Neck	1. Bleeding, pain, dysphagia, shortness of breath	1. 70/35, 60/30, 50/16, 42/12 (divided 14/4 monthly), 20–30/5–10
Gynecologic	1. Pain, vaginal bleeding, hydronephrosis, urinary outlet obstruction	1. 45/25, 44.6/12 (divided 14.8/4 monthly), 20–30/5–10, 8/1
Genitourinary	1. Hematuria, pain, urinary outlet obstruction	1. 45/25, 30–36/5-6 (weekly 6 Gy fraction), 20/5
Rectum	1. Pain, rectal bleeding, tenesmus, rectal obstruction	1. 45/25, 30/10, 30/6 (twice per week 6 Gy fractions) 20–30/5–10, 8/1
Orbit	1. Sudden onset blindness, double vision, pain	1. 30/10, 20/5
Spleen	1. Pain, early satiety, portal hypertension, limited bending at the waist	1. 2.5–5/5–10 (two doses per week)
Liver	1. Pain, early satiety	1. 30/10, 21/10, 10/2

Current Scope of the Problem

Over 1.6 million patients will be diagnosed with cancer in the United States in 2017, and more than 600 000 of those affected will die of their disease [11]. The aging of many of the populations in the Western world will increase the number of persons reaching the age where cancer incidence increases, thereby adding to the need for greater palliative oncology care. During the next ten years, the percentage of US residents aged 65 years or older will increase from 13% to more than 19% of the total population [12]. The most common manifestations of terminal cancer include painful bone metastases, brain metastases, locally advanced and metastatic lung disease, and liver metastases. These clinical situations cause physical pain, decreased functioning, and emotional distress. Although up to 40% of patients who receive radiotherapy do so for palliative intent, the radiation oncology field has devoted only a limited amount of resources towards research involving this patient group [13]. About 25% of palliative radiotherapy is given to patients with newly diagnosed disease, with nearly 50% of cancer patients going on to receive further radiotherapy at some point during their disease trajectory [14]. Recent efforts have led to the publication of palliative radiotherapy treatment guidelines, and the increased need for effective treatments will demand a greater dedication to the investigation of these matters [15–17]. Palliative radiotherapy does not exist in a vacuum, and effective palliative care including palliative radiotherapy will require efficient interdisciplinary care, including appropriate pharmacologic pain interventions.

Pharmacologic Management of Pain

The Nature of Cancer Pain

Some estimates suggest that nearly two-thirds of cancer patients suffer from pain at some point during their illness. Although radiotherapy is beneficial in the management of tumor-induced pain, radiation oncologists must be versed in the correct pharmacologic management of that pain due to the lag time between treatment initiation and pain relief, as well as the existence of patients whose pain does not respond to radiotherapy as desired. Moreover, pain flare may occur in 40% of patients immediately following palliative radiotherapy for their painful bone metastases [18]. Cancer pain is often complex, and requires consistent assessments upon nearly every visit between a patient and their physicians. The patient should be asked to describe the nature of the pain, its intensity, the time course associated with it, the effects of the pain on their daily functioning, the response to previous treatment, and the effectiveness of their current pain regimen.

Non-Steroidal Anti-Inflammatory Medications

The World Health Organization pain medicine ladder describes initiation of pharmacologic therapy for cancer pain with non-steroidal anti-inflammatory drugs (NSAIDs) [19]. Drugs in the NSAID class commonly provide analgesia, decreased inflammation, and anti-pyretic effects. While they do not cause sedation and respiratory depression that are common to opioid medications, they may cause stomach upset, increased bleeding, or decreased functioning of the liver or kidneys [20]. Although NSAIDs may have a ceiling beyond which they do not further aid in pain relief, their concurrent use with opioids may diminish the dose of narcotics required to achieve the desired degree of comfort [21].

Opioid Medications

Cancer pain commonly requires opioids in addition to NSAIDS to achieve adequate and consistent relief. Intermittent pain may be managed with short-acting opioids, while discomfort that occurs throughout the day requires a longer-acting opiate with short-acting medicine available for periods of pain exacerbation, or 'breakthrough pain.' Breakthrough pain commonly occurs several times per day, exacerbated by physical activity, ranges from moderate to severe intensity, and lasts an average of 30 min [22]. Total daily long-acting opioid doses may be titrated fairly rapidly to match whatever levels are needed to mitigate breakthrough pain experienced during the day. While side effects such as sedation and constipation are common to most opioids, the radiation oncologist must also be aware of medication-specific side effects of opioids, such as the build-up of toxic metabolites with some agents, especially in cases of renal insufficiency [23, 24]. Opioids have several routes of administration, including intravenous, intraspinal, transdermal, sublingually, and rectally, but the oral route is the easiest and therefore most desired route.

Adjuvant Pain Medications

Several adjuvant pain medications or interventions may be used in place of or in addition to NSAIDs and opioids, depending on the clinical circumstance. Steroids are potent anti-inflammatory agents whose use is best reserved for short-term pain crises due to cumulative side effects with prolonged treatment [25]. Anti-seizure

medications such as gabapentin or pregalbin can help to relieve neuropathic pain, which might be refractory to relief by other classes of drugs [26, 27]. Neuropathic pain may alternatively respond to antidepressant medications, including those either in the tricyclic or in the selective serotonin and norepinephrine reuptake inhibitor classes [28, 29]. Lastly, spinal nerve blocks may prove efficacious where other pharmacologic interventions have failed.

Clinical Indications for Palliative Radiotherapy

Painful Bone Metastases

Response Rates

About 50–75% of patients with radiologically evident bone metastases eventually come to have discomfort at the site of at least one of those lesions, and the treatment of painful bone metastases remains the most common use of palliative radiotherapy. External beam radiation therapy (EBRT) provides an overall pain response to 60–80% of patients and a complete response in 25–30% [30]. Symptoms due to bone metastases commonly present earlier in the disease course than do those due to visceral disease spread, such as lung or liver metastases. Breast and prostate cancers are the most common primary cancers that metastasize to bone. Carcinomas of the lung, thyroid, and kidney also spread to bone at a rate of up to 30–40% [31]. While tumors of kidney or soft tissue are characteristically thought to be more resistant to the beneficial effects of radiotherapy, painful bone metastases of those histologies may still respond favorably to treatment [32, 33].

Fractionation Schema

Any one of a number of EBRT fractionation schema may provide good palliative relief of pain caused by bone metastases. Nonetheless, a recent worldwide survey revealed that radiation oncologists commonly employ over 100 different dosing regimens for the treatment of this one common palliative scenario [34]. The American Society for Radiation Oncology (ASTRO) concluded in its Bone Metastases Treatment Guidelines that four regimens have been sufficiently studied to conclude that their rates of pain response are optimal and equivalent to each other: 30 Gy in 10 fractions; 24 Gy in six fractions; 20 Gy in five fractions; and a single 8-Gy fraction [15]. The guideline authors concluded that fractionated courses are associated with a lower rate of re-treatment to the same site than a single-fraction treatment (8% versus 20%, respectively). Additionally, outcomes for the treatment of neuropathic pain may be slightly worse with a single 8-Gy fraction than with 20 Gy in five fractions, although the results of one trial comparing the two regimens were inconclusive and the topic remains controversial [35, 36].

Prospective randomized data has shown that a single 8-Gy fraction constitutes a reasonable approach for some bone metastases patients with a limited life expectancy, but current survey data would suggest that this approach is less commonly employed in the United States when compared to other countries [34, 37, 38]. For instances where painful bone metastases are widely spread through the skeleton, either wide-field external beam radiotherapy, such as hemi-body irradiation, or intravenous injection of radioisotopes such as strontium-89 or samarium-153 may successfully provide relief [39, 40]. One new injectable alpha-particle-emitting radium-223-based agent may hold promise in this setting, because its dose-limiting hematologic toxicity is lower than that of other similar radiopharmaceuticals [41].

Spinal Cord/Cauda Equina Compression

Treatment Decision-Making

Malignant spinal cord/cauda equina compression (MSCC) occurs when extraosseous spread of bone metastases impinges on the thecal sac and causes pressure that leads to neurologic dysfunction distal to the impingement. The diagnosis of MSCC is an oncologic emergency that occurs in 2.5–10% of cancer patients and which requires prompt diagnosis and intervention to maximize the chances for preserving neurologic function [39]. A magnetic resonance imaging scan with IV gadolinium contrast of the affected area is the most appropriate means by which to confirm the diagnosis of MSCC. Corticosteroids must be initiated immediately and followed by surgery or radiotherapy within 24–48 h after the presentation of neurologic symptoms to maximize the chance of maintaining neurologic function [42, 43]. A randomized trial suggested that surgery plus postoperative radiotherapy for patients with sufficient performance status and prognosis improves neurologic recovery and survival when compared to patients treated with radiotherapy alone [44]. Surgery should be most strongly considered in patients with spinal instability, compression caused by a retropulsed bone fragment, who have received radiotherapy in the same location in the past, and when histologic evaluation is needed to determine the nature of a tumor arising at an unknown primary site. Factors related to the patient (age, performance status, comorbid disease, reluctance to undergo surgery) or the disease (visceral metastases, multiple levels of spinal cord compression, presence of symptoms for more than 72 h) may dissuade the use of surgery. Additionally, further analyses have concluded that radiotherapy, alone, may be equally as efficacious as surgery plus postoperative radiotherapy in patients aged >65 years [45, 46].

Fractionation Schema

While conflicting data exist regarding the best fractionation scheme for MSCC, many clinicians employ fractionated courses of radiation to 30 Gy in 10 fractions or 40 Gy in 20 fractions for patients, with the rationale that these biologically equivalent doses are sufficiently high to provide a good initial and durable response [47]. However, two prospective randomized studies failed to show a difference in pain control or ambulation in patients treated with 16 Gy in two fractions versus 30 Gy in 10 fractions or 16 Gy in two fractions versus a single 8-Gy dose [48, 49]. Two other studies suggested that there was no difference in ambulation but some improvement in local control when longer courses were given to patients with MSCC [50, 51]. While any of the studied fractionation schemes (40 Gy in 20 fractions, 30 Gy in 10 fractions, 16 Gy in two fractions, and 8 Gy in one fraction) are reasonable for the primary treatment of MSCC, the shorter courses may be more appropriate for those with poor overall prognoses, while those patients with a better prognosis may have a greater benefit with the longer course of radiotherapy. The optimal dose for postoperative radiotherapy is also unknown, although 30 Gy in 10 fractions seems to be the most commonly used and reasonable regimen.

Use of Highly Conformal Radiotherapy Techniques

Technological advances in radiation therapy have allowed for highly conformal treatment that takes advantage of multileaf collimation, real-time image guidance, and robotic technology. The resulting SBRT mechanism for delivering radiotherapy holds great interest in those who provide care for patients with spine metastases and MSCC. The goal of SBRT is to take advantage of a steep dose gradient to provide high doses to only the involved vertebral body, or even to just a portion of a vertebral body with relative sparing of the adjacent spinal cord or nerve roots [52–56]. The greatest theoretical advantages of these techniques would be to provide dose escalation for the primary treatment of spine metastases, or to safely deliver re-treatment to previously irradiated lengths of spine. The drawbacks of this approach include the need for technologically advanced machinery, a greater time dedicated to treatment planning, dependence on meticulous body immobilization, and the potential for increased side effects including myelitis, dermatitis, and vertebral compression fractures due to an incomplete understanding of normal tissue tolerance with these high-dose regimens [52,55,57]. Further research will undoubtedly better define the proper niche for SBRT in the treatment of spine metastases and MSCC.

Brain Metastases

Incidence and Prognosis

While the exact incidence of brain metastases is difficult to discern, it has been estimated that between 20% and 40% of solid tumor patients will develop intracranial metastases at some point during the trajectory of their neoplastic disease [58, 59]. Brain metastases can directly cause symptoms by the invasion of central nervous system structures or indirectly by causing cerebral edema that alters normal brain functions. Those symptoms can include headache, seizures, focal motor weakness, dysphasia, visual changes, nausea, and decreased levels of consciousness. The presence of brain disease portends a poor prognosis, and the effects of intracranial lesions commonly contribute to patient death. The Radiation Therapy and Oncology Group (RTOG) previously defined prognostic groups based on measurable variables from completed brain metastases trials. The resulting recursive partitioning analysis (RPA) prognostic factors divide patients into three groups, with the least favorable group made up of patients with a Karnofsky performance status of less than 70 and a corresponding median life expectancy of just 2.3 months [60]. Patients who make up the most favorable RPA category (Karnofsky performance of 70 or better, age <65 years, controlled primary disease, and no extracranial metastases) have a median survival expectancy of 7.2 months. The majority of patients with brain metastases fall into the intermediate risk group and have a median survival of 4.2 months. A newer prognostic tool, named the Graded Prognostic Assessment, also divides this patient group by prognostic factors, with some suggestions that it may be more predictive than the RPA tool [61]. The differentiation of patients into prognostic groups may guide treatment decision-making, given the need to balance the aggressiveness of therapy with the amount of time dedicated to receiving that treatment and possible resulting side effects.

External-Beam Whole-Brain Radiotherapy

The most established treatment methods for brain metastases include corticosteroids to diminish intracranial pressure, anti-seizure medication when a seizure heralds the presence of tumor, and EBRT [62, 63]. While standard EBRT provides only a moderate survival improvement and little chance for long-term control of metastatic brain disease, it does commonly provide a two-thirds chance for temporary improvement in neurologic symptoms [64]. Whole-brain radiation therapy (WBRT) is chosen in circumstances of multiple metastases, for a small number of metastases too large for stereotactic radiosurgery (SRS) and not amenable to resection, or for histologies such as small-cell lung carcinoma that show a tendency toward microscopic

dissemination. The acute side effects are usually mild and include alopecia and desquamation. Patients who live long enough to face the late effects of WBRT might suffer problems ranging from mild fatigue to short-term memory difficulty. The causes of these longer-term side effects likely include small-vessel damage, chronic inflammation, and cortical damage [65]. The approaches to decrease these effects currently under investigation include the concurrent administration of an anti-Alzheimer's disease drug, memantine, as well as the delivery of hippocampal-sparing radiotherapy in an effort to spare neurons that are responsible for the formation of memory (see ClinicalTrials.gov; Memantine in preventing side effects in patients undergoing whole-brain radiation therapy for brain metastases from solid tumors) [66–68]. Ongoing research aimed at enhancing the anti-tumor effects of WBRT include the concurrent administration of chemotherapy agents such as temozolomide, epidermal growth factor-inhibiting agents such as lapatinib, and angiogenic-inhibiting agents such as bevacizumab [69–84]. For patients in the least favorable RPA class, a separate trial investigated the worthiness of delivering radiation therapy, at all, by randomizing patients to supportive care plus WBRT versus supportive care alone [85].

Stereotactic Radiosurgery (SRS)

Surgical resection should be considered for a solitary lesion in a non-eloquent area of the brain, and postoperative EBRT can increase intracranial tumor control and functionality without adding a significant survival advantage [59]. However, technologic advances have allowed for a relative sparing of normal brain tissue by the delivery of high doses of radiation with (SRS) [86]. Patients with single brain metastases can be treated with either surgical resection or SRS. The value of adding WBRT to SRS in patients with one to four metastases resides in improved local control and decreased failure at other brain sites without any improvement in survival [87]. While WBRT may decrease the risk of tumor-induced neurologic decline, the addition of WBRT to SRS has been found to cause a measurable worsening of treatment-induced neurocognitive functioning [87, 88]. The correct role for postoperative SRS to the tumor bed remains unknown, with studies having suggested conflicting results with regards to local control and neurocognitive functioning [89–91].

Locally Advanced Lung Cancer

Symptoms and Rates of Palliation

Locally advanced lung cancer can cause symptoms by compression of or direct extension into structures of the respiratory system (lung, trachea, or bronchi), the vascular system (superior vena cave, pulmonary vessels), the chest wall (ribs, intercostal muscles), or aerodigestive tract (esophagus). Symptoms which may require palliative radiotherapy include cough, shortness of breath, hemoptysis, bronchial or tracheal obstruction, esophageal dysfunction, superior vena cava obstruction, or brachial plexopathy. Conversely, palliative radiotherapy may worsen fatigue and cause dysphagia leading to weight loss, so discretion must be practiced in these scenarios. Radiotherapy to the lungs may also exacerbate shortness of breath due to pre-existing chronic obstructive pulmonary disease, and appropriate patients should be counseled regarding this risk.

Fractionation Schema and Treatment Options

Numerous randomized trials have assessed appropriate palliative dose fractionation for locally advanced lung cancer, though many of those studies were completed before the advent of modern simulation and dose-planning techniques [16, 92, 93]. The studied regimens have ranged from as short as a single 10-Gy fraction to as lengthy as 50–60 Gy in 25–30 fractions. Although there is not a single defined optimal dosing schedule, shorter fractionation schedules (10 Gy in one fraction, 17 Gy in two fractions, 20 Gy in five fractions) are equally efficacious in providing palliative relief with fewer side effects than lengthier courses, and longer courses show a 5% improvement in overall survival in patients with good performance status. Palliative improvement with either short- or longer-course radiation has been shown for dyspnea (40–97%), hemoptysis (77–92%), cough (60–91%), superior vena cava syndrome (51–96%), and pain (70–78%). Consequently, decisions regarding the most appropriate fractionation scheme should take into account patient features including age, performance status, pulmonary function, presence of pleural effusion, and weight loss [16]. The addition of endobronchial brachytherapy to EBRT has not been shown to significantly improve dyspnea, though it may be considered for symptomatic recurrence of intraluminal disease that has previously been treated with EBRT [94]. Furthermore, the addition of concurrent chemotherapy with EBRT does not lead to symptom improvements and may add unwanted toxicity [16]. Lastly, the use of highly conformal therapy such as SBRT for locally advanced lung cancer holds promise but has not yet been extensively studied [95].

Liver Metastases

Liver metastases are a common site of disease spread for tumors arising in the gastrointestinal tract, lung, and breast [96]. While the most common treatment for liver metastases is system therapy, patients with a small number of non-sizeable liver metastases may undergo surgical resection or receive non-surgical ablative treatment [97–99]. The worthiness of resection of oligometastases

of the liver has been shown in studies, though the number of patients with metastases amenable to resection or radiofrequency ablation is limited [98–100].

While the data for the use of SBRT in this setting has only just started to accrue, it is intriguing to theorize about the potential value of non-surgical ablative therapy for oligometastases with the goals of improved local control and survival [101–106]. A Phase II clinical trial demonstrated improvements in symptoms in 52% of patients who received a single fraction of 8 Gy to metastatic disease in the liver [107].

In patients whose liver metastases cause symptoms but are too numerous or large for considerations of resection or non-surgical ablation, EBRT to the whole liver can provide temporary relief. Several studies have demonstrated the effectiveness of EBRT to the whole liver to total doses of 20–30 Gy at 1.5–3.0 Gy [108, 109]. Palliation was achieved in 55–95% of patients, and 49% of patients had a decrease in liver size and improvement in liver function. Care must be taken in choosing the fractionation scheme for EBRT to the liver, since the low normal tissue tolerance of the liver can result in radiation-induced liver disease which manifests as elevated liver function tests, rapid weight gain, increased abdominal firth, and ascites.

Esophageal Cancer

Esophageal cancer commonly causes dysphagia that may progress from difficulty swallowing solids to a decreased ability to swallow liquids. In the most extreme cases, the patient may have difficulty swallowing their own saliva. Even in cases where therapy is delivered with curative intent, the overall prognosis for those with esophageal cancer is poor. Concurrent palliative therapy is advised for all of these patients from the time of their initial diagnosis. EBRT can provide temporary relief from swallowing in this patient group, though the most effective dose regimens are delivered over several weeks and are commonly augmented with systemic chemotherapy [110]. The use of prolonged radiotherapy and concurrent chemotherapy is debatable in patients with very poor performance status or significant weight loss. The use of brachytherapy, photodynamic therapy, or placement of expandable stents should be evaluated as potential palliative interventions in addition to or in place of combined chemoradiotherapy [111].

Head and Neck Cancer

Locally advanced and recurrent head and neck cancer may produce severe symptoms including bleeding, pain, infection, difficulty swallowing, neck and facial edema, decreased voice quality, and shortness of breath. Even patients who are cured of their head and neck cancers suffer acute and late side effects that require palliative care interventions. For those patients whose disease is too advanced, whose performance status is too poor, or whose comorbidities are too great to be certain that cure may be achieved, palliative radiation can be delivered as a monotherapy with reasonable results. One early trial that compared palliative radiotherapy to 60–70 Gy in six to seven weeks versus 40–48 Gy over a much shorter time frame showed no obvious difference in response rates, palliation of symptoms, or side effects [112]. A separate prospective trial that evaluated the use of 50 Gy in 16 fractions for incurable squamous cell carcinoma of the head and neck revealed a response rate of 73%, excellent palliation of symptoms, median survival of 17 months, and acceptable toxicity [113]. The Radiation Therapy and Oncology Group evaluated a fractionation scheme that delivered 14 Gy in four fractions given over two consecutive days with the option to repeat that same dosing twice more at four-week intervals to a potential total dose of 42 Gy in 12 fractions. The median survival for the group was nearly six months, with quality of life found to have improved in nearly half of the patients [114]. A separate study also used the response of the tumor and tolerance of the patient to treatment to determine the total dose. Patients with locally advanced disease and poor prognosis received a hypofractionated dose of 20 Gy in five fractions over a single week, and then were switched to a more standard fractionation regimen to a total dose of 70 Gy only if the initial week of treatment provided a 50% regression in the size of the tumor. The one-third of patients who showed significant regression and completed the total dose had a median survival of 13 months, while the group with the inferior response had a median survival of only six months. However, both groups noted relatively good relief from their presenting symptoms [115].

Gynecologic Malignancies

Patients with newly discovered or recurrent gynecologic malignancies can suffer vaginal or rectal bleeding, pelvic pain, vaginal discharge, bowel obstruction, fistulas, or hydronephrosis. Radiation therapy can provide excellent rates of relief from all of these problems except for the correction of a fistula. The RTOG measured the efficacy and tolerability of a hypofractionated course of radiotherapy that delivered 14.4 Gy in four fractions given twice per day over two consecutive days. Patients who survived long enough and who tolerated the side effects of treatment were offered two additional rounds of treatment to that same dose at three- to six-week intervals up to a possible total dose of 44.6 Gy in 12 fractions. The side effects of treatment were generally well tolerated, and more than half of the patients completed all 12 planned doses. The subjective and objective response rates to treatment were found to be about 50%, with a repeat trial showing feasibility of the same approach with only two- to

four-week intervals between 14.4 Gy doses [116, 117]. Surgical excision is only useful in providing palliation to this patient group, though other possible adjuvant interventions may include vaginal packing, vaginal high-dose rate brachytherapy, placement of ureteral stents, or arterial embolization.

Locally Advanced Genitourinary Cancer

Locally advanced or recurrent genitourinary tumors might cause hematuria, pain, urinary obstruction, infection, or fistula formation. Palliative radiotherapy can provide temporary relief of these symptoms. A hypofractionated course of 6 Gy per fraction given once per week to a total of 30–36 Gy has demonstrated palliative benefit, with 91% of patients hematuria free after 10 months [118, 119]. Two trials which compared shorter- versus longer-course radiotherapy for patients with symptoms from locally advanced bladder cancer suggested similar rates of symptom relief and survival, though the longer courses correlated with a slightly longer survival than was seen with the shorter courses [120, 121]. Locally recurrent, hormone-refractory prostate cancer has been shown to respond favorably to hypofractionated doses as low as 20 Gy in five fractions, with nearly 90% of these patients noting partial or near-complete relief from their symptoms [122]. The symptoms of both locally advanced prostate and bladder cancer might be aided by ureteral stenting or use of an indwelling or intermittent urinary catheter.

Rectal Cancer

About 30% of patients with rectal cancer present with metastatic disease at the time of their initial diagnosis. Another 40% of rectal cancer patients will experience local recurrence requiring palliative treatment at some point in the trajectory of the disease [123, 124]. The symptoms caused by uncontrolled disease may include abdominal pain, nausea and vomiting, unintentional weight loss, changes in bowel habits, bleeding, tenesmus, and bowel obstruction. Decompressive surgery can relieve many of these symptoms, though emergency surgery should be avoided due to high complication and mortality rates [125]. Palliative radiotherapy has shown excellent rates of palliation for symptoms including pain (65–89%), bleeding (75–100%), mass effect (24–71%), rectal discharge (50%), and urologic symptoms (22%), with reasonable durability of response [126–129]. One of those groups utilized a hypofractionated dose of 30 Gy in six fractions given two times per week, with an excellent colostomy-free status until death from metastatic disease [127, 129]. Chemotherapy can be delivered concurrently with radiotherapy with acceptable side effects, and other adjuvant interventions such as self-expanding stents, laser ablation, high-dose rate brachytherapy, or radiofrequency ablation can be added to the treatment regimen depending on patient- and tumor-specific variables [130–132].

Blindness from Orbital Metastasis

On rare occasions, tumors may metastasize to the orbital fat, retina, uvea or extraocular muscles within the posterior orbit and cause diplopia, pain, or blindness. The most common histologies leading to ocular metastases are breast cancer, malignant melanoma, and prostate cancer. Patients commonly present with sudden onset visual field loss. Pain may not always be preceded or accompanied by vision loss. It is rare for ocular metastases to present as the first site of metastatic disease, with 75–85% of those patients suffering from this condition already having known metastatic cancer. Just as would be true for other neurologic dysfunctions caused by tumor compression (such as MSCC), the successful treatment of this condition requires prompt recognition, initiation of corticosteroids, and initiation of radiotherapy. Unfortunately, even in cases where radiotherapy palliates the symptoms of orbital metastases, their formation usually heralds an aggressive phase of metastatic progression of the disease and is associated with a poor overall prognosis [133, 134].

Splenomegaly Due to Hematologic Cancer

Patients with hematologic malignancy or myelofibrosis may develop massive splenomegaly that causes discomfort, early satiety, portal hypertension, difficulties bending at the waist, and cytopenias due to the sequestration of cells. Splenectomy is the preferred treatment for those who fail medical therapy but have adequate performance status and a relatively favorable prognosis. In cases where splenectomy is unsafe or declined by the patient, very small doses of radiotherapy can decrease the size of the spleen in 90% of those suffering from this condition. Biweekly treatments of increasing dosage (first two treatments of 50 cGy, second two treatments of 75 cGy, and third two treatments of 100 cGy) to a total dose of 4.5 Gy over 3 weeks have shown to be effective in palliating symptomatic splenomegaly. Splenic regression commonly lasts for up to six months, and re-treatment can be offered to those whose splenomegaly recurs. The patient's blood counts should be monitored meticulously during the treatments to make certain that a dangerous thrombocytopenia does not develop [135–137].

Contraindications to Palliative Radiotherapy

Though radiotherapy can be a valuable means by which to provide palliation for a myriad of end-of-life cancer

Table 7.2 Circumstances when palliative radiotherapy is contraindicated.

Category	Limiting factor
Patient-related	1. Death imminent 2. Multiple progressive symptoms
Treatment-related	1. Required treatment course too lengthy 2. Re-treatment exceeds normal tissue tolerance (relative contraindication)
Healthcare system-related	1. Radiotherapy facility or technology unavailable 2. Inappropriately late radiotherapy consultation request

symptoms, certain circumstances act as relative or absolute contraindications to its use. Given a lag time between the initiation of radiotherapy and the onset of palliation in most circumstances, treatment should not be offered to patients whose remaining lifespan is so short that they would not likely survive to experience relief. The tendency for oncology physicians to overestimate survival in terminal cancer patients can lead to futile treatment for some patients [138].

Along those same lines, it is relatively contraindicated to deliver palliative radiotherapy to address a single symptom when several other symptoms are worsening and will likely go uncontrolled (see Table 7.2). Symptoms tend to occur concurrently in what have been termed 'symptom clusters,' with the failure to recognize and base treatment upon this clustering a potential failure to improve quality of life [139, 140]. Treatments should be directed towards improving quality of life as measured by validated instruments such as the EORTC QLQ-C15-PAL tool [141]. Lastly, therapy should be offered only in a manner that does not place an undue burden on the patient or their caregiver. This goal can be met by streamlining the consultation, CT planning simulation, radiation treatment planning and treatment delivery process, while still allowing for enough time to perform quality assurance on treatment planning and delivery to ensure safe and accurate treatment [142].

Palliative Care Special Topics

Pediatric Palliative Care

Palliative care is important for the 25% of childhood cancer patients who die from their disease, and it is also

Table 7.3 Members of the Palliative Care Oncology Team.

Oncology physicians	1. Medical oncologist 2. Radiation oncologist
Palliative care nurses	1. Generalist nurse 2. Advanced practice nurse
Pain management specialists	1. Palliative care pharmacist 2. Pain service physician
Psychosocial professionals	1. General social worker or 2. Palliative care social worker 3. Psychologist
Spiritual caregivers	1. Chaplain or 2. Palliative care-certified chaplain
Home health	1. Nurse 2. Nursing assistant
Hospice	1. Hospice physician 2. Hospice nurse

meaningful for those who will survive and face the physical and emotional sequelae of the disease and treatment toxicity [143]. Most pediatric oncology cases are appropriately treated at larger academic institutions, so the provision of pediatric palliative care is also clustered in these facilities. Pediatric patients have favorable clinical response rates for painful metastases, spinal cord compression, and respiratory compromise [144, 145]. Palliative radiation dose using short-course fractionation schemes ranging from 8 to 30 Gy in one to 10 fractions have been used in pediatric patients with excellent response rates and no reported grade 3 or 4 toxicity [146, 147].

The pediatric palliative care teams in these centers should include at a minimum a trained pediatric radiation oncologist, nurse or nurse practitioner, social worker, chaplain, and home health workers [148, 149] (Table 7.3). While pediatric palliative care may be offered in community hospital settings or by adult-based palliative care and hospice programs, the potential gains of limiting these circumstances are evident. Children should be included in conversations about the diagnosis, prognosis, and treatment options for their disease, with the discussion framed in a manner appropriate for the child's level of understanding and emotional capacity. Children of all ages gain a sense of control by taking part in these conversations, while adolescents as young as 14 years old are able to help make decisions regarding the aggressiveness of treatment and code status [150, 151]. One study revealed that parents who openly discussed a poor prognosis with their child had fewer post-mortem regrets about the experience than those who did not [152].

Prognostication

A Surveillance, Epidemiology, and End Results study showed that of the 15 287 patients that initiated radiotherapy in the last month of life, 17.8% of these patients received more than 10 days of radiation treatment [153]. A life expectancy prediction model among patients receiving palliative radiotherapy was developed to aid radiation oncologists determine dose and fractionation schemes based on life expectancy. Additionally, estimating life expectancy helps patients with metastatic disease weigh the risks and benefits of further treatment with curative intent, decide on palliative cancer treatments, and initiate end-of-life conversations and planning. However, for many oncologists, this task is difficult to achieve even for the most veteran physician. Prognostic models can help stratify patients on expected life expectancy.

A prognostic model based on a cohort of patients who received palliative radiotherapy was used to help stratify patients on expected life expectancy. Using three clinical factors – namely, cancer type (breast versus non-breast), Karnofsky performance status (<70 versus ≥70), and site of metastasis (bone only versus other), patients could be separated into three groups with median survivals of 13.8 months, 6 months, and 2.1 months [154, 155]. To further enhance the model, the second predictive TEACHH model was created to help further separate patients with life expectancy less than three months and those more than one year. The TEACHH model took into account cancer type ('T') (lung and other versus breast and prostate), ECOG performance ('E') (2–4 versus 0–1), older age ('A') (>60 versus ≤60 years), prior palliative chemotherapy courses ('C') (>2 versus 0–1), hepatic metastases ('H'), and hospitalizations within three months before palliative radiotherapy ('H') (0 versus ≥1) [156]. The 'TEACHH' predictive model was able to divide patients into three groups with distinct median survivals of 19.9 months, 5 months, and 1.7 months.

Palliative Care Team

The multidisciplinary palliative care team is comprised of a specialist in palliative medicine, a palliative care nurse, social worker, physiotherapist, pastoral carer, and palliative radiation oncologists. A randomized control trial of early palliative care intervention with newly diagnosed metastatic non-small-cell lung cancer showed significant improvements in quality of life, mood, and median survival [6]. When multidisciplinary palliative care was added to regular oncology care, there was reduced likelihood of incomplete palliative radiotherapy [157]. In an outpatient palliative radiotherapy setting, the consultations of clinical pharmacist, occupational therapist, and registered dietitian improved tiredness, anxiety, depression, and drowsiness after four weeks [158].

Nurses

Palliative care nurses can be generalists or advanced practice nurses (APNs). Recently published standards having defined the scope and appropriate training of the palliative nursing practice [159]. The APN specialization requires a master's degree education, allowing the graduate to function in roles including clinical expertise, clinical consultation, administration, education, and research [160]. APNs commonly serve as one of the primary communicators between patients, their families, and the palliative service [161]. Predicted increases in the number of patients facing cancer will lead to a greater need for palliative care nurses.

Social Workers

Oncology social workers are critical members of the palliative care team, especially given that nearly three-fourths of patients report psychosocial distress over issues related to the logistics of their treatments, coping with their illness and side effects, and managing relationships with their partner or other family members [162]. Not surprisingly, psychosocial distress correlates with factors including the poor prognosis, fatigue, loss of autonomy, lack of social support, and pain [163–166]. These factors are associated with poor quality of life and requests for hastening death by cancer patients. Appropriate management of psychosocial distress by social workers as members of the palliative care team improve quality of life and, in some cases, even survival [163, 167].

Spiritual Caregivers

The majority of people in the US practice religion in their daily lives, and nearly 90% of advanced cancer patients find that their religion is important in coping with their illness [168]. The majority of cancer patients say that their spiritual needs are not adequately met by their physician or their healthcare facility [169]. Though community clergy can answer a great need in these circumstances, palliative care teams often include board-certified chaplains who lead the spiritual care for palliative oncology patients. The process of board certification for chaplains includes a graduate level degree, a minimum of at least 1600 hours of clinical training, and a code of ethics that prohibits proselytizing [170]. The growing trend has been for spiritual care to be delivered as emotional care by all members of the palliative care staff, with the chaplain acting as the leader of those efforts [171]. Screening for spiritual care needs can be carried out with a validated survey tool whose acronym is FICA, which stands for faith, importance, community, and address in care [172].

The proper assessment and management of spiritual needs can noticeably improve quality of life scores in this group [173].

Communication with Palliative Care Patients

Pitfalls in Communication

Though communication between palliative oncology patients and their physicians is critical from the diagnosis until death, very few clinicians have received formal education about the best ways to communicate with patients. Studies show that physicians often interrupt within 30 seconds after a patient begins to speak about their situation, and the result is that patients feel that their needs are unmet [174–176]. Physician domination of the conversation, often in the form of lecturing without listening, is a second type of communication gap [177]. Another suboptimal result of diminished physician listening is premature reassurance, which is typified by a physician providing an answer before the patient has had sufficient time to formulate and enunciate their question [177, 178]. Collusion is the phrase to describe the situation where both the physician and patient are reluctant to discuss uncomfortable topics, such as a poor prognosis, and they subconsciously agree to avoid the reality of the situation [177]. When the physician, alone, exhibits an inability to approach an issue raised by a patient, they may show a behavior known as 'blocking,' where they change the subject or simply ignore a question that has been raised [177]. Lastly, a provider may fall short in their ability to communicate by ignoring the affective aspects of the conversation, as one might see when a patient cries without the physician acknowledging the emotional difficulties of facing a potentially fatal cancer [175].

Optimizing Communication

Physicians can optimize communication by any number of means, with one well-known pneumonic containing the six steps necessary to optimize their conversations with patients. The acronym SPIKES stands for the following steps: (i) Prepare the Setting for the conversation in a quiet room with limited interruptions; (ii) assess the patient's Perception of their disease process; (iii) invite the patient to share their desire for how much Information they would like to be told; (iv) deliver knowledge about the situation in an understandable and Empathetic fashion; and (v) Summarize the news and make certain that the patient is comfortable with the results of the conversation [178].

Conclusions and Future Directions

Palliative radiotherapy remains an effective, safe, and efficient means by which to relieve the symptoms caused by a number of locally advanced and metastatic tumors. Though accurate survival predictions for patients with life-threatening cancer remain difficult, the increased ability to separate palliative oncology patients into those with poor prognoses who require a short course of radiotherapy versus those whose prognoses justify more aggressive radiotherapy will add greatly to the outcomes of patients with advance disease. The combination of aging populations in the developed world and decreased deaths caused by infection and malnutrition in developing countries will dramatically increase the need for worldwide palliative radiotherapy care in the coming decades. That increased attention to end-of-life issues will require a greater dedication to palliative care research, interdisciplinary collaboration between radiation oncologists and other specialists, and a streamlining of radiation therapy methodologies to maximize access and minimize costs to this enlarging group of patients.

References

1 Robbins, J. (1983) *Caring for the Dying Patient and the Family.* Taylor & Francis.

2 Connor, S. (1998) *Hospice: Practice, Pitfalls, and Promise.* Taylor & Francis.

3 Radioworks, A. (2011) *The Hospice Experiment: A Revolution in Dying.* American Public Media.

4 NHPCO (2010) *NHPCO Facts and Figures: Hospice Care in America.*

5 Connor, S.R., Pyenson, B., Fitch, K., Spence, C., Iwasaki, K. (2007) Comparing hospice and nonhospice patient survival among patients who die within a three-year window. *J. Pain Symptom Manag.*, **33**, 238–246.

6 Temel, J.S., Greer, J.A., Muzikansky, A., Gallagher, E.R., *et al.* (2010) Early palliative care for patients with metastatic non-small-cell lung cancer. *N. Engl. J. Med.*, **363**, 733–742.

7 World Health Organization (2016) *Cancer, WHO Definition of Palliative Care.*

8 Clark, D. (2000) *Total Pain: The Work of Cicely Saunders and the Hospice Movement.* APS Bulletin.

9 Stanton, A. (1895) Wilhelm Conrad Rontgen On a New Kind of Rays: translation of a paper read before the Wurzburg Physical and Medical Society. Nature.

10 Coutard, H. (1934) Principles of x-ray therapy of malignant diseases. *Lancet*, **224**, 1–8.

11 Siegel, R., Miller, K., Jemal, A. (2017) Cancer Statistics 2017. *CA Cancer J. Clin.*, **67**, 7–30.

12 Administration on Aging (2010) *A profile of older Americans.* http://www.aoa.gov/aoaroot/aging_statistics/Profile/2010/3.aspx. Most recently accessed October 6, 2015.

13 Coia, L. (1996) Palliative radiation therapy in the United States. *Cancer J. Oncol.*, **6**(Suppl 1), 62–69.

14 Lutz, S.T., Chow, E.L., Hartsell, W.F., Konski, A.A. (2007) A review of hypofractionated palliative radiotherapy. *Cancer*, **109**, 1462–1470.

15 Lutz, S., Berk, L., Chang, E., Chow, E., *et al.* (2011) Palliative radiotherapy for bone metastases: an ASTRO evidence-based guideline. *Int. J. Radiat. Oncol. Biol. Phys.*, **79**, 965–976.

16 Rodrigues, G., Videtic, G.M., Sur, R., Bezjak, A., *et al.* (2011) Palliative thoracic radiotherapy in lung cancer: An American Society for Radiation Oncology evidence-based clinical practice guideline. *Pract. Radiat. Oncol.*, **1**, 60–71.

17 Tsao, M.N., Rades, D., Wirth, A., Lo, S.S., *et al.* (2012) Radiotherapeutic and surgical management for newly diagnosed brain metastasis(es): An American Society for Radiation Oncology evidence-based guideline. *Pract. Radiat. Oncol.*, **2**(3), 210–225. doi:10.1016/j.prro.2011.12.004.

18 Hird, A., Chow, E., Zhang, L., Wong, R., *et al.* (2009) Determining the incidence of pain flare following palliative radiotherapy for symptomatic bone metastases: results from three Canadian cancer centers. *Int. J. Radiat. Oncol. Biol. Phys.*, **75**, 193–197.

19 World Health Organization (2016) *Cancer, WHO's pain ladder.*

20 Munir, M.A., Enany, N., Zhang, J.M. (2007) Nonopioid analgesics. *Med. Clin. North Am.*, **91**, 97–111.

21 Khan, M.I., Walsh, D., Brito-Dellan, N. (2011) Opioid and adjuvant analgesics: compared and contrasted. *Am. J. Hosp. Palliat. Care*, **28**, 378–383.

22 Portenoy, R.K., Payne, D., Jacobsen, P. (1999) Breakthrough pain: characteristics and impact in patients with cancer pain. *Pain*, **81**, 129–134.

23 King, S., Forbes, K., Hanks, G.W., Ferro, C.J., Chambers, E.J. (2011) A systematic review of the use of opioid medication for those with moderate to severe cancer pain and renal impairment: a European Palliative Care Research Collaborative opioid guidelines project. *Palliat. Med*, **25**, 525–552.

24 Thwaites, D., McCann, S., Broderick, P. (2004) Hydromorphone neuroexcitation. *J. Palliat. Med.*, **7**, 545–550.

25 Soares, L.G., Chan, V.W. (2007) The rationale for a multimodal approach in the management of

breakthrough cancer pain: a review. *Am. J. Hosp. Palliat. Care*, **24**, 430–439.

26 Backonja, M., Beydoun, A., Edwards, K.R., Schwartz, S.L., *et al.* (1998) Gabapentin for the symptomatic treatment of painful neuropathy in patients with diabetes mellitus: a randomized controlled trial. *JAMA*, **280**, 1831–1836.

27 Dworkin, R.H., Corbin, A.E., Young, J.P., Jr, Sharma, U., *et al.* (2003) Pregabalin for the treatment of postherpetic neuralgia: a randomized, placebo-controlled trial. *Neurology*, **60**, 1274–1283.

28 Dworkin, R.H., O'Connor, A.B., Backonja, M., Farrar, J.T., *et al.* (2007) Pharmacologic management of neuropathic pain: evidence-based recommendations. *Pain*, **132**, 237–251.

29 Laird, B., Colvin, L., Fallon, M. (2008) Management of cancer pain: basic principles and neuropathic cancer pain. *Eur. J. Cancer*, **44**, 1078–1082.

30 Chow, E., Harris, K., Fan, G., Tsao, M., Sze, W.M. (2007) Palliative radiotherapy trials for bone metastases: a systematic review. *J. Clin. Oncol.*, **25**, 1423–1436.

31 Perez, C., Brady, L.W., Halperin, E.C. (2004) Palliative of Bone Metastases – Biology and Physiology, in *Principles and Practices of Radiation Oncology*. Lippincott, Williams, and Wilkins, Philadelphia.

32 Lee, J., Hodgson, D., Chow, E., Bezjak, A., *et al.* (2005) A phase II trial of palliative radiotherapy for metastatic renal cell carcinoma. *Cancer*, **104**, 1894–1900.

33 Perry, H., Chu, F.C. (1962) Radiation therapy in the palliative management of soft tissue sarcomas. *Cancer*, **15**, 179–183.

34 Fairchild, A., Barnes, E., Ghosh, S., Ben-Josef, E., *et al.* (2009) International patterns of practice in palliative radiotherapy for painful bone metastases: evidence-based practice? *Int. J. Radiat. Oncol. Biol. Phys.*, **75**, 1501–1510.

35 Dennis, K., Chow, E., Roos, D., DeAngelis, C., *et al.* (2011) Should bone metastases causing neuropathic pain be treated with single-dose radiotherapy? *Clin. Oncol. (R. Coll. Radiol.)*, **23**, 482–484.

36 Roos, D.E., Turner, S.L., O'Brien, P.C., Smith, J.G., *et al.* and Trans-Tasman Radiation Oncology Group (2005) Randomized trial of 8 Gy in 1 versus 20 Gy in 5 fractions of radiotherapy for neuropathic pain due to bone metastases (Trans-Tasman Radiation Oncology Group, TROG 96.05). *Radiother. Oncol.*, **75**, 54–63.

37 Chow, E., Zeng, L., Salvo, N., Dennis, K., Tsao, M., Lutz, S. (2012) Update on the systematic review of palliative radiotherapy trials for bone metastases. *Clin. Oncol. (R. Coll. Radiol.)*, **24**, 112–124.

38 Hartsell, W.F., Scott, C.B., Bruner, D.W., Scarantino, C.W., *et al.* (2005) Randomized trial of short- versus long-course radiotherapy for palliation of painful bone metastases. *J. Natl Cancer Inst.*, **97**, 798–804.

39 Rades, D., Dunst, J., Schild, S.E. (2008) The first score predicting overall survival in patients with metastatic spinal cord compression. *Cancer*, **112**, 157–161.

40 Tripp, P., Kuettel, M. (2006) Radiation therapy for cancer pain management, in *Cancer Pain: Pharmacological, Interventional, and Palliative Care Approaches* (ed Oscar A. de Leon-Casasola), Elsevier, Inc., Philadelphia, pp. 465–477.

41 Liepe, K. (2009) Alpharadin, a 223Ra-based alpha-particle-emitting pharmaceutical for the treatment of bone metastases in patients with cancer. *Curr. Opin. Investig. Drugs*, **10**, 1346–1358.

42 Greenberg, H.S., Kim, J.H., Posner, J.B. (1980) Epidural spinal cord compression from metastatic tumor: results with a new treatment protocol. *Ann. Neurol.*, **8**, 361–366.

43 Prasad, D., Schiff, D. (2005) Malignant spinal-cord compression. *Lancet Oncol.*, **6**, 15–24.

44 Patchell, R.A., Tibbs, P.A., Regine, W.F., Payne, R., *et al.* (2005) Direct decompressive surgical resection in the treatment of spinal cord compression caused by metastatic cancer: a randomised trial. *Lancet*, **366**, 643–648.

45 Chi, J.H., Gokaslan, Z., McCormick, P., Tibbs, P.A., Kryscio, R.J., Patchell, R.A. (2009) Selecting treatment for patients with malignant epidural spinal cord compression-does age matter?: results from a randomized clinical trial. *Spine (Phil., Pa, 1976)*, **34**, 431–435.

46 Rades, D., Huttenlocher, S., Dunst, J., Bajrovic, A., *et al.* (2010) Matched pair analysis comparing surgery followed by radiotherapy and radiotherapy alone for metastatic spinal cord compression. *J. Clin. Oncol.*, **28**, 3597–3604.

47 Loblaw, D.A., Perry, J., Chambers, A., Laperriere, N.J. (2005) Systematic review of the diagnosis and management of malignant extradural spinal cord compression: the Cancer Care Ontario Practice Guidelines Initiative's Neuro-Oncology Disease Site Group. *J. Clin. Oncol.*, **23**, 2028–2037.

48 Maranzano, E., Bellavita, R., Rossi, R., De Angelis, V., *et al.* (2005) Short-course versus split-course radiotherapy in metastatic spinal cord compression: results of a phase III, randomized, multicenter trial. *J. Clin. Oncol.*, **23**, 3358–3365.

49 Maranzano, E., Trippa, F., Casale, M., Costantini, S., *et al.* (2009) 8Gy single-dose radiotherapy is effective in metastatic spinal cord compression: results of a phase III randomized multicentre Italian trial. *Radiother. Oncol.*, **93**, 174–179.

50 Rades, D., Fehlauer, F., Stalpers, L.J., Wildfang, I., *et al.* (2004) A prospective evaluation of two radiotherapy schedules with 10 versus 20 fractions for the treatment of metastatic spinal cord compression: final results of a multicenter study. *Cancer*, **101**, 2687–2692.

51 Rades, D., Stalpers, L.J., Veninga, T., Schulte, R., *et al.* (2005) Evaluation of five radiation schedules and prognostic factors for metastatic spinal cord compression. *J. Clin. Oncol.*, **23**, 3366–3375.

52 Chang, E.L., Shiu, A.S., Mendel, E., Mathews, L.A., *et al.* (2007) Phase I/II study of stereotactic body radiotherapy for spinal metastasis and its pattern of failure. *J. Neurosurg. Spine*, **7**, 151–160.

53 Gerszten, P.C., Burton, S.A., Ozhasoglu, C., Welch, W.C. (2007) Radiosurgery for spinal metastases: clinical experience in 500 cases from a single institution. *Spine (Phil., Pa., 1976)*, **32**, 193–199.

54 Ryu, S., Fang Yin, F., Rock, J., Zhu, J., *et al.* (2003) Image-guided and intensity-modulated radiosurgery for patients with spinal metastasis. *Cancer*, **97**, 2013–2018.

55 Ryu, S., Jin, J.Y., Jin, R., Rock, J., Ajlouni, M., Movsas, B., Rosenblum, M., and Kim, J.H. (2007). Partial volume tolerance of the spinal cord and complications of single-dose radiosurgery. *Cancer* **109**, 628-636.

56 Sahgal, A., Ames, C., Chou, D., Ma, L., *et al.* (2009) Stereotactic body radiotherapy is effective salvage therapy for patients with prior radiation of spinal metastases. *Int. J. Radiat. Oncol. Biol. Phys.*, **74**, 723–731.

57 Gibbs, I.C., Patil, C., Gerszten, P.C., Adler, J.R., Jr, Burton, S.A. (2009) Delayed radiation-induced myelopathy after spinal radiosurgery. *Neurosurgery*, **64**, A67–A72.

58 Hart, M.G., Grant, R., Walker, M., Dickinson, H. (2005) Surgical resection and whole brain radiation therapy versus whole brain radiation therapy alone for single brain metastases. Cochrane Database Syst. Rev., CD003292.

59 Posner, J.B., Chernik, N.L. (1978) Intracranial metastases from systemic cancer. *Adv. Neurol.*, **19**, 579–592.

60 Gaspar, L.E., Scott, C., Murray, K., Curran, W. (2000) Validation of the RTOG recursive partitioning analysis (RPA) classification for brain metastases. *Int. J. Radiat. Oncol. Biol. Phys.*, **47**, 1001–1006.

61 Sperduto, P.W., Chao, S.T., Sneed, P.K., Luo, X., *et al.* (2010) Diagnosis-specific prognostic factors, indexes, and treatment outcomes for patients with newly diagnosed brain metastases: a multi-institutional analysis of 4,259 patients. *Int. J. Radiat. Oncol. Biol. Phys.*, **77**, 655–661.

62 Ryken, T.C., McDermott, M., Robinson, P.D., Ammirati, M., *et al.* (2010) The role of steroids in the management of brain metastases: a systematic review and evidence-based clinical practice guideline. *J. Neurooncol.*, **96**, 103–114.

63 Vecht, C.J., Hovestadt, A., Verbiest, H.B., van Vliet, J.J., van Putten, W.L. (1994) Dose-effect relationship of dexamethasone on Karnofsky performance in metastatic brain tumors: a randomized study of doses of 4, 8, and 16 mg per day. *Neurology*, **44**, 675–680.

64 Borgelt, B., Gelber, R., Kramer, S., Brady, L.W., *et al.* (1980) The palliation of brain metastases: final results of the first two studies by the Radiation Therapy Oncology Group. *Int. J. Radiat. Oncol. Biol. Phys.*, **6**, 1–9.

65 Caselli, R.J., Dueck, A.C., Osborne, D., Sabbagh, M.N., *et al.* (2009) Longitudinal modeling of age-related memory decline and the APOE epsilon4 effect. *N. Engl. J. Med.*, **361**, 255–263.

66 Gondi, V., Hermann, B.P., Mehta, M.P., Tome, W.A. (2013) Hippocampal dosimetry predicts neurocognitive function impairment after fractionated stereotactic radiotherapy for benign or low-grade adult brain tumors. *Int. J. Radiat. Oncol. Biol. Phys.*, **85**, 348–354.

67 Raber, J., Rola, R., LeFevour, A., Morhardt, D., *et al.* (2004) Radiation-induced cognitive impairments are associated with changes in indicators of hippocampal neurogenesis. *Radiat. Res.*, **162**, 39–47.

68 Memantine in Preventing Side Effects in Patients Undergoing Whole-Brain Radiation Therapy for Brain Metastases From Solid Tumors. (2016) Retrieved from https://clinicaltrials.gov/ct2 (Identification No. NCT00566852).

69 Aboody, K.S., Brown, A., Rainov, N.G., Bower, K.A., *et al.* (2000) Neural stem cells display extensive tropism for pathology in adult brain: evidence from intracranial gliomas. *Proc. Natl Acad. Sci. USA*, **97**, 12846–12851.

70 Aboody, K.S., Najbauer, J., Schmidt, N.O., Yang, W., *et al.* (2006) Targeting of melanoma brain metastases using engineered neural stem/progenitor cells. *Neuro Oncol.*, **8**, 119–126.

71 Ceresoli, G.L., Cappuzzo, F., Gregorc, V., Bartolini, S., Crino, L., Villa, E. (2004) Gefitinib in patients with brain metastases from non-small-cell lung cancer: a prospective trial. *Ann. Oncol.*, **15**, 1042–1047.

72 Chiu, C.H., Tsai, C.M., Chen, Y.M., Chiang, S.C., Liou, J.L., Perng, R.P. (2005) Gefitinib is active in patients with brain metastases from non-small cell lung cancer and response is related to skin toxicity. *Lung Cancer*, **47**, 129–138.

73 De Braganca, K.C., Janjigian, Y.Y., Azzoli, C.G., Kris, M.G., *et al.* (2010) Efficacy and safety of bevacizumab in active brain metastases from non-small cell lung cancer. *J. Neurooncol.*, **100**, 443–447.

74 Hirsch, F.R., Herbst, R.S., Olsen, C., Chansky, K., *et al.* (2008) Increased EGFR gene copy number detected by fluorescent in situ hybridization predicts outcome in non-small-cell lung cancer patients treated with cetuximab and chemotherapy. *J. Clin. Oncol.*, **26**, 3351–3357.

75 Hotta, K., Kiura, K., Ueoka, H., Tabata, M., *et al.* (2004) Effect of gefitinib ('Iressa', ZD1839) on brain metastases in patients with advanced non-small-cell lung cancer. *Lung Cancer*, **46**, 255–261.

76 Joo, K.M., Park, I.H., Shin, J.Y., Jin, J., *et al.* (2009) Human neural stem cells can target and deliver therapeutic genes to breast cancer brain metastases. *Mol. Ther.*, **17**, 570–575.

77 Lin, N.U., Dieras, V., Paul, D., Lossignol, D., *et al.* (2009) Multicenter phase II study of lapatinib in patients with brain metastases from HER2-positive breast cancer. *Clin. Cancer Res.*, **15**, 1452–1459.

78 Namba, Y., Kijima, T., Yokota, S., Niinaka, M., *et al.* (2004) Gefitinib in patients with brain metastases from non-small-cell lung cancer: review of 15 clinical cases. *Clin. Lung Cancer*, **6**, 123–128.

79 Olson, J.J., Paleologos, N.A., Gaspar, L.E., Robinson, P.D., *et al.* (2010) The role of emerging and investigational therapies for metastatic brain tumors: a systematic review and evidence-based clinical practice guideline of selected topics. *J. Neurooncol.*, **96**, 115–142.

80 Sandler, A., Gray, R., Perry, M.C., Brahmer, J., *et al.* (2006) Paclitaxel-carboplatin alone or with bevacizumab for non-small-cell lung cancer. *N. Engl. J. Med.*, **355**, 2542–2550.

81 Schmidt, N.O., Przylecki, W., Yang, W., Ziu, M., *et al.* (2005) Brain tumor tropism of transplanted human neural stem cells is induced by vascular endothelial growth factor. *Neoplasia*, **7**, 623–629.

82 Shimato, S., Mitsudomi, T., Kosaka, T., Yatabe, Y., *et al.* (2006) EGFR mutations in patients with brain metastases from lung cancer: association with the efficacy of gefitinib. *NeuroOncol.*, **8**, 137–144.

83 Wu, C., Li, Y.L., Wang, Z.M., Li, Z., Zhang, T.X., Wei, Z. (2007) Gefitinib as palliative therapy for lung adenocarcinoma metastatic to the brain. *Lung Cancer*, **57**, 359–364.

84 Yano, S., Shinohara, H., Herbst, R.S., Kuniyasu, H., *et al.* (2000) Expression of vascular endothelial growth factor is necessary but not sufficient for production and growth of brain metastasis. *Cancer Res.*, **60**, 4959–4967.

85 Dexamethasone and Supportive Care With or Without Whole-Brain Radiation Therapy in Treating Patients With Non-Small Cell Lung Cancer That Has Spread to the Brain and Cannot Be Removed By Surgery. (2016) Retrieved from https://clinicaltrials.gov/ct2 (Identification No. NCT00403065).

86 Linskey, M.E., Andrews, D.W., Asher, A.L., Burri, S.H., *et al.* (2010) The role of stereotactic radiosurgery in the management of patients with newly diagnosed brain metastases: a systematic review and evidence-based clinical practice guideline. *J. Neurooncol.*, **96**, 45–68.

87 Aoyama, H., Shirato, H., Tago, M., Nakagawa, K., *et al.* (2006) Stereotactic radiosurgery plus whole-brain radiation therapy vs stereotactic radiosurgery alone for treatment of brain metastases: a randomized controlled trial. *JAMA*, **295**, 2483–2491.

88 Kocher, M., Soffietti, R., Abacioglu, U., Villa, S., *et al.* (2011) Adjuvant whole-brain radiotherapy versus observation after radiosurgery or surgical resection of one to three cerebral metastases: results of the EORTC 22952-26001 study. *J. Clin. Oncol.*, **29**, 134–141.

89 Hwang, S.W., Abozed, M.M., Hale, A., Eisenberg, R.L., *et al.* (2010) Adjuvant Gamma Knife radiosurgery following surgical resection of brain metastases: a 9-year retrospective cohort study. *J. Neurooncol.*, **98**, 77–82.

90 Quigley, M.R., Fuhrer, R., Karlovits, S., Karlovits, B., Johnson, M. (2008) Single session stereotactic radiosurgery boost to the post-operative site in lieu of whole brain radiation in metastatic brain disease. *J. Neurooncol.*, **87**, 327–332.

91 Tsao, M., Xu, W., Sahgal, A. (2012) A meta-analysis evaluating stereotactic radiosurgery, whole-brain radiotherapy, or both for patients presenting with a limited number of brain metastases. *Cancer*, **118**, 2486–2493.

92 Fairchild, A., Harris, K., Barnes, E., Wong, R., *et al.* (2008) Palliative thoracic radiotherapy for lung cancer: a systematic review. *J. Clin. Oncol.*, **26**, 4001–4011.

93 Tang, J.I., Shakespeare, T.P., Lu, J.J., Chan, Y.H., *et al.* (2008) Patients' preference for radiotherapy fractionation schedule in the palliation of symptomatic unresectable lung cancer. *J. Med. Imaging Radiat. Oncol.*, **52**, 497–502.

94 Langendijk, H., de Jong, J., Tjwa, M., Muller, M., *et al.* (2001). External irradiation versus external irradiation plus endobronchial brachytherapy in inoperable non-small cell lung cancer: a prospective randomized study. *Radiother. Oncol.*, **58**, 257–268.

95 Kelley, K.D., Benninghoff, D.L., Stein, J.S., Li, J.Z. *et al.* (2015). Medically inoperable peripheral lung cancer treated with stereotactic body radiation therapy. *Radiat. Oncol.*, **10**, 120.

96 Hess, K.R., Varadhachary, G.R., Taylor, S.H., Wei, W., *et al.* (2006) Metastatic patterns in adenocarcinoma. *Cancer*, **106**, 1624–1633.

97 Lo, S.S., Teh, B.S., Mayr, N.A., Olencki, T.E., Wang, J.Z., *et al.* (2010) Stereotactic body radiation therapy for oligometastases. *Discov. Med.*, **10**, 247–254.

98 Simmonds, P.C., Primrose, J.N., Colquitt, J.L., Garden, O.J., Poston, G.J., Rees, M. (2006) Surgical resection of hepatic metastases from colorectal cancer: a systematic review of published studies. *Br. J. Cancer*, **94**, 982–999.

99 Wong, S.L., Mangu, P.B., Choti, M.A., Crocenzi, T.S., *et al.* (2010) American Society of Clinical Oncology

2009 clinical evidence review on radiofrequency ablation of hepatic metastases from colorectal cancer. *J. Clin. Oncol.*, **28**, 493–508.

100 House, M.G., Ito, H., Gonen, M., Fong, Y., *et al.* (2010) Survival after hepatic resection for metastatic colorectal cancer: trends in outcomes for 1,600 patients during two decades at a single institution. *J. Am. Coll. Surg.*, **210**, 744–752.

101 Bydder, S., Spry, N.A., Christie, D.R., Roos, D., *et al.* (2003) A prospective trial of short-fractionation radiotherapy for the palliation of liver metastases. *Australas. Radiol.*, **47**, 284–288.

102 Chang, D.T., Swaminath, A., Kozak, M., Weintraub, J., *et al.* (2011) Stereotactic body radiotherapy for colorectal liver metastases: a pooled analysis. *Cancer*, **117**, 4060–4069.

103 Herfarth, K.K., Debus, J. (2005) [Stereotactic radiation therapy for liver metastases]. *Chirurgia*, **76**, 564–569.

104 Katz, A.W., Carey-Sampson, M., Muhs, A.G., Milano, M.T., Schell, M.C., Okunieff, P. (2007) Hypofractionated stereotactic body radiation therapy (SBRT) for limited hepatic metastases. *Int. J. Radiat. Oncol. Biol. Phys.*, **67**, 793–798.

105 Lee, M.T., Kim, J.J., Dinniwell, R., Brierley, J., *et al.* (2009) Phase I study of individualized stereotactic body radiotherapy of liver metastases. *J. Clin. Oncol.*, **27**, 1585–1591.

106 Swaminath, A., Dawson, L.A. (2010) Emerging role of radiotherapy in the management of liver metastases. *Cancer J.*, **16**, 150–155.

107 Soliman, H., Ringash, J., Jiang, H., Singh, K., *et al.* (2013) Phase II trial of palliative radiotherapy for hepatocellular carcinoma and liver metastases. *J. Clin. Oncol.*, **31**, 3980–3986.

108 Borgelt, B.B., Gelber, R., Brady, L.W., Griffin, T., Hendrickson, F.R. (1981) The palliation of hepatic metastases: results of the Radiation Therapy Oncology Group pilot study. *Int. J. Radiat. Oncol. Biol. Phys.*, **7**, 587–591.

109 Prasad, B., Lee, M.S., Hendrickson, F.R. (1977) Irradiation of hepatic metastases. *Int. J. Radiat. Oncol. Biol. Phys.*, **2**, 129–132.

110 Berger, B., Belka, C. (2009) Evidence-based radiation oncology: oesophagus. *Radiother. Oncol.*, **92**, 276–290.

111 Homs, M.Y., Steyerberg, E.W., Eijkenboom, W.M., Tilanus, H.W., *et al.* (2004) Single-dose brachytherapy versus metal stent placement for the palliation of dysphagia from oesophageal cancer: multicentre randomised trial. *Lancet*, **364**, 1497–1504.

112 Weissberg, J.B., Pillsbury, H., Sasaki, C.T., Son, Y.H., Fischer, J.J. (1983) High fractional dose irradiation of advanced head and neck cancer. Implications for combined radiotherapy and surgery. *Arch. Otolaryngol.*, **109**, 98–102.

113 Al-mamgani, A., Tans, L., Van Rooij, P.H., Noever, I., Baatenburg de Jong, R.J., Levendag, P.C. (2009) Hypofractionated radiotherapy denoted as the 'Christie scheme': an effective means of palliating patients with head and neck cancers not suitable for curative treatment. *Acta Oncol.*, **48**, 562–570.

114 Corry, J., Peters, L.J., Costa, I.D., Milner, A.D., Fawns, H., Rischin, D., Porceddu, S. (2005). The 'QUAD SHOT' – a phase II study of palliative radiotherapy for incurable head and neck cancer. *Radiother. Oncol.*, **77**, 137–142.

115 Mohanti, B.K., Umapathy, H., Bahadur, S., Thakar, A., Pathy, S. (2004) Short course palliative radiotherapy of 20 Gy in 5 fractions for advanced and incurable head and neck cancer: AIIMS study. *Radiother. Oncol.*, **71**, 275–280.

116 Spanos, W., Jr., Guse, C., Perez, C., Grigsby, P., Doggett, R.L., Poulter, C. (1989) Phase II study of multiple daily fractionations in the palliation of advanced pelvic malignancies: preliminary report of RTOG 8502. *Int. J. Radiat. Oncol. Biol. Phys.*, **17**, 659–661.

117 Spanos, W.J., Jr., Perez, C.A., Marcus, S., Poulter, C.A., *et al.* (1993) Effect of rest interval on tumor and normal tissue response – a report of phase III study of accelerated split course palliative radiation for advanced pelvic malignancies (RTOG-8502). *Int. J. Radiat. Oncol. Biol. Phys.*, **25**, 399–403.

118 Dirix, P., Vingerhoedt, S., Joniau, S., Van Cleynenbreugel, B., Haustermans, K. (2016) Hypofractionated palliative radiotherapy for bladder cancer. *Support. Care Cancer*, **24**, 181–186.

119 Scholten, A.N., Leer, J.W., Collins, C.D., Wondergem, J., Hermans, J., Timothy, A. (1997) Hypofractionated radiotherapy for invasive bladder cancer. *Radiother. Oncol.*, **43**, 163–169.

120 Duchesne, G.M., Bolger, J.J., Griffiths, G.O., Roberts, J., *et al.* (2000) A randomized trial of hypofractionated schedules of palliative radiotherapy in the management of bladder carcinoma: results of medical research council trial BA09. *Int. J. Radiat. Oncol. Biol. Phys.*, **47**, 379–388.

121 Srinivasan, V., Brown, C.H., Turner, A.G. (1994) A comparison of two radiotherapy regimens for the treatment of symptoms from advanced bladder cancer. *Clin. Oncol. (R. Coll. Radiol.)*, **6**, 11–13.

122 Din, O.S., Thanvi, N., Ferguson, C.J., Kirkbride, P. (2009) Palliative prostate radiotherapy for symptomatic advanced prostate cancer. *Radiother. Oncol.*, **93**, 192–196.

123 Jemal, A., Siegel, R., Ward, E., Hao, Y., Xu, J., Thun, M.J. (2009) Cancer statistics, 2009. *CA Cancer J. Clin.*, **59**, 225–249.

124 Rothenberger, D.A. (2004) Palliative therapy of rectal cancer. Overview: epidemiology, indications, goals,

extent, and nature of work-up. *J. Gastrointest. Surg.*, **8**, 259–261.

125 Leitman, I.M., Sullivan, J.D., Brams, D., DeCosse, J.J. (1992) Multivariate analysis of morbidity and mortality from the initial surgical management of obstructing carcinoma of the colon. *Surg. Gynecol. Obstet.*, **174**, 513–518.

126 Brierley, J.D., Cummings, B.J., Wong, C.S., Keane, T.J., *et al.* (1995) Adenocarcinoma of the rectum treated by radical external radiation therapy. *Int. J. Radiat. Oncol. Biol. Phys.*, **31**, 255–259.

127 Crane, C.H., Janjan, N.A., Abbruzzese, J.L., Curley, S., *et al.* (2001) Effective pelvic symptom control using initial chemoradiation without colostomy in metastatic rectal cancer. *Int. J. Radiat. Oncol. Biol. Phys.*, **49**, 107–116.

128 Mohiuddin, M., Marks, G., Marks, J. (2002) Long-term results of reirradiation for patients with recurrent rectal carcinoma. *Cancer*, **95**, 1144–1150.

129 Saltz, L.B. (2004) Palliative management of rectal cancer: the roles of chemotherapy and radiation therapy. *J. Gastrointest. Surg.*, **8**, 274–276.

130 Belfiore, G., Tedeschi, E., Ronza, F.M., Belfiore, M.P., *et al.* (2009) CT-guided radiofrequency ablation in the treatment of recurrent rectal cancer. *Am. J. Roentgenol.*, **192**, 137–141.

131 Tam, T.Y., Mukherjee, S., Farrell, T., Morgan, D., Sur, R. (2009) Endoscopic brachytherapy for obstructive colorectal cancer. *Brachytherapy*, **8**, 313–317.

132 Watt, A.M., Faragher, I.G., Griffin, T.T., Rieger, N.A., Maddern, G.J. (2007) Self-expanding metallic stents for relieving malignant colorectal obstruction: a systematic review. *Ann. Surg.*, **246**, 24–30.

133 Soysal, H.G. (2007). Metastatic tumors of the uvea in 38 eyes. *Can. J. Ophthalmol.*, **42**, 832–835.

134 Valenzuela, A.A., Archibald, C.W., Fleming, B., Ong, L., *et al.* (2009) Orbital metastasis: clinical features, management and outcome. *Orbit*, **28**, 153–159.

135 McFarland, J.T., Kuzma, C., Millard, F.E., Johnstone, P.A. (2003) Palliative irradiation of the spleen. *Am. J. Clin. Oncol.*, **26**, 178–183.

136 Mesa, R.A. (2009) How I treat symptomatic splenomegaly in patients with myelofibrosis. *Blood*, **113**, 5394–5400.

137 Paulino, A.C., Reddy, S.P. (1996) Splenic irradiation in the palliation of patients with lymphoproliferative and myeloproliferative disorders. *Am. J. Hosp. Palliat. Care*, **13**, 32–35.

138 Glare, P., Virik, K., Jones, M., Hudson, M., Eychmuller, S., Simes, J., Christakis, N. (2003) A systematic review of physicians' survival predictions in terminally ill cancer patients. *Br. Med. J.*, **327**, 195–198.

139 Chow, E., Fan, G., Hadi, S., Filipczak, L. (2007) Symptom clusters in cancer patients with bone metastases. *Support Care Cancer*, **15**, 1035–1043.

140 Dodd, M.J., Miaskowski, C., Paul, S.M. (2001) Symptom clusters and their effect on the functional status of patients with cancer. *Oncol. Nurs. Forum*, **28**, 465–470.

141 Caissie, A., Culleton, S., Nguyen, J., Zhang, L., *et al.* (2012) EORTC QLQ-C15-PAL quality of life scores in patients with advanced cancer referred for palliative radiotherapy. *Support Care Cancer*, **20**, 841–848.

142 Sunnybrook Health Sciences Centre (2011) Rapid Radiotherapy Response Program Overview.

143 Wolfe, G.J., Grier, H.E. (2002) Care of the dying child, in *Principles and Practice of Pediatric Oncology* (eds P.A. Pizzo, D.G. Poplack), Lippincott Williams & Wilkins, Philadelphia.

144 Bertsch, H., Rudoler, S., Needle, M.N., Malloy, P., *et al.* (1998) Emergent/urgent therapeutic irradiation in pediatric oncology: patterns of presentation, treatment, and outcome. *Med. Pediatr. Oncol.*, **30**, 101–105.

145 Rahn, D.A., 3rd, Mundt, A.J., Murphy, J.D., Schiff, D., Adams, J., Murphy, K.T. (2015) Clinical outcomes of palliative radiation therapy for children. *Pract. Radiat. Oncol.*, **5**, 183–187.

146 Deutsch, M., Tersak, J.M. (2004) Radiotherapy for symptomatic metastases to bone in children. *Am. J. Clin. Oncol.*, **27**, 128–131.

147 Koontz, B.F., Clough, R.W., Halperin, E.C. (2006) Palliative radiation therapy for metastatic Ewing sarcoma. *Cancer*, **106**, 1790–1793.

148 American Academy of Pediatrics Committee on Bioethics and Committee on Hospital Care (2000) Palliative care for children. *Pediatrics*, **106**, 351–357.

149 Bonanno, G.A., Bradlyn, A.S., Davies, E., Donnelly, J.P., *et al.* (2002) When children die: improving palliative care and end-of-life care for children and their families. National Academy Press, Washington, DC.

150 deCinque, N., Monterosso, L., Dadd, G., Sidhu, R., Macpherson, R., Aoun, S. (2006) Bereavement support for families following the death of a child from cancer: experience of bereaved parents. *J. Psychosoc. Oncol.*, **24**, 65–83.

151 Teno, J.M., Clarridge, B.R., Casey, V., Welch, L.C., *et al.* (2004) Family perspectives on end-of-life care at the last place of care. *JAMA*, **291**, 88–93.

152 Kreicbergs, U., Valdimarsdottir, U., Onelov, E., Henter, J.I., Steineck, G. (2004) Talking about death with children who have severe malignant disease. *N. Engl. J. Med.*, **351**, 1175–1186.

153 Guadagnolo, B.A., Liao, K.P., Elting, L., Giordano, S., *et al.* (2013) Use of radiation therapy in the last 30 days of life among a large population-based cohort of elderly patients in the United States. *J. Clin. Oncol.*, **31**, 80–87.

154 Chow, E., Abdolell, M., Panzarella, T., Harris, K., *et al.* (2008) Predictive model for survival in patients with advanced cancer. *J. Clin. Oncol.*, **26**, 5863–5869.

155 Chow, E., Abdolell, M., Panzarella, T., Harris, K., *et al.* (2009) Validation of a predictive model for survival in metastatic cancer patients attending an outpatient palliative radiotherapy clinic. *Int. J. Radiat. Oncol. Biol. Phys.*, **73**, 280–287.

156 Krishnan, M.S., Epstein-Peterson, Z., Chen, Y.H., Tseng, Y.D., *et al.* (2014) Predicting life expectancy in patients with metastatic cancer receiving palliative radiotherapy: the TEACHH model. *Cancer*, **120**, 134–141.

157 Nieder, C., Angelo, K., Dalhaug, A., Pawinski, A., *et al.* (2014) Palliative radiotherapy with or without additional care by a multidisciplinary palliative care team: A retrospective comparison. *ISRN Oncol.*, **2014**, 715396.

158 Pituskin, E., Fairchild, A., Dutka, J., Gagnon, L., *et al.* (2010). Multidisciplinary team contributions within a dedicated outpatient palliative radiotherapy clinic: a prospective descriptive study. *Int. J. Radiat. Oncol. Biol. Phys.*, **78**, 527–532.

159 Hospice and Palliative Nurses Association/American Nurses Association (2007) *Hospice and Palliative Nursing: Scope and Standards of Practice.* Silver Spring, MD.

160 Society, O.N. (2004). Statement on the Scope and Standards of Oncology Nursing Practice (Pittsburgh).

161 Coyle, N. (2010) Introduction to palliative nursing care, in *Oxford Textbook of Palliative Nursing* (eds B. Ferrell, N. Coyle), Oxford University Press, New York, pp. 3–11.

162 Muriel, A.C., Hwang, V.S., Kornblith, A., Greer, J., *et al.* (2009) Management of psychosocial distress by oncologists. *Psychiatr. Serv.*, **60**, 1132–1134.

163 Oregon Health Authority (2009) Summary of Oregon's death with dignity act.

164 Brown, L.F., Kroenke, K. (2009) Cancer-related fatigue and its associations with depression and anxiety: a systematic review. *Psychosomatics*, **50**, 440–447.

165 O'Mahony, S., Goulet, J., Kornblith, A., Abbatiello, G., *et al.* (2005) Desire for hastened death, cancer pain and depression: report of a longitudinal observational study. *J. Pain Symptom Manage.*, **29**, 446–457.

166 Zabora, J., Brintzenhofe-Szoc, K., Curbow, B., Hooker, C., Piantadosi, S. (2001) The prevalence of psychological distress by cancer site. *Psychooncology*, **10**, 19–28.

167 Peppercorn, J.M., Smith, T.J., Helft, P.R., Debono, D.J., *et al.* and American Society of Clinical Oncology (2011). American Society of Clinical Oncology statement: Toward individualized care for patients with advanced cancer. *J. Clin. Oncol.*, **29**, 755–760.

168 Davis, J.A., Smith, T.W. (2002) Summary of the 2002 General Social Survey conducted by the National Opinion Research Center.

169 Balboni, T.A., Vanderwerker, L.C., Block, S.D., Paulk, M.E., *et al.* (2007) Religiousness and spiritual support among advanced cancer patients and associations with end-of-life treatment preferences and quality of life. *J. Clin. Oncol.*, **25**, 555–560.

170 Balboni, T.A., Paulk, M.E., Balboni, M.J., Phelps, A.C., *et al.* (2010) Provision of spiritual care to patients with advanced cancer: associations with medical care and quality of life near death. *J. Clin. Oncol.*, **28**, 445–452.

171 Delgado-Guay, M.O., Hui, D., Parsons, H.A., Govan, K., *et al.* (2011) Spirituality, religiosity, and spiritual pain in advanced cancer patients. *J. Pain Symptom Manage.*, **41**, 986–994.

172 Puchalski, C., Ferrell, B., Virani, R., Otis-Green, S., *et al.* (2009) Improving the quality of spiritual care as a dimension of palliative care: the report of the Consensus Conference. *J. Palliat. Med.*, **12**, 885–904.

173 Williams, J.A., Meltzer, D., Arora, V., Chung, G., Curlin, F.A. (2011) Attention to inpatients' religious and spiritual concerns: predictors and association with patient satisfaction. *J. Gen. Intern. Med.*, **26**, 1265–1271.

174 Beckman, H.B., Frankel, R.M. (1984) The effect of physician behavior on the collection of data. *Ann. Intern. Med.*, **101**, 692–696.

175 Hallenback, J. (2003) *Palliative Care Perspectives.* Oxford University Press, New York.

176 Waitzkin, H. (1985) Information giving in medical care. *J. Health Soc. Behav.*, **26**, 81–101.

177 Back, A.L., Arnold, R.M., Baile, W.F., Tulsky, J.A., Fryer-Edwards, K. (2005) Approaching difficult communication tasks in oncology. *CA Cancer J. Clin.*, **55**, 164–177.

178 Saraiya, B., Arnold, R., Tulsky, J.A. (2010) Communication skills for discussing treatment options when chemotherapy has failed. *Cancer J.*, **16**, 521–523.

8

Patient Safety and Quality: Management for the Radiation Oncologist

Fiori Alite and Abhishek A. Solanki

Introduction

Ensuring patient safety and quality in radiation delivery are inherent requirements when delivering cancer therapy as complex as modern radiation therapy. Over the past 20 years, drastic technological advances in radiation treatment planning, treatment set-up precision and verification and delivery have been accompanied by increased requirements for complex data processing, interplay between the multiple aspects of treatment planning and delivery, specialized training of staff, and efficient and reliable communication between team members. Due to this complexity, radiation therapy represents a system exposed to a greater potential for errors.

There is no standard definition for an 'error' event, and most events do not result in clinically relevant detriment. Nonetheless, it is important to draw a distinction between error and harm. Errors cannot ever be completely eliminated, but harm may be nearly preventable or potential harm may be mitigated. Available data suggest that quality and safety events occur in 1–3% of patients receiving radiation therapy [1]. The benchmark that is commonly strived for is that of the airline industry, which boasts one death in 4.7 million passenger flights. In medicine, anesthesiologists report one death in 200 000 procedures [2]. This represents the goal of the innovations of quality and safety methodologies developed in radiation oncology.

Patient safety and quality have always been at the forefront of radiation oncologists' minds. However, over the past half-decade there has been renewed vigor in identifying systematic interventions that can minimize the risk of errors and potential harm in radiation therapy, partially prompted by several lay press articles published in 2010 describing cases of fatal radiation misadministration [3–6]. At the national level, the American Society for Radiation Oncology (ASTRO), the American College of Radiology (ACR), and the American Association of Physicists in Medicine (AAPM) have championed these efforts through participation in congressional hearings, collaboration with radiation device vendors and the Federal Drug Administration (FDA) to re-evaluate device approval processes, and collaborative consensus recommendations on quality control processes [7]. Additionally, there have been many individual practice-level efforts to re-evaluate processes and make error prevention an increasingly scientific and precise process in radiation oncology.

Defining Safety and Quality

From the clinical radiation oncologist's perspective, radiation safety and quality are two distinct but conceptually entwined ideas. Radiation safety generally deals with factors in radiation planning and delivery that can lead to errors and potential harm in patient treatment. For example, planning on the wrong patient data set, dose calculation errors, selecting the wrong energy or particle for treatment, inappropriate or misplaced compensators or wedges, and errors in image guidance and verification. *Radiation quality* refers to decisions and policies that ensure the optimal decision making in order to select, plan and deliver the correct and clinically appropriate radiation therapy. *Quality management* includes quality control, or steps made to ensure high-quality performance by a process, staff-member, or device. *Quality assurance* (QA) refers to the assessment of the quality provided by these phenomena and required interventions to maximize this. Beyond technical assurances that ensure radiation delivery, quality can also encompass decision-making earlier in the clinical patient course, for example ensuring that radiation treatment decisions conform to national clinical practice consensus guidelines [e.g., National Comprehensive Cancer Network (NCCN) guidelines, American College of Radiology (ACR) consensus statements] and that patient counseling has included all treatment options available. Ensuring that clinical target volume delineation has appropriately incorporated all surgical information (i.e., detailed gross and microscopic pathologic reports, information from the full operative report and/or clinical input from surgeon at the time of contouring), diagnostic radiographic and functional imaging findings (including direct input from subspecialty radiologist at time of contouring), and that target delineation is performed based on expert panel or consensus group contouring atlases or outlines, is critically important.

An important take-home point when discussing radiation oncology safety is that an error upstream or poor system design in the evaluation and treatment workflow process can result in downstream effects and misadministration of treatment. For example, incomplete history-taking or the acquisition of previous radiation oncology records followed by generation of a radiation plan with dose overlap in a region previously treated, resulting in overdose to a critical structure and potentially adverse clinical outcomes. A summary of radiation oncology workflow and some possible error events is provided in Figure 8.1.

Key components in quality in the radiation oncology clinic are the departmental and institutional QA practices. Most departments have standard and department-specific QA processes instituted to identify errors, but if QA steps are inadequate or not implemented sufficiently upstream in the care path, this can result in errors being picked up either too late or not at all. It is also important to note that since most external beam radiation therapy (EBRT) is delivered via a protracted fractionated scheme, errors not caught early enough in the process may recur multiple times and could be amplified throughout the treatment course.

Interestingly, radiation therapy is evolving towards more hypofractionated radiation treatment approaches. This makes accurate and reliable treatment with each fraction that much more important, and thus the magnitude of potential harm caused by errors in each fraction is amplified.

Defining and Quantifying Radiation Incidents

No consensus definition exists in the radiation oncology community when reporting radiation events and errors, but several reporting scales and instruments have been developed. Quantifying radiation safety events that affect patient care and outcomes when delivering radiation therapy procedures is important in communicating and forming a common language within the radiotherapy, general medical and lay-person communities.

Developed in 2008 by the French Nuclear Safety Authority (ASN) in collaboration with the French Society for Radiation Oncology (SFRO) and French Society for Medical Physics (SFPM), the ASN-SFRO scale classifies events into eight levels that correspond to gradable toxicity by the internationally used Common Terminology Criteria for Adverse Events (CTCAE) [8,9]. This metric has been incorporated in publications of radiation safety from incident learning systems in Europe. In addition, the scale allows for quantifying events that affect more than one patient. A summary of the ASN-SFRO scale is provided in Table 8.1. Developed by Konski and colleagues, the Radiation Error Scoring System (RESS), stratifies radiation errors into meaningful categories based on the potential clinical effect in terms of patient harm, effect on radiation prescription, and also incorporates national radiation error reporting guidelines and has been used for institutional reviews reporting error analyses [10]. A summary of the RESS system is provided in Table 8.2.

Errors can exist along a spectrum: some may lead merely to logistic issues instead of changes in treatment toxicity or efficacy, while others can have a detrimental impact on a patient's clinical outcome. Most, however, likely fall into the gray area in between the two ends of the spectrum. Error identification also is variable, as some errors can easily be identified, while others may be more silent.

Beyond actual radiation events, the identification of near-miss events also has a critical impact on workflow, provides data to guide practice quality improvement from incident learning systems, informs on the contributing factors and potential impact of errors and system defects, and further aids in building a culture of safety. ASTRO recommends that near-misses should be addressed with similar vigor as that applied to actual radiation errors [11]. Near-miss events can vary in their potential of clinical consequence, and therefore the University of Washington, together with AAPM task force guidelines, has developed a near-miss risk index (NMRI) that scores near-events on their level of workflow effect and potential for patient harm [12,13]. A summary of the NMRI scale is shown in Table 8.3.

Importance of Radiation Oncology Incident Learning Systems

The most extreme errors – those resulting in patient death or severe morbidity – are nearly always investigated thoroughly. However, errors potentially of a

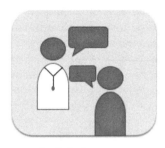

Errors in clinical assessment
- Inadequate/Inaccurate physical exam
- Incomplete assessment of radiation specific history
  - Previous radiation therapy
  - Pacemaker/Defibrillator
  - History of Connective Tissue Disease
  - Pregnancy risk assessment

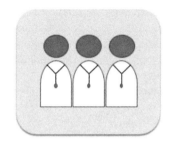

Errors In clinical management
- Incomplete discussion of treatment options
- Incomplete utilization of multidisciplinary decision making
- Incomplete/Inappropriate utilization of national treatment guidelines
- Incorrect timing or coordination of radiotherapy with surgical or systemic therapy approaches
- Incomplete use of ancillary services
  - Nutrition, Prophylactic PEG, Speech/Swallow, Dental services, Lymphedema

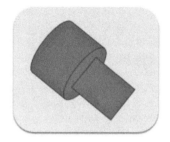

Errors in use of imaging/simulation
- Incomplete utilization of staging imaging, overutilization or misinterpretation of imaging
- Incorrect immobilization chosen
- Incorrect use of target volume enhancement with use of PO or IV contrast
  - No Renal function assessment prior to contrast enhancement
  - IV Contrast Errors
    - Administering contrast without premedication in a known allergic patient
    - Forgoing contrast without considering premedication in a known allergic patient

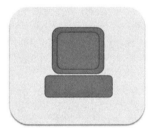

Errors in Treatment Planning
- Incorrect target and normal tissue contours
- Errors in image registration and/or fusion
- Dose information incorrectly exported to dose calculation program
- Incorrect or suboptimal beam placement
- Dose to target or normal tissues too high or too low
  - Does not meet current national standards
  - Violates Normal Tissue Thresholds
- Emergency treatment planning, dose calculation errors (i.e. using PDD to calculate MU when patient is set up SAD)

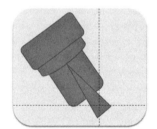

Errors in Patient Setup
- Wrong Site/Wrong Patient
- Inability to verify patient's marks are valid for treatment
- Radiation therapist shifts the patient's position based on treatment plan incorrectly
- Failing to re-mark patient after treatment shifts are made
- Emergency Clinical Setup Errors

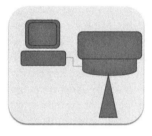

Errors in Treatment Delivery
- Treatment plan and film are exported incorrectly to treatment machine
- Incorrect dose delivered
  - Incorrect beams and energy are chosen
  - Incorrect field size, block, compensators, wedges
  - Incorrect calibration or machine QA

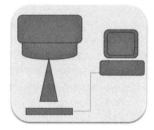

Errors in Treatment Verification
- Incorrectly exporting setup images to record and verify system
- Incorrect acquisition or interpretation of IGRT
  - Incorrect choice of IGRT or inadequate IGRT
  - Aligning to wrong contour
  - Shifting incorrectly based on bony anatomy
  - Accidental shifts made

Figure 8.1 Types of radiation oncology quality factors and errors.

Table 8.1 The ASN-SFRO scale for rating nuclear incidents and accidents and radiation protection events [8, 9]. Adapted from Autorite de Surate Nucleaire (ASN) 2007.

Level 1	Corresponding to CTCAE grade 1, covers mild effects as well as events for which no effect is expected	
Level 2*	Corresponding to CTCAE grade 2, covers acute effects or moderate late effects such as moderate radiation-induced stenosis, tissue damage causing little inconvenience (cutaneous fibrosis), or minimal or zero deterioration in quality of life	Classified as Radiation Incident
Level 3*	Corresponding to CTCAE grade 3, covers acute effects or severe late effects such as manageable and non-life-threatening tissue necrosis, with moderate deterioration in quality of life (severe proctitis, severe cystitis, etc.)	
Level 4*	Corresponding to CTCAE grade 4, covers acute effects or serious late effects such as radiation myelitis, large tissue necrosis that is unmanageable and life-threatening with severe deterioration in quality of life (e.g. serious proctitis, serious cystitis)	Classified as Radiation Accident
Level 5, 6†, 7‡	Corresponding to CTCAE grade 5 of the clinical classification, make reference to one or more cases of death	

*If more than one patient is effected by a Level 2–4 event a + sign is demarcated.
†If the event leads to more than one but less than or equal to 10 deaths it is classified as Level 6.
‡If the event leads to more than 10 deaths it is classified as Level 7.

Table 8.2 The Radiation Error Scoring System (RESS) quantifies radiation errors into categories based on clinical effect, effect on radiation prescription, and incorporates national US radiation error reporting guidelines.

Level of radiation error	Effect on patient harm	Effect on radiation prescription
I	A solitary event and no harm to patient	Requires no change
II	A solitary event and no harm to patient	Requires a change in the radiation prescription
III	Treatment errors with potential for causing permanent damage or serious injury to the patient, even if the treatment did not result in any harm and was corrected	Treatment errors requiring a change in the radiation prescription and felt to potentially harm patients or substantially missing the tumor volume on any treatment
IV	Errors involving a medical reportable event for radiation: • Wrong individual treated. • A >20% difference compared to intended dose to the target. • Total weekly dose differs from weekly prescribed dose by more than 30%. • Substantially missing the tumor volume for more than half the number of treatments. • The presence of a non-patient in the treatment room during an exposure regardless of dose received.	

Source: Konski *et al.* 2009 [10]. Reproduced with permission of Elsevier.

Table 8.3 Definitions of the near-miss risk index (NMRI), which represents the potential risk of a near-miss event.

NMRI level	Risk of potential harm to patient	Criteria	
		Effects on workflow	Clinical impact
0	None	Event does not pose downstream risk in workflow	Event is not related to patient safety or quality of treatment
1	Mild	Event may enhance the risk of other downstream errors	Event may cause emotional distress or inconvenience to patient with no clinical impact
2	Moderate	Event enhances the risk of other critical downstream errors	Temporary pain or discomfort for patient Deviations from best practices, but with no obvious clinical impact
3	Severe	Limited barriers to prevention of problem	Event with potential clinical impact that is non-critical
4	Critical	Extremely limited barriers to prevention of problem	Event with potentially critical clinical impact

Source: Nyflot *et al.* 2015 [13]. Reproduced with permission of Elsevier.

lesser magnitude can reveal a great deal regarding staff practices and risk assessment, and thereby are an important part of improving patient safety. Incident learning systems are critical for identifying and learning from these errors. In commercial aviation, the Aviation Safety Reporting System (ASRS) is a federal-backed national incident learning system, while the Aviation Safety Action Program (ASAP), is a 'local' incident learning system that many carriers have adopted [14]. Both of these are non-punitive programs for voluntary reporting of safety issues that airline staff may encounter. In medicine, many anesthesia departments have instituted an Anesthesia Information Monitoring System (AIMS), which not only facilitates workflow and in recording clinical data, but also acts as an incident learning system [15]. Additionally, the Anesthesia Incident Reporting System (AIRS) has been implemented as a nationwide voluntary incident reporting mechanism [16].

Incident learning systems are paramount to the reporting and tracking of events, concerns, and performance issues, as well as highlighting the utility of having objective quantitative data to help guide and assess improvement [12]. Both, proactive and reactive measures must be implemented in order to build a culture of safety [17, 18]. A feedback process reacting to identified incidents can be used to enhance proactive safety measures, and help guide prospective risk assessment. Both in the United States and Europe, secure online voluntary cross-institutional incident reporting and learning systems have been established in order to identify and track areas for improvement in radiation oncology. Reporting on 1074 incidents, the Radiation Oncology Safety Information System (RO-SIS) highlighted several themes in incident reporting [19]. Of the reported incidents, 51% resulted in incorrect irradiation, and when an incident is not detected prior to treatment an average of 22% of the prescribed treatment fractions were delivered incorrectly. The majority of reported errors were found by radiation therapists at the treatment unit (43%), while the physics quality control process was the second source of identifying errors (33%). When found by the quality control process, errors were more likely to be reported as near-misses than when 'found at later patient treatment' and from '*in-vivo* dosimetry.' The similarly designed ASTRO-led Radiation Oncology Incident Learning System (RO-ILS) experience was recently reported in 2015 after one year of data analysis [20]. The analysis found that conformal radiation therapy resulted in three times as many patient safety events as intensity-modulated radiotherapy (IMRT) (29% versus 11%). Of a total of 220 events analyzed, the 'treatment planning' and 'pretreatment review/verification' steps were the most commonly identified sites of error (33%). The authors concluded that incident learning systems are a powerful tool, and all radiation oncology clinics should institute

participation in a nationally validated incident learning system database. Still, it is also important to note that there are significant limitations with voluntary reporting systems, and these often are not precise measures of error or harm rates. Clearly, proactive systems assessing error rates and potential for harm are needed.

In addition to national and international incident learning systems, there are several reported experiences of departmental incident learning systems, and an increasing number of institutions are developing such programs. At the University of Seattle, Nyloft *et al.* analyzed reporting trends after a two-year experience with an incident learning system using the NMRI as a metric, and found that the highest risk events originated in 'imaging for treatment planning' and were detected in 'on-treatment quality management.' Importantly, the group found that over the two years' incorporation of the incident learning system, event reporting and staff participation both increased and the NMRI level of the reported events decreased, implying improved safety [13].

The incident learning experience in both Europe and the US point to incorporating QA earlier in the radiation workflow and 'working with awareness' as important safety layers [19, 20]. Although having vast implications in changing workplace culture, it is important to acknowledge that most studies suggest that incident learning systems suffer from under-reporting and non-random reporting that varies with the severity of the error. The reasons for this are likely multifactorial, but likely include fear of repercussion, embarrassment of self-reporting, and that a uniform quantification method for reporting does not exist. Specifically, in a survey about attitudes of physician self-reporting and attitudes toward incident learning systems, physicians were less likely to report errors and were significantly more "…concerned about getting colleagues in trouble, liability, effect on departmental reputation, and embarrassment" than their similarly surveyed colleagues [21]. Despite this limitation, incidents identified through these mechanisms can be extremely useful in developing policies for error and harm prevention. Additionally, active engagement from leadership and a nurturing departmental safety culture may improve participation.

Concepts in Quality Management

Building complex systems that rely on human interaction is an inherently error-prone process, and systematic research into the nature of when errors occur has resulted in a science and methodology of identifying system vulnerabilities in order to maximize quality. Most of these methodologies were initially implemented in the aerospace, military, and large-scale industries, but more recently they have permeated into the health and radiation oncology sector, and are currently implemented in several radiation oncology departments [2].

Developed by James Reason in 1990, the Swiss Cheese Model delineated that patient harm does not occur from a solitary event due to individual poor performance or error, but evolves through several strata of organizational, environmental, and individual failures that must all align to result in harm. Consequently, building a culture of safety relies on implementing safeguards among the various layers of the model, since a 'good catch' along any of these strata would prevent the error [7, 22]. Developed by Perrow in 1984, Normal Accident Theory (NAT) provides a framework for analyzing failure within complex healthcare systems, dividing systems where failures propagate predictably as linear, and those in which failures behave unpredictably as interactively complex [23, 24]. For example, an emergent clinical set-up on a weekend day or after normal office hours using a single posterior-anterior (PA) field delivery for palliating spinal cord compression can be considered linear. Multiple dose level, sliding window IMRT for head and neck cancer can be considered interactively complex. Second, loosely coupled systems are those that can adequately detect and respond to failure, whereas systems that cannot detect and respond to failures are considered tightly coupled. In the previous example, although the emergent treatment is technically simpler with interaction between fewer individuals, the non-standard time and less-familiar processes employed predispose workers to a larger amount of cognitive biases during decision making that increase the probability of failures, making the system likely as tightly coupled as a complex IMRT planning and delivery system. Within the framework of NAT it is possible to build QA programs in radiation oncology that decrease the probability of errors propagating and going undetected [24]. The Global Risk Analysis (GRA) method, developed by the École Centrale Paris during the 1950s, uses a semi-quantitative scale to allow the prioritization of risk mitigation measures, and has been applied in radiation oncology departments to implement corrective actions prior to incidents in order to improve patient safety [25, 26].

Quality and safety assessment can be pursued retrospectively/reactively, after an error leading to harm occurs, with the goal of remedying the contributing factors that led to the error and trying to prevent future error. But quality and safety assessment can also be pursued prospectively, with the goal of predicting the probability, severity, and ability to detect potential errors, and implement methods to prevent them. Historically, medical charts and case reviews have been the primary approach for quality improvement after errors occur. This approach has predominantly been a retrospective approach. When a radiation error occurs, every aspect of the patient's care is reviewed to identify aberrations from the standard process. The root cause for the error, and changes to prevent future errors, are then created.

There are multiple tools for prospective quality control and process improvement. Just as in retrospective approaches, prospective quality control requires multidisciplinary collaboration including at least one physician, physicist, dosimetrist, nurse, therapist and information technology (IT) staff. Process mapping is a visual depiction of the workflow of a process, with connections drawn between each step of the pathway, allowing for a comprehensive understanding of the process, as well as the role of each individual step. Process failure mode and effects analysis (FMEA) is an inductive approach used to identify the probability, severity, or detection of errors for any given step(s) of the process [27, 28]. This is then assigned a risk priority number (Probability × Severity × Detection). Fault tree analysis is a deductive approach in which a failure event in the process is identified and all of the circumstances given the environment and workflow are detected that could lead to the outcome.

Although multiple tools are available, these tools have yet to be standardized and systematically applied in radiation oncology departments throughout the country.

The Quality Management Process

It is the entire multidisciplinary group's responsibility to strive for high-quality care and to maximize patient safety. Each department is unique, with individualized staff roles, devices, processes, environments, coverage factors, and resources. Thus, the quality management program must be individualized to each center, and most centers create a quality and safety team to oversee this program. The radiation oncologist leads the group, which consists of the physician, physicist, medical dosimetrist, radiation therapist, nurse, IT specialist, resident or in-training professional and administrative staff. The physicist primarily leads the technical QA of the treatment planning system, treatment plans, and the devices used for patient care. The medical director must create policies and procedures promoting a safe environment for patients and personnel. Standard operating procedures (SOPs) must be created to allow for standardization and to potentially limit errors [11, 29]. Unfortunately, as important as departmental policies and standard operating procedures are, many errors occur due to a lapse in following standard policies and operating procedures, and consequently the creation of 'hard stops' to prevent errors is critical [11]. Ultimately, it is the entire group's responsibility to build a safe patient environment.

In developing processes and policies, several resources are available to help guide development. The ACR, ASTRO, AAPM, and American Brachytherapy Society

(ABS) have collaborated to develop several consensus recommendations for quality control processes [30–32]. In addition, there are published ASTRO 'white papers' for image-guided radiotherapy, high-dose rate brachytherapy, stereotactic radiosurgery/stereotactic body radiotherapy, IMRT, and peer review [33–37], all of which are useful resources for any QA program developing new processes or reviewing the standing processes. Additionally, federal and state regulations must be followed. Here, an excellent comprehensive resource is the '*Safety is No Accident*' publication by ASTRO, a useful manual for use in developing a quality management program [11].

The physicist usually leads the technical pre-treatment and treatment verification QA processes. Detailed discussion regarding technical QA processes for plan preparation and dose/set-up verification are outside the scope of this chapter, but guidelines are available through several task group reports from the AAPM [38–42].

The quality team is responsible for leading the retrospective and prospective quality control methods detailed in the prior section. Incident learning systems should be implemented to aid in this endeavor. The quality and patient safety committee usually meets monthly or at least quarterly to review issues that arise in the interim and assess active quality projects, as well as hold morbidity and mortality conferences.

The traditional hierarchical approach to quality management – errors leading to policies/procedures enacted by leadership and obeyed by frontline staff – is rapidly being replaced by a more collaborative approach, in which quality and safety is the culture, and each individual in the department can provide input into safety issues and projects (Figure 8.2) [43]. Many institutions have enacted safety rounds, in which departmental leadership meet with the frontline work staff in their work area to discuss present or potential safety issues periodically.

The quality improvement infrastructure in any radiation oncology department is a multicomponent system that depends on all staff members and all levels of care [37]. At each point in the workflow in radiation therapy, several quality assessment and improvement procedures must be implemented to ensure safety, with responsibilities assigned to various members of the team critical to the individual task. An example breakdown of the various QA procedures implemented in radiation oncology clinics is shown in Table 8.4.

Maximizing communication between groups within the department and outside of the department (i.e., medical oncologists and primary care physicians), is also critical. Utilizing the electronic medical record to its maximal potential is encouraged. Developing effective avenues of communication between the staff members during "hand-offs" is crucial, particularly for cases that deviate from the SOP. Additionally, guidelines for safe staffing are available, although due to variability in the number

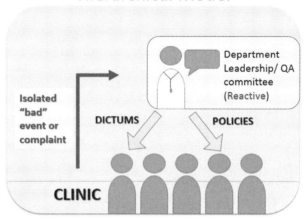

Hierarchical Model

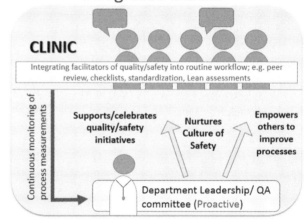

Integrated Model

Figure 8.2 Two models of departmental QA. The upper panel shows the hierarchical top-down, reactive model. The lower panel shows the Integrated, bottom-up, integrated proactive model. *Source:* Chera *et al.* 2012 [43]. Reproduced with permission of Elsevier.

of complex and less-complex cases, no one recommendation can apply to all departments [11,44].

Communication with the patient's care team outside of the radiation oncology department is as important as communication within the department. The timely generation of pertinent clinical notes is valuable in patient care (including initial consultation, on-treatment visit notes or triage notes, follow-up notes, treatment completion summary notes, etc.). Guidelines are available for the recommended data that should be provided in these documents [11,45]. There is a movement throughout healthcare towards a consolidation of information via a single electronic medical record, and many institutions are exploring ways to integrate radiation-specific documentation with the patient's hospital-wide electronic medical record [46]. At Loyola University Medical Center, efforts have been initiated to standardize all radiation oncology-specific documentation from initiation of the

Table 8.4 Examples of QA processes implemented in clinics in order to ensure patient safety and identify potential errors.

Clinical assessment	Treatment planning	Treatment delivery	Treatment monitoring	Treatment assessment and outcomes
Multi-disciplinary conferences utilizing latest national guidelines and all members of oncologic team Structured order sets and Electronic Medical Record based checklists prior to initiating simulation of patient (i.e., ensuring consent in chart, pathology confirming malignancy, pacemaker, pregnancy, etc.)	Daily, Monthly, and Yearly CT simulator QA per AAPM guidelines Peer review conferences initiated early in treatment process and having oversight on appropriateness of simulation, immobilization, target delineation, radiation treatment planning and delivery Documentation of clear clinical treatment planning note delineating intended target, prescription dose, fractionation, etc.	Daily, Monthly, yearly LINAC and Brachytherapy unit QA per AAPM guidelines Assurance of signed treatment plan, signed prescription Verbalized 2 form of identification Computerized Record and Verify System[a] Sterile cockpit rule on treatment machine ensuring professional and distraction free zone while initiating and delivering treatment	Daily, Monthly and Yearly QA of on board imaging per AAPM guidelines (i.e., portal imaging, on line electronic portal imaging devices (EPID), CBCT, kV systems, flouro) *In-vivo* dosimetry measurements (TLDs, ODLDs on a case by case scenario) Daily, Weekly assessment and feedback by Radiation Oncologist of target verification Adaptive radiotherapy	Monthly meetings of Quality Improvement Committee Institutional and national Incident Learning System reporting and assessment Initiation of individual Practice Quality Improvement projects (i.e., chart reviews evaluating treatment package time, assessing if local control and rates of failure for individual practitioner match the literature, evaluating if patient management meet cooperative group standards)

[a]Record and Verify systems area defined as computerized systems attached to individual treatment machines and designed to capture, before each beam delivery, several treatment parameters accessible through encoders (e.g., collimator opening, gantry and collimator angle, and presence of accessories such as wedge filters) and to compare them to the intended parameters, either entered manually or automatically transferred from the simulator or the treatment planning system. Adapted from International Atomic Energy Agency Human Health Report 2013 [75].

encounter with consultation, simulation, treatment documentation, completion note and follow-up. Harmonization between radiation treatment planning and delivery electronic medical record (EMR) and hospital-wide EMR in an easily accessible and interpretable fashion by all services is being accomplished through various mechanisms, including automatic transfer of treatment notes into the hospital-wide EMR, standardized completion of treatment reports that employ isodose distributions to help guide follow-up radiographic response criteria assessment, and toxicity and treatment information to be utilized in survivorship efforts.

Increased awareness of the often unmet needs of cancer survivors and their growing number has led to a movement towards the development of comprehensive survivorship care plans for patients who complete treatment in oncology based on Institute of Medicine recommendations in 2006 [47]. Historically, radiation oncologists have already instituted treatment completion summary documents that are routinely sent to primary care physicians and the patient care teams. However, this usually contains primarily of information about the radiation treatment and the treatment course and acute toxicities incurred. To help create a more comprehensive document, with information describing the long-term expected disease outcomes, late toxicities, and recommendations for surveillance of disease control and toxicities, ASTRO recently published a radiation oncology-specific template for survivorship care plans [48].

Lessons from Practice Quality Improvement Experiences

With growing experience in quality improvement using incident learning systems, there is a growing body of literature exploring potential causes of error and steps to prevent errors. In this section, some of the published data from several institutions regarding potential errors is discussed. These findings must be utilized cautiously, given that each department has unique workflows.

In an analysis of their near-miss incident learning system, Gao *et al.* reported that 29% of patients treated on an emergent basis had a near-miss event reported. When near-miss events did occur, they appeared to be of higher severity NMRI score (1.9 versus 1.4 for non-emergent reporting), as well as having a higher percentage of NMRI score of 4 when compared to non-emergent reporting (14% versus 5%). In addition, treatments that were rendered during weekends or holidays also showed higher NMRI 4 scores (see Table 8.3 for a summary of the NMRI scoring system) [49]. This indeed may be a real effect, since an NMRI score of 4 is less likely to be influenced by reporting bias, and therefore should inform each department policy when implementing off-hours emergent treatment protocols and policies. Other groups confirmed a similar predilection for increased error rate if the delivery of radiation was judged to be during the weekend and off-hours (1.3% versus 0.09% per fraction) [51]. In a multivariate logistic regression analysis of reported radiation incidents Walker *et al.* identified several factors associated with reported incidents in the planning and treatment delivery domains [50]. As the total number of fractions delivered, number of separate prescription items, and radiation beam duration increased, the risk of incident reporting was also significantly increased. In order to elucidate if time pressures to treatment leading to potential rushed planning and delivery resulted in more incidents reported, work days from plan approval to start were quantified and found to be statistically significantly associated with more incident reporting. Treatment factors which were independently found to affect reported errors included delivery on the first day of treatment, increased number of fractions delivered, treatments employing IMRT, treatments with increased number of prescriptions, and treatments with longer beam-on time (measured in minutes).

In a 10-year analysis of errors at one institution, Dominello *et al.* noted that a specifically designed 'no rush policy' employed to "…restrict large scale re-planning (LSR) if machine down time is projected to last for a single day or less…", resulted in a decrease of departmental error rates. Prior to the initiation of the no LSR policy, the overall reported error rate was 0.24%, but after implementation of the policy was significantly reduced to 0.08%. Thus, avoiding rushed, LSR may prevent radiation errors [51].

As has been documented in other fields of medicine, physician cross-coverage can lead to an increased risk of adverse events, near-misses, and medical events due to an increased need for the transfer and communication of often critical patient information to a physician who is unfamiliar with the patient case, often termed the hand-off [52]. In an analysis of perceived workload and performance on cross-covering physicians, Mosaly *et al.* used the National Aeronautics and Space Administration-Task Load Index (NASA-TLX), and objective monitoring via physiological endpoints of pupil size and blink rate to compare two scenarios of 'cross-coverage' and 'regular coverage' among eight participating physicians. The study results showed that physicians tasked with reviewing radiation plans they are cross-covering for another physician had an increased perceived workload and degraded performance [52]. In a similar analysis,

Mazur *et al.* showed that utilizing the NASA-TLX scale on nine physicians performing three radiation planning tasks that increased their workload led to an increased rate and severity of grade of errors, as judged by a pre-defined scale [53]. It appears that an increased workload, whether due to unfamiliarity with patient in a physician hand-off scenario or other stress factors, leads to a potential for greater radiation error. Policies that streamline workflow efficiency must therefore be pursued in order to minimize potential for error.

Concepts in Standardization and Workflow Efficiency

The reality of modern medicine requires an increasing demand on physicians and staff on productivity with the goal of increased value. Value in healthcare is a priority not just for payers and governmental policy-makers on a grand scale, but also for individual clinics. The nature of safety and workflow efficiency is intertwined and therefore efficient processes within the radiation oncology department represent an important component of any quality management program.

The radiation oncology workflow has changed significantly as radiation delivery has evolved over the past 20 years. In addition, the evolution of workplace tools towards electronic records and planning systems, and expanding physician workloads that include billing, insurance and regulatory demands, may have unforeseen effects on safety. Therefore, ensuring synergy among the multifaceted and hierarchical process of radiation therapy delivery is critical when implementing and evaluating radiation oncology information systems [54].

Lean philosophy, first championed due to its use and success by the Toyota manufacturing corporation, has been applied and adapted in multiple industries, including medicine and radiation oncology [55, 56]. The goal of this approach is to identify steps and processes that maximize value, while eliminating steps and processes that are wasteful. The tools used include Kaizen (translating to 'improvement' in Japanese) events, which include all staff members who play a role in a specific process collaborating to re-evaluate the process, their individual contribution to the process, and work together to improve efficiency [55], as well as the Gemba walk, which is a 'site visit' by the quality team to the location where the process is performed to observe the detailed steps of the process and to identify methods to improve the process.

Six Sigma is a system tied to Lean philosophy that uses more sophisticated statistical and quantitative methods to analyze problems and decrease variability in outcomes and thereby improve quality [57, 58]. The primary tool is the DMAIC approach, which attempts to identify a specific problem, quantify the problem using statistical analysis of collected data regarding the problem, analyze these data to help create interventions to 'solve' the problem, and then follow-up after the intervention is complete to confirm that the gains are sustained. The five steps in the DMAIC process are:

1. *Define* the problem.
2. *Measure* data related to the problem.
3. *Analyze* the data to help generate conclusions regarding the cause of the problem.
4. *Improve* the process to avoid the problem.
5. *Control* the process so interventions made are adhered to and the problem is avoided.

Clinical Targets for Standardization and Workflow Efficiency

Many institutions have created their own 'digital white board' to help with regulating workflow through the radiation treatment process from consultation to treatment. The use of electronic-based checklists integrated into oncology EMR and pathway-based EMRs has also been described to further streamline patient care and improve safety endpoints [59, 60]. These efforts may serve as the strongest defenders towards ensuring minimal treatment package time for patients from diagnosis to completion of treatment, which is a significant challenge to many departments and critical as delays have been correlated with poorer clinical outcomes [61]. Recently, commercially available software such as the Varian (Palo Alto, California) - developed ARIA® Version 11 Visual Care Path and Standard Imaging's (Middleton, Wisconsin) RT Workspace® have been developed specifically to streamline workflow efficiency, leading to a reduction in errors and an increase in staff satisfaction, by providing a task-based graphical interface which can be followed visually as patient treatment plan and delivery progresses from simulation to treatment delivery, image guidance, and possible plan, re-evaluation and adaptation [62].

Although most institutions have general agreed-upon treatment approaches for each disease site amongst the practicing physicians, some institutions have gone as far as to develop evidence-based standardized treatment pathways for the treatment of most/all of their patients. At Long Island Jewish Hospital, Potters *et al.* described their institutional experience of creating standard treatment planning pathways and found excellent physician compliance [63]. Researchers at the University of Pittsburgh demonstrated in the treatment of breast cancer that implementation of an evidence-based clinical treatment pathway to identify women who qualified for hypofractionated whole-breast irradiation (HF-WBI), resulted in a marked increased utilization, from

approximately 8–20% to more than 75% [64]. However, the clinical impact on patient outcomes of standardized treatment pathways has not yet been reported.

Standardizing treatment plan evaluation represents another avenue of streamlining workflow and potentially avoiding error. Simple-to-review and understand dosimetry plan goal sheets that are site- and tumor-specific can be integrated into the peer review process [23]. Here, an example has been provided of the treatment planning goals sheet employed by Loyola University Medical Center for patients undergoing treatment with thoracic stereotactic body radiation therapy (SBRT) (see Table 8.5). Such tables allow for the objective and efficient evaluation of dose volume endpoints for the planning target volume and normal tissues, and in the future this approach may become more seamlessly integrated into treatment planning systems. Having clearly defined department standards based on published data and cooperative group experience can help mitigate the sometimes unsystematic clinician-based review of the radiation plan. It must be stressed, however, that although digital review sheets can be used to quickly and accurately assess key dosimetric endpoints, they do not replace clinical judgment and experience. For example, quickly assessing if the volume of the combined lungs receiving at least 20 Gy (V20) has been met for a radiation plan to the lung in a binary yes/no fashion in a goal sheet cannot replace a thorough assessment of the clinical indication for treatment, a refined analysis of the various patient-specific anatomic and clinicopathological characteristics that modulate pneumonitis risk, and a thorough review of dose distribution in axial, sagittal, transverse and three-dimensional volumetric view [65].

Importance of Peer Review in Radiation Oncology

Peer review, both within the department and externally, is a vital aspect of any healthcare service department. A Cochrane-led meta-analysis found that audit and feedback is effective in improving healthcare outcomes and patient safety [66]. Robust peer review serves as an important arbiter of any safety or QA program, and radiation oncology departments rely heavily on peer review to ballast protocols resulting from experiences with incident learning, error reporting, checklist and workflow efficiency maximization.

A detailed analysis and multilevel recommendations are provided for radiation oncology departments by the landmark Marks *et al.* ASTRO white paper [37]. Peer review encompasses the "…evaluation of work and performance by other people in the same field to enhance the quality of work or the performance…" [67].

Table 8.5 Example of treatment planning dosimetric goal sheet that can be used to standardize treatment plan evaluation and peer review (bold text = goal not met), and to note when goals are not met, providing clinical acknowledgment and explanation.

Target or tissue (in order of priority)	Parameter	Target	Treatment plan	Dose criteria met?
Spinal cord	Max dose	<3000 cGy	794 cGy	Yes
	D 0.25 ml	<2250 cGy	726 cGy	Yes
	D 0.5 ml	<1350 cGy	702 cGy	Yes
Brachial plexus	Max dose	<3200 cGy	N/A	
	D 3 ml	<3000 cGy	N/A	
PTV Volume in ml 20.05	V100 (%)	≥95%	97.5%	Yes
	V95 (%)	≥99%	100%	Yes
ITV	V100 (%)	100%	100%	Yes
Conformity	Max PTV point dose	(110–130%)	118.2%	Yes
	Min PTV dose (0.03 ml)	(>95%)	96.7%	Yes
	CI @ 100% IDL	<1.2	1.03	Yes
	CI @ 50% IDL (R50)	<4.6	4.23	Yes
	PTV + 2 cm Max dose	<53	50%	Yes
Esophagus (non-adjacent wall)	Max dose	<105% of Rx	5.3%	Yes
	D 15 ml	<2750 cGy	27 cGy	Yes
Whole lung - ITV	TL V20	<10%	1.9%	Yes
	TL V12.5	<15%	4.6%	Yes
	TL V5	<37%	13%	Yes
	Spared V13.5	>1000 ml	3040 ml	Yes
	Spared V12.5	>1500 ml	3025 ml	Yes
Heart/pericardium	Max dose	<105% of Rx	92.1%	Yes
	D 15 ml	<3200 cGy	1957 cGy	Yes
Rib and chest wall	V30	<30 ml	N/A	
Trachea/bronchus	Max dose*	**<105% of Rx**	**107.4%**	**No**
	D 4 ml	<1800 cGy	295 cGy	Yes
Great vessels(non-adjacent wall)	Max dose	<105% of Rx	95.2%	Yes
	D 10 ml	<4700 cGy	1865 cGy	Yes

*The benefits of treatment clinically outweigh the risks of any dose criteria not achieved
List any special considerations: Trachea/bronchus dose clinically acceptable due to proximity of PTV; no more than two fractions per week.

Although essentially all academic radiation oncology centers have instituted prospective pretreatment 'tumor boards' for multidisciplinary clinical management decisions, and most radiation oncologists are familiar with 'chart rounds' that review each physician's cases, this report provides a more refined and comprehensive analysis of clinical targets and criteria requiring peer review. The peer review process is broken down into six broad process steps:

1. Consultation, decision planning to include radiation as part of multimodality approach.
2. Simulation, imaging, immobilization.
3. Anatomical model definition.
4. Planning, optimization.
5. Plan preparation.
6. Treatment.

For each category, the process to be performed and decision to be made is codified as well as prioritized in importance, the person who performs the task is identified, the decision to be reviewed is defined, the person or persons who must perform peer review are identified, and the ideal timing of when peer review should be performed is detailed [37].

Addressing every step benefitting from peer review can be both cost- and time-prohibitive, and therefore may negatively impact clinical efficiency. Hence, the authors emphasize that prioritizing earlier processes of peer review – particularly target contour delineation peer review after image segmentation has been performed – can have a broader impact and reduce need for re-planning. In an analysis performed by Brundage *et al.*, the most common reasons for modification after peer review related to changes to the planned target volume (PTV)

(31%), the protection of critical structures (15%), selection of treatment volumes (11%), and selection of dose (11%) [68]. Although most department have structured chart rounds to evaluate dose distribution to target by physician peers, the analysis found this to be the least reported reason for modification after peer review (6%). It appears that a transition of the peer review process earlier during the course of treatment can lead to more impactful recommendations from the peer review team and improve time-efficiency, leading to improved treatment planning and delivery. Prioritizing peer reviews to target areas of highest probability of potential error is also recommended. As highlighted by an analysis by Ford *et al.*, incorrect contours used, wrong computed tomography (CT) simulation data, wrong isocenter used, wrong markings used, and incorrect patient in the record and verify system entered, represent the top five areas of risk [69]. In a survey of academic institutions in the US, assessing the quantity and quality of peer review performed in 2011, more than 80% of institutions peer reviewed all external beam therapy courses, but only 58% and 40–47% reviewed all stereotactic radiosurgery and brachytherapy cases, respectively [70]. In addition, attendance by senior physicians – which would be expected to enhance the quality of peer review – was found to be a function of harmonized clinical schedules where time commitments did not clash with peer review attendance.

Most centers perform peer review after the patient has begun therapy, with >80% of respondents to an ASTRO-led survey on peer review practices reporting reviews of patients within the first week of treatment [70]. However, several institutions have transitioned to a prospective peer review process to be performed prior to the initiation of radiation planning and treatment, where peer review is performed after contours are completed and written directive for dose is defined [71–73]. This can be particularly important for patients who have a limited number of fractions (e.g., palliative 8 Gy in a single fraction, single-fraction radiosurgery, or SBRT of one to five fractions), where peer review after the start of treatment planning, and especially after radiation treatment delivery has been completed, is not ideal.

At Loyola University Medical Center, a prospective contouring and planning rounds has been implemented, in which patients are presented prospectively prior to the start of treatment planning and delivery whenever possible. At the time of CT simulation, patients are placed into one of four pathways to optimize review timing and workflow:

1. *Standard*– patients being treated with a definitive approach who may start treatment ≥5 days after CT simulation.
2. *Urgent* – patients being treated with a definitive approach who must start treatment ≤4 days after CT simulation.

3. *Non-emergent palliative* – patients being treated with a palliative approach who may start treatment electively at any time after CT simulation.
4. *Emergent* – patients who must be simulated, planned, and treated prior to the next peer review session.

Patients in the standard definitive group must have their physician-defined treatment targets reviewed at a peer review session prior to the dosimetrists beginning treatment planning. Urgent definitive patients may have treatment planning begun prior to peer review in order to optimize workflow, but before the patient may start treatment, the physician-defined target volumes must be reviewed in a peer review session. Non-emergent palliative cases are handled in the same way. Emergent cases, due to the need to begin treatment in the emergent setting, are reviewed after the patient has begun treatment. A summarized process map is shown in Figure 8.3. This approach to peer review allows for the prospective review of patient dose/fractionation and treatment target and normal tissue goals prior to planning and prior to any treatment in most patients.

For smaller centers, particularly those with a single or few physicians, peer review can be challenging. For these centers, developing collaborations with other centers and potentially utilizing teleconferencing for peer review is a reasonable approach to allow for adequate peer review of their patients.

External peer review of a program, or so-called 'accreditation,' is also a useful tool in re-evaluating a quality management program. Multiple organizations provide practice evaluations as part of accreditation programs. The American College of Radiology (ACR) and the American College of Radiation Oncology (ACRO) accreditation programs are utilized by many practices. In order to enhance their quality improvement initiatives in 2012, ASTRO introduced as part of its accreditation the Accreditation Program for Excellence (APEx®), which establishes standards of performance derived from white papers and consensus guidelines. By putting the recommendations of the ASTRO white papers, the target safety campaign, and *Safety is no Accident* into action and practice, the APEx program is thematically organized into five pillars of patient care and management and 16 standards that are to be objectively assessed by radiation departments and surveyors as part of the APEx accreditation (see Table 8.6) [74]. APEx® provides a mechanism for a rigorous five-phase review that involves an initial application and self-assessment based on each pillar and standard, electronic remote and on-site review of department policies, communication with key staff, followed by a review for accreditation. Highlighted among this process is a strong commitment to building a culture of safety, instituting a rigorous and robust peer review process, as well as an incident learning system that incorporates both radiation events/errors as well as near-misses.

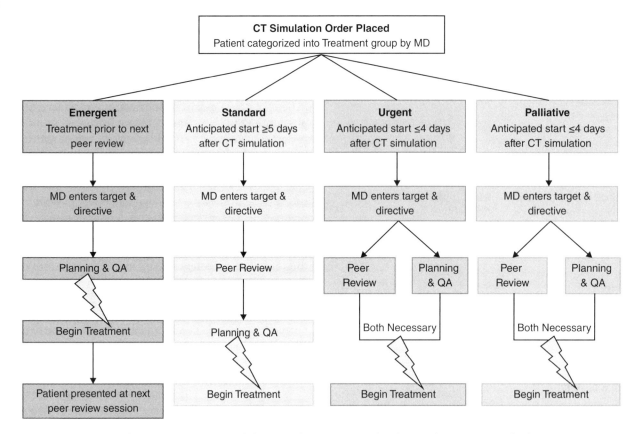

Figure 8.3 Process map of proactive contouring and chart rounds peer review utilized at Loyola University Medical Center.

Table 8.6 ASTRO Accreditation Program for Excellence program standards are thematically organized into five pillars.

Pillar 1 – Process of Care	Standard 1	• Patient evaluation
		• Care coordination
		• Follow up
	Standard 2	• Treatment planning
	Standard 3	• Patient-specific safety interventions
		• Safe practices in treatment preparation and delivery
Pillar 2 – The Radiation Oncology Team	Standard 4	• Staff roles and responsibilities
	Standard 5	• Qualifications and ongoing training of staff
	Standard 6	• Safe staffing plan
Pillar 3 – Safety	Standard 7	• Culture of safety
	Standard 8	• Radiation safety
	Standard 9	• Emergency preparation and planning
Pillar 4 – Quality Management	Standard 10	• Facility and equipment
	Standard 11	• Information management
		• Integration of systems
	Standard 12	• Quality management of treatment procedures and modalities
	Standard 13	• Peer review of clinical processes
Pillar 5 – Patient-Centered Care	Standard 14	• Patient consent
	Standard 15	• Patient education
		• Patient health management
	Standard 16	• Performance measurement
		• Outcomes reporting

References

1 Marks, L.B., Jackson, M., Xie, L., *et al.* (2011) The challenge of maximizing safety in radiation oncology. *Pract. Radiat. Oncol.*, **1** (1), 2–14.

2 Institute of Medicine (1999) *To Err is Human: Building a Safer System.* National Academy Press, Washington, DC.

3 Bogdanich, W. (2010) Safety features planned for radiation machines. *New York Times*, 2010; A19.

4 Bogdanich, W. (2010) V.A. is fined over errors in radiation at hospital. *New York Times*, 2010; A20.

5 Bogdanich, W., Ruiz, R.R. (2010) Radiation errors reported in Missouri. *New York Times*, 2010; A17.

6 Bogdanich, W. (2010) Radiation offers new cures, and ways to do harm. *New York Times*, 2010; A1.

7 Marks, L.B., Pawlicki, T.A., Hayman, J.A. (2015) Learning to Appreciate Swiss Cheese and other Industrial Engineering Concepts. *Pract. Radiat. Oncol.*, **5**, 277–281.

8 Autorite de Surate Nucleaire (ASN) (2007) ASN-SFRO Experimental scale for dealing with radiation protection events affecting patients undergoing a medical radiotherapy procedure. *Autorite de Surete Nucleaire*, Paris.

9 Common Terminology Criteria for Adverse Event, Cancer Therapy Evaluation Program, August 2006. Available at: http://ctep.cancer.gov. Accessed Nov 25, 2015.

10 Konski, A., Movsas, B., Konopka, M., Ma, C., Price, R., Pollack, A. (2009) Developing a radiation error scoring system to monitor quality control events in a radiation oncology department. *J. Am. Coll. Radiol.*, **6** (1), 45–50.

11 Zietman, A., Palta, J., Steinberg, M., *et al.* (2012) *Safety Is No Accident: A Framework for Quality Radiation Oncology and Care.* American Society for Radiation Oncology, Fairfax, VA.

12 Ford, E.C., Fong de Los Santos, L., Pawlicki, T., *et al.* (2012) Consensus recommendations for incident learning database structures in radiation oncology. *Med. Phys.*, **39**, 7272–7290.

13 Nyflot, M.J., Zeng, J., Kusano, A.S., *et al.* (2015) Metrics of success: Measuring impact of a departmental near-miss incident learning system. *Pract. Radiat. Oncol.*, **5** (5), e409–e416.

14 Barach, P., Small, S.D. (2000) Reporting and preventing medical mishaps: lessons from non-medical near miss reporting systems. *Br. Med. J.*, **320** (7237), 759–763.

15 Egger Halbeis, C.B., Epstein, R.H., Macario, A., Pearl, R.G., Grunwald, Z. (2008) Adoption of anesthesia information management systems by academic departments in the United States. *Anesth. Analg.*, **107** (4), 1323–1329.

16 Anesthesia Quality Institute (2011; updated 2015) Anesthesia Incident Reporting System (AIRS). Available at: https://www.aqihq.org/airs. Accessed Nov 24, 2015.

17 DeRosier, J., Stalhandske, E., Bagian, J.P., Nudell, T. (2002) Using Health Care Failure Mode and Effect Analysis: the VA National Center for Patient Safety's prospective risk analysis system. *J. Commun. J. Qual. Improv.*, **28**, 248–267.

18 Marx, D.A., Slonim, A.D. (2003) Assessing patient safety risk before the injury occurs: an introduction to sociotechnical probabilistic risk modelling in health care. *Qual. Safety Health Care*, **12**, ii33–ii38.

19 Cunningham, J., Coffey, M., Knöös, T., Holmberg, O. (2010) Radiation Oncology Safety Information System (ROSIS) – profiles of participants and the first 1074 incident reports. *Radiother. Oncol.*, **97** (3), 601–607.

20 Hoopes, D.J., Dicker, A.P., Eads, N.L., *et al.* (2015) RO-ILS: Radiation Oncology Incident Learning System: A report from the first year of experience. *Pract. Radiat. Oncol.*, **5** (5), 312–318.

21 Smith, K.S., Harris, K.M., Potters, L., *et al.* (2014) Physician attitudes and practices related to voluntary error and near-miss reporting. *J. Oncol. Pract.*, **10** (5), e350–e357.

22 Reason, J. (2000) Human error: Models and management. *Br. Med. J.*, **320**, 768–770.

23 Chera, B.S., Mazur, L., Marks, L.B. (2015) Applying Normal Accident Theory to radiation oncology: Failures are normal but patient harm can be prevented. *Pract. Radiat. Oncol.*, **5**, 325–327

24 Chera, B.S., Mazur, L., Buchanan, I., *et al.* (2015) Improving Patient Safety in Clinical Oncology: Applying lessons from Normal Accident Theory. *JAMA Oncol.*, **1** (7), 958–964.

25 Desroches, A. (2013) The management of risks by the global risk analysis. *Transfus. Clin. Biol.*, **20**, 198–210.

26 Mazeron, R., Aguini, N., Rivin, E., *et al.* (2014) Improving safety in radiotherapy: the implementation of the Global Risk Analysis method. *Radiother. Oncol.*, **112** (2), 205–211.

27 Ford, E.C., Gaudette, R., Myers, L., *et al.* (2009) Evaluation of safety in a radiation oncology setting using failure mode and effects analysis. *Int. J. Radiat. Oncol. Biol. Phys.*, **74**, 852–858.

28 Denny, D.S., Allen, D.K., Worthington, N., Gupta, D. (2014) The use of failure mode and effect analysis in a radiation oncology setting: the Cancer Treatment Centers of America experience. *J. Healthcare Qual.*, **36** (1), 18–28.

29 Pawlicki, T., Mundt, A.J. (2007) Quality in radiation oncology. *Med. Phys.*, **34** (5), 1529–1534.

30 American College of Radiology (2014) ACR–ASTRO Practice Parameter for the Performance of Stereotactic Radiosurgery. Available at: http://www.acr.org/~/

media/ACR/Documents/PGTS/guidelines/Stereotactic_Radiosurgery.pdf. Accessed Dec 06, 2015.

31 American College of Radiology (2015) Radiation Oncology Practice Parameters and Technical Standards. Available at: http://www.acr.org/Quality-Safety/Standards-Guidelines/Practice-Guidelines-by-Modality/Radiation-Oncology. Accessed Nov 24, 2015.

32 American College of Radiology (2015) ACR–ABS practice parameter for performance of radionuclide-based high dose rate brachytherapy. Available at: http://www.acr.org/~/media/ACR/Documents/PGTS/guidelines/High_Dose_Rate_Brachy.pdf. Accessed Nov 24, 2015.

33 Moran, J.M., Dempsey, M., Eisbruch, A., *et al.* (2011) Safety considerations for IMRT: executive summary. *Med. Phys.*, **38** (9), 5067–5072.

34 Solberg, T.D., Balter, J.M., Benedict, S.H., *et al.* (2012) Quality and safety considerations in stereotactic radiosurgery and stereotactic body radiation therapy: Executive summary. *Pract. Radiat. Oncol.*, **2** (1), 2–9.

35 Thomadsen, B.R., Erickson, B.A., Eifel, P.J., *et al.* (2014) A review of safety, quality management, and practice guidelines for high-dose-rate brachytherapy: executive summary. *Pract. Radiat. Oncol.*, **4** (2), 65–70.

36 Jaffray, D.A., Langen, K.M., Mageras, G., *et al.* (2013) Safety considerations for IGRT: Executive summary. *Pract. Radiat. Oncol.*, **3** (3), 167–170.

37 Marks, L.B., Adams, R.D., Pawlicki, T., *et al.* (2013) Enhancing the role of case-oriented peer review to improve quality and safety in radiation oncology: Executive summary. *Pract. Radiat. Oncol.*, **3** (3), 149–156.

38 Cody, D.D., Fisher, T.S., Gress, D.A., *et al.* (2013) AAPM Medical Physics Practice Guideline 1.a: CT protocol management and review practice guideline. *J. Appl. Clin. Med. Phys.*, **14** (5), 3–12.

39 Fontenot, J.D., Alkhatib, H., Garrett, J.A., *et al.* (2014) AAPM Medical Physics Practice Guideline 2.a: Commissioning and quality assurance of X-ray-based image-guided radiotherapy systems. *J. Appl. Clin. Med. Phys.*, **15** (1), 4528.

40 Seibert, J.A., Clements, J.B., Halvorsen, P.H., *et al.* (2015) AAPM Medical Physics Practice Guideline 3.a: Levels of supervision for medical physicists in clinical training. *J. Appl. Clin. Med. Phys.*, **16** (3), 5291.

41 Fong de Los Santos, L.E., Evans, S., Ford, E.C., *et al.* (2015) Medical Physics Practice Guideline 4.a: Development, implementation, use and maintenance of safety checklists. *J. Appl. Clin. Med. Phys.*, **16** (3), 5431.

42 Smilowitz, J.B., Das, I.J., Feygelman, V., *et al.* (2015) AAPM Medical Physics Practice Guideline 5.a.: Commissioning and QA of Treatment Planning Dose Calculations – Megavoltage Photon and Electron Beams. *J. Appl. Clin. Med. Phys.*, **16** (5), 5768.

43 Chera, B.S., Jackson, M., Mazur, L.M., *et al.* (2012) Improving quality of patient care by improving daily practice in radiation oncology. *Semin. Radiat. Oncol.*, **22** (1), 77–85.

44 Battista, J.J., Clark, B.G., Patterson, M.S., *et al.* (2012) Medical physics staffing for radiation oncology: a decade of experience in Ontario, Canada. *J. Appl. Clin. Med. Phys.*, **13** (1), 3704.

45 American College of Radiology (2014) ACR–ASTRO practice parameter for communication: radiation oncology. Available at: http://www.acr.org/~/media/ACR/Documents/PGTS/guidelines/Comm_Radiation_Oncology.pdf. Accessed Nov 25, 2015.

46 Russo, G.A. (2015) When Electronic Health Records (EHRs) Talk Everyone Can Win: Our experience creating a software link between hospital and radiation oncology electronic health records. *Int. J. Radiat. Oncol. Biol. Phys.*, **94** (1), 206–207.

47 Institute of Medicine and National Research Council (2006) From Cancer Patient to Cancer Survivor: Lost in Transition. Washington, DC: The National Academies Press, 2006. doi:10.17226/11468.

48 Chen, R.C., Hoffman, K.E., Sher, D.J., *et al.* (2015) Development of a standard survivorship care plan template for radiation oncologists. *Pract. Radiat. Oncol.*, **6** (1), 57–65.

49 Gao, W., Nyflot, M.J., Novak, A., *et al.* (2015) Can emergent treatments result in more severe errors?: An analysis of a large institutional near-miss incident reporting database. *Pract. Radiat. Oncol.*, **5** (5), 319–324.

50 Walker, G.V., Johnson, J., Edwards, T., *et al.* (2015) Factors associated with radiation therapy incidents in a large academic institution. *Pract. Radiat. Oncol.*, **5** (1), 21–27.

51 Dominello, M.M., Paximadis, P., Zaki, M., *et al.* (2015) Ten-Year Trends in Safe Radiotherapy Delivery and Results of a Radiation Therapy Quality Assurance Intervention. *Pract. Radiat. Oncol.*, **5** (6), e665–e671.

52 Mosaly, P.R., Mazur, L.M., Jones, E.L., *et al.* (2013) Quantifying the impact of cross coverage on physician's workload and performance in radiation oncology. *Pract. Radiat. Oncol.*, **3** (4), e179–e186.

53 Mazur, L.M., Mosaly, P., Jackson, M., *et al.* (2012) Quantitative assessment of workload and stressors in clinical radiation oncology. *Int. J. Radiat. Oncol. Biol. Phys.*, **83**, e571–e576.

54 Fong de Los Santos, L.E., Herman, M.G. (2012) Radiation oncology information systems and clinical practice compatibility: Workflow evaluation and comprehensive assessment. *Pract. Radiat. Oncol.*, **2** (4), e155–e164.

55 Ohno, T. (1988) *Toyota Production System, Beyond Large Scale Production.* Productivity Press, New York.

56 Kim, C.S., Hayman, J.A., Billi, J.E., Lash, K., Lawrence, T.S. (2007) The application of lean thinking to the care of patients with bone and brain metastasis with radiation therapy. *J. Oncol. Pract.*, **3** (4), 189–193.

57 Pande, P.S., Neuman, R.P., Cavanagh, R.R. (2001) *The Six Sigma way: How GE, Motorola, and other top companies are honing their performance.* 1st edition. McGraw-Hill Professional, New York, pp. 299–302.

58 Cima, R.R., Brown, M.J., Hebl, J.R., *et al.* (2011) Use of lean six sigma methodology to improve operating room efficiency in a high volume tertiary-care academic medical center. *J. Am. Coll. Surg.*, **213**, 83–92.

59 Sicotte, C., Lapointe, J., Clavel, S., *et al.* (2015) Benefits of improving processes in cancer care with a care pathway-based Electronic Medical Record. *Pract. Radiat. Oncol.*, **6** (1), 26–33.

60 Albuquerque, K.V., Miller, A.A., Roeske, J.C.J. (2011) Implementation of Electronic Checklists in an Oncology Medical Record: Initial Clinical Experience. *Oncol. Pract.*, **7** (4), 222–226.

61 Jensen, A.R., Nellemann, H.M., Overgaard, J. (2007) Tumor progression in waiting time for radiotherapy in head and neck cancer. *Radiother. Oncol.*, **84** (1), 5–10.

62 Kovalchuk, N., Russo, G.A., Shin, J.Y., Kachnic, L.A. (2015) Optimizing efficiency and safety in a radiation oncology department through the use of ARIA 11 Visual Care Path. *Pract. Radiat. Oncol.*, **5** (5), 295–303.

63 Potters, L., Raince, J., Chou, H., *et al.* (2013) Development, implementation, and compliance of treatment pathways in radiation medicine. *Front. Oncol.*, **3**, 105.

64 Chapman, B.V., Rajagopalan, M.S., Heron, D.E., *et al.* (2015) Clinical pathways: A catalyst for the adoption of hypofractionation for early-stage breast cancer. *Int. J. Radiat. Oncol. Biol. Phys.*, **93** (4), 854–861.

65 Bradley, J.D., Hope, A., El Naqa, I., *et al.* (2007) A nomogram to predict radiation pneumonitis, derived from a combined analysis of RTOG 9311 and institutional data. *Int. J. Radiat. Oncol. Biol. Phys.*, **69** (4), 985–992.

66 Ivers, N., Jamtvedt, G., Flottorp, S., *et al.* (2012) Audit and feedback: effects on professional practice and healthcare outcomes. *Cochrane Database Syst. Rev.*, **6**, CD000259.

67 Hulick, P.R., Ascoli, F.A. (2005) Quality assurance in radiation oncology. *J. Am. Coll. Radiol.*, **2**, 613–616.

68 Brundage, M.D., Dixon, P.F., Mackillop, W.J., *et al.* (1999) A real-time audit of radiation therapy in a regional cancer center. *Int. J. Radiat. Oncol. Biol. Phys.*, **43**, 115–124.

69 Ford, E.C., Gaudette, R., Myers, L., *et al.* (2009) Evaluation of safety in a radiation oncology setting using failure mode and effects analysis. *Int. J. Radiat. Oncol. Biol. Phys.*, **74**, 852–858.

70 Lawrence, Y.R., Whiton, M.A., Symon, Z., *et al.* (2012) Quality assurance peer review chart rounds in 2011: a survey of academic institutions in the United States. *Int. J. Radiat. Oncol. Biol. Phys.*, **84** (3), 590–595.

71 Hoopes, D.J., Johnstone, P.A., Chapin, P.S., *et al.* (2015) Practice patterns for peer review in radiation oncology. *Pract. Radiat. Oncol.*, **5** (1), 32–38.

72 Cox, B.W., Kapur, A., Sharma, A., *et al.* (2015) Prospective contouring rounds: A novel, high-impact tool for optimizing quality assurance. *Pract. Radiat. Oncol.*, **5** (5), e431–e436.

73 Matuszak, M.M., Hadley, S.W., Feng, M., *et al.* (2015) Enhancing safety and quality through pre-planning peer review for patients undergoing stereotactic body radiation therapy. *Pract. Radiat. Oncol.*, **6** (2), e39–e46.

74 ASTRO (2015) *Accreditation Program for Excellence: Safety and quality for radiation oncology practice, Program Guidance.* American Society for Radiation Oncology, Fairfax, VA.

75 International Atomic Energy Agency (2013) Human Health Report No. 7. Record and Verify Systems for Radiation Treatment of Cancer: Acceptance Testing, Commissioning and Quality Control. IAEA Publishing, Vienna, Austria.

Section 2

Cancers of the Head and Neck

Section Editor: Min Yao

9

Carcinoma of the Oral Cavity

Keith Unger, Felix Ho, James Melotek and Nancy Lee

Structure of the Oral Cavity

The oral cavity extends from the skin–vermilion junction of the lips to the junction of the hard and soft palate superiorly, laterally to the anterior tonsillar pillar, and inferiorly to the circumvallate papillae. The oral cavity is divided into subsites: lips, oral tongue, floor of mouth, buccal mucosa, upper and lower gingiva, hard palate, and retromolar trigone (Figure 9.1). The natural history and clinical presentation of primary carcinomas located in each subsite of the oral cavity vary significantly and will be discussed separately.

Lip

The lip begins at the junction of the vermilion border and includes only the vermilion surface, or the portion of the lip that comes into contact with the opposing lip. It is divided into an upper lip and a lower lip. Notable surface landmarks include the labial commissures laterally and the labial tubercles inferior to the philtrum. The motor function of the lips is controlled by the facial nerve (cranial nerve VII) and the sensory innervation is from the second and third divisions of the trigeminal nerve (cranial nerve V).

The majority of carcinomas of the lower lip are moderately to well-differentiated squamous cell carcinomas. Basal cell carcinomas arising from the skin that invade the lips secondarily should be considered carcinomas of the skin. After carcinomas of the skin, carcinoma of the lip is the next most common cancer of the head and neck. In the United States, the incidence of lip cancer is 12.7 per 100 000 annually [1]. The incidence rates are generally stable or falling among males worldwide, but are rising among females [2]. Elderly men are affected most frequently, particularly in the sixth and seventh decades of life. Lip carcinomas are rare among blacks and Asians.

Chronic exposure to sunlight appears to be a predisposing factor, and carcinoma of the lip occurs most frequently in fair-skinned persons who work outdoors [3]. Other possible etiologic factors are tobacco smoking and viruses.

Carcinoma of the lip typically spreads by direct extension to the surrounding soft tissue, skin, and bone. Regional lymph node metastases occur in fewer than 20% of patients, but are associated with increased cancer mortality [4]. The average incidence of regional lymph node metastasis is about 5–10% at presentation, and approximately an equal proportion of clinically node-negative patients subsequently develop cervical node metastasis. The risk of lymph node involvement increases with high-risk features which include increased depth of invasion, poor differentiation, commissure involvement, large tumor size, and recurrence after prior treatment [5–7]. Perineural spread occurs in 2% of cases [8]. Lower-lip carcinomas that do not involve the central one-third of the lip typically metastasize to the ipsilateral submental, submandibular, and upper cervical lymph nodes (Figure 9.2). Lower-lip carcinomas involving the central one-third of the lip can involve the bilateral neck nodes [4]. Carcinoma at or near the commissure may rarely metastasize to the facial nodes. Carcinoma of the upper lip may metastasize directly to the ipsilateral upper cervical, preauricular, or submandibular nodes; contralateral metastases are uncommon except for tumors in a midline location (Figure 9.3). Distant metastasis from carcinoma of the lip is extremely rare.

Oral Tongue

The oral tongue (anterior two-thirds of the tongue) extends anteriorly from the sulcus terminale to the undersurface of the tongue at the junction of the floor of the mouth. The circumvallate papillae are large taste buds

Clinical Radiation Oncology: Indications, Techniques, and Results, Third Edition. Edited by William Small Jr.
© 2017 John Wiley & Sons, Inc. Published 2017 by John Wiley & Sons, Inc.

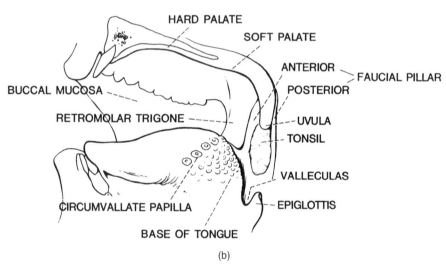

that lie anterior to the sulcus terminale. The frenulum is a ventral attachment to the floor of mouth. The extrinsic musculature of the tongue includes the genioglossus, hyoglossus, styloglossus, and palatoglossus. The extrinsic muscles originate outside of the tongue and insert into it. They are responsible for elevating, depressing, protruding, and retracting the tongue. The intrinsic musculature of the tongue is responsible for the dexterity of the tongue. The hypoglossal nerve (cranial nerve XII) is the motor nerve of the tongue. The lingual nerve, a branch of the mandibular division of cranial nerve V, provides sensation for the tongue. Taste for the anterior two-thirds of the tongue is supplied by the chorda tympani nerve, a branch of cranial nerve VII.

The majority of carcinomas of the oral tongue are moderately to well-differentiated squamous cell carcinomas. Tumors may be exophytic, papillary, or infiltrative, and

are commonly associated with leukoplakia. Carcinoma of the oral tongue is the second most common malignancy of the oral cavity, and it occurs more frequently in males than in females. The peak incidence occurs in the fifth through the seventh decades of life. Carcinomas of the oral tongue are associated with poor oral hygiene, heavy tobacco smoking, and alcoholism. The vast majority of carcinomas occur on the lateral and ventral surfaces of the tongue. In the early stages, patients may present with an ulcer which may or may not cause local pain, but in more advanced cases, patients may complain of ipsilateral otalgia, secondary to involvement of the lingual nerve, hypersalivation, or dysphagia. Careful inspection and palpation of areas adjacent to the visible tumor are necessary to identify base of tongue and floor of mouth involvement. The inability to fully protrude the tongue indicates deep musculature invasion.

Figure 9.2 Patterns of lymph node involvement from squamous cell carcinoma of the lower lip.

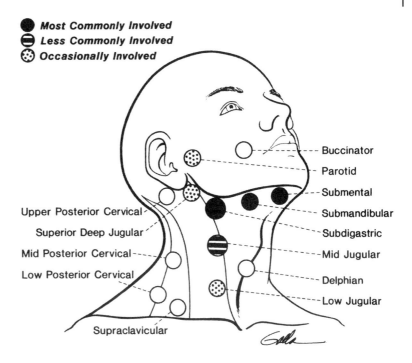

Oral tongue carcinomas spread by direct invasion into the floor of the mouth, anterior tonsillar pillar, base of tongue, and mandible. Approximately 30–45% of patients have clinically evident cervical lymph node metastasis at presentation, and 5–10% of these are bilateral. Byers *et al.* found that the risk of occult lymph node involvement in clinically node-negative patients with stage T1–2 and T3–4 disease was 19% and 32%, respectively [9]. Tumor thickness, T-stage, perineural invasion, infiltrating-type invasion, and poorly differentiated tumors have been correlated with the incidence of lymph nodal involvement [10–12]. The tumor thickness cut-off for an increasing risk of lymph node involvement varies widely, and has been reported as 2 mm to 8 mm [10, 11, 13, 14]. The subdigastric nodes are most frequently involved and the submandibular and midjugular lymph nodes are less

Figure 9.3 Patterns of lymph node involvement from squamous cell carcinoma of the upper lip.

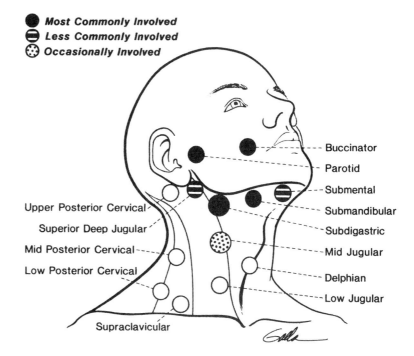

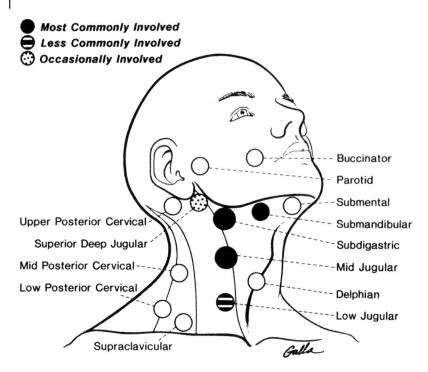

● **Most Commonly Involved**
⊖ **Less Commonly Involved**
⊙ **Occasionally Involved**

Figure 9.4 Patterns of lymph node involvement from squamous cell carcinoma of the oral tongue.

Buccinator
Parotid
Submental
Submandibular
Subdigastric
Mid Jugular
Delphian
Low Jugular

Upper Posterior Cervical
Superior Deep Jugular
Mid Posterior Cervical
Low Posterior Cervical

Supraclavicular

commonly involved (Figure 9.4). The submental, lower jugular, and posterior cervical nodes are rarely involved. Myers *et al.* found that extracapsular extension was the most important predictor of regional recurrence, distant metastasis, and overall survival [15]. The lungs, liver, and bones are the most common distant metastatic sites.

Floor of the Mouth

The floor of the mouth is a semilunar space over the mylohyoid and hyoglossus muscles, extending from the inner surface of the lower alveolar ridge to the undersurface of the tongue. The hypoglossal nerve (cranial nerve XII) passes through a gap between the mylohyoid and hyoglossus muscles. The posterior border is at the base of the anterior tonsillar pillars. The floor of the mouth is divided by the frenulum of the tongue. The submandibular glands, submandibular ducts (Wharton's ducts), and the sublingual glands are located within the floor of the mouth.

The majority of the carcinomas of the floor of the mouth are moderately to well-differentiated squamous cell carcinomas. Adenoid cystic and mucoepidermoid carcinomas arising from the minor salivary glands form a small minority of cases. Carcinoma of the floor of the mouth accounts for approximately 15% of all carcinomas of the oral cavity. Similar to carcinoma of the oral tongue, carcinoma of the floor of the mouth is often associated with tobacco smoking, heavy alcohol consumption, and poor oral hygiene. Most patients are diagnosed in the fifth to seventh decade of life. Early lesions often present as an elevated mucosal lesion with or without associated leukoplakia on routine physical examination. Invasion of the tongue is common, and it may be difficult to distinguish the origin of the primary lesion. In advanced cases, patients may complain of otalgia from referred pain, hypersalivation, altered speech, loose teeth, and bleeding. Bimanual palpation is used to determine the extent of the primary and for fixation to the mandible.

Carcinomas of the floor of the mouth spread by direct invasion into the tongue, lower alveolar ridge, and mandible. Approximately 30% of patients have clinically positive lymph nodes at presentation [16]. Shah *et al.* found occult lymph node metastasis in 26% of patients without clinical lymph node involvement on elective neck dissection [17]. The incidence of neck involvement increases with T-stage and tumor thickness [18]. The submandibular lymph nodes are most frequently involved and the subdigastric, midjugular, and submental nodes are less frequently involved (Figure 9.5). Distant metastasis occurs in approximately 10% of patients.

Buccal Mucosa

The buccal mucosa includes the membrane lining of the inner surface of the cheeks and lips, from the line of contact of the opposing lips to the line of attachment of mucosa of the upper and lower alveolar and pterygomandibular raphe. The buccinator muscle is the muscle of the cheek. Superficial to the muscle is the buccal fat pad, which gives the cheeks a rounded contour.

Figure 9.5 Patterns of lymph node involvement from squamous cell carcinoma of the floor of mouth.

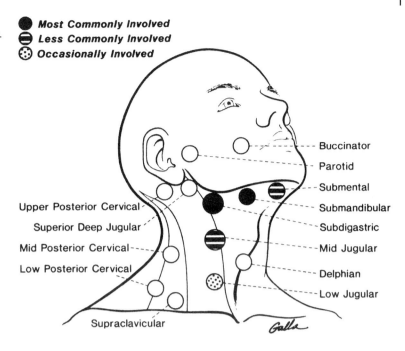

● **Most Commonly Involved**
◒ **Less Commonly Involved**
⊙ **Occasionally Involved**

Buccinator
Parotid
Submental
Submandibular
Subdigastric
Mid Jugular
Delphian
Low Jugular

Upper Posterior Cervical
Superior Deep Jugular
Mid Posterior Cervical
Low Posterior Cervical

Supraclavicular

Most carcinomas of the buccal mucosa are low-grade squamous cell carcinomas. They often occur in association with pre-existing leukoplakia, and excision of the oral leukoplakia may reduce the subsequent development of carcinoma [19]. They generally occur along the middle and posterior portions of the cheek along the occlusion line of the teeth. There are three distinct tumor types: exophytic, ulcerative, and verrucous. Verroucous carcinomas occur more frequently in the buccal mucosa than at other sites in the oral cavity [20]. After carcinoma of the lip, oral tongue, floor of the mouth, and lower gingiva, carcinoma of the buccal mucosa is the fifth most common carcinoma of the oral cavity. It is the most common carcinoma of the oral cavity in India, Malaysia, and Taiwan. It usually occurs in the sixth and seventh decades of life, and is more prevalent in males than in females. There is an association with tobacco and betel nut chewing [21,22]. Patients may present with pain, bleeding, trismus, or cervical lymphadenopathy. In advanced stages, the tumor may destroy the entire cheek and invade the adjacent bones and the neck.

Infiltrative carcinomas of the buccal mucosa typically invade the buccinator muscle early. Local spread may involve the gingivobuccal sulcus, upper and lower alveolar ridges, hard palate, maxilla, mandible, deep lobe of the parotid, and commissure of the lip. Very advanced tumors may perforate the skin of the cheek. Lymph node metastasis occurs in approximately 9% to 31% of patients [20, 23]. The submandibular and subdigastric lymph nodes are most frequently involved (Figure 9.6). The risk of subclinical lymph node metastases is 16% [24]. Distant metastases are uncommon, since patients often die of uncontrolled local disease before distant metastases are manifested clinically.

Gingiva and Hard Palate

The upper gingiva (upper alveolar ridge) includes the mucosa covering the upper ridge of the alveolar process of the maxilla. The gingiva extends from the line of attachment of the mucosa in the upper gingival buccal gutter to the junction of the hard palate. The posterior margin is the upper end of the pterygo-palatine arch. The lower gingiva (lower alveolar ridge) includes the mucosa covering the alveolar process of the mandible and extends from the line of attachment of mucosa in the buccal gutter to the line of free mucosa of the floor of the mouth. Posteriorly, it extends to the ascending ramus of the mandible. The hard palate is formed by the palatine process of the maxilla and horizontal plates of the palatine bones. It is bordered anteriorly and laterally by the upper alveolar ridge and extends to the posterior edge of the palatine bone where it is contiguous with the soft palate.

Squamous cell carcinoma is the most common histology, and the majority are well-differentiated or moderately differentiated. Approximately 80% of carcinomas arise in the lower gingiva and most occur posterior to the bicuspids. Tumors can be ulcerative, exophytic, or verrucous in their gross appearance. They are commonly associated with leukoplakia. Patients with gingival carcinoma often present with a history of ill-fitting dentures, loose teeth, bleeding upon mastication, or a non-healing

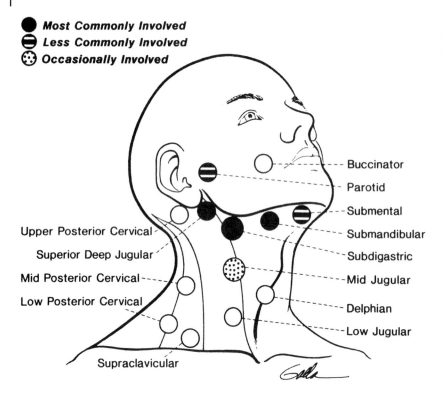

● **Most Commonly Involved**
⊜ **Less Commonly Involved**
⊙ **Occasionally Involved**

Buccinator
Parotid
Submental
Submandibular
Subdigastric
Mid Jugular
Delphian
Low Jugular

Upper Posterior Cervical
Superior Deep Jugular
Mid Posterior Cervical
Low Posterior Cervical

Supraclavicular

Figure 9.6 Patterns of lymph node involvement from squamous cell carcinoma of the buccal mucosa.

ulcer. Parathesias of the lower lip may indicate involvement of the inferior dental nerve. Trismus and pain can result from bone invasion. Primary malignancies of the hard palate are rare and account for a small minority of patients with oral cavity carcinomas [25]. Patients often complain of ill-fitting dentures, pain, intermittent bleeding, or a sore that does not heal.

Gingival carcinomas commonly invade into bone. Carcinomas of the upper gingiva may also spread by direct invasion into the maxillary sinus or the upper gingivobuccal sulcus. Radiographic studies can aid in differentiating a locally advanced upper gingival primary from a maxillary sinus primary extending into the gingiva. Carcinomas of the lower gingiva may involve the underlying mandible, retromolar trigone, buccal mucosa, or floor mouth. Tumor spreads mainly through the occlusal ridge alone or in combination with penetration of the buccal or lingual plates in edentulous patients [26, 27]. Byers *et al.* reported clinically apparent lymph node metastases in 16% of patients and subclinical node involvement in 18% of patients with carcinomas of the lower gingiva [28]. In a series of 33 patients with squamous cell carcinoma confined to the upper gingiva, the risk of lymph node involvement was 21% versus 27% for tumors that had spread to the hard palate [29]. The submandibular lymph nodes are most frequently involved in gingival carcinomas. Involvement of the subdigastric and upper cervical nodes is less common. The majority of hard palate malignant tumors are adenoid cystic carcinomas or mucoepidermoid carcinomas.

Squamous cell carcinomas are rare. Lymph node spread is present in less than 10% of patients.

Retromolar Trigone

The retromolar trigone is a triangular surface overlying the ascending ramus of the mandible from the level of the posterior surface of the last molar tooth to the apex superiorly, adjacent to the tuberosity of the maxilla. The mucous membranes blend medially with the anterior tonsillar pillar and with the buccal mucosa laterally.

Carcinomas of the retromolar trigone are rare. The majority of tumors are squamous cell carcinomas, and most are moderately to well-differentiated. Frequently, they are indistinguishable from carcinomas arising from the anterior tonsillar pillar and are often reported as a single site. The incidence of clinical lymph node involvement at diagnosis is approximately 39%, and the risk of occult node metastases is 25% [30]. The lymphatic drainage is to the ipsilateral submandibular, subdigastric, and superior jugular nodes. Retromolar carcinomas often present with pain, which can be referred to the external auditory canal and preauricular area.

Diagnosis and Staging

Patients with oral cavity cancers should be evaluated with a comprehensive oral examination, biopsy of the primary lesion, and chest imaging. Computed tomography (CT)

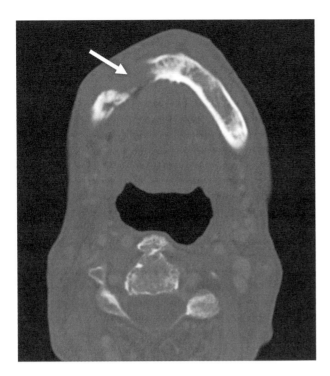

Figure 9.7 Transverse computed tomography (CT) image depicting right mandible invasion (arrow) from squamous cell carcinoma of the floor of mouth.

scanning is commonly used to evaluate the local extent of the tumor and regional spread to cervical lymph nodes. CT is particularly valuable for detecting invasion into the mandible, maxilla, and pterygopalatine fossa (Figure 9.7). MRI is widely accepted as being superior to CT in evaluating soft-tissue lesions. Several studies have reported that MRI accurately predicts the depth of invasion in oral tongue cancers (Figure 9.8) [31, 32]. Positron emission

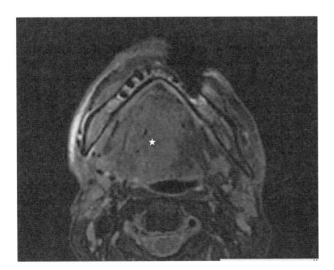

Figure 9.8 Axial T2-weighted fat-suppression MRI scan showing hyperintensity (asterisk) in the anterior and right lateral oral tongue, indicating extensive tumor infiltration.

tomography (PET) scan has been shown to be of value in oral cavity cancer staging. A prospective study of 134 patients with squamous cell carcinoma of the oral cavity and a clinically negative neck were evaluated preoperatively by PET scanning and CT/MRI scans. PET proved to be twice as sensitive as CT/MRI for detecting occult cervical nodal metastasis [33]. In a study conducted by Kovacs *et al.*, PET scanning in combination with sentinel node biopsy reduced the rate of elective node dissections in the treatment of oral and oropharyngeal cancers [34]. The role of PET in staging oral cavity cancers is the subject of further investigation.

Staging for oral cavity carcinomas from the Eighth Edition (2017) of the American Joint Committee on Cancer (AJCC) staging system is summarized in Table 9.1 [35].

Epidemiology

Currently, approximately 32,670 cases of oral cavity cancer and 6650 deaths resulting from the condition are reported each year in the United States, accounting for 30% of head and neck cancers [36]. Males have a higher incidence than females, with a ratio of 3:2 [37]. There is a strong causal relationship between oral cavity cancers and tobacco and alcohol use [38, 39]. Smoking cessation has been found to decrease the risk of subsequent oral cavity cancers [40]. In the United States, the majority of oral cavity cancers occur in older adults, though recent reports have suggested an increased incidence of oral tongue cancers in young nonsmokers and nondrinkers. The causative factor of this remains unclear [41]. In South Asia, oral cavity cancer is highly prevalent and accounts for 17% of all malignancies in India compared to less than 5% in Western countries [42]. The chewing of betel nut leaves is thought to be a leading cause of oral cavity cancers in South Asian countries [43]. Genetic abnormalities, including Fanconi's anemia and dyskeratosis congenita, are associated with a higher risk of oral cavity cancers. Fanconi's anemia is an autosomal recessive disease caused by mutations in genes involved in DNA damage repair, and is most commonly associated with hematologic abnormalities. Dyskeratosis congenita, or Zinsser–Engman–Cole syndrome, is a rare genetic disorder that results in progressive bone marrow failure and is characterized by the triad of reticulated skin hyperpigmentation, nail dystrophy, and oral leukoplakia.

Despite increasing evidence indicating an etiologic linkage between human papilloma virus (HPV) and oropharyngeal cancers, there are conflicting reports regarding an association between HPV and oral cavity cancers [44]. HPV does not infect all mucosal sites equally, and an overwhelming majority of HPV-associated cancers arise in the oropharynx [45]. HPV status was not predictive of the overall or disease-free

Table 9.1 American Joint Committee on Cancer (AJCC) TNM Staging Classification for the Lip and Oral Cavity (8th edn, 2017).

Primary Tumor (T)

TX	Primary tumor cannot be assessed
Tis	Carcinoma in situ
T1	Tumor ≤2 cm, ≤5 mm depth of invasion (DOI) DOI is depth of invasion and not tumor thickness
T2	Tumor ≤2 cm, DOI >5 mm and ≤10 mm or tumor >2 cm but ≤4 cm and ≤10 mm DOI
T3	Tumor >4 cm or any tumor >10 mm DOI
T4	Moderately advanced or very advance local disease
T4a	Moderately advanced local disease
	(lip) Tumor invades through cortical bone or involves the inferior alveolar nerve, floor of mouth, or skin of face (i.e., chin or nose).
	(oral cavity) Tumor invades adjacent structures only (e.g., through cortical bone of the mandible or maxilla or involves the maxillary sinus or skin of the face). Note: Superficial erosion of bone/tooth socket (alone) by a gingival primary is not sufficient to classify a tumor as T4
T4b	Very advanced local disease
	Tumor invades masticator space, pterygoid plates, or skull base, and/or encases the internal carotid artery

Regional Lymph Nodes
Clinical N (cN)

NX	Regional lymph nodes cannot be assessed
N0	No regional lymph node metastasis
N1	Metastasis in a single ipsilateral lymph node, 3 cm or smaller in greatest dimension ENE (−)
N2	Metastasis in a single ipsilateral lymph node, larger than 3 cm but not larger than 6 cm in greatest dimension and ENE (−); or in multiple ipsilateral lymph nodes, none larger than 6 cm in greatest dimension and ENE (−); or in bilateral or contralateral lymph nodes, none larger than 6 cm in greatest dimension and ENE (−)
N2a	Metastasis in a single ipsilateral lymph node, larger than 3 cm but not larger than 6 cm in greatest dimension and ENE (−)
N2b	Metastasis in multiple ipsilateral lymph nodes, none larger than 6 cm in greatest dimension and ENE (−)
N2c	Metastasis in bilateral or contralateral lymph nodes, none larger than 6 cm in greatest dimension and ENE (−)
N3	Metastasis in a lymph node larger than 6 cm in greatest dimension and ENE (−); or in any node(s) and clinically overt ENE (+)
N3a	Metastasis in a lymph node larger than 6 cm in greatest dimension and ENE (−)
N3b	Metastasis in any node(s) and clinically overt ENE (+)

Pathological N (pN)

NX	Regional lymph nodes cannot be assessed
N0	No regional lymph node metastasis
N1	Metastasis in a single ipsilateral lymph node, 3 cm or smaller in greatest dimension and ENE (−)
N2	Metastasis in a single ipsilateral lymph node, 3 cm or smaller in greatest dimension and ENE (+); or larger than 3 cm but not larger than 6 cm in greatest dimension and ENE (−); or metastases in multiple ipsilateral lymph nodes, none larger than 6 cm in greatest dimension and ENE (−); or in bilateral or contralateral lymph node(s), none larger than 6 cm in greatest dimension, ENE (−)
N2a	Metastasis in a single ipsilateral node, 3 cm or smaller in greatest dimension and ENE (+); or a single ipsilateral node larger than 3 cm but not larger than 6 cm in greatest dimension and ENE (−)
N2b	Metastasis in multiple ipsilateral nodes, none larger than 6 cm in greatest dimension and ENE (−)
N2c	Metastasis in bilateral or contralateral lymph node(s), none larger than 6 cm in greatest dimension and ENE (−)
N3	Metastasis in a lymph node larger than 6 cm in greatest dimension and ENE (−); or metastasis in a single ipsilateral node larger than 3 cm in greatest dimension and ENE (+); or multiple ipsilateral, contralateral, or bilateral nodes, any with ENE (+); or a single contralateral node 3 cm or smaller and ENE (+)
N3a	Metastasis in a lymph node larger than 6 cm in greatest dimension and ENE (−)
N3b	Metastasis in a single ipsilateral node larger than 3 cm in greatest dimension and ENE (+); or multiple ipsilateral, contralateral or bilateral nodes, any with ENE (+); or a single contralateral node 3 cm or smaller and ENE (+)

Distant Metastases (M)

M0	No distant metastasis
M1	Distant metastasis

Table 9.1 (*Continued*)

Stage Grouping			
Stage 0	T1s	N0	M0
Stage I	T1	N0	M0
Stage II	T2	N0	M0
Stage III	T3	N0	M0
	T1, 2, 3	N1	M0
Stage IVA	T4a	N0, N1	M0
	T1, 2, 3, 4a	N2	M0
Stage IVB	Any T	N3	M0
	T4b	Any N	M0
Stage IVC	Any T	Any N	M1

Source: AJCC Cancer Staging Manual, Eighth Edition (2017), Springer, New York, Inc.

survival in patients with non-oropharyngeal cancers in a meta-analysis [46]. To date, ongoing clinical trials studying treatment de-escalation in HPV-associated carcinomas have typically not included patients with primary tumors in the oral cavity.

Selection of Therapy

Oral cancers can be managed with surgery, radiation therapy, or a combination of modalities. Treatment strategies are dictated by the anatomic subsite, tumor stage, histologic type, and patient factors such as medical comorbidities, performance status, and patient preference. Additionally, treatment approaches can vary by institution, and are largely based on the availability of expertise, physician preference, and the patient population of the institution.

For early-stage disease, single-modality treatment involving either radiation therapy alone or surgery is preferred. Resection alone is more often the treatment of choice for properly selected T1 and T2 disease. To address potential spread to the regional lymphatics, selective or comprehensive neck dissection may be required, especially for T2 tumors. Surgery provides pathologic data and avoids the prolonged treatment course required for external beam radiation therapy (EBRT). Resections are often accomplished with preservation of speech and swallowing function, and late salivary and dental effects associated with radiation therapy can be avoided. For patients who cannot undergo surgery or if surgery were to result in an unacceptable functional loss, radiation therapy is an acceptable alternative treatment. T1 and selected cases of T2 oral cavity cancers can be treated with radiation therapy alone, including EBRT, brachytherapy, or both.

Compared to other sites in the head-and-neck region, oral cavity cancers have been found to have increased locoregional recurrence rates following surgery alone [47, 48]. For locally advanced carcinomas (T3 or T4) of the oral cavity, combination therapy with surgery and chemoradiation is recommended. Recently, there has been considerable debate regarding the optimal timing of radiation therapy and chemotherapy with respect to surgery. In the RTOG 73-03 study, patients with operable head-and-neck cancers were randomized to preoperative or postoperative radiation therapy, and improved locoregional control rates with postoperative radiation were reported [49]. In a trial conducted by Licitra *et al.*, 195 patients with advanced oral cavity cancers were randomized to cisplatin and fluorouracil followed by surgery or surgery alone; radiation therapy was reserved for high-risk patients. Preoperative chemotherapy led to fewer mandibular resections and a decreased use of postoperative radiation therapy, but there was no effect on overall survival [50]. Currently, the standard practice for advanced oral cavity cancers is postoperative radiation therapy. Chemotherapy can be added to adjuvant radiation therapy for the presence of extracapsular spread or involved surgical margins. It is strongly recommended that the selection of patients for combined modality therapy be made in a multidisciplinary fashion.

Adjuvant Therapy

The aim of postoperative radiotherapy is to improve locoregional control and possibly improve survival [51]. Indications for postoperative radiation therapy include the presence of one or more of the following pathologic factors: involved, close, or uncertain surgical margins; extracapsular extension; more than one lymph node involved; lymph node size >3 cm; advanced T-staging including soft tissue, muscle, or bone invasion; perineural or lymphovascular invasion; and inadequate lymphadenectomy [48, 52]. The conventional postoperative dose is 60 Gy to the primary site, including the entire surgical bed and involved neck areas. A boost up to 66 Gy should be considered for higher-risk patients with involved or close surgical margins and/or extracapsular nodal extension. The clinically and pathologically uninvolved neck areas receive 54 Gy [47, 53]. Postoperative radiotherapy can be started as soon as wound healing is complete, usually within three to four weeks after surgery. Hinerman *et al.* found that a prolongation of the interval between surgery and radiation therapy beyond 51 days resulted in a trend towards worse locoregional control in high-risk patients with oral cavity cancer [52].

Based largely on two randomized trials showing improved outcomes, patients at high-risk for locoregional recurrence following resection should receive postoperative chemoradiation. The landmark studies RTOG 9501 and EORTC 22931 demonstrated improved locoregional control and disease-free survival rates with concurrent cisplatin (100 mg m^{-2} on days 1, 22, and 43) and postoperative radiation therapy compared to radiation therapy alone [54, 55]. The two trials had differing eligibility criteria, but a comparative analysis by Bernier *et al.* showed that all patients with positive margins and/or extranodal extension derived the greatest benefit from postoperative chemoradiation [56].

Definitive Chemoradiation

Chemotherapy combined with radiotherapy is the preferred treatment for patients with unresectable locally advanced squamous cell carcinoma of the oral cavity. A number of randomized trials [57–59] and several meta-analyses [60, 61] have demonstrated improved outcomes with concurrent chemotherapy as compared to sequential treatment or radiation therapy alone for patients with locally advanced head-and-neck cancers. Although these results have been applied to the management of oral cavity cancers, most trials included very few patients with oral cavity cancers or excluded these patients entirely. Lo *et al.* demonstrated improved survival in patients with oral cavity and oropharynx cancers receiving 5-fluorouracil (5-FU) concurrently with radiotherapy as compared to patients receiving radiotherapy alone [62]. In an Intergroup Phase III study, chemoradiation + cisplatin was compared to radiation therapy alone in patients with unresectable locally advanced head-and-neck cancer, including 13% of those with oral cavity cancer [63]. The authors found an improved overall survival and disease-free survival with the addition of chemotherapy. Although no prospective studies have been conducted specifically investigating surgery versus chemoradiation for oral cavity cancer, the latter has been extensively been studied at the University of Chicago. In their 20-year experience of 140 patients with advanced oral cavity cancer treated with organ-preserving definitive chemoradiation, the 5-year overall and progression-free survival were 63.2% and 58.7%, respectively. The incidence of osteoradionecrosis was 19%, though satisfactory function was achieved in the majority [64].

Radiotherapeutic Management

Conventional EBRT

In the definitive and adjuvant treatment settings, EBRT techniques for oral cavity cancers traditionally have involved two-dimensional (2D) or three-dimensional (3D) planning. Patients are simulated with the head immobilized in the neutral position with a custom thermoplastic face mask. A bite block is often used to displace the tongue from the palate. Radiopaque wires are used to delineate palpable lymph nodes, commissures of the lips, and any scars in postoperative patients. When higher-energy beams (>4 MV) are utilized, bolus material may be necessary for adequate coverage of surgical scars or superficial lymph nodes. For patients with short necks, the shoulders can be lowered by pulling on a tensioning device looped under the feet. The oral cavity primary and first echelon upper-neck nodes have been traditionally treated with opposed lateral photon fields (Figure 9.9). The lateral portals typically include a 2.0 cm margin on the primary or the entire postoperative bed. The posterior cervical chain is only electively irradiated for cervical node involvement. An off-cord field reduction occurs at approximately 45 Gy. For node-positive or

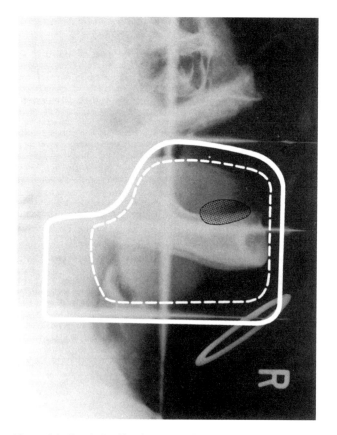

Figure 9.9 Simulation film depicting a lateral port for postoperative radiotherapy for an anterior floor of mouth cancer.

higher-risk disease, the unilateral or bilateral lower neck is treated by a half-beam blocked anterior or anterior–posterior field with a larynx block. For selected lateral tumors, a wedged-pair or mixed photon-electron technique can be used. The total dose depends on the extent of the disease and whether EBRT is used alone or in combination with brachytherapy or surgery. When definitive EBRT alone is used, the total dose is usually in the range of 70–74 Gy. In the postoperative setting, dissected areas receive 60 Gy and dissected areas with involved margins receive 66 Gy. Undissected areas at low risk for tumor involvement receive 50 Gy.

Intensity-Modulated Radiation Therapy

Intensity-modulated radiation therapy (IMRT) is an increasingly accepted treatment option for cancers of the oral cavity. IMRT can reduce the dose to normal tissues, and has been shown to improve post-treatment salivary gland function [65, 66] and quality of life [67, 68] in the treatment of head-and-neck cancers as compared to conventional techniques. Patients are simulated as described above with a mask and a bite block when appropriate. The low neck nodes can be treated either with IMRT or alternatively with anterior or anterior-posterior field(s) that is beam split to the IMRT fields; these are known as an extended-whole field (EWF) IMRT technique and a split-field (SF) IMRT technique, respectively [69–71]. If the SF technique is considered, the match typically occurs at just above the arytenoids as the larynx can be spared and shielded under the midline block in the low anterior neck field(s). If an EWF technique is utilized, the IMRT treatment volumes should be delineated to encompass the bilateral lower neck. When lymph nodes extend to the low neck, an EWF IMRT technique is preferred.

IMRT requires accurate target delineation due to its high conformality and the possibility of a marginal recurrence. Target delineation is especially challenging in the postoperative setting after distortion of the normal anatomy. Target volumes should be based on preoperative diagnostic imaging studies, surgical, and pathologic findings as well as the postoperative CT scan. For patients treated in the postoperative setting, a *high-risk* and *low-risk* clinical target volume (CTV) should be defined to encompass regions of potential microscopic disease. The *high-risk* CTV includes the preoperative gross disease; the entire postoperative bed at the primary site including the surgical scar and, in the case of extranodal extension, the sternocleidomastoid muscle. Nodal regions with pathologic involvement; and adjacent nodal regions at high risk for subclinical disease. The *low-risk* CTV should include the contralateral uninvolved neck. In patients with gross residual disease, a gross tumor volume (GTV) is also defined. A *gross disease* CTV is defined as the GTV with a 0.5 cm margin. A planned target volume (PTV) is generated for each CTV with a margin of 0.3–0.5 cm. Normal structures, including the spinal cord, brainstem, optic apparatus, mandible, cochlea, parotid glands, and larynx, should be delineated.

Several institutions have reported their experience with IMRT for oral cavity cancers [72–75], and some variability is apparent in target delineation and dose fractionation between institutions. At Memorial-Sloan Kettering, the *high-risk* PTV receives 60 Gy in 2-Gy fractions for negative surgical margins and absence of extracapsular extension. In the case of microscopically positive margins or extracapsular extension, these regions within the *high-risk* PTV receive 66 Gy in 2- to 2.2-Gy fractions. The low-risk PTV receives 54 Gy in 1.8-Gy fractions. If a separate anterior low neck field is used, it receives 50–50.4 Gy in 1.8- to 2-Gy fractions (Table 9.2; Figures 9.10

Table 9.2 Guidelines for target delineation for postoperative intensity-modulated radiation therapy (IMRT) for oral cavity malignancies.

Tumor site	Stage	High-risk PTV, 60 Gy at 2-Gy fractions*	Low-risk PTV, 54 Gy at 1.8-Gy fractions
Oral tongue; floor of mouth	T1-T4N0	Tumor bed and levels I-IV at physician's discretion**,***	Levels I-IV at physician's discretion**,***
Oral tongue; floor of mouth	T1-T4N1-3	Tumor bed and ipsilateral levels I–V or bilateral levels I–V if contralateral nodes involved	Contralateral levels I–IV if uninvolved***
Buccal mucosa; retromolar trigone; hard palate; gingiva	T1-T4N0	Tumor bed and levels I–IV at physician's discretion**,***	Levels I–IV at physician's discretion**,***
Buccal mucosa; retromolar trigone; hard palate; gingiva	T1-T4N1-3	Tumor bed and ipsilateral levels I–V or bilateral levels I–V if contralateral nodes involved	Contralateral levels I–IV if uninvolved***

*66 Gy for microscopically positive margins or extracapsular extension; 70 Gy if gross residual disease.
**Decision to include in low- or high-risk region based on tumor features and physician's discretion.
***Nodal level V can be treated at the physician's discretion.
PTV, Planned target volume.

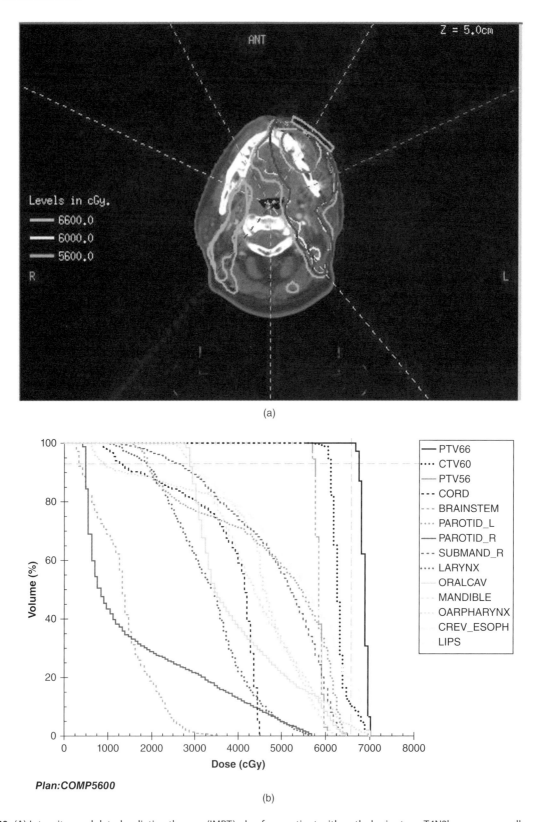

Figure 9.10 (A) Intensity-modulated radiation therapy (IMRT) plan for a patient with pathologic stage T4N2b squamous cell carcinoma of the gingiva shown in the axial plane. (B) Dose–volume histogram for the relevant structures. Note that the bolus is placed over the surgical scar. For a color version of this figure, see the color plate section.

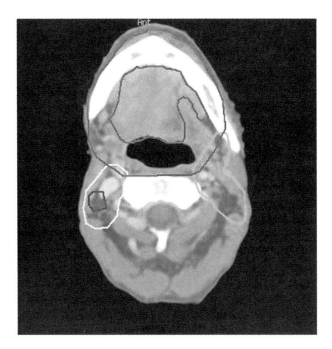

Figure 9.11 Contours for a patient with unresectable T3N2b squamous cell carcinoma of the oral tongue treated with intensity-modulated radiation therapy (IMRT). The dose levels are as follows: red (inner line), gross tumor volume (GTV); red (outer line), planning target volume (PTV) 70 Gy; blue, PTV 70 Gy; yellow, PTV 59.4 Gy; green, PTV 54 Gy. Note the coverage of the base of tongue due to the risk of subclinical spread. For a color version of this figure, see the color plate section.

and 9.11). In the case of gross residual disease, the gross disease PTV is treated to a definitive dose of 70 Gy.

Intraoral Cone Radiotherapy

Intraoral cone radiotherapy using 100–250 kVP x-rays or 6 MeV electron beams is an acceptable treatment for properly selected small lesions of the floor of the mouth or oral tongue. Phillips *et al.* reported good control rates with an acceptable risk of tissue necrosis using 55 Gy in 18 days and 60 Gy in 26 days [53]. Peroral radiotherapy can also be used in combination with EBRT to deliver a boost dose to lesions that are marginally encompassed by an intraoral cone. The boost should be given before the external beam treatment, and is usually 21–27 Gy in 3-Gy fractions. The advantages of peroral radiotherapy over interstitial radiotherapy or EBRT include: a limited irradiated volume, thus allowing for salivary gland function preservation; no hospitalization or anesthetics are necessary; and minimal risk of bone necrosis. This technique requires proper patient immobilization and cooperation to obtain adequate coverage of the lesion. Peroral radiotherapy is no longer commonly available.

Brachytherapy

Considerable experience has been acquired treating oral cavity cancers with brachytherapy, either alone or in combination with EBRT for the treatment of oral cavity carcinomas [76, 77]. The advantages of brachytherapy for oral cavity tumors include the accessibility of the tumor sites; the ability to deliver high doses while sparing surrounding normal tissues; and the short treatment duration compared to external beam irradiation. Low-dose rate (LDR) treatments using 0.3–0.6 Gy per hour have been routinely employed for oral cavity cancers, but recently there has been increased interest in high-dose rate and pulsed-dose rate brachytherapy [78]. When interstitial LDR brachytherapy is used alone for well-defined, early-stage T1 to T2N0 tumors, the usual implant dose is 60–70 Gy delivered over a period of six to seven days. LDR brachytherapy with doses of 25–30 Gy have been successfully employed in combination with EBRT in the definitive and adjuvant settings [79].

The brachytherapy technique should be based on a classic system, such as the Patterson–Parker or Quimby, or new methods using computer-based systems [80, 81]. Catheters are generally placed parallel and equidistant, with an intersource space of 1–1.5 cm, using ultrasound or fluroscopic guidance. When the tumor thickness is 1 cm or less, a single-plane implant is often adequate. When the tumor thickness is greater than 1 cm, then a double-plane implant or volume implant is necessary to deliver a uniform dose to the tumor volume. Iridium-192 is commonly used for temporary implants in the form of pins (epingles), wires, or seeds preloaded in a plastic ribbon, but iodine-125 is the isotope of choice for permanent implants. The use of high-dose rate (HDR) remote afterloading using iridium sources has recently increased. HDR techniques minimize exposure to personnel and allow the optimization of dose distribution using computer planning [82]. With improvements in surgical techniques and increasingly conformal radiation planning, however, the use of brachytherapy has diminished.

Site-Specific Treatment Recommendations and Results of Treatment

Squamous cell carcinoma of the oral cavity is a challenging subset of head and neck cancers. The five-year locoregional control and disease-specific survival rates range from 50% to 80% [52, 83, 84]. Oral cavity cancers have a high propensity to spread to cervical lymph nodes, occurring in approximately 35% of patients. Nodal metastases are also an important prognostic factor. Leyland *et al.* reported the five-year disease-specific survival rates for patients with node-negative disease as 59% versus 39%

Table 9.3 Outcomes from selected series using intensity-modulated radiation therapy (IMRT) for oral cavity cancers.

Study/Reference	Treatment	No. of patients	3-year locoregional control, %	3-year overall survival, %
Yao *et al.* (2007) [73]	Postoperative;	49	82	68
	Definitive	5		
Chen *et al.* (2009) [158]	Postoperative	22	64*	67
Gomez *et al.* (2009) [72]	Postoperative	35	77	74
Daly *et al.* (2011) [75]	Postoperative;	30	53	59
	Definitive	7	60	38

*Crude

for patients with lymph node involvement in a series of 891 patients with oral cavity cancer [85]. A number of institutions have recently reported encouraging outcomes with definitive and postoperative IMRT for oral cavity cancers (Table 9.3).

Lip

Carcinoma of the lip can be managed successfully with either radiotherapy or surgery [86]. The preferred treatment depends on the extent of disease, the functional and cosmetic results of the treatment, expediency, the patient's age, and the availability of treatment personnel and facilities [87]. Surgery is usually recommended for small lesions (<2 cm) of the lower lip, young patients, bone invasion, cervical lymph node metastases, and recurrence after radiotherapy. Radiotherapy is usually indicated for larger tumors without bone involvement, or for oral commissure involvement that would otherwise result in an unacceptable cosmetic or functional outcome following resection [86, 88]. Radiotherapy is also administered postoperatively for inadequate surgical margins, lymph node metastasis, and locally advanced disease. Prophylactic neck irradiation or neck dissection is generally indicated for T3 or T4 disease, but not for T1 or T2, clinically N0 disease [6]. Factors associated with increased risk for nodal metastasis include poorly differentiated tumors, recurrent disease, and commissure involvement [6, 7].

External beam radiotherapy for lip cancer can be delivered with orthovoltage x-rays or electrons [89]. The treatment volume should include the primary lesion with a margin of 1.0–1.5 cm for orthovoltage and 2.0–2.5 cm for electrons. A lead shield can be inserted between the inner surface of the lip and the gingiva to prevent irradiation of the intraoral structures. The electron energy should be chosen based on the thickness of the lesion. When treating the neck, parallel-opposed fields should include the primary and nodal levels 1 and 2, matched with a low anterior neck field when appropriate. For advanced upper-lip lesions, appositional electron fields (known as

'mustache fields') can be used to treat the facial lymphatics [90]. If perineural invasion is present, the field should extend to the base of skull along the course of the involved cranial nerve. The recommended dose for external beam alone for small lesions (<2 cm) is 45–50 Gy in three weeks. For larger lesions, a more protracted treatment course of 60–70 Gy in four to seven weeks is suggested. Brachytherapy with or without EBRT generally involves interstitial implants with afterloading iridium-192 [77]. When brachytherapy alone is used for T1 or T2 lesions, the dose is 60–65 Gy over five to seven days with LDR. A brachytherapy boost can be used after 40–50 Gy of external beam irradiation.

Squamous cell carcinoma of the lip can be controlled with either radiation therapy or surgery in the majority of patients. Control of the primary lesion can be achieved with external beam irradiation or interstitial implants in >90% of patients with T1 disease, and in >75% for T2 or T3 disease [88, 91–93]. The results of treatment are summarized in Table 9.4.

Oral Tongue

Surgery is the preferred treatment modality for medically operable patients with carcinoma of the oral tongue. With the excellent functional outcome of the reconstructed oral tongue after hemiglossectomy for early or moderately advanced lesions, definitive radiotherapy is reserved for patients who are medically inoperable or refuse surgery. Definitive radiotherapy for early tongue cancers can be given with an interstitial implant alone or external beam irradiation combined with an interstitial implant boost or an intraoral cone boost [94–96]. More advanced and locally infiltrative lesions are difficult to manage with radiation therapy alone, and may require total glossectomy with or without laryngectomy. For patients who are not candidates for surgery or brachytherapy, definitive external beam irradiation with concurrent chemotherapy can be attempted. Postoperative radiation therapy is indicated for T3 or T4 disease, multiple cervical lymph node metastases,

Table 9.4 Results of selected trials of radiation therapy for treatment of carcinoma of the lip.

Study (Year, Follow-up)	No. of Patients	Treatment modality	Stage	Local control, %
Jorgensen *et al.* (1973, 5 year) [159]	869	LDR interstitial brachytherapy	T1	93
			T2	87
			T3	74
De Visscher *et al.* (1996, 10 year) [88]	106	LDR interstitial brachytherapy or EBRT	T1	99*
			T2	77*
Guinot *et al.* (2003, 3 year) [160]	39	HDR interstitial brachytherapy +/- EBRT	T1-T2	95
			T4	74
Guibert *et al.* (2010, 8 year) [161]	92	LDR interstitial brachytherapy	T1-2	75

*Crude rate
EBRT, external beam radiation therapy; HDR, high dose rate; LDR, low dose rate.

close or positive margins, extracapsular extension, and lymphovascular or perineural invasion. Postoperative chemoradiation has been shown to be superior to radiation alone for patients with positive margins or extranodal extension and is now considered standard of care [54–56].

Brachytherapy may be used as part of the definitive treatment of oral tongue carcinomas [97]. Well-differentiated T1 oral tongue carcinomas with a depth of invasion of 4 mm or less can be controlled with an interstitial implant or peroral radiotherapy alone [98]. A combination of external beam irradiation or neck dissection with brachytherapy should be employed for other lesions. Lesions >1 cm in thickness require a double-plane or volume implants, while a single-plane interstitial implant can be used for more limited lesions. LDR brachytherapy dose rates of 30 to 50 cGy h^{-1} (to a dose of 65–70 Gy) have been reported to maximize local control and minimize necrosis [99]. Dose reduction for short overall treatment time may lead to an increased local recurrence rate [100, 101]. Fractionated HDR interstitial brachytherapy is an alternate treatment approach. A phase III trial of high- and low-dose interstitial radiotherapy for early oral tongue cancer showed that HDR has similar rates of local control and the added advantage of eliminating exposure to the medical staff [82, 102]. When brachytherapy alone is used, the suggested dose is 60–70 Gy over five to seven days. For larger T2 lesions, a total dose of 75–80 Gy is delivered by using both interstitial implant and EBRT, with 30–40 Gy being a typical dose delivered by external beam irradiation. The treatment volume for the boost is determined by the tumor volume prior to the initiation of external beam irradiation.

Due to the high risk of nodal metastasis from tongue carcinomas, the neck should be managed by neck dissection or radiation therapy, except for well-differentiated, T1 tumors with a minimal depth of invasion [10, 14, 103]. In the clinically node-negative neck, treatment volumes typically include the submental, submandibular, subdigastric, and mid- and low-neck nodes (levels I–IV). In patients with unilateral lymph node metastasis, the rate of contralateral occult node metastases has been found to be 35–55% [104–106]; therefore bilateral neck irradiation should be employed.

Long-term survival in carcinoma of the oral tongue is directly related to the stage of disease. Using multiple treatment modalities, Gujrathi *et al.* reported five-year overall survival rates for stages I, II, III, and IV of 64%, 46%, 42%, and 16%, respectively [107]. Shibuya *et al.* reported five-year primary tumor control rates for stages T1 and T2 treated with brachytherapy alone or in combination with external beam irradiation of 85% for superficial lesions, 70% for exophytic lesions, and 45% for infiltrative lesions. The five-year overall survivals for stages T1, T2a, and T2b were 84%, 78%, and 72%, respectively [108]. Nodal metastases in oral tongue cancers have also been shown to significantly decrease overall survival [109]. In a series of 280 patients, the five-year overall survival for patients with N0 disease was 50% compared to 11% for patients with involved necks [110].

The comparison of outcomes by treatment modality is limited by the retrospective nature of the published literature, variations in patient populations and treatment methods, and institutional biases. Several reports have failed to show any significant difference in survival when comparing modalities for the treatment of oral cavity cancers [107, 111, 112]. When adjusting for stage, Sessions *et al.* found no difference in overall survival when comparing local resection alone, composite resection, radiation therapy alone, local resection with radiation therapy, and composite resection with radiation therapy [109]. Fein *et al.* demonstrated similar control rates in T1 and T2 lesions for radiation therapy alone versus surgery alone or combined with radiation [112]. In contrast, a retrospective study from Japan demonstrated inferior outcomes with brachytherapy as compared to surgery in

Table 9.5 Outcomes from selected series for treatment for squamous cell carcinoma of the oral tongue

Study (Year)	Patient, n	Treatment modality	Stage	Local control, %
Wendt *et al.* (1990) [115]	103	EBRT and/or IB	T1N0	81
			T2N0	67
Mazeron *et al.* (1991) [99]	153	IB only	T1N0	87
			T2N0	92
Wang *et al.* (1995) [162]	112	EBRT and IOC	T1N0	93*
			T2N0	80*
Sessions *et al.* (2002) [109]	279	S, RT, or S and RT	T1-4N1-3	66
Fan *et al.* (2007) [163]	201	S then EBRT	T1-4N1-3	72

*5 year actuarial
EBRT = external beam radiation therapy; IB = interstitial brachytherapy; IOC = intraoral cone; S = surgery; RT = radiation therapy

stage I–II tumors, with five-year overall survival rates for the LDR, HDR, and surgery groups of 84.0%, 72.9%, and 95.4%, respectively [113]. Another study by Aksu *et al.* compared definitive radiation with surgery and postoperative radiation in 80 patients with stage I–IVA disease [114]. Patients who received surgery and postoperative radiation therapy had a five-year overall survival advantage versus those treated with definitive radiation alone (49% versus 16%, respectively). The optimal treatment approach for oral tongue cancers should be determined by individual institutions in a multidisciplinary setting. The local control rates from selected series are summarized in Table 9.5.

Brachytherapy is often combined with external beam irradiation for the definitive treatment of oral tongue cancers. Fein *et al.* reported a local control rate of 83% with an interstitial boost following external beam irradiation [112]. In a series from M. D. Anderson, external beam irradiation or interstitial implant alone resulted in inferior control rates for T1 or T2 disease. A high dose of interstitial therapy was found to be necessary to secure optimum local control, and >40 Gy of external beam irradiation was important for control in the neck [115]. Since definitive radiation therapy generally requires interstitial brachytherapy, a small area of the mandible usually receives a dose in excess of 75 Gy, which may lead to late mandibular complications. The incidence of osteonecrosis was 19% in the series reported by Delclos and coworkers, with 6% of patients requiring surgical management [116]. Another series reported a 38% complication rate, such as erosive ulcerations and bone exposure in patients who received brachytherapy for stage I and II disease [108]. The risks of treatment-related complications following definitive radiation therapy for oral cavity cancers have led many to advocate for primary surgical resection when feasible.

Recurrence after radiotherapy is difficult to salvage by surgery, with reported five-year survival rates of 39% for local recurrence, and 27% for locoregional recurrence [117]. Local recurrence after treatment with glossectomy alone has a similarly poor outcome, with long-term survival in less than 10% of cases [118]. Metastatic cervical lymph node metastases that develop after the primary lesion has been controlled can be successfully salvaged, though poor median overall survival of 18 months after recurrence has been reported [119].

Floor of Mouth

Radiotherapy or surgery are treatment options for early-stage floor of mouth cancers. Given the risk of osteoradionecrosis of the mandible or soft-tissue necrosis with brachytherapy, surgical resection is the preferred approach for small lesions in patients who are medically operable. Advanced-stage cancers are generally treated with surgery followed by postoperative radiotherapy, especially when there is invasion of the mandible, with large or multiple cervical lymph node metastases, or extensive involvement of the musculature of the tongue. A combination of chemotherapy and radiotherapy should be used for unresectable disease or medically inoperable patients.

Radiotherapy modalities for carcinoma of the floor of the mouth include external beam irradiation, peroral cone irradiation, and interstitial implants. Interstitial implants alone or peroral cone irradiation may be used for superficial or exophytic T1 lesions after excisional biopsy or in combination with external beam irradiation for more advanced disease biopsy [120]. LDR interstitial radiotherapy techniques are similar for oral tongue carcinoma and floor of mouth carcinoma. As with brachytherapy for other head and neck sites, HDR can be employed with the elimination of radiation exposure for the medical staff [121]. In the definitive treatment setting, external beam irradiation is delivered to 50–54 Gy with a boost to the primary lesion with 10–20 Gy using interstitial implant, peroral cone irradiation, or external beam irradiation. If IMRT is used as definitive treatment alone,

Table 9.6 Outcomes from selected series for treatment of squamous cell carcinomas of the floor of mouth

Study (year)	Patients (n)	Local control rate, %	Regional control rate, %	5 yr Disease free survival
Araki *et al.* (1990) [164]	76	84	82	
Hicks *et al.* (1997) [125]	99	80	74	76
Sessions *et al.* (2000) [122]	280	59	82	56

the entire region can be treated using a dose-painting technique, delivering 70 Gy to the primary tumor and involved lymph nodes, 59.4–63 Gy in 1.8-Gy fractions or 60 Gy in two Gy fractions to the uninvolved but high-risk regions, and 54 Gy in 1.8-Gy fractions to the low-risk regions. For postoperative treatment, the high-risk areas receive 60–66 Gy, and the low risk areas receive 50–54 Gy. The clinically negative neck should be managed with radiation therapy or surgery, except in selected T1N0 cases. Similar to carcinoma of the oral tongue, the floor of mouth is not a well-lateralized structure and thus the bilateral neck is treated.

A summary of outcomes from selected series for treatment of floor of mouth carcinomas is shown in Table 9.6. The five-year disease-specific survival for carcinoma of the floor of mouth ranges from 56% to 76% [122–125]. Survival has been shown to relate to T-stage [122, 126, 127], N-stage [122, 127], and margin status [128]. In a study conducted by Sessions *et al.* of 280 patients treated with surgery or radiation, recurrence at the primary site was the most common site of failure (primary only, 41% and all primary failures, 50%), and was more than twice as common as failures in the neck [122]. Distant metastasis occurred in 30%, while 20% of patients developed second primaries. In a series of 160 patients from France, brachytherapy alone had local control rates of 89% for T1 and T2 lesions, with a five-year survival of 76% [129]. Actuarial survival of these patients was poor, owing to a significant number of deaths from second primary cancer or intercurrent disease. Following radiation therapy, bone and soft-tissue necrosis occurs in 10–21% of patients, usually within two years after treatment with definitive radiation therapy [116, 129, 130]. Most cases of necrosis heal with conservative management, although some patients may require hemimandibulectomy.

Buccal Mucosa

Surgery is often the preferred treatment for carcinomas of the buccal mucosa. Radiotherapy alone can be considered in small (T1) lesions involving the commissure or in the mid-cheek without involvement of the gingiva. The extent of surgery is dependent on the degree of locoregional involvement. A marginal or segmental mandibulectomy, or a partial maxillectomy, should be performed when bone involvement is suspected. For

patients with clinical lymph node involvement a selective, modified radical, or radical neck dissection is recommended based on the extent of disease, while a supraomohyoid neck dissection (level I–III) can be considered in the node-negative neck [131]. Adjuvant radiation therapy is indicated for high risk disease including advanced stages or adverse pathologic features. Studies have also reported high local recurrence rates for T1,2N0 disease [132–134], and for a tumor thickness >6 mm [135]. Therefore, postoperative radiotherapy may be considered for early-stage buccal carcinoma as well. As in other sites of the oral cavity, adjuvant treatment with chemotherapy and radiation is recommended for patients with positive margins or extranodal extension. Either 3D conformal therapy or IMRT should be utilized to spare the contralateral parotid gland. The target volume should include the surgical bed and the entire buccal mucosa. For well-lateralized lesions, treatment of the ipsilateral neck alone is indicated for N0 disease. For node-positive disease, consideration should be given for treatment of the contralateral neck. Postoperative dosing regimens for buccal mucosa cancer are similar to other regions of the oral cavity. Interstitial implants with iridium wires or seeds in nylon ribbons can be used for the treatment of early, small lesions that do not involve the buccogingival sulcus, the gingiva, or bone. Usually, a minimum tumor dose of 60–70 Gy in five to eight days is delivered through a single-plane or double-plane implant, depending on the thickness of the lesion.

The primary site of relapse following treatment for squamous cell carcinoma of the buccal mucosa is local. The local failure rates ranged from 37% to 80% in retrospective series [132, 136, 137]. A prospective, randomized trial from India examined the role of postoperative radiotherapy in stage III and IV carcinoma of the buccal mucosa. The three-year actuarial disease-free survival with and without postoperative radiotherapy was 68% versus 38%, respectively [138]. Surgery can be used to salvage patients who fail radical radiotherapy. One series reported an overall five-year disease-free survival of 60% after salvage surgery [139]. A summary of selected trials for treatment of squamous cell carcinoma of the buccal mucosa is provided in Table 9.7.

Multiple studies have demonstrated the superiority of multimodality treatment versus that of surgery or radiation alone. A study by Lin *et al.* examined 121

Table 9.7 Outcomes from selected series for treatment of squamous cell carcinomas of the buccal mucosa

Study (year, follow up)	Patients, n	Stage III/IV, %	Local control, %	Locoregional control, %	Disease- specific survival, %
Pop *et al.* (1988, 5 year) [136]	49	63		45	52**
Fang *et al.* (1997, 3 year) [140]	57	89		64	62
Sieczka *et al.* (2001, 5 year) [134]	27	42	56*		73
Iyer *et al.* (2004, 3 year) [165]	147	8	88*	74*	77
Lin *et al.* (2006, 5 year) [133]	121	64		36	37

*crude
**overall survival

patients treated with either surgery alone, radiotherapy alone, or surgery plus postoperative radiation. The rate of local recurrence in patients with T1–T2N0 disease who received surgery alone was 40%. For locally advanced disease, locoregional control and overall survival were improved in patients receiving combined modality treatment [133]. Another study of combined modality therapy found the three-year locoregional control rate to be 64%. Positive surgical margins and skin infiltration were found to be negative prognostic factors [140].

Hard Palate and Gingiva

Surgery is the treatment of choice for most carcinomas of the gingiva and hard palate. Small, superficial squamous cell carcinomas can be managed with primary radiotherapy using a surface mold. Postoperative radiotherapy is indicated in high-risk patients with close/positive margins, perineural invasion, lymphovascular invasion, stage T3/T4, or node-positive disease. In the postoperative setting, doses of 60–66 Gy using 1.8–2 Gy per fraction are administered, with a dose of 66 Gy being reserved for patients with positive margins or extracapsular extension. The postoperative doses utilized are the same as outlined above for the oral tongue and floor of mouth, and IMRT can be utilized when available. When a lower anterior neck field is utilized, the dose 50–50.4 Gy. The location of the primary tumor often necessitates treatment of the bilateral neck; however, in well-lateralized alveolar ridge lesions, unilateral neck irradiation can be employed.

Squamous cell carcinoma of the hard palate is relatively rare. Evans and Shah from Memorial Sloan-Kettering Cancer Center reported their 15-year experience and demonstrated five-year disease-free survival rates for stages I, II, III, and IV disease of 75%, 46%, 40%, and 8%, respectively [141]. In a series from the University of Virginia, which included patients with squamous cell carcinoma of the hard palate, the five-year cause-specific survival was 59%. Yorozu *et al.* reported a five-year survival rate of 48% and a crude local control rate of 32% for 19 patients with squamous cell carcinoma of the hard palate treated with radiotherapy [142]. The risk of

a metachronous primary carcinoma after treatment for carcinomas of the hard palate is 28% [143, 144].

Soo *et al.* reported the outcomes of 61 patients with squamous cell carcinoma of the upper gingiva treated primarily with surgery. The five-year survival rate was 51% (31/61), and the clinical stage was the only factor associated with survival [145]. In a series from India of tumors of the superior gingival-buccal complex, 110 patients were treated with either surgery alone, radiation alone, or a combined modality approach. The five-year progression-free survival was 49% for patients treated with surgery, and 0% for patients treated with a nonsurgical approach [146].

Retromolar Trigone

T1 and early T2 carcinomas of the retromolar trigone can be managed with external beam irradiation or surgery. If there is involvement of the anterior tonsillar pillar, soft palate, or buccal mucosa and an extensive surgical resection is required, then radiation therapy is the preferred treatment. Surgical resection is necessary when there is clinical or radiographic evidence of bone invasion. When medullary bone invasion is found intraoperatively, a segmental mandibulectomy is required. Postoperative radiation is indicated for typical risk features including locally advanced tumors, close/positive margins, or multiple positive nodes. As detailed previously for other oral cavity sites, postoperative chemoradiation is used for the presence of extracapsular extension or positive margins.

For definitive treatment with external beam irradiation, a single mixed photon and electron beam lateral field or parallel opposing fields can be used. For conventional techniques, the dose is 66–74 Gy in 2-Gy fractions. IMRT can alternatively be used with a dose of 70 Gy for gross disease, 59.4–63 Gy for high-risk disease, and 54 Gy for low-risk disease. Prophylactic treatment of the ipsilateral neck is required as retromolar trigone lesions have a high propensity for occult spread to the neck. Treatment of the contralateral neck is at the physician's disrection but should be considered in node-positive cases.

Table 9.8 Outcomes from selected trials for treatment of squamous cell carcinomas of the retromolar trigone

Study (year)	Patients, n	Modality	Crude local control, %	5-year overall survival
Lo *et al.* (1987) [147]	159	RT	71	83
Huang *et al.* (2001) [150]	65	RT and S or RT	85	
Mendenhall *et al.* (2005) [149]	99	RT and S or RT	63	50
Bayman *et al.* (2010) [166]	43	RT	47*	31

*5-year actuarial rate

The results for treatment of carcinoma of the retromolar trigone from selected series are shown in Table 9.8. Some reports combine tumors of the retromolar trigone and anterior tonsillar pillar together. Lo *et al.* reported no difference in local control rates between the two sites in 137 patients treated with radiation therapy [147]. However, most of the published literature separates primary tumors of the retromolar trigone and anterior tonsillar pillar. Tumors of the retromolar trigone have a unique pattern of spread and are more susceptible to bone invasion [148]. Byers *et al.* reported the results of 110 patients with carcinoma of the retromolar trigone treated with surgery, radiation therapy, or combined modality treatment [30]. The five-year overall survival rate was only 20%, and the crude local or regional failure rates with radiation alone and combined modality treatment were 16% and 18%, respectively. In contrast, other studies have shown that combined surgery and radiation – particularly with advanced tumors – yields superior results over radiotherapy alone [149, 150]. Mendenhall *et al.* compared 36 patients treated with definitive radiation with 64 patients treated with surgery and radiation. On multivariate analysis, combined modality treatment was associated with improved local control, local-regional control, distant metastasis-free survival, cause-specific survival, and overall survival [149].

Complications of Treatment

Common acute effects of treatment for oral cavity cancers include mucositis, xerostomia, and alterations in taste. Patchy (grade 2) or confluent (grade 3) mucositis is expected during treatment, but simple erythema (grade 1) usually indicates that the treatment is too pro-tracted, allowing for tumor proliferation. Xerostomia typically occurs one week after initiation of treatment, and recovery occurs within one year if the damage to the salivary glands is not severe [151]. Salivary gland function decreases gradually between 20–40 Gy with a dramatic worsening with doses greater than 40 Gy [151,152]. Sparing of the parotid glands with IMRT reduces the incidence of xerostomia and leads to recovery of salivary function and improvements in post-treatment quality of life [153]. Other late effects after radiation therapy include osteoradionecrosis, most commonly involving the mandible [154,155]. Soft-tissue necrosis may be seen after both brachytherapy and peroral cone treatment. After recurrent tumor is ruled out, conservative management with saline irrigation, broad-spectrum antibiotics, and analgesics is usually indicated. For refractory or large necroses associated with bone necrosis, surgery may be required.

Early reports indicate that IMRT reduces toxicity associated with the treatment of oral cavity cancers. The University of Michigan reported no cases of osteoradionecrosis in 176 patients treated with IMRT for head and neck cancer [156]. The average mandibular volume receiving ≥70 Gy was 6.5%, and the average dose gradient in the axial plane was 11 Gy. The authors also attributed the lack of osteoradionecrosis to the strict use of prophylactic dental care. In a study from Memorial Sloan-Kettering Cancer Center [157] of 35 patients receiving postoperative IMRT for oral cavity cancer, the rate of chronic trismus was 17% and the rate of osteoradionecrosis was 6%. Daly *et al.* reported a grade ≥2 late complication rate of 13% after postoperative IMRT for oral cavity squamous cell carcinoma [75]. The toxicity profile of IMRT for the postoperative treatment of oral cavity cancers is favorable and further study is warranted.

References

1 Moore, S., Johnson, N., Pierce, A., Wilson, D., *et al.* (1999) The epidemiology of lip cancer: a review of global incidence and aetiology. *Oral Dis.*, 5 (3), 185–195.

2 Yako-Suketomo, H., Marugame, T. (2008) Comparison of time trends in lip cancer incidence (1973-97) in East Asia, Europe and USA, from Cancer Incidence in Five Continents, Vols IV–VIII. *Jpn. J. Clin. Oncol.*, **38** (6), 456–457.

3 Pogoda, J.M., Preston-Martin, S. (1996) Solar radiation, lip protection, and lip cancer risk in Los

Angeles County women (California, United States). *Cancer Causes Control*, **7** (4), 458–463.

4 Zitsch, R.P., 3rd, Lee, B.W., Smith, R.B. (1999) Cervical lymph node metastases and squamous cell carcinoma of the lip. *Head Neck*, **21** (5), 447–453.

5 Cross, J.E., Guralnick, E., Daland, E.M. (1948) Carcinoma of the lip: A review of 563 case records of carcinoma of the lip at Pondville Hospital. *Surg. Gynecol. Obstet.*, **81**, 153.

6 Wurman, L.H., Adams, G.L., Meyerhoff, W.L. (1975) Carcinoma of the lip. *Am. J. Surg.*, **130** (4), 470–474.

7 Vartanian, J.G., Carvalho, A.L., de Araújo Filho, M.J., Junior, M.H., *et al.* (2004) Predictive factors and distribution of lymph node metastasis in lip cancer patients and their implications on the treatment of the neck. *Oral Oncol.*, **40** (2), 223–227.

8 Byers, R.M., O'Brien, J., Waxler, J. (1978) The therapeutic and prognostic implications of nerve invasion in cancer of the lower lip. *Int. J. Radiat. Oncol. Biol. Phys.*, **4** (3-4), 215–217.

9 Byers, R.M., Wolf, P.F., Ballantyne, A.J. (1988) Rationale for elective modified neck dissection. *Head Neck Surg.*, **10** (3), 160–167.

10 Matsuura, K., Hirokawa, Y., Fujita, M., Akagi, Y., *et al.* (1998) Treatment results of stage I and II oral tongue cancer with interstitial brachytherapy: maximum tumor thickness is prognostic of nodal metastasis. *Int. J. Radiat. Oncol. Biol. Phys.*, **40** (3), 535–539.

11 Yamazaki, H., Inoue, T., Teshima, T., Tanaka, E., *et al.* (1998) Tongue cancer treated with brachytherapy: is thickness of tongue cancer a prognostic factor for regional control? *Anticancer Res.*, **18** (2B), 1261–1265.

12 Sparano, A., Weinstein, G., Chalian, A., Yodul, M., *et al.* (2004) Multivariate predictors of occult neck metastasis in early oral tongue cancer. *Otolaryngol. Head Neck Surg.*, **131** (4), 472–476.

13 Spiro, R.H., Huvos, A.G., Wong, G.Y., Spiro, J.D., *et al.* (1986) Predictive value of tumor thickness in squamous carcinoma confined to the tongue and floor of the mouth. *Am. J. Surg.*, **152** (4), 345–350.

14 Byers, R.M., El-Naggar, A.K., Lee, Y.Y., Rao, B., *et al.* (1998) Can we detect or predict the presence of occult nodal metastases in patients with squamous carcinoma of the oral tongue? *Head Neck*, **20** (2), 138–144.

15 Myers, J.N., Greenberg, J.S., Mo, V., Roberts, D. (2001) Extracapsular spread. A significant predictor of treatment failure in patients with squamous cell carcinoma of the tongue. *Cancer*, **92** (12), 3030–3036.

16 Lindberg, R. (1972) Distribution of cervical lymph node metastases from squamous cell carcinoma of the upper respiratory and digestive tracts. *Cancer*, **29** (6), 1446–1449.

17 Shah, J.P., Candela, F.C., Poddar, A.K. (1990) The patterns of cervical lymph node metastases from squamous carcinoma of the oral cavity. *Cancer*, **66** (1), 109–113.

18 Mohit-Tabatabai, M.A., *et al.* (1986) Relation of thickness of floor of mouth stage I and II cancers to regional metastasis. *Am. J. Surg.*, **152** (4), 351–353.

19 Saito, T., Sugiura, C., Hirai, A., Notani, K., *et al.* (2001) Development of squamous cell carcinoma from pre-existent oral leukoplakia: with respect to treatment modality. *Int. J. Oral Maxillofac. Surg.*, **30** (1), 49–53.

20 Bloom, N.D., Spiro, R.H. (1980) Carcinoma of the cheek mucosa. A retrospective analysis. *Am. J. Surg.*, **140** (4), 556–559.

21 Lampe, I. (1955) Radiation therapy of cancer of the buccal mucosa and lower gingiva. *Am. J. Roentgenol. Radium Ther. Nucl. Med.*, **73** (4), 628–638.

22 Zain, R.B., Ikeda, N., Gupta, P.C., Warnakulasuriya, S. *et al.* (1999) Oral mucosal lesions associated with betel quid, areca nut and tobacco chewing habits: consensus from a workshop held in Kuala Lumpur, Malaysia, November 25-27, 1996. *J. Oral Pathol. Med.*, **28** (1), 1–4.

23 Conley, J., Sadoyama, J.A. (1973) Squamous cell cancer of the buccal mucosa. A review of 90 cases. *Arch. Otolaryngol.*, **97** (4), 330–333.

24 MacComb, W.S., Fletcher, G.H., Healey. J.E.J. (1967) *Cancer of the Head and Neck*. Williams & Wilkins, Baltimore, MD.

25 New, G., Hallberg, O. (1941) The end results of the treatment of malignant tumors of the palate. *Surg. Gynecol*, **73**, 520.

26 Hong, S.X., *et al.* (2001) Mandibular invasion of lower gingival carcinoma in the molar region: its clinical implications on the surgical management. *Int. J. Oral Maxillofac. Surg.*, **30** (2), 130–138.

27 McGregor, A.D., MacDonald, D.G. (1988) Routes of entry of squamous cell carcinoma to the mandible. *Head Neck Surg.*, **10** (5), 294–301.

28 Byers, R.M., *et al.* (1981) Results of treatment for squamous carcinoma of the lower gum. *Cancer*, **47** (9), 2236–2268.

29 Beltramini, G.A., *et al.* (2011) Is neck dissection needed in squamous-cell carcinoma of the maxillary gingiva, alveolus, and hard palate? A multicentre Italian study of 65 cases and literature review. *Oral Oncol.*, **48** (2),97–101.

30 Byers, R.M., *et al.* (1984) Treatment of squamous carcinoma of the retromolar trigone. *Am. J. Clin. Oncol.*, **7** (6), 647–652.

31 Lam, P., *et al.* (2004) Correlating MRI and histologic tumor thickness in the assessment of oral tongue cancer. *Am. J. Roentgenol.*, **182** (3), 803–808.

32 Park, J.O., *et al.* (2011) Diagnostic accuracy of magnetic resonance imaging (MRI) in the assessment

of tumor invasion depth in oral/oropharyngeal cancer. *Oral Oncol.*, **47** (5), 381–386.

33 Ng, S.H., *et al.* (2006) Prospective study of [18F]fluorodeoxyglucose positron emission tomography and computed tomography and magnetic resonance imaging in oral cavity squamous cell carcinoma with palpably negative neck. *J. Clin. Oncol.*, **24** (27), 4371–4376.

34 Kovacs, A.F., *et al.* (2004) Positron emission tomography in combination with sentinel node biopsy reduces the rate of elective neck dissections in the treatment of oral and oropharyngeal cancer. *J. Clin. Oncol.*, **22** (19), 3973–3980.

35 Amin, M.B. (2017) *AJCC Cancer Staging Manual.* Springer, New York.

36 Jemal, A., *et al.* (2017) Cancer statistics. *CA Cancer J. Clin.*, **67** (1), 7–30.

37 Funk, G.F., *et al.* (2002) Presentation, treatment, and outcome of oral cavity cancer: a National Cancer Data Base report. *Head Neck*, **24** (2), 165–180.

38 Boyle, P., Macfarlane, G.J., Scully, C. (1993) Oral cancer: necessity for prevention strategies. *Lancet*, **342** (8880), 1129.

39 Hindle, I., *et al.* (2000) Is alcohol responsible for more intra-oral cancer? *Oral Oncol.*, **36** (4), 328–333.

40 Macfarlane, G.J., *et al.* (1995) Alcohol, tobacco, diet and the risk of oral cancer: a pooled analysis of three case-control studies. *Eur. J. Cancer B Oral. Oncol.*, **31B** (3), 181–187.

41 Schantz, S.P., Yu, G.P. (2002) Head and neck cancer incidence trends in young Americans, 1973-1997, with a special analysis for tongue cancer. *Arch. Otolaryngol. Head Neck Surg.*, **128** (3), 268–274.

42 Marur, S., Forastiere, A.A. (2008) Head and neck cancer: changing epidemiology, diagnosis, and treatment. *Mayo Clin. Proc.*, **83** (4), 489–501.

43 Sharma, D.C. (2003) Betel quid and areca nut are carcinogenic without tobacco. *Lancet Oncol.*, **4** (10), 587.

44 Kreimer, A.R., *et al.* (2005) Human papillomavirus types in head and neck squamous cell carcinomas worldwide: a systematic review. *Cancer Epidemiol. Biomarkers Prev.*, **14** (2), 467–475.

45 Blitzer, G.C., *et al.* (2014) Review of the clinical and biologic aspects of human papillomavirus-positive squamous cell carcinomas of the head and neck. *Int. J. Radiat. Oncol. Biol. Phys.*, **88** (4), 761–770.

46 Ragin, C.C., Taioli, E. (2007) Survival of squamous cell carcinoma of the head and neck in relation to human papillomavirus infection: review and meta-analysis. *Int. J. Cancer*, **121** (8), 1813–1820.

47 Peters, L.J., *et al.* (1993) Evaluation of the dose for postoperative radiation therapy of head and neck cancer: first report of a prospective randomized trial. *Int. J. Radiat. Oncol. Biol. Phys.*, **26** (1), 3–11.

48 Ang, K.K., *et al.* (2001) Randomized trial addressing risk features and time factors of surgery plus radiotherapy in advanced head-and-neck cancer. *Int. J. Radiat. Oncol. Biol. Phys.*, **51** (3), 571–578.

49 Tupchong, L., *et al.* (1991) Randomized study of preoperative versus postoperative radiation therapy in advanced head and neck carcinoma: long-term follow-up of RTOG study 73-03. *Int. J. Radiat. Oncol. Biol. Phys.,* **20** (1), 21–28.

50 Licitra, L., *et al.* (2003) Primary chemotherapy in resectable oral cavity squamous cell cancer: a randomized controlled trial. *J. Clin. Oncol.*, **21** (2), 327–333.

51 Huang, D.T., *et al.* (1992) Postoperative radiotherapy in head and neck carcinoma with extracapsular lymph node extension and/or positive resection margins: a comparative study. *Int. J. Radiat. Oncol. Biol. Phys.*, **23** (4), 737–742.

52 Hinerman, R.W., *et al.* (2004) Postoperative irradiation for squamous cell carcinoma of the oral cavity: 35-year experience. *Head Neck*, **26** (11), 984–994.

53 Phillips, T.L. (1968) Peroral roentgen therapy. *Radiology*, **90** (3), 525–531.

54 Cooper, J.S., *et al.* (2004) Postoperative concurrent radiotherapy and chemotherapy for high-risk squamous-cell carcinoma of the head and neck. *N. Engl. J. Med.*, **350** (19), 1937–1944.

55 Bernier, J., *et al.* (2004) Postoperative irradiation with or without concomitant chemotherapy for locally advanced head and neck cancer. *N. Engl. J. Med.*, **350** (19), 1945–1952.

56 Bernier, J., *et al.* (2005) Defining risk levels in locally advanced head and neck cancers: a comparative analysis of concurrent postoperative radiation plus chemotherapy trials of the EORTC (#22931) and RTOG (# 9501). *Head Neck*, **27** (10), 843–850.

57 Brizel, D.M., *et al.* (1998) Hyperfractionated irradiation with or without concurrent chemotherapy for locally advanced head and neck cancer. *N. Engl. J. Med.*, **338** (25), 1798–1804.

58 Merlano, M., *et al.* (1996) Five-year update of a randomized trial of alternating radiotherapy and chemotherapy compared with radiotherapy alone in treatment of unresectable squamous cell carcinoma of the head and neck. *J. Natl Cancer Inst.*, **88** (9), 583–589.

59 Calais, G., *et al.* (1999) Randomized trial of radiation therapy versus concomitant chemotherapy and radiation therapy for advanced-stage oropharynx carcinoma. *J. Natl Cancer Inst.*, **91** (24), 2081–2086.

60 Browman, G.P., *et al.* (2001) Choosing a concomitant chemotherapy and radiotherapy regimen for squamous cell head and neck cancer: A systematic review of the published literature with subgroup analysis. *Head Neck*, **23** (7), 579–589.

61 Pignon, J.P., *et al.* (2009) Meta-analysis of chemotherapy in head and neck cancer (MACH-NC): an update on 93 randomised trials and 17,346 patients. *Radiother. Oncol.*, **92** (1), 4–14.

62 Lo, T.C., *et al.* (1976) Combined radiation therapy and 5-fluorouracil for advanced squamous cell carcinoma of the oral cavity and oropharynx: a randomized study. *Am. J. Roentgenol.*, **126** (2), 229–235.

63 Adelstein, D.J., *et al.* (2003) An intergroup phase III comparison of standard radiation therapy and two schedules of concurrent chemoradiotherapy in patients with unresectable squamous cell head and neck cancer. *J. Clin. Oncol.*, **21** (1), 92–98.

64 Melotek, J.M., *et al.* (0000) Definitive Chemoradiation Therapy for Advanced Oral Cavity Cancer: A 20-Year Experience. *Int. J. Radiat. Oncol. Biol. Phys.*, **96** (2), S84.

65 Daly, M.E., *et al.* (2007) Evaluation of patterns of failure and subjective salivary function in patients treated with intensity modulated radiotherapy for head and neck squamous cell carcinoma. *Head Neck*, **29** (3), 211–220.

66 Eisbruch, A., *et al.* (1999) Dose, volume, and function relationships in parotid salivary glands following conformal and intensity-modulated irradiation of head and neck cancer. *Int. J. Radiat. Oncol. Biol. Phys.*, **45** (3), 577–587.

67 Lin, A., *et al.* (2003) Quality of life after parotid-sparing IMRT for head-and-neck cancer: a prospective longitudinal study. *Int. J. Radiat. Oncol. Biol. Phys.*, **57** (1), 61–70.

68 Parliament, M.B., *et al.* (2004) Preservation of oral health-related quality of life and salivary flow rates after inverse-planned intensity-modulated radiotherapy (IMRT) for head-and-neck cancer. *Int. J. Radiat. Oncol. Biol. Phys.*, **58** (3), 663–673.

69 Lee, N., *et al.* (2007) Choosing an intensity-modulated radiation therapy technique in the treatment of head-and-neck cancer. *Int. J. Radiat. Oncol. Biol. Phys.*, **68** (5), 1299–1309.

70 Amdur, R.J., *et al.* (2007) Matching intensity-modulated radiation therapy to an anterior low neck field. *Int. J. Radiat. Oncol. Biol. Phys.*, **69** (2 Suppl.), S46–S48.

71 Dabaja, B., *et al.* (2005) Intensity-modulated radiation therapy (IMRT) of cancers of the head and neck: comparison of split-field and whole-field techniques. *Int. J. Radiat. Oncol. Biol. Phys.*, **63** (4), 1000–1005.

72 Gomez, D.R., *et al.* (2009) Intensity-modulated radiotherapy in postoperative treatment of oral cavity cancers. *Int. J. Radiat. Oncol. Biol. Phys.*, **73** (4), 1096–1103.

73 Yao, M., *et al.* (2007) The failure patterns of oral cavity squamous cell carcinoma after intensity-modulated radiotherapy – the University of Iowa experience. *Int. J. Radiat. Oncol. Biol. Phys.*, **67** (5), 1332–1341.

74 Studer, G., *et al.* (2007) IMRT in oral cavity cancer. *Radiat. Oncol.*, **2**, 16.

75 Daly, M.E., *et al.* (2011) Intensity-modulated radiotherapy for oral cavity squamous cell carcinoma: patterns of failure and predictors of local control. *Int. J. Radiat. Oncol. Biol. Phys.*, **80** (5), 1412–1422.

76 Goffinet, D.R. (1993) Brachytherapy for head and neck cancer. *Semin. Radiat. Oncol.*, **3** (4), 250–259.

77 Harrison, L.B. (1997) Applications of brachytherapy in head and neck cancer. *Semin. Surg. Oncol.*, **13** (3), 177–184.

78 Mazeron, J.J., Noel, G., Simon, J.M. (2002) Head and neck brachytherapy. *Semin. Radiat. Oncol.*, **12** (1), 95–108.

79 Mazeron, J.J., *et al.* (2009) GEC-ESTRO recommendations for brachytherapy for head and neck squamous cell carcinomas. *Radiother. Oncol.*, **91** (2), 150–156.

80 Quimby, E. (1944) Dosage table for linear radium sources. *Radiology*, **43**, 572.

81 Johns, H.E., Cunningham, J.R. (1983) *The Physics of Radiology*. Charles C. Thomas, Springfield, Ill.

82 Inoue, T., *et al.* (1996) Phase III trial of high and low dose rate interstitial radiotherapy for early oral tongue cancer. *Int. J. Radiat. Oncol. Biol. Phys.*, **36** (5), 1201–1204.

83 Parsons, J.T., *et al.* (1997) An analysis of factors influencing the outcome of postoperative irradiation for squamous cell carcinoma of the oral cavity. *Int. J. Radiat. Oncol. Biol. Phys.*, **39** (1), 137–148.

84 Zelefsky, M.J., *et al.* (1990) Postoperative radiotherapy for oral cavity cancers: impact of anatomic subsite on treatment outcome. *Head Neck*, **12** (6), 470–475.

85 Layland, M.K., Sessions, D.G., Lenox, J. (2005) The influence of lymph node metastasis in the treatment of squamous cell carcinoma of the oral cavity, oropharynx, larynx, and hypopharynx: N0 versus N+. *Laryngoscope*, **115** (4), 629–639.

86 Stranc, M.F., Fogel, M., Dische, S. (1987) Comparison of lip function: surgery vs radiotherapy. *Br. J. Plast. Surg.*, **40** (6), 598–604.

87 de Visscher, J.G., *et al.* (1998) Surgical treatment of squamous cell carcinoma of the lower lip: evaluation of long-term results and prognostic factors – a retrospective analysis of 184 patients. *J. Oral Maxillofac. Surg.*, **56** (7), 814–820; discussion 820–821.

88 de Visscher, J.G., *et al.* (1996) Results of radiotherapy for squamous cell carcinoma of the vermilion border of the lower lip. A retrospective analysis of 108 patients. *Radiother. Oncol.*, **39** (1), 9–14.

89 Sykes, A.J., Allan, E., Irwin, C. (1996) Squamous cell carcinoma of the lip: the role of electron treatment. *Clin. Oncol. (R. Coll. Radiol.)*, **8** (6), 384–386.

90 Ang, K.K., Garden, A.S. (2006) *Radiotherapy for Head and Neck Cancer.* 3rd edition. Lippincott Williams and Wilkins, Philadelphia.

91 Petrovich, Z., *et al.* (1987) Carcinoma of the lip and selected sites of head and neck skin. A clinical study of 896 patients. *Radiother. Oncol.*, **8** (1), 11–17.

92 Cerezo, L., *et al.* (1993) Squamous cell carcinoma of the lip: analysis of the Princess Margaret Hospital experience. *Radiother. Oncol.*, **28** (2), 142–147.

93 Tombolini, V., *et al.* (1998) Brachytherapy for squamous cell carcinoma of the lip. The experience of the Institute of Radiology of the University of Rome 'La Sapienza'. *Tumori*, **84** (4), 478–482.

94 Wang, C.C. (1989) Radiotherapeutic management and results of T1N0, T2N0 carcinoma of the oral tongue: evaluation of boost techniques. *Int. J. Radiat. Oncol. Biol. Phys.*, **17** (2), 287–291.

95 Lyos, A.T., *et al.* (1999) Tongue reconstruction: outcomes with the rectus abdominis flap. *Plast. Reconstr. Surg.*, **103** (2), 442–447; discussion 448–449.

96 Salibian, A.H., *et al.* (1999) Functional hemitongue reconstruction with the microvascular ulnar forearm flap. *Plast. Reconstr. Surg.*, **104** (3), 654–660.

97 Fujita, M., *et al.* (1999) Interstitial brachytherapy for stage I and II squamous cell carcinoma of the oral tongue: factors influencing local control and soft tissue complications. *Int. J. Radiat. Oncol. Biol. Phys.*, **44** (4), 767–775.

98 Mendenhall, W.M., *et al.* (1981) Analysis of time-dose factors in squamous cell carcinoma of the oral tongue and floor of mouth treated with radiation therapy alone. *Int. J. Radiat. Oncol. Biol. Phys.*, **7** (8), 1005–1011.

99 Mazeron, J.J., *et al.* (1991) Effect of dose rate on local control and complications in definitive irradiation of T1-2 squamous cell carcinomas of mobile tongue and floor of mouth with interstitial iridium-192. *Radiother. Oncol.*, **21** (1), 39–47.

100 Burgers, J.M., Awwad, H.K., van der Laarse, R. (1985) Relation between local cure and dose-time-volume factors in interstitial implants. *Int. J. Radiat. Oncol. Biol. Phys.*, **11** (4), 715–723.

101 Awwad, H.K., Burgers, J.M., Marcuse, H.R. (1974) The influence of tumor dose specification on the early clinical results of interstitial radium tongue implants. *Radiology*, **110** (1), 177–182.

102 Inoue, T., *et al.* (2001) Phase III trial of high- vs. low-dose-rate interstitial radiotherapy for early mobile tongue cancer. *Int. J. Radiat. Oncol. Biol. Phys.*, **51** (1), 171–175.

103 Haddadin, K.J., *et al.* (1999) Improved survival for patients with clinically T1/T2, N0 tongue tumors undergoing a prophylactic neck dissection. *Head Neck*, **21** (6), 517–525.

104 Koo, B.S., *et al.* (2006) Management of contralateral N0 neck in oral cavity squamous cell carcinoma. *Head Neck*, **28** (10), 896–901.

105 O'Brien, C.J., *et al.* (2000) The use of clinical criteria alone in the management of the clinically negative neck among patients with squamous cell carcinoma of the oral cavity and oropharynx. *Arch. Otolaryngol. Head Neck Surg.*, **126** (3), 360–365.

106 Kowalski, L.P., *et al.* (1999) Factors influencing contralateral lymph node metastasis from oral carcinoma. *Head Neck*, **21** (2), 104–110.

107 Gujrathi, D., *et al.* (1996) Treatment outcome of squamous cell carcinoma of the oral tongue. *J. Otolaryngol.*, **25** (3), 145–149.

108 Shibuya, H., *et al.* (1993) Brachytherapy for stage I & II oral tongue cancer: an analysis of past cases focusing on control and complications. *Int. J. Radiat. Oncol. Biol. Phys.*, **26** (1), 51–58.

109 Sessions, D.G., *et al.* (2002) Analysis of treatment results for oral tongue cancer. *Laryngoscope*, **112** (4), 616–625.

110 Nyman, J., Mercke, C., Lindstrom, J. (1993) Prognostic factors for local control and survival of cancer of the oral tongue. A retrospective analysis of 230 cases in western Sweden. *Acta Oncol.*, **32** (6), 667–673.

111 Marks, J.E., *et al.* (1981) Carcinoma of the oral tongue: a study of patient selection and treatment results. *Laryngoscope*, **91** (9 Pt 1), 1548–1559.

112 Fein, D.A., *et al.* (1994) Carcinoma of the oral tongue: a comparison of results and complications of treatment with radiotherapy and/or surgery. *Head Neck*, **16** (4), 358–365.

113 Umeda, M., *et al.* (2005) A comparison of brachytherapy and surgery for the treatment of stage I-II squamous cell carcinoma of the tongue. *Int. J. Oral Maxillofac. Surg.*, **34** (7), 739–744.

114 Aksu, G., *et al.* (2006) Treatment results and prognostic factors in oral tongue cancer: analysis of 80 patients. *Int. J. Oral Maxillofac. Surg.*, **35** (6), 506–513.

115 Wendt, C.D., *et al.* (1990) Primary radiotherapy in the treatment of stage I and II oral tongue cancers: importance of the proportion of therapy delivered with interstitial therapy. *Int. J. Radiat. Oncol. Biol. Phys.*, **18** (6), 1287–1292.

116 Delclos, L., Lindberg, R.D., Fletcher, G.H. (1976) Squamous cell carcinoma of the oral tongue and floor of mouth. Evaluation of interstitial radium therapy. *Am. J. Roentgenol.*, **126** (2), 223–228.

117 Yuen, A.P., *et al.* (1997) Results of surgical salvage of locoregional recurrence of carcinoma of the tongue after radiotherapy failure. *Ann. Otol. Rhinol. Laryngol.*, **106** (9), 779–782.

118 Yuen, A.P., *et al.* (1998) Local recurrence of carcinoma of the tongue after glossectomy: patient prognosis. *Ear Nose Throat J.*, **77** (3), 181–184.

119 Godden, D.R., *et al.* (2002) Recurrent neck disease in oral cancer. *J. Oral Maxillofac. Surg.*, **60** (7), 748–753; discussion 753–755.

120 Ange, D.W., Lindberg, R.D., Guillamondegui, O.M. (1975) Management of squamous cell carcinoma of the oral tongue and floor of mouth after excisional biopsy. *Radiology*, **116** (1), 143–146.

121 Inoue, T., *et al.* (1998) High dose rate versus low dose rate interstitial radiotherapy for carcinoma of the floor of mouth. *Int. J. Radiat. Oncol. Biol. Phys.*, **41** (1), 53–58.

122 Sessions, D.G., *et al.* (2000) Analysis of treatment results for floor-of-mouth cancer. *Laryngoscope*, **110** (10 Pt 1), 1764–1772.

123 Fu, K.K., Lichter, A., Galante, M. (1976) Carcinoma of the floor of mouth: an analysis of treatment results and the sites and causes of failures. *Int. J. Radiat. Oncol. Biol. Phys.*, **1** (9-10), 829–837.

124 Shaha, A.R., *et al.* (1984) Squamous carcinoma of the floor of the mouth. *Am. J. Surg.*, **148** (4), 455–459.

125 Hicks, W.L., Jr, *et al.* (1997) Squamous cell carcinoma of the floor of mouth: a 20-year review. *Head Neck*, **19** (5), 400–405.

126 Pernot, M., *et al.* (1995) Epidermoid carcinomas of the floor of mouth treated by exclusive irradiation: statistical study of a series of 207 cases. *Radiother. Oncol.*, **35** (3), 177–185.

127 Shons, A.R., Magallanes, F., McQuarrie, D. (1984) The results of aggressive regional operation in the treatment of cancer of the floor of the mouth. *Surgery*, **96** (1), 29–34.

128 Loree, T.R., Strong, E.W. (1990) Significance of positive margins in oral cavity squamous carcinoma. *Am. J. Surg.*, **160** (4), 410–414.

129 Marsiglia, H., *et al.* (2002) Brachytherapy for T1-T2 floor-of-the-mouth cancers: the Gustave-Roussy Institute experience. *Int. J. Radiat. Oncol. Biol. Phys.*, **52** (5), 1257–1263.

130 Lozza, L., *et al.* (1997) Analysis of risk factors for mandibular bone radionecrosis after exclusive low dose-rate brachytherapy for oral cancer. *Radiother. Oncol.*, **44** (2), 143–147.

131 Misra, S., Chaturvedi, A., Misra, N. (2008) Management of gingivobuccal complex cancer. *Ann. R. Coll. Surg. Engl.*, **90** (7), 546–553.

132 Strome, S.E., *et al.* (1999) Squamous cell carcinoma of the buccal mucosa. *Otolaryngol. Head Neck Surg.*, **120** (3), 375–379.

133 Lin, C.S., *et al.* (2006) Squamous cell carcinoma of the buccal mucosa: an aggressive cancer requiring multimodality treatment. *Head Neck*, **28** (2), 150–157.

134 Sieczka, E., *et al.* (2001) Cancer of the buccal mucosa: are margins and T-stage accurate predictors of local control? *Am. J. Otolaryngol.*, **22** (6), 395–399.

135 Urist, M.M., *et al.* (1987) Squamous cell carcinoma of the buccal mucosa: analysis of prognostic factors. *Am. J. Surg.*, **154** (4), 411–414.

136 Pop, L.A., *et al.* (1989) Evaluation of treatment results of squamous cell carcinoma of the buccal mucosa. *Int. J. Radiat. Oncol. Biol. Phys.*, **16** (2), 483–487.

137 Krishnamurthi, S., Shanta, V., Sastri, D.V. (1971) Combined therapy in buccal mucosal cancers. *Radiology*, **99** (2), 409–415.

138 Mishra, R.C., Singh, D.N., Mishra, T.K. (1996) Post-operative radiotherapy in carcinoma of buccal mucosa, a prospective randomized trial. *Eur. J. Surg. Oncol.*, **22** (5), 502–504.

139 Cherian, T., *et al.* (1991) Evaluation of salvage surgery in heavily irradiated cancer of the buccal mucosa. *Cancer*, **68** (2), 295–299.

140 Fang, F.M., *et al.* (1997) Combined-modality therapy for squamous carcinoma of the buccal mucosa: treatment results and prognostic factors. *Head Neck*, **19** (6), 506–512.

141 Evans, J.F., Shah, J.P. (1981) Epidermoid carcinoma of the palate. *Am. J. Surg.*, **142** (4), 451–455.

142 Yorozu, A., Sykes, A.J., Slevin, N.J. (2001) Carcinoma of the hard palate treated with radiotherapy: a retrospective review of 31 cases. *Oral Oncol.*, **37** (6), 493–497.

143 Chung, C.K., *et al.* (1980) Radiotherapy in the management of primary malignancies of the hard palate. *Laryngoscope*, **90** (4), 576–584.

144 Chung, C.K., *et al.* (1979) Squamous cell carcinoma of the hard palate. *Int. J. Radiat. Oncol. Biol. Phys.*, **5** (2), 191–196.

145 Soo, K.C., *et al.* (1988) Squamous carcinoma of the gums. *Am. J. Surg.*, **156** (4), 281–285.

146 Pathak, K.A., *et al.* (2007) Squamous cell carcinoma of the superior gingival-buccal complex. *Oral Oncol.*, **43** (8), 774–779.

147 Lo, K., *et al.* (1987) Results of irradiation in the squamous cell carcinomas of the anterior faucial pillar-retromolar trigone. *Int. J. Radiat. Oncol. Biol. Phys.*, **13** (7), 969–974.

148 Hao, S.P., *et al.* (2006) Treatment of squamous cell carcinoma of the retromolar trigone. *Laryngoscope*, **116** (6), 916–920.

149 Mendenhall, W.M., *et al.* (2005) Retromolar trigone squamous cell carcinoma treated with radiotherapy alone or combined with surgery. *Cancer*, **103** (11), 2320–2325.

150 Huang, C.J., *et al.* (2001) Cancer of retromolar trigone: long-term radiation therapy outcome. *Head Neck*, **23** (9), 758–763.

151 Blanco, A.I., *et al.* (2005) Dose-volume modeling of salivary function in patients with head-and-neck cancer receiving radiotherapy. *Int. J. Radiat. Oncol. Biol. Phys.*, **62** (4), 1055–1069.

152 Chao, K.S., *et al.* (2001) A prospective study of salivary function sparing in patients with head-and-neck cancers receiving intensity-modulated or three-dimensional radiation therapy: initial results. *Int. J. Radiat. Oncol. Biol. Phys.*, **49** (4), 907–916.

153 Nutting, C.M., *et al.* (2011) Parotid-sparing intensity modulated versus conventional radiotherapy in head and neck cancer (PARSPORT): a phase 3 multicentre randomised controlled trial. *Lancet Oncol.*, **12** (2), 127–136.

154 Vanderpuye, V., Goldson, A. (2000) Osteoradionecrosis of the mandible. *J. Natl Med. Assoc.*, **92** (12), 579–584.

155 Fujita, M., *et al.* (1996) An analysis of mandibular bone complications in radiotherapy for T1 and T2 carcinoma of the oral tongue. *Int. J. Radiat. Oncol. Biol. Phys.*, **34** (2), 333–339.

156 Ben-David, M.A., *et al.* (2007) Lack of osteoradionecrosis of the mandible after intensity-modulated radiotherapy for head and neck cancer: likely contributions of both dental care and improved dose distributions. *Int. J. Radiat. Oncol. Biol. Phys.*, **68** (2), 396–402.

157 Gomez, D.R., *et al.* (2008) Intensity-Modulated Radiotherapy in Postoperative Treatment of Oral Cavity Cancers. *Int. J. Radiat. Oncol. Biol. Phys.*, **73** (4), 1096–1103.

158 Chen, W.C., *et al.* (2009) Comparison between conventional and intensity-modulated post-operative radiotherapy for stage III and IV oral cavity cancer in terms of treatment results and toxicity. *Oral Oncol.*, **45** (6), 505–510.

159 Jorgensen, K., Elbrond, O., Andersen, A.P. (1973) Carcinoma of the lip. A series of 869 patients. *Acta Otolaryngol.*, **75** (4), 312–313.

160 Guinot, J.L., *et al.* (2003) Lip cancer treatment with high dose rate brachytherapy. *Radiother. Oncol.*, **69** (1), 113–115.

161 Guibert, M., *et al.* (2010) Brachytherapy in lip carcinoma: long-term results. *Int. J. Radiat. Oncol. Biol. Phys.*, **81** (5), e839–e843.

162 Wang, C.C., *et al.* (1995) Early carcinoma of the oral cavity: a conservative approach with radiation therapy. *J. Oral Maxillofac. Surg.*, **53** (6), 687–690.

163 Fan, K.H., *et al.* (2007) Combined-modality treatment for advanced oral tongue squamous cell carcinoma. *Int. J. Radiat. Oncol. Biol. Phys.*, **67** (2), 453–461.

164 Araki, L.T., *et al.* (1990) Surgical management of squamous cell carcinoma of the floor of the mouth. *Jpn. J. Clin. Oncol.*, **20** (4), 387–391.

165 Iyer, S.G., *et al.* (2004) Surgical treatment outcomes of localized squamous carcinoma of buccal mucosa. *Head Neck*, **26** (10), 897–902.

166 Bayman, N.A., *et al.* (2010) Primary radiotherapy for carcinoma of the retromolar trigone: a useful alternative to surgery. *Clin. Oncol. (R. Coll. Radiol.)*, **22** (2), 119–124.

10

Oropharyngeal Cancer

Charles Woods, Mitchell Machtay and Min Yao

Introduction

The estimated incidence of cancers of the pharynx in the United States in 2017 is 17,000, with 3,050 deaths [1]. The oropharynx is traditionally divided into four subsites: soft palate; base of tongue; tonsillar region; and lateral and posterior pharyngeal walls. The oropharyngeal structures are critical for the normal functions of speech and swallowing, and neoplasms arising in the oropharynx often compromise these normal functions. The management of oropharyngeal cancer is best accomplished by a multidisciplinary approach with input from the head and neck surgeon, radiation oncologist, and medical oncologist. The goal of this approach is to offer the modalities that will result in the best local control of the tumor while maintaining an adequate level of oropharyngeal function. Radiation therapy often plays a central role in the management of oropharyngeal cancers due to the high radiosensitivity of squamous cell carcinoma and the goal of organ and functional preservation. Intensity-modulated radiation therapy (IMRT) is commonly used due to its ability to decrease the dose to uninvolved structures which can result in better preservation of quality of life (QOL) after treatment. Chemotherapy is frequently used in the definitive and postoperative setting to improve local-regional control. In this chapter, attention is focused on the definitive management of oropharyngeal cancer with radiation therapy.

Anatomy

The anatomy of the oropharynx and oral cavity is illustrated in Figure 10.1. The oropharynx is divided into four subsites: soft palate; base of tongue; tonsillar region; and lateral and posterior pharyngeal walls. The borders of the oropharynx are the soft palate superiorly, the hyoid bone and vallecula inferiorly, the pharyngeal walls laterally and posteriorly, and the circumvallate papillae anteriorly which separate the oral tongue from the base of tongue.

Soft Palate

The soft palate, including the uvula, separates the oropharynx from the nasopharynx and is formed from the levator veli palatine, tensor veli palatine, uvular, palatoglossus, and palatopharyngeus muscles. Its anterior border is the hard palate, and it is continuous laterally with the tonsillar pillars. Functionally, the soft palate closes off the nasopharynx during speech and swallowing so as to prevent oral contents from entering the nasopharynx and allowing for the production of certain sounds. Sensory innervation is via the lesser palatine nerve, a branch of V2. Tumors of the soft palate usually present on the oropharyngeal surface and very rarely on the nasopharyngeal surface.

Tonsillar Region

The tonsillar region includes the anterior and posterior (faucil) pillars which are formed by the palatatoglossus and palatopharyngeus muscles. Superiorly, these muscles give rise to the soft palate. Between the pillars sits the palatine tonsil, which consists of lymphoid tissue covered by a stratified squamous epithelium and laterally by a fibrous capsule. Lateral to this capsule are the medial and lateral pterygoid muscles, mandible, and superior pharyngeal constrictor muscle. Sensory innervation is via the lesser and superior palatine nerves, branches of V2. Tumors of the tonsillar region commonly present with

Clinical Radiation Oncology: Indications, Techniques, and Results, Third Edition. Edited by William Small Jr.
© 2017 John Wiley & Sons, Inc. Published 2017 by John Wiley & Sons, Inc.

Figure 10.1 Diagrams showing various anatomic sites of the oral cavity and oropharynx. (a) Anterior view. (b) Lateral view.

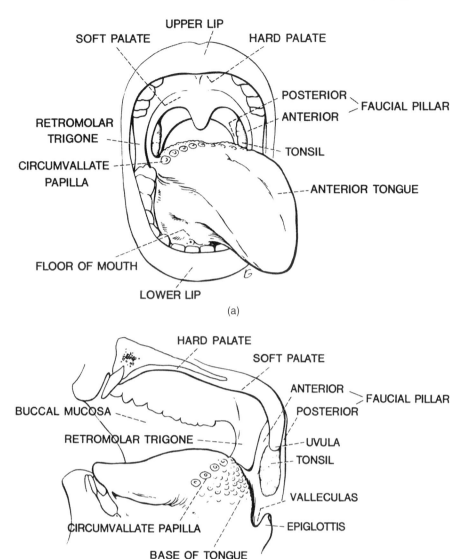

(a)

(b)

enlarged cervical lymph nodes due to lymph node metastasis. Non-Hodgkin's lymphoma may also occur in the lymphoid tissue and should be part of the differential diagnosis prior to pathologic confirmation.

Base of Tongue

The tongue is formed by the genioglossus, hyoglossus, styloglossus, and palatoglossus muscles. Its anterior border is the circumvallate papillae. Posteriorly, base of tongue (BOT) includes the vallecula with the lingual surface of the epiglottis being the posterior border. The glossopalatine sulci form the lateral borders. Taste and other sensory inputs are via the lingual branch of the glossopharyngeal nerve (IX). The BOT contains submucosal lymphoid tissue (lingual tonsil) which can be mistaken

for neoplasm on positron emission tomography (PET) due to its level metabolic activity and the uptake of ^{18}F-fluorodeoxyglucose (FDG).

Posterior and Lateral Pharyngeal Walls

The structure of the lateral and posterior pharyngeal walls is formed by the superior and middle pharyngeal constrictor muscles. Superficial to these muscles is a stratified squamous epithelium, and deep to these muscles lay the retropharyngeal space, prevertebral musculature, prevertebral fascia, and the vertebral body, respectively. The superior border is at the level of the soft palate and the inferior border is at the level of the epiglottis and is continuous with the pyriform sinuses. Sensory innervation is via the glossopharyngeal and vagus nerves.

Neck Nodal Levels

The head and neck region is rich in lymphatics and contains hundreds of lymph nodes. The oropharynx in particular has abundant lymphatic channels, and nodal metastasis is common and often the first presentation of the disease. Therefore, a thorough understanding of the neck and how nodal levels are classified by surgeons and radiation oncologists is essential.

The neck nodal levels were traditionally classified by head and neck surgeons to provide a common language about how dissections were performed. Robbins and colleagues formed a consensus statement in 2008 for the American Head and Neck Society regarding nodal levels as surgically defined [2]. However, given the increased use of three-dimensional (3D)-conformal radiotherapy, IMRT and axial imaging, there was a need to define nodal levels radiographically and this has been proposed by multiple groups [3–5]. In an effort to standardize nodal target delineation, international consensus guidelines (endorsed by DAHANCA, EORTC, GORTEC, NCIC, and RTOG) were made regarding the delineation of nodal levels and clinical target volumes (CTVs) in the node-negative neck and are presented in Table 10.1 [6]. These guidelines were recently updated mainly to modify the nodal areas in the lower and posterior neck typically involved in nasopharyngeal carcinoma, and to include the lymph node regions draining the face, the scalp, and those nodal regions close to the base of skull [7]. Thus, the updated guidelines will not greatly affect the management of oropharyngeal cancer. A digital contouring atlas is available on the RTOG website [8]. Nodal levels and important anatomic landmarks as depicted by Som and coworkers are shown in Figure 10.2 [3].

Epidemiology, Etiology, and Risk Factors

The estimated incidence of cancers of the pharynx in the United States in 2015 was 15 520, with 2660 deaths [1]. Statistics are not presented for pharyngeal subsites. While the overall incidence of head and neck cancers has been decreasing over the past several years due to declines in tobacco smoking, the incidence of oropharyngeal cancers is increasing due to human papilloma virus (HPV) infection [9]. The traditional risk factors of tobacco and alcohol use are well established. A meta-analysis by Bagnardi and coworkers demonstrated a relative risk of 6.0 for oral cavity and pharyngeal cancers with a daily ethanol consumption of 100 g [10]. Franceschi and coworkers performed a case-control study that demonstrated an odds ratio of 12.9 for pharyngeal cancer in current cigarette smokers [11].

Over the past decade, HPV has emerged as an important etiologic factor in oropharyngeal cancer. There are more than 100 subtypes of HPV, and the most common oncogenic subtypes are HPV 16 and 18. The prevalence of oral HPV infection is approximately 7% among Americans ages 14–69 years, with the prevalence of HPV type 16 being 1% [12]. Most of the molecular biology and pathogenesis of HPV-induced cancers comes from the extensive research in cervical cancer, which is also HPV-related. Viral oncoproteins E6 and E7 are thought to be responsible for increased proliferation in infected cells. These viral proteins disrupt the normal cell cycle check points and lead to unregulated division. The presence of E6 results in the degradation of p53 tumor-suppressor protein, which in turn leads to an unregulated G1/S transition in the cell cycle. Protein E7 inactivates Rb protein, leading to an increased level of E2F transcription factor which is important in turning on the transcription of S-phase genes [13].

Importantly, patients with HPV-associated squamous cell carcinoma (SCCA) of the head and neck have markedly better outcomes than HPV-negative SCCA. Analyses of the HPV status of tumors from many large prospective trials have consistently demonstrated improved local control and survival in patients with HPV-positive tumor [14–16]. A large prospective trial with de-intensified treatment in this group of patients (RTOG 1016, radiation to 70 Gy with cisplatin versus cetuximab) has been completed and the results are eagerly awaited [17]. Several other de-intensified trials are underway or in development with the goal of decreasing the morbidity of radiation treatment for HPV-positive cancers while maintaining good local control and survival outcomes.

Epidermal growth factor receptor (EGFR) is overexpressed in some SCCAs, and the present understanding of the receptor and its signaling pathways have led to effective therapies such as the monoclonal antibody, cetuximab. The overexpression of EGFR has been associated with poorer outcomes. Ang and coworkers investigated the impact of EGFR expression and found that an increased expression of EGFR was an independent prognostic indicator for survival and local control [18]. Hong *et al.* noted that both HPV status and EGFR expression are independent prognostic markers. Patients with HPV-negative/EGFR-positive tumors had an adjusted 13-fold increase in the risk of locoregional failure compared with HPV-positive/EGFR-negative tumors [19].

Pathology

Squamous cell carcinoma is the most common pathologic finding from oropharyngeal tumors (>90%). Other uncommon cancers include lymphomas (primarily non-Hodgkin's), minor salivary gland tumors, melanoma, and sarcoma.

Table 10.1 International consensus of nodal levels in the node-negative neck.

Level	Cranial	Caudal	Anterior	Posterior	Lateral	Medial
			Anatomic boundaries			
Ia	Geniohyoid m., plane tangent to basilar edge of mandible	Plane tangent to body of hyoid bone	Symphysis menti, platysma m.	Body of hyoid bone	Medial edge of ant. belly of digastric m.	n/a
Ib	Mylohyoid m., cranial edge of submandibular gland	Plane through central part of hyoid bone	Symphysis menti, platysma m.	Posterior edge of submandibular gland	Basilar edge /innerside of mandible, platysma m., skin	Lateral edge of ant. belly of digastric m.
IIa	Caudal edge of lateral process of C1	Caudal edge of the body of hyoid bone	Post. edge of sub-mandibular gland; ant. edge of int. carotid artery; post. edge of post. belly of digastric m.	Post. border of int. jugular vein	Medial edge of SCM	Medial edge of int. carotid artery, paraspinal (levator scapulae) m.
IIb	Caudal edge of lateral process of C1	Caudal edge of the body of hyoid bone	Post. border of int jugular vein	Post. border of the SCM	Medial edge of SCM	Medial edge of int. carotid artery, paraspinal (levator scapulae) m.
III	Caudal edge of the body of hyoid bone	Caudal edge of cricoid cartilage	Postero-lateral edge of the sternohyoid m.; ant. edge of SCM	Post. edge of the SCM	Medial edge of SCM	Int. edge of carotid artery, paraspinal (scalenius) m.
IV	Caudal edge of cricoid cartilage	2 cm cranial to sternoclavicular joint	Anteromedial edge of SCM	Post. edge of the SCM	Medial edge of SCM	Medial edge of internalcarotid artery, paraspinal (scalenius) m.
V	Cranial edge of body of hyoid bone	CT slice encompassing the transverse cervical vessels	Post. edge of the SCM	Ant-lateral border of the trapezius m.	Platysma m., skin	Paraspinal (levator scapulae, splenius capitis) m.
VI	Caudal edge of body of thyroid cartilage	Sternal manubrium	Skin; platysma m.	Separation between trachea and esophagus	Medial edges of thyroid gland, skin and ant.-medial edge of SCM	n/a
RP	Base of skull	Cranial edge of the body of hyoid bone	Fascia under the pharyngeal mucosa	Prevertebral m. (longus colli, longus capitis)	Medial edge of the internal carotid artery	Midline

SCM: sternocleidomastoid muscle; RP: retropharyngeal.
Source: Grégoire *et al.* 2003 [6]. Reproduced with permission of Elsevier.

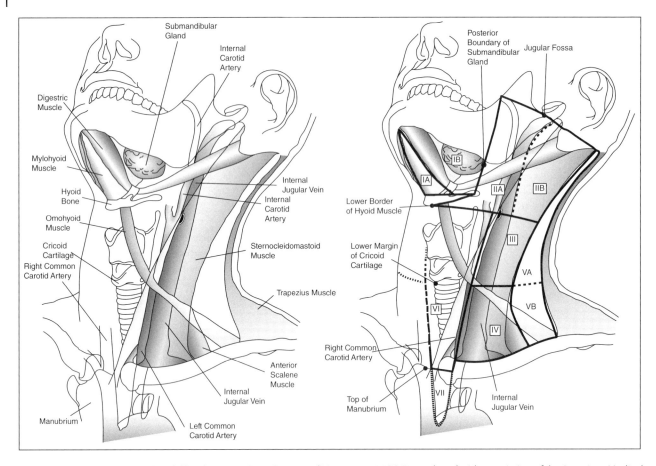

Figure 10.2 Neck anatomy and nodal levels. *Source:* Som, Curtin, and Mancuso 1999 [3]. Reproduced with permission of the American Medical Association.

The HPV status of the SCCA has become an important prognostic marker, and is routinely required for most clinical trials involving oropharyngeal cancer. HPV-positive SCCA express the viral oncoproteins E6 and E7, overexpress p16 (often used as a surrogate for HPV infection for immunohistochemistry), and usually lack p53 mutations [20]. Pathologic findings for HPV-positive SCCA include basaloid morphology, infiltrating lymphocytes, and a lack of significant keratinization. Lymph node metastases often have a cystic appearance on pathology and imaging. HPV-negative SCCA typically is keratinizing and often has mutant p53.

Patterns of Spread

Local spread of oropharyngeal tumors can lead to trismus, decreased tongue mobility, speech and swallowing deficits. Cervical lymph node involvement is also common due to the rich lymphatic system of the oropharynx. Lymphatic drainage of oropharyngeal cancers for all subsites is primarily to level II. The distribution of neck metastasis from head and neck cancers was reported by Lindberg in his landmark series of patients from

M. D. Anderson with clinically positive necks [21]. Lindbergh noted increasing nodal involvement and bilateral involvement with increasing tumor size. The percentage of patients with clinically positive necks by subsite is presented in Table 10.2.

Candela and coworkers also reported on a series of oropharyngeal cancer patients with clinically negative necks (N0) and positive necks from Memorial Sloan-Kettering Cancer Center who underwent radical neck dissection; the study results are summarized in Table 10.3 [22]. Even in patients with a clinically negative neck, metastasis to level II was common. In clinically N0

Table 10.2 Percentage of patients with clinically positive necks by subsite.

Subsite	Node-positive/total	Percentage
BOT	144/185	78
Soft palate	35/80	44
Tonsillar fossa	106/140	76
Oropharyngeal walls	88/149	59

Source: Lindberg 1972 [21]. Reproduced with permission of John Wiley & Sons.

Table 10.3 Distribution of nodal metastases in oropharyngeal cancer.

Site (level)	I	II	III	IV	V	Total
Clinically positive neck						
BOT and vallecula	17%	70%	42%	31%	9.3%	87%
Tonsillar region and LPW	10%	72%	41%	21%	8.6%	76%
Clinically negative neck (N0)						
Site (level)	I	II	III	IV	V	Total
BOT and vallecula	3.7%	30%	22%	7.4%	0	33%
Tonsillar region and LPW	0	19%	14%	9.5%	4.8%	29%

BOT, base of tongue; LPW, lateral pharyngeal wall.
Source: Candela, Kothari, and Shah 1990 [22]. Reproduced with permission of John Wiley & Sons.

patients, the involvement of levels I and V was a rare finding, occurring in only 1.4% of patients for each level. Skip metastases (e.g., from level I to III without involvement of level II) were also a rare finding.

Retropharyngeal lymph nodes, if involved, are usually clinically occult and can be assessed only by imaging studies. Retropharyngeal nodes are commonly involved in nasopharyngeal cancer, occurring in patients when assessed with computed tomography (CT) or magnetic resonance imaging (MRI) [23, 24]. While less common in other head and neck sites, any tumor originating in the pharyngeal walls, or a tumor that extends locally to the pharyngeal wall, has a high likelihood of retropharyngeal lymph node metastasis [25]. When Bussels and colleagues reported on the incidence of retropharyngeal lymph node metastasis in oropharyngeal cancer [26], the overall incidence was 16%, and was highest for posterior pharyngeal wall (38%) and soft palate (56%). Involvement of retropharyngeal lymph nodes has also been associated with higher rates of regional recurrence [27]. The retropharyngeal lymph nodes are divided into lateral and medial groups, with involvement of the medial retropharyngeal nodes being extremely rare [28].

Clinical Presentation

Presenting signs and symptoms for oropharyngeal cancer patients often vary depending on which subsite is involved. A common complaint is a persistent sore throat, or patients may have the sensation of something being stuck in their throats. A painless, enlarging, neck mass is also a common presentation, and patients have often undergone antibiotic therapy before being referred to a head and neck surgeon.

Patients with locally advanced disease can present with trismus due to pterygoid muscle invasion, odynophagia, voice changes ('hot potato voice'), or weight loss secondary to dysphagia and/or odynophagia. Detectable distant metastasis at first presentation is not common, and if it occurs is most often noted as pulmonary nodules.

Otalgia is a common complaint among patients presenting with locally advanced head and neck cancer. The otalgia is due to referred pain via the auricular (Arnold) and tympanic (Jacobson) nerves which join cranial nerves IX and X, respectively (Figure 10.3) [29].

Patient Evaluation

A complete evaluation begins with a thorough history and physical examination. Particularly helpful are questions related to difficulty with swallowing or speech, weight loss, pain, tongue and jaw mobility, as well as a review of systems that encompasses possible distant sites of disease such as the liver and lung. Physical examination should include a detailed inspection of the oral mucosa, noting the location, size and extent of the tumor as well as the state of the patient's dentition. A mirror examination is helpful in visualizing more posterior and inferior lesions such as the base of tongue. Attention to the color of the mucosa is also important as lesions may extend superficially, producing some erythematous changes that should be included in the radiation therapy treatment plan. Palpation of the oral mucosa can help identify the submucosal extent of lesions. Tongue mobility and whether trismus is present should be assessed as these can indicate involvement of the tongue musculature and the pterygoid muscles, respectively. The neck and supraclavicular region should be carefully inspected and palpated to assess for nodal metastasis with documentation of nodal size, mobility, and anatomic level. Patients should also undergo fiberoptic endoscopy for a better assessment of areas difficult to visualize directly or with a mirror examination. Fiberoptic endoscopy allows for good visualization of the nasopharynx as well as the base of tongue, vallecula, and larynx for assessment of local tumor extension, as well as possible synchronous primary tumors.

An examination under anesthesia by a head and neck surgeon is helpful in determining the extent of disease. Since many patients have a history of significant tobacco and alcohol use, head and neck surgeons may also

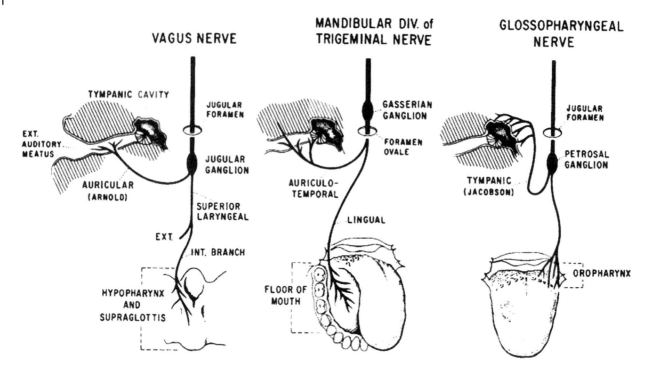

Figure 10.3 Pathways of referred otalgia related to various tumor sites.

perform a bronchoscopy and esophagoscopy to evaluate for potential synchronous primaries in other parts of the aerodigestive tract. Biopsies should be directed at suspicious lesions and fine-needle aspiration; alternately, a core biopsy should be performed with patients presenting with nodal disease without a clear primary site. HPV testing by direct or surrogate methods (e.g., p16 by immunohistochemistry) is required for a complete pathologic assessment of an oropharyngeal cancer, since evidence of an HPV-associated tumor is a good prognostic factor.

Imaging of the head and neck should at least include a contrast-enhanced CT scan. Lymph nodes that have filling defects on imaging, level II lymph nodes that are >1.5 cm in size, or lymph nodes at other levels that are >1 cm in size, should be considered malignant unless pathologic information is discordant. MRI is useful in visualizing fascial planes, muscle invasion, nerve involvement, and depth of invasion [30]. Park and colleagues showed MRI to be an accurate method for evaluating the depth of tumor invasion in the oral cavity and oropharynx, and was also predictive of nodal metastasis [31]. Metabolic imaging (e.g., PET) is increasingly being used for staging and treatment planning [32]. PET/CT imaging is more accurate than CT/MRI at detecting primary tumors, nodal metastasis, and distant disease [33–35]. A meta-analysis conducted by Al-braheem and coworkers showed that PET was able to detect the primary site of disease in 28% of patients with an unknown

primary and with an initial negative work-up [35]. Chest x-radiography is indicated in all patients and CT imaging of the chest is recommended in patients with T3/T4 lesions, nodal disease, or concerning symptoms/signs.

Basic blood parameters should be monitored, including a complete blood count, basic chemistries, and liver function tests for evaluation prior to surgery or chemotherapy. Head and neck radiotherapy often results in xerostomia, which leads to accelerated tooth decay. All patients should have a full dental evaluation prior to the start of radiation, with all necessary extractions performed prior to treatment. Fluoride treatments should begin post-treatment to prevent tooth decay. An evaluation of speech and swallowing should also be performed. Patients should be assessed for tobacco use and alcohol dependence, and provided with appropriate counseling and access to cessation programs. Patients should also be evaluated by a dietician for nutritional status.

Staging

Oropharyngeal cancer is staged according to the American Joint Commission on Cancer (AJCC), 8th edition [34]. Staging should be based on both examination findings and available imaging. Staging is based on tumor size, extent of invasion, the number, laterality, and size of regional lymph nodes, and the presence of distant metastasis (TNM staging). Changes from the AJCC

Table 10.4 AJCC 2017 staging for oropharyngeal cancer (HPV negative disease).

Primary Tumor (T)

TX	Primary tumor cannot be assessed
T0	No evidence of primary tumor
Tis	Carcinoma *in situ*
T1	Tumor ≤2 cm in greatest dimension
T2	Tumor >2 cm but ≤4 cm in greatest dimension
T3	Tumor >4 cm in greatest dimension or extension to the lingual surface of epiglottis
T4a	Moderately advanced local disease. Tumor invades the larynx, extrinsic muscle of the tongue (genioglossus, hyoglossus, styloglossus, or palatoglossus m.), medial pterygoid m., hard palate, or mandible.
T4b	Very advanced local disease. Tumor invades lateral pterygoid m., pterygoid plates, lateral nasopharynx, or skull base or encases carotid artery.

Regional Lymph Nodes (N)

NX	Regional lymph nodes cannot be assessed
N0	No regional lymph node metastasis
N1	Metastasis in a single ipsilateral lymph node, ≤3 cm in greatest dimension and ENE (−)
N2a	Metastasis in a single ipsilateral lymph node >3 cm but ≤6 cm in greatest dimension and ENE (−)
N2b	Metastasis in multiple ipsilateral lymph nodes, none >6 cm in greatest dimension and ENE (−)
N2c	Metastasis in bilateral or contralateral lymph nodes, none >6 cm in greatest dimension and ENE (−)
N3a	Metastasis in a lymph node >6 cm in greatest dimension and ENE (−)
N3b	Metastasis in any node(s) and clinically overt ENE (+)

Note: Metastases at level VII are considered regional lymph node metastasis, not distant.

Distant Metastasis (M)

M0	No distant metastasis
M1	Distant metastasis

Stage Grouping

Stage	T	N	M
0	Tis	0	0
I	T1	0	0
II	T2	0	0
III	T3	0	0
	T1-3	N1	0
IVA	T4a	N0-2	0
	T1-3	N2	0
IVB	T4b	Any N	0
	Any T	N3	0
IVC	Any T	Any N	1

Source: AJCC Cancer Staging Manual, Eighth Edition (2017), Springer, New York, Inc.

2002 staging system include the division of T4 into T4a (moderately advanced local disease) and T4b (very advanced local disease). The AJCC 2017 staging system for HPV negative disease is shown in Table 10.4.

The previous AJCC stage grouping for oropharyngeal cancer was developed mostly basing on HPV-negative disease. HPV-positive oropharyngeal cancer has a significant better local regional control and survival. Therefore, the previous AJCC stage grouping does not fit in these patients [37, 38]. Ang *et al.* [16], using data from RTOG 0129, divided oropharyngeal cancer into three risk groups based on HPV status, smoking history, T stage, and N stage. HPV-positive patients with less than 10 pack-years of smoking (PYS) were classified as the

ICON-S stage classification	T1	T2	T3	T4
N0	I	I	II	III
N1	I	I	II	III
N2	II	II	II	III
N3	III	III	III	III

Figure 10.4 Proposed ICON-S stage tabulation grid for 8th edition TNM. Note that distant metastatic disease (M1) is considered stage IV.

low-risk group. HPV-positive patients with more than 10 PYS and had N0-N2a disease were also classified as a low-risk group. The three-year overall survival (OS) for the low-risk patients was 93.0%. HPV-positive patients with more than 10 PYS and N2b-N3 disease were classified as an intermediate-risk group. HPV-negative patients with less than 10 PYS and T2-3 disease were also classified as intermediate risk. The three-year OS for the low-risk patients was 70.8%. HPV-negative patients with more than 10 PYS or with T4 tumor, regardless of their smoking history, were classified as a high-risk group, with a three-year OS of only 46.2%. Huang *et al.* [37], using recursive partitioning analysis (RPA), analyzed 573 HPV-positive oropharyngeal cancers treated at Princess Margaret Hospital from 2000 to 2010. HPV-related oropharyngeal cancers were divided into RPA-I (T1-3N0-2b), RPA-II (T1-3N2c), and RPA-III (T4 or N3; five-year OS: 82%, 76%, and 54%, respectively; $P = 0.001$). A further RPA (including RPA stage, age, and PYS) derived the following four valid prognostic groups for survival: group I (T1-3N0-N2c, and <20 PYS); group II (T1-3N0-N2c, and more than 20 PYS); group III (T4 or N3, age ≤70 years); and group IVA (T4 or N3, age >70 years; five-year OS: 89%, 64%, 57%, and 40%, respectively; $P = 0.001$). Recently, the International Collaboration on Oropharyngeal Cancer Network for Staging (ICON-S) developed and validated a staging system for HPV-related oropharyngeal cancer [38]. A total of 1907 patients with HPV+ oropharyngeal cancer were recruited, 661 at the training center and 1246 at the validation centers. They found that the 5-year overall survival was similar for 7th edition TNM stage I, II, III, and IVA, suggesting 7th AJCC edition staging is not suitable for HPV+ oropharyngeal cancer. Since 5-year overall survival was similar among N1, N2a, and N2b, they were merged into one category as ICON-S N1. They re-termed the 7th edition N categories as follows: ICON-S N0, no lymph nodes; ICON-S N1, ipsilateral lymph nodes; ICON-S N2, bilateral or contralateral lymph nodes; and ICON-S N3, lymph nodes larger than 6 cm. These new N categories are similar to those for nasopharyngeal cancer. There was no difference in 5-year overall survival between T4a and T4b tumors, they suggested that T4 was no longer subdivided. Based on these and using adjusted hazard ratios (AHR) modeling, the entire cohort of 1907 patients with HPV+

oropharyngeal cancer were divided into ICON-S stage I (n = 962; T1-T2N0-N1), ICON-S stage II (n = 564; T1-T2N2 or T3N0-N2), and ICON-S stage III (N = 381; T4 or N3). Patients who had distant metastatic disease (M1) were classified as ICON-S stage IV because of adverse prognosis irrespective of T and N category. Figure 10.4 summarizes the ICON-S stage for HPV positive oropharyngeal cancer which represents the proposed 8th edition TNM stage.

General Management Principles

Management of oropharyngeal cancer is best approached by a multidisciplinary team of surgeons, radiation oncologists, and medical oncologists. The main goals of therapy should be loco-regional tumor control and preserving the functions of the oropharynx. Early T stage lesions (T1-T2) can be successfully managed with surgery followed by post-operative radiotherapy if indicated by appropriate pathologic features or with radiation therapy alone [39]. Surgery can provide pathologic information but if the procedure is expected to result in a poor functional outcome (e.g. difficulty with speech or swallowing), radiotherapy is the preferred modality.

Locally-advanced lesions (T3-T4) are generally managed with definitive radiotherapy with concurrent chemotherapy as surgery often would result in significant morbidity and substantial loss of function. However, in appropriate-selected cases surgery can be employed followed by post-operative radiotherapy [40, 41]. Post-operative chemoradiation is indicated in patients with high-risk pathologic features (e.g. extracapsular extension or positive margins).

Brachytherapy can also be used in the definitive management of oropharyngeal cancer either as the primary treatment or a boost but is not the focus of this chapter [42–47].

These strategies are discussed in more detail in the following sections.

Early T-Stage Disease

Early T stage disease (T1–T2) can be managed with surgery alone ± adjuvant radiotherapy, or with radiotherapy alone ± neck dissection. The choice of the primary modality should be based on achieving the highest rate of tumor control while maintaining organ function as much as possible. There are no randomized trials to provide guidance on the initial choice of modality. Parsons and coworkers examined a reported series of oropharyngeal cancer that employed either surgery ± adjuvant radiotherapy or definitive radiotherapy ± neck dissection [48]. A total of 51 series including approximately 6400 patients was analyzed. For BOT tumors who underwent surgery ± adjuvant radiotherapy versus radiotherapy ± neck dissection, local control was 79% versus 76% (p = 0.087); five-year survival 49% versus 52% (p = 0.2); severe complications 32% versus 3.8% (p = 0.001); and fatal complications 3.5% versus 0.4% (p = 0.001). For patients with tonsillar cancer, the results were: local control 70% versus 68% (p = 0.2); five-year survival 47% versus 43% (p = 0.2); severe complications 23% versus 6% (p = 0.001); and fatal complications 3.2% versus 0.8% (p = 0.001). These data suggest that definitive radiotherapy ± neck dissection should be the primary modality for most patients with oropharyngeal cancer, as definitive radiotherapy provides similar local control and survival rates as surgery but with significantly less severe and fatal complications.

However, this study included series published before 2000, when most surgical patients had traditional open surgery. Recently, with the development of minimally invasive surgery with trans-oral laser microsurgery (TLM) or trans-oral robotic surgery (TORS), and with improvements in perioperative care, severe surgical complications have significantly decreased. TLM or TORS and selective neck dissection is a reasonable option for patients with a small primary tumor, especially those with HPV-positive cancer [49, 50].

Tonsillar Cancer

Early T-stage cancer of the tonsillar fossa can present as a well-lateralized lesion. If the contralateral neck is not involved at presentation, there is no significant extension towards midline or involvement of the BOT, and no advanced nodal disease (N0-N1), the patient can undergo surgery alone with ipsilateral selective neck dissection level I–IV or radiation treatment alone.

For patients treated with radiation, the treatment can be directed towards the primary site of disease and ipsilateral neck. This treatment approach spares contralateral structures and decreases morbidity. Jackson and coworkers reported on 178 patients with SCCA of the tonsil who were treated to the ipsilateral neck only [51]; patients were generally treated to 60 Gy at 2.4 Gy per fraction. The authors reported a local control rate of 84% for T1 and T2 tumors. Of the 101 patients with N0 disease, only two developed contralateral nodal recurrences. O'Sullivan reported on the Princess Margaret

Hospital experience [52], whereby 228 patients (the majority with T1 or T2 and N0 disease) were treated with an ipsilateral technique the contralateral failure rate was only 3.5%. The majority of patients were treated with a wedged-pair technique designed to encompass the primary tumor and the ipsilateral level II lymph nodes. Level III and IV lymph node levels were treated with an anterior hemi-neck matched field. The typical prescription was 50 Gy in 20 fractions to the primary tumor. The authors noted that there were no contralateral failures among patients with T1 disease. For all stages, most of the contralateral failures were in patients whose tumor extended into the soft palate or BOT. Rusthoven and colleagues reported their experience with ipsilateral treatment using more modern techniques with 3D conformal radiotherapy or IMRT [53]. In this case, 20 patients with well-lateralized disease were treated either definitively or adjuvantly. Two patients had T3 disease, 13 had N2b disease, 80% underwent tonsillectomy, and 19 patients received chemotherapy. Treatment was to the primary tumor and ipsilateral neck to 66–70 Gy for definitive treatment, and 60–66 Gy for postoperative patients. Rusthoven and coworkers reported no in-field failures or contralateral nodal failures. The two-year disease-free survival and OS were both 79.5%.

Collectively these studies demonstrate that carefully selected patients with T1-2 and N0-N1 disease can be successfully treated with ipsilateral radiation alone. However, if the tumor is noted to invade the BOT or significantly involve the soft palate, the patient should undergo comprehensive radiation. The American College of Radiology appropriateness criteria state that ipsilateral radiotherapy is appropriate only for patients with <1 cm of invasion into the BOT or soft palate and who have N0 or N1 disease [54].

Base of Tongue

The BOT is functionally important in phonation and swallowing. Patients with small primary tumor can have surgery with ipsilateral selective neck dissection level I–IV with/without adjuvant radiation, depending on the pathology or definitive radiation treatment.

Radiotherapy can provide good local control for early-stage disease while avoiding the complications of surgery. Mendenhall reported on 333 patients with BOT tumors treated with definitive radiotherapy [55], and found the local control rates at five years to be: T1, 98%; T2, 92%; T3, 82%; and T4, 53%. Seleck *et al.* summarized the M. D. Anderson experience using definitive radiotherapy in the management of T1 and T2 BOT tumors, and reported a five-year local control rate of 83% [56]. Wang *et al.* reported on 169 patients with SCCA of the BOT who were treated at Massachusetts General Hospital [57], and found that T1 and T2 tumors treated with once- or twice-daily definitive radiotherapy had five-year local control rates of 79% and 85%, respectively.

Soft Palate

The soft palate is important for phonation and swallowing, and is difficult to reconstruct after surgery. Thus, radiotherapy is often preferred in disease management as it results in less structural compromise. Chera and coworkers reported their experience with 145 patients who underwent definitive radiotherapy for soft palate tumors [58]. The median dose given to the primary site was 70.4 Gy, and 10 patients received induction or concurrent chemotherapy. Local control rates at five years by T stage were: T1, 90%; T2, 91%; T3, 67%; and T4, 57%. Seleck reported on using definitive radiotherapy in the management of T1 and T2 soft palate lesions and reported a five-year local control rate of 85% [56].

Pharyngeal Wall

The pharyngeal wall is an uncommon primary subsite. The University of Florida reported on 148 patients with SCCA of the pharyngeal wall (37% oropharynx) managed with definitive radiotherapy with or without planned neck dissection [59]. Eleven patients received induction or concurrent chemotherapy. The five-year rates of local control by T stage were: T1, 93%; T2, 82%; T3, 59%; and T4, 50%. Seleck reported the M. D. Anderson experience using definitive radiotherapy in the management of T1 and T2 lesions [56], and found that 20 patients with posterior oropharyngeal wall tumors had an 88% local control rate at five years.

Together, these data demonstrate that definitive radiotherapy can provide excellent local control for early-stage lesions, while avoiding some of the complications and functional compromise associated with surgery.

Locally Advanced Oropharyngeal Cancer

Chemoradiotherapy

For patients with large primary tumors or with extensive nodal disease, the addition of chemotherapy to radiation is needed to increase local-regional control and OS. This approach also allows for more patients to have organ preservation. Platinum-based chemotherapy is preferred, and single-agent cisplatin with concurrent radiation is the current standard of care. Platinum-based regimens combined with 5-fluorouracil (5-FU) or a taxane are also acceptable. This recommendation derives from several randomized trials incorporating concurrent chemotherapy with radiation, which demonstrated improved treatment outcomes.

The RTOG conducted a Phase I/II study (RTOG 81-17) of concurrent cisplatin and radiotherapy in patients with unresectable head and neck cancer which demonstrated the tolerability and efficacy of the regimen [60, 61]. These results led to larger Phase III randomized trials using concurrent platinum-based chemotherapy regimens and radiotherapy. Adelstein and coworkers reported the results of an intergroup study where patients with unresectable head and neck cancer were randomized to one of three arms: 70 Gy in 35 fractions of radiotherapy alone; 70 Gy with concurrent cisplatin (100 mg m^{-2}) × three cycles; or to a split course of 30 Gy + 30–40 Gy with concurrent cisplatin and 5-FU × three cycles [62]. The three-year OS was 23%, 37%, and 27%, respectively (p = 0.014, radiotherapy alone and concurrent cisplatin arms). Toxicity was increased in the concurrent chemoradiation arms when compared to the radiotherapy alone arm. The significant improvement in OS with concurrent cisplatin led to this regimen becoming the standard of care in locally advanced oropharyngeal cancer. GORTEC 94-01 was a French study of 226 patients with stage III and IV oropharyngeal cancer who were randomized to 70 Gy in 35 fractions with or without the addition of carboplatin and 5-FU × three cycles [63]. Toxicity was significantly higher in the chemoradiation arm. Concurrent chemoradiotherapy improved the three-year locoregional control from 42% to 66% (p = 0.03), and also improved OS from 31% to 51% (p = 0.02). Several groups have also reported the results of concurrent chemoradiation versus radiation alone; the details of selected studies are presented in Table 10.5.

Further evidence for the benefit of concurrent chemoradiation comes from the Meta-Analysis of Chemotherapy on Head Neck Cancer (MACH-NC), which was initially reported in 2000 and subsequently updated in 2009 [70]. The updated meta-analysis included 87 trials with a total of 16 485 patients, and showed a statistically significant benefit in survival upon the addition of chemotherapy to radiation. Concurrent chemoradiation also appeared to be superior to induction or adjuvant chemotherapy. The five-year absolute survival benefit for concurrent chemotherapy was 6.5% compared to 2.4 % with induction chemotherapy. A subsequent analysis by tumor site echoed the benefit for oropharyngeal cancer patients, with an absolute survival benefit at five years being 8.1% [71]. The timing of chemotherapy also appeared to remain important for oropharyngeal cancer patients, with the hazard ratio for death being 0.78 in the concurrent chemotherapy group and 1.00 in the induction chemotherapy subset.

Biologic Therapy and Radiation

Cytotoxic chemotherapy given concurrently with radiation is the standard of care in organ-preserving definitive

Table 10.5 Select studies of concurrent chemoradiation and/or altered fractionation for locally advanced oropharyngeal cancer.

Study/Reference	No. of patients	% with OP cancer	Treatment	Time (years)	LC/LRC (%)	DFS/PFS (%)	OS (%)
Intergroup (Adelstein et al.) [62]	295	56%	RT: 70 Gy/35 fx CRT: 70 Gy/35 fx + cisplatin × 3 cycles CRT: split 30 Gy + 30–40 Gy + cisplatin/5-FU × 3 cycles	3	NR	NR	23 37 (SS) 27
GORTEC 94-01 (Calais et al.) [63]	226	100%	RT: 70 Gy/35fx CRT: 70 Gy/35fx + carboplatin/5-FU × 3 cycles	3	42 66 (SS)	20 42 (SS)	31 51 (SS)
Brizel et al. [64]	116	49%	AFX: 75 Gy @ 1.25 Gy BID → adjuvant cisplatin/5-FU × 2 cycles AFX/CRT: 70 Gy @ 1.25 Gy BID + cisplatin/5-FU × 2 cycles → adjuvant cisplatin/5-FU × 2 cycles	3	44 70 (SS)	41 61	34 55
Huguenin et al. [65]	224	53%	AFX: 74.4 Gy @ 1.2 Gy BID AFX/CRT: 74.4 Gy @ 1.2 Gy BID + cisplatin × 2 cycles	5	33 51 (SS)	24 27	32 46
FNCLCC-GORTEC (Bensadoun et al.) [66]	163	75%	AFX: 80.4 Gy @ 1.2 Gy BID AFX/CRT: 80.4 Gy @ 1.2 Gy BID + cisplatin/5-FU × 3 cycles	2	60 79	25 48	20 38
DAHANCA 6/7 (Overgaard et al.) [67]	1485	28% pharynx	RT: 66–68 Gy/33–34 fx, 5 days/week + nimorazole AFX: 66–68/33–34 fx, 6 days/week + nimorazole	5	60 70	NR	OR 0.98
RTOG 90-03 (Fu et al.) [68]	1073	60%	RT: 70 Gy/35 fx AFX: 81.6 Gy @1.2 Gy BID AFX: 67.2 Gy @ 1.6 Gy BID – split course AFX: 72 Gy with concomitant boost	2	46 54 48 55	32 38 33 39	46 55 46 51
Bonner et al. [69]	424	60%	RT alone (daily, BID, or concomitant boost) CRT: RT + cetuximab × 8 weeks	3	34 47	31 42	45 55

AFX: altered fractionation schedule; CRT: chemoradiotherapy; DFS/PFS: disease-free survival or progression-free survival; LC/LRC: local control or loco-regional control; NR: not reported; OP: oropharyngeal; OR: odds ratio; OS: overall survival; RT, radiotherapy.

therapy for advanced oropharyngeal cancer. However, these agents add additional toxicity and morbidity to the treatment, and consequently much research has been focused on identifying specific targets for biologic therapies with the hope of increasing tumor control while minimizing adverse effects. SCCAs of the head and neck express high levels of EGFR, and the chimeric monoclonal antibody cetuximab (C225) has been shown to induce changes in the cell cycle of SCCA cell lines and act as a radiosensitizer [72, 73]. A landmark randomized clinical trial conducted by Bonner and coworkers investigated the use of cetuximab (400 mg m^{-2} loading dose followed by seven weekly doses of 250 mg m^{-2} during radiation) in patients with locally advanced head and neck cancer. Patients were treated to 70–78.6 Gy using a conventional, twice-daily, or concomitant boost fractionation schedule. The majority of patients had

oropharyngeal cancers. The addition of cetuximab to radiation demonstrated a significant improvement in locoregional control as well as OS, especially in the oropharyngeal cancer subgroup [74]. The five-year overall survival was 46% and 36% in the cetuximab + radiotherapy and radiotherapy arms, respectively (p = 0.018) [69]. Significant adverse effects were similar between the two groups, with the exception of an acneiform rash which is a common occurrence in patients treated with cetuximab. Interestingly, a more severe acneiform rash was associated with increased OS (p = 0.002).

Given that combining cetuximab or cisplatin with radiotherapy leads to improvements in survival, the RTOG conducted a randomized trial, RTOG 0522, to test the hypothesis that using the two agents simultaneously with radiotherapy could further improve treatment outcomes [75]. This Phase III trial randomized

940 patients to concurrent cisplatin × two cycles and radiotherapy (Arm A) versus concurrent cisplatin × two cycles and radiotherapy plus cetuximab (Arm B). However, the study demonstrated no advantage when cetuximab was added to the cisplatin regimen. No differences were found between arms A and B in 30-day mortality (1.8% versus 2.0%, respectively; $P = 0.81$), three-year progress-free survival (61.2% versus 58.9%, respectively; $P = 0.76$), three-year OS (72.9% versus 75.8%, respectively; $P = 0.32$), locoregional failure (19.9% versus 25.9%, respectively; $P = 0.97$), or distant metastasis (13.0% versus 9.7%, respectively; $P = 0.08$). Furthermore, the experimental arm resulted in more skin toxicity and mucositis. Hence, radiotherapy with concurrent cisplatin remains the standard of care in patients able to tolerate cytotoxic chemotherapy. Cetuximab-based therapy with radiation is reserved for patients who are not medically fit enough for traditional chemotherapies.

Altered Fractionation

Several groups have investigated altered fractionation treatment regimens (other than once daily 1.8–2.0 Gy fractionation) in an effort to improve local tumor control. Hyperfractionation has been explored as a way of exploiting differences in tumor and normal tissue biology, theoretically allowing for dose escalation without increasing late complications. In theory, accelerated fractionation (treatment schemes used to decrease the total treatment time) should minimize SCCA repopulation during treatment and result in increased tumor control.

RTOG 90-03 was a randomized study investigating altered fractionation treatment regimens [68]. Patients with locally advanced head and neck cancer were randomized to either conventional radiation to 70 Gy in 35 daily fractions or to one of three experimental arms: hyperfractionation/dose escalation to 81.6 Gy, given at 1.2 Gy per fraction, twice daily; accelerated fractionation/split-course to 67.2 Gy delivered at 1.6 Gy per fraction, twice daily with a two-week break; and accelerated radiotherapy by a concomitant boost to 72 Gy with a second treatment given daily to the boost field (1.8 Gy + 1.5 Gy to boost) for the final 12 fractions. Patients treated with hyperfractionation or the concomitant boost technique had better outcomes than those treated with conventional fractionation. The split-course regimen did not lead to improved outcomes. The two-year local-regional control for the conventional fractionation arm was 46% versus 54% (p = 0.045) for the hyperfractionation arm, and 55% (p = 0.05) for the accelerated fractionation/concomitant boost arm. Differences in OS between the trial arms were not significant. The acute affects were more severe in the experimental arms but this did not translate into increased late effects.

The Danish Head and Neck Cancer Study Group (DAHANCA) conducted trials (DAHANCA 6 and 7) examining the effect of shortening overall treatment time [67]. Patients were treated to 66–68 Gy in 33–34 fractions, but were randomized to either five treatments per week or accelerated treatment given in six treatments per week. Patients also received the hypoxic radiosensitizer nimorazole. At five years, patients in the accelerated group had significant improvement in locoregional control (70% versus 60%, p = 0.0005) and disease-specific survival (73% versus 63%, p = 0.01) compared to the conventional five-treatment-per week schedule.

Bourhis and coworkers performed a meta-analysis with over 6500 patients to compare conventional fractionation with hyperfractionation and/or accelerated fractionation regimens. Altered fractionation showed an absolute survival benefit of 3.5% at five years (p = 0.003) [76]. The absolute benefit was most pronounced for patients undergoing hyperfractionated regimens, with an absolute benefit of 8%. Locoregional control was also improved with an absolute benefit of 6.4% (p < 0.0001).

Concurrent chemotherapy and altered fractionation schemes both result in improved outcomes. Consequently, some groups have examined the possibility of combining altered fractionation schemes with concurrent chemotherapy in an effort to further improve patient outcomes. GORTEC 99-02 randomized 840 patients to one of three arms: conventional radiotherapy and concurrent chemotherapy with carboplatin/5-FU; accelerated radiotherapy (70 Gy in six weeks) and concurrent chemotherapy with carboplatin/5-FU; or very accelerated radiotherapy alone (64.8 Gy given at 1.8 Gy twice daily) [77]. The three-year progression-free survival was 37.6% after conventional chemoradiation, 34.1% after accelerated chemoradiation, and 32.2% after very accelerated radiotherapy. Accelerated radiotherapy with concurrent chemotherapy did not improve progression-free survival over conventional chemoradiation (HR 1.02, p = 0.88). More patients in the very accelerated radiotherapy arm had RTOG grade 3–4 acute mucosal toxicity compared with the accelerated chemoradiation arm or the conventional chemoradiotherapy arm. The RTOG also performed a randomized trial (RTOG 0129) of 743 patients comparing conventionally fractionated chemoradiation (70 Gy over seven weeks with three cycles of cisplatin) with a concomitant boost chemoradiation regimen (72 Gy over six weeks with two cycles of cisplatin) [78]. At a median follow-up of 7.9 years (range: 0.3 to 10.1 years) for 355 surviving patients, no differences were observed in OS (HR 0.96; 95% CI 0.79–1.18; $P = 0.37$; eight-year survival 48% versus 48%), progress-free survival (HR 1.02; 95% CI 0.84–1.24; $P = 0.52$; eight-year estimate 42% versus 41%), locoregional failure (HR 1.08; 95% CI 0.84–1.38; $P = 0.78$; eight-year estimate 37% versus 39%), or distant metastasis (HR 0.83; 95%

CI 0.56–1.24; $P = 0.16$; eight-year estimate 15% versus 13%). Taken together, the results of these trials support standard fractionation with concurrent platinum-based chemotherapy as the standard of care in locally advanced head and neck cancer. Altered fractionation combined with chemotherapy did not improve outcomes and led to increased toxicity.

Induction Chemotherapy

Many clinical trials have been previously reported with cisplatin-based induction chemotherapy. Although there were good responses of the tumor to chemotherapy, there was no benefit in final treatment outcomes, especially in OS. Recently, there has been a surge in interest in induction chemotherapy with taxane-based regimens, which have shown to be active in SCCA of the head and neck. The Eastern Cooperative Oncology Group performed a prospective Phase II trial (E2399) of induction paclitaxel and carboplatin followed by concurrent chemoradiation to 70 Gy with paclitaxel [79]. Organ preservation and OS for oropharyngeal cancer patients at two years were 84% and 83%, respectively. Also noteworthy was that data on HPV status were collected prospectively, and patients with HPV-positive cancers had better response rates to induction chemotherapy and had markedly improved two-year OS rates of 95% compared to 62% in patients with HPV-negative cancers (p = 0.005) [80].

Two large randomized trials have compared the addition of a taxane to platinum and 5-FU (TPF) to the historic platinum and 5-FU combination (PF) alone for induction chemotherapy. The TAX 323 study randomized patients to induction PF versus TPF for four cycles, followed by radiotherapy (without concurrent chemotherapy) to a dose of 66–74 Gy [81]. A significant advantage was seen for the TPF group in terms of progression-free survival and OS. The TAX 324 trial randomized patients to induction PF versus TPF for three cycles, followed by concurrent carboplatin and radiation to a dose of 70–74 Gy [82]. Posner and colleagues also reported significantly better outcomes for the TPF arm in locoregional control as well as OS. No significant difference was noted in distant failures. These studies demonstrated the benefit of adding a taxane to the traditional PF induction chemotherapy, but did not address whether the induction strategy is superior to concurrent chemoradiotherapy alone.

Two Phase III studies have been reported which compared sequential therapy (induction chemotherapy followed by concurrent chemoradiation) with the standard of care, namely upfront concurrent chemoradiation. The PARADIGM trial randomized 145 patients to either sequential therapy (induction TPF for three cycles followed by concurrent chemoradiation with either carboplatin or docetaxel), or to upfront concurrent chemoradiation alone with two cycles of cisplatin [83]. Despite the less-intensive chemotherapy regimen in the upfront concurrent chemoradiation arm, there was no difference in observed three-year OS (73% in the sequential arm versus 78% in the upfront chemoradiation arm, p = 0.77) or three-year progression-free survival (67% versus 73%, p = 0.55). In the DeCIDE study, 285 patients with N2/N3 disease were randomized to receive sequential therapy with TPF induction chemotherapy for two cycles, followed by concurrent chemoradiation with TP, and hydroxyurea with twice-daily radiotherapy versus upfront concurrent radiotherapy with the same TP and hydroxyurea regimen [84]. Patients in the sequential therapy arm experienced more hematologic toxicity. No difference in three-year OS was observed (75% in the sequential arm versus 73% in the upfront chemoradiation arm, p = 0.7). Fewer distant recurrences occurred in the sequential group, but the difference was not statistically significant (19 versus 29; $P = 0.11$). The results of these recently reported trials failed to show any improvement in outcomes with induction chemotherapy, and consequently upfront concurrent chemoradiation with cisplatin should remain the standard of care.

Postoperative Management

For appropriately selected patients, surgery may be the primary therapy undertaken in the management of oropharyngeal cancer. Modern surgical techniques, including TLM and/or TORS allow for the precise resection of tumors while maintaining a better functional status when compared to larger, more morbid, open surgical procedures [85, 86]. Surgery allows for a full assessment of the pathologic features of the tumor. Postoperative radiotherapy is indicated for patients with high-risk features to offer better locoregional control. Indications for postoperative radiotherapy include: positive, close, or uncertain margins; extracapsular extension; N2+ disease; perineural invasion; lymphovascular space invasion; or higher T-stage including extension into bone or muscle [87]. The sequencing of radiation therapy in relation to surgery was investigated in the RTOG 73-03 trial, which randomized patients to preoperative (50 Gy) or postoperative (60 Gy) radiotherapy [88, 89]. Although the locoregional control was significantly better in the postoperative arm of the trial, no significant differences were seen in OS or complication rates.

Postoperative Chemoradiation

Patients with high-risk pathologic features are at increased risk of locoregional failure even with the addition of radiotherapy. Two large randomized trials in Europe and North America investigated the benefits of adding concurrent cisplatin (100 mg m^{-2} on days 1, 22, and 43) to radiotherapy in patients with high-risk pathologic features [90, 91]. The EORTC 22931 trial demonstrated significant improvements in locoregional control (82% versus 69%, p = 0.007), progression-free survival (47% versus 36%, p = 0.04), and OS (53% versus 40% p = 0.02) with the addition of concurrent cisplatin. RTOG 95-01 also favored the concurrent chemoradiation arm with significant improvements in locoregional control (82% versus 72%, p = 0.01) but did not demonstrate a significant difference in OS. Toxicity was increased in both trials by the addition of concurrent chemotherapy. Due to the different eligibility criteria in both trials, a combined analysis was carried out to evaluate which patients would benefit most from the addition of cisplatin to radiotherapy in the postoperative setting [92]. The combined analysis concluded that positive margins and extracapsular extension were most strongly associated with the benefit from chemotherapy, and that these patients should be treated with concurrent cisplatin if medically fit.

The ongoing RTOG 0920 trial [93] is currently examining the addition of cetuximab to radiation in postoperative patients with intermediate-risk factors (lymphovascular space invasion, perineural invasion, N2+, T3, or close margins). The ongoing RTOG 1216 trial is for postoperative patients with high-risk factors including positive margins or extracapsular extension [94]. In this trial, eligible patients are randomized to radiation with either weekly cisplatin, or weekly docetaxel, or weekly cetuximab and docetaxel.

Radiation Therapy Techniques

Conventional Technique

Patients should be CT-simulated supine with the head hyperextended in a thermoplastic head/shoulder mask. A bite block can be used to depress the tongue and separate the upper jaw from the lower jaw so that the dose to the upper jaw is reduced. Intravenous contrast should be utilized. Palpable nodal disease is outlined with a wire. A three-field technique is used with a pair of parallel-opposed lateral fields (upper neck fields) covering the primary tumor and Level II lymph nodes and retropharyngeal nodes if indicated. The anterior border should be at least 2 cm anterior to the primary tumor. In the case of a tonsillar cancer the border should always be anterior to the retromolar trigone. Posteriorly, the border should be placed at the posterior edge of spinous process. The superior border is placed at the skull base. Inferiorly the field edge should be placed above the notch of the thyroid cartilage to match to the anterior lower neck field (Figure 10.5). An anterior-posterior field (lower neck field) encompassing the Level III, Level IV and supraclavicular lymph nodes is matched with the inferior border of the upper neck fields. The isocenter is set at

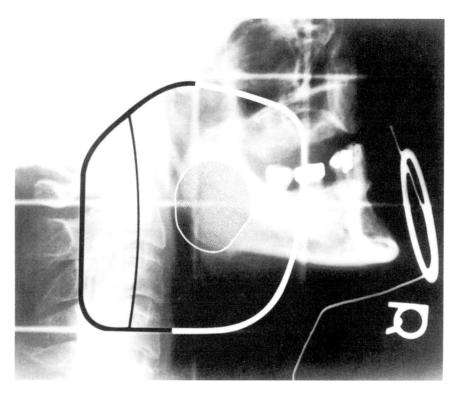

Figure 10.5 Simulation film illustrating portal arrangement and shrinking field off-cord technique with oropharyngeal cancer.

the matching line. A midline laryngeal block is placed in the lower neck field to reduce the dose to the larynx.

The opposed lateral upper neck fields are initially treated to 45 Gy at conventional fraction using 6 MV photons. Then off-cord, the posterior necks are treated with electrons to 50–54 Gy and the anterior necks continued with opposed lateral field to 54 Gy. Subsequently, the primary tumor is treated with a boost with opposed lateral fields that encompassing the primary tumor with a 2 cm margin to bring the final total dose to 70 Gy. The lower neck field is treated to 45–50 Gy. The involved nodes in the lower neck field can then be treated with 3D conformal technique to bring the dose to 70 Gy.

Intensity-Modulated Radiation Therapy (IMRT)

Advances in imaging and computing have allowed for the development of computer-controlled multi-leaf collimators (MLCs) and inverse planning. The use of IMRT techniques is now commonplace in the treatment of head and neck cancers [95]. IMRT planning generates steep dose gradients that allow for a highly conformal treatment to designated targets, and allows the sparing of normal structures uninvolved by tumor [96,97]. These steep dose gradients allow for dose escalation which can potentially lead to better tumor control while also decreasing the side effects from the treatment. The use of IMRT when compared to 3D-conformal techniques has been shown to reduce xerostomia and improve QOL [98–100], and has been confirmed by randomized trial [101]. However, highly conformal plans and steep dose gradients can result in marginal misses and failures. Therefore, IMRT requires a thorough understanding of anatomy and pathways of potential spread.

While IMRT can potentially be used for all oropharyngeal patients, it is important to consider the goals of sparing normal structures and also to understand that the ultimate goal is tumor control and patient survival. Oropharyngeal cancer patients with involvement of bilateral high-level II lymph nodes may not benefit significantly from the use of IMRT due to the adjacent parotid gland. Aggressive sparing of the parotid could lead to underdosing areas which potentially harbor microscopic disease. These patients could also be considered for conventional radiotherapy techniques. Nonetheless, IMRT still has the benefit of treating patients with one single plan and avoids tedious matching and planning multiple times for off-cord fields and boosts.

Several investigators have reported the outcomes of using IMRT in the treatment of oropharyngeal cancer (Table 10.6). RTOG performed a multi-institutional Phase II study (RTOG 0022) of moderately accelerated definitive IMRT alone without chemotherapy in patients with T1-2 and N0-1 oropharyngeal cancer [102]. The primary tumor and involved nodes received 66 Gy, and

subclinical planned target volumes (PTVs) received 54–60 Gy, both in 30 fractions. All patients received bilateral neck radiation. The two-year locoregional failure rate was 9%. It was noted that half of the patients with major protocol underdose deviations experienced locoregional failure. Toxicity with IMRT also appeared to be improved as compared to conventional radiation. A reduction in xerostomia was noted when compared with historical RTOG trials using conventional techniques.

The delineation of target volumes should be based on clinical examination as well as imaging studies. The physical examination is critical, as tumor extension may be present on examination (e.g., extension of erythema into the soft palate or the extent of induration in the BOT) that may not be detected on imaging studies. For patients treated definitively, a gross tumor volume (GTV) should be defined which incorporates the primary tumor as well as involved nodes. A clinical target volume (CTV) is then created by expanding the GTV by 0.5–1.0 cm (CTV1). Apisarnthanarax and coworkers performed a pathologic analysis of 96 dissected nodes and tried to determine the extent of extracapsular extension (ECE) of these nodes [111]. These authors noted that in 96% of the cases the extent of disease was <5 mm from the node capsule, and suggested that adding a 5 mm margin to the node should be sufficient for CTV1. A high-risk CTV is then created that includes the nodal levels that have involved lymph nodes (CTV2), as well as the soft tissue around the primary tumor that may have microscopic disease. An intermediate-risk CTV is contoured which includes levels that are not clinically or radiographically involved with disease but may harbor microscopic disease (CTV3). PPTVs are then created by expanding the CTVs by 0.3–0.5 cm, depending on set-up error(s) at the institution and whether or not daily image-guided radiotherapy (IGRT) is used.

At the present authors' institution the following dose regimen is generally used: PTV1 (70 Gy), PTV2 (63 Gy), and PTV3 (56 Gy) in 35 fractions. Figure 10.6 shows a patient with a stage T4bN2bM0 tonsillar cancer treated with an IMRT (Tomotherapy) technique with concurrent cisplatin. For HPV-related oropharyngeal cancer, lower doses can be used. In RTOG 1016, which has recently completed with the recruitment of more than 900 patients, the following dose regimen was used: PTV1 (70 Gy), PTV2 (56 Gy), and PTV3 (52.5 Gy) in 35 fractions [17]. Further dose de-escalation is under investigation, such as in NRG HN 002, a Phase II randomized trial comparing 60 Gy in six weeks with concurrent weekly cisplatin versus 60 Gy in five weeks radiation alone [112]. However, this regimen should be used only in the setting of a clinical trial.

The dose constraints used in study RTOG 0022 are shown in Table 10.7. With dose de-escalation in HPV-related oropharyngeal cancer, doses to normal structures

Table 10.6 Select studies of oropharyngeal cancer managed with IMRT.

Study (year)	No. of patients	Patient characteristics	Median f/u (months)	Time point (years)	Local control (%)	DFS (%)	DMFS (%)	OS (%)	Comments
Eisbruch *et al.* (RTOG 0022, 2010) [102]	67	T1-2 N0-1	33.6	2	91	82	NR	95.5	Prospective, multi-institutional, no chemo, DM in 1 pt, no post-op
Yao *et al.* (2006) University of Iowa [103]	66	88% Stage IV	27.3	3	92	64.4	80.4	78.1	4 post-op
Chao *et al.* (2004) Washington University [104]	74	T1-4 N0-N3, 93% Stage III or IV	33	4	87	81	90	87	43 post-op, GTV and nGTV associated with LRC
Daly *et al.* (2010) Stanford [105]	107	T1-4 N0-3, 96% Stage III or IV	29	3	92	81	92	83	22 post-op, Outcome associated with T-stage
Setton *et al.* (2011) MSKCC [106]	442	94% Stage III or IV	36.8	3	94.4	NR	NR	84.9	30 post-op, DM rate 12.5%
Garden *et al.* (2007) MDACC [107]	51	Small primaries (<4cm) N0-3	45	2	94	88	NR	94	No post-op
Huang *et al.* (2008) UCSF [108]	71	Stage III and IV	33	3	94	81	NR	83	No post-op
Mendenhall *et al.* (2010) University of Florida [109]	130	90% Stage III or IV	45.6	5	84	NR	93	76	No post-op
Shoushtari *et al.* (2010) University of Virginia [110]	112	88% Stage III or IV	26.4	3	90.5	81.7	88.4	76.5	No post-op, p16+ patients had better outcomes

DM, distant metastasis; DMFS, distant metastasis-free survival; NR, not reported; OS, overall survival.

can be further reduced. When treating with IMRT, the nodal levels in the lower neck can be addressed with one of two accepted techniques: extended-whole field (EWF) IMRT or with a split-field (SF) technique [113, 114]. The SF technique treats above the larynx with IMRT fields, and an anterior-posterior field is matched to the IMRT field at a match plane just above the arytenoids. This allows for a central block to be placed in the low neck anterior-posterior field for laryngeal sparing. The SF technique can result in a lower larynx dose, although modern and thoughtful IMRT planning can result in similar larynx dosimetry [115–117]. When there are nodes involved in the lower neck, the EWF technique is preferred since no match is required near an involved node or nodal level that could lead to dose uncertainty.

Postoperative Techniques

Within the adjuvant setting, defining postoperative target volumes can be challenging due to distortion of the anatomy from surgery. Preoperative assessment by the radiation oncologist is helpful in determining high-risk areas of disease. A thorough postoperative examination should be performed to assess for healing as well as potential recurrence during the postoperative period. The operative note and pathology reports should be thoroughly examined and the procedure discussed with the surgeon if questions regarding the extent of tumor and margin status are not clear. Both, preoperative and postoperative imaging should be incorporated into target volume delineation.

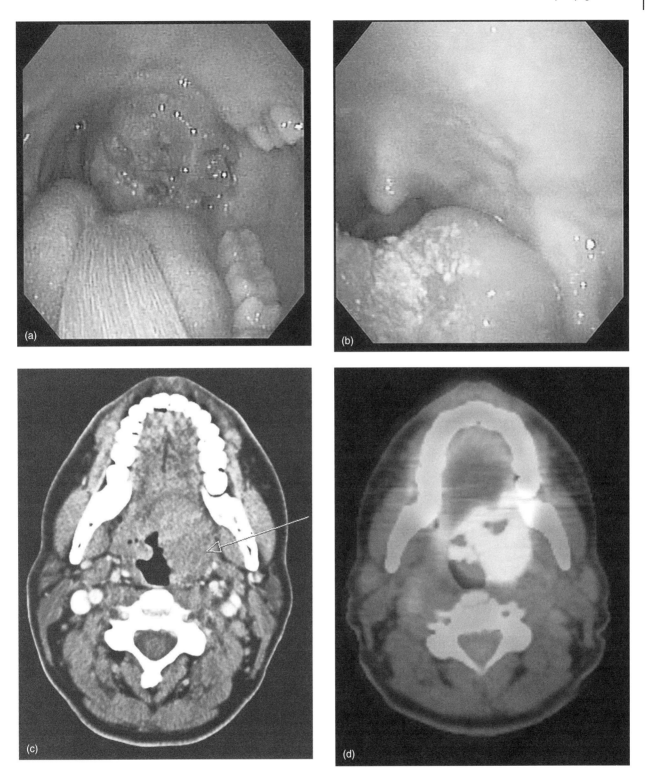

Figure 10.6 A patient with stage T4bN2bM0 left tonsillar cancer treated with an IMRT (Tomotherapy) technique with concurrent cisplatin. (a) Pretreatment. (b) At 3 months after treatment. (c) Pretreatment CT. (d) Pretreatment PET/CT. (e) 3 months post-treatment PET/CT showing resolution of abnormal FDG uptake. (f) IMRT (Tomotherapy) plan demonstrating the 70 Gy (red), 63 Gy (green), and 56 Gy (blue) dose regions. For a color version of this figure, see the color plate section. For a color version of this figure, see the color plate section.

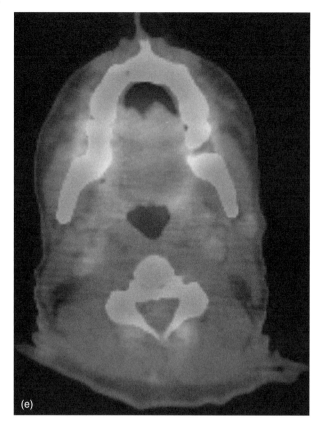

Figure 10.6 (*Continued*)

Radiation therapy should begin when healing is complete, approximately three to four weeks after surgery, and not be unnecessarily delayed since prolonged treatment periods have been associated with local failure [118, 119]. Rosenthal and coworkers [118] noted that a treatment package time (the time from surgery to the end of radiotherapy) greater than 100 days was associated with increased local failure.

Patients are simulated supine with the head hyperextended in a thermoplastic head/shoulder mask with a

bite block. Intravenous contrast should be used for CT-simulation to aid in vessel delineation. Generally, patients should be treated with an IMRT technique, with 60 Gy given to the primary site including the surgical bed and involved neck regions. Areas with ECE or involved/close surgical margins should be considered for a boost to 66 Gy. The uninvolved neck should receive 54–56 Gy [120]. A PTV is generated for each CTV a by an expansion of 0.3–0.5 cm.

Figure 10.7 is an example of a T1N2aM0 tonsillar cancer status post trans-oral laser resection and right neck dissection treated with an IMRT (Tomotherapy) technique postoperatively.

Table 10.7 IMRT dose constraints used in RTOG 0022.

Glottic larynx:	2/3 <50 Gy
Brainstem	max. 54 Gy
Spinal cord	max. 45 Gy
Mandible	max. 70 Gy
Parotid	Mean dose to either parotid <26 Gy or at least 50% of either parotid gland will receive <30 Gy or at least 20 ml of the combined volume of both parotid glands will receive <20 Gy.

Source: Eisbruch *et al.* 2010 [102]. Reproduced with permission of Elsevier.

Conclusions

Radiation therapy plays a principal role in the management of oropharyngeal cancers. Over the past decade, advances in imaging and therapy delivery have led to modern radiation techniques such as IMRT that allow for better normal tissue sparing and have become the standard of care. The incorporation of chemotherapy into treatment regimens for advanced disease has also led to improved outcomes. Targeted, biologic agents

Figure 10.7 A patient with stage T1N2aM0 right tonsillar cancer status after trans-oral laser resection of the primary tumor and right neck dissection treated with postoperative IMRT (Tomotherapy) according to protocol RTOG 0920. (a) Preoperative CT demonstrating right Level II lymphadenopathy. (b) IMRT (Tomotherapy) plan showing the 66 Gy (red), 60 Gy (yellow), and 56 Gy (blue) dose regions. For a color version of this figure, see the color plate section. For a color version of this figure, see the color plate section.

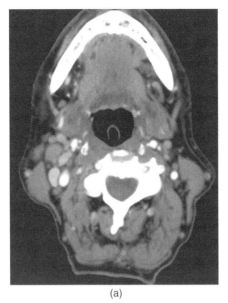

(a)

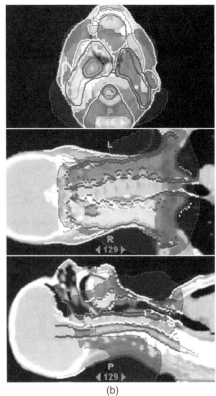

(b)

such as cetuximab will likely play a larger role in the future and allow for effective therapies with less toxicity. Finally, HPV is now known as the etiologic factor in many cases of oropharyngeal cancer. Clinical trials with de-escalation of treatment are under way that may redefine how radiation oncologists effectively treat this subclass of disease, hopefully resulting in excellent outcomes while minimizing morbidity.

References

1 Siegel, L.R., Miller, K.D., Jemal, A. (2017) Cancer Statistics. *CA Cancer J. Clin.*, **67**, 7–30.

2 Robbins, K.T., Shaha, A.R., Medina, J.E., *et al.* (2008) Consensus statement on the classification and terminology of neck dissection. *Arch. Otolaryngol. Head Neck Surg.*, **134** (5), 536–538.

3 Som, P.M., Curtin, H.D., Mancuso, A.A. (1999) An imaging-based classification for the cervical nodes designed as an adjunct to recent clinically based nodal classifications. *Arch. Otolaryngol. Head Neck Surg.*, **125** (4), 388–396.

4 Gregoire, V., Coche, E., Cosnard, G., *et al.* (2000) Selection and delineation of lymph node target volumes in head and neck conformal radiotherapy. Proposal for standardizing terminology and procedure based on the surgical experience. *Radiother. Oncol.*, **56** (2), 135–150.

5 Nowak, P.J., Wijers, O.B., Lagerwaard, F.J., Levendag, P. (1999) A three dimensional CT-based target definition for elective irradiation of the neck. *Int. J. Radiat. Oncol. Biol. Phys.*, **45**, 33–39.

6 Grégoire, V., Levendag, P., Ang, K.K., *et al.* (2003) CT-based delineation of lymph node levels and related CTVs in the node-negative neck: DAHANCA, EORTC, GORTEC, NCIC, RTOG consensus guidelines. *Radiother. Oncol.*, **69** (3), 227–236.

7 Grégoire, V., Ang, K.K., Budach, W., *et al.* (2014) Delineation of the neck node levels for head and neck tumors: A 2013 update. DAHANCA, EORTC, HKNPCSG, NCIC CTG, NCRI, RTOG, TROC consensus guidelines. *Radiother. Oncol.*, **110**, 172–181.

8 Grégoire, V., Levendag, P. (2013) RTOG Head and Neck Contouring Atlas. Available at: https://www.rtog.org/LinkClick.aspx?fileticket=uQmTaI3efxE%3d&tabid=229. Accessed August 30, 2015.

9 Chaturvedi, A.K., Engels, E.A., Pfeiffer, R.M., *et al.* (2011) Human papillomavirus and rising

oropharyngeal cancer incidence in the United States. *J. Clin. Oncol.*, **29**, 4294–4301.

10 Bagnardi, V., Blangiardo, M., La Vecchia, C., Corrao, G. (2001) A meta-analysis of alcohol drinking and cancer risk. *Br. J. Cancer*, **85** (11), 1700–1705.

11 Franceschi, S., Talamini, R., Barra, S., *et al.* (1990) Smoking and drinking in relation to cancers of the oral cavity, pharynx, larynx, and esophagus in northern Italy. *Cancer Res.*, **50** (20), 6502–6507.

12 Gillison, M.L., Broutian, T., Pickard, R.K., *et al.* (2012) Prevalence of oral HPV infection in the United States, 2009-2010. *JAMA*, **307** (7), 693–703.

13 Feller, L., Wood, N.H., Khammissa, R.A., Lemmer, J. (2010) Human papillomavirus-mediated carcinogenesis and HPV-associated oral and oropharyngeal squamous cell carcinoma. Part 1: human papillomavirus-mediated carcinogenesis. *Head Face Med.*, **6**, 14.

14 Lassen, P., Eriksen, J.G., Krogdahl, A., *et al.* (2011) The influence of HPV-associated p16-expression on accelerated fractionated radiotherapy in head and neck cancer: evaluation of the randomised DAHANCA 6&7 trial. *Radiother. Oncol.*, **100** (1), 49–55.

15 Posner, M.R., Lorch, J.H., Goloubeva, O., *et al.* (2011) Survival and human papillomavirus in oropharynx cancer in TAX 324: a subset analysis from an international phase III trial. *Ann. Oncol.*, **22** (5), 1071–1077.

16 Ang, K.K., Harris, J., Wheeler, R., *et al.* (2010) Human papillomavirus and survival of patients with oropharyngeal cancer. *N. Engl. J. Med.*, **363** (1), 24–35.

17 Trotti, A., Gillison, M. RTOG 1016 Protocol Information (2016) Available at: https://www.rtog.org/ ClinicalTrials/ProtocolTable/StudyDetails.aspx?study =1016. Accessed August 30, 2015.

18 Ang, K.K., Berkey, B.A., Tu, X., *et al.* (2002) Impact of epidermal growth factor receptor expression on survival and pattern of relapse in patients with advanced head and neck carcinoma. *Cancer Res.*, **62** (24), 7350–7356.

19 Hong, A., Dobbins, T., Lee, C.S., *et al.* (2011) Relationships between epidermal growth factor receptor expression and human papillomavirus status as markers of prognosis in oropharyngeal cancer. *Eur. J. Cancer*, **46** (11), 2088–2096.

20 Westra, W.H. (2009) The changing face of head and neck cancer in the 21st century: the impact of HPV on the epidemiology and pathology of oral cancer. *Head Neck Path.*, **3** (1), 78–81.

21 Lindberg, R. (1972) Distribution of cervical lymph node metastases from squamous cell carcinoma of the upper respiratory and digestive tracts. *Cancer*, **29** (6), 1446–1449.

22 Candela, F.C., Kothari, K., Shah, J.P. (1990) Patterns of cervical node metastases from squamous carcinoma of the oropharynx and hypopharynx. *Head Neck*, **12** (3), 197–203.

23 Chua, D.T., Sham, J.S., Kwong, D.L., *et al.* (1997) Retropharyngeal lymphadenopathy in patients with nasopharyngeal carcinoma: a computed tomography-based study. *Cancer*, **79** (5), 869–877.

24 Liu, L.Z., Zhang, G.Y., Xie, C.M., *et al.* (2006) Magnetic resonance imaging of retropharyngeal lymph node metastasis in nasopharyngeal carcinoma: patterns of spread. *Int. J. Radiat. Oncol. Biol. Phys.*, **66** (3), 721–730.

25 McLaughlin, M.P., Mendenhall, W.M., Mancuso, A.A., *et al.* (1995) Retropharyngeal adenopathy as a predictor of outcome in squamous cell carcinoma of the head and neck. *Head Neck*, **17** (3), 190–198.

26 Bussels, B., Hermans, R., Reijnders, A., *et al.* (2006) Retropharyngeal nodes in squamous cell carcinoma of oropharynx: incidence, localization, and implications for target volume. *Int. J. Radiat. Oncol. Biol. Phys.*, **65** (3), 733–738.

27 Dirix, P., Nuyts, S., Bussels, B., *et al.* (2006) Prognostic influence of retropharyngeal lymph node metastasis in squamous cell carcinoma of the oropharynx. *Int. J. Radiat. Oncol. Biol. Phys.*, **65** (3), 739–744.

28 Chong, V.F., Fan, Y.F., Khoo, J.B. (1995) Retropharyngeal lymphadenopathy in nasopharyngeal carcinoma. *Eur. J. Radiol.*, **21** (2), 100–105.

29 Wang, C.C. (1997) *Radiation Therapy for Head and Neck Neoplasms*, 3rd edition. Wiley-Liss, New York, p. 331.

30 Rumboldt, Z., Day, T.A., Michel, M. (2006) Imaging of oral cavity cancer. *Oral Oncol.*, **42** (9), 854–865.

31 Park, J.O., Jung, S.L., Joo, Y.H., *et al.* (2011) Diagnostic accuracy of magnetic resonance imaging (MRI) in the assessment of tumor invasion depth in oral/oropharyngeal cancer. *Oral Oncol.*, **47** (5), 381–386.

32 Woods, C., Sohn, J., Yao, M. (2011) *PET Clinics: The Application of PET in Radiation Treatment Planning for Head and Neck Cancer.* Elsevier.

33 Roh, J., Yeo, N., Kim, J.S., *et al.* Utility of 2-[18F] fluoro-2-deoxy-D-glucose positron emission tomography and positron emission tomography/computed tomography imaging in the preoperative staging of head and neck squamous cell carcinoma. *Oral Oncol.*, **43**, 887–893.

34 Ng, S., Yen, T., Liao, C., *et al.* (2005) 18F-FDG PET and CT/MRI in oral cavity squamous cell carcinoma: a prospective study of 124 patients with histologic correlation. *J. Nucl. Med.*, **46**, 1136–1143.

35 Al-Ibraheem, A., Buck, A., Krause, B.J., *et al.* (2009) Clinical applications of FDG PET and PET/CT in head and neck cancer. *J. Oncol.*, **2009**, 208725.

36 Amin, M.B., *et al.* (eds) (2017) *AJCC Cancer Staging Manual, 8th Edition.* Springer.

37 Huang, S.H., Xu, W., Waldron, J., *et al.* (2015) Refining American Joint Committee on Cancer/Union for International Cancer Control TNM stage and prognostic groups for human papillomavirus-related oropharyngeal carcinomas. *J. Clin. Oncol.*, **33**, 836–845.

38 O'Sullivan, B., Huang, S.H., Su, J., *et al.* (2016) Development and validation of a staging system for HPV-related oropharyngeal cancer by the International Collaboration on Oropharyngeal cancer Network for Staging (ICON-S): a multicenter cohort study. *Lancet Oncol.*, **17**, 440–451.

39 Karatzanis, A.D., Psychogios, G., Waldfahrer, F., *et al.* (2012) Surgical management of T1 oropharyngeal carcinoma. *Head Neck*, **34**, 1277–1282.

40 Rich, J.T., Liu, J., Haughey, B.H. (2011) Swallowing function after transoral laser microsurgery (TLM) ± adjuvant therapy for advanced-stage oropharyngeal cancer. *Laryngoscope*, **121** (11), 2381–2390.

41 Haughey, B.H., Hinni, M.L., Salassa, J.R., *et al.* (2011) Transoral laser microsurgery as primary treatment for advanced-stage oropharyngeal cancer: A United States multicenter study. *Head Neck*, **33** (12), 1683–1694

42 Mazeron, J.J., Ardiet, J.M., Haie-Méder, C., *et al.* (2009) GEC-ESTRO recommendations for brachytherapy for head and neck squamous cell carcinomas. *Radiother. Oncol.*, **91** (2), 150–156.

43 Nag, S., Cano, E.R., Demanes, D.J., *et al.* (2001) The American Brachytherapy Society recommendations for high-dose-rate brachytherapy for head-and-neck carcinoma. *Int. J. Radiat. Oncol. Biol. Phys.*, **50** (5), 1190–1198.

44 Strnad, V. (2004) Treatment of oral cavity and oropharyngeal cancer. Indications, technical aspects, and results of interstitial brachytherapy. *Strahlenther. Onkol.*, **180** (11), 710–717.

45 Le Scodan, R., Pommier, P., Ardiet, J.M., *et al.* (2005) Exclusive brachytherapy for T1 and T2 squamous cell carcinomas of the velotonsillar area: results in 44 patients. *Int. J. Radiat. Oncol. Biol. Phys.*, **63** (2), 441–448.

46 Strnad, V., Melzner, W., Geiger, M., *et al.* (2005) Role of interstitial PDR brachytherapy in the treatment of oral and oropharyngeal cancer. A single-institute experience of 236 patients.*Strahlenther. Onkol.*, **181** (12), 762–767.

47 Pernot, M., Hoffstetter, S., Peiffert, D., *et al.* (1996) Role of interstitial brachytherapy in oral and oropharyngeal carcinoma: reflection of a series of 1344 patients treated at the time of initial presentation. *Otolaryngol. Head Neck Surg.*, **115** (6), 519–526.

48 Parsons, J.T., Mendenhall, W.M., Stringer, S.P., *et al.* (2002) Squamous cell carcinoma of the oropharynx: surgery, radiation therapy, or both. *Cancer*, **94** (11), 2967–2980.

49 Hinni, M.K., Nagel, T., Howard, B. (2015) Oropharyngeal cancer treatment: the role of transoral surgery. *Curr. Opin. Otolaryngol. Head Neck Surg.*, **23** (2), 132–138.

50 Zevallos, J.P., Mitra, N., Swisher-McClure, S. (2016) Patterns of care and perioperative outcomes in transoral endoscopic surgery for oropharyngeal squamous cell carcinoma. *Head Neck*, **38** (3), 402–409.

51 Jackson, S.M., Hay, J.H., Flores, A.D., *et al.* (1999) Cancer of the tonsil: the results of ipsilateral radiation treatment. *Radiother. Oncol.*, **51** (2), 123–128.

52 O'Sullivan, B., Warde, P., Grice, B., *et al.* (2001) The benefits and pitfalls of ipsilateral radiotherapy in carcinoma of the tonsillar region. *Int. J. Radiat. Oncol. Biol. Phys.*, **51** (2), 332–343.

53 Rusthoven, K.E., Raben, D., Schneider, C., *et al.* (2009) Freedom from local and regional failure of contralateral neck with ipsilateral neck radiotherapy for node-positive tonsil cancer: results of a prospective management approach. *Int. J. Radiat. Oncol. Biol. Phys.*, **74** (5), 1365–1370.

54 Yeung, A.R., Garg, M.K., Lawson, J., *et al.* (2012) ACR appropriateness criteria: ipsilateral radiation for squamous cell carcinoma of the tonsil. *Head Neck*, **34**, 613–616.

55 Mendenhall, W.M., Morris, C.G., Amdur, R.J., *et al.* (2006) Definitive radiotherapy for squamous cell carcinoma of the base of tongue. *Am. J. Clin. Oncol.*, **29** (1), 32–39.

56 Selek, U., Garden, A.S., Morrison, W.H., *et al.* (2004) Radiation therapy for early-stage carcinoma of the oropharynx. *Int. J. Radiat. Oncol. Biol. Phys.*, **59** (3), 743–751.

57 Wang, C.C., Montgomery, W., Efird, J. (1995) Local control of oropharyngeal carcinoma by irradiation alone. *Laryngoscope*, **105** (5 Pt 1), 529–533.

58 Chera, B.S., Amdur, R.J., Hinerman, R.W., *et al.* (2008) Definitive radiation therapy for squamous cell carcinoma of the soft palate. *Head Neck*, **30** (8), 1114–1119.

59 Hull, M.C., Morris, C.G., Tannehill, S.P., *et al.* (2003) Definitive radiotherapy alone or combined with a planned neck dissection for squamous cell carcinoma of the pharyngeal wall. *Cancer*, **98** (10), 2224–2231.

60 Al-Sarraf, M., Pajak, T.F., Marcial, V.A., *et al.* (1987) Concurrent radiotherapy and chemotherapy with cisplatin in inoperable squamous cell carcinoma of the head and neck. An RTOG Study. *Cancer*, **59** (2), 259–265.

61 Marcial, V.A., Pajak, T.F., Mohiuddin, M., *et al.* (1990) Concomitant cisplatin chemotherapy and radiotherapy in advanced mucosal squamous cell carcinoma of the head and neck. Long-term results of the Radiation Therapy Oncology Group study 81-17. *Cancer*, **66** (9), 1861–1868.

62 Adelstein, D.J., Li, Y., Adams, G.L., *et al.* (2003) An intergroup phase III comparison of standard radiation therapy and two schedules of concurrent chemoradiotherapy in patients with unresectable squamous cell head and neck cancer. *J. Clin. Oncol.*, **21** (1), 92–98.

63 Calais, G., Alfonsi, M., Bardet, E., *et al.* (1999) Randomized trial of radiation therapy versus concomitant chemotherapy and radiation therapy for advanced-stage oropharynx carcinoma. *J. Natl Cancer Inst.*, **91** (24), 2081–2086.

64 Brizel, D.M., Albers, M.E., Fisher, S.R., *et al.* (1998) Hyperfractionated irradiation with or without concurrent chemotherapy for locally advanced head and neck cancer. *N. Engl. J. Med.*, **338** (25), 1798–1804.

65 Huguenin, P., Beer, K.T., Allal, A., *et al.* (2004) Concomitant cisplatin significantly improves locoregional control in advanced head and neck cancers treated with hyperfractionated radiotherapy. *J. Clin. Oncol.*, **22** (23), 4665–4673.

66 Bensadoun, R.J., Bénézery, K., Dassonville, O., *et al.* (2006) French multicenter phase III randomized study testing concurrent twice-a-day radiotherapy and cisplatin/5-fluorouracil chemotherapy (BiRCF) in unresectable pharyngeal carcinoma: Results at 2 years (FNCLCC-GORTEC). *Int. J. Radiat. Oncol. Biol. Phys.*, **64** (4), 983–994.

67 Overgaard, J., Hansen, H.S., Specht, L., *et al.* (2003) Five compared with six fractions per week of conventional radiotherapy of squamous-cell carcinoma of head and neck: DAHANCA 6 and 7 randomised controlled trial. *Lancet*, **362** (9388), 933–940.

68 Fu, K.K., Pajak, T.F., Trotti, A., *et al.* (2000) A Radiation Therapy Oncology Group (RTOG) phase III randomized study to compare hyperfractionation and two variants of accelerated fractionation to standard fractionation radiotherapy for head and neck squamous cell carcinomas: first report of RTOG 9003. *Int. J. Radiat. Oncol. Biol. Phys.*, **48** (1), 7–16.

69 Bonner, J.A., Harari, P.M., Giralt, J., *et al.* (2010) Radiotherapy plus cetuximab for locoregionally advanced head and neck cancer: 5-year survival data from a phase 3 randomised trial, and relation between cetuximab-induced rash and survival. *Lancet Oncol.*, **11** (1), 21–28.

70 Pignon, J.P., le Maître, A., Maillard, E., *et al.* (2009) Meta-analysis of chemotherapy in head and neck cancer (MACH-NC): an update on 93 randomised trials and 17,346 patients. *Radiother Oncol.*, **92** (1), 4–14.

71 Blanchard, P., Baujat, B., Holostenco, V., *et al.* (2011) Meta-analysis of chemotherapy in head and neck cancer (MACH-NC): a comprehensive analysis by tumour site. *Radiother. Oncol.*, **100** (1), 33–40.

72 Harari, P.M., Huang, S.M. (2001) Head and neck cancer as a clinical model for molecular targeting of therapy: combining EGFR blockade with radiation. *Int. J. Radiat. Oncol. Biol. Phys.*, **49** (2), 427–433.

73 Huang, S.M., Harari, P.M. (2000) Modulation of radiation response after epidermal growth factor receptor blockade in squamous cell carcinomas: inhibition of damage repair, cell cycle kinetics, and tumor angiogenesis. *Clin. Cancer Res.*, **6** (6), 2166–2174.

74 Bonner, J.A., Harari, P.M., Giralt, J., *et al.* (2006) Radiotherapy plus cetuximab for squamous-cell carcinoma of the head and neck. *N. Engl. J. Med.*, **354** (6), 567–578.

75 Ang, K.K., Zhang, Q., Rosenthal, D.I., *et al.* (2014) Randomized Phase III trial of concurrent accelerated radiation plus cisplatin with or without cetuximab for stage III to IV head and neck carcinoma: RTOG 0522. *J. Clin. Oncol.*, **32**, 2940–2450.

76 Bourhis, J., Overgaard, J., Audry, H., *et al.* (2006) Hyperfractionated or accelerated radiotherapy in head and neck cancer: a meta-analysis. *Lancet*, **368** (9538), 843–854.

77 Bourhis, J., Sire, C., Graff, P., *et al.* (2012) Concomitant chemoradiotherapy versus acceleration of radiotherapy with or without concomitant chemotherapy in locally advanced head and neck carcinoma (GORTEC 99-02): an open-label phase 3 randomised trial. *Lancet Oncol.*, **13** (2), 145–153.

78 Nguyen-Tan, P.F., Zhng, Q., Ang, K.K. (2014) Randomized phase III trial to test accelerated versus standard fractionation in combination with concurrent cisplatin for head and neck carcinomas in the Radiation Therapy Oncology Group 0129 Trial: Long-term report of efficacy and toxicity. *J. Clin. Oncol.*, **32**, 3858–3867.

79 Cmelak, A.J., Li, S., Goldwasser, M.A., Murphy, B., *et al.* (2007) Phase II trial of chemoradiation for organ preservation in resectable stage III or IV squamous cell carcinomas of the larynx or oropharynx: results of Eastern Cooperative Oncology Group Study E2399. *J. Clin. Oncol.*, **25** (25), 3971–3977.

80 Fakhry, C., Westra, W.H., Li, S., *et al.* (2008) Improved survival of patients with human papillomavirus-positive head and neck squamous cell carcinoma in a prospective clinical trial. *J. Natl Cancer Inst.*, **100** (4), 261–269.

81 Vermorken, J.B., Remenar, E., van Herpen, C., *et al.* (2007) Cisplatin, fluorouracil, and docetaxel in unresectable head and neck cancer. *N. Engl. J. Med.*, **357** (17), 1695–1704.

82 Posner, M.R., Hershock, D.M., Blajman, C.R., *et al.* (2007) Cisplatin and fluorouracil alone or with docetaxel in head and neck cancer. *N. Engl. J. Med.*, **357** (17), 1705–1715.

83 Haddad, R., O'Neill, A., Rabinowits, G., *et al.* (2013) Induction chemotherapy followed by concurrent chemoradiotherapy (sequential chemoradiotherapy) versus concurrent chemoradiotherapy alone in locally advanced head and neck cancer (PARADIGM): a randomised phase 3 trial. *Lancet Oncol.*, **14** (3), 257–264.

84 Cohen, E.E., Karrison, T.G., Kocherginsky, M., *et al.* (2014) Phase III randomized trial of induction chemotherapy in patients with N2 or N3 locally advanced head and neck cancer. *J. Clin. Oncol.*, **32** (25), 2735–2743.

85 Hartl, D.M., Ferlito, A., Silver, C.E., *et al.* (2011) Minimally invasive techniques for head and neck malignancies: current indications, outcomes and future directions. *Eur. Arch. Otorhinolaryngol.*, **268** (9), 1249–1257.

86 Silver, C.E., Beitler, J.J., Shaha, A.R., *et al.* (2009) Current trends in initial management of laryngeal cancer: the declining use of open surgery. *Eur. Arch. Otorhinolaryngol.*, **266** (9), 1333–1352.

87 Ang, K.K., Trotti, A., Brown, B.W., *et al.* (2001) Randomized trial addressing risk features and time factors of surgery plus radiotherapy in advanced head-and-neck cancer. *Int. J. Radiat. Oncol. Biol. Phys.*, **51** (3), 571–578.

88 Kramer, S., Gelber, R.D., Snow, J.B., *et al.* (1987) Combined radiation therapy and surgery in the management of advanced head and neck cancer: final report of study 73-03 of the Radiation Therapy Oncology Group. *Head Neck Surg.*, **10** (1), 19–30.

89 Tupchong, L., Scott, C.B., Blitzer, P.H., *et al.* (1991) Randomized study of preoperative versus postoperative radiation therapy in advanced head and neck carcinoma: long-term follow-up of RTOG study 73-03. *Int. J. Radiat. Oncol. Biol. Phys.*, **20** (1), 21–28.

90 Bernier, J., Domenge, C., Ozsahin, M., *et al.* (2004) Postoperative irradiation with or without concomitant chemotherapy for locally advanced head and neck cancer. *N. Engl. J. Med.*, **350** (19), 1945–1952.

91 Cooper, J.S., Pajak, T.F., Forastiere, A.A., *et al.* (2004) Postoperative concurrent radiotherapy and chemotherapy for high-risk squamous-cell carcinoma of the head and neck. *N. Engl. J. Med.*, **350** (19), 1937–1944.

92 Bernier, J., Cooper, J.S., Pajak, T.F., *et al.* (2005) Defining risk levels in locally advanced head and neck cancers: a comparative analysis of concurrent postoperative radiation plus chemotherapy trials of the EORTC (#22931) and RTOG (# 9501). *Head Neck*, **27** (10), 843–850.

93 Machtay, M. RTOG 0920 Protocol Information. https://www.rtog.org/ClinicalTrials/ProtocolTable/StudyDetails.aspx?study=0920. Accessed August 30, 2015.

94 Harari, P.M., Rosenthal, D.I. RTOG 1216 Protocol Information. https://www.rtog.org/ClinicalTrials/ProtocolTable/StudyDetails.aspx?study=1216. Accessed August 30, 2015.

95 Mell, L.K., Mehrotra, A.K., Mundt, A.J. (2005) Intensity-modulated radiation therapy use in the U.S., 2004. *Cancer*, **104** (6), 1296–1303.

96 Lee, N., Puri, D.R., Blanco, A.I., Chao, K.S. (2007) Intensity-modulated radiation therapy in head and neck cancers: an update.*Head Neck*, **29** (4), 387–400.

97 Grégoire, V., De Neve, W., Eisbruch, A., *et al.* (2007) Intensity-modulated radiation therapy for head and neck carcinoma. *Oncologist*, **12** (5), 555–564.

98 Chao, K.S., Deasy, J.O., Markman, J., *et al.* (2001) A prospective study of salivary function sparing in patients with head-and-neck cancers receiving intensity-modulated or three-dimensional radiation therapy: initial results. *Int. J. Radiat. Oncol. Biol. Phys.*, **49** (4), 907–916.

99 Lin, A., Kim, H.M., Terrell, J.E., *et al.* (2003) Quality of life after parotid-sparing IMRT for head-and-neck cancer: a prospective longitudinal study. *Int. J. Radiat. Oncol. Biol. Phys.*, **57** (1), 61–70.

100 Yao, M., Karnell, L.H., Funk, G.F., *et al.* (2007) Health-related quality-of-life outcomes following IMRT versus conventional radiotherapy for oropharyngeal squamous cell carcinoma. *Int. J. Radiat. Oncol. Biol. Phys.*, **69** (5), 1354–1360.

101 Nutting, C.M., Morden, J.P., Harrington, K.J., *et al.* (2011) Parotid-sparing intensity modulated versus conventional radiotherapy in head and neck cancer (PARSPORT): a phase 3 multicentre randomised controlled trial. *Lancet Oncol.*, **12**, 127–136.

102 Eisbruch, A., Harris, J., Garden, A.S., *et al.* (2010) Multi-institutional trial of accelerated hypofractionated intensity-modulated radiation therapy for early-stage oropharyngeal cancer (RTOG 00-22). *Int. J. Radiat. Oncol. Biol. Phys.*, **76** (5), 1333–1338.

103 Yao, M., Nguyen, T., Buatti, J.M., *et al.* (2006) Changing failure patterns in oropharyngeal squamous cell carcinoma treated with intensity modulated radiotherapy and implications for future research. *Am. J. Clin. Oncol.*, **29** (6), 606–612.

104 Chao, K.S., Ozyigit, G., Blanco, A.I., *et al.* (2004) Intensity-modulated radiation therapy for oropharyngeal carcinoma: impact of tumor volume. *Int. J. Radiat. Oncol. Biol. Phys.*, **59** (1), 43–50.

105 Daly, M.E., Le, Q.T., Maxim, P.G., Loo, B.W., *et al.* (2010) Intensity-modulated radiotherapy in the treatment of oropharyngeal cancer: clinical outcomes and patterns of failure. *Int. J. Radiat. Oncol. Biol. Phys.*, **76** (5), 1339–1346.

106 Setton, J., Caria, N., Romanyshyn, J., *et al.* (2012) Intensity-modulated radiotherapy in the treatment of oropharyngeal cancer: an update of the Memorial Sloan-Kettering Cancer Center experience. *Int. J. Radiat. Oncol. Biol. Phys.*, **82** (1), 291–298.

107 Garden, A.S., Morrison, W.H., Wong, P.F., *et al.* (2007) Disease-control rates following intensity-modulated radiation therapy for small primary oropharyngeal carcinoma. *Int. J. Radiat. Oncol. Biol. Phys.*, **67** (2), 438–444.

108 Huang, K., Xia, P., Chuang, C., *et al.* (2008) Intensity-modulated chemoradiation for treatment of stage III and IV oropharyngeal carcinoma: the University of California-San Francisco experience. *Cancer*, **113** (3), 497–507.

109 Mendenhall, W.M., Amdur, R.J., Morris, C.G., *et al.* (2010) Intensity-modulated radiotherapy for oropharyngeal squamous cell carcinoma. *Laryngoscope*, **120** (11), 2218–2222.

110 Shoushtari, A., Meeneghan, M., Sheng, K., *et al.* (2010) Intensity-modulated radiotherapy outcomes for oropharyngeal squamous cell carcinoma patients stratified by p16 status. *Cancer*, **116** (11), 2645–2654.

111 Apisarnthanarax, S., Elliott, D.D., El-Naggar, A.K., *et al.* (2006) Determining optimal clinical target volume margins in head-and-neck cancer based on microscopic extracapsular extension of metastatic neck nodes. *Int. J. Radiat. Oncol. Biol. Phys.*, **64** (3), 678–683.

112 Yom, S. (2015) Reduced-dose intensity-modulated radiation therapy with or without cisplatin in treating patients with advanced oropharyngeal cancer. Available at: https://clinicaltrials.gov/ct2/show/NCT02254278?term=HN002&rank=1. Accessed August 30, 2015.

113 Amdur, R., Liu, C., Li, J., *et al.* (2007) Matching intensity-modulated radiation therapy to an anterior low neck field. *Int. J. Radiat. Oncol. Biol. Phys.*, **69** (2), S46–S48.

114 Lee, N., Mechalakos, J., Puri, D.R., Hunt, M. (2007) Choosing an intensity-modulated radiation therapy technique in the treatment of head-and-neck cancer. *Int. J. Radiat. Oncol. Biol. Phys.*, **68** (5), 1299–1309.

115 Dabaja, B., Salehpour, M., Rosen, I., *et al.* (2005) Intensity-modulated radiation therapy (IMRT) of cancers of the head and neck: comparison of split-field and whole-field techniques. *Int. J. Radiat. Oncol. Biol. Phys.*, **63** (4), 1000–1005.

116 Amdur, R., Li, J., Liu, C., *et al.* (2004) Unnecessary laryngeal irradiation in the IMRT era. *Head Neck*, **26** (3), 257–263

117 Galloway, T., Amdur, R., Liu, C., *et al.* (2011) Revisiting unnecessary larynx irradiation with whole-neck IMRT. *Pract. Radiat. Oncol.*, **1** (1), 27–32.

118 Rosenthal, D.I., Liu, L., Lee, J.H., *et al.* (2002) Importance of the treatment package time in surgery and postoperative radiation therapy for squamous carcinoma of the head and neck. *Head Neck*, **24** (2), 115–126.

119 Parsons, J.T., Mendenhall, W.M., Stringer, S.P., *et al.* (1997) An analysis of factors influencing the outcome of postoperative irradiation for squamous cell carcinoma of the oral cavity. *Int. J. Radiat. Oncol. Biol. Phys.*, **39** (1), 137–148.

120 Peters, L.J., Goepfert, H., Ang, K.K., *et al.* (1993) Evaluation of the dose for postoperative radiation therapy of head and neck cancer: first report of a prospective randomized trial. *Int. J. Radiat. Oncol. Biol. Phys.*, **26** (1), 3–11.

11

Larynx and Hypopharynx

Changhu Chen

Introduction

The human larynx is divided into three portions, the supraglottis, the glottis, and the subglottis (Figure 11.1). The supraglottis is composed of the epiglottis, aryepiglottic folds, arytenoids, and false vocal cords. The glottis consists of true vocal cords, including the anterior and posterior commissures, while the subglottis extends from the lower boundary of the glottis to the inferior aspect of the cricoid cartilage.

The hypopharynx is the lowest portion of the pharynx, which is contiguous superiorly with the oropharynx and inferiorly with the cervical esophagus. Anatomically, it extends from the superior border of the hyoid bone to the inferior border of the cricoid cartilage. The hypopharynx is divided into three subsites including the pyriform sinus, posterior hypopharyngeal wall, and postcricoid area (Figure 11.2). Unlike cancers of the larynx, hypopharyngeal cancers typically present in locally advanced stages with extensive cervical lymph node metastases, often bilaterally. The majority of hypopharyngeal cancers (60–70%) arises from pyriform sinus, and approximately one-fourth arise from the posterior pharyngeal wall. Postcricoid tumors are the least common type.

Lymph Node Metastasis

Lymphatic drainage from each of the subsites of the larynx is different and unique. Because of this, patterns of spread can vary significantly depending on the location of the primary lesion. For example, the glottis has a sparse lymphatic network and incidence of lymph node metastases in primary glottic cancer is relatively low [1].

For T1 tumors, the incidence ranges from 0% to 2%, but for T2 and T3 lesions the incidence increases to 10% and 15%, respectively. Carcinomas arising from the supraglottic region tend to develop lymph node metastases frequently. As the lesions arise further from the glottis and more towards the base of tongue, or further towards the esophagus, there is a higher incidence of lymph node metastases given the richer lymphatics in these areas. The difference in incidence may vary from 30% to 75%, depending on the stage of the primary tumors. Bilateral cervical lymph node metastases are common and occur in one-fourth to one-third of patients. The most frequently involved lymph nodes are the upper jugular (level II) and mid-jugular (level III) nodes. The retropharyngeal/Rouviere nodes are occasionally involved. The subglottis can drain to lower jugular nodes (level IV) and paratracheal nodes (level VI). The precricoid node is traditionally also called the Delphian node.

The hypopharynx has ample lymphatics, which drain to the upper jugular, midjugular, lower jugular/ supraclavicular (level II–IV), and retropharyngeal nodes (Rouviere nodes). When tumors involve the lower portion of the hypopharynx and the postcricoid area, paratracheal and paraesophageal lymph nodes (level VII) can be involved. A report from M. D. Anderson Cancer Center showed a 75% incidence of nodal metastases in patients with hypopharyngeal tumors [2].

Patient Evaluation

The clinical evaluation of all patients should include a detailed history and physical examination. Examination under anesthesia with directed laryngoscopy for the evaluation of tumor size, morphology, invasion of adjacent

Clinical Radiation Oncology: Indications, Techniques, and Results, Third Edition. Edited by William Small Jr.
© 2017 John Wiley & Sons, Inc. Published 2017 by John Wiley & Sons, Inc.

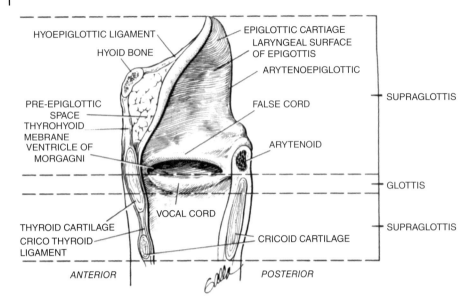

Figure 11.1 Anatomy of the larynx.

structures, mobility of the vocal cords, and for tumor biopsy should be performed. For patients with T1-2 glottic tumors, further work-up with imaging studies may not be necessary due to a low incidence of lymphatic or distant metastasis. However, when deep infiltration is suspected a neck computed tomography (CT) or magnetic resonance imaging (MRI) might be useful for the evaluation of tumor invasion into soft tissues or the thyroid cartilage. For all other patients, imaging studies should include head and neck CT scan or MRI and chest x-radiography or chest CT. Positron emission tomography (PET) scans may be informative for stage III–IV disease. Esophagoscopy and bronchoscopy with

biopsy of suspicious areas should also be performed. Laboratory tests should include a complete blood count, a comprehensive metabolic panel, and thyroid function tests. Baseline speech, swallowing, and nutrition evaluation by the appropriate specialist is important. Additionally, evaluation and preventive dental care should occur at least two to three weeks prior to starting radiation.

Staging

The TNM staging (8th edition) for squamous cell carcinoma of the larynx and hypopharynx is as follows [3]:

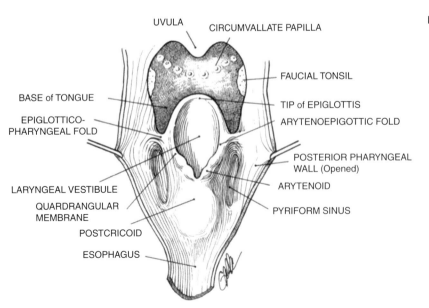

Figure 11.2 Anatomy of the hypopharynx.

Primary tumor (T) staging

TX   Primary tumor cannot be assessed.

Tis   Carcinoma *in situ.*

Supraglottis

T1   Tumor limited to one subsite of supraglottis with normal vocal cord mobility

T2   Tumor invades mucosa of more than one adjacent subsite of supraglottis or glottis or region outside the supraglottis (e.g., mucosa of base of tongue, vallecula, medial wall of pyriform sinus) without fixation of the larynx

T3   Tumor limited to larynx with vocal cord fixation and/or invades any of the following: postcricoid area, pre-epiglottic space, paraglottic space, and/or inner cortex of thyroid cartilage

T4   Moderately advanced or very advanced

T4a   Moderately advanced local disease
Tumor invades through the outer cortex of the thyroid cartilage and/or invades tissues beyond the larynx (e.g., trachea, soft tissues of neck including deep extrinsic muscle of the tongue, strap muscles, thyroid, or esophagus)

T4b   Very advanced local disease
Tumor invades prevertebral space, encases carotid artery, or invades mediastinal structures.

Glottis

TX   Primary tumor cannot be assessed

Tis   Carcinoma in situ

T1   Tumor limited to the vocal cord(s) (may involve anterior or posterior commissure) with normal mobility.

T1a   Tumor limited to one vocal cord.

T1b   Tumor involves both vocal cords.

T2   Tumor extends to supraglottis and/or subglottis, and/or with impaired vocal cord mobility.

T3   Tumor limited to the larynx with vocal cord fixation and/or invasion of paraglottic space and/or inner cortex of the thyroid cartilage.

T4   Moderately advanced or very advanced

T4a   Moderately advanced local disease
Tumor invades through the outer cortex of the thyroid cartilage and/or invades tissues beyond the larynx (e.g., trachea, soft tissues of neck including deep extrinsic muscle of the tongue, strap muscles, thyroid, or esophagus).

T4b   Very advanced local disease
Tumor invades prevertebral space, encases carotid artery, or invades mediastinal structures.

Subglottis

TX   Primary tumor cannot be assessed

Tis   Carcinoma in situ

T1   Tumor limited to the subglottis.

T2   Tumor extends to vocal cord(s) with normal or impaired mobility.

T3   Tumor limited to larynx with vocal cord fixation and/or invasion of paraglottic space and/or inner cortex of the thyroid cartilage

T4   Moderately advanced or very advanced

T4a   Moderately advanced local disease
Tumor invades cricoid or thyroid cartilage and/or invades tissues beyond the larynx (e.g., trachea, soft tissues of neck including deep extrinsic muscles of the tongue, strap muscles, thyroid, or esophagus)

T4b   Very advanced local disease
Tumor invades prevertebral space, encases carotid artery, or invades mediastinal structures.

Hypopharynx

TX   Primary tumor cannot be assessed

Tis   Carcinoma in situ

T1   Tumor limited to one subsite of hypopharynx and/or 2 cm or smaller in greatest dimension

T2   Tumor invades more than one subsite of hypopharynx or an adjacent site, or measures larger than 2 cm but not larger than 4 cm in greatest dimension without fixation of hemilarynx

T3   Tumor larger than 4 cm in greatest dimension or with fixation of hemilarynx or extension to esophagus

T4   Moderately advanced and very advanced local disease

T4a   Moderately advanced local disease
Tumor invades thyroid/cricoid cartilage, hyoid bone, thyroid gland, or central compartment soft tissue including prelaryngeal strap muscles and subcutaneous fat

T4b   Very advanced local disease
Tumor invades prevertebral fascia, encases carotid artery, or involves mediastinal structures

Regional Lymph Node (N)

NX   Regional lymph nodes cannot be assessed.

N0   No regional lymph node metastasis.

N1   Metastasis in a single ipsilateral lymph node, 3 cm or smaller in greatest dimension and ENE (−)

N2   Metastasis in a single ipsilateral lymph node larger than 3 cm but not larger than 6 cm in greatest dimension and ENE (−); or metastases in multiple ipsilateral lymph nodes, none larger than 6 cm in greatest dimension and ENE (−); or in bilateral or contralateral lymph nodes, none larger than 6 cm in greatest dimension and ENE (−)

N2a   Metastasis in a single ipsilateral lymph node, larger than 3 cm but not larger than 6 cm in greatest dimension and ENE (−)

N2b   Metastasis in multiple ipsilateral lymph nodes, none larger than 6 cm in greatest dimension.

N2c   Metastasis in bilateral or contralateral lymph nodes, none larger than 6 cm in greatest dimension and ENE (−)

N3   Metastasis in a lymph node, larger than 6 cm in greatest dimension and ENE (−); or metastasis in any node(s) and clinically overt ENE [ENE(+)]

N3a   Metastasis in a lymph node larger than 6 cm in greatest dimension and ENE (−)

N3b   Metastasis in any node(s) and ENE (+)

Note: A designation of "U" or "L" may be used for any N category to indicate metastasis above the lower border of the cricoid (U) or below the lower border of the cricoid (L). Similarly, clinical and pathological ENE should be recorded as ENE (−) or ENE (+).

Distant Metastasis (M)

M0   No distant metastasis

M1   Distant metastasis.

Anatomic Stage – Larynx

GROUP	T	N	M
0	Tis	N0	M0
I	T1	N0	M0
II	T2	N0	M0
III	T3	N0	M0
	T1, T2, T3	N1	M0
IVA	T4a	N0, N1	M0
	T1, T2, T3, T4a	N2	M0
IVB	T4b	Any N	M0
	Any T	N3	M0
IVC	Any T	Any N	M1

Anatomic Stage – Hypopharynx

GROUP	T	N	M
0	Tis	N0	M0
I	T1	N0	M0
II	T2	N0	M0
III	T3	N0	M0
	T1, T2, T3	N1	M0
IVA	T4a	N0, N1	M0
	T1, T2, T3, T4a	N2	M0
IVB	T4b	Any N	M0
	Any T	N3	M0
IVC	Any T	Any N	M1

Selection of Treatment

Radiation therapy and surgery have been used in the treatment of early-stage laryngeal and hypopharyngeal cancer. Early disease often can be cured with either surgery alone or radiation alone, and the use of combined modality should be avoided.

Advanced disease, however, often requires combined-modality therapies. For selected patients with T3 and early T4 disease, laryngeal preservation with radiation and concurrent chemotherapy is the treatment of choice. Surgery can be reserved for salvage. For advanced diseases with thyroid cartilage erosion, which are not suitable for laryngeal preservation, total laryngectomy followed by postoperative radiotherapy is standard treatment for laryngeal cancers. In contrast, advanced hypopharyngeal cancers require both laryngectomy and partial pharyngectomy followed by postoperative radiation therapy [4–8]. For patients with positive margins and/or extracapsular extension, postoperative radiation with concurrent chemotherapy has been shown to be superior to radiation alone in randomized studies. For patients with unresectable diseases or who are medically inoperable, radiation treatment with or without chemotherapy is appropriate.

Carcinoma of the Glottis

Carcinoma *In Situ* (CIS)

Conservative surgical procedures are usually used for the initial treatment of CIS. Microexcision, laser ablation, or vocal cord stripping are the most frequently used modalities [9–11]. Repeated stripping or laser excisions may lead to a worsening of voice quality. Radiation therapy is usually reserved for recurrences after surgical treatment and for diffuse disease not suitable for initial surgical management. Nevertheless, primary radiation therapy is an effective treatment for CIS [12–14].

T1 and T2 Tumors

Both, T1 and T2 glottic tumors can be treated either with radiation therapy or with surgery. T1 tumors respond well to radiation and above 90% local control rate can be achieved [1], whereas for T2 tumors a 75–85% local control rate can be achieved with radiation. Conservative surgical approaches including laser excision, laryngofissure or partial laryngectomy can control early glottic lesions [15–21], but this usually results in poor voice quality. In addition, partial laryngectomy is not suitable for patients of advanced age, poor surgical candidates, or those with poor lung function. For many patients with T2 tumors, voice-preserving surgeries are not feasible and total laryngectomy may be necessary [22, 23]. Thus, radiation therapy is the treatment of choice for T1 and T2 glottic tumors. Salvage surgery is often successful for patients who fail radiation therapy. When using radiation only the primary tumor is treated and neck lymphatics usually do not need to be covered.

T3 Tumors

Historically, T3 glottic tumors were treated with total laryngectomy, followed by postoperative radiation therapy for patients with high-risk pathologic features. The landmark Department of Veterans Affairs (VA) larynx preservation trial randomized stage III or IV laryngeal cancer patients to induction chemotherapy followed by radiation versus total laryngectomy, followed by postoperative radiation. The authors reported similar overall survival (OS) rates, but the induction chemotherapy and radiation group had more local recurrences and fewer distant metastases, and 64% of patients retained their larynx in two years [6]. Subsequently, the Radiation Therapy Oncology Group (RTOG) Phase III larynx preservation trial (RTOG 91-11) compared induction chemotherapy followed by radiation, concurrent chemoradiation, and radiation alone, and showed a higher rate of larynx preservation and equivalent survival rate with concurrent chemoradiation therapy compared to radiation alone, or induction chemotherapy followed by radiation [7]. Concurrent chemoradiation therapy is considered to be the standard of care for patients with T3 tumors. In planning radiation therapy for T3 tumors, the primary tumor and the level II, III, and IV lymph nodes are usually treated.

T4 Tumors

Total laryngectomy followed by postoperative radiation therapy remains the standard care for patients with T4 tumors [24]. Primary radiation therapy, often with concurrent chemotherapy or cetuximab, is an option for patients who cannot or are unwilling to undergo total laryngectomy. Radiation fields cover the primary tumor and bilateral neck lymph nodes including levels II, III, and IV/supraclavicular lymph nodes.

Carcinoma of the Supraglottis

T1 and T2 Disease

Both, radiation therapy and surgery are reasonable treatment options for patients with T1 and T2 supraglottic cancer. Transoral laser microsurgery (TLM) has been used to remove early lesions at some centers [25, 26], while larger lesions can be removed with supraglottic laryngectomy. As aspiration can be a severe problem with the removal of the epiglottis, extensive rehabilitation is required after surgery. Appropriate patient selection is critical when using a surgical approach. Those patients with poor pulmonary function are not good candidates for supraglottic laryngectomy.

Radiation therapy is often the treatment of choice for patients with early T stage disease. Local control rates with radiation are comparable to those achieved with supraglottic laryngectomy [27]. Radiation therapy has also often been used for patients who are medically inoperable or whose tumors are not amenable to partial laryngectomy.

As there is a high risk of lymph node involvement even with a small primary tumor, both necks must be addressed in addition to management of the primary tumor in the treatment of supraglottic cancer. In patients with clinically node-negative disease, the neck is usually managed with the same modality that has been decided for treating the primary tumor. If the primary tumor is treated with a surgical approach, then neck dissection should be carried out. For midline tumors such as those in epiglottis, bilateral neck dissection is necessary. Postoperative radiation is indicated for those with high-risk pathology features. For patients treated with radiation as definitive therapy, both necks must be included in the radiation fields.

Patients with clinically positive lymph nodes usually require combined-modality therapy, either surgery followed by postoperative radiation or definitive radiation with concurrent chemotherapy. For patients treated with definitive radiotherapy, a neck dissection is necessary if nodal disease persists after radiation. Planned neck dissection for patients with N2 and N3 neck disease is controversial. Many consider that a neck dissection after radiation is necessary, but some argue for observation and neck dissection not being needed in patients with resolution of nodal disease after radiation, especially in those who present with N2 neck disease [28].

T3 Disease

The optimal treatment of T3 supraglottic tumors is controversial. Larynx-preservation with concurrent chemoradiation therapy has become the standard treatment for many patients with T3 tumors. More than two-thirds of the patients enrolled in the RTOG 91-11 trial had supraglottic cancer [7]. However, total laryngectomy is still performed for T3 supraglottic cancer in many centers. A partial laryngectomy can be performed in patients with disease involving the pre-epiglottic space, but with no significant subglottic involvement, and one arytenoid cartilage can be spared [29]. Unfortunately, these patients often require postoperative radiation therapy due to inadequate margins, perineural or vascular invasion, or the involvement of multiple lymph nodes.

T4 Disease

T4 supraglottic disease is usually managed with total laryngectomy followed by postoperative radiation. For patients with close or positive margins, or extracapsular extension, concurrent chemotherapy with postoperative radiation has shown to be superior to radiation alone [30, 31]. In medically inoperable patients, concurrent chemoradiation therapy may be a reasonable option.

Carcinoma of the Subglottis

Subglottic cancer is rare and is often managed with total laryngectomy. A partial laryngectomy is usually not possible. Postoperative radiation is indicated for positive or close margins, cartilage invasion, and multiple lymph node involvement. Small tumors may be treated with radiation therapy [32, 33]. The outcomes are usually poorer than that of the other sites in the larynx.

Carcinoma of the Hypopharynx

Most patients with hypopharyngeal cancer present with advanced disease. Early-stage tumors are relatively uncommon. T1-2 tumors can be treated with partial pharyngectomy without or with partial laryngectomy [34–36], or definitive radiation therapy [37]. Radiation therapy usually results in better speech and swallowing function. Because of the high risk of lymph node involvement, both necks need to be addressed even in patients with clinically negative nodes. Since it is difficult to achieve negative margins by the prevertebral fascia, lesions arising from posterior pharyngeal wall should be treated with radiation therapy. Concurrent chemotherapy with radiation was reported in early-stage hypopharyngeal cancer, although this may not be a standard occurrence [38].

For patients with T3 hypopharyngeal cancer, concurrent chemoradiation for larynx preservation is the treatment of choice. In the European Organization for Research and Treatment of Cancer phase III trial (EORTC 24891), which randomized operable pyriform sinus cancer to surgery followed by radiation versus induction chemotherapy (if complete response), followed by radiation, over one-third of patients in the induction chemotherapy arm preserved their larynx and the OS was not compromised [8]. Most patients enrolled in this trial had T2 or T3 tumors, with only a few having T4 tumors. Although no Phase III randomized trial has been completed to compare induction chemotherapy versus concurrent chemotherapy in hypopharyngeal cancer, in general concurrent chemoradiation is more effective than induction chemotherapy followed by radiation therapy in head and neck cancer [39, 40].

Patients with T4 tumors should be treated with surgery followed by postoperative radiation therapy [41], or concurrent chemoradiation for patients with high-risk pathologic features. For patients who are medically inoperable, or with unresectable disease, concurrent chemoradiation is a reasonable option [42]. If a patient cannot tolerate concurrent chemotherapy, radiation alone is the only choice, but usually with poor outcomes [43].

Radiation Therapy Techniques

Patient Set-Up and Virtual Simulation

Currently, virtual simulation on a CT scanner (CT simulation) is used almost in every practice. CT simulation allows for target delineation and virtual radiation field arrangement, and also provides a direct review of radiation dose distribution and evaluation of tumor coverage and normal structure-sparing before radiation is started.

Patients are simulated in the supine position with the head extended. The head and neck is immobilized with a thermoplastic mask (Figures 11.3 and 11.4) to minimize movement during the treatment. This also allows reproduction of the treatment position during multifraction radiation therapy. The patient's shoulders are pulled down to avoid lateral beams. A mouthpiece is usually not necessary for most laryngeal cancer or hypopharyngeal cancer patients.

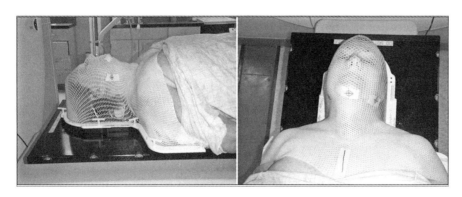

Figure 11.3 A thermoplastic mask for head and neck immobilization. For a color version of this figure, see the color plate section.

Figure 11.4 A patient in the treatment position fitted with an immobilization mask. For a color version of this figure, see the color plate section.

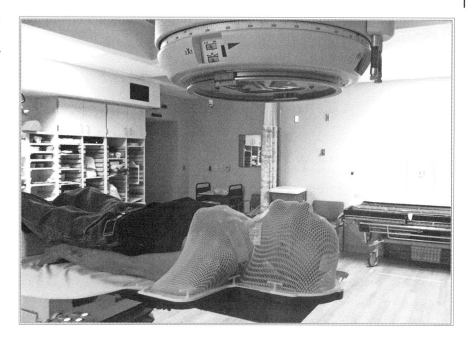

Fiducials are placed for isocenter localization, or in most practices the isocenter is marked on the immobilization mask. Axial CT images are then obtained, normally using an intravenous contrast agent. The target volumes and normal structures are contoured on the CT image set. These targets and normal structures can then be used for conventional three-dimensional (3D) conformal or intensity-modulated radiation therapy (IMRT) planning.

Radiation Fields, Treatment Volumes, Dose and Fractionation

Carcinoma of the Glottis

Radiation Fields and Treatment Volumes

For T1 and T2 glottic tumors, a pair of small lateral opposed photon fields is used to encompass the larynx only (Figure 11.5a). Typical field sizes are 5 × 5 cm or 6 × 6 cm. The isocenter is placed at the middle of the true vocal cord. The fields are defined by anatomic landmarks: anteriorly, the fields should flash the skin surface, often 1.5–2.0 cm anterior to the skin. The posterior border is the anterior edge of the vertebral bodies for the tumors in the anterior two-thirds of the vocal cords, and splitting the vertebral bodies for the tumors in the posterior one-third of the vocal cords. The superior border is placed above the thyroid notch, and the inferior border is inferior to the cricoid cartilage. For patients with T2 lesions, the borders are adjusted appropriately to cover the tumor. The superior border should be raised for patients with supraglottic involvement, and the inferior border is lowered for patients with subglottic disease

extension, often to encompass the upper trachea. The neck lymphatics do not need to be treated unless there is extensive supraglottic involvement. The radiation fields for CIS are the same as that for T1 tumors.

Because of the triangular shape of the larynx and anterior neck, a pair of wedges is usually needed to optimize the dose distribution (Figure 11.5b). Treating without wedges or under-wedging results in 'hot spots' in the anterior area of the neck, but this may be advantageous for anterior lesions. Special attention should be paid to the tumor arising in the anterior commissure. Occasionally, a tissue-equivalent bolus is needed to bring the radiation dose close to the skin surface for adequate dose coverage of the tumor (Figure 11.5b).

Cobalt 60 (^{60}Co) allows a better dose coverage of superficial tissue that is ideal for treating early-stage laryngeal cancer. However, ^{60}Co units are not available to most radiation therapy practices today. Concerns have been

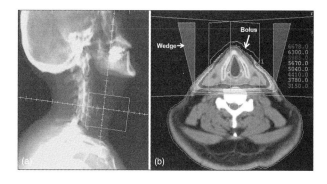

Figure 11.5 (a) Digitally reconstructed radiograph (DRR) showing a lateral field for a patient with a T1 laryngeal carcinoma. (b) Wedge pair and bolus are used to optimize dose distribution. For a color version of this figure, see the color plate section.

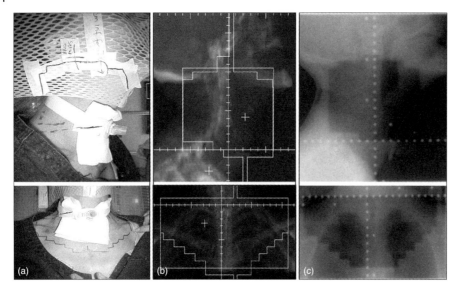

Figure 11.6 Three-field technique with upper neck opposed lateral fields (upper row) and lower neck anterior-posterior field (lower row). (a) Photographs for patient set-up. (b) Digitally reconstructed radiographs. (c) X-ray portals. For a color version of this figure, see the color plate section.

raised regarding 6 MV photons, which have a relatively large build-up region that may result in under-dosing the superficial tissue, especially in patients with a tumor in the anterior commissure. A tissue-equivalent bolus placed on the anterior neck can be used in those patients (Figure 11.5b) [44,45].

For T3-4 glottic tumors, both the primary tumor and the neck lymphatics need to be treated, even in patients with a clinically negative neck. Traditionally, a three-field technique is used with a pair of parallel-opposed lateral fields (upper-neck fields) covering the primary tumor and upper- and mid-jugular lymph nodes (Figure 11.6, upper row). The superior border is placed 2.0 cm above the angle of the mandible, while the inferior border is placed at the bottom of the cricoid. Anteriorly, the fields should flash the skin surface, often 1.5–2.0 cm anterior to the skin. The posterior border is placed behind the spinous processes. An anterior-posterior field (lower-neck field) encompassing the lower jugular and supraclavicular lymph nodes is matched with the inferior border of the upper-neck fields (Figure 11.6, lower row). The isocenter is set at the matching line.

The field design for postoperative radiation therapy of T3 and T4 glottic tumor is similar to that used for the definitive treatment. The operative bed and neopharynx are included in the upper-neck fields, and the stoma in the lower-neck field. Every effort should be taken to not match fields through the stoma. High-risk areas (positive or close margins, neck lymph nodes) can be boosted with additional dose using the 3D technique. Indications for stoma boost include emergent tracheostomy, subglottic tumor extension, tumor invasion into the soft tissue of the neck, extranodal extension in level VI, close or positive margin and surgical scar across the stoma.

The use of IMRT in locally advanced laryngeal cancer is controversial. The superior border of upper-neck fields in patients with N0 disease often does not encompass a significant amount of the parotid gland. However, IMRT can certainly spare more parotid tissue compared to the conventional radiation technique, especially in patients with positive neck nodes and the upper level II lymph node region needs to be treated. For patients with a low-lying larynx, IMRT is superior to the three-field technique, which often has difficulty to avoid radiating through the shoulders. In addition, IMRT can be delivered in one single dose-painting plan, that avoids the tedious matching and boosting used in three-field conventional technique. In cases of postoperative radiation therapy, IMRT can avoid matching radiation fields through the stoma.

In IMRT planning, accurate target delineation is critical. The gross tumor volume (GTV) should include the gross tumor and enlarged lymph nodes. In general, the clinical target volumes (CTVs) are defined on each slice of the axial CT images. CTV1 usually includes GTV with a 1–2 cm margin, depending on the risk of tumor spread. CTV2 is the high-risk regions that harbor microscopic disease, and includes the whole larynx and cervical lymphatics surrounding the grossly involved lymph nodes. CTV3 is the intermediate-risk regions encompassing the rest of the neck lymphatics. This includes the contralateral neck that receives elective radiation (Figures 11.7 and 11.8) For patients with N0 neck, the superior level II are contoured up to the C1–C2 junction. For patients with node-positive disease, level II lymphatics are contoured to the jugular fossa on the involved side, and the ipsilateral levels IB and V should also be included in CTV2 or CTV3, depending on the risk of involvement. The contralateral level II is contoured up to the C1–C2 junction. Normal structures including parotids, oral cavity, mandible, spinal cord, and cervical esophagus are also delineated.

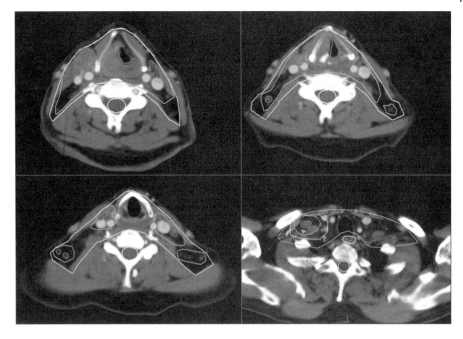

Figure 11.7 Target volume contouring, axial view, gross tumor volumes (GTV in red) including the primary tumor and gross lymph nodes, and clinical target volumes, CTV1 (light red), CTV2 (light green) and CTV3 (light blue). The spinal cord and esophagus are also delineated. For a color version of this figure, see the color plate section.

When planning IMRT in a postoperative setting, all available clinical information should be reviewed, including preoperative clinical and radiographic findings, operative and pathologic evaluations, and postoperative clinical and radiographic findings. CTV1 is the tumor bed including all sites of known disease before surgery; CTV2 encompasses the entire operative bed and any high-risk regions; and CTV3 includes undissected areas that may harbor microscopic disease.

To account for daily set-up variations, planning target volumes (PTVs) are created by adding a 3- to 5-mm margin around the CTVs.

Dose and Fractionation

T1 glottic tumors are treated to doses of 60–66 Gy, with 60 Gy most likely adequate for patients in whom the diagnostic procedure has removed all visible tumors. Higher doses are used for visible gross disease. Occasionally, a

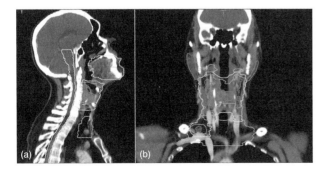

Figure 11.8 Target volume contouring, sagittal (a) and coronal (b) views. Parotids, oral cavity and spinal cord as well as the esophagus are also contoured. For a color version of this figure, see the color plate section.

dose as high as 70 Gy may be needed for large lesions. It has become clear that the radiation fraction size should not be less than 2 Gy, as fractions less than 2 Gy result in lower control rates. A small randomized trial showed that the use of 2.25-Gy fractions with a shorter overall treatment time resulted in superior local control compared to the conventional use of 2-Gy fractions for T1 glottic carcinoma, without adverse reactions from the greater fraction [46]. A total dose of 63 Gy in fractions of 2.25 Gy is a reasonable regimen for T1 tumors.

For T2 glottic tumors, 66–70 Gy in 33-35 fractions are often delivered. As for T1 tumors, fractions less than 2 Gy lead to poorer local control. A total dose of 65.25 Gy in fractions of 2.25 Gy is widely used. Some advocate twice-daily hyperfractionation in treating T2 tumors to a total dose of 76.6–79.2 Gy at 1.2 Gy per fraction. However, this has not been confirmed to have any significant improvement on local control. In RTOG 9512, patients with T2 squamous cell carcinoma of the vocal cord were randomized to hyperfractionation to 79.2 Gy in 66 fractions of 1.2 Gy given twice daily, or standard fractionation to 70 Gy in 35 daily fractions. The five-year local control rate was 78% versus 70% for hyperfractionation and conventional fractionation, respectively, but the difference was not statistically significant [78]. For T3 and T4 glottic tumors, definitive radiation therapy regimen is usually 70 Gy in 35 fractions. The appropriate radiation dose and fractionation to be used with chemotherapy is not entirely clear. In the RTOG 91-11 larynx-preservation trial, all patients received 70 Gy in 35 fractions. No data exist to support reducing the dose after induction chemotherapy, even in the cases of complete response. Although efficacy is expected to increase with concurrent chemoradiation therapy, the reduction of total radiation

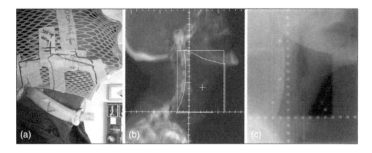

Figure 11.9 Reduction of the initial opposed lateral upper neck fields in order to be off the spinal cord after 45–46 Gy. (a) Photograph of the patient set-up. (b) Digitally reconstructed radiograph. (c) X-ray portal. For a color version of this figure, see the color plate section.

dose in concurrent chemoradiation setting is unproven. In concurrent chemoradiation therapy the standard dose and fractionation is still 70 Gy in 35 fractions.

If a patient is to be treated with a conventional three-field technique, the initial upper-neck fields must be reduced from the posterior border at around 45 Gy to be off the spinal cord (Figure 11.9). The posterior necks are then treated with electron fields to bring the dose to 50–54 Gy and avoid overdosing the spinal cord. When 50–54 Gy has been delivered to the primary tumor and the bilateral necks, a final boost dose of 16–20 Gy is delivered to the primary tumor and gross lymph nodes with adequate margins. The boost dose is usually delivered by 3D radiation techniques with a 1- to 2-cm margin around the gross disease (Figure 11.10).

In the postoperative radiation therapy setting, a total dose of 60–66 Gy in 30–33 fractions is widely accepted. The operative bed and the neck are treated to 50–54 Gy, coming off the spinal cord at 42–44 Gy with a final 3D boost to the high-risk areas (close or positive margins, multiple nodes involvement, extracapsular extension, soft-tissue extension of the primary tumor) to 60–66 Gy. The uninvolved lower neck and supraclavicular fossa included in the lower-neck field is treated to 50 Gy at 2 Gy per fraction, with the dose prescribed to 3 cm from skin surface. The stoma is treated to 50–54 Gy. When stoma boost is indicated, the stoma is boosted to a total dose of 60–66 Gy, usually with *en face* electrons.

When IMRT with integrated boost is used, all volumes are treated simultaneously in one single plan with dose painting. All target volumes are radiated during each radiation session, but a lower dose is delivered to the subclinical disease volume at each fraction. The overall treatment time for subclinical disease is prolonged from the conventional five weeks (50 Gy in 25 fractions) up to 6.5–7 weeks (33–35 fractions). It is important to adjust the dose to electively radiated regions to correct for this change. In definitive IMRT with integrated boost, the dose to PTV1 is typically 70 Gy, to PTV2 59–63 Gy, and to PTV3 54–56 Gy. IMRT is usually delivered once daily in 33–35 fractions (Figure 11.11). Postoperative IMRT is usually delivered in 30 daily fractions with 60–66 Gy to PTV1, 57–60 Gy to PTV2, and 54–56 Gy to PTV3 (Figure 11.12). The treatment is so delivered that at least 95% of the PTVs receive the prescribed doses. IMRT with conventional 2-Gy fractions to all target volumes to 50–54 Gy, followed by sequential IMRT or 3D conformal boost to PTV1 and PTV2, has also been used by some radiation oncologists. This approach delivers a conventional daily fraction dose of 2 Gy to all target volumes, but requires multiple plans to complete a course of radiation therapy. Currently, no definitive data are available to indicate that one technique is superior to the other. The choice of these different IMRT techniques/approaches is a matter of the physician's experience and preference. Dose constraints to normal structures are as follows: The maximum point dose to the spinal cord is limited to 48–50 Gy; the mean dose to each parotid is <26 Gy, or 50% of the parotid receives <30 Gy. For the oral cavity and esophagus, 70% of the volumes should receive less than 45–50 Gy to minimize the toxicities.

Carcinoma of the Supraglottis

Radiation Fields and Treatment Volumes

Bilateral necks need to be treated in all supraglottic carcinoma because of the high risk of lymph node metastasis. In patients with T1 N0 lesions, the lower

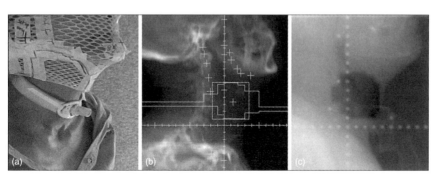

Figure 11.10 Final boost with three-dimensional (3D) technique. A right oblique field is showing. (a) Photograph of the patient set-up; (b) Digitally reconstructed radiograph. (c) X-ray portal. For a color version of this figure, see the color plate section.

Figure 11.11 IMRT plan showing radiation dose distribution for a patient with a T3N2cM0 squamous cell carcinoma of the glottis. 6930 cGy (green) to the PTV1, 5940 cGy (blue) to the PTV2, and 5610 cGy (light green) to the PTV3 in 33 fractions. For a color version of this figure, see the color plate section.

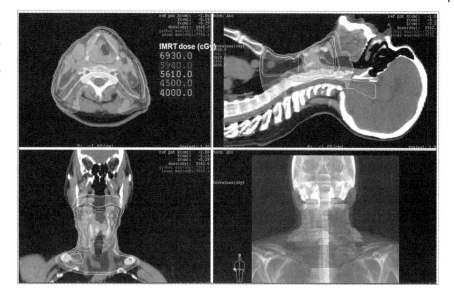

jugular and supraclavicular nodes do not need be included and two upper-neck opposed lateral fields are usually used without a lower-neck field. The superior border is placed at about 1–2 cm above the angle of mandible to encompass the subdigastric nodes. The inferior border is set at 1–2 cm below the cricoid. The fields flash the skin surface 1.5–2.0 cm anteriorly, and the posterior border is at the posterior spinal processes.

The radiation field design for T2 and more advanced supraglottic lesion is similar to that used to T3-4 glottic cancer. The low neck is treated with a matching anterior-posterior lower-neck field, while the superior border of the upper-neck field is adjusted according to lymphadenopathy, and covers the entire jugular chain and follows the inner table of the skull posteriorly.

Radiation fields used in patients after a supraglottic laryngectomy are similar to those used in definitive radiotherapy. The techniques for postoperative radiation therapy after total laryngectomy for supraglottic tumors are similar to those employed for postoperative radiation therapy for glottic cancers. However, in treating supraglottic tumors the draining lymphatics need to be covered more comprehensively. When lymph nodes are involved, the superior border of the field must cover up to the jugular foramen. Boost fields are more generous superiorly when the base of the tongue is involved.

For IMRT planning, the delineation of target volumes for supraglottic cancer is essentially the same as for advanced glottic cancer. Neck nodes, at levels II and III, are contoured as CTV2 in patients with T1 N0 disease,

Figure 11.12 Postoperative IMRT plan showing radiation dose distribution for a patient with a T4N2bM0 Squamous cell carcinoma of the glottis after total laryngectomy and bilateral neck dissection. 6300 cGy (green) to the PTV1 and 5400 cGy (blue) to the PTV2 in 30 fractions. PTV3 was not needed in this case. For a color version of this figure, see the color plate section.

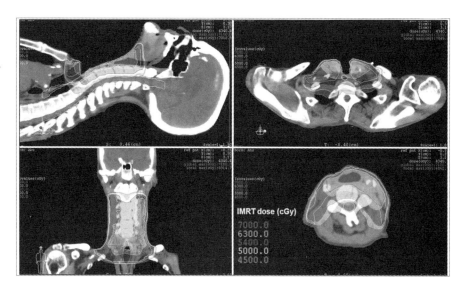

and levels IV and VI are included in CTV2 for patients with T2 N0 disease. Otherwise, the guidelines for target delineation are similar to those for advanced glottic cancer. IMRT in postoperative supraglottic cancer is also similar to that used in postoperative glottic tumor IMRT.

Dose and Fractionation

For T1 supraglottic carcinoma, 66 Gy in 2 Gy per fraction is used in definitive radiation therapy, while for T2 and more advanced lesions 70 Gy in 35 fractions is the standard. Altered fractionation regimens such as hyperfractionated schedules and concomitant boost technique were proven to be superior in local disease control compared to conventional once-daily schedules in patients treated with radiation alone [47]. At present, locally advanced disease is often treated with concurrent chemotherapy, and the efficacy of altered fractionation radiation schedules in the concurrent chemoradiation setting is not entirely clear. As it stands, 70 Gy in 35 fractions remains the standard radiation regimen for concurrent chemoradiation therapy.

When a conventional three-field technique is used, the principles are the same as in T3-4 glottic cancer radiation therapy. If IMRT is to be used, the rules are also the same for supraglottic carcinomas as for T3-4 glottic carcinomas. The dose and fractionation for postoperative radiation therapy after total laryngectomy for supraglottic carcinoma are similar to those for glottic carcinomas. In patients who undergo postoperative radiation after supraglottic laryngectomy, 60 Gy in six weeks to the larynx area is reasonable. A higher dose may be needed if there is a positive margin or residual disease. The risk of significant complications, particularly laryngeal necrosis, may increase after partial laryngectomy with a high radiation dose. Both necks also need to be addressed in the postoperative setting.

Carcinoma of the Hypopharynx

Radiation Fields and Treatment Volumes

Radiation fields used in the treatment of hypopharyngeal carcinomas should encompass the primary tumor and bilateral cervical lymphatics, regardless of the primary tumor stage because of the high risk of lymph node metastasis. The nodal levels at risk include the retropharyngeal nodes and levels II through V. When a conventional three-field technique is used, the upper-neck fields should encompass the primary tumor, the retropharyngeal nodes, the upper jugular and mid-jugular nodes and posterior cervical nodes. The retropharyngeal nodes lie anterior to C1 and C2. The superior border of the upper-neck fields should extend to the base of the sphenoid sinus. For pyriform sinus tumors, the inferior border of the upper-neck lateral fields must cover the entire cricoid cartilage with a 1–2 cm margin. For tumors in the postcricoid area and those arising in posterior pharyngeal wall, the upper-neck fields need to include the upper cervical esophagus. The challenge is that the shoulders are often in the way of upper lateral fields, and this may require a different field arrangement, such as turning the gantry anterior-posteriorly by 5–15°. Occasionally, the couch also needs to be turned so that the beams are arriving superior-inferiorly. The posterior border of the upper-neck lateral fields is adjusted to cover the posterior cervical nodes. A matching lower-neck field encompassing the lower jugular and supraclavicular lymph nodes is always needed. For postoperative radiation, the tumor bed and all cervical lymphatics – including the retropharyngeal nodes – need to be encompassed in the radiation fields. The stoma can be included in the upper-neck lateral fields, or in the lower-neck field.

Because of the extent of the radiation fields and the technical challenging in matching the upper-neck and lower-neck fields in conventional radiation, IMRT is preferred in the treatment of hypopharyngeal cancer. In IMRT planning for definitive treatment, coverage of the neck is similar to that for T3-4 glottic and supraglottic cancers, except that retropharyngeal and levels II to V lymph nodes are covered in all patients, even those with node-negative disease. CTV1 includes the primary tumor and grossly involved lymph nodes with a 1–2 cm margin, while CTV2 should include the whole hypopharynx and upper esophagus in addition to the lymphatics surrounding the grossly involved nodes. CTV3 includes the rest of the cervical lymphatics and the contralateral neck, which is to be radiated electively. Postoperative target volumes are similar to those for advanced laryngeal cancer, except that the retropharyngeal nodes are contoured as CTV3.

Dose and Fractionation

Dose and fractionation in the radiation treatment of hypopharyngeal cancer are almost the same as in supraglottic cancer radiation treatment. T1 disease is treated to 66 Gy in 33 fractions, while T2 and more advanced diseases are usually treated with concurrent chemotherapy and radiation to 70 Gy in 35 fractions. When IMRT is to be used for definitive treatment, the doses and fraction sizes to the PTVs are as described in IMRT for T3-4 supraglottic cancer.

Postoperative radiation dose and fractionation in hypopharyngeal cancer radiation therapy are essentially the same as in supraglottic cancer postoperative radiation. If the lower neck is not involved, it is treated to 50 Gy, and if portions of the operative bed are within the lower-neck field, these areas are boosted to 54–56 Gy. Postoperative IMRT is delivered as for tumors of the glottis in 30 fractions. PTV1 receives 60–66 Gy, PTV2 receives 57 Gy, and PTV3 receives 54 Gy.

Figure 11.13 (a) A patient with CIS involving both true vocal cords. (b) Five months after radiation therapy of 63 Gy in 2.25 Gy per fraction. For a color version of this figure, see the color plate section.

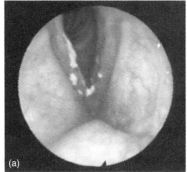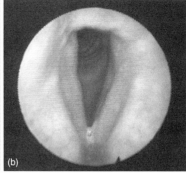

Results of Radiation Therapy

Carcinoma of the Glottis

Carcinoma *In Situ*

Local control rates with primary radiation therapy for CIS of the glottis are over 90% (Figure 11.13) [12–14], similar to the local control rates achieved with radiation in T1 invasive disease. It should be noted that many CIS series might have included patients with invasive carcinoma due to limited tissue sampling. The voice quality of patients treated with radiation therapy is at least as good as, and often superior to, that in patients treated with surgery [48, 49].

T1 Disease

The local control rates for T1 tumors treated with radiation are 85–95% (Figure 11.14; see Table 11.1) [1, 50–55]. For patients who have local failure after radiation, salvage surgery is usually successful, with ultimate control rates above 95%. Salvage surgery usually requires a total laryngectomy, although voice preservation with partial laryngectomy for selected patients is possible [56–62]. Re-radiation is not standard, but can be used in those patients who decline surgery, reportedly with reasonable outcomes [63].

Voice quality usually improves after radiation therapy [64], and the majority of patients treated with radiation maintain good voice quality [65, 66]. In general, the voice quality of patients treated with radiotherapy is

Table 11.1 Results of radiation therapy for T1-2 glottic carcinomas.

Author(s)/Reference	No. of patients	Local Control Rate for T1 tumors (%)	Local Control Rate for T2 tumors (%)
Chera *et al.*, 2010 [1]	585	93.5	75
Smee *et al.*, 2010 [50]	522	94.7	84.5
Jørgensen *et al.*, 2002 [51]	1005	88	67
Le *et al.*, 1997 [52]	398	85	70
Wang, 1997 [53]	665	93	71-77
Hendrickson, 1985 [54]	364	90	73
Lustig *et al.*, 1984 [55]	342	90	78

superior to that in those who have undergone surgery [67–69].

T2 Disease

Local control rates for T2 glottic cancer treated with radiation range from 65% to 80%, and the ultimate local control rate with salvage surgery is about 90% (Table 11.2; Figure 11.15). The wide variation in local control rates

Figure 11.14 (a) A patient with a T1b squamous cell carcinoma arising from CIS involving both true vocal cords. (b) Six months after radiation therapy of 63 Gy in 2.25 Gy per fraction. For a color version of this figure, see the color plate section.

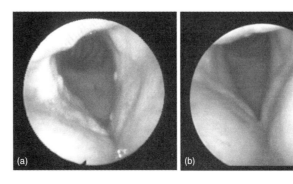

Table 11.2 Results of radiation therapy for T3 glottic carcinomas.

Author(s)/Reference	No. of patients	Local Control Rate (%)
Hinerman *et al.*, 2007 [79]	87	67
Mendenhall *et al.*, 1997 [80]	75	63
Wang, 1997 [53]	65	57
Bryant *et al.*, 1995 [4]	55	55
Terhaard *et al.*, 1991 [81]	104	53
Croll *et al.*, 1989 [82]	30	70
Lundgren *et al.*, 1988 [83]	141	44
Hendrickson, 1985 [54]	39	56
Lustig *et al.*, 1984 [55]	47	65

treated with radiation is probably due to relatively inaccurate disease staging. Some patients might have more advanced disease, which was not detected by clinical examination but may be revealed if a CT had been obtained. In addition, tumor volumes have not been taken into consideration in regard to the local control in most early reports.

Vocal cord mobility as a prognostic indicator is controversial. It has been reported in some series that patients who had T2 tumors with impaired vocal cord mobility had an inferior local control rate than those who had normal vocal cord mobility [70–72]. However, others have not seen a difference in local disease control based on impairment of vocal cord mobility [73–76].

Hyperfractionated radiation therapy has been used to improve control rates for T2 glottic tumors. Studies from the University of Florida [77], M. D. Anderson Cancer Center [73], and the RTOG [78] showed only trends of improved local control for patients with T2 disease treated with hyperfractionation, but with no statistically significant difference.

T3-4 Disease

Local control rates for patients with T3 glottic cancer treated with radiation alone are in the range of 44%

to 70% (Table 11.2) [4, 53–55, 79–83]. Most of these series had relatively small patient numbers. The salvage rate with surgery for patients who recur after radiation therapy is about 50%. Bryant *et al.* reported that the disease-specific survival of patients treated with radiation and salvage surgery was not statistically different from that of patients who had laryngectomy and postoperative radiation therapy [4]. A report from the University of Florida showed that the disease-free survival and overall survival were comparable in patients treated with radiation therapy and those who had undergone laryngectomy [84].

Patients with T3 tumors are usually candidates for larynx-preservation therapy. In the VA larynx-preservation trial and in the RTOG 91-11 trial, the majority of patients had T3 tumors. In the VA trial, about two-thirds of patients were able to preserve their larynx after induction chemotherapy followed by radiation, and the overall survival was not compromised compared to that of patients who had laryngectomy and postoperative radiation [6]. Results from the RTOG 91-11 trial showed no significant differences in laryngeal preservation rates between patients who received induction chemotherapy followed by radiation compared with radiation only. However, those patients who received concurrent cisplatin and radiotherapy had a significantly higher larynx-preservation rate (72%, 67%, and 84%, respectively). The five-year overall survivals were almost the same in all three arms, however [7]. Laryngectomy followed by radiation therapy or chemoradiation therapy for patients with high-risk pathologic features is the treatment of choice for patients with T4 glottic tumors, with reported local control rates of 60–70%. Although the VA larynx trial suggested that induction chemotherapy might be appropriate for advanced laryngeal cancer [6], a report from M. D. Anderson Cancer Center suggested that patients with T4 disease do not benefit from this approach [85], and total laryngectomy should be the standard of care. RTOG 91-11 excluded patients with T4 tumors which penetrated through the thyroid cartilage or invaded >1 cm into the base of tongue.

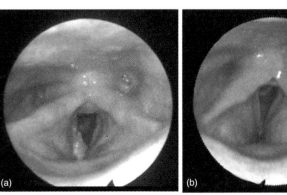

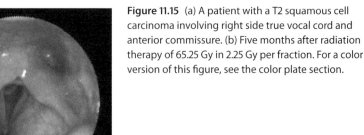

Figure 11.15 (a) A patient with a T2 squamous cell carcinoma involving right side true vocal cord and anterior commissure. (b) Five months after radiation therapy of 65.25 Gy in 2.25 Gy per fraction. For a color version of this figure, see the color plate section.

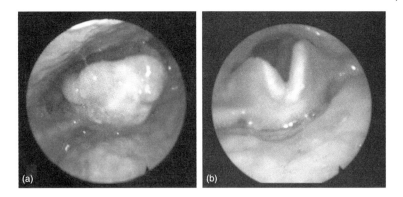

Figure 11.16 (a) A patient with a T1N0 squamous cell carcinoma in the epiglottis. (b) Three months after radiation therapy of 66 Gy in 2.2 Gy per fraction with concurrent chemotherapy. For a color version of this figure, see the color plate section.

Carcinoma of the Supraglottis

T1 supraglottic tumor is relatively rare. With radiation therapy alone, the local control rates range from 80% to 100% (Figure 11.16) [27,86–88].

Local control rates for T2 tumors have been reported in the range of 60% to 90%. Reports from single-institution experiences indicated that twice-daily fractionation might improve the control rate in this group of patients [27,86–88].

Control rates with radiation therapy alone for T3 tumors range from 40% to 75%. Twice-daily fractionation may also be beneficial in T3 disease [27,53,86–88].

Most patients with bulky or infiltrative T3 supraglottic tumors, especially those with vocal cord fixation, are treated with surgery. Some patients have lesions that are amenable to supraglottic laryngectomy, but others require total laryngectomy. Local disease control rates with supraglottic laryngectomy range from 80% to 90% [89–91]. Many patients require postoperative radiation therapy due to inadequate margins or the presence of nodal disease. Induction chemotherapy followed by radiation therapy and concurrent chemoradiation therapy for larynx preservation has been tested in Phase III trials. As noted above, concurrent chemoradiation results in a higher laryngectomy-free survival, whereas the overall survival is similar with radiation alone, induction chemotherapy followed by radiation therapy or concurrent chemoradiation (Figure 11.17) [7].

Patients with T4 tumors may not respond as well to chemoradiation therapy as T2-3 tumors, and often need salvage laryngectomy [92]. The response of T4 tumors to chemoradiation is usually not durable. Total laryngectomy, followed by postoperative radiation or chemoradiation yields better locoregional control [24].

Carcinoma of the Hypopharynx

Early-stage disease is rare. Local disease control rates with radiation alone are in the range of 70% to 90% for T1 disease, and 60% to 80% for T2 disease [37,38,53,93–96].

For patients with T3-4 tumors, surgery with postoperative radiation results in locoregional control rates in the range of 50% to 90%. However, the five-year survival rates have been consistently low, from 22% to 43% [97–99]. Patients who are treated with surgery and postoperative radiation therapy have significantly higher local control and survival rates than those who undergo surgery alone. Frank *et al.* found that patients with hypopharyngeal cancer who received postoperative irradiation had only 14% locoregional failure rate, compared to 57% for those treated with surgery only, despite the fact that patients treated with combined modalities had more advanced disease and addition of postoperative radiotherapy was associated with improved disease-free and adjusted overall cancer-specific survival [100].

In the EORTC larynx-preservation study for patients with hypopharyngeal cancer, induction chemotherapy – followed by radiation therapy for complete responders

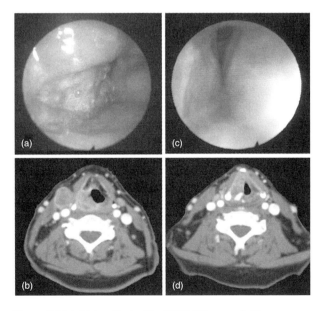

Figure 11.17 (a,b) A patient with a T3N2aM0 supraglottic squamous cell carcinoma. (a) Photograph. (b) Axial CT image. (c,d) At four months after concurrent cisplatin chemotherapy and IMRT to 69.3 Gy in 2.1 Gy per fraction. (c) Photograph. (d) Axial CT image. For a color version of this figure, see the color plate section.

or surgery for incomplete responders – was compared with immediate pharyngolaryngectomy and postoperative radiation. Survival rates were equivalent in the two groups, but 35% of the patients in the chemotherapy and radiation group preserved their larynx [8].

IMRT for Laryngeal and Hypopharyngeal Cancer

The use of IMRT in head and neck cancer radiotherapy has increased significantly during the past decade [101]. Parotid-sparing with IMRT reduces xerostomia, which is usually permanent with three-field conventional radiation techniques, and improves xerostomia-related quality of life [102, 103]. IMRT offers excellent outcomes in locoregional control and overall survival in patients with head and neck cancer, especially in those with oropharyngeal cancer.

A report of the University of Iowa experience showed that, with IMRT, the two-year overall survival, local progression-free survival and locoregional progression-free survival were 85%, 94%, and 92%, respectively. Patients with oropharyngeal cancer did significantly better than patients with oral cavity and laryngeal cancer, with a two-year local-regional control rate of 98%, compared to 78% for oral cavity cancer and 85% for laryngeal cancer (p = 0.005) [104].

Series of retrospective studies on IMRT in patients with locally advanced laryngeal and hypopharyngeal cancers showed that IMRT is at least as effective as conventional radiation therapy, but with reduced toxicities [105, 106]. Lee *et al.* showed two-year local progression-free, regional progression-free and laryngectomy-free survivals of 86%, 89%, and 92%, respectively, in 31 patients with advanced stage laryngeal and hypopharyngeal cancer (most with stage IV disease) treated with IMRT. There was no grade 2 or higher xerostomia observed at the time of data analysis [107]. Daly *et al.* reported the outcomes of 42 patients with squamous cell carcinoma of the hypopharynx ($n = 23$) and larynx ($n = 19$) who underwent IMRT (36 patients received systemic therapy). The median follow-up was 30 months among surviving patients, and the three-year actuarial locoregional control, freedom from distant metastasis, and overall survival rates were 80%, 72%, and 46%, respectively. Patients with hypopharyngeal tumors fared worse than those with laryngeal tumors [108].

Early data showed that treatment with IMRT in patients with advanced hypopharyngeal cancer resulted in excellent locoregional control, overall survival, and larynx preservation [109–111]. Hypopharyngeal cancer is notorious with regards to high rates of local and distant failure [112]. IMRT improves target coverage while sparing the salivary glands as well as the spinal cord. This potentially allows radiation dose escalation, which may result in a higher local control rate in laryngo-hypopharyngeal cancers, especially in advanced hypopharyngeal cancers [113, 114].

Larynx Preservation in Laryngeal and Hypopharyngeal Cancer

The goal of larynx-preservation therapy in patients with laryngeal or hypopharyngeal cancer is to control the tumor and preserve a functional larynx. Since the VA larynx trial which showed that induction chemotherapy of cisplatin and 5-fluorouracil (5-FU) followed by definitive radiation therapy can preserve the larynx in about two-thirds of patients with locally advanced laryngeal cancer, the EORTC subsequently demonstrated the safety and efficacy of this approach in patients with hypopharyngeal cancer [6, 8]. The RTOG 91-11 larynx trial showed that concurrent cisplatin chemotherapy and radiation therapy is more effective in larynx preservation than sequential induction chemotherapy followed by radiation therapy or radiation therapy alone [7]. More recent randomized studies demonstrated that three-drug induction chemotherapy (docetaxel, cisplatin and 5-FU; TPF) followed by radiation or concurrent chemoradiation increases overall response rate, larynx preservation rate and prolongs survival in patients with locally advanced laryngeal and hypopharyngeal cancer, compared to the classic two-drug induction chemotherapy (cisplatin and 5-FU; PF) [115, 116]. However, controversy persists regarding patient selection for larynx preservation.

Patients with a functional larynx and a T3 tumor that requires a total laryngectomy if treated by a surgical approach are the main candidates for larynx-preservation chemoradiation therapy (Figures 11.17 and 11.18).

Patients with T4 disease are probably not good candidates for larynx preservation. An analysis of data from the VA larynx trial demonstrated a poorer response to chemotherapy and more frequent salvage laryngectomy in patients with T4 disease [117]. The odds ratio of achieving a response to chemotherapy for patients with T1 to T3 versus T4 disease was 5.6 (95% CI 1.5–20.8; p = 0.0108). In those patients who did respond to chemotherapy and received radiation therapy for larynx preservation, salvage laryngectomy was required in 56% of patients with T4 tumors compared to 28% of those with T1 to T3 tumors (p = 0.001). Patients with T4 disease with tumor penetrating through the cartilage or extending more than 1 cm into the base of the tongue were not eligible for RTOG 91-11 [7]. These patients should undergo surgery with total laryngectomy and neck dissection, followed by postoperative radiation or chemoradiation therapy, if they have positive/close surgical margin or extracapsular extension of involved lymph nodes.

Patients with T2 tumors are generally good candidates for laryngeal preservation chemoradiation therapy.

For those patients whose tumors are amenable for partial laryngectomy, surgery is also a reasonable option of treatment. Patients who were eligible for partial laryngectomy were actually excluded from the EORTC larynx-preservation trial in hypopharyngeal cancer patients, and also from the RTOG 91-11 trial [7, 8]. However, patients with an endophytic T2 tumor, which is not suitable for partial laryngectomy, as well as those with lymphadenopathy and at high risk for extracapsular extension (ECE), should be considered for nonsurgical larynx preservation approach. In these cases, if patients undergo surgery, postoperative chemoradiation therapy is usually required because of high-risk pathologic features [30, 31]. The functional outcome of tri-modality therapy might be worse than chemoradiotherapy as primary therapy.

Patients with laryngeal dysfunction are not good candidates for larynx preservation [118]. Indicators of baseline laryngeal dysfunction include a tracheotomy, tumor-related dysphagia requiring a gastric tube, and a recent history of aspiration pneumonia. In addition, patients with a history of recurring pneumonia and chronic obstructive pulmonary disease should probably also be excluded from larynx-preservation approach [116].

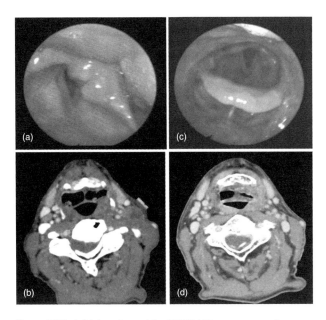

Figure 11.18 (a,b) A patient with a T3N2bM0 squamous cell carcinoma of the hypopharynx involving the left aryepiglottic fold and arytenoids. (a) Photograph. (b) Axial CT image. (c,d) At three months after concurrent chemotherapy and IMRT of 69.3 Gy in 2.1 Gy per fraction. (c) Photograph. (d) Axial CT image. For a color version of this figure, see the color plate section.

References

1 Chera, B.S., Amdur, R.J., Morris, C.G., *et al.* (2010) T1N0 to T2N0 squamous cell carcinoma of the glottic larynx treated with definitive radiotherapy. *Int. J. Radiat. Oncol. Biol. Phys.*, **78**, 461–466.

2 Lindberg, R. (1972) Distribution of cervical lymph node metastases from squamous cell carcinoma of the upper respiratory and digestive tracts. *Cancer*, **29**, 1446–1449.

3 AJCC (2017) Cancer Staging Manual, 8th edition. Springer.

4 Bryant, G.P., Poulsen, M.G., Tripcony, L., *et al.* (1995) Treatment decision in T3N0M0 glottic carcinoma. *Int. J. Radiat. Oncol. Biol. Phys.*, **31**, 285–293.

5 Parsons, J., Mendenhall, W., Stringer, S., *et al.* (1998) T4 laryngeal carcinoma: radiotherapy alone with surgery reserved for salvage. *Int. J. Radiat. Oncol. Biol. Phys.*, **40**, 549–552.

6 Department of Veterans Affairs Laryngeal Cancer Study Group (1992) Induction chemotherapy plus radiation compared with surgery plus radiation in patients with advanced laryngeal cancer. *N. Engl. J. Med.*, **324**, 1685–1690.

7 Forastiere, A.A., Goepfert, H., Maor, M., *et al.* (2003) Concurrent chemotherapy and radiotherapy for organ preservation in advanced laryngeal cancer. *N. Engl. J. Med.*, **349**, 2091–2098.

8 Lefebvre, J.L., Chevalier, D., Luboinski, B., *et al.* (1996) Larynx preservation in pyriform sinus cancer: preliminary results of a European Organization for Research and Treatment of Cancer phase III trial. EORTC Head and Neck Cancer Cooperative Group. *J. Natl Cancer Inst.*, **88**, 890–899.

9 Maran, A.G., Mackenzie, I.J., Stanley, R.E. (1984) Carcinoma in situ of the larynx. *Head Neck Surg.*, **7**, 28–31.

10 Wolfensberger, M., Dort, J.C. (1990) Endoscopic laser surgery for early glottic carcinoma: a clinical and experimental study. *Laryngoscope*, **100**, 1100–1105.

11 McGuirt, W.F., Browne, J.D. (1991) Management decisions in laryngeal carcinoma in situ. *Laryngoscope*, **101**, 125–129.

12 Smitt, M.C., Goffinet, D.R. (1994) Radiotherapy for carcinoma-in-situ of the glottic larynx. *Int. J. Radiat. Oncol. Biol. Phys.*, **28**, 251–255.

13 Spayne, J.A., Warde, P., O'Sullivan, B., *et al.* (2001) Carcinoma-in-situ of the glottic larynx: results of treatment with radiation therapy. *Int. J. Radiat. Oncol. Biol. Phys.*, **49**, 1235–1238.

14 Sengupta, N., Morris, C.G., Kirwan, J., *et al.* (2010) Definitive radiotherapy for carcinoma in situ of the true vocal cords. *Am. J. Clin. Oncol.*, **33**, 94–95.

15 Strong, M.S. (1975) Laser excision of carcinoma of the larynx. *Laryngoscope*, **85**, 1286–1289.

16 Sessions, D., Maness, G., Mcswain, B. (1964) Laryngofissure in the treatment of carcinoma of the vocal cord. *Laryngoscope*, **75**, 490–502.

17 Soo, K.C., Shah. J.P., Gopinath. K.S., *et al.* (1988) Analysis of prognostic variables and results after supraglottic partial laryngectomy. *Am. J. Surg.*, **156**, 301–305.

18 Laccourreye, O., Weinstein, G., Brasnu, D., *et al.* (1991) Vertical partial laryngectomy: a critical analysis of local recurrence. *Ann. Otol. Rhinol. Laryngol.*, **100**, 68–71.

19 Peretti, G., Nicolai, P., Redaelli De Zinis, L.O., *et al.* (2000) Endoscopic CO_2 laser excision for T1, T1, and T2 glottic carcinomas: cure rate and prognostic factors. *Otolaryngol. Head Neck Surg.*, **123**, 124–131.

20 Puxeddu, R., Argiolas, F., Bielamowicz, S., *et al.* (2000) Surgical therapy of T1 and selected cases of T2 glottic carcinoma: cordectomy, horizontal glottectomy and CO_2 laser endoscopic resection. *Tumori*, **86**, 277–282.

21 Grant, D.G., Salassa, J.R., Hinni, M.L., *et al.* (2007) Transoral laser microsurgery for untreated glottic carcinoma. *Otolaryngol. Head Neck Surg.*, **137**, 482–486.

22 Mendenhall, W.M., Parsons, J.T., Stringer, S.P., *et al.* (1988) T1-T2 vocal cord carcinoma: a basis for comparing the results of radiotherapy and surgery. *Head Neck Surg.*, **10**, 373–377.

23 Hartl, D.M., Ferlito, A., Brasnu, D.F., *et al.* (2011) Evidence-based review of treatment options for patients with glottic cancer. *Head Neck*, **33**, 1638–1648.

24 Patel, U.A., Howell, L.K. (2011) Local response to chemoradiation in T4 larynx cancer with cartilage invasion. *Laryngoscope*, **121**, 106–110.

25 Steiner, W. (1993) Results of curative laser microsurgery of laryngeal carcinomas. *Am. J. Otolaryngol.*, **14**, 116–121.

26 Grant, D.G., Salassa, J.R., Hinni, M.L., *et al.* (2007) Transoral laser microsurgery for carcinoma of the supraglottic larynx. *Otolaryngol. Head Neck Surg.*, **136**, 900–906.

27 Hinerman, R.W., Mendenhall, W.M., Amdur, R.J., *et al.* (2002) Carcinoma of the supraglottic larynx: treatment results with radiotherapy alone or with planned neck dissection. *Head Neck*, **24**, 456–467.

28 Corry, J., Smith, J.G., Peters, L.J. (2001) The concept of a planned neck dissection is obsolete. *Cancer J.*, **7**, 472–474.

29 Robbins, K.T., Davidson, W., Peters, L.J., *et al.* (1988) Conservation surgery for T2 and T3 carcinomas of the supraglottic larynx. *Arch. Otolaryngol. Head Neck Surg.*, **114**, 421–426.

30 Bernier, J., Domenge, C., Ozsahin, M., *et al.* (2004) Postoperative irradiation with or without concomitant chemotherapy for locally advanced head and neck cancer. *N. Engl. J. Med.*, **350**, 1945–1952.

31 Cooper, J.S., Pajak, T.F., Forastiere, A.A., *et al.* (2004) Postoperative concurrent radiotherapy and chemotherapy for high-risk squamous-cell carcinoma of the head and neck. *N. Engl. J. Med.*, **350**, 1937–1944.

32 Garas, J., McGuirt, W.F., Sr (2006) Squamous cell carcinoma of the subglottis. *Am. J. Otolaryngol.*, **27**, 1–4.

33 Paisley, S., Warde, P.R., O'Sullivan, B., *et al.* (2002) Results of radiotherapy for primary subglottic squamous cell carcinoma. *Int. J. Radiat. Oncol. Biol. Phys.*, **52**, 1245–1250.

34 Makeieff, M., Mercante, G., Jouzdani, E., *et al.* (2004) Supraglottic hemipharyngolaryngectomy for the treatment of T1 and T2 carcinomas of laryngeal margin and piriform sinus. *Head Neck*, **26**, 701–705.

35 Holsinger, F.C., Motamed, M., Garcia, D., *et al.* (2006) Resection of selected invasive squamous cell carcinoma of the pyriform sinus by means of the lateral pharyngotomy approach: the partial lateral pharyngectomy. *Head Neck*, **28**, 705–711.

36 Vilaseca, I., Blanch, J.L., Bernal-Sprekelsen, M., *et al.* (2004) CO_2 laser surgery: a larynx preservation alternative for selected hypopharyngeal carcinomas. *Head Neck*, **26**, 953–959.

37 Rabbani, A., Amdur, R.J., Mancuso, A.A., *et al.* (2008) Definitive radiotherapy for T1-T2 squamous cell carcinoma of pyriform sinus. *Int. J. Radiat. Oncol. Biol. Phys.*, **72**, 351–355.

38 Nakamura, K., Shioyama, Y., Sasaki, T., *et al.* (2005) Chemoradiation therapy with or without salvage surgery for early squamous cell carcinoma of the hypopharynx. *Int. J. Radiat. Oncol. Biol. Phys.*, **62**, 680–683.

39 Brizel, D., Albers, M., Fisher, S., *et al.* (1998) Hyperfractionated irradiation with or without concurrent chemotherapy for locally advanced head and neck cancer. *N. Engl. J. Med.*, **338**, 1798–1804.

40 Pignon, J., Bourhis, J., Domenge, C., *et al.* (2000) Chemotherapy added to locoregional treatment for head and neck squamous-cell carcinoma: three meta-analyses of updated individual data. *Lancet*, **355**, 949–955.

41 Tsou, Y.A., Lin, M.H., Hua, C.H., *et al.* (2007) Survival outcome by early chemoradiation therapy salvage or early surgical salvage for the treatment of hypopharyngeal cancer. *Otolaryngol. Head Neck Surg.*, **137**, 711–716.

42 Prades, J.M., Schmitt, T.M., Timoshenko, A.P., *et al.* (2002) Concomitant chemoradiotherapy in pyriform sinus carcinoma. *Arch Otolaryngol Head Neck Surg.*, **128**, 384–388.

43 Wei, W.I. (2002) The dilemma of treating hypopharyngeal carcinoma: more or less: Hayes Martin Lecture. *Arch Otolaryngol Head Neck Surg.*, **128**, 229–232.

44 Foote, R.L., Grado, G.L., Buskirk, S.J., *et al.* (1996) Radiation therapy for glottic cancer using 6-MV photons. *Cancer*, **77**, 381–386.

45 Sombeck, M.D., Kalbaugh, K.J., Mendenhall, W.M., *et al.* (1996) Radiotherapy for early vocal cord cancer: a dosimetric analysis of 60-Co versus 6 MV photons. *Head Neck*, **18**, 167–173.

46 Yamazaki, H., Nishiyama, K., Tanaka, E., *et al.* (2006) Radiotherapy for early glottic carcinoma (T1N0M0): results of prospective randomized study of radiation fraction size and overall treatment time. *Int. J. Radiat. Oncol. Biol. Phys.*, **64**, 77–82.

47 Fu, K.K., Pajak, T.F., Trotti, A., *et al.* (2000) A Radiation Therapy Oncology Group (RTOG) phase III randomized study to compare hyperfractionation and two variants of accelerated fractionation to standard fractionation radiotherapy for head and neck squamous cell carcinomas: first report of RTOG 9003. *Int. J. Radiat. Oncol. Biol. Phys.*, **48**, 7–16.

48 Smith, J.C., Johnson, J.T., Cognetti, D.M., *et al.* (2003) Quality of life, functional outcome, and costs of early glottic cancer. *Laryngoscope*, **113**, 68–76.

49 Loughran, S., Calder, N., MacGregor, F.B., *et al.* (2005) Quality of life and voice following endoscopic resection or radiotherapy for early glottic cancer. *Clin. Otolaryngol.*, **30**, 42–47.

50 Smee, R.I., Meagher, N.S., Williams, J.R., *et al.* (2010) Role of radiotherapy in early glottic carcinoma. *Head Neck*, **32**, 850–859.

51 Jørgensen, K., Godballe, C., Hansen, O., *et al.* (2002) Cancer of the larynx – treatment results after primary radiotherapy with salvage surgery in a series of 1005 patients. *Acta Oncol.*, **41**, 69–76.

52 Le, Q.T., Fu, K.K., Kroll, S., *et al.* (1997) Influence of fraction size, total dose, and overall time on local control of T1-T2 glottic carcinoma. *Int. J. Radiat. Oncol. Biol. Phys.*, **39**, 115–126.

53 Wang, C.C. (1997) Carcinoma of the larynx, in *Radiation Therapy for Head and Neck Neoplasms*, 3rd edition (ed. C.-C. Wang), Wiley-Liss, New York, pp. 221–255.

54 Hendrickson, F.R. (1985) Radiation therapy treatment of larynx cancers. *Cancer*, **55**, 2058–2061.

55 Lustig, R.A., MacLean, C.J., Hanks, G.E., *et al.* (1984) The patterns of care outcome studies: results of the national practice in carcinoma of the larynx. *Int. J. Radiat. Oncol. Biol. Phys.*, **10**, 2357–2362.

56 Puxeddu, R., Piazza, C., Mensi, M.C., *et al.* (2004) Carbon dioxide laser salvage surgery after radiotherapy failure in T1 and T2 glottic carcinoma. *Otolaryngol. Head Neck Surg.*, **130**, 84–88.

57 Crampette, L., Garrel, R., Gardiner, Q., *et al.* (1999) Modified subtotal laryngectomy with cricohyoidoepiglottopexy – long term results in 81 patients. *Head Neck*, **21**, 95–103.

58 Shvero, J., Koren, R., Zohar, L., *et al.* (2003) Laser surgery for the treatment of glottic carcinomas. *Am. J. Otolaryngol.*, **24**, 28–33.

59 Watters, G.W., Patel, S.G., Rhys-Evans, P.H. (2000) Partial laryngectomy for recurrent laryngeal carcinoma. *Clin. Otolaryngol. Allied Sci.*, **25**, 146–152.

60 Rodríguez-Cuevas, S., Labastida, S., Gonzalez, D., *et al.* (1998) Partial laryngectomy as salvage surgery for radiation failures in T1-T2 laryngeal cancer. *Head Neck*, **20**, 630–633.

61 Marioni, G., Marchese-Ragona, R., Pastore, A., *et al.* (2006) The role of supracricoid laryngectomy for glottic carcinoma recurrence after radiotherapy failure: a critical review. *Acta Otolaryngol.*, **126**, 1245–1251.

62 Ganly, I., Patel, S.G., Matsuo, J., *et al.* (2006) Results of surgical salvage after failure of definitive radiation therapy for early-stage squamous cell carcinoma of the glottic larynx. *Arch Otolaryngol Head Neck Surg.*, **132**, 59–66.

63 Wang, C., McIntyre, J. (1993) Re-irradiation of laryngeal carcinoma – techniques and results. *Int. J. Radiat. Oncol. Biol. Phys.*, **26**, 783–785.

64 Agarwal, J.P., Baccher, G.K., Waghmare, C.M., *et al.* (2009) Factors affecting the quality of voice in the early glottic cancer treated with radiotherapy. *Radiother Oncol.*, **90**, 177–182.

65 Lesnicar, H., Smid, L., Zakotnik, B. (1996) Early glottic cancer: the influence of primary treatment on voice preservation. *Int. J. Radiat. Oncol. Biol. Phys.*, **36**, 1025–1032.

66 Harrison, L.B., Solomon, B., Miller, S., *et al.* (1990) Prospective computer-assisted voice analysis for patients with early stage glottic cancer: a preliminary report of the functional result of laryngeal irradiation. *Int. J. Radiat. Oncol. Biol. Phys.*, **19**, 123–127.

67 Jones, A.S., Fish, B., Fenton, J.E., *et al.* (2004) The treatment of early laryngeal cancers (T1-T2 N0): surgery or irradiation? *Head Neck*, **26**, 127–135.

68 Bron, L.P., Soldati, D., Zouhair, A., *et al.* (2001) Treatment of early stage squamous-cell carcinoma of the glottic larynx: endoscopic surgery or cricohyoidoepiglottopexy versus radiotherapy. *Head Neck*, **23**, 823–829.

69 Kennedy, J.T., Paddle, P.M., Cook, B.J., *et al.* (2007) Voice outcomes following transoral laser microsurgery for early glottic squamous cell carcinoma. *J. Laryngol. Otol.*, **121**, 1184–1188.

70 Klintenberg, C., Lundgren, J., Adell, G., *et al.* (1996) Primary radiotherapy of T1 and T2 glottic carcinoma-analysis of treatment results and prognostic factors in 223 patients. *Acta Oncol.*, **35** (Suppl. 8), 81–86.

71 Harwood, A.R., Beale, F.A., Cummings, B.J., *et al.* (1981) T2 glottic cancer: an analysis of dose-time-volume factors. *Int. J. Radiat. Oncol. Biol. Phys.*, **7**, 1501–1505.

72 Kelly, M.D., Hahn, S.S., Spaulding, C.A., *et al.* (1989) Definitive radiotherapy in the management of stage I and II carcinomas of the glottis. *Ann. Otol. Rhinol. Laryngol.*, **98**, 235–239.

73 Garden, A.S., Forster, K., Wong, P.F., *et al.* (2003) Results of radiotherapy for T2N0 glottic carcinoma: does the '2' stand for twice-daily treatment? *Int. J. Radiat. Oncol. Biol. Phys.*, **55**, 322–328.

74 Wiggenraad, R.G., Terhaard, C.H., Horidjik, G.J., *et al.* (1990) The importance of vocal cord mobility in T2 laryngeal cancer. *Radiother. Oncol.*, **18**, 321–327.

75 Howell-Burke, D., Peters, L.J., Goepfert, H., *et al.* (1990) T2 glottic cancer. *Arch. Otolaryngol. Head Neck Surg.*, **116**, 830–835.

76 Karim, A.B., Kralendonk, J.H., Yap, L.Y., et al. (1987) Heterogeneity of stage II glottic carcinoma and its therapeutic implications. *Int. J. Radiat. Oncol. Biol. Phys.*, **13**, 313–317.

77 Mendenhall, W.M., Amdur, R.J., Morris, C.G., *et al.* (2001) T1-T2N0 squamous cell carcinoma of the glottic larynx treated with radiation therapy. *J. Clin. Oncol.*, **19**, 4029–4036.

78 Trotti, A., 3rd, Zhang, Q., Bentzen, S.M., Emami, B., *et al.* (2014) Randomized trial of hyperfractionation versus conventional fractionation in T2 squamous cell carcinoma of the vocal cord (RTOG 9512). *Int. J. Radiat. Oncol. Biol. Phys.*, **89**, 958–963.

79 Hinerman, R., Mendenhall, W., Morris, C., *et al.* (2007) T3 and T4 true vocal cord squamous carcinomas treated with external beam irradiation: a single institution's 35-year experience. *Am. J. Clin. Oncol.*, **30**, 181–185.

80 Mendenhall, W.M., Parsons, J.T., Mancuso, A.A., *et al.* (1997) Definitive radiotherapy for T3 squamous cell carcinoma of the glottic larynx. *J. Clin. Oncol.*, **15**, 2394–2402.

81 Terhaard, C.H.F., Karim, A.B.M.F., Hoogenraad, W.J., *et* al. (1991) Local control in T3 laryngeal cancer treated with radical radiotherapy, time dose relationship: the concept of nominal standard dose and linear quadratic model. *Int. J. Radiat. Oncol. Biol. Phys.*, **20**, 1207–1214.

82 Croll, G.A., Gerritsen, G.J., Tiwari, R.M., *et al.* (1989) Primary radiotherapy with surgery in reserve for advanced laryngeal carcinoma Results and complications. *Eur. J. Surg. Oncol.*, **15**, 350–356.

83 Lundgren, J.A.V., Gilbert, R.W., Van Nostrand, A.W.P., *et al.* (1988) T3N0M0 glottic carcinoma – a failure analysis. *Clin. Otolaryngol.*, **13**, 455–465.

84 Mendenhall, W.M., Parsons, J.T., Stringer, S.P., *et al.* (1992) Stage T3 squamous cell carcinoma of the glottic larynx: a comparison of laryngectomy and irradiation. *Int. J. Radiat. Oncol. Biol. Phys.*, **23**, 725–732.

85 Shirinian, M.H., Weber, R.S., Lippman, S.M., *et al.* (1994) Laryngeal preservation by induction chemotherapy plus radiotherapy in locally advanced head and neck cancer: the M.D. Anderson Cancer Center experience. *Head Neck*, **16**, 39–44.

86 Sykes, A.J., Slevin, N.J., Gupta, N.K., *et al.* (2000) 331 cases of clinically node-negative supraglottic carcinoma of the larynx: a study of a modest size fixed field radiotherapy approach. *Int. J. Radiat. Oncol. Biol. Phys.*, **46**, 1109–1115.

87 Nakfoor, B.M., Spiro, I.J., Wang, C.C., *et al.* (1998) Results of accelerated radiotherapy for supraglottic carcinoma: a Massachusetts General Hospital and Massachusetts Eye and Ear Infirmary experience. *Head Neck*, **20**, 379–384

88 Garden, A.S., Morrison, W.H., Ang, K.K., *et al.* (1995) Hyperfractionated radiation in the treatment of squamous cell carcinomas of the head and neck: a comparison of two fractionation schedules. *Int. J. Radiat. Oncol. Biol. Phys.*, **31**, 493–502.

89 Lee, N.K., Goepfert, H., Wendt, C.D. (1990) Supraglottic laryngectomy for intermediate stage cancer: U.T.M.D. Cancer Center experience with combined therapy. *Laryngoscope*, **100**, 831–836.

90 Bocca, E., Pignatarom O., Oldinim C. (1983) Supraglottic laryngectomy: 30 years of experience. *Ann. Otol. Rhinol. Laryngol.*, **92**, 14–18.

91 Ogura, J.H., Marks, J.E., Freeman, R.B. (1980) Results of conservation surgery for cancers of the supraglottis and pyriform sinus. *Laryngoscope*, **90**, 591–600.

92 Bradford, C.R., Wolf, G.T., Carey, T.E., *et al.* (1999) Predictive markers for response to chemotherapy, organ preservation, and survival in patients with advanced laryngeal carcinoma. *Otolaryngol Head Neck Surg.*, **121**, 534–538.

93 Garden, A.S., Morrison, W.H., Clayman, G.L., *et al.* (1996) Early squamous cell carcinoma of the hypopharynx: outcomes of treatment with radiation alone to the primary disease. *Head Neck*, **18**, 317–322.

94 Amdur, R., Mendenhall, W., Stringer, S., *et al.* (2001) Organ preservation with radiotherapy for T1-T2 carcinoma of the pyriform sinus. *Head Neck*, **23**, 353–362.

95 Nakamura, K., Shioyama, Y., Kawashima, M., *et al.* (2006) Multi-institutional analysis of early squamous cell carcinoma of the hypopharynx treated with radical radiotherapy. *Int. J. Radiat. Oncol. Biol. Phys.*, **65**, 1045–1050.

96 Nakajima, A., Nishiyama, K., Morimoto, M., *et al.* (2012) Definitive radiotherapy for T1-2 hypopharyngeal cancer: A single-institution experience. *Int. J. Radiat. Oncol. Biol. Phys.*, **82**, e129–e135.

97 Vandenbrouck, C., Sancho, H., Le Fur, R., *et al.* (1977) Results of a randomized clinical trial of preoperative irradiation versus postoperative in treatment of tumors of the hypopharynx. *Cancer*, **39**, 1445–1449.

98 El Badawi, S.A., Goepfert, H., Fletcher, G.H., *et al.* (1982) Squamous cell carcinoma of the pyriform sinus. *Laryngoscope*, **92**, 357–364.

99 Hinerman, R.W., Morris, C.G., Amdur, R.J., *et al.* (2006) Surgery and postoperative radiotherapy for squamous cell carcinoma of the larynx and pharynx. *Am. J. Clin. Oncol.*, **29**, 613–621

100 Frank, J.L., Garb, J.L., Kay, S., *et al.* (1994) Postoperative radiotherapy improves survival in squamous cell carcinoma of the hypopharynx. *Am. J. Surg.*, **168**, 476–480.

101 Sher, D.J., Neville, B.A., Chen, A.B., *et al.* (2011) Predictors of IMRT and Conformal Radiotherapy Use in Head and Neck Squamous Cell Carcinoma: A SEER-Medicare Analysis. *Int. J. Radiat. Oncol. Biol. Phys.*, **81**, e179–e206.

102 Braaksma, M.M., Wijers, O.B., van Sörnsen de Koste, J.R., *et al.* (2003) Optimisation of conformal radiation therapy by intensity modulation: cancer of the larynx and salivary gland function. *Radiother Oncol.*, **66**, 291–302.

103 van Rij, C.M., Oughlane-Heemsbergen, W.D., Ackerstaff, A.H., *et al.* (2008) Parotid gland sparing IMRT for head and neck cancer improves xerostomia related quality of life. *Radiat Oncol.*, **3**, 41.

104 Yao, M., Dornfeld, K.J., Buatti, J.M., *et al.* (2005) Intensity-modulated radiation treatment for head-and-neck squamous cell carcinoma – the University of Iowa experience. *Int. J. Radiat. Oncol. Biol. Phys.*, **63**, 410–421.

105 Dirix, P., Nuyts, S. (2010) Value of intensity-modulated radiotherapy in Stage IV head-and-neck squamous cell carcinoma. *Int. J. Radiat. Oncol. Biol. Phys.*, **78**, 1373–1380.

106 Studer, G., Peponi, E., Kloeck, S, *et al.* (2010) Surviving hypopharynx-larynx carcinoma in the era of IMRT. *Int. J. Radiat. Oncol. Biol. Phys.*, **77**, 1391–1396.

107 Lee, N.Y., O'Meara, W., Chan, K., *et al.* (2007) Concurrent chemotherapy and intensity-modulated radiotherapy for locoregionally advanced laryngeal and hypopharyngeal cancers. *Int. J. Radiat. Oncol. Biol. Phys.*, **69**, 459–468

108 Daly, M.E., Le, Q.T., Jain, A.K., *et al.* (2011) Intensity-modulated radiotherapy for locally advanced cancers of the larynx and hypopharynx. *Head Neck*, **33**, 103–111.

109 Liu, W.S., Hsin, C.H., Chou, Y.H., *et al.* (2010) Long-term results of intensity-modulated radiotherapy concomitant with chemotherapy for hypopharyngeal carcinoma aimed at laryngeal preservation. *BMC Cancer*, **10**, 102.

110 Huang, W.Y., Jen, Y.M., Chen, C.M., *et al.* (2010) Intensity modulated radiotherapy with concurrent chemotherapy for larynx preservation of advanced resectable hypopharyngeal cancer. *Radiat. Oncol.*, **5**, 37.

111 Studer, G., Lütolf, U.M., Davis, J.B., *et al.* (2006) IMRT in hypopharyngeal tumors. *Strahlenther. Onkol.*, **182**, 331–335.

112 Kotwall, C., Sako, K., Razack, M.S., *et al.* (1987) Metastatic patterns in squamous cell cancer of the head and neck. *Am. J. Surg.*, **154**, 439–442 .

113 Clark, C.H., Bidmead, A.M., Mubata, C.D., *et al.* (2004) Intensity-modulated radiotherapy improves target coverage, spinal cord sparing and allows dose escalation in patients with locally advanced cancer of the larynx. *Radiother. Oncol.*, **70**, 189–198.

114 Miah, A.B., Bhide, S.A., Guerrero-Urbano, M.T., *et al.* (2012) Dose-Escalated Intensity-Modulated Radiotherapy Is Feasible and May Improve Locoregional Control and Laryngeal Preservation in Laryngo-hypopharyngeal Cancers. *Int. J. Radiat. Oncol. Biol. Phys.*, **82**, 539–547.

115 Posner, M.R., Hershock, D.M., Blajman, C.R., *et al.* (2007) Cisplatin and fluorouracil alone or with docetaxel in head and neck cancer. *N. Engl. J. Med.*, **357**, 1705–1715.

116 Pointreau, Y., Garaud, P., Chapet, S., *et al.* (2009) Randomized trial of induction chemotherapy with cisplatin and 5-fluorouracil with or without docetaxel for larynx preservation. *J. Natl Cancer Inst.*, **101**, 498–506.

117 Bradford, C.R., Wolf, G.T., Carey, T.E., *et al.* (1999) Predictive markers for response to chemotherapy, organ preservation, and survival in patients with advanced laryngeal carcinoma. *Otolaryngol. Head Neck Surg.*, **121**, 534–538.

118 Lefebvre, J.L., Rolland, F., Tesselaar, M., *et al.* (2009) EORTC Radiation Oncology Group. Phase 3 randomized trial on larynx preservation comparing sequential vs alternating chemotherapy and radiotherapy. *J. Natl Cancer Inst.*, **101**, 142–152.

12

Carcinoma of the Nasopharynx

Keith Unger, Felix Ho, James Melotek and Nancy Lee

Anatomy

The nasopharynx consists of three regions, namely the vault, lateral walls, and posterior wall. The floor of the nasopharynx is formed by the superior surface of the soft palate. The lateral walls include the mucosa covering the torus tubarius, which forms the eustachian tube orifice, and the fossa of Rosenmuller, a recess that lies posterior to the torus. Anteriorly, the nasopharynx is continuous with the nasal cavity via the posterior choanae. The relative positions of the structures of the nasopharynx, as seen in the sagittal projection, are shown in Figure 12.1.

The posterior wall of the nasopharynx contains four anatomic layers: (i) the mucous membrane of the pharynx; (ii) the pharyngobasilar fascia; (iii) the superior pharyngeal constrictor muscle; and (iv) the buccopharyngeal fascia. The pharyngobasilar fascia extends superiorly, encircling the space between the upper border of the superior constrictor muscle and the skull base. The eustachian tube pierces the pharyngobasilar fascia at the sinus of Morgagni, a common site for tumor infiltration. The American Joint Committee on Cancer (AJCC) defines three anatomic spaces that are in close proximity to the nasopharynx and are relevant for staging of nasopharyngeal carcinoma (NPC): the parapharyngeal space; the carotid space; and the masticator space [1]. The parapharyngeal space lies lateral and posterior to the nasopharynx. It extends from the skull base down to the level of the angle of the mandible, and is anterior to the styloid process and medial to the masticator space. The carotid space is an enclosed fascial space that lies posterior to the styloid process and contains the internal carotid artery, internal jugular vein, and cranial nerves IX–XII. The masticator space includes the muscles of mastication and is enclosed by the superficial layer of the deep cervical fascia.

Patterns of Spread

The lateral walls are the most common sites of origin for NPC (Figure 12.2). Lateral and posterior spread into the parapharyngeal space occurs early, while invasion of the pterygoid muscles and plates occurs in more advanced disease. The degree of parapharyngeal extension has been correlated with overall survival [2]. Direct tumor extension or lateral retropharyngeal lymph node metastases in the parapharyngeal space can lead to compression or invasion of several cranial nerves, including cranial nerve XII as it exits through the hypoglossal canal, cranial nerves IX to XI as they exit from the jugular foramen, and the cervical sympathetic nerves. Compression or direct invasion of the internal carotid artery can also occur in advanced disease. Anterior spread to the nasal cavity and inferior spread to the oropharynx are common and have comparable outcomes to tumor confined to the nasopharynx [3,4]. In advanced cases tumor may spread to adjacent maxillary or ethmoid sinuses. Tumor can also involve the orbital apex through the inferior orbital fissure, or invade the C1 vertebral body posteriorly and inferiorly. Superiorly, tumor can invade directly through the base of skull, sphenoid sinus, and clivus. Tumor spread through the foramen lacerum provides easy access to the cavernous sinus and can lead to the involvement of cranial nerves III to VI. Perineural spread along the maxillary and mandibular branches of the trigeminal nerve can lead to intracranial extension from spread through the foramina rotundum and ovale, respectively (Figure 2D).

The nasopharynx has a rich supply of submucosal lymphatics and has a high incidence of node involvement. At presentation, 90% of patients have clinically involved neck nodes; bilateral spread occurs in about 50% of cases, but metastasis to the contralateral nodes only is uncommon [5,6]. The primary lymphatic drainage

Clinical Radiation Oncology: Indications, Techniques, and Results, Third Edition. Edited by William Small Jr.
© 2017 John Wiley & Sons, Inc. Published 2017 by John Wiley & Sons, Inc.

Figure 12.1 Diagram of a sagittal view of the nasopharynx.

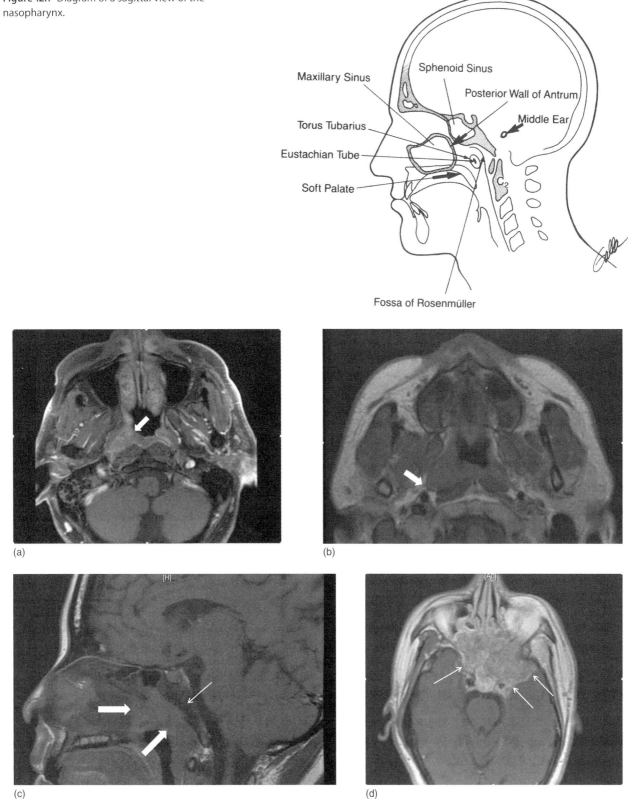

Figure 12.2 (A) Axial contrast-enhanced magnetic resonance scan (MRI) of a patient with carcinoma of the nasopharynx, demonstrating tumor in the right fossa of Rosenmuller (arrow). (B) Axial T1-weighted MRI of a patient with stage T2 carcinoma of the nasopharynx, demonstrating tumor invasion into the right parapharyngeal space (arrow). (C) Sagittal T1-weighted MRI scan demonstrating a soft-tissue mass in the nasopharynx (thick arrows) with invasion into the clivus. Note the abnormal low signal intensity in the marrow of the clivus (thin arrow). (D) Axial contrast-enhanced T1-weighted MRI scan demonstrating tumor invasion into the skull base and cavernous sinus (arrows).

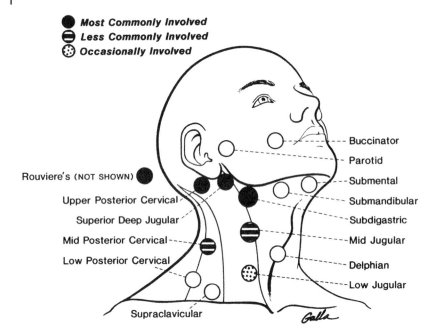

Figure 12.3 Diagram depicting patterns of lymph node involvement from nasopharyngeal carcinoma.

of the nasopharynx is to the lateral retropharyngeal lymph nodes and to the junctional and jugulodigastric lymph nodes (level II) (Figure 12.3). The lateral retropharyngeal nodes lie near the lateral border of the posterior pharyngeal wall and medial to the carotid artery in the retropharyngeal space. The uppermost of this group of nodes is the lateral retropharyngeal node of Rouvière. The incidence of retropharyngeal lymphadenopathy ranges from 37% to 86% with clinically involved cervical lymph nodes, and from 16% to 40% for no clinical cervical lymph node involvement [7–9]. Another direct path of spread is to the deep nodes of the posterior triangle, the spinal accessory nodes (level V). From the primary groups of nodes, further spread can occur down the jugular and posterior cervical chains. Contralateral or bilateral lymph node involvement is a result of lymphatic channels crossing the midline. Spread to the submaxillary and submental nodes occurs rarely. Spread to the parotid nodes can occur via the lymphatics of the eustachian tube, draining to the lymphatics of the tympanic membrane and external auditory canal.

The incidence of distant metastasis at diagnosis is 3% and it may occur in 18–50% or more of cases during the course of the disease [10–14]. Advanced neck node disease [10,15–17], particularly in the low neck [18,19], correlates strongly with the incidence of distant metastasis. The most common sites of distant metastasis are bone, followed by the lungs and liver.

Clinical Presentation

The most common presenting symptom from NPC is a painless neck mass [16]. The neck mass may enlarge

rapidly due to necrosis or hemorrhage, and it may be tender to palpation. Other common symptoms include epistaxis, decreased hearing, nasal obstruction, pain, and cranial nerve deficits. Unilateral serous otitis media can occur as a result of obstruction, usually by compression rather than direct extension of the eustachian tube orifice. A sore throat can occur when the tumor involves the oropharynx. Trismus results from invasion of the pterygoid muscles or involvement of the motor branches of the fifth nerve. Direct extension into the posterior orbit can result in proptosis. Pain from lifting the head and extending the neck can result from posterior invasion of the prevertebral muscles or retropharyngeal lymph nodes.

Cranial nerve involvement occurs in 12–24% of patients at presentation [17,20,21]. Cranial nerve III to VI involvement can result from intracranial extension to the cavernous sinus, usually by tumor extension through the foramen lacerum. Lateral retropharyngeal lymph node metastases in the retroparotid space can result in involvement of cranial nerves IX to XII and the cervical sympathetic chain. Cranial nerves V and VI are most frequently involved, while cranial nerves I, VII, and VIII are rarely involved. Two syndromes can be seen in association with NPC, including the petrosphenoidal syndrome of Jacod and the syndrome of retroparotid space of Villaret. The petrosphenoidal syndrome presents with unilateral trigeminal neuralgia (cranial nerve V), unilateral ptosis (III), complete ophthalmoplegia (III, IV, and VI) and amaurosis (II). The syndrome of retroparotid space presents with dysphagia (IX and X); perversion of taste in the posterior third of the tongue (IX); hyperesthesias, hypoesthesias, or anesthesias of the mucous membrane of the soft palate, pharynx, and larynx; respiratory and salivary problems (X); hemiparesis of the soft palate;

Table 12.1 Pretreatment diagnostic and staging evaluation for nasopharyngeal carcinoma.

History

Physical examination

Comprehensive head and neck examination including assessment of cranial nerve function

Endoscopy

Fiberoptic nasopharyngoscopy

Nasopharyngeal biopsy

Routine laboratory studies

Imaging

  Head and neck

    Head and neck including base of skull

    MRI scan with gadolinium (preferred)

    CT scan with contrast ± PET scan

  Distant sites

    Chest imaging

    CT chest, abdomen, pelvis ± PET scan for Stage III/IV disease

Dental, audiology, speech pathology, and nutrition evaluations

paralysis and atrophy of the trapezius and sternocleido-mastoid muscles (XI); and unilateral paralysis and atrophy of the tongue (XII). Compression of the cervical sympathetic nerve may result in Horner's syndrome.

Diagnosis and Staging

The recommended pretreatment evaluation is summarized in Table 12.1. Fiberoptic nasoscopes and laryngoscopes are important tools for examining the nasopharynx. Early lesions usually occur on the lateral walls but often are not visible and may only be identified as submucosal fullness in the fossa of Rosenmuller. A diagnosis of NPC is established by biopsy of a primary tumor in the nasopharynx. When there is no visible tumor, random biopsies should be taken from Rosenmuller's fossa on each of the lateral walls and the superior posterior wall of the nasopharynx. Fine-needle aspiration of a neck mass may establish the presence of metastatic NPC in cervical lymph nodes.

Magnetic resonance imaging (MRI) and computed tomography (CT) scans are the main imaging modalities for diagnosis, radiation treatment planning, and follow-up of NPC. Compared to CT, MRI has better tissue contrast and multiplanar capacity, allowing for more accurate evaluation of the primary tumor extent [22–24]. In a large series involving 420 patients, the use of MRI changed the T stage in 50% of cases and

the clinical stage in 40% [25]. Studies have shown that MRI is superior in detecting early skull base involvement and subtle intracranial extension [26, 27]. Additionally, MRI more accurately discriminates between metastatic retropharyngeal lymphadenopathy and direct tumor extension. Fluorodeoxyglucose positron emission tomography (FDG-PET) can provide valuable functional information on the extent of the tumor and presence of regional lymph node metastasis [28, 29] and aid in the detection of distant metastasis [30]. However, in one series MRI was shown to be superior to FDG-PET in delineating the extent of the primary tumor [31]. The exact role of FDG-PET in the management of NPC is the subject of continued research.

Staging

The Eighth Edition (2017) of the American Joint Committee on Cancer (AJCC) staging system for NPC is detailed in Table 12.2 [32]. It is important to understand changes to the staging system over time for interpretation of older studies which use prior classifications. The designation "T0" has been added in the Eighth Edition for an EBV-positive unknown primary with cervical lymph node involvement. Tumors confined to the nasopharynx have similar outcomes to tumors that extend to the nasal cavity and oropharynx [3, 4]. In the Seventh Edition (2010) system, T2a was therefore downstaged to T1, which is defined as tumor confined to the nasopharynx, or tumor that extends to the nasal cavity and/or oropharynx. Tumors with parapharyngeal involvement were classified as T2 in the 2010 system and were no longer subdivided as T2b. Tumors with parapharyngeal space involvement are at higher risk for local and regional recurrence, as well as a high rate of distant metastasis [33]. In the Eighth Edition, adjacent muscle involvement (including medial pterygoid, lateral pterygoid, and prevertebral) is now designated as T2. Cranial nerve involvement has been shown to carry a worse prognosis than skull base involvement [17, 18, 34, 35]; as such, T3 disease includes involvement of the bony structures of the skull base, whereas T4 includes involvement of the cranial nerves. The previous T4 criteria of extension to the "masticator space" or "infratemporal fossa" have been replaced in the Eighth Edition by a specific description of soft tissue involvement to avoid ambiguity. NPC has a unique pattern of nodal spread as compared to other sites in the head and neck region, which is reflected in the nodal staging classification. Retropharyngeal nodes are the first echelon of nodal metastases [36], and retropharyngeal lymph node involvement independent of laterality and without cervical lymph node involvement was defined as N1 beginning in the 2010 system. Spread to the low neck correlates strongly with the development of distant metastasis [18, 19]. The previous N3b criterion of

Table 12.2 (A) American Joint Committee on Cancer (AJCC) TNM staging system for nasopharyngeal carcinoma.

2017 8th ed. AJCC Staging†

Primary Tumor (T)

TX — Primary tumor cannot be assessed

T0 — No tumor identified, but EBV-positive cervical node(s) involvement

T1 — Tumor confined to nasopharynx, or extension to oropharynx and/or nasal cavity without parapharyngeal involvement

T2 — Tumor with extension to parapharengeal space, an/or adjacent soft tissue involvement (medial pterygoig, lateral pterygoid, prevertebral muscles)

T3 — Tumor with infiltration of bony structures at skull base, cervical vertebra, pterygoid structures, and/or paranasal sinuses

T4 — Tumor with intracranial extension, involvement of cranial nerves, hypopharynx, orbit, parotid gland, and/or extensive soft tissue infiltration beyond the lateral surface of the lateral pterygoid muscle

Regional Lymph Nodes (N)

NX — Regional lymph nodes cannot be assessed

N0 — No regional lymph node metastasis

N1 — Unilateral metastasis in cervical lymph node(s), an/or unilateral or bilateral metastasis in retropharyngeal lymph node(s), 6 cm or smaller in greatest dimension, above the caudal border of cricoid cartilage

N2 — Bilateral metastasis in cervical lymph node(s), 6 cm or smaller in greatest dimension, above the caudal border of cricoid cartilage

N3 — Unilateral or bilateral metastasis in cervical lymph node(s), larger than 6 cm in greatest dimension, and/or extension below the caudal border of cricoid cartilage

Distant Metastasis (M)

M0 — No distant metastasis

M1 — Distant metastasis

supraclavicular fossa extension was changed to lower neck involvement (as defined by nodal extension below the caudal border of the cricoid cartilage) in the Eighth Edition. Additionally, N3a and N3b have been merged into a single N3 category. Lastly, the previous sub-stages IVA (T4 N0-2 M0) and IVB (any T N3 M0) are now merged to form IVA, whereas the previous IVC (any T any N M1) is now upstaged to IVB.

Table 12.2 (B) Stage grouping.

2017 8th ed. AJCC Staging† Anatomic Stage/ Prognostic Groups			
Stage 0	Tis	N0	M0
Stage I	T1	N0	M0
Stage II	T1, T0	N1	M0
	T2	N0	M0
	T2	N1	M0
Stage III	T1, T0	N2	M0
	T2	N2	M0
	T3	N0	M0
	T3	N1	M0
	T3	N2	M0
Stage IVA	T4	N0	M0
	T4	N1	M0
	T4	N2	M0
	Any T	N3	M0
Stage IVB	Any T	Any N	M1

† Amin, M.B. (ed) (2017) *AJCC Cancer Staging Manual*, 8th edition, Spring, New York.

Epidemiology

The incidence of NPC varies dramatically by geographic region. It is endemic in southeast China (Guangdong Province), southeast Asia, and regions of Alaska. NPC is of intermediate incidence in North Africa and in the Philippines, and is rare among Japanese and whites. The age-adjusted incidence rate (per 100 000 population per year) is 28.8 in Hong Kong, 17.2 in Eskimos, Indians, and Aleuts in Alaska, 16.8 in Singapore, 4.6 in the Philippines, 2.8 in Algeria, and 0.6 in the United States and Japan [37, 38]. The peak incidence of NPC occurs in the fourth and fifth decades of life, and the male-to-female ratio is 3:1 [39].

Epidemiologic and experimental observations suggest that the causes of NPC are multifactorial and likely related to environmental factors, viral infection, and genetics. There is a decreased incidence of NPC in successive generations of Chinese who have migrated to Western Countries, though their incidence is still higher than among the indigenous populations [3, 40]. Environmental factors such as poor ventilation, cigarette smoking, occupational exposures, and diet have been associated with NPC. The ingestion of salted fish during early childhood has been implicated as an important environmental factor among the Southern Chinese [39, 41, 42].

Epstein–Barr virus (EBV) has long been associated with non-keratinizing NPC, irrespective of ethnic or geographic origin. This association is reflected by elevated EBV antibody profiles, increased circulating EBV DNA levels, and expression of the EBV genome in tumor cells [43–45]. Epidemiological studies have provided substantial evidence for a hereditable component of the risk for NPC [46, 47]. In a large case-control study from Guangdong, China, family history was the strongest predictor for NPC, with a 3.4-fold higher risk compared to the matched controls [48]. Highly significant differences in histocompatibility human leukocyte antigen (HLA) patterns have been found between Chinese NPC patients and control subjects, suggesting a genetically determined susceptibility related to the presentation of viral antigens to the immune system [49].

Pathology

Carcinomas account for 80–99% of the malignant tumors of the nasopharynx. Electron microscopy studies have demonstrated that the malignant epithelial cells of the nasopharynx are of squamous origin, and that undifferentiated carcinoma is a variant of squamous cell carcinoma [50, 51]. The World Health Organization (WHO) classification divides NPC into three histological types:

squamous cell carcinoma (type 1); non-keratinizing carcinoma (type 2); and basaloid squamous cell carcinoma (type 3). Non-keratinizing carcinoma is subdivided into differentiated (type 2a) and undifferentiated carcinomas (type 2b) [52]. Basaloid squamous carcinoma is a high-grade variant of squamous cell carcinoma, and rarely occurs as a primary tumor in the nasopharynx. The prior WHO terminology is widely cited in the literature and uses the following designations: squamous cell carcinoma (type I); non-keratinizing carcinoma or transitional cell carcinoma (type II); and undifferentiated carcinoma or lymphoepithelial carcinoma (type III). The term lymphoepithelial carcinoma or lymphoepithelioma is a variant of undifferentiated NPCs and describes numerous lymphocytes found among the tumor cells. The distribution of WHO histopathologic types varies with geography, race, and national origin [53]. In southern China, the rates of squamous cell carcinoma, differentiated carcinoma, and undifferentiated carcinoma are approximately 3%, 9%, and 88%, while in the United States the rates are 20%, 10%, and 70%, respectively [54, 55]. Other uncommon malignant tumors found in the nasopharynx include adenocarcinoma, lymphoma, plasmacytoma, melanoma, and sarcomas.

Selection of Therapy

The mainstay of treatment for NPC is external beam radiation therapy (EBRT). NPC has a high propensity for early cervical and retropharyngeal lymph node involvement, either unilaterally or bilaterally. Additionally, there is often local spread to adjacent soft tissue, sinuses, cranial nerves, or to the skull base. Radiation therapy allows for the comprehensive coverage of both clinically apparent disease and areas at risk for subclinical spread. Several trials have demonstrated improved outcomes with sequential or concurrent chemotherapy in locally advanced NPC. Although surgery is not used in the primary management of NPC, neck dissection is utilized for persistent disease after definitive radiation treatment. Surgery can also be used in the management of local or regional recurrence.

Early-stage disease is treated with radiation alone, while locally advanced NPC (T2 or higher or N+) is treated with a combination of chemotherapy and radiation. Currently, the standard treatment approach for locally advanced NPC is based on a phase III trial by the Head and Neck Intergroup [56]. In this trial, chemotherapy consisted of cisplatin (CDDP) 100 mg m^{-2} every three weeks during radiotherapy, and three cycles of CDDP 80 mg m^{-2} plus 5-fluorouracil (5-FU) infusion 1000 mg m^{-2} per day, for four days every four weeks after

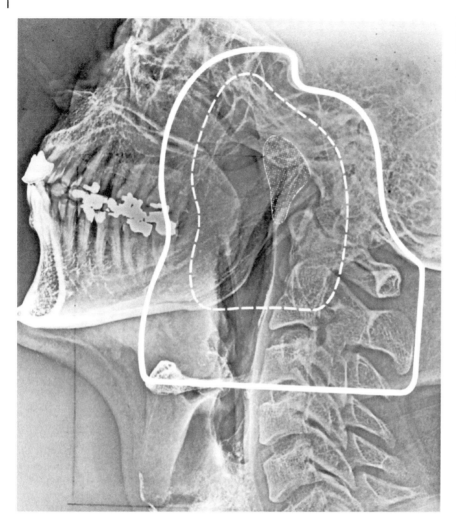

Figure 12.4 Lateral radiograph depicting portals for irradiation of the primary and bilateral upper cervical lymph nodes for treatment of nasopharyngeal carcinoma. The dashed line depicts the off-cord portal boosting dose to the primary site.

the completion of radiotherapy. Radiation was delivered to a total dose of 70 Gy.

Radiotherapeutic Management

The treatment of NPC is technically challenging given the close proximity of the tumor to critical structures, including the brainstem, optic apparatus, and temporal lobes. It has been recognized that conventional head and neck irradiation leads to substantial impairments in the patient's quality of life. Increasingly, conformal radiation therapy techniques such as intensity-modulated radiation therapy (IMRT) have been successfully utilized in the management of NPC, allowing for the delivery of adequate tumoricidal doses while respecting normal tissue tolerances. Additionally, advances in imaging have improved target delineation. As a result, the use of conformal techniques improves the post-treatment quality of life by reducing dose to normal tissues such as the parotids, cochlea, and temporo-mandibular joints.

Two-Dimensional and Three-Dimensional Radiation Therapy

Two-dimensional (2D) radiation therapy planning for NPC typically involves a three-field technique, using opposed lateral fields and a low anterior neck field with a midline block to shield the larynx and spinal cord (Figure 12.4). Areas of subclinical spread generally receive a dose of 50–54 Gy, with a field reduction off the spinal cord at 42 Gy. The dose to the posterior cervical areas is supplemented with electron beams. The primary and involved neck nodes can be boosted to a total dose of 66–70 Gy with opposed laterals in 33–35 fractions. These techniques are especially challenging when there is parapharyngeal extension or large retropharyngeal lymph nodes, due to dose limitations of the brainstem and upper cervical spinal cord. The advent of three-dimensional (3D) computerized planning techniques addressed poor tumor dose coverage for tumors volumes that are often concave. Dosimetric studies have demonstrated better target coverage and reduction in normal tissue dose as compared to conventional 2D plans [57, 58].

Intensity-Modulated Radiation Therapy (IMRT)

IMRT has mostly replaced conventional 2D and 3D techniques for the treatment of NPC in the centers where this technology is available. With IMRT, radiation beams can be modulated such that a high dose can be delivered to the tumor while significantly reducing the dose to the surrounding normal tissues [59–61]. When compared to 2D and 3D techniques, IMRT improves tumor volume coverage while reducing dose to the ipsilateral parotid gland, optic nerve, and brainstem [62]. Two recent randomized trials have shown improvements in salivary function after treatment with IMRT compared to conventional radiation therapy for early-stage NPC [63, 64]. Early clinical experience with IMRT at the University of San Francisco (UCSF) and several other centers have demonstrated the feasibility of IMRT [65–68]. High rates of local and regional control with limited late treatment-related side effects have been confirmed in a multi-institutional Radiation Therapy Oncology Group trial [69]. All NPC patients should be treated with IMRT whenever possible.

Simulation and Treatment Planning

The patient should be simulated with the head in a hyper-extended position so that there is adequate separation between the primary and retropharyngeal lymph nodes and the upper neck field [65]. The tip of the uvula and the base of the occiput should be on a plane parallel to the beam axis. The head, neck – and in some cases, the shoulders – are immobilized using a thermoplastic mask. CT scan slice thickness should be 3 mm or less through the region that contains the primary target volume. The regions above and below the target volume may be scanned with a slice thickness of 3–5 mm. Pretreatment MRI assists in delineation of the gross tumor volume (GTV) in the area of the base of skull as well as surrounding critical normal structures, and should be obtained, unless medically contraindicated. If possible, the treatment planning MRI scan should be obtained with the patient in the treatment position; otherwise, image fusion methods should be employed to correlate the CT and MRI scans.

The treatment volume should encompass the GTV as well as regions of microscopic disease and potential spread of disease, known as the clinical target volume (CTV). Due to the high dose conformality produced by IMRT and the potential for a marginal or out-of-field recurrence, accurate GTV and CTV delineation is required. Clinical information, endoscopic findings, CT, and MRI should be used to delineate the GTV. Grossly

positive lymph nodes are defined as any lymph nodes >1 cm or nodes with a necrotic center. Retropharyngeal nodes are considered to be positive if >0.5 cm. The GTV should include the primary tumor in the nasopharynx, gross retropharyngeal lymphadenopathy, and gross nodal disease.

A *gross disease CTV* should be defined as the GTV plus an additional margin of 5 mm to account for areas of microscopic spread. The margin can be reduced for tumors in close proximity to critical structures, such as for tumors abutting the brainstem.

The *high-risk subclinical CTV* encompasses the GTV plus all potential areas of microscopic spread of disease, including, bilaterally: upper deep jugular (junctional, parapharyngeal) nodes; submandibular nodes; subdigastric (jugulodigastric) nodes; midjugular nodes; low jugular and supraclavicular nodes; posterior cervical nodes; and retropharyngeal nodes. CT-based anatomic atlases of the head and neck lymph node regions aid in target delineation [70–73]. The high-risk subclinical CTV should be at least 10 mm from the GTV, except when the CTV is in air, bone, or abutting critical structures. The high-risk subclinical CTV also includes at least the entire nasopharynx, clivus, the base of skull (including the foramen ovale and foramen rotundum), pterygoid fossae, parapharyngeal space, inferior sphenoid sinus (the entire sphenoid sinus covered for T3 or T4 disease) and posterior third of the nasal cavity and maxillary sinuses (ensuring coverage of the pterygopalatine fossae). The cavernous sinus is included in high-risk patients (T3–T4 disease or when there is bulky disease in the roof of the nasopharynx). For node-negative or low-risk node-positive patients, level I may be omitted at the discretion of the physician. The planning target volume (PTV) is created by adding an additional margin of 3–5 mm to all CTVs to compensate for variations in treatment setup and internal organ motion. Studies should be implemented by each institution to determine the magnitude of setup uncertainty and define the PTV margin. In the area of critical structures such as the brainstem, the PTV margin may be reduced to respect normal tissue constraints. Adjacent normal structures, including the brainstem, spinal cord, optic nerves, chiasm, parotid glands, oral cavity, temporo-mandibular (T-M) joints, mandible, eyes, lens, temporal lobe, and glottic larynx should be outlined.

The midjugular, low jugular, and supraclavicular nodes can be treated either with IMRT, or alternatively with an anteroposterior (AP) field that is beam-split to the IMRT fields, known as an extended-whole field (EWF) IMRT technique and a split-field (SF) IMRT technique, respectively [74–76]. If a SF technique is considered, the match typically occurs at just above the arytenoids as the larynx can be spared and shielded under the midline block in the low anterior neck field(s). If an EWF technique is utilized, a *low risk subclinical CTV* should also be defined which encompasses the bilateral lower neck and supraclavicular nodal regions. If there is gross nodal disease in the low neck, the entire ipsilateral low neck should be included in the *high-risk subclinical CTV.* When EWF IMRT is used, the brachial plexus should be contoured to ensure that there are no undesired hotspots.

Investigators have utilized various dose fractionation schemes for the treatment of NPC with IMRT [66–68]. At Memorial Sloan-Kettering, as well as multiple other centers, a simultaneous integrated boost technique is employed. For patients receiving concurrent chemoradiation, the prescribed dose to the PTV of the *gross disease CTV* is 70 Gy in 33 fractions at 2.12 Gy per fraction. The PTV of the *high-risk subclinical CTV* receives 59.4 Gy in 33 fractions at 1.8 Gy per fraction. If the patient is treated using EWF IMRT, the prescribed dose to the *low-risk subclinical CTV* is 54 Gy in 33 fractions at 1.64 Gy per fraction. If a SF IMRT technique is utilized, the low neck will receive 50.4 Gy in 28 fractions of 1.8 Gy per fraction using conventional AP or AP/posteroanterior (PA) fields. Recommended dose constraints are detailed in Table 12.3. An IMRT treatment plan is shown in Figure 12.5.

Table 12.3 Recommended dose constraints for normal structures using intensity-modulated radiation therapy for the treatment of nasopharyngeal carcinoma.

Structure	Dose constraint
Critical normal structures	
Brainstem	≤54 Gy or 60 Gy to 1% of the PRV
Optic nerves, chiasm	≤50 Gy or ≤54 Gy
Spinal cord	≤45 Gy or 50 Gy to 1% of the PRV
Brachial plexus	≤66 Gy
Mandible and T-M Joints	≤ 70 Gy or 75 Gy to 1 cc
Other normal structures*	
Parotid glands	≤Mean dose of 26 Gy (at least in one gland)
Submandibular glands	Dose as low as possible
Cochlea	≤55 Gy to 5% of the volume
Oral cavity	≤Mean dose of 40 Gy
Eyes	≤50 Gy
Lens	≤25 Gy
Glottic larynx, post cricoids pharynx, esophagus	≤Mean dose of 45 Gy

PRV, planning organ at risk; this is defined as an expansion of the organ at risk.
*Coverage of the gross tumor volume or clinical target volume should not be compromised to meet planning goals.

Brachytherapy

Brachytherapy has been used to provide an additional conformal boost in the primary treatment of NPC and for the definitive treatment of recurrent or persistent disease. A variety of brachytherapy applicators and techniques have been used for the delivery of intracavitary [77–85] and interstitial treatments [77–85]. Levendag *et al.* [33] described a technique using high-dose rate irradiation, whereby the mucosa is anesthetized and the Rotterdam Nasopharynx Applicator is then inserted, remaining in place for the duration of treatment. Dose prescriptions are based on anatomic points identified on AP and lateral localization x-ray films. For T1 to T2 tumors, the prescribed boost dose is 17 Gy given as 3- or 4-Gy treatments, ≥6 h apart, after completion of 60 Gy of external beam irradiation. The three-year local control rate was 97% for patients with T1 or T2 disease with minimal complications [78]. Permanent interstitial implantation techniques have also been reported using gold-198 seeds [35] and iodine-125 [86]. Brachytherapy techniques are limited by the extent of disease, operator experience, and the patient's anatomy. With the availability of IMRT, the use of brachytherapy has diminished.

Results of Treatment

Definitive Radiation Therapy

Treatment outcomes with radiation therapy alone using conventional planning techniques are summarized in Table 12.4. T- and N-stage have been shown to affect outcomes. The five-year survivals for T1, T2, T3, and T4 treated with radiation therapy alone range from 60–76%, 48–68%, 27–55%, and 0–29%, respectively. The five-year survival for N0, N1, and N2 or N3 patients was 42–78%, 27–70%, and 32–52%, respectively [12, 87].

A number of factors appear to affect local control rates, including T-stage, N-stage, presence of cranial nerve deficits, tumor histology, and use of prophylactic comprehensive nodal irradiation. Local control is worse with increasing T-stage: 67–97% for T1, 54–94% for T2, 34–78% for T3, and 40–71% for T4 [6, 11, 12, 17, 87–89]. Among patients with T4 disease, cranial nerve II–VI deficits have been associated with decreased local control [90]. The control rate of cervical lymph node metastasis for N0, N1, and N2 or N3 was 82–100%, 86–92%, and 78–89%, respectively [6, 12, 17]. Tumor histology has also been shown to affect locoregional control, with lower rates observed in patients with keratinizing squamous cell carcinoma in Western series [15,16,91]. In several Asian studies, in which the vast majority of patients have undifferentiated tumors, tumor histology was not associated with locoregional control rates [92–94].

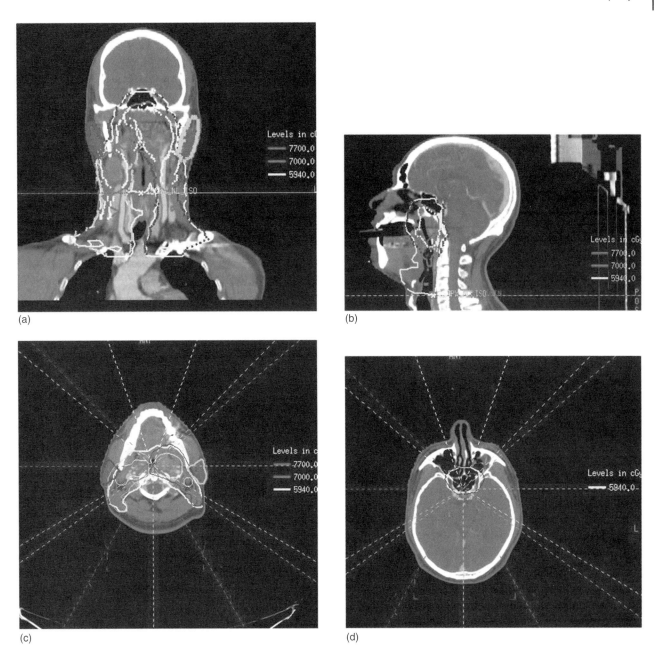

(a)

(b)

(c)

(d)

Figure 12.5 Intensity-modulated radiation therapy (IMRT) plan for a patient with T2N2 carcinoma of the nasopharynx displayed in the (A) coronal, (B) sagittal, and (C–E) axial planes. (F) Dose-volume histogram for the relevant structures. For a color version of this figure, see the color plate section.

The importance of comprehensive nodal irradiation as a prognostic factor for patients with clinically negative necks was demonstrated in a large retrospective series involving over 5000 patients treated with definitive radiation. The incidence of nodal relapse in node-negative patients was 11% after prophylactic nodal irradiation, but 40% for those who did not receive it [95].

Studies using conventional radiation therapy techniques for the treatment of NPC suggest a correlation between local control and the dose delivered to the tumor [89, 96, 97]. Stereotactic radiosurgery (SRS)

has been employed to boost the dose after fractionated external beam irradiation. At Stanford University, 82 patients, including 31 with T4 tumors, received a planned SRS boost of 7–15 Gy in one fraction after completion of 66 Gy using conventional external beam irradiation [98, 99]. The local control rate at five years was 98%, though there were 10 cases of temporal lobe necrosis. A recent randomized trial tested dose escalation using low dose rate (LDR) or high dose rate (HDR) brachytherapy boost after conventional EBRT in patients with locally advanced NPC. There was no difference in three-year

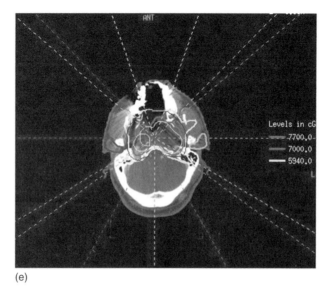

(e)

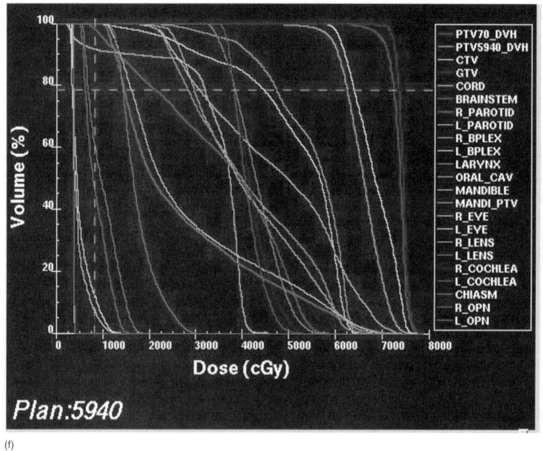

(f)

Figure 12.5 *(Continued)*

local recurrence-free survival, disease-free survival, or overall survival with the addition of brachytherapy [100]. The role of altered fractionation in the treatment of NPC using conventional techniques has been shown to be of limited benefit. Teo et al. conducted a trial with 159 patients randomized to conventional radiotherapy (60 Gy in 24 fractions over 30 days) versus hyperfractionated radiotherapy (71 Gy in 40 fractions over 30 days) using 2D planning techniques [101]. There was no difference in local control or survival rates, and hyperfractionated

Table 12.4 Radiation therapy alone for the treatment of nasopharyngeal carcinoma.

Study/Reference	No. of patients	Five-year actuarial survival (%)	Five-year actuarial local control (%)
Hoppe *et al.*, 1976 [12]	82	62	79 (crude)
Huang, 1980 [34]	1605	32	84
Vikram *et al.*, 1985 [89]	107	56 (estimate)	69 (crude)
Lee *et al.*, 1992 [95]	5037	52	66
Bailet *et al.*, 1992 [88]	103	58	68 (crude)
Sanguineti *et al.*, 1997 [146]	378	48	71

treatment resulted in increased central nervous system toxicity. NPC-9002 was a multi-institutional randomized trial with treatment five days per week versus an accelerated schedule of six days of treatment per week [102]. Accelerated treatment did not improve outcomes after adjusting for the use of concurrent chemotherapy.

Chemotherapy

Concurrent chemotherapy and radiation therapy is the standard treatment for NPC, with the exception of T1 disease. Randomized trials of chemoradiation with

or without adjuvant chemotherapy are summarized in Table 12.5. The Intergroup-0099 study was a seminal phase III trial which demonstrated a survival benefit for chemoradiation over radiotherapy alone [56]. Patients were randomized to cisplatin (100 mg m^{-2} on days 1, 21, and 43) with concurrent radiotherapy (70 Gy in 35 fractions) followed by three cycles of adjuvant cisplatin (80 mg m^{-2} on day 1) and fluorouracil (1000 mg m^{-2} per day on days 1 through 4) versus radiotherapy alone. The three-year progression-free survival rate with chemoradiation was significantly improved (69% versus 24%; p < 0.01). There also were improvements in overall

Table 12.5 Concurrent chemotherapy and radiation therapy with or without adjuvant chemotherapy for the treatment of nasopharyngeal carcinoma.

Study/Reference	No. of patients	Treatment	Time (years)	Locoregional control*	Disease-free survival*
Intergroup-0099, 1998 [56]	193	RT 70 Gy RT + 3 cycles P then 3 cycles PF	3	59% vs. 86% (p = 0.05)	24% vs. 69% (p < 0.001)
Lin *et al.*, 2003 [147]	284	RT 70–74 Gy RT + 2 cycles P	5	73% vs. 89% (p < 0.01)	53% vs. 72% (p = 0.01)
Kwong *et al.*, 2004 [108]	222	RT 62.5–68 Gy RT + UT then 6 cycles F/VBM	3	72% vs. 82% (p = 0.39)	77% vs 87% (p = 0.06)
Chan *et al.*, 2005 [148]	350	RT 66 Gy RT + 6–8 cycles P	5	59% vs. 70% (p = 0.065)	54% vs 60% (p = 0.16)
Zhang *et al.*, 2005 [149]	115	RT 70–74 Gy RT + 6 cycles Ox	2	NR	83% vs. 96% (p =0.02)
Wee *et al.*, 2005 [105]	221	RT 70 Gy RT + 3 cycles P then 3 cycles PF	3	NR	53% vs. 72% (p = 0.01)
NPC-9901, 2005 [150]	348	RT ≥66 Gy RT + 3 cycles P then 3 cycles PF	3	82% vs. 92% (p = 0.01)	62% vs. 72% (p = 0.03)

* Control arms versus experimental arms;
AJCC, American Joint Committee on Cancer; F, 5-flurouracil; NR, not reported; Ox, oxaliplatin; P, cisplatin; RT, radiation therapy; UT, uracil and tegafur; VBM, vincristine, bleomycin, methotrexate.

survival, locoregional control, and distant control with concurrent therapy. This trial has been criticized for the poor outcomes observed in patients treated with radiotherapy alone compared to historical controls, but two large meta-analyses have corroborated the improvement in overall survival with concurrent chemotherapy and radiation [103, 104].

The role of adjuvant chemotherapy remains undefined. The Intergroup-0099 and Singapore studies, using concurrent and adjuvant chemotherapy, demonstrated improved survival and reduction in distant metastasis with the addition of chemotherapy [56,105]. However, no individual trial testing the role of adjuvant chemotherapy has demonstrated an improvement in survival [106–108]. Additionally, patients are often unable to complete all cycles of adjuvant chemotherapy. In the Intergroup and Singapore studies, compliance with the three cycles of adjuvant chemotherapy was only 55% and 57%, respectively. Since the current treatment recommendations for NPC are largely based on the Intergroup study, many clinicians consider adjuvant chemotherapy the standard of care. However, patients should be advised of the increased risks of treatment-related toxicity and that the overall benefit may be relatively limited.

Recent Advances

Several large institutions have published locoregional control rates greater than 90% using IMRT for the treatment of NPC [66–68] (Table 12.6). UCSF reported a local control rate of 97% and a regional control rate of 98% [65]. However, distant metastasis remained high; the distant metastasis-free rate was 66% at four years and the overall survival was 88%. Building on the excellent local control rates from individual centers, the Radiation Therapy Oncology Group conducted a Phase II trial (RTOG 0225) to test whether IMRT could successfully be delivered in a multi-institutional setting [69]. Patients with Stage I to IVB NPC were treated using IMRT with concurrent chemotherapy for stage ≥T2b and/or node-positive disease. Chemotherapy consisted

of concurrent cisplatin and adjuvant cisplatin and fluorouracil as per the Intergroup-0090 study [56]. A total of 68 patients was enrolled from 17 centers. The compliance rate with the IMRT specified in the protocol was 84%. Compliance with the concurrent chemotherapy was higher in the RTOG study compared to the Intergroup study (83% versus 63%), but slightly fewer patients completed three cycles of adjuvant chemotherapy in the RTOG study (46% versus 55%). The two-year local progression-free, regional progression-free, and distant metastasis-free rates were 93%, 91%, and 85%, respectively. The RTOG study validated the excellent locoregional control rates reported by large institutions and demonstrated the transportability of IMRT to the multi-institutional setting.

With the high rates of locoregional control obtained using IMRT and chemotherapy, 21–34% of patients will ultimately develop distant metastasis [65, 66, 68, 109]. Since the predominant site of failure is distant, recent clinical research efforts have focused on improving systemic therapy. The RTOG has reported the results of a phase II trial (RTOG 0615) of the anti-angiogenic monoclonal antibody, bevacizumab, added to the concurrent and adjuvant phases of treatment [110]. In this case, 44 patients with stage ≥T2b and/or node-positive disease received concurrent and adjuvant bevacizumab (15 mg m−2) with chemotherapy. The two-year distant metastases-free and overall survival rates were each 91%. When comparing RTOG 0615 to RTOG 0225 and Intergroup-0099, the progression-free survival rates were similar (72% versus 73% and 69%, respectively), but the overall survival was higher in RTOG 0615 (91% versus 80% and 78%, respectively) [56,69]. The results of RTOG 0615 suggest a possible role for bevacizumab, although these findings need to be confirmed in the setting of a randomized trial.

There is current interest in using EBV DNA as a biomarker for treatment selection, since levels of post-treatment plasma EBV are strongly associated with outcomes [45]. NRG HN001 is a currently accruing international phase III trial randomizing patients with undetectable post-chemoradiation EBV DNA to adjuvant chemotherapy or surveillance. Additionally, there is

Table 12.6 Selected series of intensity modulated radiation therapy for the treatment of nasopharyngeal carcinoma.

Study/Reference	No of patients	Local control (%)	Regional control (%)	Distant metastasis-free survival (%)	Overall survival (%)
Lee *et al.*, (2002, 4-year) [65]	67	97	98	66	88
Kam *et al.*, (2004, 3-year) [68]	63	92	98	79	90
RTOG 0025, (2009, 2-year) [69]	68	93	91	85	80
RTOG 0615, (2011, 2-year) [110]	44	NR	NR	91	91

NR, not reported.

renewed interest in the role of induction chemotherapy for improving systemic control with the recent publication of a phase III randomized trial demonstrating significant improvements in distant failure and survival with the use of a reduced-dose docetaxel, cisplatin, and fluorouracil induction chemotherapy regimen [111].

Retreatment for Persistent Disease or Local Failure

Local failure following definitive treatment for NPC remains a challenging problem. Survival is poor without treatment, and chemotherapy alone offers limited palliation but no chance of cure [112, 113]. Experience with retreatment has included nasopharyngectomy, external beam irradiation, brachytherapy, particle beam radiotherapy, and stereotactic radiosurgery [79, 84–86, 113–125]. Historically, five-year actuarial survival rates have been poor: 38% for recurrent stage T1 to T2 and 15% for recurrent stage T3 to T4 disease [79]. Salvage nasopharyngectomy is typically only used for superficial recurrences, since it is difficult to perform en bloc resection with skull base involvement. Long-term local control rates of 58% with T1 disease and 28% with T2 disease have been reported following salvage nasopharyngectomy [126]. The outcomes for retreatment of recurrent or persistent NPC are summarized in Table 12.7.

The delivery of adequate tumoricidal doses is often limited using conventional irradiation techniques, given the tolerance of previously irradiated normal tissue and the proximity of the tumor to adjacent critical structures. Importantly, multiple studies have demonstrated superior disease control with a dose of 60 Gy or greater for the retreatment of NPC [125, 127, 128]. Superficial disease may be treated with brachytherapy alone, or combined with EBRT for more advanced recurrences. Local

control rates approaching 90% following brachytherapy alone for superficial recurrences have been reported [129]. The addition of brachytherapy to EBRT has not been shown to improve local control rates in recurrence [125, 130]. However, treatment with external beam radiation combined with brachytherapy results in decreased grade 3 or greater late complications, compared to external beam radiation alone [130]. Single-fraction stereotactic radiosurgery [131] or fractionated stereotactic radiation therapy [132, 133] have been utilized for recurrent or persistent NPC. When the tumor is not amenable to brachytherapy or stereotactic radiotherapy, IMRT is the preferred modality [134–136]. In one study using IMRT with or without stereotactic radiosurgery, the one-year local control rate was 56%, but was 100% for recurrent stage T1-3 [134]. Once-a-day fractionation using IMRT to 60–70 Gy with concurrent chemotherapy may be used for re-treatment if an acceptable radiotherapy plan is achieved. High-dose brachytherapy or stereotactic boost can be employed for residual disease after EBRT.

Complications of Therapy

The large volumes required for appropriate treatment of NPC commonly result in acute reactions such as dermatitis and mucositis, and late reactions such as xerostomia and fibrosis. Using conventional radiation techniques, the overall complication rate ranges from 31% to 66%, of which 6–15% are severe and 1–3% fatal [6, 12, 17, 95]. With modern radiation therapy techniques, these complication rates have decreased [65–68, 137]. Xerostomia is the most common sequela following treatment. Dental problems, a consequence of decreased saliva and altered salivary consistency, occurred in 4–17% of patients treated with conventional radiotherapy [6, 12]. Salivary gland function decreases gradually between 20

Table 12.7 Results of reirradiation for recurrent or persistent nasopharyngeal carcinoma.

Study/Reference	No. of patients	Technique	Five-year local control (%)	Five-year survival (%)	Severe complications (%)
Pryzant *et al.*, 1992 [85]	53	EBRT ± B	35 (crude)	21	15
Hwang *et al.*, 1998 [84]	34	Multiple approaches	63 (crude)	33	20
Pai *et al.*, 2002 [151]	36	FSRT	58*	31	0
Chua *et al.*, 2005 [134]	31	IMRT	65	63	19
Wu *et al.*, 2007 [132]	90	FSRT	75–89*	58†	19
Koutcher *et al.*, 2010 [130]	29	EBRT/IMRT ± B	52	60	39

*3 years.
†3-year disease-specific survival.
B, intracavitary or interstitial brachytherapy; EBRT, conventional external beam radiation therapy; FSRT, fractionated stereotactic radiation therapy; IMRT, intensity-modulated radiation therapy.

and 40 Gy, with a dramatic worsening with doses greater than 40 Gy [138, 139]. Two randomized trials of patients with early NPC have shown improved salivary function with IMRT compared to conventional techniques. In a study of 51 patients with NPC, patients were randomized to IMRT or conventional radiation therapy [64]. The use of IMRT resulted in improved post-treatment stimulated whole salivary flow rates and improved patient reported quality of life. Kam *et al.* reported a reduction in observer-rated severe xerostomia (RTOG grade 2 or greater) with IMRT in 60 patients with early-stage NPC [63]. In RTOG 0225, there was a minimal difference between pre-treatment and post-treatment objective salivary function at 12 months, which indicated a recovery of salivary flow after treatment with IMRT [69].

Hearing loss is a common sequela of treatment, especially in patients receiving cisplatin-based regimens. Using conventional techniques, hearing loss occurs in 6–8% of patients [6, 12, 19]. The incidence of sensorineural hearing impairment is related to the mean dose to the cochlea, and several investigators have recommended limiting the mean dose to ≤45 Gy [140, 141]. Chronic otitis media is another common late complication of radiation therapy that affects hearing, occurring in between 3% and 18% of patients [6, 12, 19]. Following chemoradiation, Eisbruch *et al.* correlated the development of aspiration and dysphagia with dose to the pharyngeal constrictor muscles and the supraglottic larynx [142]. The use of SF IMRT with central shielding for the treatment of NPC may decrease dose to the pharyngoesphageal axis as compared to EWF IMRT, resulting in lower rates of severe dysphagia [143].

Neurologic sequelae of treatment can be the most severe and debilitating complications. Temporal lobe necrosis occurs in approximately 3% of patients, often resulting in epilepsy and cognitive impairment [12, 19, 144]. Cranial nerve dysfunction, usually affecting cranial nerves IX to XII, may result from a combination of fibrosis, vascular injury, and direct neuronal damage. Following treatment of locally advanced NPC, blindness may occur; however, limiting the doses to the optic nerves and chiasm to ≤54 Gy significantly reduces the probability of optic neuropathy. Improvements in tumor localization and treatment planning, including the use of IMRT, may reduce the incidence of these devastating treatment complications. Indeed, a recent prospective randomized trial comparing 2D-radiotherapy versus IMRT including patients with locally advanced NPC demonstrated significant reductions in the occurrence of temporal lobe necrosis and cranial nerve palsy in patients treated with IMRT, as well as lower rates of xerostomia, hearing loss, trismus, and neck fibrosis [145]. Symptomatic hypothalamic–pituitary dysfunction can occur following radiation to treat NPC. Regular post-treatment evaluation of endocrine function may be indicated, particularly of thyroid-stimulating hormone levels.

References

1 Edge, S., *et al.* (eds) (2010) *AJCC Cancer Staging Manual.* Springer, New York.

2 Kalogera-Fountzila, A., *et al.* (2006) Prognostic factors and significance of the revised 6th edition of the AJCC classification in patients with locally advanced nasopharyngeal carcinoma. *Strahlenther. Onkol.,* **182** (8), 458–466.

3 Dickson, R.I., Flores, A.D. (1985) Nasopharyngeal carcinoma: an evaluation of 134 patients treated between 1971-1980. *Laryngoscope,* **95** (3), 276–283.

4 Bedwinek, J.M., Perez, C.A., Keys, D.J. (1980) Analysis of failures after definitive irradiation for epidermoid carcinoma of the nasopharynx. *Cancer,* **45** (11), 2725–2729.

5 Fletcher, G.H., Million, R.R. (1965) Malignant Tumors of the Nasopharynx. *Am. J. Roentgenol. Radium Ther. Nucl. Med.,* **93**, 44–55.

6 Mesic, J.B., Fletcher, G.H., Goepfert, H. (1981) Megavoltage irradiation of epithelial tumors of the nasopharynx. *Int. J. Radiat. Oncol. Biol. Phys.,* **7** (4), 447–453.

7 Chong, V.F., Fan, Y.F., Khoo, J.B. (1995) Retropharyngeal lymphadenopathy in nasopharyngeal carcinoma. *Eur. J. Radiol.,* **21** (2), 100–105.

8 Chua, D.T., *et al.* (1997) Retropharyngeal lymphadenopathy in patients with nasopharyngeal carcinoma: a computed tomography-based study. *Cancer,* **79** (5), 869–877.

9 McLaughlin, M.P., *et al.* (1995) Retropharyngeal adenopathy as a predictor of outcome in squamous cell carcinoma of the head and neck. *Head Neck,* **17** (3), 190–198.

10 Bedwinek, J.M., *et al.* (1981) Analysis of failures following local treatment of isolated local-regional recurrence of breast cancer. *Int. J. Radiat. Oncol. Biol. Phys.,* **7** (5), 581–585.

11 Chu, A.M., *et al.* (1984) Irradiation of nasopharyngeal carcinoma: correlations with treatment factors and stage. *Int. J. Radiat. Oncol. Biol. Phys.,* **10** (12), 2241–2249.

12 Hoppe, R.T., Goffinet, D.R., Bagshaw, M.A. (1976) Carcinoma of the nasopharynx. Eighteen years'

experience with megavoltage radiation therapy. *Cancer*, **37** (6), 2605–2612.

13 McNeese, M.D., Fletcher, G.H. (1981) Retreatment of recurrent nasopharyngeal carcinoma. *Radiology*, **138** (1), 191–193.

14 Moench, H.C., Phillips, T.L. (1972) Carcinoma of the nasopharynx. Review of 146 patients with emphasis on radiation dose and time factors. *Am. J. Surg.*, **124** (4), 515–518.

15 Frezza, G., *et al.* (1986) Patterns of failure in nasopharyngeal cancer treated with megavoltage irradiation. *Radiother. Oncol.*, **5** (4), 287–294.

16 Johansen, L.V., Mestre, M., Overgaard, J. (1992) Carcinoma of the nasopharynx: analysis of treatment results in 167 consecutively admitted patients. *Head Neck*, **14** (3), 200–207.

17 Perez, C.A., *et al.* (1992) Carcinoma of the nasopharynx: factors affecting prognosis. *Int. J. Radiat. Oncol. Biol. Phys.*, **23** (2), 271–280.

18 Teo, P., *et al.* (1992) Prognostic factors in nasopharyngeal carcinoma investigated by computer tomography – an analysis of 659 patients. *Radiother. Oncol.*, **23** (2), 79–93.

19 Lee, A.W., *et al.* (1992) Retrospective analysis of nasopharyngeal carcinoma treated during 1976-1985: late complications following megavoltage irradiation. *Br. J. Radiol.*, **65** (778), 918–928.

20 Leung, S.F., *et al.* (1990) Cranial nerve involvement by nasopharyngeal carcinoma: response to treatment and clinical significance. *Clin. Oncol. (R. Coll. Radiol.)*, **2** (3), 138–141.

21 Neel, H.B., 3rd (1985) Nasopharyngeal carcinoma. Clinical presentation, diagnosis, treatment, and prognosis. *Otolaryngol. Clin. North Am.*, **18** (3), 479–490.

22 Ng, S.H., *et al.* (1997) Nasopharyngeal carcinoma: MRI and CT assessment. *Neuroradiology*, **39** (10), 741–746.

23 Poon, P.Y., Tsang, V.H., Munk, P.L. (2000) Tumour extent and T stage of nasopharyngeal carcinoma: a comparison of magnetic resonance imaging and computed tomographic findings. *Can. Assoc. Radiol. J.*, **51** (5), 287–295, quiz 286.

24 Sakata, K., *et al.* (1999) Prognostic factors of nasopharynx tumors investigated by MR imaging and the value of MR imaging in the newly published TNM staging. *Int. J. Radiat. Oncol. Biol. Phys.*, **43** (2), 273–278.

25 Liao, X.B., *et al.* (2008) How does magnetic resonance imaging influence staging according to AJCC staging system for nasopharyngeal carcinoma compared with computed tomography? *Int. J. Radiat. Oncol. Biol. Phys.*, **72** (5), 1368–1377.

26 Chung, N.N., *et al.* (2004) Impact of magnetic resonance imaging versus CT on nasopharyngeal carcinoma: primary tumor target delineation for radiotherapy. *Head Neck*, **26** (3), 241–246.

27 Nishioka, T., *et al.* (2000) Skull-base invasion of nasopharyngeal carcinoma: magnetic resonance imaging findings and therapeutic implications. *Int. J. Radiat. Oncol. Biol. Phys.*, **47** (2), 395–400.

28 Di Martino, E., *et al.* (2000) Diagnosis and staging of head and neck cancer: a comparison of modern imaging modalities (positron emission tomography, computed tomography, color-coded duplex sonography) with panendoscopic and histopathologic findings. *Arch. Otolaryngol. Head Neck Surg.*, **126** (12), 1457–1461.

29 Scarfone, C., *et al.* (2004) Prospective feasibility trial of radiotherapy target definition for head and neck cancer using 3-dimensional PET and CT imaging. *J. Nucl. Med.*, **45** (4), 543–552.

30 Chang, J.T., *et al.* (2005) Nasopharyngeal carcinoma staging by (18)F-fluorodeoxyglucose positron emission tomography. *Int. J. Radiat. Oncol. Biol. Phys.*, **62** (2), 501–507.

31 King, A.D., *et al.* (2008) The impact of 18F-FDG PET/CT on assessment of nasopharyngeal carcinoma at diagnosis. *Br. J. Radiol.*, **81** (964), 291–298.

32 Amin, M.B. (ed) (2017) *AJCC Cancer Staging Manual*, 8th edition. Springer, New York.

33 Xiao, G.L., Gao, L., Xu, G.Z. (2002) Prognostic influence of parapharyngeal space involvement in nasopharyngeal carcinoma. *Int. J. Radiat. Oncol. Biol. Phys.*, **52** (4), 957–963.

34 Huang, S.C. (1980) Nasopharyngeal cancer: a review of 1605 patients treated radically with cobalt 60. *Int. J. Radiat. Oncol. Biol. Phys.*, **6** (4), 401–407.

35 Sham, J.S., *et al.* (1991) Cranial nerve involvement and base of the skull erosion in nasopharyngeal carcinoma. *Cancer*, **68** (2), 422–426.

36 King, A.D., *et al.* (2000) Neck node metastases from nasopharyngeal carcinoma: MR imaging of patterns of disease. *Head Neck*, **22** (3), 275–281.

37 Parkin D.M., Muir C.S. (1992) Cancer Incidence in Five Continents. Comparability and quality of data. *IARC Sci. Publ.*, **120**, 45–173.

38 Lanier, A., *et al.* (1980) Nasopharyngeal carcinoma in Alaskan Eskimos Indians, and Aleuts: a review of cases and study of Epstein-Barr virus, HLA, and environmental risk factors. *Cancer*, **46** (9), 2100–2106.

39 Ho, J.H. (1978) An epidemiologic and clinical study of nasopharyngeal carcinoma. *Int. J. Radiat. Oncol. Biol. Phys.*, **4** (3-4), 182–198.

40 Buell, P. (1974) The effect of migration on the risk of nasopharyngeal cancer among Chinese. *Cancer Res.*, **34** (5), 1189–1191.

41 Tai, T.M. (2001) Descriptive epidemiology of nasopharyngeal cancer. *Curr. Opin. Oncol.*, **8**, 114.

42 Teo, P.M., *et al.* (1991) A comparison of Ho's, International Union Against Cancer, and American Joint Committee stage classifications for nasopharyngeal carcinoma. *Cancer*, **67** (2), 434–439.

43 Brooks, L., *et al.* (1992) Epstein-Barr virus latent gene transcription in nasopharyngeal carcinoma cells: coexpression of EBNA1, LMP1, and LMP2 transcripts. *J. Virol.*, **66** (5), 2689–2697.

44 Henle, G., Henle, W. (1976) Epstein-Barr virus-specific IgA serum antibodies as an outstanding feature of nasopharyngeal carcinoma. *Int. J. Cancer*, **17** (1), 1–7.

45 Chan, K.C., Lo, Y.M. (2002) Circulating EBV DNA as a tumor marker for nasopharyngeal carcinoma. *Semin. Cancer Biol.*, **12** (6), 489–496.

46 Feng, B.J., *et al.* (2002) Genome-wide scan for familial nasopharyngeal carcinoma reveals evidence of linkage to chromosome 4. *Nat. Genet.*, **31** (4), 395–399.

47 Jia, W.H., *et al.* (2005) Complex segregation analysis of nasopharyngeal carcinoma in Guangdong, China: evidence for a multifactorial mode of inheritance (complex segregation analysis of NPC in China). *Eur. J. Hum. Genet.*, **13** (2), 248–252.

48 Ren, Z.F., *et al.* (2010) Effect of family history of cancers and environmental factors on risk of nasopharyngeal carcinoma in Guangdong, China. *Cancer Epidemiol.*, **34** (4), 419–424.

49 Simons, M.J., *et al.* (1977) Immunogenetic aspects of nasopharyngeal carcinoma. V. Confirmation of a Chinese-related HLA profile (A2, Singapore 2) associated with an increased risk in Chinese for nasopharyngeal carcinoma. *Natl Cancer Inst. Monogr.*, **47**, 147–151.

50 Svoboda, D., Kirchner, F., Shanmugaratnam, K. (1965) Ultrastructure of nasopharyngeal carcinomas in American and Chinese patients; an application of electron microscopy to geographic pathology. *Exp. Mol. Pathol.*, **28**, 189–204.

51 Michaels, L., Hyams, V.J. (1977) Undifferentiated carcinoma of the nasopharynx: a light and electron microscopical study. *Clin. Otolaryngol. Allied Sci.*, **2** (2), 105–114.

52 Chan, J., Bray, F., McCarron, P. (2005) Nasopharyngeal carcinoma, in *World Health Organization Classification of Tumors* (eds J.W. Eveson, L. Barnes, P. Reichart), IARC Press, Lyon, France, pp. 87–99.

53 Marks, J.E., Phillips, J.L., Menck, H.R. (1998) The National Cancer Data Base report on the relationship of race and national origin to the histology of nasopharyngeal carcinoma. *Cancer*, **83** (3), 582–588.

54 McGuire, L.J., Lee, J.C. (1990) The histopathologic diagnosis of nasopharyngeal carcinoma. *Ear Nose Throat J.*, **69** (4), 229–236.

55 Neel, H.B., 3rd (1992) Nasopharyngeal carcinoma: diagnosis, staging, and management. *Oncology (Williston Park)*, **6** (2), 87–95; discussion 99–102.

56 Al-Sarraf, M., *et al.* (1998) Chemoradiotherapy versus radiotherapy in patients with advanced nasopharyngeal cancer: phase III randomized Intergroup study 0099. *J. Clin. Oncol.*, **16** (4), 1310–1317.

57 Chau, R.M., *et al.* (2001) Three-dimensional dosimetric evaluation of a conventional radiotherapy technique for treatment of nasopharyngeal carcinoma. *Radiother. Oncol.*, **58** (2), 143–153.

58 Kutcher, G.J., *et al.* (1991) Three-dimensional photon treatment planning for carcinoma of the nasopharynx. *Int. J. Radiat. Oncol. Biol. Phys.*, **21** (1), 169–182.

59 Nutting, C., Dearnaley, D.P., Webb, S. (2000) Intensity modulated radiation therapy: a clinical review. *Br. J. Radiol.*, **73** (869), 459–469.

60 Butler, E.B., *et al.* (1999) Smart (simultaneous modulated accelerated radiation therapy) boost: a new accelerated fractionation schedule for the treatment of head and neck cancer with intensity modulated radiotherapy. *Int. J. Radiat. Oncol. Biol. Phys.*, **45** (1), 21–32.

61 Eisbruch, A., *et al.* (1999) Dose, volume, and function relationships in parotid salivary glands following conformal and intensity-modulated irradiation of head and neck cancer. *Int. J. Radiat. Oncol. Biol. Phys.*, **45** (3), 577–587.

62 Xia, P., *et al.* (2000) Comparison of treatment plans involving intensity-modulated radiotherapy for nasopharyngeal carcinoma. *Int. J. Radiat. Oncol. Biol. Phys.*, **48** (2), 329–337.

63 Kam, M.K., *et al.* (2007) Prospective randomized study of intensity-modulated radiotherapy on salivary gland function in early-stage nasopharyngeal carcinoma patients. *J. Clin. Oncol.*, **25** (31), 4873–4879.

64 Pow, E.H., *et al.* (2006) Xerostomia and quality of life after intensity-modulated radiotherapy vs. conventional radiotherapy for early-stage nasopharyngeal carcinoma: initial report on a randomized controlled clinical trial. *Int. J. Radiat. Oncol. Biol. Phys.*, **66** (4), 981–991.

65 Lee, N., *et al.* (2002) Intensity-modulated radiotherapy in the treatment of nasopharyngeal carcinoma: an update of the UCSF experience. *Int. J. Radiat. Oncol. Biol. Phys.*, **53** (1), 12–22.

66 Wolden, S.L., *et al.* (2006) Intensity-modulated radiation therapy (IMRT) for nasopharynx cancer: update of the Memorial Sloan-Kettering experience. *Int. J. Radiat. Oncol. Biol. Phys.*, **64** (1), 57–62.

67 Kwong, D.L., *et al.* (2004) Intensity-modulated radiotherapy for early-stage nasopharyngeal carcinoma: a prospective study on disease control and preservation of salivary function. *Cancer*, **101** (7), 1584–1593.

68 Kam, M.K., *et al.* (2004) Treatment of nasopharyngeal carcinoma with intensity-modulated radiotherapy: the

Hong Kong experience. *Int. J. Radiat. Oncol. Biol. Phys.*, **60** (5), 1440–1450.

69 Lee, N., *et al.* (2009) Intensity-modulated radiation therapy with or without chemotherapy for nasopharyngeal carcinoma: radiation therapy oncology group phase II trial 0225. *J. Clin. Oncol.*, **27** (22), 3684–3690.

70 Som, P.M., Curtin, H.D., Mancuso, A.A. (2000) Imaging-based nodal classification for evaluation of neck metastatic adenopathy. *Am. J. Roentgenol.*, **174** (3), 837–844.

71 Nowak, P.J., *et al.* 91999) A three-dimensional CT-based target definition for elective irradiation of the neck. *Int. J. Radiat. Oncol. Biol. Phys.*, **45** (1), 33–39.

72 Gregoire, V., *et al.* (2000) Selection and delineation of lymph node target volumes in head and neck conformal radiotherapy. Proposal for standardizing terminology and procedure based on the surgical experience. *Radiother. Oncol.*, **56** (2), 135–150.

73 Gregoire, V., *et al.* (2003) CT-based delineation of lymph node levels and related CTVs in the node-negative neck: DAHANCA, EORTC, GORTEC, NCIC,RTOG consensus guidelines. *Radiother. Oncol.*, **69** (3), 227–236.

74 Lee, N., *et al.* (2997) Choosing an intensity-modulated radiation therapy technique in the treatment of head-and-neck cancer. *Int. J. Radiat. Oncol. Biol. Phys.*, **68** (5), 1299–1309.

75 Amdur, R.J., *et al.* (2007) Matching intensity-modulated radiation therapy to an anterior low neck field. *Int. J. Radiat. Oncol. Biol. Phys.*, **69** (2 Suppl.), S46–S48.

76 Dabaja, B., *et al.* (2005) Intensity-modulated radiation therapy (IMRT) of cancers of the head and neck: comparison of split-field and whole-field techniques. *Int. J. Radiat. Oncol. Biol. Phys.*, **63** (4), 1000–1005.

77 Levendag, P.C., *et al.* (1998) Fractionated high-dose-rate brachytherapy in primary carcinoma of the nasopharynx. *J. Clin. Oncol.*, **16** (6), 2213–2220.

78 Levendag, P.C., *et al.* (2002) Role of endocavitary brachytherapy with or without chemotherapy in cancer of the nasopharynx. *Int. J. Radiat. Oncol. Biol. Phys.*, **52** (3), 755–768.

79 Wang, C.C. (1987) Re-irradiation of recurrent nasopharyngeal carcinoma–treatment techniques and results. *Int. J. Radiat. Oncol. Biol. Phys.*, **13** (7), 953–956.

80 Wang, C.C. (1991) Improved local control of nasopharyngeal carcinoma after intracavitary brachytherapy boost. *Am. J. Clin. Oncol.*, **14** (1), 5–8.

81 Zhang, Y.W., Liu, T.F., Fi, C.X. (1989) Intracavitary radiation treatment of nasopharyngeal carcinoma by the high dose rate afterloading technique. *Int. J. Radiat. Oncol. Biol. Phys.*, **16** (2), 315–318.

82 Lee, N., *et al.* (2002) Managing nasopharyngeal carcinoma with intracavitary brachytherapy: one institution's 45-year experience. *Brachytherapy*, **1** (2), 74–82.

83 Teo, P., *et al.* (1994) Afterloading radiotherapy for local persistence of nasopharyngeal carcinoma. *Br. J. Radiol.*, **67** (794), 181–185.

84 Hwang, J.M., Fu, K.K., Phillips, T.L. (1998) Results and prognostic factors in the retreatment of locally recurrent nasopharyngeal carcinoma. *Int. J. Radiat. Oncol. Biol. Phys.*, **41** (5), 1099–1111.

85 Pryzant, R.M., *et al.* (1992) Re-treatment of nasopharyngeal carcinoma in 53 patients. *Int. J. Radiat. Oncol. Biol. Phys.*, **22** (5), 941–947.

86 Vikram, B. (1997) Permanent iodine-125 (I-125) boost after teletherapy in primary cancers of the nasopharynx is safe and highly effective: long-term results. *Int. J. Radiat. Oncol. Biol. Phys.*, **38** (5), 1140.

87 Wang, C. (1990) Carcinoma of the nasopharynx, in *Radiation Therapy for Head and Neck Neoplasms: Indications, Techniques, and Results* (ed. C.-C. Wang), Year Book Medical Publishers, Chicago, pp. 261–283.

88 Bailet, J.W., *et al.* (1992) Nasopharyngeal carcinoma: treatment results with primary radiation therapy. *Laryngoscope*, **102** (9), 965–972.

89 Vikram, B., *et al.* (1985) Patterns of failure in carcinoma of the nasopharynx: I. Failure at the primary site. *Int. J. Radiat. Oncol. Biol. Phys.*, **11** (8), 1455–1459.

90 Geara, F.B., *et al.* (1997) Carcinoma of the nasopharynx treated by radiotherapy alone: determinants of distant metastasis and survival. *Radiother. Oncol.*, **43** (1), 53–61.

91 Santos, J.A., *et al.* (1995) Impact of changes in the treatment of nasopharyngeal carcinoma: an experience of 30 years. *Radiother. Oncol.*, **36** (2), 121–127.

92 Saw, D., *et al.* (1985) Prognosis and histology in Stage I nasopharyngeal carcinoma (NPC). *Int. J. Radiat. Oncol. Biol. Phys.*, **11** (5), 893–898.

93 Chua, D.T., *et al.* (1996) Prognostic value of paranasopharyngeal extension of nasopharyngeal carcinoma. A significant factor in local control and distant metastasis. *Cancer*, **78** (2), 202–210.

94 Teo, P.M., *et al.* (1991) A proposed modification of the Ho stage-classification for nasopharyngeal carcinoma. *Radiother. Oncol.*, **21** (1), 11–23.

95 Lee, A.W., *et al.* (1992) Retrospective analysis of 5037 patients with nasopharyngeal carcinoma treated during 1976-1985: overall survival and patterns of failure. *Int. J. Radiat. Oncol. Biol. Phys.*, **23** (2), 261–270.

96 Marks, J.E., *et al.* (1982) Dose-response analysis for nasopharyngeal carcinoma: an historical perspective. *Cancer*, **50** (6), 1042–1050.

97 Teo, P.M., *et al.* (2006) Dose-response relationship of nasopharyngeal carcinoma above conventional tumoricidal level: a study by the Hong Kong nasopharyngeal carcinoma study group (HKNPCSG). *Radiother. Oncol.*, **79** (1), 27–33.

98 Le, Q.T., *et al.* (2003) Improved local control with stereotactic radiosurgical boost in patients with nasopharyngeal carcinoma. *Int. J. Radiat. Oncol. Biol. Phys.*, **56** (4), 1046–1054.

99 Hara, W., *et al.* (2008) Excellent local control with stereotactic radiotherapy boost after external beam radiotherapy in patients with nasopharyngeal carcinoma. *Int. J. Radiat. Oncol. Biol. Phys.*, **71** (2), 393–400.

100 Rosenblatt, E., *et al.* (2011) Brachytherapy Boost in Loco-regionally Advanced Nasopharyngeal Carcinoma: A Prospective Randomized Trial of the International Atomic Energy Agency. *Int. J. Radiat. Oncol. Biol. Phys.*, **81** (2 Suppl.), S4–S5.

101 Teo, P.M., *et al.* (2000) Final report of a randomized trial on altered-fractionated radiotherapy in nasopharyngeal carcinoma prematurely terminated by significant increase in neurologic complications. *Int. J. Radiat. Oncol. Biol. Phys.*, **48** (5), 1311–1322.

102 Lee, A.W., *et al.* (2006) Preliminary results of a randomized study (NPC-9902 Trial) on therapeutic gain by concurrent chemotherapy and/or accelerated fractionation for locally advanced nasopharyngeal carcinoma. *Int. J. Radiat. Oncol. Biol. Phys.*, **66** (1), 142–151.

103 Baujat, B., *et al.* (2006) Chemotherapy in locally advanced nasopharyngeal carcinoma: an individual patient data meta-analysis of eight randomized trials and 1753 patients. *Int. J. Radiat. Oncol. Biol. Phys.*, **64** (1), 47–56.

104 Langendijk, J.A., *et al.* (2004) The additional value of chemotherapy to radiotherapy in locally advanced nasopharyngeal carcinoma: a meta-analysis of the published literature. *J. Clin. Oncol.*, **22** (22), 4604–4612.

105 Wee, J., *et al.* (2005) Randomized trial of radiotherapy versus concurrent chemoradiotherapy followed by adjuvant chemotherapy in patients with American Joint Committee on Cancer/International Union against cancer stage III and IV nasopharyngeal cancer of the endemic variety. *J. Clin. Oncol.*, **23** (27), 6730–6738.

106 Rossi, A., *et al.* (1988) Adjuvant chemotherapy with vincristine, cyclophosphamide, and doxorubicin after radiotherapy in local-regional nasopharyngeal cancer: results of a 4-year multicenter randomized study. *J. Clin. Oncol.*, **6** (9), 1401–1410.

107 Chi, K.H., *et al.* (2002) A phase III study of adjuvant chemotherapy in advanced nasopharyngeal

carcinoma patients. *Int. J. Radiat. Oncol. Biol. Phys.*, **52** (5), 1238–1244.

108 Kwong, D.L., *et al.* (2004) Concurrent and adjuvant chemotherapy for nasopharyngeal carcinoma: a factorial study. *J. Clin. Oncol.*, **22** (13), 2643–2653.

109 Hara, W., Loo, B.W., Goffinet, D.R. (2008) Excellent local control with sterotactic radiotherapy boost after external beam radiotherapy in patients with nasopharyngeal carcinoma. *Int. J. Radiat. Oncol. Biol. Phys.*, **71** (2), 393–400.

110 Lee, N.Y., *et al.* (2011) Phase II study of chemoradiation plus bevacizumab (BV) for locally/regionally advanced nasopharyngeal carcinoma (NPC): Preliminary clinical results of RTOG 0615. *J. Clin. Oncol.*, **29** (Suppl.), Abstract 5516.

111 Sun, Y., *et al.* (2016) Induction chemotherapy plus concurrent chemoradiotherapy versus concurrent chemoradiotherapy alone in locoregionally advanced nasopharyngeal carcinoma: a phase 3, multicentre, randomised controlled trial. *The Lancet Oncol.*, **17** (11), 1509–1520.

112 Decker, D.A., *et al.* (1983) Chemotherapy for nasopharyngeal carcinoma. A ten-year experience. *Cancer*, **52** (4), 602–605.

113 Yan, J.H., Hu, Y.H., Gu, X.Z. (1983) Radiation therapy of recurrent nasopharyngeal carcinoma. Report on 219 patients. *Acta Radiol. Oncol.*, **22** (1), 23–28.

114 Harrison, L.B., *et al.* (1992) Nasopharyngeal brachytherapy with access via a transpalatal flap. *Am. J. Surg.*, **164** (2), 173–175.

115 Feehan, P.E., *et al.*, (1992) Recurrent locally advanced nasopharyngeal carcinoma treated with heavy charged particle irradiation. *Int. J. Radiat. Oncol. Biol. Phys.*, **23** (4), 881–884.

116 Chua, D.T., *et al.* (2001) Salvage treatment for persistent and recurrent T1-2 nasopharyngeal carcinoma by stereotactic radiosurgery. *Head Neck*, **23** (9), 791–798.

117 Chua, D.T., *et al.* (1999) Stereotactic radiosurgery as a salvage treatment for locally persistent and recurrent nasopharyngeal carcinoma. Head Neck, **21** (7), 620–626.

118 Kondziolka, D., Lunsford, L.D. (1991) Stereotactic radiosurgery for squamous cell carcinoma of the nasopharynx. *Laryngoscope*, **101** (5), 519–522.

119 Wei, W.I. (2003) Cancer of the nasopharynx: functional surgical salvage. *World J. Surg.*, **27** (7), 844–848.

120 Syed, A.M., *et al.* (2000) Brachytherapy for primary and recurrent nasopharyngeal carcinoma: 20 years' experience at Long Beach Memorial. *Int. J. Radiat. Oncol. Biol. Phys.*, **47** (5), 1311–1321.

121 Kwong, D.L., *et al.* (2001) Long term results of radioactive gold grain implantation for the treatment

of persistent and recurrent nasopharyngeal carcinoma. *Cancer*, **91** (6), 1105–1113.

122 Lee, N., *et al.* (2007) Salvage re-irradiation for recurrent head and neck cancer. *Int. J. Radiat. Oncol. Biol. Phys.*, **68** (3), 731–740.

123 Dawson, L.A., *et al.* (2001) Conformal re-irradiation of recurrent and new primary head-and-neck cancer. *Int. J. Radiat. Oncol. Biol. Phys.*, **50** (2), 377–385.

124 Hwang, H.N. (1983) Nasopharyngeal carcinoma in the People's Republic of China: incidence, treatment, and survival rates. *Radiology*, **149** (1), 305–309.

125 Lee, A.W., *et al.* (1997) Reirradiation for recurrent nasopharyngeal carcinoma: factors affecting the therapeutic ratio and ways for improvement. *Int. J. Radiat. Oncol. Biol. Phys.*, **38** (1), 43–52.

126 Hao, S.P., *et al.* (2008) Nasopharyngectomy for recurrent nasopharyngeal carcinoma: a review of 53 patients and prognostic factors. *Acta Otolaryngol.*, **128** (4), 473–481.

127 Leung, T.W., *et al.* (2000) Salvage radiation therapy for locally recurrent nasopharyngeal carcinoma. *Int. J. Radiat. Oncol. Biol. Phys.*, **48** (5), 1331–1338.

128 Oksuz, D.C., *et al.* (2004) Reirradiation for locally recurrent nasopharyngeal carcinoma: treatment results and prognostic factors. *Int. J. Radiat. Oncol. Biol. Phys.*, **60** (2), 388–394.

129 Law, S.C., *et al.* (2002) Reirradiation of nasopharyngeal carcinoma with intracavitary mold brachytherapy: an effective means of local salvage. *Int. J. Radiat. Oncol. Biol. Phys.*, **54** (4), 1095–1113.

130 Koutcher, L., *et al.* (2010) Reirradiation of locally recurrent nasopharynx cancer with external beam radiotherapy with or without brachytherapy. *Int. J. Radiat. Oncol. Biol. Phys.*, **76** (1), 130–137.

131 Cmelak, A.J., *et al.* (1997) Radiosurgery for skull base malignancies and nasopharyngeal carcinoma. *Int. J. Radiat. Oncol. Biol. Phys.*, **37** (5), 997–1003.

132 Wu, S.X., *et al.* (2007) Outcome of fractionated stereotactic radiotherapy for 90 patients with locally persistent and recurrent nasopharyngeal carcinoma. *Int. J. Radiat. Oncol. Biol. Phys.*, **69** (3), 761–769.

133 Unger, K.R., *et al.* (2010) Fractionated stereotactic radiosurgery for reirradiation of head-and-neck cancer. *Int. J. Radiat. Oncol. Biol. Phys.*, **77** (5), 1411–1419.

134 Chua, D.T., *et al.* (2005) Re-irradiation of nasopharyngeal carcinoma with intensity-modulated radiotherapy. *Radiother. Oncol.*, **77** (3), 290–294.

135 Lu, T.X., *et al.* (2004) Initial experience using intensity-modulated radiotherapy for recurrent nasopharyngeal carcinoma. *Int. J. Radiat. Oncol. Biol. Phys.*, **58** (3), 682–687.

136 Hsiung, C.Y., *et al.* (2002) Intensity-modulated radiotherapy versus conventional three-dimensional conformal radiotherapy for boost or salvage treatment of nasopharyngeal carcinoma. *Int. J. Radiat. Oncol. Biol. Phys.*, **53** (3), 638–647.

137 Eisbruch, A., *et al.* (1996) Parotid gland sparing in patients undergoing bilateral head and neck irradiation: techniques and early results. *Int. J. Radiat. Oncol. Biol. Phys.*, **36** (2), 469–480.

138 Chao, K.S., *et al.* (2001) A prospective study of salivary function sparing in patients with head-and-neck cancers receiving intensity-modulated or three-dimensional radiation therapy: initial results. *Int. J. Radiat. Oncol. Biol. Phys.*, **49** (4), 907–916.

139 Blanco, A.I., *et al.* (2005) Dose-volume modeling of salivary function in patients with head-and-neck cancer receiving radiotherapy. *Int. J. Radiat. Oncol. Biol. Phys.*, **62** (4), 1055–1069.

140 Pan, C.C., *et al.* (2005) Prospective study of inner ear radiation dose and hearing loss in head-and-neck cancer patients. *Int. J. Radiat. Oncol. Biol. Phys.*, **61** (5), 1393–1402.

141 Chen, W.C., *et al.* (2006) Sensorineural hearing loss in combined modality treatment of nasopharyngeal carcinoma. *Cancer*, **106** (4), 820–829.

142 Eisbruch, A., *et al.* (2004) Dysphagia and aspiration after chemoradiotherapy for head-and-neck cancer: which anatomic structures are affected and can they be spared by IMRT? *Int. J. Radiat. Oncol. Biol. Phys.*, **60** (5), 1425–1439.

143 Fua, T.F., *et al.* (2007) Intensity-modulated radiotherapy for nasopharyngeal carcinoma: clinical correlation of dose to the pharyngo-esophageal axis and dysphagia. *Int. J. Radiat. Oncol. Biol. Phys.*, **67** (4), 976–981.

144 Lee, A.W., *et al.* (2002) Factors affecting risk of symptomatic temporal lobe necrosis: significance of fractional dose and treatment time. *Int. J. Radiat. Oncol. Biol. Phys.*, **53** (1), 75–85.

145 Peng, G., *et al.* (2012) A prospective, randomized study comparing outcomes and toxicities of intensity-modulated radiotherapy vs. conventional two-dimensional radiotherapy for the treatment of nasopharyngeal carcinoma. *Radiat. Oncol.*, **104** (3), 286–293.

146 Sanguineti, G., *et al.* (1997) Carcinoma of the nasopharynx treated by radiotherapy alone: determinants of local and regional control. *Int. J. Radiat. Oncol. Biol. Phys.*, **37** (5), 985–996.

147 Lin, J.C., *et al.* (2003) Phase III study of concurrent chemoradiotherapy versus radiotherapy alone for advanced nasopharyngeal carcinoma: positive effect on overall and progression-free survival. *J. Clin. Oncol.*, **21** (4), 631–637.

148 Chan, A.T., *et al.* (2005) Overall survival after concurrent cisplatin-radiotherapy compared with

radiotherapy alone in locoregionally advanced nasopharyngeal carcinoma. *J. Natl Cancer Inst.*, **97** (7), 536–539.

149 Zhang, L., *et al.* (2005) Phase III study comparing standard radiotherapy with or without weekly oxaliplatin in treatment of locoregionally advanced nasopharyngeal carcinoma: preliminary results. *J. Clin. Oncol.*, **23** (33), 8461–8468.

150 Lee, A.W., *et al.* (2005) Preliminary results of a randomized study on therapeutic gain by concurrent chemotherapy for regionally-advanced nasopharyngeal carcinoma: NPC-9901 Trial by the Hong Kong Nasopharyngeal Cancer Study Group. *J. Clin. Oncol.*, **23** (28), 6966–6975.

151 Pai, P.C., *et al.* (2002) Stereotactic radiosurgery for locally recurrent nasopharyngeal carcinoma. *Head Neck*, **24** (8), 748–753.

13

Carcinoma of the Paranasal Sinuses and Nasal Cavity

Farzan Siddiqui, Nicholas Galanopoulos and Min Yao

Introduction

Carcinomas of the paranasal sinuses are rare malignancies which account for only 3–5% of all head and neck cancers, and 1% of all cancers [1–3]. They are generally asymptomatic in their early stages and are often not diagnosed until they are locally advanced. Due to their rarity and heterogeneous histology, limited data are available as to the best treatment approach for these tumors.

The paranasal sinuses consist of the maxillary sinus, ethmoid sinus, sphenoid sinus, and frontal sinus. Of these, the maxillary sinus is the most common site of paranasal sinus cancers, followed by the ethmoid sinus. Carcinomas of the sphenoid and frontal sinuses are very rare.

The predominant cell type is squamous cell carcinoma, which accounts for over 80% of paranasal sinus cancers [1, 2]. Other histologic types include adenocarcinoma, adenoid cystic carcinoma, esthesioneuroblastoma, lymphoma, melanoma, sarcoma, sinonasal undifferentiated carcinoma, and neuroendocrine tumors.

Anatomy

The anatomy of the nasal cavity and paranasal sinus is illustrated in Figure 13.1. The nasal cavity itself is centrally located and is divided into two halves by the nasal septum. Superiorly, it is bounded by the base of the skull (the frontal sinuses and cribriform plate). The floor of the nasal cavity consists of the soft and hard palate. Laterally, it is bounded by the maxillary sinus, anteriorly by the nasal vestibule, and posteriorly by the nasopharynx.

The *paranasal sinuses* are unique in that they largely consist of air-filled spaces. This allows for an insidious growth of tumor with relatively few obvious symptoms until the tumor reaches an advanced stage. Involvement of the surrounding structures of the paranasal sinuses are often the first symptoms of the disease. In particular, the orbit, vascular structures, and brain parenchyma can be involved in advanced stages.

The *maxillary sinus* is the largest of the paranasal sinuses. It is bounded by the floor of the orbit superiorly, the lateral wall of nasal cavity medially, the zygomatic process laterally, and the alveolar processes inferiorly. Anteriorly, it forms the facial wall located behind the cheek, while posteriorly it forms the infratemporal wall bordered by the infratemporal and pterygopalatine fossae. The maxillary sinus can be divided into two portions by an imaginary line drawn from the medial canthus to the angle of the mandible; this line is known as Ohngren's line, and separates the maxillary sinus into suprastructure (posterosuperior portion) and infrastructure (anteroinferior portion). Lesions located in the suprastructure have a worse prognosis since they are much more difficult to resect due to early invasion by these tumors into critical structures, including the pterygopalatine fossa, orbit, infratemporal fossa, and skull base.

The *ethmoid sinuses* consist of small air cells that are in close proximity to critical structures such as the orbit and base of skull. They are surrounded by the frontal sinus and the base of the skull superiorly, by the nasal cavity medially, by the orbits laterally, and by the maxillary sinus inferiorly. They are separated from the orbit by a thin bone called the lamina papyracea, and are in close proximity to the optic nerve laterally and the optic chiasm posteriorly.

The *sphenoid sinus* is a midline structure with the pituitary gland and optic chiasm sitting above it and cavernous sinuses lateral to it. It is superior to the nasopharynx and posterior to the ethmoid sinuses and nasal cavity.

Clinical Radiation Oncology: Indications, Techniques, and Results, Third Edition. Edited by William Small Jr.
© 2017 John Wiley & Sons, Inc. Published 2017 by John Wiley & Sons, Inc.

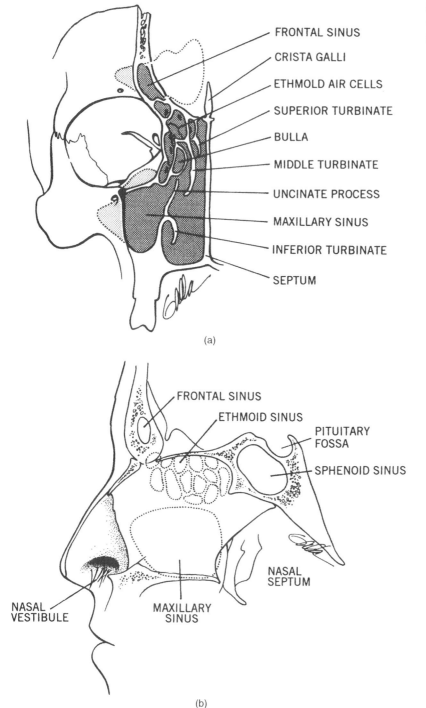

FRONTAL SINUS

CRISTA GALLI

ETHMOLD AIR CELLS

SUPERIOR TURBINATE

BULLA

MIDDLE TURBINATE

UNCINATE PROCESS

MAXILLARY SINUS

INFERIOR TURBINATE

SEPTUM

(a)

FRONTAL SINUS

ETHMOID SINUS

PITUITARY FOSSA

SPHENOID SINUS

NASAL SEPTUM

NASAL VESTIBULE

MAXILLARY SINUS

(b)

Figure 13.1 Diagram showing nasal cavity, vestibule, and paranasal sinuses in (a) anteroposterior and (b) lateral view.

Patterns of Tumor Spread

Maxillary Sinus

For maxillary sinus cancers, location plays an important role in the natural history of the disease. Lesions originating in the suprastructure (superior to Ohngren's line) have the potential to invade the nasal cavity, ethmoid sinus, orbit, pterygopalatine fossa, infratemporal fossa, and base of skull. Lesions inferior to Ohngren's line tend to invade the soft palate, mandible, buccal mucosa, nasal cavity, and pterygopalatine space. The latter lesions therefore carry a much better prognosis as they are more easily resectable with less morbidity as compared to suprastructural lesions. In advanced stages, suprastructural tumors can invade the orbit, leading to proptosis, diplopia, and other visual changes. Infrastructure lesions can lead to trismus, facial swelling, and tooth pain as lesions spread into the infratemporal and pterygopalatine fossae.

Lymph node involvement at the time of diagnosis is rare for most paranasal sinus malignancies. However, in patients with squamous cell and poorly differentiated carcinoma of the maxillary sinus, the cumulative macroscopic and microscopic incidence of nodal disease can be as high as 30%. From the M.D. Anderson Cancer Center experience, among those who did not receive elective neck treatment, nine of 24 patients (38%) with squamous cell and poorly differentiated carcinoma had regional recurrences [4]. The most commonly involved lymph nodes are ipsilateral level II and level Ib lymph node groups. Contralateral nodal involvement is rare. Le *et al.* also reported that the overall risk of nodal involvement at diagnosis and on follow-up was 28% for squamous cell carcinomas of the maxillary sinus [5]. The risk of lymph node involvement is correlated with T stage. All patients with nodal involvement had T3-4 disease, and none had T2 tumors.

Nasoethmoidal Complex

This structure includes the nasal cavity and ethmoidal sinuses, given their close proximity to each other. The nasal cavity is divided into left and right halves by the nasal septum. The pattern of tumor spread is typically determined by where within the nasal cavity the tumor originates. For example, lesions in the superior portion of the nasal cavity can invade the orbit through the lamina papyracea and the anterior cranial fossa through the cribriform plate, whereas more inferior lesions can invade the maxillary sinuses and the palate. Anteriorly, they can grow into subcutaneous tissue and the overlying skin.

The small air cells that comprise the ethmoid sinus lie in close proximity to the orbit and are only separated from it by a thin bone, the lamina papyracea. This allows for easy access to the orbit, which may result in diplopia and proptosis in advanced stages. It can also extend into the anterior cranial fossa through the cribriform plate. Ethmoid sinus cancer often extends to involve the adjacent maxillary sinus.

Lymph node involvement is exceedingly rare. In one series of primary nasal cavity cancer, the rate of subsequent neck failure in patients not receiving elective neck radiation was only 7% [6].

Clinical Presentation

For sinonasal malignancies, presenting symptoms are usually non-specific and may mimic sinusitis until the lesions become very advanced. Common symptoms include nasal obstruction, nasal discharge, and facial discomfort. The diagnosis requires a high index of suspicion [7].

In advanced stages, the symptoms and signs result from extension of the tumor to adjacent soft tissues and organs. For example, when the tumor extends anteriorly to involve the subcutaneous tissue it can cause facial swelling and pain. Patients can present with proptosis, diplopia and orbital pain when the tumor invades into the orbit. For inframaxillary tumor, patients often present with toothache, unhealed tooth socket after teeth extraction, or a mass in the upper gum.

Patient Evaluation and Work-Up

A full history and physical examination should be performed with emphasis on careful examination of cranial nerve function. Flexible fiberoptic scope examination allows the assessment of local extension of the disease, especially when it involves the nasal cavity and nasopharynx. Radiographic studies include dedicated computed tomography (CT) and magnetic resonance imaging (MRI) of the sinuses. CT offers better information on bony invasion, while MRI offers better information on the involvement of soft tissues, nerves, skull base, brain, and a better differentiation of fluid from solid tumor. Tissue biopsy should be performed for definitive pathologic diagnosis.

Staging

The American Joint Committee on Cancer (AJCC) 8th Edition Staging for cancers of the maxillary sinus and nasoethmoidal complex (including nasal cavity and ethmoid sinus) is outlined in Table 13.1. Each subsite has a unique T-stage, but the N-stage follows that of the other head and neck subsites (except for nasopharyngeal cancers). Clinical staging is based on information obtained during patient evaluation. Pathology staging includes information from clinical staging and histologic study of the surgically resected specimen.

Principles of Management

The management of nasal cavity and paranasal sinus malignancies typically involves a multimodality approach. Surgery is the 'gold standard' for resectable early-stage lesions, with radiation added in the adjuvant setting depending on pathologic risk factors. Indications for postoperative radiation include positive or close surgical margins, high-grade tumor, perineural invasion, piecemeal resection, or concern regarding the surgical margins [8–12].

Table 13.1 Staging for nasal cavity and paranasal sinus cancers.

AJCC, 8th edition	Maxillary sinus
T1	Tumor limited to maxillary sinus mucosa with no erosion or destruction of bone.
T2	Tumor causing bone erosion or destruction including extension into the hard palate and/or middle nasal meatus, except extension to posterior wall of maxillary sinus and pterygoid plates.
T3	Tumor invades any of the following: bone of the posterior wall of maxillary sinus; subcutaneous tissues; floor or medial wall of orbit; pterygoid fossa; ethmoid sinuses.
T4a	Moderately advanced local disease. Tumor invades anterior orbital contents, skin of cheek, pterygoid plates, infratemporal fossa, cribriform plate, sphenoid or frontal sinuses.
T4b	Very advanced local disease. Tumor invades any of the following: orbital apex; dura; brain; middle cranial fossa; cranial nerves other than maxillary division of trigeminal nerve (V2); nasopharynx; or clivus.

AJCC, 8th edition	Nasal cavity and ethmoid sinus
T1	Tumor restricted to any one subsite, with or without bony invasion.
T2	Tumor invading two subsites in a single region or extending to involve an adjacent region within the nasoethmoidal complex, with or without bony invasion.
T3	Tumor extends to invade the medal wall or floor of the orbit, maxillary sinus, palate, or cribriform plate.
T4a	Moderately advanced local disease. Tumor invades any of the following: anterior orbital contents; skin of nose or cheek; minimal extension to anterior cranial fossa; pterygoid plates; sphenoid; or frontal sinuses.
T4b	Very advanced local disease. Tumor invades any of the following: orbital apex; dura; brain; middle cranial fossa; cranial nerves other than maxillary division of trigeminal nerve (V2); nasopharynx; or clivus.

N Stage
- NX - Cannot be assessed
- N0 - No regional lymph nodes metastasis
- N1 - Single ipsilateral lymph node, ≤3 cm in greatest dimension and ENE (−)
- N2
  - N2a - Single ipsilateral lymph node, 3–6 cm in greatest dimension and ENE (−)
  - N2b - Multiple ipsilateral lymph nodes, ≤6 cm in greatest dimension and ENE (−)
  - N2c - Bilateral or contralateral lymph nodes, ≤6 cm in greatest dimension and ENE (−)
- N3
  - N3a - Lymph node(s) >6 cm in greatest dimension and ENE (−)
  - N3b - any node(s) with clinically overt ENE (+)

Stage Grouping
- Stage I - T1N0
- Stage II - T2N0
- Stage III - T3N0, T1-3N1
- Stage IVA - T4aN0 or N1 or T1-4aN2
- Stage IVB - T4b or N3
- Stage IVC - M1

Source: AJCC Cancer Staging Manual, Eighth Edition (2017), Springer, New York, Inc.

Most patients present with advanced diseases. A combination of surgery and radiation therapy is the treatment of choice for resectable advanced disease. In this situation, radical surgery is performed first, and radiation therapy is then used in the adjuvant setting, targeting the tumor bed, resection cavity, any areas of residual disease, and areas with a high risk of harboring microscopic diseases. Postoperative chemoradiation can be considered for patients with high-risk factors for recurrence, such as a positive margin or extracapsular extension of involved lymph nodes. However, data on this approach are limited and are largely based on extrapolation from studies performed on head and neck cancer of other subsites [13,14].

For patients with borderline resectable disease, neoadjuvant chemotherapy followed by surgery and postoperative radiation, or neoadjuvant chemoradiation followed by surgery, can be used. Neoadjuvant treatment can downstage the tumor and thus make surgery easier. This approach can also increase the possibility for orbital preservation. Lee *et al.* reported 19 patients treated at the University of Chicago with induction chemotherapy [15], and noted an 87% response rate to chemotherapy, while in half of these patients a complete pathologic response was noted at the time of surgery. Local control at five and 10 years was 76% each. The overall survival at five and 10 years was 73% and 54%, respectively. The disease-free survival at five and 10 years was 67%, respectively.

Induction chemotherapy followed by definitive concurrent chemoradiation for organ preservation is under investigation. Hanna *et al.* presented their experience at the M. D. Anderson Cancer center of 46 patients treated with induction chemotherapy [16]. Of these patients, 31 (67%) had a partial response to the chemotherapy. Subsequently, 14 patients received definitive radiation, five with chemoradiation and eight with chemoradiation followed by planned surgery for any residual disease. The remainder underwent surgery, usually followed by postoperative radiation. The authors reported a two-year overall survival for all patients of 67%; notably, the two-year overall survival for those with a partial response was significantly better than those with progressive disease (77% versus 36%, p = 0.05). As illustrated by the case in Figure 13.4 (see below), after induction chemotherapy it is feasible to deliver a high-dose radiation (70 Gy) to the postchemotherapy tumor volume, thereby increasing the chance of tumor control without damage to the optics.

In patients with unresectable disease or who refused surgery, primary radiation therapy is typically used. However, the results are inferior to combined modality therapy with surgery and adjuvant radiation. Attempts have been made to improve treatment outcomes by the addition of induction chemotherapy and/or concurrent chemotherapy with radiation. Cisplatin-based chemotherapy is often used which is extrapolated from the results of clinical trials in head and neck cancers of other subsites [13, 14]. Stereotactic body radiation therapy (SBRT) can be used as a boost to deliver additional radiation to residual tumor after radiation. However, this approach should be performed with care as it may lead to severe late complications such as brain necrosis [17] (see also the case illustrated in Figure 13.5).

Treatment of Cervical Lymph Node

Elective neck irradiation in clinically N0 necks in nasal and paranasal sinus cancer has been controversial. There are conflicting reports regarding the risk of regional failures without elective neck irradiation. Dirix *et al.* noted that only four of 122 (3%) originally N0 patients developed a regional failure in the neck [18]. Others have

reported higher incidences ranging from 10% to 30% [4, 5]. In general, routine elective neck irradiation may not be necessary in patients with clinically N0 necks. However, for patients with stage T3-4 squamous cell and poorly differentiated carcinoma of the maxillary sinus, elective neck irradiation has been shown to improve regional control, distant metastasis, and potentially overall survival [4, 5, 13].

Le *et al.* described 97 patients with maxillary sinus cancer treated at Stanford University and at the University of California, San Francisco, and noted that the five-year nodal recurrence was 20% for patients without elective neck irradiation and 0% for those who received neck irradiation [5]. Patients with neck recurrence had a significantly higher risk for distant metastasis. The five-year distant failure rate was 81% for patients with neck failure versus 29% for those with neck control (p = 0.02). There was a trend for decreased survival with nodal failure. The five-year overall survival was 37% for patients with neck control and 0% for patients with neck failure. Jiang *et al.* reviewed their M.D. Anderson Cancer Center experience of 73 patients with maxillary sinus cancer treated between 1969 and 1985 [4]. Among these patients, 49 had T3/4N0 carcinoma and 36 had squamous cell and undifferentiated carcinoma. The overall regional recurrence rate for those without neck radiation was 33% for squamous cell and undifferentiated carcinoma. None of 16 patients who received elective neck irradiation failed in the neck nodes. Following this report, the authors changed their radiation techniques and now include elective neck irradiation for patients with T2-T4 maxillary sinus squamous cell and undifferentiated carcinoma. Bristol *et al.* updated the experience and compared patients treated before and after this change [19]. Among patients with squamous cell and undifferentiated carcinoma, 13 of 36 (36%) without neck radiation developed regional recurrence, compared to three of 45 patients (7%) with the neck radiated (p < 0.001). Those receiving elective neck irradiation had a significant reduction in distant metastasis, namely 3% in those treated versus 20% in those untreated at five years (p = 0.045). There was also a significant increase in recurrence-free survival (67% in treated versus 45% in untreated at five years, p = 0.025). However, there was no significant difference in overall survival.

For patients with N0 neck who did not receive elective neck irradiation, most failed at the ipsilateral level II and level Ib when they had nodal failure. Therefore, elective neck irradiation to the ipsilateral neck should be sufficient.

Radiation Therapy Techniques

Many radiation dose-limiting structures occur in the vicinity of nasal cavity and paranasal sinuses, including orbits, optic nerves, optic chiasm, pituitary gland, parotid glands, brain, and brainstem. Hence, intensity-modulated radiotherapy (IMRT) should be used to allow the delivery of high-dose radiation to the tumor targets while sparing these critical structures.

Patient Set-Up and Simulation

The patient is immobilized with a custom headrest and a thermoplastic mask. When elective neck irradiation is needed, a head and shoulder mask that extends to the upper thorax should be used. An intraoral stent can be used to depress the oral tongue, which can help to reduce radiation dose to the oral cavity. CT images are obtained from vertex to the upper mediastinum at 3-mm intervals, and transferred to the computer for treatment planning. MRI can be obtained and co-registered to the planning CT, especially when there is residual tumor after surgery or after neoadjuvant chemotherapy. In addition, the co-registration of pre-treatment images such as CT, MRI and/or fluorodeoxyglucose positron emission tomography (FDG-PET) images to the planning CT images can help to facilitate accurate target delineation.

Target Delineation

Target delineation and radiation treatment planning should be based on physical examination, pre-treatment imaging studies (preoperative or pre-chemotherapy imaging studies for patients treated with neoadjuvant chemotherapy), intraoperative findings, pathologic findings, and post-treatment imaging studies. Therefore, it is necessary to take a multidisciplinary approach. All these findings should be carefully reviewed before target delineation by a multidisciplinary tumor board that includes surgeons, neuroradiologists, and pathologists. In the present authors' practice the surgeons and neuroradiologists are routinely asked to review the treatment planning CT and indicate the areas of concern, especially when there are positive margins.

In general, three clinical target volumes (CTVs) can be defined and outlined on each slice of the planning CT. For definitive radiation, CTV1 is the gross tumor volume (GTV) with 3–5 mm expansion. CTV2 is the high-risk areas with microscopic disease, and often includes the entire involved sinus. If the tumor invades through bone into soft tissue, a wider margin of 0.5–1.0 cm over the involved area is necessary. CTV3 is the elective lymphatic regions. For patients with positive lymph nodes, the involved lymph nodes with 5 mm are also defined as CTV1, and the high-risk lymphatic regions as CTV2. For high-risk postoperative patients, CTV1 is defined as the residual tumor plus 3–5 mm margins, and CTV2 is the surgical bed and adjacent soft tissue with margins, similar to CTV2 defined for definitive radiation. CTV3 is the

elective lymphatic regions. For intermediate-risk postoperative patients who have negative surgical margins and no extracapsular extension of adenopathy, two CTVs are generally sufficient.

Critical structures are also defined, including orbits, lens, retina, optic nerves, optic chiasm, brainstem, spinal cord, brain, parotid glands, and mandible. The optic nerve, optic chiasm and brainstem are expanded 3 mm, and the spinal cord 5 mm, to create planned organ at risk volumes (POARs).

PTVs are created by expanding the CTVs by 3–5 mm. If any PTV overlaps the POAR, the PTVs can be subtracted from the POAR to generate planning-PTVs which are used for dose calculations. However, the original PTVs should also be used in evaluation of the final treatment plan.

Dose Prescription

For definitive radiation, PTV1 is prescribed to 70 Gy at 2.0 Gy per fraction, PTV2 to 63 Gy at 1.8 Gy per fraction, and PTV3 to 56 Gy at 1.6 Gy per fraction. All volumes are treated simultaneously in total 35 fractions. For high-risk postoperative radiation, PTV1 is prescribed to 66 Gy at 2.0 Gy per fraction, PTV2 to 60 Gy at 1.82 Gy per fraction, and PTV3 to 56 Gy at 1.7 Gy per fraction. All volumes are treated simultaneously in total 33 fractions. For intermediate-risk postoperative radiation, PTV1 is prescribed to 60 Gy at 2.0 Gy per fraction, and PTV2 to 54 Gy at 1.8 Gy per fraction. Both volumes are treated simultaneously in a total of 30 fractions. Doses are prescribed to 95% of the PTV volumes.

In patients receiving treatment with sequential radiation plans in phases, the first phase delivers 50 Gy in 25 fractions to all target volumes, followed by a boost for additional dose up to 60–66 Gy to areas of intermediate-risk or positive margins. Finally, areas with gross involvement by disease receive 70 Gy in phase 3.

Recommended doses to normal structures are summarized in Table 13.2.

Case Studies

Case #1

A 62-year-old female presented with pain in the left face and bleeding from the left upper gum. An ulcerated mass was noted in the left upper gum, with biopsy revealing moderately differentiated squamous cell carcinoma. MRI of the sinus revealed a large mass in the left maxillary sinus and left masticator space, invading the floor of the left orbit. CT showed extensive bony destruction of the maxillary sinus and left maxillary alveolar ridge. The patient underwent a left extended maxillectomy with

Table 13.2 Recommended doses to normal structures.

Structure	Volume at dose	Tolerance dose (Gy)	
		1.8 Gy per fr	2.0 Gy per fr
Optic nerves	100%	<56.8	<54
Optic chiasm	100%	<56.8	<54
Eyes	100%	<21.1	<20
Brainstem	100%	<56.8	<54
Cochlea	Mean dose	<46.9	<45
Inner ear	100%	<41.7	<40
Lens of eye	100%	<3.2	<3
Spinal cord	100%	<47.4	<45
Spinal cord + 0.5 cm	100%	<52.6	<50
Parotid glands (unilateral)	Mean dose	<27.1	<26
	<50%	<31.3	<30
Parotid glands (bilateral)	Mean dose	<26	<25

left orbital exenteration and free flap reconstruction. Pathology revealed microscopic positive margins in several areas. She received postoperative radiation with concurrent cisplatin given weekly at a dose of 40 mg m^{-2}. The preoperative MRI was co-registered to the planning CT and the CTV1 was defined as the tumor bed and the postoperative changes. CTV2 was defined as the adjacent sinus and soft tissue as well as left level Ib and level II. CTV1 was treated to 66 Gy at 2 Gy per fraction, and CTV2 to 59.4 Gy at 1.8 Gy per fraction in total 33 fractions using simultaneous integrated boost technique. The isodose distribution is shown in Figure 13.2a, and the dose–volume histogram (DVH) with selected critical structures in Figure 13.2b.

Case #2

Radiation can also be delivered as a sequential boost with additional dose to the residual tumor or high risk areas. A 75-year-old female with advanced right maxillary squamous cell carcinoma underwent surgical resection which revealed a tumor measuring 4.9 × 4.6 × 2.6 cm in size, with extensive invasion into the right maxillary bone and adjacent soft tissues including invasion of the floor of orbit and soft tissues, medial cranial fossa, palate, zygomatic bone, and subcutaneous tissues (Figure 13.3). Because of invasion of the orbital floor and medial wall, she also underwent a right orbital exenteration and right selective neck dissection levels I through IV. The patient had a pathology stage of pT4a pN0. She underwent adjuvant external beam radiation therapy (EBRT) to a dose of 60 Gy to the site of primary disease (tumor bed) and 54 Gy to the ipsilateral level Ib and II in 30 fractions using a simultaneous integrated boost technique. This

was followed by a boost of 6 Gy in three fractions to the preoperative GTV plus margin.

Case #3

Induction chemotherapy can reduce the tumor size and allows the delivery of a high-radiation dose to the postchemotherapy tumor volume. A 57-year-old male presented with right facial swelling and a non-healing wound after extraction of his right upper molar. A large mass in the right maxillary sinus was found with erosion of maxillary sinus wall, extension into soft tissue and right orbit. A FDG-PET scan revealed intense FDG uptake of this mass. A biopsy of the mass showed moderately differentiated squamous cell carcinoma. The patient refused to have orbital exenteration, and was treated with induction chemotherapy using a TPF regimen (taxotere, cisplatin and 5-fluorouracil). He had a good response after three cycles of TPF, with a significant reduction in the size of the tumor. The patient then received definitive radiation with concurrent chemotherapy. Both, the pre-chemotherapy MRI scans (Figure 13.4a) and post-chemotherapy MRI scans (Figure 13.4b) were co-registered to the treatment planning CT for target delineation. The CTV1, including the residual tumor after chemotherapy (postchemotherapy tumor volume) with margin, was treated to 70 Gy. CTV2, the pre-chemotherapy tumor volume and adjacent soft tissue with margin was treated to 63 Gy. CTV3, the adjacent sinus and soft tissue with risk of tumor extension, was treated to 56 Gy (Figure 13.4c). All these volumes were treated simultaneously with dose painting. A PET-CT obtained three months after radiation revealed resolution of the hypermetabolic mass but with mild diffuse FDG uptake in the right maxillary sinus, possibly due to inflammation. A repeat PET scan obtained four months later showed no further FDG uptake in the right maxillary sinus.

Case #4

SBRT can be used as a boost to deliver additional radiation to residual tumor, but should be done carefully to avoid severe late complications [17]. A 49-year-old male presented with unresectable squamous cell carcinoma in the sphenoid sinus and nasal cavity (Figure 13.5a). The patient received IMRT to 50.4 Gy at 1.8 Gy per fraction in 28 fractions (Figure 13.5b). A higher radiation dose was difficult to deliver due to the tolerance of optic structures. He also received concurrent weekly carboplatin and taxol with radiation. The response was good (Figure 13.5c), but a biopsy of the sphenoid sinus revealed residual invasive carcinoma. The patient was treated with SBRT using a Cyberknife for an additional 18 Gy at 6 Gy per fraction in three fractions (Figure 13.5d). He has been doing well

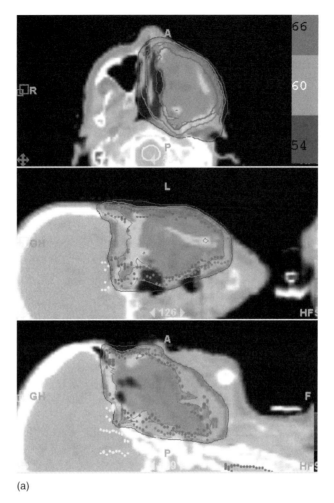

(a)

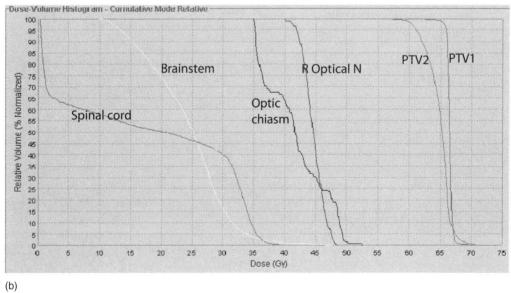

(b)

Figure 13.2 A patient with stage T4AN0 left maxillary sinus squamous cell carcinoma treated with postoperative radiotherapy. (a) Isodose distribution of the treatment plan. (b) Dose–volume histogram for the relevant structures. For a color version of this figure, see the color plate section.

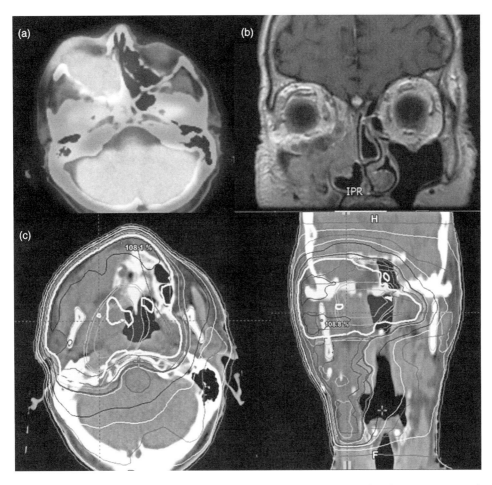

Figure 13.3 A patient with stage T4AN0 right maxillary sinus squamous cell carcinoma treated with postoperative radiotherapy. (a) Preoperative PET scan showing FDG avid lesion in the right maxillary sinus involving the orbit and causing bone instruction. (b) Coronal MRI image showing disease in the right maxillary sinus with disruption of the floor of orbit. (c) Axial and coronal images of the planning CT scan showing the dose distribution. Green line, 66 Gy isodose; yellow line, 60 Gy isodose; blue line, 54 Gy isodose. For a color version of this figure, see the color plate section.

almost four years after the initial treatment, with MRI revealing enhancement in the right frontal lobe and both temporal lobes (Figure 13.5e) which has been stable in a series of repeated MRI over two years. These were suspicious for brain necrosis induced by radiation. Currently, the patient is asymptomatic and is under close observation with repeated MRI imaging.

Treatment Outcomes

The treatment of paranasal sinus and nasal cavity tumors is challenging for several reasons: (i) the lack of large prospective or randomized trials; (ii) varied subsites and histology; and (iii) the proximity to critical normal tissues such as optic nerves, optic chiasm, eyes, pituitary, brainstem and temporal lobes of the brain. Most of these tumors present in advanced stages with destruction of bone and involvement of some of the critical structures

listed above. This makes surgical resection difficult or impossible, and may result in a resection with positive margins.

Due to the relative rarity of these cancers and lack of large randomized trials to guide their therapy, most of the treatment recommendations are based on retrospective studies. Unfortunately, these reports have included a mix of disease sites and varied histologies, as well as different radiation techniques and doses. Hence, definitive treatment recommendations regarding a specific paranasal subsite with a specific histology are difficult to ascertain.

Blanco *et al.* reported one of the largest series on patients treated for maxillary sinus and ethmoid tumors [20] in which the majority of 206 patients was treated using conventional EBRT to a median dose of 60 Gy (range: 30–81 Gy). Radiation was delivered preoperatively (26.4%), postoperatively (38.7%), or as a single modality (28.3%). At a median follow-up of 60 months, 82% of the patients had died, 58% with recurrent or

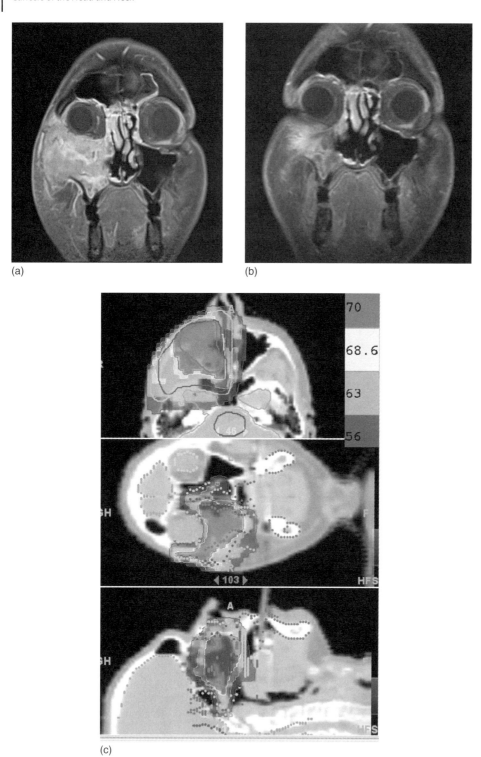

(a)

(b)

(c)

Figure 13.4 A patient with stage T4AN0 right maxillary sinus squamous cell carcinoma treated with induction chemotherapy followed by definitive concurrent chemoradiation. (a) MRI at diagnosis. (b) MRI after induction chemotherapy. (c) Isodose distribution of the treatment plan. Note that the postchemotherapy tumor volume was delivered to 70 Gy. For a color version of this figure, see the color plate section.

Figure 13.5 A patient with unresectable squamous cell carcinoma of sphenoid sinus and nasal cavity. (a) MRI at diagnosis. (b) IMRT plan to 50.4 Gy at 1.8 Gy per fraction. (c) MRI at one month after IMRT. (d) SBRT using Cyberknife for additional 18 Gy at 6 Gy per fraction. (e) MRI at three years after the initial treatment. Enhancement (arrow) was noted in the right temporal lobe suspicious for brain necrosis. For a color version of this figure, see the color plate section.

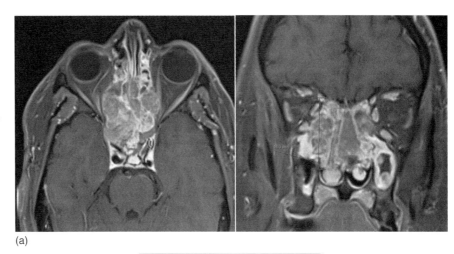

(a)

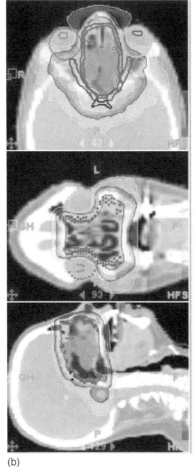

(b)

persistent primary tumor. This resulted in a five-year disease-free rate and an overall survival rate of 33% and 27%, respectively. An analysis of prognostic factors identified the presence of intracranial extension, high tumor grade, nodal involvement at diagnosis and radiation alone as poor prognostic factors.

Investigators at the Ghent University Hospital treated 105 patients with sinonasal malignancies using IMRT and reported the outcomes of 84 patients with adenocarcinoma, squamous cell carcinoma, esthesioneuroblastoma, and adenoid cystic carcinoma [21]. CT- and MRI-based planning was used to deliver 70 Gy (range: 42–70 Gy). With a median follow-up of 40 months, the five-year local control and overall survival rates were 70.7% and 58.5%, respectively. The IMRT dose–volume constraints on the optic nerves and chiasms were set at

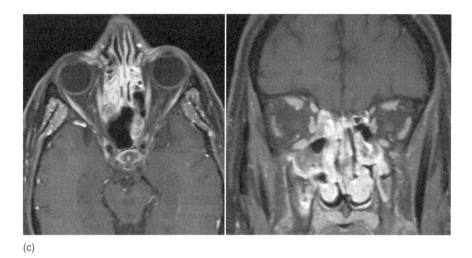

(c)

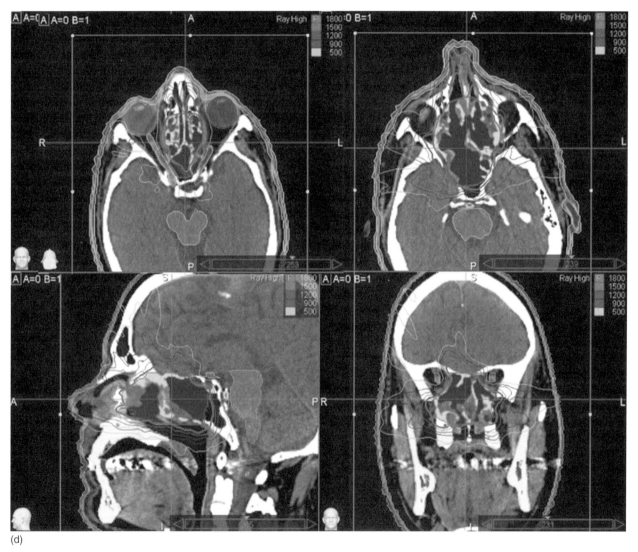

(d)

Figure 13.5 (*Continued*)

Figure 13.5 (*Continued*)

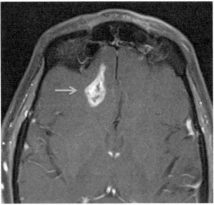 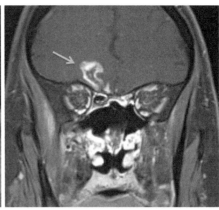

(e)

60 Gy to <5% of the volume. The retina was allowed to receive 55 Gy to <5% of the volume, and the dose to 50% of the lacrimal gland was to be kept below 30 Gy. With these dose limits only one patient developed grade III radiation-induced visual impairment. Temporal lobe necrosis was noted in three patients on long-term follow-up.

A very interesting analysis on sinonasal carcinoma was performed by Chen *et al.* [22], who analyzed outcomes in 127 patients treated between 1960 and 2005. Treatment techniques included conventional radiation therapy, 3D conformal radiotherapy and IMRT in 59, 45, and 23 patients, respectively. While no improvement in overall survival was noted, a significant reduction in late grade 3 and 4 toxicities was noted during in the recent decades with improvements in radiation treatment delivery techniques which allowed a better sparing of normal structures.

Due to the complex anatomy, and the proximity of critical normal tissues and advanced stages at presentation, complete resection with negative margins is very difficult to achieve. Resto *et al.* evaluated the impact of the extent of surgical resection in 102 patients with various histology [11]. Patients were characterized as having had a complete resection with negative margins (20%), partial resection with positive margins (49%), or biopsy only (31%). Radiation therapy was delivered using a combination of protons and photons, with approximately half the dose being delivered using protons. Complete resection was found to be associated with better treatment outcomes. Although a higher radiation dose was delivered to patients with positive margins (75 Gy versus 68 Gy for those with negative margins), there was a strong trend towards improved local control with greater extent of surgery. Statistically significant improvements in disease-free survival and overall survival were also noted in patients who had undergone a complete resection. The five-year disease-free survival was 90%, 49%, and 39% for complete resection, partial resection, and biopsy-only

patients, respectively (p = 0.009). The five-year overall survival was 90%, 53%, and 49% for complete resection, partial resection, and biopsy-only patients, respectively (p = 0.02).

When evaluating the role of concurrent radiation and chemotherapy in patients with unresectable stage IVB paranasal sinus and nasal cavity tumors, Hoppe *et al.* reported their results in 39 patients (four received radiation alone without chemotherapy due to comorbidities) [23]. These patients received a median radiation dose of 70 Gy with platinum-based chemotherapy given either as induction therapy, concurrently with, or after radiation, with most (*n* = 32; 82%) being treated concurrently. Unfortunately, even with this aggressive treatment, tumors recurred within the radiation field in 22 patients, which resulted in a five-year local progression-free survival of 21% and an overall survival of 15%.

A novel chemoradiotherapeutic approach involves infusing cisplatin directly into the tumor bed via an intra-arterial route; this is the so-called the RADPLAT protocol. Experience reported from a single institution in Japan showed very promising results [24]. Radiation was delivered to a dose of 65–70 Gy using a conventional wedge pair technique. All patients received intra-arterial cisplatin chemotherapy to a dose of 100–120 mg m^{-2} per week for four weeks concurrent with radiation. A total of 47 patients was treated, and the five-year local progression-free survival was 78.4% (69% for patients with unresectable disease and 83.2% for those with resectable disease). Similarly, the five-year overall survival rate was 69.3% for all patients, and 61.1% and 71.1% for unresectable and resectable cases, respectively. Acute toxicity was conservatively managed and there were no treatment-related deaths. Late toxicities included osteonecrosis (*n* = 7) and brain necrosis (*n* = 2). Unfortunately, severe ocular/vision problems occurred in 16 of 38 patients who were followed for two years. The local control and overall survival results of the RADPLAT approach are definitely superior compared to those of other reported series. It is likely that the late radiation-related toxicities can be minimized using IMRT techniques. This approach is worthy of further study with larger series to confirm its superiority.

Proton beam radiation therapy offers a physically advantageous dose distribution that is characterized by a sharp drop-off in dose at the end of its range – a phenomenon called the 'Bragg peak'. Proton beams also possess the property of having a sharp lateral penumbra [25]. These two physical properties result in a rapid dose reduction beyond the target area, allowing better sparing of normal tissues. Dosimetry studies comparing photon versus proton radiation for paranasal sinus tumors have been performed. The target volume coverage is comparable with both radiation techniques, but the homogeneity of dose distribution and sparing of normal tissues is better with protons [26,27]. Clinical experience with protons in these cancers is still in its infancy. However, two recent reports from Japan have demonstrated the ability to escalate doses beyond 80 GyE, with acceptable toxicity. Zenda *et al.* treated patients with unresectable paranasal sinus and nasal cavity cancers, and noted a five-year overall survival of 55% [28]. In another study, however, such high rates of survival with unresectable carcinomas were not noted, with Fukumitsu *et al.* reporting only 16% survival and 17.5% local control at five years with proton therapy [29].

The details of treatment outcomes in selected series of patients with paranasal sinus and nasal cavity cancers using different radiation techniques are summarized in Table 13.3. A review of literature over the past few decades points to some important findings and general observations regarding these uncommon cancers:

1) Surgical resection improves outcomes. Multiple reports have demonstrated the superiority of surgery followed by adjuvant radiation therapy versus radiation therapy alone [8, 20, 30, 31], and patients who had negative surgical margins did better that those with positive margins [16]. Although there is the inherent selection bias in retrospective studies that patients treated with radiation alone had more advanced diseases and poor performance status, if feasible, surgery should be attempted with the intent of complete resection with negative margins. Other advantages of an upfront surgical approach include the ability to reduce the dose of radiation needed in adjuvant setting, resulting in a lower incidence of side effects. Also, correct surgical staging of the primary disease and lymph nodal status allows better designing of the radiation fields. An additional radiation boost can be delivered to areas with close or positive margins.
2) Improvements in radiation delivery techniques reduce radiation-induced toxicities. A review of the literature shows a definite reduction in late radiation-induced toxicities with the use of IMRT as compared to 2D or 3D conformal techniques (see Table 13.3). Serious side effects included vision loss, and brain and bone necrosis. The incidence of visual impairment was in the range of 15–50% with the use of 2D techniques, but when using IMRT (which can better spare normal structures) this complication occurred rarely. A better understanding of dose-fractionation and dose-volume parameters [32] with regards to the optic structures has further contributed to reducing the incidence of long-term morbidity. The use of proton therapy for these cancers is increasing, and hopefully will allow further dose escalation while minimizing toxicities. A trial using carbon-12 ion radiation therapy in combination with IMRT is also under way [33].
3) The role of chemotherapy is undefined. Chemotherapy has been used concurrently with radiation therapy in paranasal sinus and nasal cavity cancer, but the exact role is undefined, as there is no randomized study in these rare cancers. Cisplatin-based chemotherapy is often used in patients with unresectable disease, positive margins or lymph nodes with extracapsular extension, based on the results of randomized trials conducted for head and neck cancer of other subsites [13, 14, 34, 35].
4) Elective neck node radiation of N0 neck is generally not necessary unless in patients with T3-4 squamous cell carcinoma and poorly differentiated carcinoma.

Rare Histology

Esthesioneuroblastoma

Esthesioneuroblastoma (olfactory neuroblastoma) is a rare pathology arising in the superior nasal cavity and anterior skull base in the region of the cribriform plate [42, 43]. The exact site of its origin is unknown, but it is thought to arise from the basal neural cells of the olfactory epithelium. These cancers most commonly present in the sixth decade of life. The clinical presentation is similar to that described above for tumors of the nasoethmoidal complex. Common presenting symptoms include nasal obstruction, epistaxis, headaches, facial pain, or changes in vision. One unique symptom noted is anosmia, which may precede the diagnosis by a few months. Diagnosis is established by imaging using CT or MRI scans, followed by a biopsy obtained through nasal endoscopy.

Esthesioneuroblastoma are staged using the Kadish [44] staging system which is divided into groups A (tumor limited to nasal cavity), B (tumor limited to nasal cavity and paranasal sinuses), and C (tumor extends beyond the

Table 13.3 Treatment outcomes for paranasal sinus and nasal cavity cancer.

Author/Reference	No. of patients	Site	Treatment	RT dose	Local Control (5 year)	Overall Survival (5 years)	Toxicities/complications
2D and 3D-conformal RT							
Karim *et al.* [36]	45	Nasal cavity Ethmoid	Sx→RT RT + brachy boost	65–82 Gy	DFS-68%		Loss of visual acuity- 16%
Allen *et al.* [6]	68	Nasal cavity + Septum	Sx→RT RT ± brachy	58–70 Gy	86%	82%	Visual impairment- 7%; epiphora- 15%; epistaxis- 10%; dental problems- 7%
Jiang *et al.* [4]	73	Maxillary sinus	Sx→RT	42–66 Gy	78%	48%	Vision impairment- 60%; brain necrosis; bone necrosis; soft-tissue necrosis; trismus; pituitary insufficiency; hearing loss
Jiang *et al.* [37]	34	Ethmoid	Sx→RT RT alone	50–70 Gy 2D before 1984 3D after 1984	71%	55%	All complications seen before 1984 Visual pathway injuries- 12%; brain injury- 6%; bone necrosis- 6%; pituitary insufficiency- 9%
Jansen *et al.* [31]	73	PNS	Sx→RT RT alone	39–70 Gy	65% 47%	60% 9%	Serious complications- 35%; vision loss- 20%
Katz *et al.* [30]	78	Nasal cavity/PNS	Sx→RT RT alone	55–72.6 Gy 55.8–77.2 Gy	79% 49%	68% 48%	Blindness- 41%; bone necrosis/exposure- 17%; hypopituitarism- 5%
Blanco *et al.* [20]	106	Maxillary/Ethmoid	RT Sx→RT RT→Sx	61.7 ± 8.9 60.9 ± 8.2 55.7 ± 9.6	58%	27%	Brain necrosis; conjunctivitis; keratitis; late mucositis; retinopathy; trismus
IMRT							
Daly *et al.* [38]	36	PNS/Nasal cavity	Sx→RT	63–72 Gy	58%	45%	Xerophthalmia (*n* = 1); lacrimal stenosis (*n* = 1); cataract (1 patient)
Dirix *et al.* [39]	40	PNS/Nasal cavity	Sx→RT	60–66 Gy	70%	70%	Xerophthalmia- 8%; No visual impairment
Madani *et al.* [21]	84	PNS/Nasal cavity	Sx→RT	70 Gy	71%	59%	No vision loss
Wiegner *et al.* [40]	52	PNS/Nasal cavity	Sx→RT	66 Gy	64% @2 years	66% @2y	1 grade 3 optic neuropathy related to herpes zoster
Protons							
Chera *et al.* [41]	1	maxillary Sinus	Sx→RT	74.4 CGE	Case report		Lower doses with protons as compared to IMRT photon plan
Resto *et al.* [11]	120	PNS/Nasal cavity	RT Sx→RT	55.4–79.4 Gy, Proton + photon	95%- complete resection 82%- partial resection 87%- biopsy only	90%- complete resection 53%- partial resection 49%- biopsy only	
Fukumitsu *et al.* [29]	17	Unresectable PNS/Nasal cavity	RT	70–89.6 GyE	17.5%	15.7%	Brain necrosis (*n* = 1); bone fracture (*n* = 1); unilateral blindness (*n* = 1)
Zenda *et al.* [28]	39	Unresectable PNS/Nasal cavity	RT	60–70 GyE	39%	55%	One RT- related death due to CSF leakage; Cranial nerve II and VI damage- 1 each

CGE, - Cobalt Gray Equivalent; DFS, - disease- free survival; GyE, - Gray Equivalent; PNS, - paranasal sinuses; RT, - radiation therapy; Sx, - surgery.

nasal cavity and paranasal sinuses including base of skull, intracranial compartment, orbit, distant metastatic disease). Most patients present with Kadish stage C disease, with an incidence of up to 77% of 151 patients in a study conducted by Patel *et al.* [45].

The management paradigms of this entity are similar to those described in the general principles above. Surgery plays a major role, and most centers recommend initial surgical resection followed by EBRT. The surgical technique to be employed could be either endoscopic resection or open craniofacial resection. A meta-analysis of 361 patients treated over a 16-year period compared these two approaches, and concluded that endoscopic surgery for esthesioneuroblastoma is a viable treatment option with survival comparable to that of open surgery [46]. A review article also examined this issue and concluded that currently available evidence suggests equivalent short-term outcomes with either surgical approach, as long as the resection is complete [47]. Investigators from the University of Virginia have reported on the use of preoperative radiotherapy [48] or radiotherapy with concurrent chemotherapy [49], the aim being to shrink the tumor and allow better or easier surgical resection. Preoperative radiotherapy allows the delivery of a lower dose of radiation (50 Gy in 25 fractions) to the tumor, so that the surrounding critical optic pathway structures and the brain can be spared of the high-dose radiation that is often required postoperatively (60–70 Gy), depending on pathologic margin status. Additionally, after radiation, the tumor edges are better visualized on the MRI or CT scans.

The role of elective neck irradiation and the use of chemotherapy in esthesioneuroblastoma are still unclear. One series of 77 patients had a nodal only failure rate of 7% in the untreated N0 neck (local and nodal failure rate was noted in 11 of 68 patients with initially N0 neck) [50], while another report noted a decrease in nodal recurrence from 44% to 0% following elective nodal irradiation [51]. This issue was examined in a review by Zanation *et al.* [52], but no definite consensus could be reached about how to manage initial N0 disease. The role of chemotherapy is also not well defined, with a variety of agents reported. Cisplatin is often employed in combination with etoposide, vincristine, ifosfamide, or other agents [49, 53].

Sinonasal Undifferentiated Carcinoma

Sinonasal undifferentiated carcinoma (SNUC) is another rare entity that has recently been described, with approximately 200 cases being reported [54]. A male predominance is noted with a wide range of age at presentation, the median being in the sixth decade. Most SNUCs arise in the ethmoid and maxillary sinuses [55]. Patients present with signs and symptoms similar

to those for other sinonasal malignancies, including nasal obstruction, epistaxis, proptosis, cranial nerve involvement, and facial pain [56], and these symptoms are usually of short duration. Radiographic evaluation frequently reveals a large, locally advanced malignancy invading into the orbits or intracranially. The gross pathology, histology, and immunohistochemical profile has been described by Ejaz and Wenig [56]. Due to the rarity of SNUC, no staging system has been developed specifically, although the Kadish system has been used in many publications. The prognostic factors for SNUC are not well understood, as most reported series include small numbers of patients. Chen *et al.* [57] evaluated multiple disease- and treatment-related parameters including clinical T-stage, age, primary site, dural involvement, orbit invasion, cranial nerve involvement, radiation dose and technique, and the use of chemotherapy. None of these was found to be predictive for overall survival.

A meta-analysis was recently published with individual data on 167 patients from 30 previously published series [58]. The mean age of patients was 53 years (range: 12–84 years), and 73% were males. In 60% of patients, disease extension was beyond the paranasal sinuses. At presentation, approximately 8–9% had cervical lymph node metastases, and 25% of Kadish group C patients had distant metastases. A majority of patients underwent surgical resection (53%), either alone or followed by adjuvant radiotherapy with or without chemotherapy. Radiation was part of the treatment in more than 80% of patients. As noted with other histopathologic subtypes, surgical resection offered a survival advantage, and metastases in the neck nodes and Kadish group C were poor prognostic factors. Overall, trimodality therapy appeared to be the best treatment option. The role of elective nodal irradiation (ENI) is also undefined in SNUC. In a report from the University of Florida, seven of 13 patients with clinically N0 neck at presentation received elective nodal irradiation, while six did not. None of the seven irradiated patients failed regionally, while two of the six patients who did not receive ENI failed in the neck [59]. In another series, 15 of 19 patients received ENI and no neck nodal failures were noted on follow-up [57].

Conclusions

Paranasal sinus and nasal cavity cancers are a very diverse group of malignancies, both anatomically and histologically. They are characterized by advanced stages at presentation, difficult surgical resection, and a high risk of radiation-related complications due to the proximity of critical normal tissues. The lack of randomized controlled trials makes it difficult to recognize definite treatment recommendations. However, general recommendations can be summarized from retrospective studies and extrapolated from randomized studies on head and neck cancers of other sites. In general, surgery followed by radiation therapy using IMRT offers the best possible treatment outcomes in terms of local control and minimizing treatment-related complications. Concurrent radiation and chemotherapy are recommended in cases of unresectable cancers and patients with positive/close margins or involved lymph nodes with extracapsular extension.

Currently, data are emerging on newer radiation modalities such as proton therapy, which has been shown to reduce treatment-related morbidities. Induction chemotherapy followed by concurrent chemoradiation treatment for organ preservation is also under investigation. This may reduce the high dose target volume if there is good response to the chemotherapy. However, further studies are needed to improve local control and overall survival, as well as preservation of the quality of life for patients.

References

1 Goldenberg, D., Golz, A., Fradis, M., Martu, D., Netzer, A., Joachims, H.Z. (2001) Malignant tumors of the nose and paranasal sinuses: a retrospective review of 291 cases. *Ear Nose Throat J.*, **80**, 272–277.

2 Roush, G.C. (1979) Epidemiology of cancer of the nose and paranasal sinuses: current concepts. *Head Neck Surg.*, **2**, 3–11.

3 Ansa, B., Goodman, M., Ward, K., *et al.* (2013) Paranasal sinus squamous cell carcinoma incidence and survival based on Surveillance, Epidemiology, and End Results data, 1973 to 2009. *Cancer*, **119**, 2602–2610.

4 Jiang, G.L., Ang, K.K., Peters, L.J., Wendt, C.D., Oswald, M.J., Goepfert, H. (1991) Maxillary sinus carcinomas: natural history and results of postoperative radiotherapy. *Radiother. Oncol.*, **21**, 193–200.

5 Le, Q.T., Fu, K.K., Kaplan, M.J., Terris, D.J., Fee, W.E., Goffinet, D.R. (2000) Lymph node metastasis in maxillary sinus carcinoma. *Int. J. Radiat. Oncol. Biol. Phys.*, **46**, 541–549.

6 Allen, M.W., Schwartz, D.L., Rana, V., *et al.* (2008) Long-term radiotherapy outcomes for nasal cavity and septal cancers. *Int. J. Radiat. Oncol. Biol. Phys.*, **71**, 401–406.

7 Ang, K.K., Jiang, G.L., Frankenthaler, R.A., *et al.* (1992) Carcinomas of the nasal cavity. *Radiother. Oncol.*, **24**, 163–168.

8 Mendenhall, W.M., Amdur, R.J., Morris, C.G., *et al.* (2009) Carcinoma of the nasal cavity and paranasal sinuses. *Laryngoscope*, **119**, 899–906.

9 Dulguerov, P., Jacobsen, M.S., Allal, A.S., Lehmann, W., Calcaterra, T. (2001) Nasal and paranasal sinus carcinoma: are we making progress? A series of 220 patients and a systematic review. *Cancer*, **92**, 3012–3129.

10 Guntinas-Lichius, O., Kreppel, M.P., Stuetzer, H., Semrau, R., Eckel, H.E., Mueller, R.P. (2007) Single modality and multimodality treatment of nasal and paranasal sinuses cancer: a single institution experience of 229 patients. *Eur. J. Surg. Oncol.*, **33**, 222–228.

11 Resto, V.A., Chan, A.W., Deschler, D.G., Lin, D.T. (2008) Extent of surgery in the management of locally advanced sinonasal malignancies. *Head Neck*, **30**, 222–229.

12 Choussy, O., Ferron, C., Vedrine, P.O., *et al.* (2008) Adenocarcinoma of ethmoid: a GETTEC retrospective multicenter study of 418 cases. *Laryngoscope*, **118**, 437–443.

13 Bernier, J., Domenge, C., Ozsahin, M., *et al.* (2004) Postoperative irradiation with or without concomitant chemotherapy for locally advanced head and neck cancer. *N. Engl. J. Med.*, **350**, 1945–1952.

14 Cooper, J.S., Pajak, T.F., Forastiere, A.A., *et al.* (2004) Postoperative concurrent radiotherapy and chemotherapy for high-risk squamous-cell carcinoma of the head and neck. *N. Engl. J. Med.*, **350**, 1937–1944.

15 Lee, M.M., Vokes, E.E., Rosen, A., Witt, M.E., Weichselbaum, R.R., Haraf, D.J. (1999) Multimodality therapy in advanced paranasal sinus carcinoma: superior long-term results. *Cancer J. Sci. Am.*, **5**, 219–223.

16 Hanna, E.Y., Cardenas, A.D., DeMonte, F., *et al.* (2011) Induction chemotherapy for advanced squamous cell carcinoma of the paranasal sinuses. *Arch. Otolaryngol. Head Neck Surg.*, **137**, 78–81.

17 Lee, D.S., Kim, Y.S., Cheon, J.S., *et al.* (2012) Long-term outcome and toxicity of hypofractionated stereotactic body radiotherapy as a boost treatment for head and neck cancer: the importance of boost volume assessment. *Radiat. Oncol.*, **7**, 85

18 Dirix, P., Nuyts, S., Geussens, Y., *et al.* (2007) Malignancies of the nasal cavity and paranasal sinuses: long-term outcome with conventional or three-dimensional conformal radiotherapy. *Int. J. Radiat. Oncol. Biol. Phys.*, **69**, 1042–1050.

19 Bristol, I.J., Ahamad, A., Garden, A.S., *et al.* (2007) Postoperative radiotherapy for maxillary sinus cancer: long-term outcomes and toxicities of treatment. *Int. J. Radiat. Oncol. Biol. Phys.*, **68**, 719–730.

20 Blanco, A.I., Chao, K.S., Ozyigit, G., *et al.* (2004) Carcinoma of paranasal sinuses: long-term outcomes with radiotherapy. *Int. J. Radiat. Oncol. Biol. Phys.*, **59**, 51–58.

21 Madani, I., Bonte, K., Vakaet, L., Boterberg, T., De Neve, W. (2009) Intensity-modulated radiotherapy for sinonasal tumors: Ghent University Hospital update. *Int. J. Radiat. Oncol. Biol. Phys.*, **73**, 424–432.

22 Chen, A.M., Daly, M.E., Bucci, M.K., *et al.* (2007) Carcinomas of the paranasal sinuses and nasal cavity treated with radiotherapy at a single institution over five decades: are we making improvement? *Int. J. Radiat. Oncol. Biol. Phys.*, **69**, 141–147.

23 Hoppe, B.S., Nelson, C.J., Gomez, D.R., *et al.* (2008) Unresectable carcinoma of the paranasal sinuses: outcomes and toxicities. *Int. J. Radiat. Oncol. Biol. Phys.*, **72**, 763–769.

24 Homma, A., Oridate, N., Suzuki, F., *et al.* (2009) Superselective high-dose cisplatin infusion with concomitant radiotherapy in patients with advanced cancer of the nasal cavity and paranasal sinuses: a single institution experience. *Cancer*, **115**, 4705–4714.

25 Urie, M.M., Sisterson, J.M., Koehler, A.M., Goitein, M., Zoesman, J. (1986) Proton beam penumbra: effects of separation between patient and beam modifying devices. *Med. Phys.*, **13**, 734–741.

26 Lomax, A.J., Goitein, M., Adams, J. (2003) Intensity modulation in radiotherapy: photons versus protons in the paranasal sinus. *Radiother. Oncol.*, **66**, 11–18.

27 Mock, U., Georg, D., Bogner, J., Auberger, T., Potter, R. (2004) Treatment planning comparison of conventional, 3D conformal, and intensity-modulated photon (IMRT) and proton therapy for paranasal sinus carcinoma. *Int. J. Radiat. Oncol. Biol. Phys.*, **58**, 147–154.

28 Zenda, S., Kohno, R., Kawashima, M., *et al.* (2011) Proton beam therapy for unresectable malignancies of the nasal cavity and paranasal sinuses. *Int. J. Radiat. Oncol. Biol. Phys.*, **81**, 1473–1478.

29 Fukumitsu, N., Okumura, T., Mizumoto, M., *et al.* (2011) Outcome of T4 (International Union Against Cancer Staging System, 7th edition) or Recurrent Nasal Cavity and Paranasal Sinus Carcinoma Treated with Proton Beam. *Int. J. Radiat. Oncol. Biol. Phys.*, **83**, (2), 704–711.

30 Katz, T.S., Mendenhall, W.M., Morris, C.G., Amdur, R.J., Hinerman, R.W., Villaret, D.B. (2002) Malignant tumors of the nasal cavity and paranasal sinuses. *Head Neck*, **24**, 821–829.

31 Jansen, E.P., Keus, R.B., Hilgers, F.J., Haas, R.L., Tan, I.B., Bartelink, H. (2000) Does the combination of radiotherapy and debulking surgery favor survival in paranasal sinus carcinoma? *Int. J. Radiat. Oncol. Biol. Phys.*, **48**, 27–35.

32 Mayo, C., Martel, M.K., Marks, L.B., Flickinger, J., Nam, J., Kirkpatrick, J. (2010) Radiation dose-volume effects of optic nerves and chiasm. *Int. J. Radiat. Oncol. Biol. Phys.*, **76**, S28–S35.

33 Jensen, A.D., Nikoghosyan, A.V., Windemuth-Kieselbach, C., Debus, J., Munter, M.W. (2011) Treatment of malignant sinonasal tumours with intensity-modulated radiotherapy (IMRT) and carbon ion boost (C12). *BMC Cancer*, **11**, 190.

34 Adelstein, D.J., Li, Y., Adams, G.L., *et al.* (2003) An intergroup phase III comparison of standard radiation therapy and two schedules of concurrent chemoradiotherapy in patients with unresectable squamous cell head and neck cancer. *J. Clin. Oncol.*, **21**, 92–98.

35 Forastiere, A.A., Goepfert, H., Maor, M., *et al.* (2003) Concurrent chemotherapy and radiotherapy for organ preservation in advanced laryngeal cancer. *N. Engl. J. Med.*, **349**, 2091–2098.

36 Karim, A.B., Kralendonk, J.H., Njo, K.H., Tabak, J.M., Elsenaar, W.H., van Balen, A.T. (1990) Ethmoid and upper nasal cavity carcinoma: treatment, results and complications. *Radiother. Oncol.*, **19**, 109–120.

37 Jiang, G.L., Morrison, W.H., Garden, A.S., *et al.* (1998) Ethmoid sinus carcinomas: natural history and treatment results. *Radiother. Oncol.*, **49**, 21–27.

38 Daly, M.E., Chen, A.M., Bucci, M.K., *et al.* (2007) Intensity-modulated radiation therapy for malignancies of the nasal cavity and paranasal sinuses. *Int. J. Radiat. Oncol. Biol. Phys.*, **67**, 151–157.

39 Dirix, P., Vanstraelen, B., Jorissen, M., Vander Poorten, V., Nuyts, S. (2010) Intensity-modulated radiotherapy for sinonasal cancer: improved outcome compared to conventional radiotherapy. *Int. J. Radiat. Oncol. Biol. Phys.*, **78**, 998–1004.

40 Wiegner, E.A., Daly, M.E., Murphy, J.D., *et al.* (2011) Intensity-modulated radiotherapy for tumors of the nasal cavity and paranasal sinuses: Clinical outcomes and patterns of failure. *Int. J. Radiat. Oncol. Biol. Phys.*, **83** (1), 243–251.

41 Chera, B.S., Malyapa, R., Louis, D., *et al.* (2009) Proton therapy for maxillary sinus carcinoma. *Am. J. Clin. Oncol.*, **32**, 296–303.

42 Faragalla, H., Weinreb, I. (2009) Olfactory neuroblastoma: a review and update. *Adv. Anat. Pathol.*, **16**, 322–331.

43 Ow, T.J., Bell, D., Kupferman, M.E., Demonte, F., Hanna, E.Y. (2013) Esthesioneuroblastoma. *Neurosurg. Clin. North Am.*, **24**, 51–65.

44 Kadish, S., Goodman, M., Wang, C.C. (1976) Olfactory neuroblastoma. A clinical analysis of 17 cases. *Cancer*, **37**, 1571–1576.

45 Patel, S.G., Singh, B., Stambuk, H.E., *et al.* (2012) Craniofacial surgery for esthesioneuroblastoma: report of an international collaborative study. *J. Neurol. Surg. B Skull Base*, **73**, 208–220.

46 Devaiah, A.K., Andreoli, M.T. (1009) Treatment of esthesioneuroblastoma: a 16-year meta-analysis of 361 patients. *Laryngoscope*, **119**, 1412–1416.

47 Soler, Z.M., Smith, T.L. (2012) Endoscopic versus open craniofacial resection of esthesioneuroblastoma: what is the evidence? *Laryngoscope*, **122**, 244–245.

48 Polin, R.S., Sheehan, J.P., Chenelle, A.G., *et al.* (1998) The role of preoperative adjuvant treatment in the management of esthesioneuroblastoma: the University of Virginia experience. *Neurosurgery*, **42**, 1029–1037.

49 Sohrabi, S., Drabick, J.J., Crist, H., Goldenberg, D., Sheehan, J.M., Mackley, H.B. (2011) Neoadjuvant concurrent chemoradiation for advanced esthesioneuroblastoma: a case series and review of the literature. *J. Clin. Oncol.*, **29**, e358–e361.

50 Ozsahin, M., Gruber, G., Olszyk, O., *et al.* (2010) Outcome and prognostic factors in olfactory neuroblastoma: a rare cancer network study. *Int. J. Radiat. Oncol. Biol. Phys.*, **78**, 992–997.

51 Monroe, A.T., Hinerman, R.W., Amdur, R.J., Morris, C.G., Mendenhall, W.M. (2003) Radiation therapy for esthesioneuroblastoma: rationale for elective neck irradiation. *Head Neck*, **25**, 529–534.

52 Zanation, A.M., Ferlito, A., Rinaldo, A., *et al.* (2010) When, how and why to treat the neck in patients with esthesioneuroblastoma: a review. *Eur. Arch. Otorhinolaryngol.*, **267**, 1667–1671.

53 Resto, V.A., Eisele, D.W., Forastiere, A., Zahurak, M., Lee, D.J., Westra, W.H. (2000) Esthesioneuroblastoma: the Johns Hopkins experience. *Head Neck*, **22**, 550–558.

54 Frierson, H.F., Jr, Mills, S.E., Fechner, R.E., Taxy, J.B., Levine, P.A. (1986) Sinonasal undifferentiated carcinoma. An aggressive neoplasm derived from schneiderian epithelium and distinct from olfactory neuroblastoma. *Am. J. Surg. Pathol.*, **10**, 771–779.

55 Al-Mamgani, A., van Rooij, P., Mehilal, R., Tans, L., Levendag, P.C. (2013) Combined-modality treatment improved outcome in sinonasal undifferentiated carcinoma: single-institutional experience of 21 patients and review of the literature. *Eur. Arch. Otorhinolaryngol.*, **270**, 293–299.

56 Ejaz, A., Wenig, B.M. (2005) Sinonasal undifferentiated carcinoma: clinical and pathologic features and a discussion on classification, cellular differentiation, and differential diagnosis. *Adv. Anat. Pathol.*, **12**, 134–143.

57 Chen, A.M., Daly, M.E., El-Sayed, I., *et al.* (2008) Patterns of failure after combined-modality approaches incorporating radiotherapy for sinonasal undifferentiated carcinoma of the head and neck. *Int. J. Radiat. Oncol. Biol. Phys.*, **70**, 338–343.

58 Reiersen, D.A., Pahilan, M.E., Devaiah, A.K. (2012) Meta-analysis of treatment outcomes for sinonasal undifferentiated carcinoma. *Otolaryngol. Head Neck Surg.*, **147**, 7–14.

59 Tanzler, E.D., Morris, C.G., Orlando, C.A., Werning, J.W., Mendenhall, W.M. (2008) Management of sinonasal undifferentiated carcinoma. *Head Neck*, **30**, 595–599.

14

Salivary Gland Carcinomas
Allen M. Chen

Introduction

Malignant neoplasms of the salivary glands account for a small minority of head and neck cancers. Traditionally, these tumors have been divided into those of the major and minor salivary glands, with the former consisting of the paired parotid, submandibular, and sublingual glands, and the latter involving the hundreds of mucus-secreting glands beneath the mucosal lining of the entire upper aerodigestive tract. Although relatively uncommon, salivary gland cancers are notable for their remarkable heterogeneity, not only with respect to primary site of origin, but also with respect to histology. The World Health Organization (WHO) has identified nearly 40 histological subtypes of salivary gland neoplasms, with the majority of them being benign [1]. The most common malignant tumors include mucoepidermoid carcinoma, adenoid cystic carcinoma, carcinoma ex pleomorphic adenoma, and adenocarcinoma. In view of the tremendous histologic diversity of these tumors, which results in varying clinical and pathological presentations, unique challenges exist in the management of patients with newly diagnosed salivary gland carcinoma. The propensity of these malignancies for insidious local growth, perineural spread, and disease recurrence over prolonged periods of time also has significant implications with respect to diagnosis, treatment, and follow-up.

Anatomy and Natural History

The vast majority of salivary gland cancers occur in the parotid gland, with lesser numbers occurring in the submandibular and minor salivary glands. Sublingual gland cancers are exceedingly rare, comprising less than 1% of all salivary gland tumors. Interestingly, an inverse

relationship has been observed between the anatomic size of the salivary gland and its ratio of malignant to benign tumors. Only about 20% of cancers arising from the parotid gland are malignant; in comparison, approximately 90% of cancers from the sublingual and minor salivary glands are malignant.

Salivary gland carcinomas can manifest in a variety of fashions, which reflects the considerable heterogeneity of these tumors with respect to the primary site of origin and histologic features. Patients with major salivary gland neoplasms typically present with an enlarging mass prompting the seeking of medical attention (Figure 14.1). Episodic pain, which can develop from suppuration or hemorrhage into a mass or from local infiltration into adjacent tissue, is relatively uncommon and may be associated with both benign and malignant tumors. However, facial paralysis, which occurs in a small percentage of patients with a parotid gland mass, generally indicates malignancy with involvement of the facial nerve (cranial nerve, CN VII) [2]. More advanced cases can invade the parapharyngeal space and/or skull base, resulting in the potential compromise of the glossopharyngeal, vagus, accessory, and hypoglossal nerves (CN IX–XII) and produce such symptoms as dysphagia, sore throat, referred earache, trismus, numbness, and headache. For patients with submandibular cancers, local spread can result in involvement of the trigeminal nerve (CN V) and, less commonly, CN VII and XII. Sublingual cancers usually present as a palpable fullness in the floor of mouth. Minor salivary gland cancers have a varied presentation because they can potentially occur anywhere in the upper aerodigestive tract. Most arise within the oral cavity (particularly the hard palate) or oropharynx, and present as a submucosal, painless lump with indolent growth. Salivary gland carcinomas arising from the nasal cavity or paranasal sinuses can present

Clinical Radiation Oncology: Indications, Techniques, and Results, Third Edition. Edited by William Small Jr.
© 2017 John Wiley & Sons, Inc. Published 2017 by John Wiley & Sons, Inc.

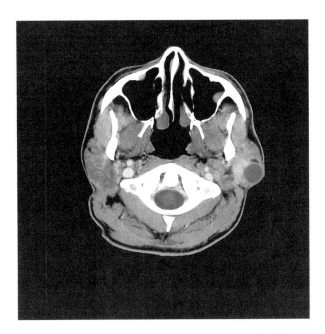

Figure 14.1 CT scan with contrast demonstrating a left-sided superficial parotid lesion in a 50-year-old male who presented with a painless, enlarging mass. Subsequent work-up showed low-grade mucoepidermoid carcinoma.

with facial pain and nasal obstruction or epistaxis. Those arising from the larynx are less common but can produce voice and/or swallowing changes.

The natural history of salivary gland carcinoma depends largely on the specific histologic subtype. In general, low-grade tumors are more likely to behave similarly to benign neoplasms, whereas high-grade tumors tend to act more aggressively with respect to both local and distant spread. Local growth is characterized by infiltration into the gland and adjacent soft tissues such as skin, muscle, and bone. Once neural invasion occurs, salivary gland cancers are notorious for insidious extension along nerve sheaths, often traversing lengthy distances without clinical symptoms [2]. Base of skull and/or intracranial involvement from salivary gland cancer has been well-described [3]. Hematogenous spread is more common than regional lymph node metastasis for both major and minor salivary gland cancers. The reported incidence of distant metastasis at presentation varies based on histology, with the highest rates observed in patients with adenoid cystic carcinoma, adenocarcinoma, and carcinoma ex pleomorphic adenoma. In general, distant metastasis is more common than for patients with squamous cell carcinomas of the head and neck, and typically involves the lungs, bones, and liver. However, several studies have demonstrated that patients with distant disease – especially those with adenoid cystic carcinoma – can potentially survive for long periods of time due to the indolent growth rates of their cancers [5].

As a group, salivary gland carcinomas have a lower incidence of regional lymph node involvement than for squamous cell carcinomas of the head and neck. Data from the Memorial Sloan-Kettering Cancer Center demonstrated that 14 of 474 patients (14%) had clinically positive lymph nodes at presentation, with the highest rates observed in those with adenocarcinoma (22%), primary squamous cell carcinoma (21%), and carcinoma ex pleomorphic adenoma (16%) [6]. These same authors reported that the incidence of pathologically positive lymph nodes was 12%, as determined by neck dissection, among 407 patients with clinically N0 necks at the time of their diagnosis of salivary gland carcinoma. On multivariate analysis, primary tumor size greater than 4 cm and histologic grade were identified as independent predictors of subclinical nodal involvement. Other studies have since confirmed that the incidence of regional lymph node metastasis varies according to the histologic features, primary tumor stage at presentation, site of origin, and grade. In general, the highest rates are generally seen for locally advanced (T3–T4), high-grade tumors, and those involving areas with a high density of lymphatics.

Knowledge of the patterns of lymphatic drainage is critical to tailoring subsequent therapy for patients believed to be at risk for nodal involvement. The lymphatics of the parotid gland drain to the intraparotid, periparotid, submandibular, upper jugular, subdigastric, middle and low jugular, and posterior triangle lymph nodes. The lymphatics of the submandibular gland drain to the adjacent submandibular and upper/middle jugular lymph nodes. Lymphatic drainage of the sublingual gland is to the submental and submandibular lymph nodes, then to the deep cervical lymph nodes. Lymphatic drainage to the contralateral neck for patients with carcinoma of the major salivary gland is rare, but is more common among those with minor salivary gland carcinomas, which drain to varying stations based on their respective sites of origin [7].

Evaluation and Staging

Evaluation of the patient with a malignant salivary gland tumor includes a thorough history and physical examination, with detailed attention being paid to symptoms and findings associated with local tumor extension, regional lymphadenopathy, and distant metastasis. Meticulous testing of the cranial nerves is mandatory. For patients with a palpable abnormality, the size, mobility, and extent of the mass should be documented. Although fine-needle aspiration (FNA) biopsy has historically been the initial diagnostic procedure in a patient suspected of having a salivary gland malignancy, its routine use – particularly for those patients with parotid and sublingual masses – is somewhat controversial as many clinicians assert that FNA findings rarely alter the usual recommendation for surgical resection and may be associated with high false-negative rates [8]. For patients presenting with submandibular masses, there is less controversy surrounding FNA as it may be useful for distinguishing between primary malignancies and secondary or reactive processes not requiring surgery. Core-needle biopsy as an alternative to FNA may be appropriate, but concerns of potential tumor seeding may complicate this method, although this issue has never been formally analyzed. Incisional or excisional biopsies have little role in diagnosis, as such procedures can increase the likelihood of tumor spillage and nerve injury. Due to their relative rarity and their varying sites of presentation, minor salivary gland cancers are typically diagnosed incidentally during the work-up for suspected squamous cell cancers at those respective sites.

Computed tomography (CT) and magnetic resonance imaging (MRI) of the head and neck are recommended to fully evaluate tumor extent and the status of the regional lymph nodes. The latter technique is particularly useful for evaluating subclinical neural or perineural involvement which may have implications regarding the surgical approach and/or the design of radiation therapy fields. There is also increasing evidence that MRI may be useful in distinguishing between benign and malignant processes in the salivary glands [9]. The use of positron emission tomography (PET) is currently under active investigation. A research team from the University of Pennsylvania recently demonstrated the superiority of PET compared to CT and/or MRI for initial staging at both primary and regional sites among 48 patients with salivary gland cancer [10]. Additionally, the sensitivity, specificity, and positive and negative predictive values of PET for detecting metastatic disease were 93%, 96%, 82%, and 99%, respectively, compared to 80%, 95%, 75%, and 96% when using CT. Since the lungs are the most common site of distant metastasis from salivary carcinoma, a chest radiograph should be routinely obtained.

Accurate staging of malignant salivary gland tumors is important for predicting prognosis, directing subsequent therapy, and for accurate comparison of treatment results. The current 2017 American Joint Committee for Cancer (AJCC) staging system is based on the tumor, node, and metastases (TNM) characteristics for major salivary gland cancers [11]. Notably, the T4 designation was recently divided based on general operative criteria: T4a indicates lesions that are potentially resectable with clear margins, while T4b reflects tumors in which resection would unlikely result in clear margins, including those invading the skull base, pterygoid plates, and/or the carotid artery. Malignancies of the minor salivary glands are staged using the AJCC criteria for squamous cell carcinomas associated with the site of the primary lesion.

Prognostic Variables

Multiple studies have analyzed potential prognostic variables for patients undergoing definitive therapy for localized salivary gland cancer [12–14]. Most of these have confirmed the utility of the TNM- based AJCC system in predicting outcome. This method of staging was in fact developed using long-term survival data as determined by Spiro *et al.* from the Memorial Sloan-Kettering Cancer Center, who initially reported 10-year survival rates of 83% for stage I tumors, 76% for stage II tumors, and 32% for stage III tumors [13]. The most consistently demonstrated prognostic factor across single-institutional series appears to be T-stage, as made evident by a recently published analysis of 181 patients treated for localized salivary carcinoma at the University of Florida reporting 10-year survival rates of 80%, 71%, 59%, and 22% for those with T1, T2, T3, and T4 disease, respectively [14].

The major limitation of the current AJCC staging system is its failure to account for histology, which quite possibly represents the most important prognosticator for patients diagnosed with salivary gland carcinoma. Furthermore, due to the relative rarity of this disease, very little – if any – data are available which has directly evaluated the potential impact of histology as it relates to the traditional AJCC staging system in predicting clinical outcome. As a result, substantial uncertainty exists regarding whether TNM stage or histologic subtype takes precedence in prognostic stratification.

The presence of cervical lymph node involvement at the time of diagnosis among patients with salivary gland carcinoma has been demonstrated to be an important prognostic predictor of outcome [15]. In an analysis of the SEER database, lymph node metastasis was reported to be the most valuable determinant of overall survival among 903 patients treated for parotid gland carcinomas [16]. As alluded to previously, however, it must be recognized that strong associations exist between regional nodal involvement, T-stage, and histology among patients with salivary gland carcinoma, and it remains unclear which of these factors has the greatest influence in determining overall prognosis.

Role of Radiation Therapy

Surgical resection, if possible, should be the initial step in the therapeutic management of patients with localized salivary gland carcinoma. For those who are medically or surgically inoperable, primary radiation therapy is a feasible alternative. The recommendation for adjuvant radiation therapy should be made on an individualized basis and after thorough review of preoperative, intraoperative, and postoperative disease findings, preferably as part of a multidisciplinary team approach. The use of radiation therapy, either in the postoperative or definitive setting, in the treatment of salivary gland carcinomas was historically believed to be of limited value because of the widespread belief that these neoplasms were inherently radioresistant. Due to its relatively long cell-cycle time, as well as the high proportion of cells in the non-mitotic and inactive phases, salivary gland carcinomas were hypothesized to possess an intrinsic ability to repair the potentially lethal damage induced by conventional photon radiation therapy [17]. It was not until the publication of several single-institutional series during the 1970s demonstrating improved rates of local control among patients treated with the addition of postoperative radiation therapy for salivary gland carcinomas that this prevailing viewpoint began to change [18–20].

Investigators from the M. D. Anderson Cancer Center published their preliminary experiences in 1971 and 1972, and reported local control rates in excess of 90% among small cohorts of salivary gland carcinoma patients treated with postoperative radiation therapy [19,20]. Although non-randomized data, these findings compared so favorably to those of historical controls treated by surgery alone at the authors' institution that postoperative radiation therapy was adopted thereafter in selected cases. As importantly, their experiences questioned the notion that salivary gland carcinomas were radioresistant, and led to the initiation of trials at other institutions across the country.

Fu *et al.* published the initial experience in 1977 of 100 patients treated at the University of California, San Francisco (UCSF) for salivary gland carcinomas, and confirmed that postoperative radiation therapy decreased the rates of local recurrence from 54% to 14% among patients with close or positive microscopic margins after surgery for salivary gland carcinoma [21]. These authors also showed that the benefits of postoperative radiation therapy were most evident in patients with adenoid cystic carcinoma and other high-grade histologies. These findings were corroborated by a 1978 report of outcomes among 52 patients treated by initial surgery for salivary gland carcinoma at Rush Medical College [22]. Among the 17 patients who received postoperative radiation therapy, only one patient (6%) experienced local recurrence, compared to 30–50% (depending on histologic subtype) of the patients treated by surgery alone.

Although these early retrospective reports were criticized for the relatively small sample sizes and for possible imbalances in the distribution of potentially important prognostic variables, they were instrumental in altering the patterns of care for patients with salivary gland carcinoma. While the exact indications for the use of postoperative radiation therapy remained unclearly defined, and apparently differed both within and between institutions, an increasing number of patients were being offered a combined-modality approach based on its apparent efficacy and tolerability.

More recently published data with longer follow-up continues to confirm that postoperative radiation therapy improves outcome among selected patients with carcinomas of the salivary gland [23–25]. These findings, though non-randomized, are particularly noteworthy in spite of the obvious selection bias against those patients treated with postoperative radiation therapy. Typically, such patients tend to have more advanced tumors and a higher incidence of characteristics that are generally believed to predict for adverse outcome such as positive margins, unfavorable histology, perineural invasion, and lymph node metastasis. For these reasons, a matched-pair analysis was retrospectively performed by investigators at Memorial Sloan-Kettering Cancer Center in 1990 to evaluate the efficacy of postoperative radiation therapy compared to controls treated by surgery alone for major salivary gland carcinoma [26]. The group's findings showed that the addition of postoperative radiation therapy improved local control from 17% to 51% among patients with locally advanced (stage III and IV) disease, from 40% to 69% among patients with lymph node metastasis, and from 44% to 63% among those with high-grade tumors.

The UCSF experience with salivary gland carcinoma was recently updated with particular attention being paid to histologic subtype. A review of 140 surgically treated patients with adenoid cystic carcinoma identified the omission of postoperative radiation therapy as an independent predictor of local recurrence [27]. Although patients treated with a combined modality approach had more advanced tumors and higher rates of positive surgical margins and perineural invasion, their rates of local control were significantly better than those treated by surgery alone (84% versus 61% at 10 years). Lastly, among 63 patients with carcinoma ex pleomorphic adenoma, the addition of postoperative radiation therapy improved the five-year local control from 49% to 75%, and was associated with a significant survival advantage among patients without evidence of lymph node metastasis (five-year overall survival, 71% versus 52%) [28]. These findings are consistent with those of contemporary single-institutional studies (as outlined in Table 14.1), demonstrating encouraging outcomes for patients treated with surgery and postoperative radiation therapy for salivary gland carcinomas. In reviewing these series, it is important to recognize that differences in selection criteria vary with respect to potentially important prognostic variables such as extent of surgery, presentation (primary versus recurrent disease), tumor histology, and radiation dose.

Table 14.1 Selected single-institutional series reporting on surgery and postoperative radiation therapy for salivary cancer.

Reference	Site	No. of patients	Median dose (Gy)	Control	Endpoint
Harrison *et al.* [25]	Major	46	60	73%	LC at 5 years
Garden *et al.* [23]	Parotid	166	60	90%	LC at 15 years
Spiro *et al.* [52]	Parotid	62	58	84%	LC at 10 years
Garden *et al.* [53]	Minor	160	60	86%	LC at 10 years
Storey *et al.* [54]	Submandibular	83	60	88%	LRC at 10 years
Mendenhall *et al.* [14]	Major/minor	160	66	81%	LRC at 10 years
Le *et al.* [7]	Minor	54	60	88%	LC at 10 years
Terhaard *et al.* [12]	Major/minor	538	62	91%	LC at 10 years
Cianchetti *et al.* [51]	Minor	76	70	76%	LRC at 10 years

Although prospective data are lacking, this information – in aggregate – strongly suggests that postoperative radiation therapy should be considered in patients believed to be at high risk for local recurrence after surgery alone. In general, this includes patients for which there is uncertainty about the completeness or adequacy of the surgical resection based on intraoperative and pathological findings. Commonly cited indications for postoperative radiation are listed in Table 14.2. An especially instructive analysis was recently performed of 207 patients treated by surgery alone at UCSF for major salivary gland cancers [29]. Based on multivariate analysis, patients with T3–T4 disease, positive surgical margins, high-grade tumor histology, or regional lymph node metastases were shown to have excessively high local recurrence rates after surgery alone, and were thought to have benefited from postoperative radiation therapy. These findings were of particular relevance because a randomized trial comparing surgery with or without postoperative radiation therapy for salivary gland carcinoma will likely never be conducted due to existing treatment biases and the infrequency of this disease.

Despite the preponderance of evidence attesting to the efficacy of postoperative radiation therapy in improving local control, few studies have demonstrated an overall survival advantage with its use. Due to the high rates of

Table 14.2 Common indications for postoperative radiation therapy.

- Close/positive surgical margins
- Lymph node involvement
- Lymphovascular invasion
- Perineural involvement
- Soft-tissue extension
- T3–T4 disease
- High histological grade
- Recurrent cancer

distant metastasis among patients with salivary gland carcinomas, it is likely that improvements in systemic therapy are needed before a survival advantage for postoperative radiation therapy will ever be established. At the present author's institution, postoperative radiation therapy is routinely recommended for patients with T3–T4 disease, close/positive margins, high-grade tumor histology (including adenoid cystic carcinoma), perineural invasion, and/or regional lymph node involvement.

Primary Radiation Therapy

A proportion of newly diagnosed patients with salivary gland carcinoma are either deemed inoperable because of technical issues related to the extent and/or location of the primary tumor, or because of pre-existing medical comorbidities placing them at high risk for perioperative complications. Although definitive radiation therapy as an alternative to surgery in this setting was once thought to convey palliative benefits only, it is becoming increasingly evident that cure may be possible in appropriately selected patients [30–33]. These findings perhaps serve as the strongest indication that carcinomas of the salivary glands are not as radioresistant to conventional photon therapy as once believed.

In an analysis of 45 patients with newly diagnosed salivary gland carcinoma treated with primary radiation therapy at UCSF, the reported five- and ten-year rates of local control were 70% and 57%, respectively [30]. On multivariate analysis, T3–T4 disease and a radiation dose lower than 66 Gy were associated with lower rates of local control. Other investigators have similarly demonstrated a dose–response relationship for patients treated by radiation alone [14,31]. A research team from the University of Florida reported a local control rate of 75% among patients with T1–T3 salivary gland carcinoma treated with radiation therapy alone, and demonstrated that doses >70 Gy resulted in a better outcome than

Table 14.3 Selected series reporting on radiotherapy alone using photons for salivary gland carcinoma.

Reference	No. of patients	Site	Median dose (Gy)	Control rate	Endpoint
Mendenhall *et al.* [14]	64	Major/minor	74	42%	LC at 10 years
Chen *et al.* [30]	45	Major/minor	66	57%	LC at 10 years
Cianchetti *et al.* [51]	64	Minor	74	46%	LC at 10 years
Wang *et al.* [34]	24	Major/minor	68	85%	LC at 5 years
Laramore *et al.* [50]	15	Major/minor	55–70	17%	LC at 10 years

those >70 Gy [14]. The results of several retrospective series are listed in Table 14.3. In analyzing these data, it is important to recognize that comparisons between patients treated by primary radiation versus the standard surgically based approach are confounded by selection bias and are not particularly justifiable. This is because patients referred for primary radiation therapy typically have a worse performance status, are less rigorously staged, and are of more advanced age with comorbid illnesses. Finally, although techniques such as altered fractionation, particle therapy, hyperthermia, stereotactic radiosurgery and brachytherapy have been proposed as a means of improving outcome for patients treated by primary radiation therapy, these experiences are limited to single-institutional data which requires validation before they are adopted in the generalized setting [34–40].

Neutron Therapy

Neutrons have long been proposed as a means of improving outcome for patients undergoing radiation therapy on the basis of their higher relative biological effectiveness (RBE). Because neutrons are less dependent on the cell cycle phase of the target elements than conventional x-rays, many have hypothesized that neutrons are well-suited to overcome the sublethal damage repair which is believed to be responsible for the radioresistance of slow-growing tumors such as salivary gland carcinoma [41–44]. The use of neutrons dates back to the pre-World War II era, when Lawrence at the

University of California, Berkeley began clinical trials for a short period until the facility shifted its focus towards the war effort. It was not until the late 1960s, when research was re-initiated in both the United States and Europe, that preclinical studies suggested that the unique biological properties of neutrons could potentially be exploited in the clinical setting. In an elegant experiment, investigators from Denmark measured the RBE of neutrons to cobalt-60 for human tumors metastatic to the lung by documenting growth delay after treatment [45]. Their observation that metastatic adenoid cystic carcinoma had an RBE of 8 compared with 2.5 to 4 for most other tumors fueled considerable enthusiasm for the use of neutrons in the treatment of localized salivary carcinomas, and helped prompt the initiation of clinical trials.

Several single-institutional experiences have reported encouraging results with the use of neutrons for the treatment of salivary gland carcinomas, both in the definitive and postoperative setting [46–49]. Local control rates for patients treated with primary radiation therapy have ranged from 45% to 67%, with the observed discrepancies presumably related to the varying selection criteria across series. Results of selected studies reporting on neutrons are listed in Table 14.4.

The only randomized trial investigating the efficacy of primary radiation therapy for salivary gland carcinomas reported to date was conducted jointly by the Radiation Therapy Oncology Group (RTOG) and Medical Research Council (MRC) during the late 1980s, and compared neutron therapy to conventional radiation therapy with photons for unresectable primary and recurrent tumors [50].

Table 14.4 Selected series reporting on the use of neutron therapy for salivary gland carcinoma.*

Reference	Histology	No. of patients	Control rate	Endpoint
Douglas *et al.* [46]	All	279	59%	LRC at 6 years
Potter *et al.* [48]	ACC	72	73%	LC at 3 years
Krull *et al.* [47]	All	33	43%	LRC at 3 years
Laramore *et al.* [50]	All	17	67%	LRC at 2 years
Douglas *et al.* [55]	ACC	151	57%	LRC at 5 years
Huber *et al.* [56]	ACC	29	75%	LC at 2 years

*Most series included patients treated by both definitive and postoperative radiation to a variety of sites.

Although a local control advantage was demonstrated with the use of neutrons (56% versus 17%), the small number of evaluable patients (13 and 12 patients on the neutron and photon arms, respectively) made drawing conclusions difficult because of notable imbalances in the distribution of important prognostic variables between the groups. For instance, 33% of patients on the photon therapy arm had salivary gland tumors of squamous cell histology, a relatively rare and aggressive cancer, as compared to 8% on the neutron therapy arm. Similarly, none of the patients treated with photons had acinic cell histology, as compared to 23% of those treated with neutrons. Moreover, the median tumor size for patients treated with photons was 7.0 cm, with one patient having a tumor measuring 16.0 cm, compared to 4.0 cm for patients treated on the neutrons arm. Lastly, a significant proportion of patients treated on the photon therapy arm was treated to a total dose of 55 Gy, which may have been suboptimal. Despite the local control advantage associated with neutrons, no survival difference was demonstrated, and toxicity was significantly higher in the neutrons arm.

Although the results of the RTOG/MRC trial were hailed by some as direct proof of the superiority of neutrons in the treatment of salivary gland cancer, the aforementioned concerns regarding the design and execution of this trial must be recognized. As such, the validity of this analysis should be interpreted with concern, and further prospective investigations are needed before it can be said that neutrons are the preferred form of radiation therapy. At present, no convincing clinical evidence exists that they are superior to conventional photon radiation therapy for the treatment of salivary gland malignancies.

Technique

Radiation therapy plays a major role as an adjunct to surgery and is usually administered postoperatively, although definitive treatment may be considered in medically or surgically inoperable cases. For tumors of the parotid bed, the minimum treatment volume includes the surgical bed to include all clips. In general, this is defined as the area bounded superiorly by the zygomatic arch; anteriorly by the masseter muscle, lateral pterygoid muscle, and mandibular ramus; posteriorly by the mastoid process; and inferiorly by the posterior belly of the digastric muscle (Figure 14.2). The ipsilateral neck is electively irradiated for high-grade lesions or when tumor is found in lymph nodes in the neck dissection specimen. For tumors with extensive perineural invasion and/or named nerve involvement, as is frequently observed in adenoid cystic carcinoma, it is reasonable to consider irradiating the nerve pathways to the foramina of the base of skull.

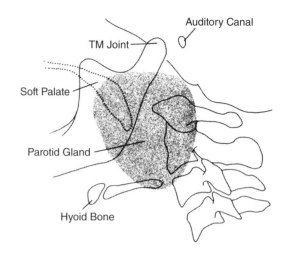

Figure 14.2 Diagram showing anatomic position of a normal parotid gland from a sialogram related to the bony landmarks of the mandible and skull base. Every attempt should be made to spare the contralateral parotid gland during irradiation.

Although intensity-modulated radiotherapy (IMRT) is increasingly used for parotid and submandibular tumors, treatment has historically been administered by one of three non-IMRT external-beam techniques. One technique involves a wedge pair, with the portals aimed either superiorly and inferiorly (to direct the exit dose away from the orbits and oral cavity), or anteriorly and posteriorly (with the portals angled so that the beams pass below the level of the eyes). The latter technique facilitates matching the low-neck portal to the primary fields and is preferred. The wedge pair technique can treat a generous portion of the base of skull in a homogeneous manner, and is particularly useful when perineural spread is present or suspected, as in adenoid cystic carcinoma. An *en-face* electron field is often used to supplement to superficial dose (Figure 14.3). Fields are best designed with the aid of CT simulation and treatment planning. A second basic technique uses ipsilateral portals shaped to fit the anatomy. A treatment scheme using a combination of photons and high-energy electrons produces a homogeneous dose distribution and delivers 30 Gy or less to the opposite salivary glands. The advantages of the technique are the ability to shape and reduce the fields easily, and the ease with which an ipsilateral low-neck field may be adjoined to the primary portal. A disadvantage – especially in patients with adenoid cystic carcinoma – is an underdosage of possible perineural tumor extensions deep in the temporal bone because of inadequate penetration of electrons in dense bone. Because electrons are so subject to perturbations from tissue inhomogeneity, the risk of deep target miss must always be borne in mind. When tumor involves the deep lobe, or otherwise extends near the midline, the use of a third technique – parallel opposed photon

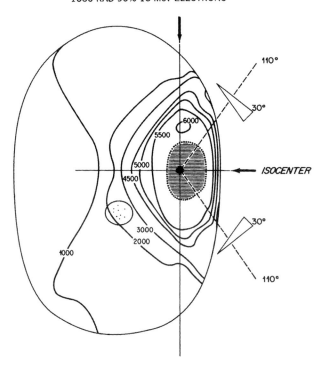

ISODOSE FOR PAROTID TUMORS
4500 RAD ⁶⁰Co WEDGE PAIR
1000 RAD 90% 15 MeV ELECTRONS

Figure 14.3 Diagram showing composite isodose for irradiating parotid tumor, using 45 Gy ipsilateral oblique wedge paired fields and 10 Gy appositional 15 MeV electron beam boost (90% isodose line).

portals weighted to the side of the lesion – may be necessary.

As illustrated in Figure 14.4, IMRT is increasingly used in the management of parotid tumors. Dosimetric studies have shown that IMRT can significantly reduce dose to normal structures compared to traditional techniques. IMRT is also useful when it is necessary to treat the nerve pathways to the foramina in the base of skull, in the event of extensive perineural involvement or named nerve invasion. Regardless of the chosen technique, care must be taken to limit inadvertent dose to the temporal lobes, ocular structures, middle/inner ears, swallowing structures (constrictor muscles), larynx, and contralateral parotid gland. Limiting and carefully monitoring dose to the anterior mucosal structures, including the oral cavity, lips, and hard palate, may be useful in decreasing acute toxicity. Lastly, the contralateral (and ipsilateral submandibular gland, if clinically appropriate) should be delineated and spared whenever possible.

Role of Chemotherapy

In general, salivary gland neoplasms respond poorly to chemotherapy, and there is no established role for its use

at present, other than for palliation. Doxorubicin- and platinum-based agents have been the most commonly studied, and nearly all of the limited data available applies only for patients treated with recurrent or metastatic disease. A prospective study from the Northern California Oncology Group demonstrated a response rate of 35% with a combination of cisplatin, doxorubicin, and 5-fluorouracil [57]. Another series from the Mayo Clinic revealed a 38% response rate using cisplatin-based chemotherapy for recurrent and advanced salivary gland cancer [58]. Notably, a current trial being conducted by the Radiation Therapy Oncology Group (RTOG) is investigating the use of concurrent cisplatin with radiation therapy after initial surgery for patients with high-risk pathological features [59]. The results of this trial are eagerly awaited.

Toxicity

Acute and late skin reactions involving the pinna, external auditory canal, and periauricular region are commonly described side effects of radiation therapy to the parotid region. Acute events, including erythema, desquamation and rarely, ulceration of the skin, can be managed conservatively with skin creams and anti-inflammatory medication. Otitis media and externa often require the use of antibiotics. Late skin changes including atrophy, fibrosis, and external canal stenosis have also been reported. Although rare, temporal bone necrosis is a potentially devastating complication after radiation therapy to this region. To minimize this complication, it is recommended to limit the volume of total bone exposed to greater than 70 Gy, whenever possible.

Problems with hearing and balance represent the most serious side effects of radiation therapy to the region of the parotid gland. In view of several recently published studies identifying a dose–response relationship for the inner and middle ear, the importance of minimizing dose to these organs at risk is becoming increasingly recognized among those undergoing treatment for head and neck cancer [60–64]. Sensorineural hearing loss, traditionally defined as a clinically significant increase in bone conduction threshold at the key human speech frequencies (0.5–4.0 kHz), has been shown to occur in approximately one-third of patients treated by definitive radiation with fields including the inner ear [65,66]. In a prospective study of 40 patients, Pan *et al.* showed that a clinically apparent hearing loss greater than 10 dB occurred when the cochlea received mean doses in excess of 45 Gy [60]. Honore *et al.* similarly developed a model predictive of sensorineural hearing loss based on pre-therapy dosimetric and clinical outcomes data of 20 patients treated with radiotherapy for nasopharyngeal carcinoma [61]. Notably, when the model was adjusted

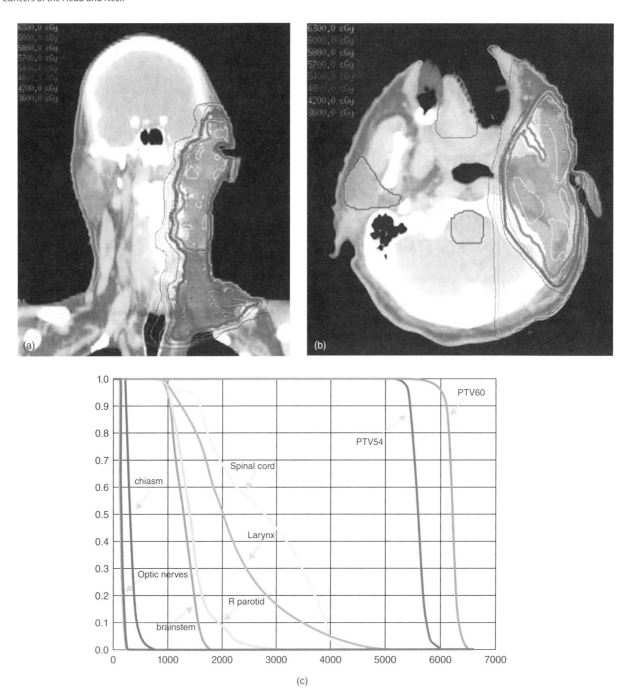

Figure 14.4 A 70-year-old male status post left-sided superficial parotidectomy and ipsilateral neck dissection for T2N1, high-grade mucoepidermoid carcinoma. The IMRT plan, shown in (a) coronal and (b) axial dimensions was designed to deliver a dose of 6000 cGy to the parotid bed and level II/III neck and 5400 cGy to the ipsilateral supraclavicular fossa, using a simultaneous-integrated boost technique. Visualized avoidance structures include the oral cavity (green), contralateral right parotid gland (light green), brainstem with margin (purple), and mandible (orange). (c) Dose–volume histogram illustrating the ability of IMRT to maximize dose to the 6000 cGy and 5400 cGy planning target volume (PTV) while minimizing dose to avoidance structures. For a color version of this figure, see the color plate section.

for age and pre-therapy hearing level, a steep dose–response curve emerged with a threshold at approximately 40 Gy. Although questions persist regarding the time course of hearing loss after irradiation and whether the dose–response relationship for toxicity to the auditory structures is linear or sigmoid shaped, a general agreement exists that doses to the inner and middle ear should be closely monitored [62–65]. The Quantitative

Analysis of Normal Tissue Effects in the Clinic (QUAN-TEC) reviews, published in 2010, recommends limiting the mean cochlear dose to less than 45 Gy so as to minimize the risk for sensorineural hearing loss [66]. The results of a prospective study from Italy, in which patients underwent audiometric evaluation consisting of pure tone audiometry and tympanometry before 3D-conformal radiation therapy and at three, six, and 24 months after treatment were recently published [67]. Among the 17 patients enrolled, the mean dose to the cochlea was 19 Gy, and none of the patients showed any evidence of permanent hearing impairment.

References

1 Seifert, G., Sobin, L.H. (1992) Histological typing of salivary gland tumors, in *World Health Organization International classification of tumors* (2nd edition). Springer-Verlag, New York.

2 Kumar, P.P., Patil, A.A., Ogren, F.P., *et al.* (1993) Intracranial skip metastasis from parotid and facial skin tumors: mechanism, diagnosis, and treatment. *J. Natl. Med. Assoc.*, **85**, 369–374.

3 Eneroth, C.M., Hamberger, C.A. (1974) Principles of treatment of different types of parotid tumors. *Laryngoscope*, **84**, 1732–1740.

4 Vrielinck, L.J., Ostyn, F., van Damme, B., *et al.* (1988) The significance of perineural spread in adenoid cystic carcinoma of the major and minor salivary glands. *Int. J. Oral Maxillofac. Surg.*, **17**, 190–193.

5 van der Wal, J.E., Becking, A.G., Snow, G.B., *et al.* (2002) Distant metastases of adenoid cystic carcinoma of the salivary glands and the value of diagnostic examinations during follow-up. *Head Neck*, **24**, 779–783.

6 Armstrong, J.G., Harrison, L.B., Thaler, H.T., *et al.* (1992) The indications for elective treatment of the neck in cancer of the major salivary glands. *Cancer*, **69**, 615–619.

7 Le, Q.T., Birdwell, S., Terris, D.J., *et al.* (1999) Postoperative irradiation of minor salivary gland malignancies of the head and neck. *Radiother. Oncol.*, **52**, 165–171.

8 Bartels, S., Talbot, J.M., DiTomasso, J., *et al.* (2000) The relative value of fine-needle aspiration and imaging in the preoperative evaluation of parotid masses. *Head Neck*, **22**, 781–786.

9 Freling, N.J., Molenaar, W.M., Vermey, A., *et al.* (1992) Malignant parotid tumors: clinical use of MR imaging and histologic correlation. *Radiology*, **185**, 691–696.

10 Cermik, T.F., Mayi, A., Acikgoz, G., *et al.* (2009) FDG PET in detecting primary and recurrent malignant salivary gland tumors. *Clin. Nucl. Med.*, **32**, 286–291.

11 Amin, M.B., *et al.* (2017) *AJCC Cancer Staging Manual*, 8th edition. Springer-Verlag, New York.

12 Terhaard, C.H., Lubsen, H., Van der Tweel, I., *et al.* (2004) Salivary gland carcinoma: independent prognostic factors for locoregional control, distant metastases, and overall survival: results of the Dutch head and neck oncology cooperative group. *Head Neck*, **26**, 681–692.

13 Spiro, R.H. (1986) Salivary neoplasms: Overview of a 35-year experience with 2807 patients. *Head Neck Surg.*, **8**, 177–184.

14 Mendenhall, W.M., Morris, C.G., Amdur, R.J., *et al.* (2005) Radiotherapy alone or combined with surgery for salivary gland carcinoma. *Cancer*, **103**, 2544–2550.

15 Lima, R.A., Tavares, M.R., Dias, F.L., *et al.* (2005) Clinical prognostic factors in malignant parotid gland tumors. *Otolaryngol. Head Neck Surg.*, **133**, 702–708.

16 Bhattacharrya, N., Fried, M.P. (2005) Determinants of survival in parotid gland carcinoma: a population-based study. *Am. J. Otolaryngol.*, **26**, 39–44.

17 Gibson, T. (1964) Locally malignant and radioresistant tumors of the face. *Plast. Reconstr. Surg.*, **34**, 491–500.

18 Tapley, N.D. (1977) Irradiation treatment of malignant tumors of the salivary glands. *Ear Nose Throat J.*, **56**, 110–114.

19 Guillamondegui, O.M., Byers, R.M., Luna, M.A., *et al.* (1975) Aggressive surgery in treatment for parotid cancer: the role of adjunctive postoperative radiotherapy. *Am. J. Roentgenol. Radium Ther. Nucl. Med.*, **123**, 49–54.

20 King, J.J., Fletcher, G.H. (1971) Malignant tumors of the major salivary glands. *Radiology*, **100**, 381–384.

21 Fu, K.K., Leibel, S.A., Levine, M.L., *et al.* (1977) Carcinoma of the major and minor salivary glands. *Cancer*, **40**, 2882–2890.

22 Elkon, D., Colman, M., Hendrickson, F.R. (1978) Radiation therapy in the treatment of malignant salivary gland tumors. *Cancer*, **41**, 502–506.

23 Garden, A.S., El-Naggar, A.K., Morrison, W.H., *et al.* (1997) Postoperative radiotherapy for malignant tumors of the parotid gland. *Int. J. Radiat. Oncol. Biol. Phys.*, **37**, 79–85.

24 North, C.A., Lee, D.J., Piantadosi, S., *et al.* (1990) Carcinoma of the major salivary glands treated by surgery or surgery plus postoperative radiotherapy. *Int. J. Radiat. Oncol. Biol. Phys.*, **18**, 1319–1326.

25 Harrison, L.B., Armstrong, J.G., Spiro, R.H., *et al.* (1990) Postoperative radiation therapy for major salivary gland malignancies. *J. Surg. Oncol.*, **45**, 52–55.

26 Armstrong, J.G., Harrison, L.B., Spiro, R.H., *et al.* (1990) Malignant tumors of major salivary gland origin. A matched-pair analysis of the role of combined surgery and postoperative radiotherapy. *Arch. Otolaryngol. Head Neck Surg.*, **116**, 290–293.

27 Chen, A.M., Bucci, M.K., Weinberg, V., *et al.* (2006) Adenoid cystic carcinoma of the head and neck treated by surgery with or without postoperative radiation therapy: prognostic features of recurrence. *Int. J. Radiat. Oncol. Biol. Phys.*, **66**, 152–159.

28 Chen, A.M., Garcia, J., Bucci, M.K., *et al.* (2007) The role of postoperative radiation therapy in carcinoma ex pleomorphic adenoma of the parotid gland. *Int. J. Radiat. Oncol. Biol. Phys.*, **67**, 138–143.

29 Chen, A.M., Granchi, P.J., Garcia, J., *et al.* (2007) Local-regional recurrence after surgery without postoperative irradiation for carcinomas of the major salivary glands: implications for adjuvant therapy. *Int. J. Radiat. Oncol. Biol. Phys.*, **67**, 982–987.

30 Chen, A.M., Bucci, M.K., Quivey, J.M., *et al.* (2006) Long-term outcome of patients treated by radiation therapy alone for salivary gland carcinomas. *Int. J. Radiat. Oncol. Biol. Phys.*, **66**, 1044–1050.

31 Terhaard, C.H., Lubsen, H., Rasch, C.R., *et al.* (2005) The role of radiotherapy in the treatment of malignant salivary gland tumors. *Int. J. Radiat. Oncol. Biol. Phys.*, **61**, 103–111.

32 Huber, P.E., Debus, J., Latz, D., *et al.* (2001) Radiotherapy for advanced adenoid cystic carcinoma: neutrons, photons, or mixed beam? *Radiother. Oncol.*, **59**, 161–167.

33 Hosokawa, Y., Ohomori, K., Kaneko, M., *et al.* (1992) Analysis of adenoid cystic carcinoma treated by radiotherapy. *Oral Surg. Oral Med. Oral Path.*, **74**, 251–255.

34 Wang, C.C., Goodman, M. (1991) Photon irradiation of unresectable carcinomas of the salivary glands. *Int. J. Radiat. Oncol. Biol. Phys.*, **21**, 569–576.

35 Douglas, J.G., Sibergeld, D.L., Laramore, G.E. (2004) Gamma knife stereotactic radiosurgical boost for patients treated primarily with neutron radiotherapy for salivary gland neoplasms. *Stereotact. Funct. Neurosurg.*, **82**, 84–85.

36 Barnett, T.A., Kapp, D.S., Goffinet, D.R. (1990) Adenoid cystic carcinoma of the salivary glands: management of recurrent, advanced, or persistent disease with hyperthermia and radiation therapy. *Cancer*, **65**, 2648–2656.

37 Douglas, J.G., Goodkin, R., Laramore, G.E. (2008) Gamma knife stereotactic radiosurgery for salivary gland neoplasms with base of skull invasion following neutron radiotherapy. *Head Neck*, **30**, 492–496.

38 Jensen, A.D., Nikoghosyan, A., Windemuth-Kieselbach, C., *et al.* (2010) Combined treatment of malignant salivary gland tumors with intensity-modulated radiation therapy and carbon ions: COSMIC. *BMC Cancer*, **10**, 546.

39 Zhang, J., Zhang, J.G., Song, T.L., *et al.* (2008) [125]I seed implant brachytherapy-assisted surgery with preservation of the facial nerve for treatment of malignant parotid gland tumors. *Int. J. Oral Maxillofac. Surg.*, **37**, 515–520.

40 Schulz-Ertner, D., Nikoghosyan, A., Jäkel, O., *et al.* (2003) Feasibility and toxicity of combined photon and carbon ion radiotherapy for locally advanced adenoid cystic carcinomas. *Int. J. Radiat. Oncol. Biol. Phys.*, **56**, 391–398.

41 Jereczek-Fossa, B.A., Krengli, M., Orecchia, R. (2006) Particle beam radiotherapy for head and neck tumors: radiobiological basis and clinical experience. *Head Neck*, **28**, 750–760.

42 Laramore, G.E. (1997) The use of neutrons in cancer therapy: a historical perspective through the modern era. *Semin. Oncol.*, **24**, 672–685.

43 Wamersie, A., Richard, F., Breteau, N. (1994) Development of fast neutron therapy worldwide. Radiobiological, clinical and technical aspects. *Acta Oncol.*, **33**, 261–264.

44 Catterall, M., Errington, R.D. (1987) The implications of improved treatment of malignant salivary gland tumors by fast neutron radiotherapy. *Int. J. Radiat. Oncol. Biol. Phys.*, **13**, 1313–1318.

45 Battermann, J.J., Breuer, K., Hart, G.A., *et al.* (1981) Observations on pulmonary metastases in patients after single doses and multiple fractions of fast neutrons and cobalt-60 gamma rays. *Eur. J. Cancer*, **17**, 539–548.

46 Douglas, J.G., Koh, W.J., Auston-Seymour, M., *et al.* (2003) Treatment of salivary gland neoplasms with fast neutron radiotherapy. *Arch. Otolaryngol. Head Neck Surg.*, **129**, 944–948.

47 Krull, A., Schwarz, R., Brackrock, S., *et al.* (1998) Neutron therapy in malignant salivary gland tumors: results at European centers. *Recent Results Cancer Res.*, **150**, 88–99.

48 Potter, R., Prott, F.J., Micke, O., *et al.* (1999) Results of fast neutron therapy of adenoid cystic carcinoma of the salivary glands. *Strahlenther. Onkol.*, **175S**, 65–68.

49 Saroja, K.R., Mansell, J., Hendrickson, F.R., *et al.* (1987) An update on malignant salivary gland tumors treated with neutrons at Fermilab. *Int. J. Radiat. Oncol. Biol. Phys.*, **13**, 1319–1325.

50 Laramore, G.E., Krall, J.M., Griffin, T.W., *et al.* (1993) Neutron versus photon irradiation for unresectable salivary gland tumors: final report of an RTOG-MRC randomized clinical trial. Radiation Therapy Oncology Group. Medical Research Council. *Int. J. Radiat. Oncol. Biol. Phys.*, **27**, 235–240.

51 Cianchetti, M., Sandow, P.S., Scarborough, L.D., *et al.* (2009) Radiation therapy for minor salivary gland carcinoma. *Laryngoscope*, **119**, 1334–1338.

52 Spiro, I.J., Wang, C.C., Montgomery, W.W. (1993) Carcinoma of the parotid gland: Analysis of treatment results and patterns of failure after combined surgery and radiation therapy. *Cancer*, **71**, 2699–2705.

53 Garden, A.S., Weber, R.S., Ang, K.K., *et al.* (1994) Postoperative radiation therapy for malignant tumors of minor salivary glands. Outcome and patterns of failure. *Cancer*, **73**, 2563–2569.

54 Storey, M.R., Garden, A.S., Morrison, W.H., *et al.* (2001) Postoperative radiotherapy for malignant tumors of the submandibular gland. *Int. J. Radiat. Oncol. Biol. Phys.*, **51**, 952–958.

55 Douglas, J.G., Laramore, G.E., Austin-Seymour, M., *et al.* (2000) Treatment of locally advanced adenoid cystic carcinoma of the head and neck with neutron radiotherapy. *Int. J. Radiat. Oncol. Biol. Phys.*, **46**, 551–557.

56 Huber, P.E., Debus, J., Latz, D., *et al.* (2001) Radiotherapy for advanced adenoid cystic carcinoma: neutrons, photons or mixed beam? *Radiother. Oncol.*, **59**, 161–167.

57 Venook, A.P., Tseng, A., Jr, Meyers, F.J., *et al.* (1987) Cisplatin, doxorubicin, and 5-fluorouracil chemotherapy for salivary gland malignancies: a pilot study of the Northern California Oncology Group. *J. Clin. Oncol.*, **5**, 951–955.

58 Creagan, E.T., Woods, J.E., Rubin, J., *et al.* (1988) Cisplatin-based chemotherapy for neoplasms arising from salivary glands and contiguous structures in the head and neck. *Cancer*, **62**, 2313–2319.

59 RTOG 1008. A randomized phase II study of adjuvant concurrent radiation and chemotherapy versus radiation alone in resected high-risk malignant salivary gland tumors. http://www.rtog.org/ClinicalTrials/ProtocolTable/StudyDetails.aspx?study = 1008.

60 Pan, C.C., Eisbruch, A., Lee, J.S., *et al.* (2005) Prospective study of inner ear radiation dose and hearing loss in head-and-neck cancer patients. *Int. J. Radiat. Oncol. Biol. Phys.*, **61**, 1393–1402.

61 Honore, H.B., Bentzen, S.M., Moller, K., *et al.* (2002) Sensorineural hearing loss after radiotherapy for nasopharyngeal carcinoma: individualized risk estimation. *Radiother. Oncol.*, **65**, 9–16.

62 Chen, W.C., Jackson, A., Budnick, A.S., *et al.* (2006) Sensorineural hearing loss in combined modality treatment of nasopharyngeal carcinoma. *Cancer*, **106**, 820–829.

63 Ho, W.K., Wei, W.I., Kwong, D.L., *et al.* (1996) Long-term sensorineural hearing loss in patients treated for nasopharyngeal carcinoma: a prospective study of the effect of radiation and cisplatin treatment. *Int. J. Radiat. Oncol. Biol. Phys.*, **36**, 281–289.

64 Ondrey, F.G., Greig, J.R., Herscher, L. (2000) Radiation dose to otologic structures during head and neck cancer radiation therapy. *Laryngoscope*, **110**, 217–221.

65 Kwong, D., Wei, W., Sham, J., *et al.* (1996) Sensorineural hearing loss in patients treated for nasopharyngeal cancer: a prospective study of the effect of radiation and cisplatin treatment. *Int. J. Radiat. Oncol. Biol. Phys.*, **36**, 281–289.

66 Bhandare, N., Jackson, A., Eisbruch, A., *et al.* (2010) Radiation therapy and hearing loss. *Int. J. Radiat. Oncol. Biol. Phys.*, **76**, S50–S57.

67 Jereczek-Fossa, B.A., Rondi, E., Zarowski, A., *et al.* (2011) Prospective study on dose distribution to the acoustic structures during postoperative 3D conformal radiotherapy for parotid tumors: dosimetric and audiometric aspects. *Strahlenther. Onkol.*, **187**, 350–356.

15

Cervical Nodes with Unknown Primary Carcinomas

Min Yao, Pierre Lavertu and Mitchell Machtay

Introduction

Cervical lymph node metastases with unknown primary, also called head and neck cancer with unknown primary (HNCUP), is uncommon. With a thorough work-up including advanced imaging and examination under anesthesia with directed biopsies, the incidence of HNCUP is in the range of 3% to 7% [1, 2]. Most patients have squamous cell carcinoma and poorly differentiated carcinoma, which is the focus of this chapter. Adenocarcinoma is rare and when present, arises from the salivary glands or from sources below the clavicles. The most commonly involved lymph node region is level II, followed by level III [1]. The distribution of the involved lymph nodes in 352 consecutive patients with squamous cell carcinoma and poorly differentiated carcinoma seen between 1975 and 1995 in a national survey by the Danish Society for Head and Neck Oncology [1] is shown in Figure 15.1. For lymphadenopathy presenting only in the lower neck and supraclavicular fossa, a primary below the clavicles should be considered.

Diagnostic Work-Up

When patients are presenting with enlarged cervical lymph nodes, a thorough history should be obtained and a physical examination performed. The skin and scalp should be carefully examined to rule out cutaneous squamous cell carcinoma that occasionally can present with a metastatic node. Office-based flexible nasopharyngolaryngoscopy is performed to visualize the nasopharynx, oropharynx, larynx, and hypopharynx. A fine-needle aspiration (FNA) of the enlarged lymph node can be performed in the office to provide a pathologic diagnosis. In the presence of squamous cell carcinoma or poorly differentiated carcinoma, the status of human papilloma virus (HPV) in the nodal biopsy should be checked. This can be achieved using immunohistochemistry (IHC) for p16, a known surrogate marker for HPV infection. HPV positivity suggests a primary site in the oropharynx, often tonsil or tongue base [3, 4]. In areas of high incidence of nasopharyngeal cancer, detection of the Epstein–Barr virus (EBV) DNA in the metastatic nodes by *in-situ* hybridization or polymerase chain reaction would indicate a nasopharyngeal origin [5, 6]. If the FNA is not diagnostic and the search for a primary is negative on endoscopy with biopsy (with or without tonsillectomy), an open biopsy or excisional biopsy of the involved lymph node will need to be done. This is only recommended as the last resort since these procedures could complicate or delay appropriate treatment. A neck dissection at the same setting may also be considered.

Computed tomography (CT) with contrast or magnetic resonance imaging (MRI) with gadolinium of the head and neck is obtained for detection of the primary tumor. Suspicious areas identified on CT/MRI scanning can guide biopsy sampling. CT/MRI can also determine the extent and size of the lymph nodes. CT of the chest is obtained to rule out primary lung cancer or lung metastases, especially in patients with bulky lymph nodes in lower neck and those with N2B or higher stage.

The usefulness of fluorodeoxyglucose positron emission tomography (FDG-PET) in the diagnostic work-up of HNCUP has been controversial. Recent studies have confirmed the role of FDG-PET in identification of the primary tumor and detection of distant metastases. Rusthoven *et al.* [7] summarized 16 retrospective studies using FDG-PET in HNCUP in a total of 302 patients, and found the technique to have a detection rate of 24.5% for tumors that were not detected by other modalities after conventional work-up (CT/MRI, and panendoscopy). In

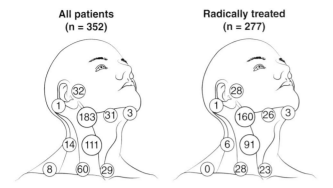

Figure 15.1 Involved lymph node levels in all patients (left) and patients treated with radical intent (right). *Source:* Grau 2000 [1]. Reproduced with permission of Elsevier.

four studies with a total of 107 patients, 17 patients were found to have new cervical lymph node metastases (15.9%) and 12 had distant metastases (11.2%). Therapeutic changes secondary to FDG-PET findings were reported in 24.7% of patients because of detection of a primary tumor or the detection of previously unknown metastases. The Danish Head and Neck Cancer Study Group published their prospective study (DAHANCA-13) using FDG-PET in HNCUP [8]. The group found that FDG-PET was able to detect a primary tumor or previously unknown distant metastases in 18 of 60 patients, with a detection rate of 30%. In 15 of these 18 patients (25%), the treatment was modified either with reduction of the radiation treatment volumes when a primary was identified, or a change to palliative treatment in the cases of distant metastases. Recently, Rudmik *et al.* [9] also conducted a prospective study of FDG-PET in the diagnostic work-up of HNCUP, enrolling 20 patients all of whom had no primary tumors identified after standard clinical evaluation. FDG-PET/CT was performed within seven days before panendoscopy and directed biopsies, and the surgeons were blinded to the results. The PET/CT results were compared with the panendoscopic findings. Additional biopsies were performed if the PET/CT was reported to be positive. The authors reported that the traditional work-up identified the primary site in five patients (25%), whereas PET/CT-directed biopsy identified the primary site in 11 patients (55%), with a crude difference in identification rate of 30%. There was one false-negative PET/CT. The PET/CT-directed biopsy was found to have a statistically significant advantage over the traditional approach.

FDG-PET should be performed before panendoscopy and directed biopsies to avoid false-positive results caused by the biopsy. In the DAHANCA-13 study, PET was performed either before (19/60 patients) or after (41/60 patients) Panendoscopy. A false-positive result was found in one of eight patients in the pre-endoscopy group, compared to 11 of 22 patients in the post-endoscopy group [8]. When the PET is performed before the panendoscopy, it allows for PET-directed biopsy which is superior to the traditional random biopsy approach [9].

Examination under anesthesia (EUA) and panendoscopy are performed, while directed biopsies are obtained from suspicious areas identified from the examination and/or imaging studies. If no suspicious areas are found, biopsies should be obtained from the nasopharynx and oropharynx. Ipsilateral tonsillectomy should also be performed in patients with intact tonsil as the tonsil is a common site for primary tumor [10, 11]. Tonsillectomy was shown to have a significantly higher yield in detecting an occult tonsilar tumor than a deep tonsil biopsy [12]. Koch *et al.* [13] noted that the rate of contralateral spread of metastatic cancer from occult tonsil lesions approached 10%, and advocated bilateral tonsillectomy as a routine step for HNCUP with intact palatine tonsils, which is controversial.

Recently, several reports have been made regarding the use of transoral laser microsurgery (TLM) or transoral robotic surgery (TORS) in identification of the primary tumor [14–17]. Nagel *et al.* [14] described their experience in 52 patients who did not have obvious primary tumor at complete head and neck examination, including flexible endoscopy. A TLM approach was used in 36 of these patients, and 31 had a primary tumor detected with a success rate of 86.1%. In this study the Carl Zeiss microscope (Oberkochen, Germany) was used with modified xenon illumination that allows for microscopic mucosal inspection to identify subtle mucosal changes. Patel *et al.* [15] reported a multi-institutional experience of 47 patients when using TORS to identify the primary sites. Of note, some of these patients had suspicious physical examination findings or imaging findings. The primary tumor was identified in 34 patients with a detection rate of 72.3%, with primary tumor as small as 0.2 cm. The diagnostic work-up for HNCUP in sequence is summarized in Figure 15.2.

As for all head and neck cancer patients, dental, audiology, speech pathology with swallow evaluation, and nutrition evaluations are necessary, especially for those who will need to receive radiation treatment.

Principles of Management

The optimal treatment of HNCUP has not yet been defined. Because of the low incidence of the lesion, no data from randomized clinical trials are yet available. All published studies have been related to retrospective series with heterogeneous patient populations and various treatment approaches. Although the main treatment modalities are surgery and radiotherapy, recent studies have also included chemotherapy as radiosensitizers

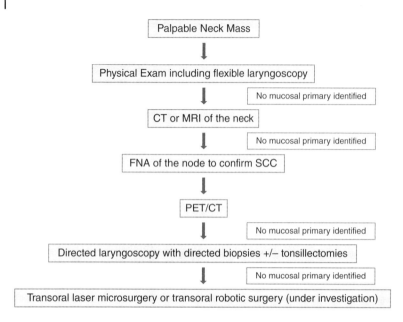

Figure 15.2 Proposed algorithm in the work-up of head and neck cancer with unknown primary. *Source:* Adapted from Keller *et al.* 2014 [49].

given concurrently with radiation. Recently, Demiroz *et al.* (18) summarized the data from 41 patients treated at the University of Michigan, and showed there to be no differences between patients treated with neck dissection and adjuvant radiotherapy ($n = 22$) or definitive radiotherapy ± concurrent chemotherapy ($n = 19$) in overall survival, progression-free survival, local-regional control, or distant metastases.

Surgery

Depending on the extent of the disease, a selective or modified radical neck dissection can be performed. This can be done either before radiation or as salvage for persistent disease after definitive radiation. Neck dissection alone may be sufficient only for selected patients with N1 disease with no extracapsular extension and no history of open biopsy [19]. Open biopsy, both incisional and excisional, may cause seeding of cancer cells and postoperative radiation treatment is indicated [20, 21].

Chemotherapy

Cisplatin-based chemotherapy is used concurrently with radiation either as definitive radiation before neck dissection, or postoperatively in patients with high-risk features such as extracapsular extension, soft-tissue tumor deposit, or positive margins [22–24]. Again, no randomized studies have been conducted supporting the role of chemotherapy in HNCUP. The uses of concurrent chemotherapy with radiation are extrapolated from randomized studies in other head and neck cancer series with known primary sites [25–27].

Radiation

Radiotherapy is a critical modality in the management of HNCUP. Grau *et al.* [1] reported the details of 352 HNCUP patients from five cancer centers in Denmark. Of 277 patients who were treated with curative intent, 23 had a neck dissection alone. These patients had significantly worse mucosal control, cause-specific survival and overall survival as compared to those who received radiotherapy. The five-year actuarial mucosal control rate for neck dissection alone was 46%, versus 84% for those with radiotherapy alone and 95% for those who had radiotherapy plus surgery (p = 0.00001).

Controversies persist regarding the sequence of radiotherapy and surgery. Some authors [28] have suggested radiation first followed by neck dissection because: (i) the target tissues are better oxygenated, making radiotherapy more effective; (ii) radiation is not delayed due to possible surgical complications; and (iii) if the mucosal primary emerges before surgery, this can be removed when the patient has neck dissection in one single definitive surgery. However, some authors have suggested that such a sequence would have a poorer survival and higher postoperative complications as compared to surgery followed by radiotherapy [29, 30]. These conclusions were derived from retrospective studies with patient selection bias. Those patients who had received radiation first might have more advanced disease, and more inoperable diseases. The best treatment sequence should be individualized and decided using a multidisciplinary approach. The disease extent, the patient's performance status, the patient's choice and the expertise of the team should all be taken into account. For patients with N1 and small N2A disease, radiation treatment after FNA or

Figure 15.3 Simulation film showing portal arrangement for a large squamous cell carcinoma in the neck with an occult primary, presumably in Waldeyer's ring.

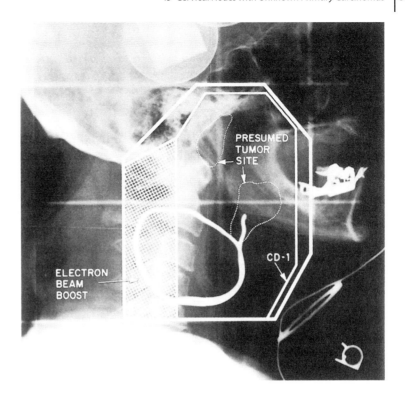

excisional biopsy may be sufficient [31]. Patients with more advanced diseases treated with definitive chemoradiation may not need to have neck dissection if they have complete response with no residual diseases on post-treatment CT scans or PET scans [32–34].

Controversies also exist regarding the radiation volumes. Some groups irradiate the ipsilateral neck only, while others recommend comprehensive irradiation to both the neck and the pharyngeal axis. In a study conducted by Grau *et al.* [1], of 250 patients who underwent radiotherapy with curative intent, 224 received comprehensive irradiation and 26 to the ipsilateral neck only. There was a significant twofold reduction in local regional recurrence by using extensive radiotherapy fields. Patients treated with comprehensive radiation also had a higher disease-specific survival. Nieder *et al.* [35] reviewed studies using ipsilateral radiotherapy versus those with comprehensive radiotherapy, and found there to be no difference in median mucosal primary emergence rate (8% versus 9.5%). However, there was a much higher median neck relapse rate in the group treated with unilateral neck radiotherapy compared to those treated with comprehensive radiotherapy (51.5% versus 19%). The median distant metastases rate was also higher in patients treated with unilateral neck radiation (38% versus 19%). The median five-year overall survival rate was 36.5% in the unilateral radiotherapy group, compared to 50% in the comprehensive radiotherapy group. In recent publications, most patients were treated with comprehensive radiotherapy. Ipsilateral neck

radiation should be reserved for those who cannot tolerate comprehensive radiation because of age and medical comorbidities.

A simulation film showing the portal arrangement for a patient with HNCUP, which include bilateral necks and the whole pharyngeal axis, is shown in Figure 15.3. As most patients may have occult primary in the oropharynx, Mendenhall *et al.* [36] proposed to spare the larynx and include necks, the oropharynx and nasopharynx in the radiation field. The upper neck was treated with parallel-opposed fields to 64.8 Gy at 1.8 Gy per fraction with radiation off spinal cord at 45 Gy. This portal included the nasopharynx, oropharynx, and the jugular and spinal accessory lymph nodes to the skull base, with inferior border at the thyroid notch. The lower neck was treated with an anterior-posterior field with a mid-line block to spare the larynx to 50 Gy at 2.0 Gy per fraction. A boost of 10–20 Gy was delivered to any involved portion of the lower neck. This treatment technique significantly reduces the radiation dose to the larynx and the hypopharynx, and thus reduces the acute and late toxicities, especially those related to speech and swallowing. In another study, the details were reported of 17 patients treated in such manner for a curative intent [37]. No patient failed at the primary mucosal site or developed distant metastases, though one patient had neck recurrence one year after treatment and one patient had persistent nodal disease and died four months after treatment. The five-year cause-specific and overall survival rates were 88% and 82%, respectively.

Intensity-Modulated Radiotherapy

Comprehensive head and neck radiation including both necks and the whole pharyngeal axis causes significant acute and late toxicities. Even with the larynx-sparing technique proposed by Mendenhall, the parotids are treated to full dosage and results in long-term xerostomia. Intensity-modulated radiotherapy (IMRT) allows sparing of the parotids and preserves salivary function. Depending on the level of lymph node involvement, IMRT also allows targeting radiation to the high-risk potential primary sites and sparing other mucosal areas. Such risk-adapted personalized radiotherapeutic plans should be adopted to maximize tumor control and preserve quality of life.

Personalized Target Volume Delineation for IMRT

Head and neck cancer has a predictable pattern of lymph node metastases [38]. Hence, the potential primary site can be suggested by the level of the lymphadenopathy. For example, a level 1 adenopathy suggests mainly an oral cavity primary, while a level II adenopathy indicates a probable oropharyngeal primary, especially when HPV is positive. Lymphadenopathies localized to level V are commonly of nasopharyngeal or cutaneous origin. Therefore, depending on the adenopathy level and the HPV status, the radiation fields can be tailored and unnecessary radiation can be avoided to normal mucosal structures unlikely to harbor occult disease. The following section illustrates the IMRT technique used by the present authors for several common presentations of HNCUP.

Definitive IMRT for Patient with Level II Lymphadenopathy

Three target volumes are defined (Figure 15.4). The involved lymph node(s) is (are) defined as GTV, which is expanded with 5–10 mm margin to create CTV1. CTV2 includes the high-risk lymphatic regions, that is, ipsilateral levels II and III, and the oropharynx (and nasopharynx) which are the most likely potential primary sites. When HPV is positive, the nasopharynx can be spared. CTV3 includes lymphatic regions in the ipsilateral lower neck and the contralateral neck. The retropharyngeal lymph nodes are also included in CTV3. CTVs are expanded 3–5 mm to create planned target volumes (PTVs). The parotids, larynx, hypopharynx and the cervical esophagus are contoured as critical structures, as well as the spinal cord and the brainstem.

PTV1 is treated to 70 Gy at 2.0 Gy per fraction, PTV2 to 60–64 Gy, and PTV3 to 54–56 Gy using a simultaneously integrated boost technique. Sequential boost can also be used. The patient can also be treated with split-field IMRT, with IMRT to the upper neck and the

potential mucosal sites (oropharynx and/or nasopharynx) and with the lower neck treated with an anterior-posterior field matched to the IMRT field at the thyroid notch. A laryngeal block is placed in the lower-neck field. This technique may reduce the dose to the larynx and hypopharynx [39, 40].

Concurrent chemotherapy should be considered for patients with N2 or N3 disease who are able to tolerate chemotherapy. Neck dissection is performed for persistent disease after radiation treatment.

Postoperative IMRT for Patients with Level II Lymphadenopathy

Again, three target volumes are defined (Figure 15.5). CTV1 is the tumor bed of the resected lymph nodes. CTV2 includes the high-risk lymphatic regions (ipsilateral level II and level III) and the oropharynx (and nasopharynx), which are the most likely potential primary sites. When the tumor is HPV-positive, the nasopharynx can be spared. CTV3 includes the ipsilateral lower neck, contralateral neck, and retropharyngeal nodes. CTVs are expanded 3–5 mm to create PTVs. The parotids, larynx, hypopharynx and the cervical esophagus are contoured as critical structures, as well as the spinal cord and the brainstem.

For patients without extracapsular nodal extension, the PTV1 and PTV2 are treated to 60 Gy at 2.0 Gy per fraction, and PTV3 to 54 Gy at 1.8 Gy per fraction. For patients with extracapsular nodal extension, PTV1 is treated to 60–66 Gy at 2.0 Gy per fraction, PTV2 to 60–64 Gy, and PTV3 to 54–56 Gy. (PTV1 and PTV2 can be combined when treated to the same radiation dose.) Concurrent chemotherapy should be considered for patients with extracapsular nodal extension, soft-tissue deposits, or positive margins.

Definitive IMRT for Patients with Multi-Level Lymphadenopathies

For patients with lymphadenopathies involving level II to level IV, the larynx and hypopharynx are not spared and should be included in CTV2 as potential primary sites, especially the portion of larynx and hypopharynx ipsilateral to the involved neck (Figure 15.6). Again, CTV1 includes involved lymph nodes with 5–10 mm margins, CTV2 includes the ipsilateral neck, and the ipsilateral pharyngeal axis, while the contralateral neck and contralateral pharyngeal axis, supraclavicular fossae, and retropharyngeal nodes are defined as CTV3.

PTV1 is treated to 70 Gy at 2.0 Gy per fraction, PTV2 to 60–64 Gy, and PTV3 to 54–56 Gy. Concurrent chemotherapy is often offered.

IMRT for Patients with Lower-Neck Level Lymphadenopathy

The IMRT technique for patients with level III or level IV lymph nodes is similar to that for patients with

Figure 15.4 This patient received definitive IMRT with concurrent chemotherapy. (a) CTV1 included the lymphadenopathy with margin and was treated to 70 Gy. CTV2 included the nasopharynx, oropharynx and the high-risk lymphatic region, and was treated to 63 Gy. CTV3 was treated to 56 Gy. This was done with one plan using simultaneously integrated boost technique and delivered in 35 fractions. The segment of esophagus in the radiation field was also outlined as a dose-limiting structure. (b) Dose–volume histogram. Note acceptable doses to the parotids, larynx, and supraglottis. *Source:* Lu, Yao, and Tan 2009 [43]. Reproduced with permission of Elsevier. (c) Representative axial slices of the IMRT plan for this patient. For a color version of this figure, see the color plate section.

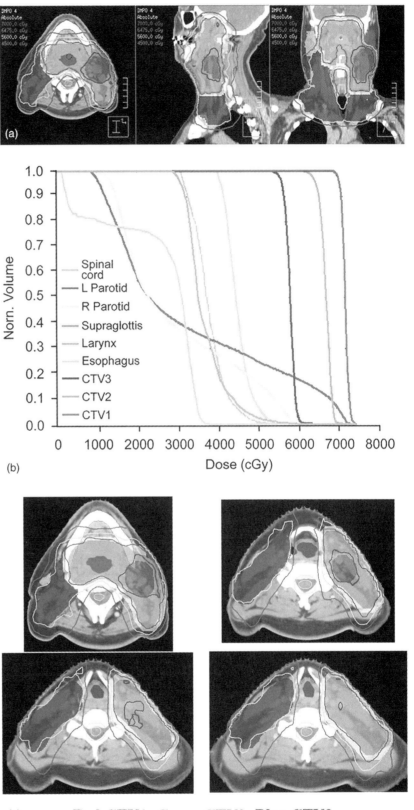

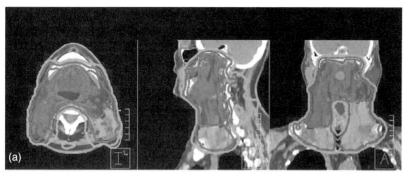

Absolute Dose (cGy): 6400 5440 4600

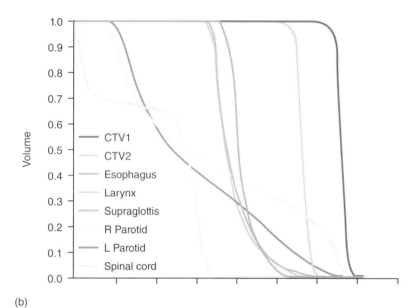

(b)

Figure 15.5 This patient with bulky level II lymph node with extracapsular extension after neck dissection received postoperative IMRT with concurrent cisplatin. (a) CTV1 included the surgical bed, the high-risk lymphatic regions, the oropharynx and nasopharynx; CTV2 included the lower-risk cervical lymphatic regions. These were treated to 64 Gy (2 Gy per fraction) and 54.4 Gy (1.7 Gy per fraction) in 32 fractions in one plan using simultaneously integrated boost technique. The segment of esophagus in the radiation field was also outlined as a dose-limiting structure. (b) Dose–volume histogram. Note acceptable doses to the parotids, larynx, and supraglottis. *Source:* Lu, Yao, and Tan 2009 [43]. Reproduced with permission of Elsevier. (c) Representative axial slices of the IMRT plan for this patient. For a color version of this figure, see the color plate section.

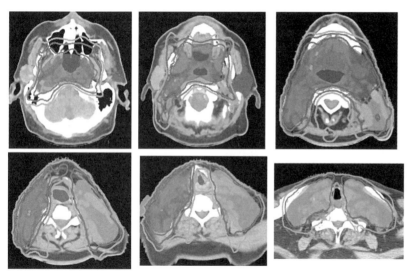

(c)   Red CTV1 and CTV2; Green CTV3

Figure 15.6 A patient with multiple lymphadenopathy at right level II to level IV. (a) FDG-PET scan of the patient. (b) IMRT plan. CTV1 included the all involved lymph nodes with margin and was treated to 70 Gy. CTV2 included the nasopharynx, oropharynx, ipsilateral larynx and hypopharynx, and the high-risk lymphatic region and was treated to 63 Gy. CTV3 was treated to 56 Gy. This was done with one plan using simultaneously integrated boost technique and delivered in 35 fractions. The segment of esophagus in the radiation field was also outlined as a dose-limiting structure. (c) Dose–volume histogram. For a color version of this figure, see the color plate section.

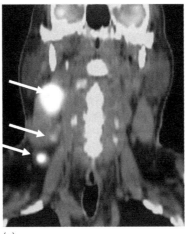
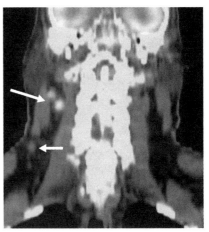

(a)

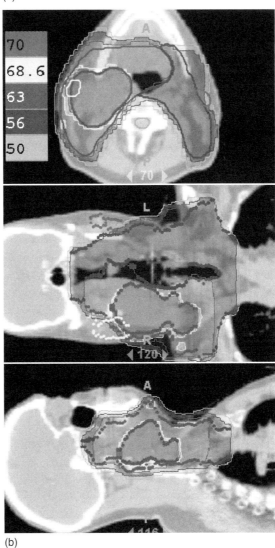

(b)

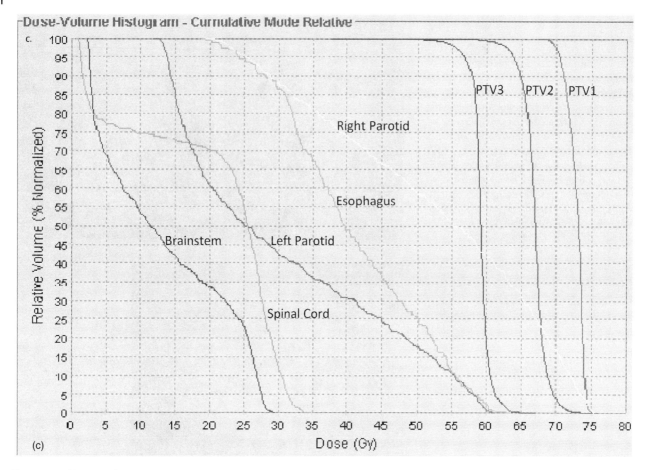

Figure 15.6 (*Continued*)

multi-level lymphadenopathies. The ipsilateral larynx and the hypopharynx should be included in CTV2, as above.

IMRT for Patients with Level I Lymphadenopathy

This is not common. The occult primary is possibly in the oral cavity, especially when only level IA is involved. As suggested by the National Comprehensive Cancer Network guideline [41], radiation should be delivered to the oral cavity, Waldeyer's ring, the oropharynx, and to both sides of the neck. The larynx and hypopharynx can be spared.

IMRT for Patients with Level V Lymphadenopathy

This is also not common. For a patient with only level V node, it is necessary to first rule out skin cancer. For patients from geographic regions where there is a high incidence of nasopharyngeal cancer (e.g., China) the radiation will need to include the nasopharynx.

Treatment Outcomes by IMRT

The results of several single-institution retrospective studies have been published (Table 15.1). Klem *et al.* [42] summarized the details of 21 patients treated at Memorial Sloan-Kettering Cancer Center, of whom 16 were treated with postoperative IMRT and five with definitive IMRT. In this case, bilateral nodal regions and mucosal sites were included, such as the oropharynx, larynx, hypopharynx and, in 90% of cases, the nasopharynx. Three patients had regional failure and two had distant failure. The most common acute toxicities were mucositis, skin toxicity, fatigue, xerostomia, and nausea. No Grade 3 or 4 xerostomia was seen on follow-up, and three patients developed esophageal stricture.

Lu *et al.* [43] reported the details of 18 patients treated at the University of Iowa, of whom eight had a neck dissection and four had an excisional biopsy before radiation. Six patients were treated with definitive IMRT, and most patients had laryngeal-sparing IMRT. Two patients had persistent lymphadenopathy after definitive radiation without chemotherapy. One patient had a salvage neck dissection, and another also had lung metastases treated with chemotherapy. The estimated two-year overall survival, regional recurrence-free survival and distant metastasis-free survival were 74.2%, 88.5%, and 88.2%, respectively.

Frank *et al.* [44] reported their experience at the M.D. Anderson Cancer Center. Of 52 patients treated, 13 had a

Table 15.1 Summary of published studies using intensity-modulated radiotherapy in head and neck cancer of unknown primary.

Institute	No. of patients	LRFS (%)	RRFS (%)	LRRFS (%)	DDFS (%)	OS (%)
Klem *et al.* [42]	21	–	90	–	90	85
Madani *et al.* [46]	23	–	–	–	76.3	74.8
Lu *et al.* [43]	18	–	88.5	–	88.2	74.2
Frank *et al.* [44]	52	98	94	–	–	89
Chen *et al.* [45]	27	–	–	92	84	87

DDFS, distant disease- free survival; LRFS, local recurrence- free survival; LRRFS, local-regional recurrence- free survival; OS, overall survival; RRFS, regional recurrence- free survival.

neck dissection, 14 had an excisional biopsy prior to radiation, and 14 also received chemotherapy, either given before radiation or concurrently with radiation. One patient had mucosal recurrence and three patients had neck recurrences; five patients failed distantly. The five-year disease-free survival and overall survival were 88% and 81%, respectively. Grade 1 xerostomia was reported as the most common complication. No Grade 4 complications were noted, and two patients developed Grade 3 esophageal toxicity.

Chen *et al.* [45] compared 27 patients treated with IMRT with 24 patients treated with conventional radiation. The necks and the mucosal axis, including the nasopharynx, oropharynx, larynx, and hypopharynx, were treated in the radiation field. A similar local-regional control was reported for patients treated with IMRT (92%) compared to those treated with conventional radiation (87%). Patients treated with IMRT experienced more Grade 3+ acute mucositis (28%) than those treated with conventional radiation (12%). However, IMRT patients had significant less Grade 3+ late toxicity (29%) than patients treated with conventional radiation (63%) (p <0.001). Grade 3+ late dysphagia occurred in 17% and 42% of patients treated by IMRT and conventional radiation, respectively. Grade 3+ late xerostomia occurred in 11% and 58% of patients treated by IMRT and conventional radiation, respectively. Significantly more patients were G-tube-dependent in the conventional radiation group than in the IMRT group (42% versus 11% at six months and 33% versus 0% at one year after treatment).

Madani *et al.* [46] compared 23 patients treated with IMRT to 18 patients treated with conventional radiation. No inter-group difference was found in terms of overall survival and distant disease-free survival, though patients treated with conventional radiotherapy had a significantly higher incidence and severity of acute dysphagia compared to the IMRT group. Patients treated with conventional radiotherapy also had significantly worse late toxicity in regards to dysphagia, xerostomia, and skin complications.

Recently, Mourad *et al.* [47] described 68 HNCUP patients treated with radiation techniques directed to bilateral necks and oropharynx only. Of these patients, 40% were treated with IMRT using a technique similar to that described above for patients with level II lymphadenopathy; 56% of the patients also received concurrent chemotherapy. At a median follow-up of 3.5 years, the local-regional control was 95.5%. One patient developed a primary tumor, and two patients failed in the neck. A three-year overall survival of 100% was reported.

Future Perspectives

During the past decade there has been a significant increase in the incidence of HPV-related oropharyngeal cancer [48]. Many of these patients present with significant cervical lymphadenopathy, but with a small oropharyngeal primary, which can be difficult to detect due to lymphoid tissue in the oropharynx, and is thus categorized as unknown primary. In Patel's series, using TORS in HNCUP [15], many detected tumors were less than 1.0 cm in size, with some as small as 0.2 cm.

It has been reported that HPV-related HNCUP patients had significantly better treatment outcomes [49, 50]. Clinical trials in treatment de-escalation with HPV-related oropharyngeal cancer are presently ongoing [51], and such an approach may be applicable to HPV-related HNCUP. De-escalation treatment with transoral surgery and neck dissection, followed by limited field radiation, has been proposed [52], but this approach should be attempted in a clinical trial setting.

Conclusions

Head and neck squamous cell carcinoma of unknown primary is not common. The diagnostic evaluation of these patients should focus on identification of the primary tumor and the determination of the extent of disease, including the presence or absence of distant metastases. This includes imaging studies, such as CT and FDG-PET, as well as examination under anesthesia with endoscopy and directed biopsies. All patients should be managed by a multidisciplinary head and neck cancer team. The sequence and combination of surgery, radiotherapy and chemotherapy should be discussed at the head and neck tumor board, and tailored to individual patients. Comprehensive radiotherapy including bilateral necks and pharyngeal axis offers better local regional control as compared to ipsilateral neck radiation, but tends to result in a greater toxicity and side effects. IMRT allows sparing of the parotids, and the radiation treatment plan can be personalized based on the level of nodal involvement. This radiation technique should be considered as the standard of care in the management of HNCUP. Currently, there is an increase in the incidence of HPV-related HNCUP. These patients have a significantly better prognosis. Treatment de-escalation in these patients has been proposed and will hopefully offer similar tumor control and survival with reduced toxicities, especially in the long term. However, this approach is currently under investigation and multicenter prospective clinical trials are needed because of the rarity of HNCUP.

References

1 Grau, C., Johansen, L.V., Jakobsen, J., *et al.* (2000) Cervical lymph node metastases from unknown primary tumors. Results from a national survey by the Danish Society of Head and Neck Oncology. *Radiother. Oncol.*, **55**, 121–129.

2 Jereczek-Fossa, B.A., Jassem, J., Orecchia, R. (2004) Cervical lymph node metastases of squamous cell carcinoma from an unknown primary. *Cancer Treat. Rev.*, **30**, 153–164.

3 Weiss, D., Koopmann, M., Rudack, C. (2011) Prevalence and impact on clinicopathological characteristics of human papillomavirus-16 DNA in cervical lymph node metastases of head and neck squamous cell carcinoma. *Head Neck*, **33**, 856–862.

4 Zhang, M.Q., El-Mofty, S.K., Davila, R.M. (2008) Detection of human papillomavirus-related squamous cell carcinoma cytologically and by in situ hybridization in fine-needle aspiration biopsies of cervical metastasis: a tool for identifying the site of an occult head and neck primary. *Cancer*, **114**, 118–123.

5 Macdonald, M.R., Freeman, J.L., Hui, M.F., *et al.* (1995) Role of Epstein–Barr virus in fine-needle aspirates of metastatic neck nodes in the diagnosis of nasopharyngeal carcinoma. *Head Neck*, **17**, 487–493.

6 Lee, W.Y., Hsiao, J.R., Jin, Y.T., *et al.* (2000) Epstein–Barr virus detection in neck metastases by in-situ hybridization in fine-needle aspiration cytologic studies: An aid differentiating the primary site. *Head Neck*, **22**, 336–340.

7 Rusthoven, K.E., Koshy, M., Paulino, A.C. (2004) The role of fluorodeoxyglucose positron emission tomography in cervical lymph node metastases from an unknown primary. *Cancer*, **101**, 2641–2649.

8 Johansen, J., Buus, S., Loft, A., *et al.* (2008) Prospective study of 18FDG-PET in the detection and management of patients with lymph node metastases to the neck from an unknown primary tumor. Results from the DAHANCA-13 study. *Head Neck*, **30**, 471–478.

9 Rudmik, L., Lau, H.Y., Matthews, T.W., *et al.* (2011) Clinical utility of PET/CT in the evaluation of head and neck squamous cell carcinoma with an unknown primary: A prospective clinical trial. *Head Neck*, **33**, 935–940.

10 Randall, D.A., Johnstone, P.A., Foss, R.D., *et al.* (2000) Tonsillectomy in diagnosis of the unknown primary tumor of the head and neck. *Otolaryngol. Head Neck Surg.*, **122**, 52–55.

11 Lapeyre, M., Malissard, L., Peiffert, D., *et al.* (1997) Cervical lymph node metastasis from an unknown primary: is a tonsillectomy necessary? *Int. J. Radiat. Oncol. Biol. Phys.*, **39**, 291–296.

12 Waltonen, J.D., Ozer, E., Schuller, D.E., *et al.* (2009) Tonsillectomy vs. deep tonsil biopsies in detecting occult tonsil tumors. *Laryngoscope*, **119**, 102–106.

13 Koch, W.M., Bhatti, N., Williams, M.F., *et al.* (2001) Oncologic rationale for bilateral tonsillectomy in head and neck squamous cell carcinoma of unknown primary source. *Otolaryngol. Head Neck Surg.*, **124**, 331–333.

14 Nagel, T.H., Hinni, M.L., Hayden, R.E., *et al.* (2014) Transoral laser microsurgery for the unknown primary: Role for the lingual tonsillectomy. *Head Neck*, **36**, 942–946.

15 Patel, S.A., Magnuson, J.S., Holsinger, F.C., *et al.* (2013) Robotic surgery for the primary head and neck squamous cell carcinoma of unknown site. *JAMA Otolaryngol. Head Neck Surg.*, **139**, 1203–1211.

16 Durmus, K., Rangarajan, S.V., Old, M.O., *et al.* (2014) Transoral robotic approach to carcinoma of unknown primary. *Head Neck*, **36**, 848–852.

17 Mehta, V., Johnson, P., Tassler, A., *et al.* (2013) A new paradigm for the diagnosis and management of unknown primary tumors of the head and neck: A role for transoral robotic surgery. *Laryngoscope*, **123**, 146–151.

18 Demiroz, C., Vainshtein, J.M., Koukourakis, G.V., *et al.* (2014) Head and neck squamous cell carcinoma of unknown primary: neck dissection and radiotherapy or definitive radiotherapy. *Head Neck*, **36**, 1589–1595.

19 Coster, J.R., Foote, R.L., Olsen, K.D., *et al.* (1992) Cervical nodal metastasis of squamous cell carcinoma of unknown origin: Indications for withholding radiation therapy. *Int. J. Radiat. Oncol. Biol. Phys.*, **23**, 743–749.

20 Ellis, E.R., Mendenhall, W.M., Rao, P.V., *et al.* (1991) Incisional or excisional neck-node biopsy before definitive radiotherapy. *Head Neck*, **13**, 177–183.

21 Mack, Y., Parsons, J.T., Mendenhall, W.M., *et al.* (1993) Squamous cell carcinoma of the head-and-neck: Management after excisional biopsy of a solitary metastatic neck node. *Int. J. Radiat. Oncol. Biol. Phys.*, **25**, 619–622.

22 Argiris, A., Smith, S.M., Stenson, K., *et al.* (2003) Concurrent chemoradiotherapy for N2 or N3 squamous cell carcinoma of the head and neck from an occult primary. *Ann. Oncol.*, **14**, 1306–1311.

23 Shehadeh, N.J., Ensley, J.F., Kucuk, O., *et al.* (2006) Benefit of postoperative chemoradiotherapy for patients with unknown primary squamous cell carcinoma of the head and neck. *Head Neck*, **28**, 1090–1098.

24 Chen, A.M., Farwell, D.G., Lau, D.H., *et al.* (2011) Radiation therapy in the management of head-and-neck cancer of unknown primary origin: How does the addition of concurrent chemotherapy affect the therapeutic ration? *Int. J. Radiat. Oncol. Biol. Phys.*, **81**, 346–352.

25 Pignon, J.P., le Maitre, A., Maillard, E., *et al.* MACH-NC Collaborative Group (2009) Meta-analysis of chemotherapy in head and neck cancer (MACH-NC): An update on 93 randomized trials and 17,346 patients. *Radiother. Oncol.*, **92**, 4–14.

26 Cooper, J.S., Pajak, T.F., Forastiere, A.A., *et al.* (2004) Postoperative concurrent radiotherapy and chemotherapy for high-risk squamous-cell carcinoma of the head and neck. *N. Engl. J. Med.*, **350**, 1937–1944.

27 Bernier, J., Domenge, C., Ozsahin, M., *et al.* (2004) Postoperative irradiation with or without concomitant chemotherapy for locally advanced head and neck cancer. *N. Engl. J. Med.*, **350**, 1945–1952.

28 Chepeha, D., Koch, W., Pitman, K. (2003) Management of unknown primary. *Head Neck*, **25**, 499–504.

29 Friesland, S., Lind, M.G., Lundgren, J., *et al.* (2001) Outcome of ipsilateral treatment for patients with metastases to neck nodes of unknown origin. *Acta Oncol.*, **40**, 24–28.

30 Erkal, H.S., Mendenhall, W.M., Amdur, R.J., *et al.* (2001) Squamous cell carcinoma metastatic to cervical lymph nodes from an unknown head-and-neck mucosal site treated with radiation therapy alone or in combination with neck dissection. *Int. J. Radiat. Oncol. Biol. Phys.*, **50**, 55–63.

31 Aslani, M., Sultanem, K., Voung, T., *et al.* (2007) Metastatic carcinoma to the cervical nodes from unknown head and neck primary site: Is there a need for neck dissection? *Head Neck*, **29**, 585–590.

32 Yao, M., Smith, R.B., Graham, M.M., *et al.* (2005) The role of FDG PET in management of neck metastasis from head-and-neck cancer after definitive radiation treatment. *Int. J. Radiat. Oncol. Biol. Phys.*, **63**, 991–999.

33 Porceddu, S.V., Pryor, D.I., Burmeister, E., *et al.* (2011) Results of a prospective study of positron emission tomography-directed management of residual nodal abnormalities in node-positive head and neck cancer after definitive radiotherapy with or without systemic therapy. *Head Neck*, **33**, 1675–1682.

34 Liauw, S.L., Mancuso, A.A., Amdur, R.J., *et al.* (2006) Postradiotherapy neck dissection for lymph node-positive head and neck cancer: The use of computed tomography to manage the neck. *J. Clin. Oncol.*, **24**, 1421–1427.

35 Nieder, C., Gregoire, V., Ang, K.K. (2001) Cervical lymph node metastases from occult squamous cell carcinoma: Cut down a tree to get an apple? *Int. J. Radiat. Oncol. Biol. Phys.*, **50**, 727–733.

36 Mendenhall, W.M., Mancuso, A.A., Amdur, R.J., *et al.* (2001) Squamous cell carcinoma metastatic to the neck from an unknown head and neck primary site. *Am. J. Otolaryngol.*, **22**, 261–267.

37 Barker, C.A., Morris, C.G., Mendenhall, W.M. (2005) Larynx-sparing radiotherapy for squamous cell carcinoma from an unknown head and neck primary site. *Am. J. Clin. Oncol.*, **28**, 445–448.

38 Werner, J.A., Dunne, A.A., Myers, J.N. (2003) Functional anatomy of the lymphatic drainage system of the upper aerodigestive tract and its role in metastasis of squamous cell carcinoma. *Head Neck*, **25**, 322–332.

39 Lee, N., Mechalakos, J., Puri, D.R., *et al.* (2007) Choosing an intensity-modulated radiation therapy technique in the treatment of head-and-neck cancer. *Int. J. Radiat. Oncol. Biol. Phys.*, **68**, 1299–1309.

40 Dabaja, B., Salehpour, M.R., Rosen, I., *et al.* (2005) Intensity-modulated radiation therapy (IMRT) of cancers of the head and neck: Comparison of split-field and whole-field techniques. *Int. J. Radiat. Oncol. Biol. Phys.*, **63**, 1000–1005.

41 http://www.nccn.org/professionals/physician_gls/pdf/head-and-neck.pdf.

42 Klem, M.L., Mechalakos, J.G., Wolden, S.L., *et al.* (2008) Intensity-modulated radiotherapy for head and neck cancer of unknown primary: Toxicity and preliminary efficacy. *Int. J. Radiat. Oncol. Biol. Phys.*, **70**, 1100–1107.

43 Lu, H., Yao, M., Tan, H. (2009) Unknown primary head and neck cancer treated with intensity-modulated radiation therapy: To what extent the volume should be irradiated. *Oral Oncol.*, **45**, 474–479.

44 Frank, S.J., Rosenthal, D.I., Petsuksiri, J., *et al.* (2010) Intensity-modulated radiotherapy for cervical node squamous cell carcinoma metastases from unknown head-and-neck primary site: M.D. Anderson Cancer Center outcomes and patterns of failure. *Int. J. Radiat. Oncol. Biol. Phys.*, **78**, 1005–1010.

45 Chen, A.M., Li, B.Q., Farwell, D.G., *et al.* (2011) Improved dosimetric and clinical outcomes with intensity-modulated radiotherapy for head-and-neck cancer of unknown primary origin. *Int. J. Radiat. Oncol. Biol. Phys.*, **79**, 756–762.

46 Madani, I., Vakaet, L., Bonte, K., *et al.* (2008) Intensity-modulated radiotherapy for cervical lymph node metastases from unknown primary cancer. *Int. J. Radiat. Oncol. Biol. Phys.*, **71**, 1158–1166.

47 Mourad, W.F., Hu, K., Shasha, D., *et al.* (2014) Initial experience with oropharynx-targeted radiation therapy for metastatic squamous cell carcinoma of unknown primary of the head and neck. *Anticancer Res.*, **34**, 243–248.

48 Chaturvedi, A.K., Engels, E.A., Pfeiffer, R.M., *et al.* (2011) Human papillomavirus and rising oropharyngeal cancer incidence in the united states. *J. Clin. Oncol.*, **29**, 4294–4301.

49 Keller, L.M., Galloway, T.J., Holdbrook, T., *et al.* (2014) P16 status, pathologic and clinical characteristics, biomolecular signature, and long-term outcomes in head and neck squamous cell carcinoma of unknown primary. *Head Neck*, **36**, 1677–1684.

50 Fotopoulos, G., Pavlidis, N. (2015) The role of human papilloma virus and p16 in occult primary of the head and neck: A comprehensive review of the literature. *Oral Oncol.*, **51**, 119–123.

51 Mirghani, H., Amen, F., Blanchard, P. *et al.* (2015) Treatment de-escalation in HPV-positive oropharyngeal carcinoma: ongoing trials, critical issues and perspectives. *Int. J. Cancer*, **136**, 1494–1503.

52 Graboyes, E.M., Sinha, P., Thorstad, W.L., *et al.* (2015) Management of human papilloma-related unknown primaries of the head and neck with a transoral surgical approach. *Head Neck*, **37**, 1603–1611.

16

Temporal Bone Tumors

Allen M. Chen

Introduction

The temporal bones are situated at the sides and base of the skull, and immediately lateral to the temporal lobes of the brain. Supporting the part of the face known as the temple, each temporal bone consists of five parts: the squama temporalis; petrous portion; mastoid portion; tympanic part; and the styloid process. The temporal bone is intimately associated with the structures forming the ear including the external auditory canal, cochlea, and inner ear.

Malignant tumors arising from the temporal bone (i.e., external auditory canal, middle ear, or mastoid) are extremely rare. Their incidence is estimated to be approximately one case per 10 000–20 000 otologic pathologic conditions [1]. Notably, chronic otitis externa and otorrhea are often associated with carcinoma of the external auditory canal. Additionally, approximately one-fourth of carcinomas of the middle ear and mastoid are superimposed with cholesteatoma formation [2]. Various histological types are diagnosed, including squamous cell carcinoma, basal cell carcinoma, adenoid cystic carcinoma, myoepithelioma, adenocarcinoma, and poorly differentiated carcinoma. Squamous cell carcinoma is the most common malignant tumor of the external auditory canal (EAC). Benign tumors adjacent to the temporal area are also common and include paraganglioma, schwannoma, meningioma, and vascular tumors.

Lymphatic Drainage

The lymphatic drainage of tumors arising over the temporal bone or ear structures are to the level II cervical lymph nodes, periparotid and facial lymph nodes, pre- and post-auricular lymph nodes, and less commonly to the mastoid region and inferior cervical lymph nodes (levels III and IV).

In squamous cell carcinoma of the EAC, the reported incidence of lymph node metastasis ranged from 10% to 23% [3–5]. Lymph node metastasis is a poor prognostic factor, indicating aggressiveness of the tumors.

Diagnosis and Staging

The most common presenting symptoms are offensive otorrhea, pain, and bleeding [5]. Patients are often treated as having chronic external otitis or chronic otitis, and often have an average six-month delay in diagnosis. Therefore, a high suspicion is necessary for early diagnosis, especially in patients with prolonged external otitis despite routine measures. Patients may have a polypoid lesion or ulcerative lesion in the EAC, with poor hearing due to obstruction of the canal. A full head and neck examination is performed, including an assessment of cranial nerve function and cervical lymphadenopathy, and nasopharyngolaryngoscopy with special attention paid to assess the nasopharynx. Computed tomography (CT) and magnetic resonance imaging (MRI) of the head and neck are recommended to fully evaluate tumor extent and the status of the regional lymph nodes. In addition, a dedicated fine-cut temporal bone CT with soft tissue and bone protocol will provide further information of the tumor extent.

Tumors of the temporal bone are not included in the American Joint Committee on Cancer (AJCC) staging system, although the criteria designed for skin carcinomas is often used in this capacity [6]. However, the AJCC staging system for skin cancers is of limited utility since the overwhelming majority of patients with temporal bone tumors would be classified as T4. Hence, various other staging systems are in use today, the two most popular being the Stell–McCormick and Arriga systems [3,7]. As outlined in Tables 16.1 and 16.2, both of these

Clinical Radiation Oncology: Indications, Techniques, and Results, Third Edition. Edited by William Small Jr.
© 2017 John Wiley & Sons, Inc. Published 2017 by John Wiley & Sons, Inc.

Table 16.1 The Stell–McCormick staging system.

T stage	Description
T1	Tumor limited to site of origin (*i.e.*, with no facial nerve paralysis and no bone destruction on radiography)
T2	Tumor extending beyond the site of origin indicated by facial paralysis or radiologic evidence of bone destruction, but no extension beyond the organ of origin
T3	Clinical or radiologic evidence of extension to surrounding structures (*i.e.*, dura, base of the skull, parotid gland, temporomandibular joint)
TX	Patients with insufficient data for classification, including patients previously treated elsewhere

Source: Moody, Hirsch, and Myers [4]. Reproduced with permission of Elsevier.

staging systems account for the degree of local tumor infiltration and correlate roughly with the extent of surgical resection required for gross tumor clearance.

Selection of Therapy

Because of the rarity of these tumors, treatments vary greatly across institutions. For example, radical surgery and radiation therapy are employed, alone or in combination. Although limited to relatively small single institutional series, most published data suggest that most malignant lesions benefit from a combined modality approach incorporating surgery and postoperative radiation therapy. Except in early lesions without evidence of bone destruction, primary radiation therapy is generally not recommended as first-line treatment. The type

Table 16.2 The Arriaga staging system.

T stage	Description
T1	Tumor limited to the external auditory canal without bony erosion or evidence of soft tissue extension
T2	Tumor with limited external auditory canal bony erosion (not full thickness) or radiographic finding consistent with limited (<0.5 cm) soft tissue involvement
T3	Tumor eroding the osseous external auditory canal (full thickness) with limited (<0.5 cm) soft tissue involvement, or tumor involving middle ear and/or mastoid, or patients presenting with facial paralysis
T4	Tumor eroding the cochlea, petrous apex, medial wall of middle ear, carotid canal, jugular foramen, or dura, or with extensive (>0.5 cm) soft tissue involvement

Source: Moffat, Wagstaff, and Hardy 2005 [5]. Reproduced with permission of John Wiley & Sons, Inc.

of surgery generally depends on the extent of tumor, with T1 cancers often amenable to partial temporal bone resection, and larger more destructive lesions requiring subtotal/total temporal bone resections with mastoidectomy. Some authors have also suggested superficial parotidectomy as a component of all *en-bloc* resections due to the relatively high likelihood of tumor spreading to the preauricular soft tissue (via the fissures of Santorini), periparotid lymph nodes, and the glenoid fossa of the temporomandibular joint [8–10]. Moffat *et al.* [5] advocated including a supraomohyoid neck dissection for all patients with squamous cell carcinoma for staging and facilitation of the resection and flap reconstruction, as well as postoperative radiation treatment. Regardless of the type of surgery utilized, the ability to achieve a gross total tumor resection appears to convey an improved prognosis [11–13].

However, due to the location of many of these tumors in the temporal bone, gross total resection can often be difficult to achieve. Even for benign tumors such as paraganglioma limited to the middle ear, surgical removal may be possible, but it is often incomplete and followed by local recurrence or disease persistence [14]. Furthermore, large tumors extending intracranially are rarely amenable to curative treatment by surgical removal. In these cases, definitive radiation therapy may be an option for patients with residual or recurrent disease after radical mastoidectomy and/or temporal bone resection, or for inoperable lesions.

Radiation Technique

Due to the proximity of the temporal bone to several critical structures in the head and neck region – including the eyes, ears, and brain – radiation therapy calls for meticulous technique. Although ipsilateral wedge-paired or anteroposterior (AP)-posteroanterior (PA) portals with megavoltage radiation and appositional electron boost was historically employed in delivering a uniform dosage throughout the entire tumor-bearing volume in the temporal bone, the use of intensity-modulated radiation therapy (IMRT) has largely supplanted this technique due to its ability to achieve a superior dose distribution and spare designated organs at risk. When electrons are utilized, a customized water bolus placed in the external ear canal can decrease the dose heterogeneity caused by auricular surface irregularities [15].

Regardless of the chosen technique, attention must be directed to sufficiently covering all potential paths of tumor spread. CT is imperative to delineate the petrosal bone, periparotid lymph nodes, retroauricular, upper jugular, and spinal accessory lymph nodes. In the setting of perineural invasion, consideration should also be given to covering the facial nerve to the stylomastoid foramen.

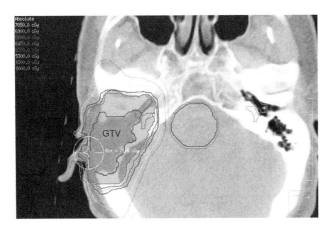

Figure 16.1 Intensity-modulated radiation therapy plan for a 75-year-old male who presented with a large squamous cell carcinoma involving the skin of the right temporal face. Notably, the patient had previously been treated to a dose of 70 Gy with cisplatin for squamous cell carcinoma of the oropharynx four years previously. He refused surgical resection for his new primary cancer and was treated with radiation to a dose of 66 Gy delivered to 95% of the planning target volume encompassing gross disease. Visible organs at risk on this axial section include the ipsilateral auditory structures (in the high-dose planning target volume), contralateral auditory structures, and brainstem. GTV, gross tumor volume. For a color version of this figure, see the color plate section.

For postoperative patients, a careful review of all preoperative imaging, operative notes, and pathology reports is crucial to appropriately ensure coverage of all target tissue. The use of MRI fusion is highly recommended to visualize all areas at highest risk for recurrence in the skull base.

When IMRT is selected, the planning target volume encompasses all gross tumor (or the surgical bed in postoperative patients) with margin to account for microscopic disease extension and daily set-up error (Figures 16.1–16.2). The ipsilateral upper neck (level II) and periparotid region is typically included in the field. In selected cases (e.g., positive cervical lymph nodes), the targets should be expanded to include the remainder of the ipsilateral neck to the supraclavicular fossa. Organs at risk should include the brainstem, temporal lobes, spinal cord, optic apparatus, oral cavity, larynx, and brachial plexus. Attention should particularly focus on sparing the contralateral parotid gland and ear structures. The use of image-guided radiotherapy (IGRT) may be particularly useful for temporal bone tumors, given its ability to visualize soft tissue during treatment and accurately verify dose delivery [16].

For patients treated postoperatively, the recommended dose ranges from 60 Gy (negative margins) to 66 Gy (positive microscopic margins) to 70 Gy (gross residual disease). For patients treated definitively, the minimum dose that should be used is 70 Gy. However, care must be taken to balance the potential benefits of aggressive radiotherapeutic treatment with possible toxicity.

The role of *chemotherapy* in the absence of distant metastatic disease is considered largely investigational. Results from a recently published prospective Phase II trial from France suggested that single-agent cetuximab has efficacy as first-line treatment of unresectable squamous cell carcinoma of the skin [17]. Among 36 patients treated with cetuximab monotherapy, an encouraging 69% had their disease controlled at six weeks. These results suggest that combining cetuximab with radiation therapy may be of value and should be tested in future trials.

Outcomes

Prabhu *et al.* reported on 30 patients with squamous cell carcinoma of the external auditory canal treated either with radiation therapy alone or combined with surgical resection between 1976 and 2003 [18]. Wedge-pair fields were used for all patients, with a median dose of 70 Gy. Patients with advanced tumors also received ipsilateral elective neck irradiation. The local-regional control at five years was 48%, and complications included two cases of osteoradionecrosis involving the temporal bone. In another analysis of 87 patients treated with radiation therapy, Ogawa *et al.* reported five-year disease-free survival rates of 83%, 55% and 38% among those with negative surgical margins, those with positive margins, and those with macroscopic residual disease, respectively [19]. Most recently, Chen *et al.* examined patterns of failure among 11 patients treated with postoperative IMRT for squamous cell carcinoma of the external auditory canal and middle ear [20]. Although the two-year local-regional rate was 71%, three cases of marginal recurrences were observed due to inadequate delineation of the clinical target volume. These were spatially located near the preauricular space and glenoid fossa of the temporomandibular joint, adjacent to the apex of the ear canal and glenoid fossa of the temporomandibular joint, and in the postauricular subcutaneous area and ipsilateral parotid nodes.

Complications

Acute and late skin reactions involving the pinna, external auditory canal, and periauricular region are commonly described side effects of radiation therapy to the region of the temporal bone. Acute events, including erythema, desquamation and, rarely, ulceration of the skin, can be managed conservatively with skin creams and

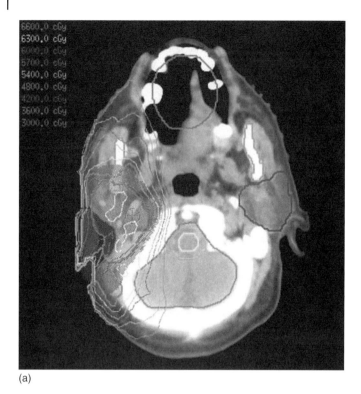

(a)

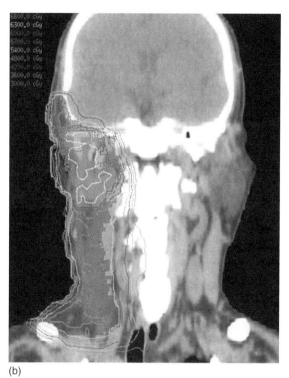

(b)

Figure 16.2 Intensity-modulated radiation therapy (IMRT) plan for a 55-year-old male who was status post gross total resection consisting of partial temporal bone resection and auriculectomy for squamous cell carcinoma of the external ear canal. The patient was subsequently treated to a total dose of 60 Gy to the tumor bed and 54 Gy to high-risk ipsilateral neck, respectively, using a simultaneous-integrated boost technique. Water bolus was employed to fill the surgical defect. (a) Visible organs at risk on this axial section include the oral cavity, spinal cord, brain, brainstem, and contralateral parotid gland. (b) Coronal view of the IMRT plan. For a color version of this figure, see the color plate section.

anti-inflammatory medication. Otitis media and externa often require the use of antibiotics. Late skin changes including atrophy, fibrosis, and external canal stenosis have also been reported. Although rare, temporal bone necrosis is a potentially devastating complication after radiation therapy to this region. Due to the location of the temporal bone within the skull base, necrosis is rarely amenable to surgical intervention and may lead to death of the patient [21]. To minimize this complication, it is recommended to limit the volume of total bone exposed to greater than 70 Gy, whenever possible.

Problems with hearing and balance represent the most serious side effects of radiation therapy to the region of the temporal bone. Although the use of IMRT can likely minimize dose to the auditory and vestibular structures, exposure to these areas are frequently unavoidable (Figure 16.1). However, in view of several recently published studies identifying a dose–response relationship for the inner and middle ear, the importance of minimizing dose to these organs at risk is becoming increasingly recognized among those undergoing radiotherapy for head and neck cancer [22–25]. Sensorineural hearing loss, traditionally defined as a clinically significant increase in bone conduction threshold at the key

human speech frequencies (0.5 to 4.0 kHz), has been shown to occur in approximately one-third of patients treated by definitive radiation with fields, including the inner ear [26,27]. In a prospective study of 40 patients, Pan *et al.* showed that clinically apparent hearing loss greater than 10 dB occurred when the cochlea received mean doses in excess of 45 Gy [22]. Honore *et al.* similarly developed a model predictive of sensorineural hearing loss based on pre-therapy dosimetric and clinical outcomes data of 20 patients treated with radiotherapy for nasopharyngeal carcinoma [23]. Notably, when the model was adjusted for age and pre-therapy hearing level, a steep dose–response curve emerged with a threshold at approximately 40 Gy. Although questions exist regarding the time course of hearing loss after radiotherapy and whether the dose–response relationship for toxicity to the auditory structures is linear or sigmoid shaped, general agreement exists that doses to the inner and middle ear should be closely monitored [24–27]. The Quantitative Analysis of Normal Tissue Effects in the Clinic (QUANTEC) reviews, published in 2010, recommends limiting the mean cochlear dose to less than 45 Gy to minimize the risk for sensorineural hearing loss [28].

References

1 Lewis, J.S. (1981) Cancer of the external auditory canal, middle ear, and mastoid, in *Cancer of the Head and Neck* (eds J.Y. Suen, E.N. Myers). Churchill-Livingstone, New York, pp. 561–562.

2 Lewis, J.S. (1972) Squamous cell carcinoma of the ear. *Arch. Otolaryngol.*, **97**, 41–42.

3 Stell, P.M., McCormick, M.S. (1985) Carcinoma of the external auditory meatus and middle ear. Prognostic factors and a suggested staging system. *J. Laryngol. Otol.*, **99**, 847–850.

4 Moody, S.A., Hirsch, B.E., Myers, E.N. (2000) Squamous cell carcinoma of the external auditory canal: an evaluation of a staging system. *Am. J. Otol.*, **21**, 582–588.

5 Moffat, D.A., Wagstaff, S.A., Hardy, D.G. (2005) The outcome of radical surgery and postoperative radiotherapy for squamous carcinoma of the temporal bone. *Laryngoscope*, **115**, 341–347.

6 Edge, S.B., Byrd, D.R., Compton, C.C., et al. (2010) *AJCC Cancer Staging Manual*, 7th edition. Springer-Verlag, New York.

7 Arriaga, M., Curtin, H., Takahashi, H., et al. (1990) Staging proposal for external auditory meatus carcinoma based on preoperative clinical examination and computed tomography findings. *Ann. Otol. Rhinol. Laryngol.*, **99**, 714–721.

8 Choi, J.Y., Choi, E.C., Lee, H.K., et al. (2003) Mode of parotid involvement in external auditory canal carcinoma. *J. Laryngol. Otol.*, **117**, 951–954.

9 Leonetti, J.P., Smith, P.G., Kletzker, G.R., et al. (1996) Invasion patterns of advanced temporal bone malignancies. *Am. J. Otol.*, **17**, 438–442.

10 Gacek, R.R., Goodman, M. (1977) Management of malignancy of the temporal bone. *Laryngoscope*, **87**, 1622–1634.

11 Pfreundner, L., Schwager, K., Willner, J., et al. (1999) Carcinoma of the external auditory canal and middle ear. *Int. J. Radiat. Oncol. Biol. Phys.*, **44**, 777–788.

12 Chang, C., Shu, M., Lee, J., et al. (2009) Treatments and outcomes of malignant tumors of external auditory canal. *Am. J. Otol.*, **30**, 44–48.

13 Nyrop, M., Grontved, A. (2002) Cancer of the external auditory canal. *Arch. Otolaryngol. Head Neck Surg.*, **128**, 834–847.

14 Simko, T.G., Griffin, T.W., Gerdes, A.J., et al. (1978) The role of radiation therapy in the treatment of glomus jugulares tumors. *Cancer*, **42**, 104–106.

15 Morrison, W.H., Wong, P.F., Starkschall, G., et al. (1995) Water bolus for electron irradiation of the ear. *Int. J. Radiat. Oncol. Biol. Phys.*, **33**, 479–483.

16 Chen, A.M., Cheng, S., Farwell, D.G., et al. (2012) Utility of daily image guidance with intensity-modulated radiotherapy for tumors of the base of skull. *Head Neck*, **34**, 763–770.

17 Maubec, E., Petrow, S., Scheer-Senyarich, I., et al. (2011) Phase II study of cetuximab as first-line single drug therapy in patients with unresectable squamous cell carcinoma of the skin. *J. Clin. Oncol.*, **29**, 3419–3426.

18 Prabhu, R., Hinerman, R.W., Indelicato, D.J., et al. (2009) Squamous cell carcinoma of the external auditory canal: Long term clinical outcomes using surgery and external-beam radiotherapy. *Am. J. Clin. Oncol.*, **32**, 401–404.

19 Ogawa, K., Nakamura, K., Hatano, K., et al. (2007) Treatment and prognosis of squamous cell carcinoma of the external auditory canal and middle ear: A multi-institutional retrospective review of 87 patients. *Int. J. Radiat. Oncol. Biol. Phys.*, **68**, 1326–1334.

20 Chen, W.Y., Kuo, S.H., Chen, Y.H., et al. (2012) Postoperative intensity-modulated radiotherapy for squamous cell carcinoma of the external auditory canal and middle ear: Treatment outcomes, marginal misses, and perspective on target delineation. *Int. J. Radiat. Oncol. Biol. Phys.*, **15**, 1485–1493.

21 Wang, C.C., Doppke, K. (1976) Osteoradionecrosis of the temporal bone: Consideration of nominal standard dose. *Int. J. Radiat. Oncol. Biol. Phys.*, **1**, 881–883.

22 Pan, C.C., Eisbruch, A., Lee, J.S., et al. (2005) Prospective study of inner ear radiation dose and hearing loss in head-and-neck cancer patients. *Int. J. Radiat. Oncol. Biol. Phys.*, **61**, 1393–1402.

23 Honore, H.B., Bentzen, S.M., Moller, K., et al. (2002) Sensorineural hearing loss after radiotherapy for nasopharyngeal carcinoma: individualized risk estimation. *Radiother. Oncol.*, **65**, 9–16.

24 Chen, W.C., Jackson, A., Budnick, A.S., et al. (2006) Sensorineural hearing loss in combined modality treatment of nasopharyngeal carcinoma. *Cancer*, **106**, 820–829.

25 Ho, W.K., Wei, W.I., Kwong, D.L., et al. (1999) Long-term sensorineural hearing loss in patients treated for nasopharyngeal carcinoma: a prospective study of the effect of radiation and cisplatin treatment. *Int. J. Radiat. Oncol. Biol. Phys.*, **21**, 547–553.

26 Ondrey, F.G., Greig, J.R., Herscher, L. (2000) Radiation dose to otologic structures during head and neck cancer radiation therapy. *Laryngoscope*, **110**, 217–221.

27 Kwong, D., Wei, W., Sham, J., et al. (1996) Sensorineural hearing loss in patients treated for nasopharyngeal cancer: a prospective study of the effect of radiation and cisplatin treatment. *Int. J. Radiat. Oncol. Biol. Phys.*, **36**, 281–289.

28 Bhandare, N., Jackson, A., Eisbruch, A., et al. (2010) Radiation therapy and hearing loss. *Int. J. Radiat. Oncol. Biol. Phys.*, **76**, S50–S57.

17

Thyroid Cancer

Roi Dagan and Robert J. Amdur

Background and Epidemiology

Thyroid cancer is the most commonly diagnosed endocrine malignancy, with an estimated 56 870 new diagnoses and 2010 deaths in the United States in 2017 [1]. The overall incidence is 7.7 per 100 000 person-years [2]. It is the fifth most common malignancy in women, accounting for approximately 5% of all new female cancer diagnoses [3]. The incidence of thyroid cancer has increased in the United States from a rate of 3.6 per 100 000 in 1973 to 8.7 per 100 000 in 2002. This increase is due to a rise in the diagnosis of small (1- to 2-cm) papillary thyroid carcinomas (PTCs) [4]. Thyroid nodules, the most common presenting symptom of thyroid cancer, affect 3–4% of the normal population, and the incidence at autopsy has been reported as high as 50% [5–7]. There is a wide spectrum of benign and malignant thyroid neoplasms, including benign cysts, colloid nodules, adenomas, carcinomas, lymphomas, sarcomas, and metastatic tumors. Thyroid sarcomas and lymphomas are best managed under paradigms that are addressed in the chapters dedicated to these tumors, and will not be addressed here. The remainder of this chapter will focus strictly on thyroid carcinoma.

Anatomy and Physiology of the Thyroid

Gross Anatomy

The average adult thyroid gland measures approximately 5×5 cm and weighs 10–20 g. It is located in the central anterior neck at the cervical–thoracic junction. There are two lateral lobes connected by a central isthmus, and 50% of individuals have a pyramidal lobe that extends superiorly from the central aspect of the gland. The lateral lobes extend superiorly to the level of the mid-thyroid cartilage overlying the larynx and inferiorly to the 6th tracheal ring. The thyroid gland wraps around 75% of the tracheal circumference and encroaches on the esophagus at its posterior extent. It is bordered laterally by the common carotid arteries. The recurrent laryngeal nerves, sympathetic trunk, vagus, and phrenic nerves are all found immediately posterior to the gland, and anteriorly it is bordered by the strap muscles. Parathyroid glands are located posterior to the thyroid gland and vary in location and number. The location of the thyroid gland, and its relationship to adjacent structures, is shown in Figure 17.1.

Microscopic Anatomy

Most of the normal thyroid tissue is comprised of follicles, which form the structural and functional unit of the gland. The follicular surface epithelium produces thyroid hormone and thyroglobulin (Tg), which are stored as colloid in a central lumen within each follicle. The follicular epithelial cell is the cell of origin for 95% of all thyroid carcinomas. Parafollicular, or C cells, are neural crest-derived cells containing granules of calcitonin, which are the cell of origin for medullary thyroid carcinoma (MTC).

Lymphatics

A dense network of capillary lymphatics drains the thyroid gland to the central and bilateral cervical lymph nodes. The first-echelon nodes for thyroid cancer metastases are located in level 6 (the central or 'visceral' compartment) between the hyoid bone and the thoracic inlet. Specifically, these are the paralaryngeal, paratracheal, and prelaryngeal (Delphian) nodes. Second-echelon nodal spread is to the mid and lower cervical nodes (levels 3 and 4), supraclavicular nodes, anterior and posterior upper mediastinal nodes, and to a lesser extent the upper cervical nodes (level 2). Retropharyngeal node involvement is unusual but can be

Clinical Radiation Oncology: Indications, Techniques, and Results, Third Edition. Edited by William Small Jr.
© 2017 John Wiley & Sons, Inc. Published 2017 by John Wiley & Sons, Inc.

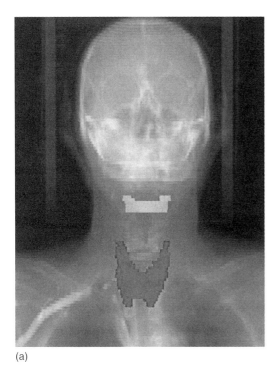
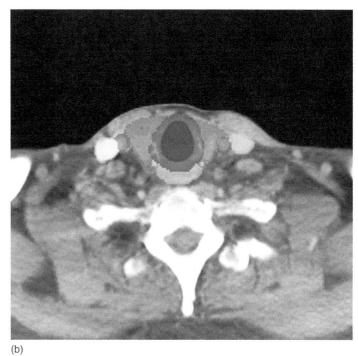

(a)   (b)

Figure 17.1 Anatomy of the thyroid gland. (a) Digitally reconstructed radiograph of a patient's head and neck showing the relative position of the thyroid gland (blue) to the hyoid bone (green) and bottom of the cricoid cartilage (purple). (b) Contrast-enhanced axial computed tomography (CT) slice at the level of the bottom of the cricoid cartilage (purple) showing the position of the thyroid gland (blue) relative to the esophagus (orange), carotid arteries (red), jugular vein (lavender) and the approximate position of the recurrent laryngeal nerves (yellow-green). *Source:* Halperin *et al.* 2013. Reproduced with permission of Wolters Kluwer Health. For a color version of this figure, see the color plate section.

encountered in the setting of advanced nodal disease. Level 1 (submental and submandibular) lymph nodes are rarely involved [8].

Physiology

The thyroid serves a critical endocrine function essential for development as well as metabolic and calcium homeostasis. The primary physiologic role is the production of thyroid hormone. A secondary role is the production of calcitonin, a hormone essential in calcium homeostasis. The follicular cells of the thyroid gland synthesize and secrete Tg and thyroid hormone, the latter of which targets virtually all cells in the body. In target cells, thyroid hormone is transported to the nucleus, where it binds to specific nuclear receptors and interacts with regulatory genes, influencing their expression. The gene products ultimately increase the cell's basal metabolic rate, protein synthesis, catecholamine effects, growth of long bones and plays an essential role in protein, fat, and carbohydrate metabolism.

Iodine is a critical component of thyroid hormone and is essential for thyroid function. The follicular cells of the thyroid gland possess a unique ability to actively uptake and concentrate iodine through the action of a sodium iodine symporter (NaIS). Thyrotropin, otherwise known as thyroid-stimulating hormone (TSH), which is synthesized and secreted by the anterior pituitary, stimulates the activity of NaIS. Functional NaIS is retained in malignant follicular cells seen in most forms of differentiated thyroid cancer (DTC). The iodine-concentrating capacity of these cells makes radioactive iodine (RAI) a potent targeted cytotoxic therapy. NaIS is also present in the parotid glands, breast tissues, gastric mucosa, and nasolacrimal ducts, placing them at risk for injury from RAI.

As previously mentioned, thyroid follicular epithelial cells also produce Tg, a large (660-kDa) glycoprotein which binds and stores iodine. Iodinated Tg is the main component of colloid. The vast majority of DTC retains the ability to synthesize and secrete Tg, making serum Tg a valuable tumor marker.

Classification of Thyroid Carcinomas

Appropriate pathologic classification is fundamental to managing thyroid carcinoma. The various classes are associated with a unique biology, natural history, and prognosis, and largely influence the available therapeutic

Table 17.1 A system of pathological classification for thyroid carcinoma.

I. Arising from follicular epithelial cell
  A. Differentiated Thyroid Carcinoma
    1. Papillary and mixed papillary variants
      a. Classic papillary carcinoma
      b. Papillary microcarcinoma
      c. Encapsulated variant
      d. Follicular variant
      e. Aggressive variants
        i. Diffuse sclerosing
        ii. Tall Cell variant
        iii. Columnar cell variant
    2. Follicular Carcinoma
      a. Classic morphology – Follicular carcinoma
      b. Hurthle Cell variant
  B. Poorly differentiated thyroid carcinoma
    a. Insular Carcinoma
  C. Undifferentiated thyroid carcinoma (Anaplastic carcinoma)
II. Arising from parafollicular Cell (C-cell)
  A. Medullary carcinoma

Source: Halperin *et al.* 2013. Reproduced with permission of Wolters Kluwer Health.

options. A system of classification based on the cell of origin, cytological features, and growth morphology is presented in Table 17.1.

Differentiated (Follicular-derived) Thyroid Carcinoma (DTC)

The two major subgroups comprising DTC are papillary thyroid carcinoma (PTC) and follicular carcinoma (FC), which are distinguished by architectural and cytological features.

Papillary Thyroid Carcinoma

This is the most common class of thyroid cancer, comprising 80–90% of all diagnoses [9]. The diagnosis is based on nuclear cytological characteristics, including nuclear enlargement, hypochromasia, intranuclear cytoplasmic inclusions (nuclear pseudoinclusions), nuclear grooves, and distinct nucleoli. All PTCs stain strongly for Tg and concentrate iodine [9–12].

The term papillary 'microcarcinoma' is used to describe incidentally identified papillary carcinomas measuring <1.0 cm in diameter; these have the most favorable prognosis of all thyroid carcinomas. Follicular-type PTC differs from the classic variant by its follicular growth pattern; however, it retains the hallmark nuclear features of PTC and has a similarly good prognosis. A less-favorable prognosis is associated with diffuse sclerosing, tall cell, and columnar cell PTC.

Follicular Carcinoma (FC)

Like classic PTC, FC bears a favorable prognosis. FC presents a diagnostic challenge since this cancer lacks the cytological features of PTC and is often grossly indistinguishable from benign follicular adenomas. The diagnosis is dependent on invasion through the entire tumor capsule or into a blood vessel located in the tumor capsule or immediately outside of the tumor capsule.

Hürthle Cell Carcinoma

Also referred to as oncocytic carcinoma, this follicular epithelial-derived carcinoma is characterized by large cells with abundant granular eosinophilic cytoplasms. Hürthle cells may be present in both benign thyroid lesions and non-Hürthle cell cancers. They must comprise at least 75% of tumor cells for the designation of Hürthle cell carcinoma. While Hürthle cell carcinoma is classically considered a variant of FC, it is now apparent that there are both follicular and papillary types. Hürthle cell carcinoma carries a relatively poor prognosis and usually presents with large tumor size, more invasive features, and early regional and distant metastatic spread. These tumors are also less likely to concentrate RAI.

Poorly Differentiated Thyroid Carcinoma (Insular Carcinoma)

These are follicular epithelial cell-derived tumors that display a more-aggressive histological appearance and biological behavior than DTC, although not as aggressive as anaplastic thyroid carcinoma (ATC). Histologically, the tumor cells are usually arranged in discrete nests separated by a fibrous stroma. These tumors are usually solid with some evidence of follicle formation and possibly gross extraglandular extension. Mitoses and necrosis are often present.

Undifferentiated (Anaplastic) Thyroid Carcinoma (ATC)

ATC is rare, accounting for less than 5% of all thyroid cancers mostly affecting patients aged over 65 years. These tumors are the most aggressive form of thyroid carcinoma and are implicated in up to 50% of all thyroid cancer deaths [13]. ATC originates from the thyroid follicular epithelium but shows little to no differentiation. Gross pathologic evaluation is characterized by widely infiltrative disease with areas of necrosis and hemorrhage. There are several different microscopic patterns described, including small cell, spindle cell, giant cell, squamoid, or pleomorphic variants. This tumor is defined as much by its clinical behavior as its histologic appearance with most patients presenting with widely invasive disease replacing most, if not all, of the normal-appearing gland and freely infiltrating into surrounding

Table 17.2 A system of classification for thyroid cancer based on the ability to concentrate RAI.

A. Usually concentrate RAI
    I. Classic papillary carcinoma
    II. Encapsulated papillary carcinoma
    III. Follicular variant and mixed follicular-papillary carcinoma
    IV. Follicular carcinoma
B. Frequently do not concentrate RAI
    I. Tall cell and columnar cell variants of papillary carcinoma
    II. Hürthle cell carcinoma
    III. Poorly differentiated (insular) carcinoma
C. Never concentrate RAI
    I. Anaplastic carcinoma
    II. Medullary carcinoma

RAI, Radioactive iodine
Source: Halperin *et al.* 2013. Reproduced with permission of Wolters Kluwer Health.

tissues. Bulky metastatic lymphadenopathy and distant metastatic spread is usually seen at the time of diagnosis.

Medullary Thyroid Carcinoma (MTC)

MTC originates from the parafollicular C cells and comprises less than 5–10% of all thyroid cancers. The presentation can be either sporadic (80%) or in association with familial multiple endocrine neoplasia syndromes (MEN IIa, IIb, and pure familial MTC), which are histologically indistinguishable. Grossly, these tumors are often encapsulated. Microscopically, the tumor may display a solid or nested growth pattern and may contain amyloid. Calcitonin stains are usually positive and are specific for MTC, but up to 20% of cases may not stain for calcitonin. In such cases, other neuroendocrine markers such as chromogrannin may be useful.

Classification Based on the Capacity to Concentrate RAI

Since RAI plays a central role in the management of thyroid cancer, it is also useful to distinguish classes of thyroid carcinoma based on their ability to concentrate iodine (Table 17.2).

Diagnostic Evaluation of Thyroid Cancer

Laboratory Studies

During the evaluation of thyroid nodules, all patients should have serum TSH level determined. Serum levels of Tg, T3, and T4 are commonly monitored, but are rarely useful in the initial management of thyroid cancer. Serum

calcitonin can be measured during the initial evaluation of patients with MTC, and is essential during follow-up for these patients. Otherwise, all patients should have a basic metabolic panel and blood counts drawn before therapy.

Imaging Studies

Thyroid and Cervical Ultrasound

Ultrasound (US) with Doppler and US-guided fine-needle aspiration (FNA) biopsy are the most appropriate studies for evaluation of thyroid nodules. Features suggestive of malignancy that warrant FNA include size (>1 cm), rounding, hypoechoiety, microcalcifications, indistinct or irregular margins, increased Doppler flow, invasion of surrounding tissue, or presence of suspicious lymph nodes. Growing lesions lacking these features should also be biopsied. For a detailed discussion on US in the evaluation of thyroid nodules, reference should be made to a consensus statement by the Society of Radiologists in Ultrasound [14] and the recently updated American Thyroid Association's (ATA) management guidelines for patients with thyroid nodules and DTC [15].

FNA is favored as a means of establishing tissue diagnosis of thyroid nodules over more invasive biopsies, since most cancers will contain definitive cytologic features. The sensitivity and specificity range from 87% to 100% and 67% to 98%, respectively [16,17]. The major limitation of FNA is its inability to distinguish malignant follicular lesions from benign adenomas. FNA cytology is classified into four categories: (i) insufficient for diagnosis; (ii) benign; (iii) positive for cancer; and (iv) suspicious or indeterminate for diagnosis, sometimes referred to as 'follicular neoplasm' or 'follicular tumor.' Between 15% and 20% of FNAs are classified as 'suspicious' or indeterminate for diagnosis; about 20% of these will ultimately show FC or Hürthle cell carcinoma on surgical specimens [18].

Cervical US is also an important staging tool as it can be used to identify lymph node metastases based on the presence of increased node size, calcification, and irregular diffuse intranodular blood flow [19,20]. Preoperative cervical US-identified lymph node metastases were occult on physical examination in 33–39% of patients in large retrospective series [21,22], and could alter the surgical approach in 14–24% of patients [19,22].

Computed Tomography and Magnetic Resonance Imaging
Computed tomography and magnetic resonance imaging (MRI) of the neck are not necessary in the evaluation of thyroid nodules or thyroid cancer except when there are symptoms, such as hoarseness, stridor, or dysphagia, or US findings suggestive of locally advanced disease. In

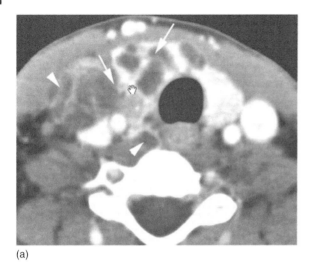
(a)

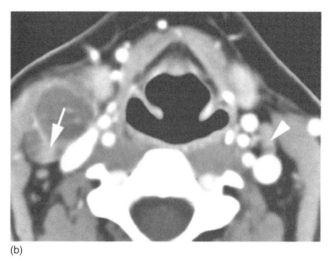
(b)

Figure 17.2 A patient presenting with a neck mass. (a) Computed tomography (CT) study showing the mass to be due to a primary papillary thyroid carcinoma coming into contact with a related level IV metastatic lymph node (arrows). The lymph node at level IV and in the tracheoesophageal groove is shown by the arrowheads. (b) A section more superiorly shows level III adenopathy that is multicystic in a pattern typical but not necessarily diagnostic of papillary thyroid carcinoma. There is upper level IV cystic adenopathy with an enhancing mural nodule (arrow) – a morphology suggestive of thyroid carcinoma. A contralateral enhancing positive node with a focal low-density defect (arrowhead) is also present. *Source:* Mancuso 2010 [23]. Reproduced with permission of Wolters Kluwer Health.

this situation, the results of these studies may be useful in surgical planning by defining the extent of extrathyroidal extension and/or lymph node metastases (Figures 17.2 and 17.3). MRI is preferred over CT because it will better show any esophageal or tracheal invasion [23]. CT should be avoided because useful imaging of the neck requires contrast enhancement, which will interfere with subsequent RAI therapy. A non-contrasted chest CT should be performed based on symptoms or clinical suspicion of mediastinal and lung metastases.

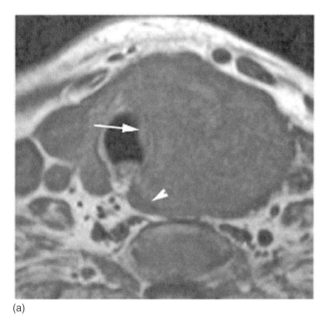
(a)

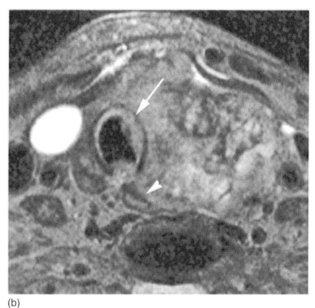
(b)

Figure 17.3 Demonstration of the value of magnetic resonance imaging (MRI) in the detection of invasion of the trachea and cervical esophagus, especially as it pertains to treatment planning. This patient has anaplastic carcinoma of the thyroid gland. (a) T1-weighted (T1W) image showing distortion of the trachea (arrow) and esophagus (arrowhead), but it is difficult to determine whether invasion is present. (b) T2-weighted (T2W) image showing obvious growth of tumor replacing the normal signal of cartilage of the trachea with growth on both sides of the cartilage (arrow) as well as replacement of the normal muscular wall signal of the cervical esophagus (arrowhead), indicating esophageal wall invasion. *Source:* Mancuso 2010 [23]. Reproduced with permission of Wolters Kluwer Health.

Nuclear Medicine Studies

Several types of nuclear medicine imaging studies are utilized in the management of thyroid cancer. Two radioactive isotopes of iodine (^{131}I and ^{123}I) are used in RAI studies, and 18-fluorodeoxyglucose is used in positron emission tomography (PET). A summary of each of these studies, the isotope utilized, and the purpose of each test is shown in Table 17.3.

Prognostic Factors

Pathologic classification and stage are the most important prognostic factors for thyroid carcinoma. As previously discussed within the classification of DTC, certain variants such as diffuse sclerosing, tall-cell, columnar cell and Hürthle cell carcinoma are associated with a poor prognosis relative to classic PTC. Additional

Table 17.3 Nuclear imaging studies used in the management of differentiated thyroid carcinomas.

Study	Isotope	Diagnostics	Results	Purpose	Comment
Radioactive uptake study (RAIU)	I-123 or I-131*	Counts are measured over the low neck 2 to 24 h after administration	Not an image but a number. Normal findings after near total thyroidectomy are 0.5% to 5%.	Quantifies the ability of thyroid tissue to concentrate iodine and estimate the amount of remaining thyroid tissue after thyroidectomy; required by federal regulation for outpatient therapy with I-131	Ideally should be done after restricting dietary iodine for 2 weeks and elevating serum TSH to >30 U ml^{-1} with levothyroxine deprivation or rhTSH administration
Thyroid scan	I-123, I-131, or Tc-99	Same basic procedures as RAIU, but the thyroid is imaged with a gamma camera	Results are given as an image	Used in the evaluation of thyroid nodules to determine if the nodule is functional (i.e., 'hot' or 'cold')	Contributes little information to justify routine use in evaluating most thyroid nodules[71] In the setting of suppressed TSH, a 'hot' nodule rarely harbors malignancy and cytology is not necessary [72]
Diagnostic whole-body scan (DxWBS)	Usually I-131 (2–5 mCi)	The entire body is imaged with a gamma camera ~3 days after RAI is administered (a delay allows washout of RAI from normal tissues)	Records images of the distribution of RAI throughout the entire body	To detect residual cancer	Patients are prepared with a low-iodine diet and TSH elevation. Some experts do not use this study in cancer management
Post-treatment whole-body scan (RxWBS)	I-131, 30 to 250 mCi (therapeutic dose range)	Same as DxWBS but performed ~7 days after RAI is administered	Same as DxWBS	Evaluates the quality of therapy for thyroid remnant ablation and identifies metastases	False positives are the only downside and their impact is mitigated when interpreted in the appropriate clinical context

*The present authors currently use I-123 at doses of 200–300 μCi.
Source: Halperin *et al.* 2013. Reproduced with permission of Wolters Kluwer Health.

Table 17.4 Prognostic factors in differentiated thyroid cancer (DTC).

Variable	Favorable	Unfavorable	Comment
Age	15 to 44 years	<15 or ≥45 years	Older age is accounted for in the AJCC staging system, but children (aged <15 years) have a 30–40% risk of recurrence
Gender	Female	Male	Twofold increase in distant metastases [73]
Family history	Absent	Present	Increased incidence of multifocality and aggressive tumors in patients with first-degree family members with DTC [66]
Tumor size	≤4 cm (<1 cm, very favorable)	>4 cm	A linear relationship exists between primary tumor size and thyroid cancer mortality [26]
Focality/ laterality	Unifocal or unilateral	Multifocal or bilateral	Twofold increase in rate of nodal metastases and threefold increase in the distant metastases with multifocal tumors
Extrathyroid extension	Organ confined	Extrathyroidal extension	1.5-fold increase in 10-year recurrence and fivefold increase in mortality
Histologic grade	Low-grade	High-grade	Tumors with increased necrosis, nuclear atypia, and vascular invasion have a worse prognosis
Lymph node metastases	Absent	Present	–
Distant metastases	Absent	Present	50% mortality with distant metastases
RAI concentration	Concentrate RAI	Inability/low capacity to concentrate RAI	–

AJCC, American Joint Committee on Cancer; DTC, differentiated thyroid cancer; RAI, radioactive iodine.
Source: Halperin *et al.* 2013. Reproduced with permission of Wolters Kluwer Health.

important prognostic factors in DTC are shown in Table 17.4.

Staging

The Eighth Edition of the AJCC staging system for thyroid cancer is shown in Table 17.5 [8]. The anatomic extent of disease, patient age, and tumor histology are used in staging. Separate staging groups are recommended for differentiated, medullary, and anaplastic carcinomas.

Treatment of Thyroid Cancer

Treatment of thyroid carcinoma in most situations requires a multimodality approach including surgery, medical therapy with TSH suppression, RAI therapy, and sometimes external-beam radiotherapy (EBRT). Most patients with DTC benefit from the administration of supratherapeutic doses of T4 in an effort to drive down the TSH level below detectable limits (<0.1 mIU l^{-1}), thereby decreasing the stimulation of residual benign and malignant thyroid cells [24–26]. Traditional systemic cytotoxic therapies have had a limited role in the management of DTC, and have mostly been limited to

patients with metastatic or recurrent disease, which is not responsive to RAI. Doxorubicin as single-agent therapy or in combination with other chemotherapies is most commonly used, and response rates of 25–40% have been reported [27]. Newer agents targeting specific pathways involved in cellular proliferation and vasculogenesis (axitinib, motesanib, sorafenib, and sunitinib) are being explored and early results have yielded limited success [28].

Surgical Management of Thyroid Cancer

Surgical excision of all gross disease is the most important treatment of localized thyroid cancer, regardless of histology, and is usually defined as total thyroidectomy with or without neck dissection. It is critical to understand that even a total thyroidectomy leaves residual thyroid tissue. The presence of residual thyroid tissue does not indicate incomplete surgery, but is necessary to reduce the risk of operative morbidity since more radical surgery would likely injure the trachea or recurrent laryngeal nerve. The most common complications of total thyroidectomy are recurrent laryngeal nerve injury (temporary 30% and permanent 2%) and hypoparathyroidism (temporary 5% and permanent 0.5%) [29]. Other complications include injury to the vagus, spinal accessory and

Table 17.5 AJCC 8th edition TNM staging system for thyroid cancer.

Primary Tumor (T)		
TX		Primary tumor cannot be assessed
T0		No evidence of primary tumor
T1		Tumor 2 cm or less in greatest dimension and limited to the thyroid gland
	T1a	Tumor 1 cm or less in greatest dimension and limited to the thyroid gland
	T1b	Tumor more than 1 cm but not more than 2 cm in greatest dimension and limited to the thyroid gland
T2		Tumor more than 2 cm but not more than 4 cm in greatest dimension and limited to the thyroid gland
T3		Tumor more than 4 cm in greatest dimension limited to the thyroid, or gross extrathyroidal extension invading only strap muscles
	T3a	Tumor more than 4 cm limited to the thyroid
	T3b	Gross extrathyroidal extension invading only strap muscles from a tumor of any size
T4		Advanced disease defined as more than minimal extrathyroidal extension
	T4a	Moderately advanced disease
		Tumor of any size extending beyond the thyroid capsule to invade subcutaneous soft tissues, larynx, trachea, esophagus, or recurrent laryngeal nerve
	T4b	Very advanced disease
		Tumor invades prevertebral fascia, encases carotid artery or mediastinal vessels
All anaplastic carcinomas are considered T4 tumors		
T4a		Intrathyroidal anaplastic carcinoma
T4b		Anaplastic carcinoma with gross extrathyroidal extension

Regional Lymph Nodes (N)		
NX		Regional lymph nodes cannot be assessed
N0		No evidence of regional lymph node metastasis
	N0a	One or more cytologically or histologically confirmed benign lymph nodes
	N0b	No radiologic or clinical evidence of locoregional lymph node metastasis
N1		Regional lymph node metastasis
	N1a	Metastasis to level VI or VII (pretracheal, paratracheal, and prelaryngeal/Delphian or upper mediastinal lymph nodes)
	N1b	Metastasis to unilateral, bilateral, contralateral cervical (Levels I, II, III, IV, or V) or retropharyngeal lymph nodes

Distant Metastasis (M)	
M0	No distant metastasis
M1	Distant metastasis

Overall Staging Groups

(DTC) Papillary or Follicular Carcinoma
Under 55 years

Stage I	Any T	Any N	M0
Stage II	Any T	Any N	M1
55 years and older			
Stage I	T1	N0/NX	M0
	T2	N0/NX	M0
Stage II	T1	N1	M0
	T2	N1	M0
	T3a/T3b	Any N	M0
Stage III	T4a	Any N	M0
Stage IVA	T4b	Any N	M0
Stage IVB	Any T	Any N	M1

Table 17.5 *(Continued)*

Medullary Carcinoma (all age groups)			
Stage I	T1	N0	M0
Stage II	T2	N0	M0
	T3	N0	M0
Stage III	T1	N1a	M0
	T2	N1a	M0
	T3	N1a	M0
Stage IVA	T4a	Any N	M0
	T1	N1b	M0
	T2	N1b	M0
	T3	N1b	M0
	T4a	N1b	M0
Stage IVB	T4b	Any N	M0
Stage IVC	Any T	Any N	M1
Anaplastic carcinoma (all stage IV)			
Stage IVA	T1-T3a	N0/NX	M0
Stage IVB	T1-T3a	N1	M0
	T3b	Any N	M0
	T4	Any N	M0
Stage IVC	Any T	Any N	M1

Source: AJCC Cancer Staging Manual, Eighth Edition (2017), Springer, New York, Inc.

superior laryngeal nerves, trachea, esophagus, thoracic duct, and carotid arteries [30].

While total thyroidectomy is considered the standard surgical approach for nearly all resectable thyroid carcinomas, published clinical guidelines consider lobectomy appropriate in certain clinical situations. As per the 2011 National Comprehensive Cancer Network (NCCN) guidelines, lobectomy is acceptable in patients with PTC if all of the following are present: (i) age 15–45 years; (ii) no prior radiotherapy; (iii) no apparent distant metastasis; (iv) no clinical evidence of cervical lymph node metastasis; (v) no extrathyroidal extension; (vi) tumor size <4 cm; and (vii) no aggressive histologic variants [31]. The 2009 ATA guidelines consider lobectomy only in tumors with the above features and are <1 cm [15]. Advocates for lobectomy argue that operative morbidity is reduced over total thyroidectomy [32]. In general, total thyroidectomy is the appropriate operation for most patients with localized DTC, because it increases the effectiveness of adjuvant RAI, removes occult intrathyroidal cancer, reduces recurrences, and increases the effectiveness of surveillance imaging and serum Tg.

There is general agreement that clinically apparent thyroid cancer lymph metastases should be surgically removed, but there is significant controversy over the role of elective neck dissection. Despite a high incidence of subclinical lymph node involvement in even small PTCs, elective neck dissection is not routinely performed because it has not shown a clear benefit in reducing recurrences and improving survival benefit and is associated with increased operative morbidity [33–36]. A recent meta-analysis with over 1200 patients showed no improvement in recurrences with the addition of prophylactic central neck dissection [37].

According to the 2009 ATA guidelines, central-compartment (level VI) dissection is recommended for all patients with clinically involved lymph nodes; however, for small T1 or T2 tumors without adverse clinical or pathologic features, a prophylactic central neck dissection can be omitted. In clinically N0 patients with other adverse features (T3 or T4), a prophylactic central neck dissection can be considered. A lateral level II–IV neck dissection is indicated only for patients with clinically apparent and biopsy-proven metastatic lymph nodes in these regions [15]. When neck dissection is indicated, *en bloc* removal of the entire level is favored in lieu of removing only abnormal lymph nodes [38–40]. Levels I, V, and VII should not be dissected unless clinically suspicious. Central and lateral neck dissections are recommended for all patients with sporadic and hereditary forms of MTC [41,42].

Management of Differentiated Thyroid Carcinoma (DTC) with RAI

The iodine-concentrating capacity of benign and malignant thyroid tissue makes an overwhelming majority of thyroid carcinomas amenable to RAI therapy. The goals of RAI are: (i) thyroid remnant ablation that facilitates the use of post-treatment serum Tg as a tumor marker; (ii) adjuvant targeted cytotoxic therapy for residual microscopic disease; and (iii) a whole-body scan to provide important staging and prognostic information.

Iodine-131 is taken up by thyroid tissue, including DTC of follicular epithelial origin, at a rate 6.6-fold higher than most tissues in the body [43]. Iodine-131 has a dual role in the management of thyroid cancer: first, β-decay to xenon (Xe)-131 results in the emission of β-particles with energy ranges of 250 to 800 keV. β-particles of this energy range will deposit their radiation dose within a millimeter of their origin, therefore providing highly targeted therapy limited to the cells which take up the iodine. A second step in the radioactive decay of iodine-131 is the transition of unstable Xe-131 into stable xenon, releasing a photon with the energy of 364 keV that easily transverses through the patient's body. Although this is undesirable from a therapeutic perspective, this property forms the basis of RAI studies that yield important prognostic information in diagnostic imaging and after RAI therapy.

Most patients with thyroid cancer should undergo RAI after total thyroidectomy. There are no randomized controlled trials showing a benefit to RAI after total thyroidectomy; however, several large retrospective series have shown improvements in recurrence rates and at least one series showed a survival benefit [26,44–47]. The 2009 ATA guidelines recommend RAI for all patients with known distant metastases, gross extrathyroidal extension of the tumor regardless of tumor size, or primary tumor size >4 cm, even in the absence of other higher risk features. RAI is recommended for selected patients with 1- to 4-cm thyroid cancers confined to the thyroid who have lymph node metastases or other high-risk features, such as age >45 years, intrathyroidal vascular invasion, multifocal disease, or aggressive histologic variants (tall cell, columnar cell, or insular carcinoma). Follicular and Hürthle cell variants are considered high risk and are, in nearly all cases, recommended for RAI, except for the smallest unifocal FCs manifesting as only capsular invasion (without vascular invasion). These so-called minimally invasive carcinomas are treated effectively with surgery alone and RAI can be avoided. RAI is not recommended for unifocal PTCs <1 cm without high-risk features or when all the foci in multifocal disease are <1 cm [15].

There are three methods of selecting the isotope activity for RAI therapy: the empiric method; the dosimetry-guided method; and the tumor-site dosimetry method. There is no consensus on the optimal method of iodine-131, and the empiric method is most often used due to its simplicity. For a detailed discussion of this issue, readers are referred to 'Choosing the Activity of I-131 for Therapy' in *Essentials of Thyroid Cancer Management* [48].

If RAI therapy is given for the first time after total thyroidectomy, the following dose schedule is recommended. For the lowest-risk patients (aged 15–45 years, stage T1N0M0 without positive margins, or aggressive histologies), 50 mCi is administered for thyroid remnant ablation. High-risk patients (stage T4, M1, or gross positive nodes with extracapsular extension) receive 200 mCi. All other patients are considered intermediate-risk and receive 150 mCi.

To obtain the maximal effect for RAI, patients must be adequately prepared for therapy. The goal of preparation is to increase the level of TSH to maximize the activity of NaIS and therefore iodine uptake into thyroid tissue. There are two basic schemes used for RAI preparation: (i) thyroid hormone deprivation; and (ii) administration of recombinant human TSH (rhTSH). All patients should also be placed on an iodine-deficient diet. It is imperative that the patient has not had iodine administered as contrast for a CT scan, cardiac catheterization, or any other medical intervention during the six months before administering RAI. Monitoring of 24-h urinary iodine excretion may help to ensure that the patient is appropriately iodine-deficient before therapy. Finally, lithium carbonate can be administered, when not contraindicated, to augment the effect of RAI.

Adverse effects of RAI therapy include acute temporary side effects such as nausea, taste disturbances, salivary gland inflammation, and menstrual cycle disturbances. When high-dose (>200 mCi) therapy is used, temporary bone marrow suppression, facial nerve weakness, and stomatitis have been reported. Rare permanent late complications include second malignancies, dry mouth and dental decay, early menopause, and infertility. When multiple courses of RAI are required for the management of recurrent disease and the total cumulative lifetime dose exceeds 500 mCi, other late toxicities can occur, such as permanent bone marrow suppression, salivary or nasolacrimal gland obstruction, and chronic dry eye.

After RAI, all patients with DTC should be followed at least every six months with clinical examinations, serum Tg measurement, and with neck US for the first few years after treatment. There is no need to follow patients with RAI diagnostic imaging. Gross recurrent tumor should be excised when feasible and patients can often be retreated with RAI with some success.

External-Beam Radiotherapy (EBRT) for Thyroid Cancer Indications

It is clear that patients with symptomatic metastatic disease benefit from palliative EBRT; the role of EBRT in non-metastatic DTC is controversial, however. An ambitious European randomized controlled trial (the Multicentre Study on Differentiated Thyroid Cancer) attempted to define the role of EBRT in patients at high risk of local-regional failure despite maximal surgery and RAI. In this trial, patients with pT4 disease with

Table 17.6 Indications for EBRT.

Age	University of Florida	2009 ATA guidelines	2011 NCCN Guidelines
Age ≤18 years	Painful metastases or impending normal tissue damage from a growing tumor not amenable to other therapies	Metastases that are symptomatic or in critical location that are otherwise untreatable	No child-specific guidelines Consider EBRT for: T4 primary, tumors not likely to concentrate iodine, or tumors with a high risk of residual disease (T4, positive margins, ECE)
Age 19–45 years	Gross tumor on an imaging study that is unresectable and known to be resistant to I-131 (resistance means recurrence after one administration of >100 mCi I-131 treatment under optimal conditions) EBRT not used if RAI may be curative or elevated Tg is the only sign of disease	Metastases that are symptomatic or in a critical location and are otherwise untreatable	
Age >45 years	Adjuvant treatment after thyroidectomy: Patients at high risk for local-regional recurrence: T4 primary, nodal metastases with extensive extracapsular extension, or gross residual disease Salvage of recurrent disease following thyroidectomy and RAI: Gross tumor that on an imaging study is unresectable and known to be resistant to I131 (resistance means recurrence after at least 1 > 100 mCi I-131 treatment under optimal conditions). We do not use EBRT if RAI may be curative or elevated Tg is the only sign of disease	Gross ETE; high likelihood of microscopic residual gross residual tumor not amenable to further surgery	

RAI, radioactive iodine; EBRT, external beam radiotherapy; ETE, extrathyroidal extension.
Source: Halperin *et al.* 2013. Reproduced with permission of Wolters Kluwer Health.

or without lymph node metastases and no known distant metastases who underwent total thyroidectomy, RAI, and TSH suppression were to be randomized to EBRT or observation. The trial closed prematurely since only 16% of patients consented to be randomized to EBRT. The trial was converted to a prospective cohort study and subsequent results failed to demonstrate a benefit to EBRT in this population [49–51]. Given the lack of level I evidence, the recommendations for EBRT are based on institutional retrospective experiences and published clinical guidelines, which are summarized in Table 17.6. A benefit from EBRT in localized DTC has been demonstrated in several series of patients treated for high-risk disease. These results are summarized in Table 17.7.

When treating metastatic tumors with palliative intent, the EBRT techniques will vary by site, tumor burden, and clinical situation; therefore, only the technique used to treat local and regional disease will be described at this point. When both RAI therapy and EBRT are indicated, the preference is to give RAI first since EBRT may result in thyroid stunning, so as to decrease the effectiveness of subsequent RAI.

Historically, thyroid cancer was planned based on simulation radiographs. Most patients were treated with simple, heavily anteriorly weighted anterior-posterior:posterior-anterior (AP:PA) fields. Alternatively, lateral fields were used, but this required using a customized bolus to deal with the issue of treating about the level of the shoulder. Superiorly, the initial fields encompassed cervical lymph node stations in the upper neck; inferiorly, the fields included lymph nodes in the upper mediastinum (to the level of the carina). At spinal cord tolerance, the fields were reduced to encompass the areas previously involved with gross disease or lymph nodes with extracapsular extension using anterior wedge pairs, *en-face* electrons, or other simple beam arrangements that were individualized depending on the clinical situation and anatomic considerations. These techniques have essentially been abandoned in lieu of three-dimensional (3D) conformal RT and IMRT.

Table 17.7 Retrospective series showing a benefit from external-beam radiotherapy (EBRT) in patients with differentiated thyroid carcinoma (DTC) routinely treated with RAI [46].

Study/Reference	No. of patients	Patients receiving EBRT (%)	Benefit of EBRT	Subset benefiting from EBRT
Farahati *et al.* [67]	169	59	Local-regional control, distant failure	Papillary tumors Node-positive
Chow *et al.* [68]	842	12	Local-regional control	Gross residual tumor after thyroidectomy
Kim *et al.* [70]	91	25	Local-regional control	pT4 or node-positive
Phlips *et al.* [72]	94	40	Local control	ETE or microscopic/gross residual tumor after thyroidectomy
Brierley *et al.* [69]	729	44	Local-regional control, cause-specific survival	Microscopic residual, ETE Age >60 years, microscopic residual, ETE

ETE, extrathyroidal extension.
Source: Halperin *et al.* 2013. Reproduced with permission of Wolters Kluwer Health.

Currently, treatment planning is performed using CT simulation. Patients are positioned supine with arms at their side and the neck extended. The head and neck should be immobilized with a custom head holder and a thermoplastic mask. Bolus material is applied over neck scars. Intravenous contrast may be helpful in defining target volumes and normal-tissue structures, but is contraindicated if RAI is likely within the next six months. Planning images are acquired from above the skull base through the entire chest. Preoperative images may be fused to the treatment planning CT to aid in target definitions, but are not necessary. Because the target volume straddles the level of the shoulder and usually contains concavities with envaginated critical normal tissues, IMRT is useful in most cases. The present authors use seven to nine coplanar axially-oriented IMRT beams. The multileaf-collimator sequencing, segment, and beam weighting are optimized by the inverse planning system based on parameters specified by the planner in order to meet specific goals for target coverage, limitations on dose heterogeneity, and normal-tissue sparing.

Target Volumes and Dose

Target volumes are delineated according to the definitions from the International Commission on Radiation Units. The gross tumor volume (GTV) represents residual gross disease. Two clinical target volumes (CTVs) are defined to represent areas at varying risk for subclinical disease beyond any GTV. The high-risk CTV is defined as the region at highest risk for residual disease, including any area of positive margins, extrathyroidal extension, lymph node station involved with gross extracapsular disease, or any residual gross disease. The standard-risk CTV includes the high-risk CTV as well as additional areas at moderate risk for residual disease; essentially,

this refers to cervical and upper mediastinal lymph node stations at risk for microscopic disease. In nearly all situations, the standard-risk CTV would encompass bilateral cervical levels II–V, levels VI (central compartment), and level VII upper mediastinal lymph nodes. Additional lymph node regions are addressed on a case-by-case basis, including levels IB, retropharyngeal lymph nodes, and the retrostyloid lymph nodes. Level Ib and retropharyngeal lymph nodes are included when there is bulky adenopathy, and the retrostyloid lymph nodes are treated when there is gross involvement of level II lymph nodes. A contouring atlas is provided in Figure 17.4 which shows the high-risk and standard-risk CTV. PTVs are created by 3D symmetric expansions of the CTVs to account for treatment set-up uncertainty and organ motion based on institutional policies. These typically range from 3 to 5 mm. Typically, 66–70 Gy is prescribed to cover 95% of the high-risk PTV, and 54–56 Gy to cover 95% of the standard-risk PTV in 33–35 fractions using a single IMRT plan with a simultaneous integrated boost.

Volumes of organs at risk should include the spinal cord, brainstem, trachea, esophagus, parotid glands, mandible, oral cavity, cochleae, pharyngeal constrictors, brachial plexus, and lungs. Planning organs at risk volumes are created by 3D symmetric expansions in similar fashion to the PTV expansion. Daily image guidance may be used to ensure target localization and reduce the set-up uncertainties in the low neck.

External-Beam Radiotherapy Outcomes

Several retrospective series have reported outcomes of patients treated with EBRT for thyroid cancer. These data should be interpreted with consideration of the patients included. That is, most series contain patients at very high risk for recurrence owing to either aggressive

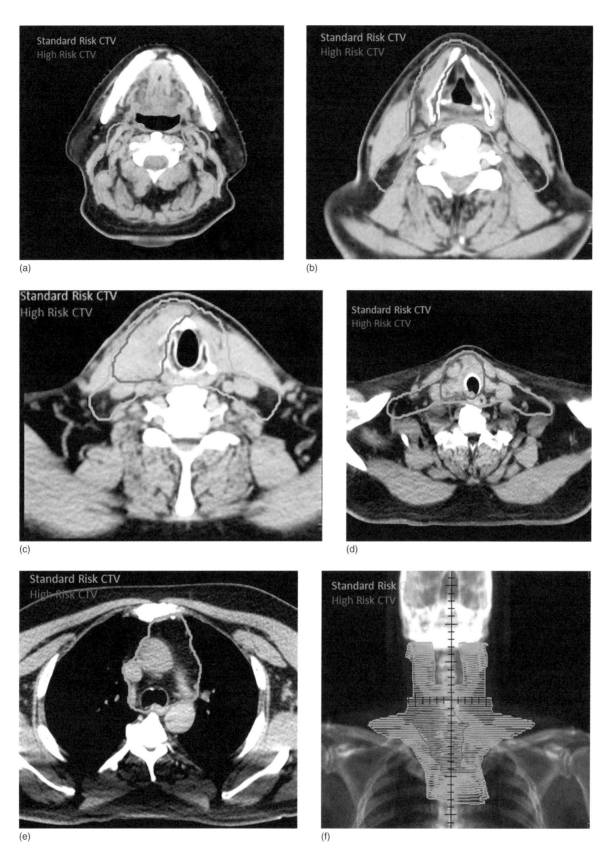

Figure 17.4 Intensity-modulated radiation therapy (IMRT) clinical target volume (CTV) contouring atlas for a patient with T2N0M0 insular thyroid carcinoma status-post total thyroidectomy and radioactive iodine (RAI). (a) Highest level of CTV for elective nodal irradiation where the posterior belly of the digastric muscle crosses the jugular vein. (b) CTV contours at the level of the thyroid notch. (c) CTV contours through the level of the cricoid cartilage. (d) CTV contours through the level of the first tracheal ring. (e) Lowest level of CTV contours covering the upper mediastinal lymph nodes at the level of the carina. (f) Digital reconstructed radiograph depicting the CTV volumes. Indications for external-beam radiation therapy (EBRT) were insular carcinoma (poorly differentiated) and positive margin. For a color version of this figure, see the color plate section.

histologies, recurrent disease, poor or no response to RAI therapy, or gross unresectable tumor. Schwartz *et al.* described 131 patients treated at the M.D. Anderson Cancer Center (Houston, TX) who had received EBRT to treat DTC between 1996 and 2005 [52]. Some 96% of patients had extrathyroidal extension of the primary tumor, and 47% had positive operative margins. The median dose to the high-risk PTV was 60 Gy (range: 38–72 Gy). IMRT was used in most patients treated in the most recent era of the series. With a median follow-up of 38 months, the four-year local-regional control and overall survival rates were 79% and 73%, respectively. Tereza-kis *et al.* reported the outcomes of 86 patients treated with EBRT for DTC at the Memorial Sloan-Kettering Cancer Center (New York, NY) between 1989 and 2006 [53]. Of these patients, 79% had extrathyroidal extension of the primary tumor and 53% had positive operative margins. With a median follow-up of 35 months, the four-year local-regional control and overall survival rates were 72% and 55%, respectively. In the University of Florida (Gainesville, FL) series published by Mead-ows *et al.* [54], 42 patients were treated with EBRT for DTC between 1962 and 2003. Most patients were treated with conventional techniques, with approximately half the patients being treated for recurrent and/or gross residual disease. The median dose was 64.9 Gy. With a median follow-up of 49 months, the five-year local-regional control and overall survival rates were 89% and 60%, respectively.

External-Beam Radiotherapy-Related Toxicity

It is recommended that EBRT is avoided in all patients with DTC who are amenable to curative therapy with RAI, especially the very young, in order to spare patients significant acute and late morbidity. The acute toxicities of EBRT are likely to be quite severe and include mucositis, taste changes, xerostomia, pharyngitis, dysphagia, hoarseness, radiation dermatitis, weight loss, and malnutrition. One series reported the rate of a need for acute and subacute percutaneous feeding tubes of 29% [53]. Late complications include fibrosis and atrophy of the skin, lung apices; fibrosis of the neck musculature, and trachea, and esophageal stenosis. The latter is the most commonly reported severe late complications [52]. Late severe dysphagia requiring a permanent feeding tube is expected in less than 5% of patients [52].

Management of Medullary Thyroid Carcinoma (MTC)

Whether MTC is in sporadic form, associated with MEN, or a pure familial MTC syndrome, it is treated the same. All patients with MTC should be tested for *RET* mutations and undergo genetic screening. The initial primary management of localized MTC is total thyroidectomy with prophylactic central neck dissection and compartment-oriented lateral neck dissection when clinically involved. RAI therapy has no role in MTC. EBRT is indicated for MTC in adult patients with unresectable gross disease, or when there is a high risk of residual microscopic disease after surgery for positive margins, T4 primary tumors, or nodal metastases with extensive extracapsular extension. EBRT simulation, planning, and delivery are the same for MTC as described in the section on EBRT for DTC. All patients should be followed by monitoring serum calcitonin levels, as this presents a sensitive and specific marker for the extent of residual disease. In patients with refractory or metastatic disease, therapies targeting RET-tyrosine kinase receptors have shown promising preclinical and early clinical results [55–59].

Management of Anaplastic Thyroid Carcinoma (ATC)

Most patients with ATC present with local-regionally advanced or metastatic disease. Unfortunately, for most patients it is not clear that any form of therapy improves outcomes, and the best supportive case should be the sole course of action. In rare situations when complete surgical excision is feasible, a multimodality approach with surgery, chemotherapy, and EBRT is a potentially curable approach. However, given the aggressiveness of the tumor and the limited life expectancy of these patients, surgery should be avoided when complete excision is not possible, since debulking does not improve outcomes. ATCs do not concentrate RAI. EBRT is the standard of care for palliation of local symptoms from unresectable disease and is given with concurrent chemotherapy postoperatively when complete resection is achieved. Several institutional series have reported outcomes of patients treated once daily or with hyperfractionated EBRT and concomitant chemotherapy with agents such as docetaxel, paclitaxel, vincristine, cisplatin, or doxorubicin [60–65]. Despite these aggressive approaches, few patients (9–44%) survive beyond two years.[66-70]

References

1 Siegel, R.L., Miller, K.D., Jemal, A. (2017) Cancer statistics, 2017. *CA: Cancer J. Clin.*, **67**, 7–30.

2 Aschebrook-Kilfoy, B., Ward, M.H., Sabra, M.M., *et al.* (2011) Thyroid cancer incidence patterns in the United States by histologic type, 1992–2006. *Thyroid*, **21**, 125–134.

3 Siegel, R., Ward, E., Brawley, O., *et al.* (2011) Cancer statistics, 2011: the impact of eliminating

socioeconomic and racial disparities on premature cancer deaths. *CA Cancer J. Clin.*, **61**, 212–236.

4 Davies, L., Welch, H.G. (2006) Increasing incidence of thyroid cancer in the United States, 1973–2002. *JAMA*, **295**, 2164–2167.

5 Mortensen, J.D., Woolner, L.B., Bennett, W.A. (1055) Gross and microscopic findings in clinically normal thyroid glands. *J. Clin. Endocrinol. Metab.*, **15**, 1270–1280.

6 Vander, J.B., Gaston, E.A., Dawber, T.R. (1968) The significance of nontoxic thyroid nodules. Final report of a 15-year study of the incidence of thyroid malignancy. *Ann. Intern. Med.*, **69**, 537–540.

7 Nixon, I.J., Ganly, I., Hann, L.E., *et al.* (2010) Nomogram for predicting malignancy in thyroid nodules using clinical, biochemical, ultrasonographic, and cytologic features. *Surgery*, **148**, 1120–1127; discussion 1127–1128.

8 American Joint Committee on Cancer (2017) *AJCC Cancer Staging Handbook*, 8th edition. Springer, New York.

9 Boone, R.T., Fan, C.Y., Hanna, E.Y. (2003) Well-differentiated carcinoma of the thyroid. *Otolaryngol. Clin. North Am.*, **36**, 73–90, viii.

10 Hay, I.D. (1990) Papillary thyroid carcinoma. *Endocrinol. Metab. Clin. North Am.*, **19**, 545–576.

11 Pacini, F., Elisei, R., Capezzone, M., *et al.* (2001) Contralateral papillary thyroid cancer is frequent at completion thyroidectomy with no difference in low- and high-risk patients. *Thyroid*, **11**, 877–881.

12 Kawaura, M., Pathak, I., Gullane, P.J., *et al.* (2001) Multicentricity in papillary thyroid carcinoma: analysis of predictive factors. *J. Otolaryngol.*, **30**, 102–105.

13 Nagaiah, G., Hossain, A., Mooney, C.J., *et al.* (2011) Anaplastic thyroid cancer: a review of epidemiology, pathogenesis, and treatment. *J. Oncol.*, **2011**, 542358.

14 Frates, M.C., Benson, C.B., Charboneau, J.W., *et al.* (2005) Management of thyroid nodules detected at US: Society of Radiologists in Ultrasound consensus conference statement. *Radiology*, **237**, 794–800.

15 Cooper, D.S., Doherty, G.M., Haugen, B.R., *et al.* (2009) Revised American Thyroid Association management guidelines for patients with thyroid nodules and differentiated thyroid cancer. *Thyroid*, **19**, 1167–1214.

16 Yang, G.C., Liebeskind, D., Messina, A.V. (2001) Ultrasound-guided fine-needle aspiration of the thyroid assessed by Ultrafast Papanicolaou stain: data from 1135 biopsies with a two- to six-year follow-up. *Thyroid*, **11**, 581–589.

17 Ko, H.M., Jhu, I.K., Yang, S.H., *et al.* (2003) Clinicopathologic analysis of fine needle aspiration cytology of the thyroid. A review of 1,613 cases and correlation with histopathologic diagnoses. *Acta Cytol.*, **47**, 727–732.

18 Mazzaferri, E.L. (2005) The Diagnosis of Thyroid Cancer, in *Essentials of Thyroid Cancer Management (Cancer Treatment and Research)* (eds R.J. Amdur, E.L. Mazzaferri), 1st edition. Springer, New York, pp. 39–48.

19 Gomez, N.R., Kouniavsky, G., Tsai, H.L., *et al.* (2011) Tumor size and presence of calcifications on ultrasonography are pre-operative predictors of lymph node metastases in patients with papillary thyroid cancer. *J. Surg. Oncol.*, **104**, 613–616.

20 Mazzaferri, E.L. (2005) Neck Ultrasonography in Patients with Thyroid Cancer, in *Essentials of Thyroid Cancer Management (Cancer Treatment and Research)* (eds R.J. Amdur, E.L. Mazzaferri), 1st edition. Springer, New York, pp. 101–120.

21 Kouvaraki, M.A., Shapiro, S.E., Fornage, B.D., *et al.* (2003) Role of preoperative ultrasonography in the surgical management of patients with thyroid cancer. *Surgery*, **134**, 946–954; discussion 954–945.

22 Stulak, J.M., Grant, C.S., Farley, D.R., *et al.* (2006) Value of preoperative ultrasonography in the surgical management of initial and reoperative papillary thyroid cancer. *Arch. Surg.*, **141**, 489–494; discussion 494–486.

23 Mancuso, A.A., Mendenhall, W.M., Vaysberg, M. (2010) Thyroid: Nodules and Malignant Tumors, in *Head and Neck Radiology* (ed. A.A. Mancuso), Vol. **1**. Lippincott Williams & Wilkins, Philadelphia, PA, pp. 1457–1481.

24 Pujol, P., Daures, J.P., Nsakala, N., *et al.* (1996) Degree of thyrotropin suppression as a prognostic determinant in differentiated thyroid cancer. *J. Clin. Endocrinol. Metab.*, **81**, 4318–4323.

25 Ludgate, M., Gire, V., Crisp, M., *et al.* (1999) Contrasting effects of activating mutations of GalphaS and the thyrotropin receptor on proliferation and differentiation of thyroid follicular cells. *Oncogene*, **18**, 4798–4807.

26 Mazzaferri, E.L., Jhiang, S.M. (1994) Long-term impact of initial surgical and medical therapy on papillary and follicular thyroid cancer. *Am. J. Med.*, **97**, 418–428.

27 Haugen, B.R. (1999) Management of the patient with progressive radioiodine non-responsive disease. *Semin. Surg. Oncol.*, **16**, 34–41.

28 Romagnoli, S., Moretti, S., Voce, P., *et al.* (2009) Targeted molecular therapies in thyroid carcinoma. *Arq. Bras. Endocrinol. Metab.*, **53**, 1061–1073.

29 Mazzaferri, E.L. (2005) Potential Complications of Thyroid Cancer Surgery, in *Essentials of Thyroid Cancer Management (Cancer Treatment and Research)* (eds R.J. Amdur, E.L. Mazzaferri), 1st edition. Springer, New York, pp.153–160.

30 Sosa, J.A., Udelsman, R. (2006) Total thyroidectomy for differentiated thyroid cancer. *J. Surg. Oncol.*, **94**, 701–707.

31 National Comprehensive Cancer Network (2011) NCCN Guidelines for Thyroid Carcinoma.

32 Udelsman, R., Lakatos, E., Ladenson, P. (1996) Optimal surgery for papillary thyroid carcinoma. *World J. Surg.*, **20**, 88–93.

33 Dionigi, G., Dionigi, R., Bartalena, L., *et al.* (2006) Surgery of lymph nodes in papillary thyroid cancer. *Expert Rev. Anticancer. Ther.*, **6**, 1217–1229.

34 Shah, M.D., Hall, F.T., Eski, S.J., *et al.* (2003) Clinical course of thyroid carcinoma after neck dissection. *Laryngoscope*, **113**, 2102–2107.

35 Zuniga, S., Sanabria, A. (2009) Prophylactic central neck dissection in stage N0 papillary thyroid carcinoma. *Arch. Otolaryngol. Head Neck Surg.*, **135**, 1087–1091.

36 Rosenbaum, M.A., McHenry, C.R. (2009) Central neck dissection for papillary thyroid cancer. *Arch. Otolaryngol. Head Neck Surg.*, **135**, 1092–1097.

37 Zetoune, T., Keutgen, X., Buitrago, D., *et al.* (2010) Prophylactic central neck dissection and local recurrence in papillary thyroid cancer: a meta-analysis. *Ann. Surg. Oncol.*, **17**, 3287–3293.

38 Fritze, D., Doherty, G.M. (2010) Surgical management of cervical lymph nodes in differentiated thyroid cancer. *Otolaryngol. Clin. North Am.*, **43**, 285–300, viii.

39 Bardet, S., Malville, E., Rame, J.P., *et al.* (2008) Macroscopic lymph-node involvement and neck dissection predict lymph-node recurrence in papillary thyroid carcinoma. *Eur. J. Endocrinol.*, **158**, 551–560.

40 Noguchi, S., Murakami, N., Yamashita, H., *et al.* (1998) Papillary thyroid carcinoma: modified radical neck dissection improves prognosis. *Arch. Surg.*, **133**, 276–280.

41 Moley, J.F., DeBenedetti, M.K. (1999) Patterns of nodal metastases in palpable medullary thyroid carcinoma: recommendations for extent of node dissection. *Ann. Surg.*, **229**, 880–887; discussion 887–888.

42 Oskam, I.M., Hoebers, F., Balm, A.J., *et al.* (2008) Neck management in medullary thyroid carcinoma. *Eur. J. Surg. Oncol.*, **34**, 71–76.

43 Amdur, R.J., Mazzaferri, E.L. (2005) Half-life and Emission Products of I-131, in *Essentials of Thyroid Cancer Management (Cancer Treatment and Research)* (eds R.J. Amdur, E.L. Mazzaferri), 1st edition. Springer, New York, pp. 165–198.

44 Samaan, N.A., Schultz, P.N., Hickey, R.C., *et al.* (1992) The results of various modalities of treatment of well differentiated thyroid carcinomas: a retrospective review of 1599 patients. *J. Clin. Endocrinol. Metab.*, **75**, 714–720.

45 DeGroot, L.J., Kaplan, E.L., McCormick, M., *et al.* (1990) Natural history, treatment, and course of papillary thyroid carcinoma. *J. Clin. Endocrinol. Metab.*, **71**, 414–424.

46 Tsang, R.W., Brierley, J.D., Simpson, W.J., *et al.* (1998) The effects of surgery, radioiodine, and external radiation therapy on the clinical outcome of patients with differentiated thyroid carcinoma. *Cancer*, **82**, 375–388.

47 Taylor, T., Specker, B., Robbins, J., *et al.* (1998) Outcome after treatment of high-risk papillary and non-Hurthle-cell follicular thyroid carcinoma. *Ann. Intern. Med.*, **129**, 622–627.

48 Amdur, R.J., Mazzaferri, E.L. (2005) Choosing the Activity of I-131 for Therapy, in *Essentials of Thyroid Cancer Management (Cancer Treatment and Research)* (eds R.J. Amdur, E.L. Mazzaferri), 1st edition. Springer, New York, pp. 169–176.

49 Biermann, M., Pixberg, M.K., Schuck, A., *et al.* (2003) Multicenter study differentiated thyroid carcinoma (MSDS). Diminished acceptance of adjuvant external beam radiotherapy. *Nuklearmedizin*, **42**, 244–250.

50 Biermann, M., Pixberg, M., Riemann, B., *et al.* (2009) Clinical outcomes of adjuvant external-beam radiotherapy for differentiated thyroid cancer – results after 874 patient-years of follow-up in the MSDS-trial. *Nuklearmedizin*, **48**, 89–98; quiz N15.

51 Powell, C., Newbold, K., Harrington, K.J., *et al.* (2010) External beam radiotherapy for differentiated thyroid cancer. *Clin. Oncol. (R. Coll. Radiol.)*, **22**, 456–463.

52 Schwartz, D.L., Lobo, M.J., Ang, K.K., *et al.* (2009) Postoperative external beam radiotherapy for differentiated thyroid cancer: outcomes and morbidity with conformal treatment. *Int. J. Radiat. Oncol. Biol. Phys.*, **74**, 1083–1091.

53 Terezakis, S.A., Lee, K.S., Ghossein, R.A., *et al.* (2009) Role of external beam radiotherapy in patients with advanced or recurrent nonanaplastic thyroid cancer: Memorial Sloan-Kettering Cancer Center experience. *Int. J. Radiat. Oncol. Biol. Phys.*, **73**, 795–801.

54 Meadows, K.M., Amdur, R.J., Morris, C.G., *et al.* (2006) External beam radiotherapy for differentiated thyroid cancer. *Am. J. Otolaryngol.*, **27**, 24–28.

55 Lam, E.T., Ringel, M.D., Kloos, R.T., *et al.* (2010) Phase II clinical trial of sorafenib in metastatic medullary thyroid cancer. *J. Clin. Oncol.*, **28**, 2323–2330.

56 Wells, S.A., Jr, Gosnell, J.E., Gagel, R.F., *et al.* (2010) Vandetanib for the treatment of patients with locally advanced or metastatic hereditary medullary thyroid cancer. *J. Clin. Oncol.*, **28**, 767–772.

57 Ye, L., Santarpia, L., Gagel, R.F. (2009) Targeted therapy for endocrine cancer: the medullary thyroid carcinoma paradigm. *Endocr. Pract.*, **15**, 597–604.

58 Torino, F., Paragliola, R.M., Barnabei, A., *et al.* (2010) Medullary thyroid cancer: a promising model for targeted therapy. *Curr. Mol. Med.*, **10**, 608–625.

59 Schlumberger, M.J., Elisei, R., Bastholt, L., *et al.* (2009) Phase II study of safety and efficacy of motesanib in patients with progressive or symptomatic, advanced or

metastatic medullary thyroid cancer. *J. Clin. Oncol.*, **27**, 3794–3801.

60 Tennvall, J., Lundell, G., Wahlberg, P., *et al.* (2002) Anaplastic thyroid carcinoma: three protocols combining doxorubicin, hyperfractionated radiotherapy and surgery. *Br. J. Cancer*, **86**, 1848–1853.

61 De Crevoisier, R., Baudin, E., Bachelot, A., *et al.* (2004) Combined treatment of anaplastic thyroid carcinoma with surgery, chemotherapy, and hyperfractionated accelerated external radiotherapy. *Int. J. Radiat. Oncol. Biol. Phys.*, **60**, 1137–1143.

62 Haigh, P.I., Ituarte, P.H., Wu, H.S., *et al.* (2001) Completely resected anaplastic thyroid carcinoma combined with adjuvant chemotherapy and irradiation is associated with prolonged survival. *Cancer*, **91**, 2335–2342.

63 Sherman, E.J., Lim, S.H., Ho, A.L., *et al.* (2011) Concurrent doxorubicin and radiotherapy for anaplastic thyroid cancer: A critical re-evaluation including uniform pathologic review. *Radiother. Oncol.*, **101**, 425–430.

64 Troch, M., Koperek, O., Scheuba, C., *et al.* (2010) High efficacy of concomitant treatment of undifferentiated (anaplastic) thyroid cancer with radiation and docetaxel. *J. Clin. Endocrinol. Metab.*, **95**, E54–E57.

65 Heron, D.E., Karimpour, S., Grigsby, P.W. (2002) Anaplastic thyroid carcinoma: comparison of conventional radiotherapy and hyperfractionation chemoradiotherapy in two groups. *Am. J. Clin. Oncol.*, **25**, 442–446.

66 Xu, L., Li, G., Wei, Q., *et al.* (2012) Family history of cancer and risk of sporadic differentiated thyroid carcinoma. *Cancer*, **118**, 1228–1235.

67 Farahati, J., Parlowsky, T., Mader, U., *et al.* (1998) Differentiated thyroid cancer in children and adolescents. *Langenbecks Arch. Surg.*, **383**, 235–239.

68 Chow, S.M., Law, S.C., Mendenhall, W.M., *et al.* (2002) Papillary thyroid carcinoma: prognostic factors and the role of radioiodine and external radiotherapy. *Int. J. Radiat. Oncol. Biol. Phys.*, **52**, 784–795.

69 Brierley, J., Tsang, R., Panzarella, T., *et al.* (2005) Prognostic factors and the effect of treatment with radioactive iodine and external beam radiation on patients with differentiated thyroid cancer seen at a single institution over 40 years. *Clin. Endocrinol. (Oxf)*, **63**, 418–427.

70 Kim, T.H., Yang, D.S., Jung, K.Y., *et al.* (2003) Value of external irradiation for locally advanced papillary thyroid cancer. *Int. J. Radiat. Oncol. Biol. Phys.*, **55**, 1006–1012.

71 Mancuso, A.A. (2011) Thyroid and Parathyroid Glands: Introduction, in *Head and Neck Radiology*, Vol. **2**. Lippincott Williams & Wilkins, Philadelphia, pp. 1428–1433.

72 Phlips, P., Hanzen, C., Andry, G., *et al.* (1993) Postoperative irradiation for thyroid cancer. *Eur. J. Surg. Oncol.*, **19**, 399–404.

73 Shah, J.P., Loree, T.R., Dharker, D., *et al.* (1992) Prognostic factors in differentiated carcinoma of the thyroid gland. *Am. J. Surg.*, **164**, 658–661.

18

Head and Neck Radiation Therapy Sequelae and Late Complications and the Role of IMRT

Xiaoshen Wang and Avraham Eisbruch

Introduction

Head and neck cancer is a prevalent cancer site, with a yearly rates of 50 000 cases and 10 000 related deaths in the United States [1]. Due to the complicated anatomic relationship between the tumor and normal structures in the head and neck, and the importance of organ preservation in maintaining the patient's quality of life (QoL), considerations of intensifying therapy must be balanced with increased toxicity of intense treatment regimens. Radiotherapy has always played an important role in the treatment of head and neck cancers (HNC), and in recent years an increasing role of systemic chemotherapy and molecular targeted therapy for locally advanced disease has evolved [2–10]. The intensification of radiotherapy for locally advanced HNC has led to significantly improved locoregional control and survival compared with conventional radiotherapy [3–10]. However, these improvements are accompanied with increased toxicity [8–10].

Currently, besides improving tumor control rate, another important goal is to reduce the probability of radiation-induced complications in order to improve the survivors' QoL. The application of three-dimensional (3D) conformal radiation therapy (3D-CRT) and intensity-modulated radiotherapy (IMRT) signified the major improvement over conventional two-dimensional (2D) radiotherapy. Using a 3D treatment planning system (TPS), both the target volume and organs at risk (OARs) can be contoured on the planning computed tomography (CT), and the spatial relationship between target volume and OARs can be clearly demonstrated in three dimensions. Using IMRT, the radiation beams can be optimized to deliver a higher dose to specified target volumes, while reducing the dose to adjacent OARs. Using IMRT to treat HNC is especially attractive due to its unique ability to treat the concave target shapes, the close vicinity of the targets and many dose-limiting and non-involved OARs, and because of the lack of breathing-related motion in these tumors.

As IMRT allows highly conformal dose distributions to target volumes of almost any shape, appropriate selection and accurate delineation of the target volumes and the avoidable organs become of critical importance [11]. Over the past few years, some groups have developed recommendation guidelines for the selection of a clinical target volume (CTV) for both the primary tumors and neck nodal areas [12–16]. Besides an appropriate selection of normal organs, the other important point is to set dose constraints when designing IMRT plans so as to spare OARs. At present, most available data about the tolerance dose of normal tissues are based on retrospective analyses or expert opinion [17, 18], but because of such drawbacks these analyses might not allow definitive conclusions to be drawn. OARs in HNC include the brainstem, spinal cord, salivary glands, the optic nerves, chiasm, swallowing structures, inner ear, mandible and bilateral temporal lobes. Exceeding the tolerances of the above-mentioned structures can result in serious late complications.

Xerostomia and dysphagia are both the main acute and late complications which result in decreased QoL during and after radiotherapy. In addition, cerebral radiation necrosis, radiation-induced cranial nerve palsy, hearing loss and osteoradionecrosis might be the main potential late complications that have debilitating impact on long-term survivors. In this chapter, the efforts to prevent the above-mentioned therapy-related complications

Clinical Radiation Oncology: Indications, Techniques, and Results, Third Edition. Edited by William Small Jr.
© 2017 John Wiley & Sons, Inc. Published 2017 by John Wiley & Sons, Inc.

are described by presenting state-of-the art evidence regarding organ-sparing by advanced radiation therapy technology.

Complications of Radiation and Chemo-Irradiation

Xerostomia

Xerostomia (dry mouth) is the most common and prominent complication during and after radiotherapy for HNC as a result of damage to the salivary glands. Radiation-induced injury to the salivary glands alters the volume, consistency, and pH of secreted saliva [19]. Because the severity of the damage to the salivary glands is dependent both on the total radiation dose and on the volume of irradiated tissue, current studies on organ-preserving radiotherapy have focused on sparing the salivary glands from unnecessary irradiation [20].

Parotid Glands

Limiting the volume of the parotid glands from receiving a high radiation dose has long been recognized as a major factor in reducing the severity of xerostomia. For most HNCs, especially squamous cell carcinoma, the necessity of treating bilateral level II lymph nodes makes it difficult to spare the parotid glands using standard, laterally opposed radiotherapy techniques. However, with 3D-CRT or IMRT, it is possible to partly spare at least one parotid gland in selected patients. A high dose is delivered to only a small part of the parotid gland that is located closest to the target volumes, while the rest of the parotid receives a low dose or no dose at all [20, 21].

Thus, the salivary function is partially preserved and can increase over time via a compensatory response of the part of the parotid that received a low dose [20, 22].

Over the past ten years, an increasing body of data has demonstrated the ability of 3D-CRT and IMRT to deliver dose distributions that allow partial preservation of parotid function, assessed by either salivary flow measurements or salivary gland scintigraphy (Table 18.1). A growing number of prospective clinical trials have demonstrated that parotid-sparing IMRT is sufficient to reduce long-term xerostomia without jeopardizing local-regional control for nasopharyngeal cancer (NPC) (Table 18.2). Although IMRT for HNC is promising in terms of local tumor control and improvement of salivary function according to single-institution studies, these data need to be validated in randomized multi-institutional studies. Recently, several randomized clinical trials have further confirmed that IMRT for NPC could reduce the severity of xerostomia without jeopardizing tumor control rate compared with conventional radiotherapy [39, 43, 44]. In oropharyngeal cancer, it has also been shown that IMRT preserved salivary flow in two prospective multi-institutional studies [32, 45].

The practice guidelines must be made for appropriate preservation of parotid function, because overemphasis on parotid sparing might lead to geographical miss and unexpected patterns of failure. During recent years, emerging data on locoregional failures after 3D-CRT or IMRT has facilitated the development of practice guidelines for parotid-sparing IMRT for HNC. In patients with negative lymph nodes, at least one (but usually both) parotid glands can be safely spared, depending on the location of the primary cancer. In patients with unilateral neck disease, sparing of the contralateral parotid gland

Table 18.1 Overview of prospective trials on parotid-sparing radiotherapy.

Author/Reference	No. of patients	Site	Stage	RT technique	Constraint (mean dose, Gy)	Objective endpoint	Subjective endpoint
Eisbruch (1996) [21]	15	All	I–IV	3D	21 ± 8	SF	XQ
Eisbruch (1999) [33]	88	All	I–IV	3D	≤26 (stimulated) ≤24 (unstimulated)	SF	NS
Chao (2001) [23]	41	All	II–IV	3D/IMRT	≤32	SF	XQ
Eisbruch (2001) [24]	84	All	I–IV	3D/IMRT	≤26	SF	XQ
Henson (2001) [25]	20	All	II–IV	3D	≤26	SF	NS
Maes (2002) [26]	39	All	I–IV	3D	≤20	SGS	VAS
Munter (2004) [27]	18	All	I–IV	IMRT	≤26	SGS	NS
Parliament (2004) [28]	23	All	I–IV	IMRT	≤26	SF	XQ
Saarilahti (2005) [29]	17	OP/NP	II–IV	IMRT	≤25.5	SF	NS
Blanco (2005) [30]	65	All	I–IV	3D/IMRT	≤25.8	SF	NS
Scrimger (2007) [31]	47	All	I–IV	IMRT	≤26	SF	XQ
Eisbruch (2010) [32]	69	OP	I–II	IMRT	<26	SF	XQ

IMRT, intensity-modulated radiotherapy; NP, nasopharynx; NS, not stated; OP, oropharynx; RT, radiotherapy; SF, salivary flow; SGS, salivary gland scintigraphy; VAS, visual analog scale; XQ, xerostomia questionnaire.

Table 18.2 Results of non-randomized studies on IMRT in the treatment of NPC.

Author/Reference	No. of patients	Stages III + IV (%)	CT (%)	Follow-up (months)	LRC/RC	OS	DMFS	Xerostomia (%)
Sultanem (2000) [34]	35	72	91	21.8	100 (4 years)	94 (4 years)	57 (4 years)	(At 2 years) Grade 0: 50, Grade 1: 50
Lee (2002) [35]	67	70	75	31	98 (4 years)	88 (4 years)	66 (4 years)	(At 2 years) Grade 0: 66, Grade 1: 32, Grade 2: 2
Kam (2004) [36]	63	57	30	29	92 (3 years)	90 (3 years)	79 (3 years)	(At 2 years) Grade 1–2: 23
Wu (2006) [37]	75	56	NA	23.8	87 (2 years)	87 (2 years)	82 (2 years)	(In 39 months) Grade 1: 24, Grade 2: 18.6, Grade 3: 1
Wolden (2006) [38]	74	77	93	35	91 (3 years)	83 (3 years)	78 (3 years)	(At 1 year) Grade 0: 25, Grade 1: 42, Grade 2: 32
Lee (2009) [39]	68	59	84	31	93 (2 years)	80 (2 years)	85 (2 years)	(At 1 year) Grade 2: 13.5, Grade 3: 3.1
Tham (2009) [40]	195	63	57	36.5	93 (3 years)	94.3 (3 years)	89.2 (3 years)	Grade 0–2:97, Grade 3: 3
Lin (2009) [41]	323	80.5	91.3	30	95 (3 years)	90 (3 years)	90 (3 years)	(At 24 months) Grade 0: 5.4, Grade 1: 86.8, Grade 2: 7.8
Lin (2009) [42]	370	83.2	90.3	31	95 (3 years)	86 (3 years)	89 (3 years)	(At 24 months) Detectable xerostomia: 7.8%, Grade 3–4: 0

CT, chemotherapy; DMFS, distant metastatic-free survival; LRC/RC, locoregional control/ regional control; NA, not available; OS, overall survival.

dose not result in increased marginal failures [46, 47]. However, sparing of the ipsilateral parotid gland should be given lower priority, especially if there are involved lymph nodes at level II [14, 20, 48]. In patients with extensively involved bilateral nodal disease, meaningful preservation of the parotid function should never be considered at the cost of under-dosing of the target volume, because locoregional failure is the worst treatment outcome. In addition, more detailed proposals have been given about the cranial border of level II, as it has clear relevance to the possibility of sparing the parotid [49]. For patients without nodal disease, the upper boundary of level II is placed at the caudal edge of the lateral process of the first vertebra [16]. For patients with involved nodal disease, level II on the involved neck side is extended to the skull base and includes the retrostyloid space [50].

Nowadays, definitions of dose/volume–response relationships for the parotid glands have been established from data regarding the correlation of residual salivary function with radiation dose. The consensus has been reached that xerostomia can be substantially reduced by limiting the mean parotid gland dose of less than 26–30 Gy as a planning criterion [51]. By reducing the mean dose to at least one parotid gland, salivary function can be partially preserved and improves gradually over time. Thus, both the prevalence and extent of dry mouth can be greatly reduced over time. Although this effect has been demonstrated in several clinical studies [25, 28, 37, 43], the improvement in objective parotid function as measured by salivary flow is not always accompanied with improved patient-reported xerostomia [28, 31, 44]. In one study it was shown that the observer-based grades underestimated the severity of xerostomia compared with the patient self-reported scores [52]. It is suggested that not only the objective parotid function but also patient's subjective scores should be the main end points in evaluating xerostomia. Because xerostomia is mainly an issue of QoL, symptoms reported by patients are more suggestive of its true severity.

Submandibular Glands

Under stimulated status, 60–65% of saliva is produced by the parotid glands, 20–30% by the submandibular glands (SMGs), and 2–5% by the sublingual glands. However, in the non-stimulated state the SMGs contribute up to 90% of salivary output [53]. Moreover, the saliva secreted by the parotid glands is purely serous, whereas saliva from the SMGs also contains mucins, which chiefly contribute to the patient's subjective sense of moisture [20]. Therefore, it is also important to protect the function of the SMGs.

In one study it was shown that surgical transfer of the SMG to the submental space before radiotherapy avoided the gland being irradiated, and can significantly prevent xerostomia, thus confirming the important role of the SMGs [54]. However, this surgical technique has not been widely applied due to its drawbacks. It is reasonable to infer that the severity of xerostomia can be reduced by sparing the SMGs from radiation. A prospective non-randomized study has revealed the feasibility of sparing the SMGs without compromising local tumor control [55].

Data regarding dose–response relationships of the SMGs were gathered by Tsujii [56], who used ^{99m}Tc-pertechnetate scintigraphy to measure salivary gland function and reported an unexpected improvement in SMG function as the dose increased from 10 to 30 Gy, followed with a steep decline after 50 Gy. Tsujii also showed that the parotid glands were more sensitive to radiation than the SMGs at 0–3 months after dosing with 20–70 Gy. Recently, the dose–response relationship for SMGs has been established on the basis of patients who underwent salivary flow measurements selectively from Wharton's duct before and after radiotherapy. The function of SMGs was shown to depend on the mean radiation dose, with recovery over time up to a mean dose of 39 Gy [57]. A recent study showed a clinical benefit from sparing the contralateral submandibular glands [57a].

Reduction of the radiation dose to the SMG might be potentially dangerous owing to its close proximity to the base of tongue, tonsil, and level IIa lymph nodes. Therefore, when trying to preserve the function of the SMGs it is important to take into account the potential risk of reducing local regional tumor control. At present, available evidence regarding the efficacy and safety of SMGs-sparing IMRT is extremely limited.

Oral Cavity and Minor Salivary Glands

The minor salivary glands, which are dispersed throughout the oral cavity, produce up to 70% of the total mucins secreted by the salivary glands [55]. Thus, it is reasonable to anticipate that limiting the radiation dose to the oral cavity might contribute to the reduction of patient-reported xerostomia. Moreover, sparing the oral cavity from unnecessary radiation might have additional benefits in preventing mucositis and taste loss [58]. Therefore, the uninvolved oral cavity should be delineated as an OAR, and be given dose constraint when designing the IMRT plan whenever possible. Currently, the mean non-involved oral cavity dose has been set at ≤30 Gy in the Department of Radiation Oncology, University of Michigan, although with very low priority.

Dysphagia

Dysphagia has a devastating effect on patient daily life, and can even lead to life-threatening complications, such as aspiration pneumonia [59]. Radiotherapy for HNC inevitably results in an appreciable dose delivery to some of the critical structures necessary for normal deglutition, such as the tongue, soft palate, pharyngeal and laryngeal muscles, which leads to unavoidable mucositis and swallowing difficulties [8–10].

Dysphagia can be evaluated by both objective and subjective methods. As with xerostomia, it was shown in one study that patient-reported symptoms were not representative of findings from the objective evaluation of swallowing [60]. To date, many research groups have carried out clinical trials to analyze the relationship between irradiated structures and dysphagia, and the findings of published studies are nearly consistent regarding the crucial structures associated with swallowing dysfunction (Table 18.3). Both, the mean dose to the pharyngeal constrictor muscles and the larynx, as well as the volume of these structures receiving 50–60 Gy, have been shown to remarkably correlate with the prevalence of dysphagia [60–69]. These findings imply that limiting the dose to the crucial swallowing structures might decrease both the incidence and severity of radiation-induced dysphagia.

In order to reduce dysphagia when using IMRT, it is important to identify and delineate any dysphagia and aspiration-related structure (DARS). Eisbruch *et al.* [69] first reported that radiation damage to the pharyngeal constrictors and the glottic/supraglottic larynx were implicated in post-radiotherapy dysphagia, and suggested that reducing the radiation dose to the DARS may lead to improved swallowing outcomes. Subsequently, a series of trials has been initiated to establish whether dose reduction to DARS can improve swallowing outcomes for HNC treated by IMRT. The results of these

Table 18.3 Overview of studies assessing crucial structures for late dysphagia.

Author/Reference	Sample	Site	Dysphagia endpoint	Dosimetric factors correlated with dysphagia
Feng (2007) [61]	36	OP/NP	VF, UW QOL	PCMs (mean dose, V50, V60, V65) and larynx (mean dose, V50)
Levendag (2007) [62]	56	OP	H&N 35	Superior and middle PCMs (mean dose)
Jensen (2007) [60]	25	Pharynx	H&N 35	Supraglottic larynx (mean dose, median dose, V60, V65)
Teguh (2008) [63]	81	OP/NP	H&N 35	Superior and middle PCMs (mean dose)
Teguh (2008) [64]	20	OP	FEES	Superior PCMs (mean dose)
Caglar (2008) [65]	96	All	VF	Inferior PCMs (mean dose, V50, D60) and larynx (mean dose, V50, D60)
Caudell (2009) [66]	83	All	VF	Inferior PCMs (V60, V65) and larynx (mean dose, V55, V60, V65, V70)
Dirix (2009) [67]	53	All	H&N 35	Middle PCMs (mean dose, V50) and supraglottic larynx (mean dose)
Feng (2010) [68]	73	OP	VF, UW QOL	PCMs (mean dose, V50, V60, V65) and larynx (mean dose, V50)
Eisbruch (2004) [69]	26	All	VF	PCMs (V50) and the glottic and supraglottic larynx (V50)

OP, oropharynx; NP, nasopharynx; VF, videofluoroscopy; UW QOL, University of Washington Quality of Life Scale; PCMs, pharyngeal constrictor muscles; V50, volume receiving ≥50 Gy; V60, volume receiving ≥60 Gy; V65, volume receiving ≥65 Gy; H&N 35, EORTC Head and Neck 35 swallowing symptom score; FEES, fiberoptic endoscopic evaluation of swallowing; D60, minimum dose received by 60% of a structure; V70, volume receiving ≥70 Gy.

studies are consistent and showed that an increased radiation dose to a larger volume of the pharyngeal constrictors resulted in worse dysphagia [60–70]. A dose–risk ratio has been suggested by several investigators. Levendag et al. [62] reported a 19% increase in the probability of dysphagia with every additional 10 Gy to the superior and middle constrictor muscles, while Li et al. [70] suggested that in order to reduce the risk of prolonged gastrostomy feeding tube use, the dose constraint should be a mean dose <55 Gy to the inferior constrictor muscle, and a maximum dose <60 Gy to the cricopharyngeal inlet.

Currently, no clear volume or dose constraints are apparent from published data, and the best approach seems to be to keep the radiation dose to these structures as low as possible. Prospective, longitudinal studies, including baseline evaluation with predetermined follow-up assessment at different time points, are still needed to better understand the relationship between dose/volume and swallowing outcomes. In a study conducted by Feng, significant correlations were observed between aspirations and the mean doses to the pharyngeal constrictor (PC) and glottic supraglottic larynx (GSL), as well as the partial volumes of these structures receiving 50–65 Gy [61]. Using these dose–volume parameters as initial IMRT optimization goals, a prospective clinical trial was carried out, the results of which suggested that chemo-IMRT aiming to reduce dysphagia can be performed safely for oropharyngeal cancer [68]. At present, at the University of Michigan, attempts are made to keep the mean dose to the non-involved PC and GSL ≤50 Gy. However, avoiding under-dosing to the targets in the vicinity of the swallowing structures should be the highest priority.

Another approach to spare the swallowing structures is a selective delineation of the nodal volume, especially avoiding delineation of the medial retropharyngeal lymph nodes. These nodes are located between the pharyngeal constrictor muscles and the prevertebral fascia near the midline, and their exclusion from the elective nodal target volume might significantly contribute to sparing the pharyngeal constrictor muscles [20, 61].

Recently, the results of a multicenter prospective study showed that radiotherapy in conjunction with cetuximab improved tumor control without increasing common radiotherapy-associated toxicities, such as dysphagia, and did not have a negative effect on the patients' QoL compared to radiotherapy alone [4, 71]. Therefore, it is inferred that cetuximab could potentially decrease treatment-related toxicity by replacing more toxic chemotherapy without jeopardizing survival. However, to date no Phase III clinical trials have been conducted that directly compare cetuximab and radiotherapy to standard chemotherapy and radiotherapy. Moreover, cetuximab is not without toxicity; according to a retrospective study, concomitant cetuximab with IMRT resulted in an approximately 10-fold increase in the rate of grade 3/4 transient dermatitis compared to the use of concomitant cisplatin (34% versus 3%) [72]. The currently available data are insufficient to warrant changing the standard practice of concurrent chemoradiotherapy to cetuximab and radiotherapy in order to reduce dysphagia.

Cerebral Radiation Necrosis

External-beam radiotherapy with opposed lateral fields has traditionally been used in treating nasopharyngeal carcinoma (NPC). Due to a tendency to spread to the skull base and cavernous sinus, traditional radiation fields usually cover the medial and inferior temporal lobes of the brain. In addition, more than 66 Gy is delivered in order to eradicate the tumor, a dose which exceeds the tolerance of the temporal lobes that might lead to cerebral necrosis. The development of cerebral radiation necrosis (CRN) is a function of dose per fraction, total dose, and time after completion of radiotherapy. The higher the dose per fraction or total dose, the sooner brain necrosis would appear [73]. Whilst there is no effective treatment to reverse this process, it can be prevented by lowering the radiation dose to the temporal lobes. Before the application of IMRT to NPC, CRN was common with the reported incidence varying from 1.6% to 22% [74, 75]. Lee *et al.* noted that 64 Gy at the conventional fraction of 2 Gy per day would lead to a CRN rate of 5% in 10 years [76]. IMRT has been used to treat NPC since the mid-1990s, and the first clinical report by Sultanem *et al.* in 2000 found no occurrence of CRN [34]. Since then, IMRT has been widely applied to treat NPC with an excellent local regional control rate, and no reports have been made of CRN to date [35–42, 77, 78]. This finding can be attributed to the dosimetric advantages of IMRT in sparing temporal lobes compared to conventional radiotherapy. In a dosimetric study aimed at comparing IMRT to conventional radiotherapy, Hunt *et al.* [79] showed that the maximum dose to the temporal lobes was 58.7 Gy with IMRT compared to 67.0 Gy with a conventional radiotherapy plan. Currently, the reported dose constraint to the temporal lobes is a maximum dose <60 Gy, or no more than 1% of the temporal lobe volume exceeding 65 Gy [39, 40, 77].

Hearing Loss

Hearing loss is a common complication of head and neck radiotherapy. The reported post-radiotherapy hearing loss rates vary between 0% and 54%, based on audiometric evaluation [80–83]. It is well known that the incidence of hearing loss increases significantly with increasing dose to the cochlea, and a combination of radiotherapy with cisplatin-based chemotherapy may increase the degree of hearing loss [84]. Published information on the dose–response relationship of hearing loss is listed in Table 18.4. Pan *et al.* [85] performed a prospective study to determine the relationship between the radiotherapy dose to the inner ear and long-term hearing loss in HNC patients treated with 3D-CRT. The results showed that an increase in the mean dose to the inner ear was associated with increased hearing loss at high-frequency (>2000 Hz), and that clinically apparent hearing loss started at a threshold dose of 45 Gy. Based on these findings, a dose ≤45 Gy to the inner ear was suggested if without underdosing the tumor targets [85, 93].

The application of IMRT may further decrease the radiation dose to the inner ear. It has been proven that IMRT is effective in reducing the incidence of hearing loss in non-NPC disease compared with conventional radiotherapy. According to a retrospective study of 26 patients with medulloblastoma, when compared to conventional

Table 18.4 Published data regarding radiation doses causing cochlear damage.

Author/Reference	Sample	Treatment	Threshold dose (Gy)	Clinically significant cochlear damage
Pan (2005) [85]	31	RT	45	≥2000 Hz
Merchant (2004) [86]	72	RT or CRT	32	Low and intermediate frequency (<32 Gy, shunt only); high-frequency (>32 Gy, with or without shunt)
Johannesen (2002) [87]	33	RT or CRT	54	>4000 Hz
Grau (1991) [88]	22	RT	50	SNHL at high frequencies (2–4 kHz)
Oh (2004) [89]	24	CRT	63.4 ± 9.1	High-frequency
Honore (2002) [90]	20	RT	15	Hearing impairment 0.3 dB/Gy and 15% risk of SNHL with 15 Gy
Chen (1999) [82]	21	RT	60	SNHL
Anteunis (1994) [91]	18	RT	50	Conductive and/or SNHL
Herrmann (2006) [92]	32	RT	20–25	ED_{50} in range of 20–25 Gy
Hitchcock (2009) [84]	62	RT or CRT	40 for RT alone 10 for CRT	SNHL High-frequency SNHL

CRT, chemoradiotherapy; RT, radiation therapy; SNHL, sensorineural hearing loss.
ED_{50}, dose at which 50% incidence is expected.

radiotherapy, IMRT delivered 68% of the radiation dose to the auditory apparatus, while still delivering full doses to the desired target volume. Grade 3 or 4 hearing loss was 64% in the conventional radiotherapy group versus 13% in the IMRT group [94]. Similarly, hearing loss in NPC treated with IMRT was relatively uncommon and less severe, although the majority of patients also received concurrent and adjuvant cisplatin-based chemotherapy [34, 38]. Using 3D-CRT, Oh *et al.* [89] observed a reduction in the dose to the inner ear from 69.6 Gy to 63.4 Gy and its resultant reduction in the incidence of hearing loss from 68.2% to 0%, even though no attempt was made to limit the radiation dose to the inner ear structure on the radiation planning.

Accurate delineation of the middle and inner ear is a prerequisite to achieve dose constraint to these structures. However, due to the small size and its close proximity of the inner ear to the target volume, even a small deviation in contouring may pose a profound impact on the quality of the IMRT plan and the risk of post-treatment sequelae. Pacholke *et al.* [95] established the first guidelines for contouring the middle ear and the two major components of the inner ear. The guidelines have been of practical help to radiation oncologists in the process of radiotherapy planning.

Radiation-Induced Nerve Palsy

It is generally believed that the cranial nerves are relatively resistant to radiation, and the incidence of cranial nerve palsy (CNP) is rare after radiotherapy. Depending on dose per fraction, total dose, and time of follow-up, the reported incidence of radiation-induced CNP is 0–5% [96,97]. However, Kong *et al.* [98] recently reported a series of 317 NPC patients with a median follow-up of 11.4 years after radiotherapy, and found 30.9% experienced radiation-induced CNP. The median time to the development of CNP after radiation was 7.6 years, and the average annual rate of developing CNP was 2.2% in long-term survivors. In theory, every cranial nerve might suffer injury from radiation. The following discussions focus on radiation-induced optic neuropathy and brachial plexopathy.

Radiation-Induced Optic Neuropathy

Radiation-induced optic neuropathy (RION) was defined as a sudden and profound irreversible visual loss due to radiation damage to the optic nerve or chiasm [99]. The incidence of RION after external photon beam radiation therapy for head and neck cancer is not well-studied. The latency to the onset of symptoms is correlated to the radiation dose, with the latency being shorter with higher doses [100]. A maximum total dose of 50 Gy delivered by fractionated radiotherapy is associated with a very low risk of RION [101–103], though the risk of RION increases with increasing doses above 50 Gy. A retrospective review of 219 patients receiving radiotherapy for paranasal sinus and nasal cavity tumors reported no cases of RION when the dose was below 50 Gy. The 10-year actuarial risks for RION following doses of 50–60 Gy and 61–78 Gy were 5% and 30%, respectively [104].

IMRT can significantly spare the optic structures as compared to conventional radiotherapy [105,106]; hence, the incidence of RION will be further reduced without compromising local tumor control. To date, RION has not been reported with regards to NPC and paranasal cavity cancers treated with IMRT [34–42, 107–109]. The common dose constraint of the optic nerve and chiasm is a maximum dose of 54 Gy or not more than 1% of the volume exceeding 60 Gy.

Radiation-Induced Brachial Plexopathy

Radiation-induced brachial plexopathy (RIBP) is a relatively common late complication after postoperative radiotherapy for breast cancer, with a reported prevalence of 1–6% at five years after 45–54 Gy irradiation [110–112]. Since the brachial plexus (BP) is adjacent to metastatic lymph nodes and high-risk nodal volume in the neck and supraclavicular area, it is inevitably covered in the radiation portals using conventional techniques. When irradiated to 54–70 Gy, RIBP is also a potential complication in HNC. This has prompted the Radiation Therapy Oncology Group (RTOG) to include the BP as an OAR in many recent protocols.

RIBP correlates with several factors, including total dose, dose per fraction, treatment technique, irradiated volume or length of the brachial plexus, and the addition of chemotherapy or surgery [113]. Owing to the dosimetric advantage of IMRT, the total dose, dose per fraction and irradiated volume to the BP can be reduced, thus leading to a reduced probability of RIBP in long-term survivors. To date, no RIBP has been reported in HNC treated with IMRT, although the BP was not defined as a dose-constraint OAR in these reports. With an increasing awareness of the debilitating effect of RIBP on the patients' QoL, guidelines for contouring the BP on axial CT or MRI scans have been proposed for radiotherapy planning [114,115]. At present, dose constraints to the BP ranging from 60 to 66 Gy are usually suggested in most RTOG protocols [116]. Recently, Platteaux *et al.* [117] performed a retrospective analysis of 43 cases of HNC treated with IMRT. The mean and maximum doses to the BP were 44.1 Gy and 64.2 Gy, respectively. With a median follow-up of 24 months, no RIBP was found. Whether delineation of the BP as an avoidance structure prior to IMRT planning improves the result of treatment in HNC and reduces long-term toxicity in this structure need to be tested in large prospective studies.

Osteoradionecrosis of the Mandible

Osteoradionecrosis (ORN) of the mandible is a well-documented late complication after radiotherapy for HNC [118, 119]. In general, bones are radioresistant and will sustain any overt damage as long as the overlying soft tissue remains intact and the bone is not subjected to excessive stress or trauma [120]. A number of risk factors are associated with the development of ORN, such as age, general health, dentition status, oral hygiene, proximity of or invasion of the tumor to mandible, treatment type, total radiation dose, and associated trauma, such as teeth extraction before or after radiotherapy [118].

Despite increasing intensity in therapy in recent years, there has been a reduction in the incidence of ORN. In a recent report of 176 cases of HNC treated with IMRT, no case with ORN was identified with a median follow-up of 35 months [120]. In this study, the following dose constraints were used for plan optimization: maximal mandibular dose <72 Gy; mean parotid gland dose ≤26 Gy; and mean non-involved oral cavity dose ≤30 Gy. Patients were instructed to receive dental care such as extraction of decaying or non-restorable teeth before radiotherapy, mouth wash with fluoride gel during and after radiotherapy, or using radiation guards during radiotherapy. The reduction in the incidence of ORN was attributed to two factors: (i) a more conformal dose distribution which spared part of the mandible that might have received a higher dose had conventional radiotherapy techniques been used; and (ii) better prophylactic and on-going dental care [120]. Which factor plays the more important role has not yet been determined. Overall, it is believed that the reductions in dose to the salivary glands and mandible are likely to translate into reduced incidences of xerostomia and osteoradionecrosis [121–124]. At present, the recommended dose constraint to the mandible is a maximum of 70 Gy in most clinical trials and published reports.

Table 18.5 Suggested dose limits for organs at risk.

Organ	Mean dose (Gy)	Maximal dose (Gy)
Parotid glands	<26[a]	–
Submandibular glands	<39[a]	–
Non-involved oral cavity	≤30	–
Optic nerves/chiasma	<54	<54
Brachial plexus	<70	<70
Larynx	<20[b]	–
Pharyngeal constrictors	<50[c]	–
Upper esophagus	<20[2]	

[a]There is no threshold; lower doses are likely to result in further improved salivary output.
[b]In cases where the lower-neck targets are at low-risk and the neck is treated with whole-field technique (this dose is equivalent to laryngeal/esophageal doses delivered by split-field IMRT using laryngeal block).
[c]The inferior constrictor means dose in cases where the lower neck is at low risk may be limited to 20 Gy, equivalent to the dose delivered by split-field IMRT using laryngeal block.

Conclusions

Quality of life may be improved by the application of IMRT without compromising tumor control for HNC. When treating HNC with IMRT or 3D-CRT, it is important to contour the target volume accurately, as well as to delineate all relevant normal structures at risk, and the available radiation-dose constraints must be taken into account (Table 18.5). Currently, xerostomia can be successfully prevented or reduced by holding a mean dose threshold of 26 Gy to at least one parotid gland. Late dysphagia can be reduced by keeping the mean dose to the non-involved pharyngeal constrictor muscles and the larynx ≤50 Gy. Late radiation-induced optic neuropathy risk can be minimized by limiting a maximum dose of 54 Gy to the optic nerve and chiasm. By lowering the dose to the inner ear, temporal lobe and mandible, the incidence of hearing loss, brain necrosis and osteonecrosis of the mandible is likely to decline. However, a prospective collection of dosimetric data along with the corresponding functional outcomes is still needed in order to establish more precise dose–response curves.

References

1 Siegel, R., Miller, K., Jemal, A. (2017) Cancer statistics, 2017. *CA Cancer J. Clin.*, **67** (1), 7–30.
2 Argiris, A., Karamouzis, M.V., Raben, D., Ferris, R.L. (2008) Head and neck cancer. *Lancet*, **371**, 1695–1709.
3 Pignon, J.P., le Maître, A., Maillard, E., Bourhis, J. (2009) (Meta-analysis of chemotherapy in head and neck cancer (MACH-NC): an update on 93 randomised trials and 17,346 patients. *Radiother. Oncol.*, **92** (1), 4–14.
4 Bonner, J.A., Harari, P.M., Giralt, J., *et al.* (2006) Radiotherapy plus cetuximab for squamous-cell carcinoma of the head and neck. *N. Engl. J. Med.*, **354**, 567–578.

5 Cohen, E.E., Haraf, D.J., Kunnavakkam, R., *et al.* (2010) Epidermal growth factor receptor inhibitor gefitinib added to chemoradiotherapy in locally advanced head and neck cancer. *J. Clin. Oncol.*, **28** (20), 3336–3343.

6 Brizel, D.M., Esclamado, R. (2006) Concurrent chemoradiotherapy for locally advanced, nonmetastatic, squamous carcinoma of the head and neck: consensus, controversy, and conundrum. *J. Clin. Oncol.*, **24** (17), 2612–2617.

7 Posner, M.R., Hershock, D.M., Blajman, C.R., *et al.* (2007) Cisplatin and fluorouracil alone or with docetaxel in head and neck cancer. *N. Engl. J. Med.*, **357** (17), 1705–1715.

8 Nuyts, S., Dirix, P., Clement, P.M., *et al.* (2009) Impact of adding concomitant chemotherapy to hyperfractionated accelerated radiotherapy for advanced head and neck squamous cell carcinoma. *Int. J. Radiat. Oncol. Biol. Phys.*, **73**, 1088–1095.

9 Garden, A.S., Harris, J., Trotti, A., *et al.* (2008) Long-term results of concomitant boost radiation plus concurrent cisplatin for advanced head and neck carcinomas: a phase II trial of the radiation therapy oncology group (RTOG 99-14). *Int. J. Radiat. Oncol. Biol. Phys.*, **71** (5), 1351–1355.

10 Manikantan, K., Khode, S., Sayed, S.I., *et al.* (2009) Dysphagia in head and neck cancer. *Cancer Treat. Rev.*, **35** (8), 724–732.

11 Harari, P.M. (2008) Beware the swing and a miss: baseball precautions for conformal radiotherapy. *Int. J. Radiat. Oncol. Biol. Phys.*, **70**, 657–659.

12 Cannon, D.M., Lee, N.Y. (2008) Recurrence in region of spared parotid gland after definitive intensity-modulated radiotherapy for head and neck cancer. *Int. J. Radiat. Oncol. Biol. Phys.*, **70**, 660–665.

13 Chao, K.S., Wippold, F.J., Ozyigit, G., Tran, B.N., Dempsey, J.F. (2002) Determination and delineation of nodal target volumes for head-and-neck cancer based on patterns of failure in patients receiving definitive and postoperative IMRT. *Int. J. Radiat. Oncol. Biol. Phys.*, **53**, 1174–1184.

14 Eisbruch, A., Marsh, L.H., Dawson, L.A., *et al.* (2004) Recurrences near base of skull after IMRT for head-and-neck cancer: Implications for target delineation in high neck and for parotid gland sparing. *Int. J. Radiat. Oncol. Biol. Phys.*, **59**, 28–42.

15 Eisbruch, A., Foote, R.L., O'Sullivan, B., Beitler, J.J., Vikram, B. (2002) Intensity-modulated radiation therapy for head and neck cancer: Emphasis on the selection and delineation of the targets. *Semin. Radiat. Oncol.*, **12**, 238–249.

16 Grégoire, V., Levendag, P., Ang, K.K., *et al.* (2003) CT-based delineation of lymph node levels and related CTVs in the node negative neck: AHANCA, EORTC, GORTEC, RTOG consensus guidelines. *Radiother. Oncol.*, **69**, 227–236.

17 Marks, L.B., Yorke, E.D., Jackson, A., *et al.* (2010) Use of normal tissue complication probability models in the clinic. *Int. J. Radiat. Oncol. Biol. Phys.*, **76**, S10–S19.

18 Emami, B., Lyman, J., Brown, A., *et al.* (1991) Tolerance of normal tissue to therapeutic irradiation. *Int. J. Radiat. Oncol. Biol. Phys.*, **21** (1), 109–122.

19 Dirix, P., Nuyts, S., Van den Bogaert, W. (2006) Radiation-induced xerostomia in patients with head and neck cancer: a literature review. *Cancer*, **107**, 2525–2534.

20 Dirix, P., Nuyts, S. (2010) Evidence-based organ-sparing radiotherapy in head and neck cancer. *Lancet Oncol.*, **11** (1), 85–91.

21 Eisbruch, A., Ship, J.A., Martel, M.K., *et al.* (1996) Parotid gland sparing in patients undergoing bilateral head and neck irradiation: techniques and early results. *Int. J. Radiat. Oncol. Biol. Phys.*, **36**, 469–480.

22 Li, Y., Taylor, J.M., Ten Haken, R.K., Eisbruch, A. (2007) The impact of dose on parotid salivary recovery in head and neck cancer patients treated with radiation therapy. *Int. J. Radiat. Oncol. Biol. Phys.*, **67**, 660–669.

23 Chao, K.S., Deasy, J.O., Markman, J., *et al.* (2001) A prospective study of salivary function sparing in patients with head-and-neck cancers receiving intensity-modulated or three-dimensional radiation therapy: initial results. *Int. J. Radiat. Oncol. Biol. Phys.*, **49**, 907–916.

24 Eisbruch, A., Kim, H.M., Terrell, J.E., *et al.* (2001) Xerostomia and its predictors following parotid-sparing irradiation of head-and-neck cancer. *Int. J. Radiat. Oncol. Biol. Phys.*, **50**, 695–704.

25 Henson, B.S., Inglehart, M.R., Eisbruch, A., Ship, J.A. (2001) Preserved salivary output and xerostomia-related quality of life in head and neck cancer patients receiving parotid-sparing radiotherapy. *Oral Oncol.*, **37**, 84–93.

26 Maes, A., Weltens, C., Flamen, P., *et al.* (2002) Preservation of parotid function with uncomplicated conformal radiotherapy. *Radiother. Oncol.*, **63**, 203–211.

27 Münter, M.W., Karger, C.P., Hoffner, S.G., *et al.* (2004) Evaluation of salivary gland function after treatment of head-and-neck tumors with intensity-modulated radiotherapy by quantitative pertechnetate scintigraphy. *Int. J. Radiat. Oncol. Biol. Phys.*, **58**, 175–184.

28 Parliament, M.B., Scrimger, R.A., Anderson, S.G., *et al.* (2004) Preservation of oral health-related quality of life and salivary flow rates after inverse-planned intensity-modulated radiotherapy (IMRT) for head-and-neck cancer. *Int. J. Radiat. Oncol. Biol. Phys.*, **58**, 663–673.

29 Saarilahti, K., Kouri, M., Collan, J., *et al.* (2005) Intensity modulated radiotherapy for head and neck cancer: evidence for preserved salivary gland function. *Radiother. Oncol.*, **74**, 251–258.

30 Blanco, A.I., Chao, K.S., El Naqa, I., *et al.* (2005) Dose-volume modelling of salivary function in patients with head-and-neck cancer receiving radiotherapy. *Int. J. Radiat. Oncol. Biol. Phys.*, **62**, 1055–1069.

31 Scrimger, R., Kanji, A., Parliament, M., *et al.* (2007) Correlation between saliva production and quality of life measurements in head and neck cancer patients treated with intensity-modulated radiotherapy. *Am. J. Clin. Oncol.*, **30**, 271–277.

32 Eisbruch, A., Harris, J., Garden, A.S., *et al.* (2010) Multi-institutional trial of accelerated hypofractionated intensity-modulated radiation therapy for early-stage oropharyngeal cancer (RTOG 00-22). *Int. J. Radiat. Oncol. Biol. Phys.*, **76** (5), 1333–1338.

33 Eisbruch, A., Ten Haken, R.K., Kim, H.M., *et al.* (1999) Dose, volume, and function relationships in parotid salivary glands following conformal and intensity-modulated irradiation of head and neck cancer. *Int. J. Radiat. Oncol. Biol. Phys.*, **45** (3), 577–587.

34 Sultanem, K., Shu, H.K., Xia, P., *et al.* (2000) Three-dimensional intensity-modulated radiotherapy in the treatment of nasopharyngeal carcinoma: the University of California-San Francisco experience. *Int. J. Radiat. Oncol. Biol. Phys.*, **48**, 711–722.

35 Lee, N., Xia, P., Quivey, J.M., *et al.* (2002) Intensity-modulated radiotherapy in the treatment of nasopharyngeal carcinoma: An update of the USCF experience. *Int. J. Radiat. Oncol. Biol. Phys.*, **53**, 12–22.

36 Kam, M.K., Teo, P.M., Chau, R.M., *et al.* (2004) Treatment of nasopharyngeal carcinoma with intensity-modulated radiotherapy: the Hong Kong experience. *Int. J. Radiat. Oncol. Biol. Phys.*, **60**, 1440–1450.

37 Wu, S., Xie, C.Y., Jin, X., Zhang, P. (2006) Simultaneous modulated accelerated radiation therapy in the treatment of nasopharyngeal cancer: a local center's experience. *Int. J. Radiat. Oncol. Biol. Phys.*, **66**, S40–S46.

38 Wolden, S.L., Chen, W.C., Pfister, D.G., Kraus, D.H., Berry, S.L., Zelefsky, M.J. (2006) Intensity-modulated radiation therapy (IMRT) for nasopharyngeal cancer: update of the Memorial Sloan-Kettering experience. *Int. J. Radiat. Oncol. Biol. Phys.*, **64**, 57–62.

39 Lee, N., Harris, J., Garden, A.S., *et al.* (2009) Intensity-modulated radiation therapy with or without chemotherapy for nasopharyngeal carcinoma: radiation therapy oncology group phase II trial 0225. *J. Clin. Oncol.*, **27** (22), 3684–3690.

40 Tham, I.W., Hee, S.W., Yeo, R.M., *et al.* (2009) Treatment of nasopharyngeal carcinoma using intensity-modulated radiotherapy – the National Cancer Centre Singapore experience. *Int. J. Radiat. Oncol. Biol. Phys.*, **75** (5), 1481–1486.

41 Lin, S., Pan, J., Han, L., Zhang, X., Liao, X., Lu, J.J. (2009) Nasopharyngeal carcinoma treated with reduced-volume intensity-modulated radiation therapy: report on the 3-year outcome of a prospective series. *Int. J. Radiat. Oncol. Biol. Phys.*, **75** (4), 1071–1078.

42 Lin, S., Lu, J.J., Han, L., Chen, Q., Pan, J. (2010) Sequential chemotherapy and intensity-modulated radiation therapy in the management of locoregionally advanced nasopharyngeal carcinoma: experience of 370 consecutive cases. *BMC Cancer*, **10**, 39.

43 Pow, E.H., Kwong, D.L., McMillan, A.S., *et al.* (2006) Xerostomia and quality of life after intensity-modulated radiotherapy vs. conventional radiotherapy for early-stage nasopharyngeal carcinoma: initial report on a randomized controlled clinical trial. *Int. J. Radiat. Oncol. Biol. Phys.*, **66** (4), 981–991.

44 Kam, M.K., Leung, S.F., Zee, B., *et al.* (2007) Prospective randomized study of intensity-modulated radiotherapy on salivary gland function in early-stage nasopharyngeal carcinoma patients. *J. Clin. Oncol.*, **25**, 4873–4879.

45 Braam, P.M., Terhaard, C.H., Roesink, J.M., Raaijmakers, C.P. (2006) Intensity-modulated radiotherapy significantly reduces xerostomia compared with conventional radiotherapy. *Int. J. Radiat. Oncol. Biol. Phys.*, **66**, 975–980.

46 Feng, M., Jabbari, S., Lin, A., *et al.* (2005) Predictive factors of local-regional recurrences following parotid sparing intensity modulated or 3D conformal radiotherapy for head and neck cancer. *Radiother. Oncol.*, **77**, 32–38.

47 Daly, M.E., Lieskovsky, Y., Pawlicki, T., *et al.* (2007) Evaluation of patterns of failure and subjective salivary function in patients treated with intensity modulated radiotherapy for head and neck squamous cell carcinoma. *Head Neck*, **29**, 211–220.

48 David, M.B., Eisbruch, A. (2007) Delineating neck targets for intensity-modulated radiation therapy of head and neck cancer. What have we learned from marginal recurrences? *Front. Radiat. Ther. Oncol.*, **40**, 193–207.

49 Astreinidou, E., Dehnad, H., Terhaard, C.H., Raaijmakers, C.P. (2004) Level II lymph nodes and radiation-induced xerostomia. *Int. J. Radiat. Oncol. Biol. Phys.*, **58**, 124–131.

50 Grégoire, V., Eisbruch, A., Hamoir, M., Levendag, P. (2006) Proposal for the delineation of the nodal CTV in the node-positive and the post-operative neck. *Radiother. Oncol.*, **79**, 15–20.

51 Chambers, M.S., Garden, A.S., Rosenthal, D., *et al.* Intensity-modulated radiotherapy: is xerostomia still prevalent? *Curr. Oncol. Rep.*, **7** (2), 131–136.

52 Meirovitz, A., Murdoch-Kinch, C.A., Schipper, M., Pan, C., Eisbruch, A. (2006) Grading xerostomia by physicians or by patients after intensity-modulated radiotherapy of head-and-neck cancer. *Int. J. Radiat. Oncol. Biol. Phys.*, **66** (2), 445–453.

53 Eisbruch, A., Rhodus, N., Rosenthal, D., *et al.* (2003) How should we measure and report radiotherapy-induced xerostomia? *Semin. Radiat. Oncol.*, **13**, 226–234.

54 Jha, N., Seikaly, H., McGaw, T., Coulter, L. (2000) Submandibular salivary gland transfer prevents radiation-induced xerostomia. *Int. J. Radiat. Oncol. Biol. Phys.*, **46**, 7–11.

55 Saarilahti, K., Kouri, M., Collan, J., *et al.* (2006) Sparing of the submandibular glands by intensity modulated radiotherapy in the treatment of head and neck cancer. *Radiother. Oncol.*, **78**, 270–275.

56 Tsujii, H. (1985) Quantitative dose-response analysis of salivary function following radiotherapy using sequential RI-sialography. *Int. J. Radiat. Oncol. Biol. Phys.*, **11**, 1603–1612.

57 Murdoch-Kinch, C.A., Kim, H.M., Vineberg, K.A., Ship, J.A., Eisbruch, A. (2008) Dose-effect relationships for the submandibular glands and implications for their sparing by intensity modulated radiotherapy. *Int. J. Radiat. Oncol. Biol. Phys.*, **72**, 373–382.

57a Wang, Z.H., Yan, C., Zhang, Z.Y., *et al.* (2011) Impact of salivary gland dosimetry on post-IMRT recovery of saliva output and xerostomia grade for head and neck cancer patients treated with or without contralateral submandibular gland sparing. *Int. J. Radiat. Oncol. Biol. Phys.*, **81**, 1479–1487.

58 Sciubba, J.J., Goldenberg, D. (2006) Oral complications of radiotherapy. *Lancet Oncol.*, **7**, 175–183.

59 Eisbruch, A., Lyden, T., Bradford, C.R., *et al.* (2002) Objective assessment of swallowing dysfunction and aspiration after radiation concurrent with chemotherapy for head and neck cancer. *Int. J. Radiat. Oncol. Biol. Phys.*, **53**, 23–28.

60 Jensen, K., Lambertsen, K., Grau, C. (2007) Late swallowing dysfunction and dysphagia after radiotherapy for pharynx cancer: frequency, intensity and correlation with dose and volume parameters. *Radiother. Oncol.*, **85** (1), 74–82.

61 Feng, F.Y., Kim, H.M., Lyden, T.H., *et al.* (2007) Intensity-modulated radiotherapy of head and neck cancer aiming to reduce dysphagia: early-dose effect relationships for the swallowing structures. *Int. J. Radiat. Oncol. Biol. Phys.*, **68**, 1289–1298.

62 Levendag, P.C., Teguh, D.N., Voet, P., *et al.* (2007) Dysphagia disorders in patients with cancer of the oropharynx are significantly affected by the radiation therapy dose to the superior and middle constrictor muscle: a dose-effect relationship. *Radiother. Oncol.*, **85**, 64–73.

63 Teguh, D.N., Levendag, P.C., Noever, I., *et al.* (2008) Treatment techniques and site considerations regarding dysphagia-related quality of life in cancer of the oropharynx and nasopharynx. *Int. J. Radiat. Oncol. Biol. Phys.*, **72**, 1119–1127.

64 Teguh, D.N., Levendag, P.C., Sewnaik, A., *et al.* (2008) Results of fiberoptic endoscopic evaluation of swallowing vs radiation dose in the swallowing muscles after radiotherapy of cancer in the oropharynx. *Radiother. Oncol.*, **89**, 57–64.

65 Caglar, H.B., Tishler, R.B., Othus, M., *et al.* (2008) Dose to larynx predicts for swallowing complications after intensity-modulated radiotherapy. *Int. J. Radiat. Oncol. Biol. Phys.*, **72**, 1110–1118.

66 Caudell, J.J., Schaner, P.E., Desmond, R.A., *et al.* (2010) Dosimetric factors associated with long-term dysphagia after radiotherapy for squamous cell carcinoma of the head and neck. *Int. J. Radiat. Oncol. Biol. Phys.*, **76** (2), 403–409.

67 Dirix, P., Abbeel, S., Vanstraelen, B., Hermans, R., Nuyts, S. (2009) Dysphagia after chemoradiotherapy for head-and-neck squamous cell carcinoma: dose-effect relationships for the swallowing structures. *Int. J. Radiat. Oncol. Biol. Phys.*, **75** (2), 385–392.

68 Feng, F.Y., Kim, H.M., Lyden, T.H., *et al.* (2010) Intensity-modulated chemoradiotherapy aiming to reduce dysphagia in patients with oropharyngeal cancer: clinical and functional results. *J. Clin. Oncol.*, **28** (16), 2732–2738.

69 Eisbruch, A., Schwartz, M., Rasch, C., *et al.* (2004) Dysphagia and aspiration after chemoradiotherapy for head-and-neck cancer: which anatomic structures are affected and can they be spared by IMRT? *Int. J. Radiat. Oncol. Biol. Phys.*, **60** (5), 1425–1439.

70 Li, B., Li, D., Lau, D.H., *et al.* (2009) Clinical-dosimetric analysis of measures of dysphagia including gastrostomy-tube dependence among head and neck cancer patients treated definitively by intensity-modulated radiotherapy with concurrent chemotherapy. *Radiat. Oncol.*, **4**, 52.

71 Bonner, J.A., Harari, P.M., Giralt, J., *et al.* (2010) Radiotherapy plus cetuximab for locoregionally advanced head and neck cancer: 5-year survival data from a phase 3 randomised trial, and relation between cetuximab-induced rash and survival. *Lancet Oncol.*, **11** (1), 21–28.

72 Studer, G., Brown, M., Salgueiro, E.B., *et al.* (2011) Grade 3/4 dermatitis in head and neck cancer

patients treated with concurrent cetuximab and IMRT. *Int. J. Radiat. Oncol. Biol. Phys.*, **81** (1), 110–117.

73 Marks, J.E., Wong, J. (1985) The risk of cerebral radiation necrosis in relation to dose, time, and fractionation. *Prog. Exp. Tumor Res.*, **29**, 210–218.

74 Lee, A.W., Ng, S.H., Ho, J.H., Tse, V.K., *et al.* (1988) Clinical diagnosis of late temporal lobe necrosis following radiation therapy for nasopharyngeal carcinoma. *Cancer*, **61**, 1535–1542.

75 Leung, S.F., Kreel, L., Tsao, S.Y. (1992) Asymptomatic temporal lobe injury after radiotherapy for nasopharyngeal carcinoma: incidence and determinants. *Br. J. Radiol.*, **65**, 710–714.

76 Lee, A.W., Foo, W., Chappell, R., *et al.* (1998) Effect of time, dose, and fractionation on temporal lobe necrosis following radiotherapy for nasopharyngeal carcinoma. *Int. J. Radiat. Oncol. Biol. Phys.*, **40**, 35–42.

77 Ng, W.T., Lee, M.C., Hung, W.M., *et al.* (2011) Clinical outcomes and patterns of failure after intensity-modulated radiotherapy for nasopharyngeal carcinoma. *Int. J. Radiat. Oncol. Biol. Phys.*, **79** (2), 420–428.

78 Lai, S.Z., Li, W.F., Chen, L., *et al.* (2011) How does intensity-modulated radiotherapy versus conventional two-dimensional radiotherapy influence the treatment results in nasopharyngeal carcinoma patients? *Int. J. Radiat. Oncol. Biol. Phys.*, **80** (3) 661–668.

79 Hunt, M.A., Zelefsky, M.J., Wolden, S., *et al.* (2001) Treatment planning and delivery of intensity-modulated radiation therapy for primary nasopharynx cancer. *Int. J. Radiat. Oncol. Biol. Phys.*, **49** (3), 623–632.

80 Ho, W.K., Wei, W.I., Kwong, D.L., *et al.* (1999) Long-term sensorineural hearing deficit following radiotherapy in patients suffering from nasopharyngeal carcinoma: a prospective study. *Head Neck*, **21**, 547–553.

81 Kwong, D.L., Wei, W.I., Sham, J.S., *et al.* (1996) Sensorineural hearing loss in patients treated for nasopharyngeal carcinoma: a prospective study of the effect of radiation and cisplatin treatment. *Int. J. Radiat. Oncol. Biol. Phys.*, **36** (2), 281–289.

82 Raaijmakers, E., Engelen, A.M. (2002) Is sensorineural hearing-loss a possible side effect of nasopharyngeal and parotid irradiation? A systematic review of the literature. *Radiother. Oncol.*, **65**, 1–7.

83 Yeh, S.A., Tang, Y., Lui, C.C., Huang, Y.J., Huang, E.Y. (2005) Treatment outcomes and late complications of 849 patients with nasopharyngeal carcinoma treated with radiotherapy alone. *Int. J. Radiat. Oncol. Biol. Phys.*, **62** (3), 672–679.

84 Hitchcock, Y.J., Tward, J.D., Szabo, A., Bentz, B.G., Shrieve, D.C. (2009) Relative contributions of radiation and cisplatin-based chemotherapy to sensorineural hearing loss in head-and-neck cancer patients. *Int. J. Radiat. Oncol. Biol. Phys.*, **73** (3), 779–788.

85 Pan, C.C., Eisbruch, A., Lee, J.S., *et al.* (2005) Prospective study of inner ear radiation dose and hearing loss in head-and-neck cancer patients. *Int. J. Radiat. Oncol. Biol. Phys.*, **61**, 1393–1402.

86 Merchant, T.E., Gould, C.J., Xiong, X., *et al.* (2004) Early neuro-otologic effects of three-dimensional irradiation in children with primary brain tumors. *Int. J. Radiat. Oncol. Biol. Phys.*, **58**, 1194–1207.

87 Johannesen, T.B., Rasmussen, K., Winther, F.Ø., Halvorsen, U., Lote, K. (2002) Late radiation effects on hearing, vestibular function, and taste in brain tumor patients. *Int. J. Radiat. Oncol. Biol. Phys.*, **53**, 86–90.

88 Grau, C., Møller, K., Overgaard, M., Overgaard, J., Elbrønd, O. (1991) Sensorineural hearing loss in patients treated with irradiation for nasopharyngeal carcinoma. *Int. J. Radiat. Oncol. Biol. Phys.*, **21**, 723–728.

89 Oh, Y.T., Kim, C.H., Choi, J.H., *et al.* (2004) Sensory neural hearing loss after concurrent cisplatin and radiation therapy for nasopharyngeal carcinoma. *Radiother. Oncol.*, **72**, 79–82.

90 Honoré, H.B., Bentzen, S.M., Møller, K., Grau, C. (2002) Sensori-neural hearing loss after radiotherapy for nasopharyngeal carcinoma: Individualized risk estimation. *Radiother. Oncol.*, **65**, 9–16.

91 Anteunis, L.J., Wanders, S.L., Hendriks, J.J., *et al.* (1994) A prospective longitudinal study on radiation-induced hearing loss. *Am. J. Surg.*, **168**, 408–411.

92 Herrmann, F., Dörr, W., Müller, R., Herrmann, T. (2006) A prospective study on radiation-induced changes in hearing function. *Int. J. Radiat. Oncol. Biol. Phys.*, **65**, 1338–1344.

93 Chen, W.C., Jackson, A., Budnick, A.S., *et al.* (2006) Sensorineural hearing loss in combined modality treatment of nasopharyngeal carcinoma. *Cancer*, **106**, 820–829.

94 Huang, E., The, B.S., Strother, D.R., *et al.* (2002) Intensity-modulated radiation therapy for pediatric medulloblastoma: early report on the reduction of ototoxicity. *Int. J. Radiat. Oncol. Biol. Phys.*, **52** (3), 599–605.

95 Pacholke, H.D., Amdur, R.J., Schmalfuss, I.M., Louis, D., Mendenhall, W.M. (2005) Contouring the middle and inner ear on radiotherapy planning scans. *Am. J. Clin. Oncol.*, **28** (2), 143–147.

96 Lee, A.W.M., Law, S.C.K, Ng, S.H., *et al.* (1992) Retrospective analysis of nasopharyngeal carcinoma

treated during 1976–1985: late complications following megavoltage irradiation. *Br. J. Radiol.*, **65**, 918–928.

97 Qin, D.X., Hu, Y.H., Yan, J.H., *et al.* (1988) Analysis of 1379 patients with nasopharyngeal carcinoma treated by radiation. *Cancer*, **61**, 1117–1124.

98 Kong, L., Lu, J.J., Liss, A.L., *et al.* (2011) Radiation-induced cranial nerve palsy: a cross-sectional study of nasopharyngeal cancer patients after definitive radiotherapy. *Int. J. Radiat. Oncol. Biol. Phys.*, **79** (5), 1421–1427.

99 van den Bergh, A.C., Schoorl, M.A., Dullaart, R.P., *et al.* (2004) Lack of radiation optic neuropathy in 72 patients treated for pituitary adenoma. *J. Neuroophthalmol.*, **24** (3), 200–205.

100 Borruat, F.-X., Schatz, N.J., Glaser, J.S., *et al.* (1996) Radiation optic neuropathy: Report of cases, role of hyperbaric oxygen therapy and literature review. *Neuroophthalmology*, **16**, 255–266.

101 Parsons, J.T., Fitzgerald, C.R., Hood, C.I., *et al.* (1983) The effects of irradiation on the eye and optic nerve. *Int. J. Radiat. Oncol. Biol. Phys.*, **9** (5), 609–622.

102 Mayo, C., Martel, M.K., Marks, L.B., *et al.* (2010) Radiation dose-volume effects of optic nerves and chiasm. *Int. J. Radiat. Oncol. Biol. Phys.*, **76** (3 Suppl.), S28–S35.

103 Lessell, S. (2004) Friendly fire: neurogenic visual loss from radiation therapy. *J. Neuroophthalmol.*, **24** (3), 243–250.

104 Jiang, G.L., Tucker, S.L., Guttenberger, R., *et al.* (1994) Radiation-induced injury to the visual pathway. *Radiother. Oncol.*, **30**, 17–25.

105 Mock, U., Georg, D., Bogner, J., *et al.* (2004) Treatment planning comparison of conventional, 3D conformal, and intensity-modulated photon (IMRT) and proton therapy for paranasal sinus carcinoma. *Int. J. Radiat. Oncol. Biol. Phys.*, **58**, 147–154.

106 Kam, M.K., Chau, R.M., Suen, J., *et al.* (2003) Intensity-modulated radiotherapy in nasopharyngeal carcinoma: Dosimetric advantage over conventional plans and feasibility of dose escalation. *Int. J. Radiat. Oncol. Biol. Phys.*, **56**, 145–157.

107 Madani, I., Bonte, K., Vakaet, L., *et al.* (2009) Intensity-modulated radiotherapy for sinonasal tumors: Ghent University Hospital update. *Int. J. Radiat. Oncol. Biol. Phys.*, **73** (2), 424–432.

108 Dirix, P., Vanstraelen, B., Jorissen, M., *et al.* (2010) Intensity-modulated radiotherapy for sinonasal cancer: improved outcome compared to conventional radiotherapy. *Int. J. Radiat. Oncol. Biol. Phys.*, **78** (4), 998–1004.

109 Hoppe, B.S., Wolden, S.L., Zelefsky, M.J., *et al.* (2008) Postoperative intensity-modulated radiation therapy for cancers of the paranasal sinuses, nasal cavity, and lacrimal glands: technique, early outcomes, and toxicity. *Head Neck*, **30** (7), 925–932.

110 Powell, S., Cooke, J., Parsons, C. (1990) Radiation-induced brachial plexus injury: follow-up of two different fractionation schedules. *Radiother. Oncol.*, **18** (3), 213–220.

111 Bowen, B.C., Verma, A., Brandon, A.H., Fiedler, J.A. (1996) Radiation-induced brachial plexopathy: MR and clinical findings. *Am. J. Neuroradiol.*, **17** (10), 1932–1936.

112 Johansson, S., Svensson, H., Denekamp, J. (2002) Dose response and latency for radiation-induced fibrosis, edema, and neuropathy in breast cancer patients. *Int. J. Radiat. Oncol. Biol. Phys.*, **52** (5), 1207–1219.

113 Gosk, J., Rutowski, R., Reichert, P., Rabczyński, J. (2007) Radiation-induced brachial plexus neuropathy - aetiopathogenesis, risk factors, differential diagnostics, symptoms and treatment. *Folia Neuropathol.*, **45** (1), 26–30.

114 Hall, W.H., Guiou, M., Lee, N.Y., *et al.* (2008) Development and validation of a standardized method for contouring the brachial plexus: preliminary dosimetric analysis among patients treated with IMRT for head-and-neck cancer. *Int. J. Radiat. Oncol. Biol. Phys.*, **72** (5), 1362–1367.

115 Truong, M.T., Nadgir, R.N., Hirsch, A.E., *et al.* (2010) Brachial plexus contouring with CT and MR imaging in radiation therapy planning for head and neck cancer. *Radiographics*, **30** (4), 1095–1103.

116 McGary, J.E., Grant, W.H., The, B.S., *et al.* Dosimetric evaluation of the brachial plexus in the treatment of head and neck cancer. *Int. J. Radiat. Oncol. Biol. Phys.*, **69**, S464–S465.

117 Platteaux, N., Dirix, P., Hermans, R., Nuyts, S. (2010) Brachial plexopathy after chemoradiotherapy for head and neck squamous cell carcinoma. *Strahlenther. Onkol.*, **186** (9), 517–520.

118 Mendenhall, W.M. (2004) Mandibular osteoradionecrosis. *J. Clin. Oncol.*, **22**, 4867–4868.

119 Sciubba, J.J., Goldenberg, D. (2006) Oral complications of radiotherapy. *Lancet Oncol.*, **7** (2), 175–183.

120 Ben-David, M.A., Diamante, M., Radawski, J.D., *et al.* (2007) Lack of osteoradionecrosis of the mandible after intensity-modulated radiotherapy for head and neck cancer: likely contributions of both dental care and improved dose distributions. *Int. J. Radiat. Oncol. Biol. Phys.*, **68** (2), 396–402.

121 Parliament, M., Alidrisi, M., Munroe, M., *et al.* (2005) Implications of radiation dosimetry of the mandible in patients with carcinomas of the oral cavity and nasopharynx treated with intensity modulated radiation therapy. *Int. J. Oral Maxillofac. Surg.*, **34**, 114–121.

122 Kielbassa, A.M., Hinkelbein, W., Hellwig, E., *et al.* (2006) Radiation-related damage to dentition. *Lancet Oncol.*, **7**, 326–335.

123 Studer, G., Studer, S.P., Zwahlen, R.A., *et al.* (2006) Osteoradionecrosis of the mandible: Minimized risk profile following intensity-modulated radiation therapy (IMRT). *Strahlenther. Onkol.*, **182**, 283–288.

124 de Arruda, F.F., Puri, D.R., Zhung, J., *et al.* (2006) Intensity-modulated radiation therapy for the treatment of oropharyngeal carcinoma: The Memorial Sloan-Kettering Cancer Center experience. *Int. J. Radiat. Oncol. Biol. Phys.*, **64**, 363–373.

Section 3

Cancer of the Intrathorax

Section Editor: Minesh P. Mehta

19

Lung Cancer

Deepak Khuntia, Pranshu Mohindra and Minesh P. Mehta

Introduction

Lung cancer remains one of the greatest global oncologic challenges. Despite advances in early diagnosis,
novel chemotherapeutic agents and the recent advent of
immune check point inhibitors, minimally invasive surgical techniques, and advanced radiation delivery methods, outcomes continue to be suboptimal with very little
change in overall survival during the past 15 years. In this
chapter, a contemporary review is presented for the treatment of both non-small-cell and small-cell lung cancer
from a radiation oncology perspective, including a general discussion on the incidence, epidemiology, staging,
and work-up.

Epidemiology

With an incidence exceeding 1.6 million cases worldwide, and mortality of about 1.4 million per year, lung
cancer has the dubious distinction of having the highest incidence and mortality of all cancers [1]. According to the American Cancer Society, it is estimated that
approximately 222 500 cases of lung and bronchial cancers occur annually, with nearly 156 000 deaths predicted for 2017 in the United States [2,3]. Approximately
80% of these are non-small-cell lung cancers (NSCLCs).
Recently, a slight decrease in the incidence has been
observed, largely related to the decrease of tobacco use in
the United States (US). This, however, is not a worldwide
trend, and even within the US, certain subpopulations
are increasing their tobacco consumption. Currently, an
increase is being seen in the use of tobacco in emerging
economies such as China, where it is estimated that today
there are nearly 300 million smokers. Given that there is
typically a latency of two to three decades for the development of lung cancer, a major future epidemic is forecast.

Given the difficulty in screening (until the recent
data from the large National Cancer Institute (NCI) CT
screening project [4]), lung cancers are often discovered
in very advanced stages. Stage I and II cancers represent
only 30% of NSCLCs, with approximately 30% and 40%
presenting with stage III and IV disease, respectively.

Small-cell lung cancer (SCLC) is the most aggressive
histologic type of lung cancer, characterized by a high
mitotic and proliferative index, rapid tumor doubling
times, and increased propensity for systemic metastases,
while maintaining very high initial sensitivity to both
chemotherapy and radiotherapy. The incidence of SCLC
in the US is diminishing, and it now accounts for <15%
of all bronchogenic carcinomas [5]. A Surveillance, Epidemiologic, and End Results (SEER) database analysis
showed a decline in proportion of SCLC among all lung
cancer histologies, from >17% in 1986 to about 13% in
2002 [6]. In contrast, there has been a relative rise in
the proportion of women with SCLC, who accounted
for half of all patients with SCLC in 2002 as against
28% in 1973. These trends reflect changing incidences of
men and women who smoke, in addition to changes in
cigarette composition itself [7,8]. The survival of patients
with SCLC continues to remain poor, with a median survival of only two to four months for untreated patients
[9]. Stage is the dominant prognostic factor and con-
founds the impact of performance status [10]. Over the
past thirty years, very modest improvements in survival
have been noted for this disease [6]. In a SEER database
analysis, the two-year survival in patients with extensive-
stage-SCLC (ES-SCLC) increased from 1.5% in 1973 to a
mere 4.6% in 2000. In contrast, there was a relative doubling of five-year survival for limited-stage-SCLC (LS-
SCLC), from 4.9% in 1973 to 10% in 1998. In general,
women had a slightly longer survival. With concurrent
chemoradiotherapy in LS-SCLC, a median survival of
18–26 months, two-year survival of 35–45% and five-
year survival of 23–26% is expected [11–14].

Clinical Radiation Oncology: Indications, Techniques, and Results, Third Edition. Edited by William Small Jr.
© 2017 John Wiley & Sons, Inc. Published 2017 by John Wiley & Sons, Inc.

Risk Factors

Smoking is the leading cause of lung cancer and is responsible for approximately 90% of cases. Carcinogens within cigarette smoke lead to numerous genetic and epigenetic alterations consequential to the formation of DNA adducts, and these result in both oncogenic events and tumor suppressor genetic losses. There does appear to be a dose–response relationship with smoking, and this decreases with time after cessation, but probably never returns to baseline. Indeed, substantial gender-based and possible ethnicity-based susceptibility factors are being identified which considerably alter the dose–response relationship. Radon exposure is the second most common cause of lung cancer in the US. Less commonly implicated carcinogens include asbestos, bis(chloromethyl)ether, polycyclic aromatic hydrocarbons, chromium, and arsenic. It is also thought that a diet low in carotenoids and lycopene may also contribute to lung cancer formation.

Presentation

Patients with lung cancer usually present with a background history of chronic obstructive pulmonary symptoms related to longstanding smoking. Recent worsening of respiratory function, including increasing dyspnea, cough, expectoration, hemoptysis and chest pain/heaviness are common presenting symptoms. In addition, patients can present with local compressive symptoms due to pressure or involvement of the mediastinal structures. This includes superior vena cava syndrome, characterized by symptoms of head fullness, facial swelling with signs of venous distention in the neck and chest wall, plethora and cyanosis. The involvement of neural structures can result in the development of Horner's syndrome (inferior sympathetic chain or inferior cervical stellate ganglion; presenting with ipsilateral ptosis, miosis, anhidrosis, enophthalmos and ipsilateral face flushing), Pancoast's syndrome (invasion of C8, T1–2 nerve roots, presenting with pain along medial scapula and upper extremity, atrophy of intrinsic muscles of hand in the C8, T1–2 distribution), hoarseness of voice (recurrent laryngeal nerve involvement), spinal cord compression (vertebral body/neural foramina involvement; presenting with motor/sensory deficits over the chest wall, lower extremities, incontinence, gait changes) or reflex sympathetic dystrophy with distal extremity burning pain and edema. Advanced nodal involvement can result in presentation with enlarging lump/fullness in the lower neck or axilla. Patients can also present with symptoms of metastatic disease to the brain, bone and liver, or with systemic symptoms of weight loss and a general failure to thrive.

Apart from the usual respiratory and local invasive or compressive symptoms noted with lung cancers in general, SCLC has a predilection for systemic effects labeled as paraneoplastic syndromes. Typical presentations include syndrome of inappropriate secretion of anti-diuretic hormone (SIADH), Cushing syndrome due to secretion of adrenocorticotropic hormone (ACTH), cerebellar degeneration (Hu syndrome), and Lambert–Eaton myasthenic syndrome [10]. These are mediated by the ectopic production of hormones or serum immune responses to self-antigens. The Hu family of DNA-binding proteins and SOX proteins are known immunogenic antigens in SCLC [15,16]. The impact of these paraneoplastic syndromes on survival is still not clear, but in general, with the exception of certain neurodegenerative conditions, they resolve as the disease responds. It has been proposed that in the setting of symptomatic antibody-mediated Lambert–Eaton syndrome, survival is superior [17]. Patients with asymptomatic increase in the titers of various antibodies and/or hormones have survival similar to those without the antibodies. Some dermatological conditions are also described specifically in relation to SCLC [18]. Patients with NSCLC can present with humoral hypercalcemia of malignancy (HHM), which is the mechanism responsible for 80% of cases with hypercalcemia in lung cancer. The vast majority of HHM is caused by tumor-produced parathyroid hormone-related protein, followed by infrequent tumor production of 1,25-dihydroxyvitamin D and parathyroid hormone. In the remaining 20% of lung cancer patients presenting with hypercalcemia, the etiology is related to advanced metastatic disease to bone [19].

Additional serum biomarkers have been studied in SCLC. These include neuron-specific enolase, chromogranin A, gastrin-releasing peptide (GRP) and pro-GRP and pro-opiomelanocortin (POMC), none of which have shown consistent clinical significance [20]. Circulating tumor cells (CTCs) are also seen in more than 80% cases of SCLC, with a higher number of these cells associated with poor outcomes [21]. It is also noted that CTCs can often form tumor microemboli, which are responsible for invasion through tissues and may in fact be a more specific marker of metastatic burden [22].

Staging and Work-Up

The typical work-up for a patient suspected of having a lung cancer includes a thorough history and physical examination, which addresses aspects such as weight loss, the possibility of paraneoplastic syndromes, a thorough chest examination with emphasis on neck and axillary adenopathy, air ventilation, and musculoskeletal anomalies. Special attention is also given to the neurologic examination, as many of these patients present with brain metastases. For patients with clinical suspicion of lung cancer, laboratory studies should be performed, including a complete blood count, comprehensive metabolic panel including lactate dehydrogenase (LDH), liver and renal function tests. Histopathological confirmation of malignancy and the histological subtype is an essential component of work-up for a suspected lung cancer (see 'Pathology' below). However, patients who are likely early stage and medically operable can be directly planned for surgery with the idea of obtaining an intraoperative tissue diagnosis through needle biopsy, wedge resection or bronchoscopic biopsy before proceeding with a definitive surgery.

For patients in whom initial imaging investigations have identified advanced disease not amenable to surgical resection, biopsy is required before initiating therapy. The choice of biopsy technique is guided by multiple factors, including the patient's performance status, the extent of disease, availability of easily accessible sites, and institutional practices/expertise. As a general approach, the least invasive and most distant site is biopsied to establish the stage. In the current era of targeted therapies, obtaining sufficient tissue for testing molecular markers is critical in planning systemic therapy. This needs effective communication with the interventional radiology or pulmonology team as part of a multidisciplinary approach towards the management of lung cancer. Thoracentesis of pleural effusion with evaluation of cytology is essential to confirm malignant involvement. Bone marrow biopsy is usually required in patients with SCLC only if hematological evaluation identifies cytopenias or nucleated red blood cells without an obvious presence of metastatic disease noted on radiological evaluations. Baseline pulmonary function tests provide useful data to help guide therapy decisions especially for surgical and radiotherapy planning. All patients who are actively smoking should be provided with smoking cessation advice, counseling, and therapy as appropriate.

Imaging

Imaging continues to play a greater role in the diagnosis and management of patients with lung cancer. Imaging is used primarily for detection, staging, and also assessing response and recurrence. The most frequently used initial modality for evaluation of symptoms related to the cardiopulmonary system includes chest radiography (CXR). Unfortunately, tumors less than 1 cm in diameter can be very difficult to diagnose using CXR, and many studies have shown poor detection rates for smaller lung cancers via chest radiographic screening. One of the better-known studies includes the Male Chest Radiography Lung Cancer Screening Project, which showed that 45 of 50 peripheral lung cancers were initially missed, and 12 of the 16 central cancers were visualized in retro-

spect but were overlooked initially [23]. Given these data, more sensitive radiographic measures have been investigated, and the recently reported National Cancer Institute (NCI) lung cancer screening study with low-dose CT showed that smaller tumors can be identified earlier, resulting in stage migration, and improved survival [4]. In this study, which involved more than 50 000 persons at high risk for lung cancer (current or former smokers who quit up to 15 years before enrollment with ≥30 pack–year smoking history, aged 55–74 years with no history of lung cancer), the annual low-dose CT scan was compared to standard CXR. A 20% relative reduction in risk of mortality was noted in the low-dose CT group, with projections suggesting that this differential is continuing to increase with time (95% CI, 6.8 to 26.7; $p = 0.004$).

The most common radiographic tool incorporated in the definitive diagnosis and work-up of patient suspected of having lung cancer is the contrast-enhanced CT scan. This test is quick, minimally invasive, and able to identify subcentimeter lesions. A variety of criteria may help to elucidate tumors that are more likely to be malignant. One of the most important factors is whether or not the tumor is growing. Tumors with a doubling time less than 400 days are considered suspicious [24]. The morphology of the nodule as visualized on imaging is also important. Tumors with spiculated margins may represent a more aggressive adenocarcinoma, while tumors with multiple strands extending from the lesion may also have a more aggressive behavior. Calcifications are present in up to 10% of carcinomas, and those that are variable in size are more suspicious. Other factors include invasion within the pulmonary vasculature, while necrosis or cavitation may suggest a likely diagnosis of cancer. Adenocarcinoma tends to be more peripherally located, while squamous cell carcinomas and small-cell carcinomas tend to be more central. A metastatic work-up should be performed in all patients; this includes contrast-enhanced CT scanning of upper abdomen to evaluate for hepatic and adrenal metastases, magnetic resonance imaging of the brain, and a bone scan, although positron emission tomography (PET) imaging is increasingly replacing the bone scan (see below).

The presence of ground-glass opacities continues to be a diagnostic challenge. Nodules less than 3 cm with a >50% ground-glass component have a lower incidence of vessel invasion and malignant lymphadenopathy. These patients also have a better prognosis compared to those with >50% solid component [25]. These tumors often have very low metabolic activity on PET imaging.

Mediastinal staging is an integral part of the work-up for any early-stage lung cancer patient being considered for surgery. Endoscopic ultrasound is now recognized as a very sensitive tool for the assessment of nodal disease. Stations that can be assessed with endobronchial ultrasound (EBUS) include 2R/2L, 4R/4L,

Table 19.1 Staging definitions. Changes are shown in **bold** text.

Tis	**Carcinoma in situ; Squamous- SCIS or Adenocarcinoma- AIS (adenocarcinoma with pure lepidic pattern, ≤3 cm in greatest dimension)**		
T1	≤3 cm surrounded by lung or visceral pleura. No evidence of invasion more proximal than the lobar bronchus **T1mi – Minimally invasive adenocarcinoma ≤3 cm dimension with a predominant lepidic pattern and ≤5 mm invasion** **T1a – ≤1 cm** **T1b – >1 cm but ≤2 cm** **T1c – >2 cm but ≤3 cm**	N1	Ipsilateral peribronchial or ipsilateral hilar lymph nodes or intrapulmonary nodes, including involvement by direct extension
T2	>3 cm and ≤5 cm OR involves main bronchus regardless of distance to the carina OR invades the visceral pleura OR associated with atelectasis or obstructive pneumonitis that extends to the hilar region involving part or all of the lung **T2a – >3 cm and ≤4 cm** **T2b – >4 cm and ≤5 cm**	N2	Ipsilateral mediastinal or subcarinal nodes
T3	**>5 cm but ≤7 cm OR directly invading the any of the following: parietal pleura, chest wall, phrenic nerve, parietal pericardium, or separate tumor nodule(s) in the same lobe as the primary.**	N3	Contralateral mediastinal, contralateral hilar, ipsilateral or contralateral scalene, or supraclavicular nodes.
T4	**>7 cm or any size with invasion of one or more of the diaphragm, mediastinum, heart, great vessels, trachea, recurrent laryngeal nerve, esophagus, vertebral body or carina; separate tumor nodules in a different ipsilateral lobe**	M1a	Separate tumor nodules in a contralateral lobe; tumors with pleural nodules; malignant pleural or pericardial effusion
		M1b	**Single extrathoracic metastasis in a single organ**
		M1c	**Multiple extrathoracic metasteses in single or multiple organs**

Source: AJCC Cancer Staging Manual, Eighth Edition (2017), Springer, New York, Inc.

level 7, and 10. Esophageal ultrasound can be used for visualizing as well as sampling nodes from stations 4, 7, 8, and 9 [26]. The role of mediastinoscopy is decreasing with increased use of PET-CT and EBUS. It is noteworthy that SCLC is usually submucosal in location, necessitating deep biopsy via bronchoscopy. As per the National Comprehensive Cancer Network (NCCN) guidelines (2016) for patients scheduled for surgery of a presumed early-stage lung cancer, invasive mediastinal staging is preferably performed during the same procedure prior to the planned resection. This minimizes delays, patient inconvenience, procedure risks, and treatment costs.

PET/CT is the newest modality incorporated in the routine staging of lung cancer. The most commonly used tracer, FDG (^{18}F-fluoro-2-deoxyglucose), preferentially accumulates in tumors with increased metabolic activity. Since PET is a functional measure, it can identify disease that is independent of anatomy, although as FDG avidity is not tumor-specific there can be false positives, which makes the confirmation of histology paramount. Other tracers that are considered experimental at this time include FLT-PET, which evaluates proliferation, and Cu-ATSM, which measures hypoxia. These modalities, along with dynamic contrast-enhanced image sequences for measuring perfusion, may become important in tailoring treatment pathways through therapy to assist in identifying regions that are potentially radioresistant or radiosensitive, thereby permitting alterations of radiation dose and/or fractionation parameters.

Staging

The staging for lung cancer is typically assessed in accordance with the tumor (T), lymph nodes (N), and metastases (M) system which has recently been updated in the American Joint Committee on Cancer (AJCC) 8th Edition [27]. The major changes with the new staging system are clarification of carcinoma in situ by histological type, addition of T1mi, split of T1 into T1a, b and c, T2 includes ateleactasis of all of the lung (previously T3), T2a and b size cut-off changes, distance to carina no longer relevant as long as carina is uninvolved (previously 2 cm or more for T2), Diaphragm involvement now T4, inclusion of pericardial nodule as M1a, Split into M1b and M1c. These changes have resulted in considerable modifications of stage grouping the introduction of new stratifications within the T stage. Further, there is recognition of the poor prognosis associated with malignant pleural effusions as being metastatic disease. A summary of the staging system and associated outcomes is presented in Tables 19.1 and 19.2.

For decades, the Veterans Administration Lung Study Group's proposed binary staging system has been employed in SCLC [28]. The classification is primarily

Table 19.2 Stage and grouping based on estimated outcomes.

Grouping	T stage	N stage	M stage	5- year OS
IA1	T1mi-T1a	N0	M0	92%
IA2	T1b	N0	M0	83%
IA3	T1c	N0	M0	77%
IB	T2a	N0	M0	68%
IIA	T2b	N0	M0	60%
IIB	T1a-c, T2a-b	N1	M0	53%
	T3	N0	M0	
IIIA	T1a-c, T2a-b	N2	M0	36%
	T3	N1	M0	
	T4	N0-1	M0	
IIIB	T1a-c, T2a-2b	N3	M0	26%
	T3-4	N2	M0	
IIIC	T3-4	N3	M0	13%
IVA	Any T	Any N	10%	1%
IVB	Any T	Any N	M1c	0%

Source: AJCC Cancer Staging Manual, Eighth Edition (2017), Springer, New York, Inc.

based on the ability to cover all known disease in one radiation portal. This 'hemithorax' field includes bilateral mediastinal, ipsilateral hilar, supraclavicular and/or scalene lymph nodes. The patients are divided into limited and extensive stage SCLC (LS-SCLC and ES-SCLC). The significance of pleural effusion and contralateral hilar and supraclavicular lymph nodes was not clearly defined in this system, but was analyzed in the limited stage definition of the International Association for the Study of Lung Cancer (IASLC) consensus report [29]. The IASLC TNM staging is based on an analysis of 8088 patients [30]. Higher clinical T and N categories of the 6th edition TNM staging system were associated with progressive decrements in survival, but differences in cN0 and cN1 were non-significant. Survival of patients with clinical stage I–II disease was significantly superior to patients with stage III with N2 or N3 disease. LS-SCLC patients, who also had pleural effusion, had an intermediate prognosis between LS-SCLC with negative effusion and ES-SCLCL, irrespective of cytology results. This analysis could still not definitively define the impact of supraclavicular nodal involvement or pericardial effusion. It was recommended that patients with both ipsilateral and contralateral supraclavicular nodes should be still included in LS though prophylactic treatment of these sites is usually not recommended. In the modern, era, it is strongly recommended to document AJCC stage grouping.

Pathology

Histology

As the current knowledge of pathology grows, it is now recognized that lung cancer is a much more heterogeneous group of tumors. There is evidence that lung cancer is likely derived from pluripotent epithelial stem cells capable of expressing a variety of phenotypes. Historically, lung cancer was categorized as either NSCLC or SCLC. Squamous cell, adenocarcinoma, and large cell carcinoma – the three subtypes of NSCLC – account for approximately 90% of the lung cancers in the US.

Squamous cell carcinoma typically arises from the proximal bronchi and is often associated with pathogenesis initiated through squamous metaplasia, carcinoma *in situ*, and subsequent invasive carcinoma. Several well-differentiated tumors demonstrate keratin pearl formation. Poorly differentiated squamous cell tumors often will have positive keratin staining as well. In the US, adenocarcinoma is the most frequent tumor, accounting for approximately 40% of all lung cancers. The majority of these tumors are more peripheral in location and arise from the surface epithelium or bronchial mucosal glands. During recent years there has been an increasing understanding of the heterogeneity in outcomes noted within the histological classification of 'adenocarcinoma.' This led to development of International Association for the Study of Lung Cancer (IASLC)/American Thoracic Society (ATS)/European Respiratory Society (ERS) sponsored 'International Multidisciplinary Classification of Lung Adenocarcinoma' [31]. Amongst important changes, bronchoalveolar carcinoma, a type of adenocarcinoma that arises from type II pneumocytes that grow along the alveolar septa, was replaced by use of terms such as adenocarcinoma *in situ* (AIS) and minimally invasive adenocarcinoma (MIA) as 3 cm or smaller nodules with either pure lepidic growth or predominant lepidic growth with ≤5 mm invasion, respectively. These lesions show little desmoplastic glandular change, and can present as a spectrum of conditions ranging from solitary peripheral nodule (most common), multifocal disease, or a progressive pneumonic form that spreads from lobe to lobe, ultimately encompassing both lungs. These tumors generally have a more indolent course. Large-cell carcinoma is the least common, accounting for approximately 15% of lung cancers. The incidence of large-cell carcinoma has been decreasing largely because of better identification with increased use of immunohistochemical staining and electron microscopy. As a result, many tumors that were felt to be large-cell carcinoma have been re-categorized as poorly differentiated adenocarcinoma or squamous cell carcinoma.

In small specimens and in poorly differentiated tumors, pathologists need to integrate morphology based on hematoxylin and eosin examination, immunohistochemical stains [thyroid transcription factor (TTF-1) and novel aspartic proteinase of the pepsin family (Napsin A) for adenocarcinoma and p63, p40 and cytokeratin (CK) 5/6 for squamous cell carcinoma], histochemical stains (e.g., mucin staining for adenocarcinoma), and molecular studies to make a correct diagnosis. An immunohistochemical cocktail comprising adenocarcinoma and squamous cell carcinoma markers (nuclear and cytoplasmic marker combinations) is sometimes performed on poorly differentiated tumors to improve the diagnostic subtyping. The new classification system strongly discourages use of NSCLC-'not otherwise'-specified or NOS.

Histopathologically, small-cell lung cancer is characterized by the presence of small, round cells with scanty cytoplasm, nuclear molding and irregular borders. These cells demonstrate a high Ki-67 index. The specific immunohistochemistry markers that aid the diagnosis of SCLC include various neuroendocrine molecules such as chromogranin, synaptophysin, neuron-specific enolase (NSE), and neural cell adhesion molecule (NCAM)/CD56. TTF-1 staining is positive in nearly all cases of SCLC. The presence of CK can help in the differentiation from other, non-bronchogenic small round tumors [10].

Molecular Biology

Lung adenocarcinoma is a heterogeneous disease with diverse somatic mutations associated with carcinogenesis. During recent years, some molecular subtypes of NSCLC have been well elucidated, and at least two distinct molecular pathways in lung carcinogenesis are now proposed: (i) a pathway associated with smoking and activation of KRAS (Kirsten rat sarcoma); and (ii) a pathway associated with never-smokers and sensitizing EGFR (epidermal growth factor receptor) mutations. Further, KRAS mutations and mutations in the EGFR tyrosine-kinase domain are mutually exclusive. Although sensitizing EGFR mutations are most frequently observed in females, never-smokers with what used to be referred to as BAC, and invasive adenocarcinoma with a predominant BAC component, also have a higher likelihood of

harboring these mutations, as do the higher proportions which have also been noted in acinar and papillary variants of adenocarcinoma. All patients with adenocarcinoma, large-cell carcinoma, NSCLC-NOS or NSCLC-favor adenocarcinoma should undergo mutation testing for KRAS and EGFR. Only <1% of lung cancers may have both EGFR and KRAS positive, with KRAS mutations typically mediating resistance to EGFR tyrosine kinase inhibitors [32]. In KRAS-negative patients, who are also negative for EGFR mutations, testing for ALK (anaplastic lymphoma kinase) gene rearrangements can be helpful. The clinical profile of ALK mutation-positive patients is similar to those with EGFR mutation, though even ALK and EGFR mutations are mutually exclusive. Further, though this may not be recommended routinely since immune checkpoint inhibitors have been approved without need for PD-L1 testing in metastatic NSCLC. In contrast to NSCLC, no easily targetable somatic 'driver mutations' have been identified for SCLC [33]. However, certain genetic aberrations are very common [34], including a loss of the tumor-suppressor retinoblastoma gene RB1, TP53 and FHIT, amongst others. Mutations in tyrosine-kinase signaling genes such as KRAS and EGFR are only rarely identified. The genetic profiling of lung cancer is now becoming commonplace, and significant changes may be made to a patient's management based on these studies. Although these discussions are beyond the scope of this chapter, they are summarized in Table 19.3.

Treatment

Early-Stage NSCLC

Surgery has been the mainstay of treatment for early-stage lung cancer, particularly for non-small-cell lung cancer. Surgery offers not only pathological verification of the primary but also confirmation of lymph node status, which may impact local radiation recommendations as well as systemic therapy recommendations. In the past, primary radiation for stage I lung cancer resulted in unacceptably low rates of local control, and therefore surgery has been the preferred primary treatment option. Recently, new advances have been made in both conformal external beam radiotherapy (EBRT) and also brachytherapy that are resulting in the conduct of clinical trials of primary radiotherapeutic approaches for early-stage NSCLC.

Early-stage NSCLC in today's practice is often identified as an incidental pulmonary nodule, the precise histologic diagnosis of which may or may not always be available. Some have recommended observation and close surveillance as a reasonable strategy for a single pulmonary nodule less than 1 cm, although in most academic centers such patients are often evaluated with PET,

Table 19.3 Genetic markers used in lung cancer diagnosis.

Marker	Description
RAS Oncogene	Family of three major oncogenes (*HRAS, KRAS, NRAS*). Typically found in smokers. Rarely found in small-cell lung cancer. Encode membrane associated proteins involved in signal transduction.
MYC Gene	Nuclear transcription factors that is over expressed primarily in small cell lung cancer and large-cell neuroendocrine tumors. Amplification is often associated with chemotherapy resistance.
TP53	This mutation is found in 90% of small-cell lung cancer and 50% of non-small-cell lung cancer. Normal TP53 plays in a central role in determining the cells response to genetic damage. This may affect chemotherapy responsiveness.
RB1	In codes a nuclear protein, RB, that undergoes phosphorylation and dephosphorylation commanded by G1 cyclins. The RB product regulates E2F1 transcription factor activation. This is common in most small-cell lung cancer as but occurs in less than 10% of non-small-cell lung cancer cases.
CDKN2A	Previously referred to as p16. Regulates phosphorylation of the RB1 protein via transcription. This is common in non-small-cell lung cancer and rare in small-cell lung cancer.
EGFR	Mediate several signal pathways critical for growth and survival in response to stress is on the micro-environment. Stresses include radiation and chemotherapies. Generally correlated with a poor prognosis and radiation resistance. It is a target of multiple monoclonal antibodies. Found in 10% of non-small-cell lung cancer cases. Typically found in non-smoking patient's, especially Asian women. More common in adenocarcinoma and squamous cell carcinoma.
ERBB2	Previously referred to as HER2. Particularly common in adenocarcinoma. Associated with decreased survival. Patients with overexpression of wild-type ERBB2 may benefit from targeted therapy directed against ERBB2-mediated signaling.
EML4-ALK	EML4-ALK fused genes are occasionally found in young patients that are non-smokers or light smokers and may benefit from inhibitors of ALK kinase.

and almost all of the hypermetabolic nodules are resected (with the exception being those where a non-malignant diagnosis is suspected based on a combination of clinical history, CT appearance, and degree of FDG-PET uptake, and temporal changes in the imaging findings) [35].

The standard treatment for the medically operable patient is lobectomy, which has been found to be equivalent to pneumonectomy and has shown in a randomized trial to reduce local recurrence from 17% with a limited resection (wedge resection or segmentectomy) [36] to 6% (p = 0.008) [36,37]. Generally, good surgical candidates have an FEV_1 greater than 1.2 liters, or predicted postoperative FEV_1 >0.8 liter with diffusing lung capacity for carbon monoxide (DLCO) >50–60%. Patients with an FEV_1/FVC of less than 75% are reported to experience higher rates of postoperative complications. When the FEV_1/FVC drops below 50%, postoperative morbidity and mortality increase significantly. Video-assisted thoracoscopic surgery (VATS) may decrease postoperative pain, shorten the time to initiation of systemic therapy, and allow for greater doses/intensity of chemotherapy to be delivered [38]. As noted above, a definitive surgical procedure is preceded by intraoperative invasive mediastinal staging and obtaining a tissue diagnosis from the primary tumor. In patients with N0 nodal group or non-hilar N1 nodal group early-stage (T1/2) NSCLC, there is no survival benefit with complete mediastinal lymph node dissection if adequate multi-level sampling has been performed (ACOSOG Z0030 trial) [39]. A minimum of three N2 stations should be evaluated [40].

Brachytherapy

In patients who have borderline pulmonary reserve where a full lobectomy would yield an oxygen-dependent or ventilator-dependent outcome, alternate approaches are necessary. A novel technique involves the incorporation of radioactive iodine-125 or cesium-131 embedded within a Vicryl mesh placed on the wedge-resection staple line. This technology offers the ability of pathologic confirmation of the tumor, as well as staging of the lymph nodes while potentially minimizing adverse effects on pulmonary reserve that could be associated with a more elaborate operation such as a lobectomy or pneumonectomy, and also minimizing radiation-induced pulmonary damage associated with external beam approaches. This procedure can also be performed with assistance from the da Vinci robot, as popularized by Khuntia and Dunnington [41].

Brachytherapy is performed with either a mesh or a double-suture technique. Prior to the procedure, the radiation oncologist and thoracic surgeon estimate the surface area of the implant to ensure that the entire length of the stapled margin of resection will be covered, with at least a 2 cm lateral margin along its linear course. Typically, a 10-cm strand of radioactive iodine-125 or

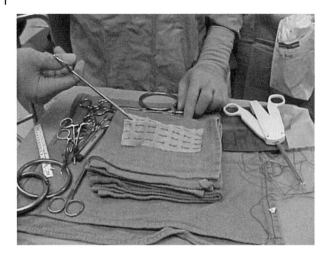

Figure 19.1 Mesh brachytherapy implant showing four rows of seeds (10 seeds per row) embedded within the vicryl mesh.

cesium-131 is utilized. Each seed generally has an activity of 0.4–0.6 mCi for I-125, and about 1.8–2.0 mCi for Cs-131. The radioactive sources come within a polyglycolic acid suture with 1-cm spacing between sources. These sutures are sewn within the mesh at specific distances to achieve the desired dose of approximately 100–120 Gy for iodine and 85 Gy for cesium (Figures 19.1–19.3a,b) [42].

With a double-suture technique, two single rows, each usually containing 10 sources are placed 0.5 cm on either side of the resection margin and affixed with several sutures, 1–2 cm apart on either side of the staple line. The activity with this double-suture technique is approximately 50% higher than what is used in the mesh technique. Appropriate measurements are taken at the surface and 1 m by the radiation physicist or radiation

oncologist at completion of surgery, and also prior to hospital discharge to ensure that the patient meets legal radiation exposure requirements.

In a matched-paired analysis performed by Santos and colleagues, a significant improvement in local control with the use of mesh brachytherapy after sublobar resection versus sublobar resection alone (18.6 versus 2%, p < 0.0001) was described [43]. A Phase III study, ACOSOG Z4032, was recently reported which randomized patients to either wedge resection alone versus wedge resection plus mesh brachytherapy [44]. With a median follow-up of nearly 4.4 years and 222 evaluable patients, no differences in time to or types of local recurrences were seen. While the outcomes were negative, this study sets up contemporary benchmarks for local recurrence following sublobar resections, with a little less than 13% of patients developing local recurrences at three years. This could have been a result of better attention to surgical margin despite sublobar surgeries, with nearly 60% of patients having a >1 cm surgical margin. The low event rates could have also resulted in underpowering of the study to detect lesser differences. On an unplanned subgroup analysis, a strong trend towards reduction in local recurrences was seen in patients with positive staple line cytology ($n = 14$). Adjuvant intraoperative brachytherapy in conjunction with sublobar resection did not significantly worsen pulmonary function, and there was no increase in perioperative pulmonary complications. It was found, however, that 22% of patients with lower-lobe tumors and 9% with upper-lobe tumors demonstrated a 10% decline in $FEV_{1\%}$ (odds ratio, 2.79; 95% confidence interval, 1.07-7.25; P = 0.04).

Typical candidates for sublobar resection include patients with an FEV_1 and/or a DLCO ≤50% predicted. Other minor criteria include patients aged over 75 years, and FEV_1 and/or DLCO between 51–60% of predicted value. Pulmonary hypertension, poor left ventricular function with an ejection fraction ≤40%, pO_2 ≤55 mmHg, or SpO_2 ≤80%, pCO_2 >45 mmHg and a dyspnea scale score ≥3 are relative indications (Table 19.4). Based on the results of the ACOSOG Z4032 study described above, the use of adjuvant mesh brachytherapy may not be necessary, especially if a wide surgical margin can be achieved or an anatomic segmentectomy is performed [45]. For those patients in whom this is not achievable, an alternate approach that is increasingly becoming standard of care for medically inoperable patients is stereotactic body radiotherapy (SBRT) as described below. SBRT is also being considered in some patients that fail mesh brachytherapy [46].

Stereotactic Body Radiotherapy and 3D Conformal Radiation

In the past, patients with medically inoperable early-stage NSCLC would undergo conventional radiation

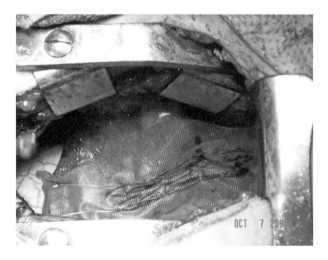

Figure 19.2 Intraoperative placement of the mesh on top of the staple line.

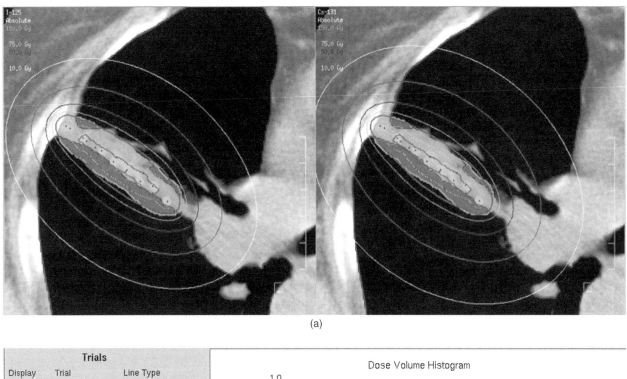

(a)

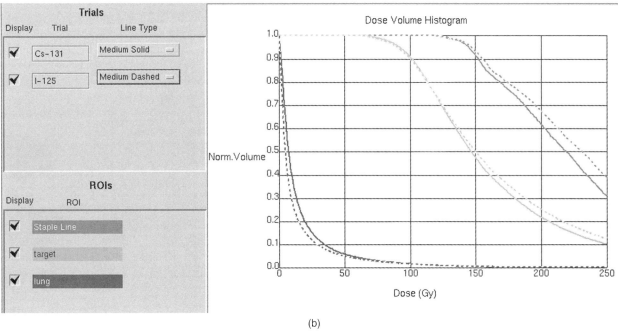

(b)

Figure 19.3 (a) Isodose lines for ^{125}I permanent implant on the left and [131]Cs permanent implant on the right. Very similar physical dose distributions are obtained. (b) Dose–volume histogram of the lung, target, and staple line for ^{125}I and [131]Cs permanent implants. Excellent coverage of the staple line is obtained with 100% of the staple line receiving the prescription dose. There is a over 90% coverage of the staple line plus 5 mm margin with both isotopes, yielding similar physical DVHs. For a color version of this figure, see the color plate section.

therapy, resulting in 30% or lower survival at 3 years [47]. Stage-matched comparisons show that conventional radiotherapy has far inferior results than surgical series [48,49]. This low rate of local control and inferior survival was largely due to inadequate tumor doses. Stereotactic body radiotherapy (SBRT) has significantly improved local control rates, which now approach those of resection. The four key technologies that have

made this feasible include aggressive immobilization to reduce motion and ensure day-to-day accuracy, four-dimensional (4D) planning CT to account for motion, image-guided techniques to verify delivery accuracy, and more sophisticated collimators which allow for conformal, as well as intensity-modulated, planning. In 2000, less than 5% of radiation oncology practices had incorporated SBRT into clinical practice, but by 2010 this number

Table 19.4 Modified Medical Research Council dyspnea scale.

Grade	Description
0	No breathlessness except for with strenuous exercise
1	Breathlessness when hurrying on level or walking on a slight hill
2	Walk slower than people the same age on the level because of breathlessness or has to stop for breath when walking at own pace on the level
3	Stopped for breath after walking about 100 meters or a few minutes on the level
4	Too breathless to leave the house or breathless when dressing or undressing

had exceeded 60%, with most of the remaining practices likely to add this capability in the near future [50].

A safe and successful SBRT program must include multiple minimum requirements, such as a multidisciplinary, well-coordinated team functioning within a process of high alert for possible error occurrence and having the ability to communicate this without reprimand or recrimination, appropriate personnel training, 4D imaging, immobilization devices to restrict patient motion during the course of radiation (Figure 19.4a,b),

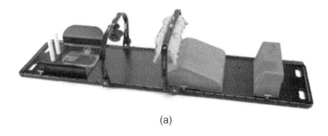

(a)

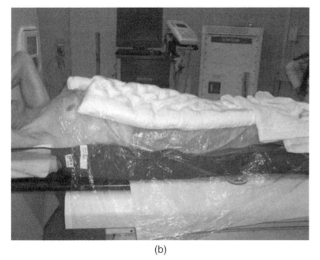

(b)

Figure 19.4 (a) Body Pro-Lok system sold by Civco. The technology utilizes strategic immobilization fixtures to compress the diaphragm to minimize chest motion. Illustration courtesy of Alonso Gutierrez, PhD. (b) Bodyfix system sold by Elekta, Inc. A vacuum bag system is utilized to immobilize the chest and abdomen to reduce tumor motion.

accurate dose calculation algorithms, and image guidance to ensure the patient is appropriately positioned and the treatment is being delivered to the intended target. A variety of technologies, such as Cyberknife, Novalis, Synergy, Trilogy, Tomotherapy, and TruBeam can achieve this. With the incorporation of MR onboard radiation-delivery systems, further accuracy in SBRT has been achieved because of the ability to perform true 4D volumetric tumor motion assessment. The correct use of the technology and physician expertise is far more important than the delivery vehicle. SBRT program requirements and guidelines have been reviewed by the American Association of Physicist in Medicine (AAPM) Task Group 101, as well as by ASTRO, and the interested reader is directed to these reports [51,52]. The most significant observation from these reports is that quality assurance programs with rigorous double checks for every aspect of the program are a necessary component.

Most of the early SBRT studies were initiated during the early 2000s and are summarized in Table 19.5. This information suggests that a dose of 45 Gy in three fractions or higher (BED >100 Gy_{10}) results in local control rates in excess of 90%. In a Japanese multi-institutional experience, a biologic effective dose (BED) of $\geq$100 Gy for tumor control resulted in lower local recurrence rates (8.1% versus 26.4%; $p < 0.05$) and improved three-year overall survival (88.4% versus 69.4%, $p < 0.05$) [53]. RTOG 0915, a randomized Phase II study, compared two fractionation schedules (34 Gy in one fraction versus 48 Gy in four fractions) for patients with early-stage NSCLC with tumor size $\leq$2 cm, non-central in location. At a median follow-up of 2.5 years, no increase in toxicity with excellent local control rates were seen with 34 Gy in one fraction [54]. Early studies also showed that the treatment of more centrally located tumors results in significant morbidity and mortality, and an ongoing RTOG protocol is exploring the appropriate doses for these tumors [55]. The starting dose level in the RTOG study (0813) was 50 Gy in five fractions (10 Gy per fraction), and this was escalated to 60 Gy in five fractions, each of 12 Gy. The DLT rates for 50, 52.5, 55,

Table 19.5 SBRT lung results. Data from prospective studies are shown in **bold** text.

Study/Reference	No. of patients	Dose (Gy)	No. of fractions	Local control	Overall survival
RTOG [108]	**55**	**54**	**3**	**98% (3 yr)**	**56% (3 Yr)**
Indiana [109]	**70**	**60–66**	**3**	**88% (3 yr)**	**43% (3 Yr)**
Nordic Group [110]	**57**	**45**	**3**	**92% (3 yr)**	**60% (3 Yr)**
Torino [111]	**62**	**45**	**3**	**88% (3 yr)**	**57% (3 Yr)**
Kyoto [112]	**45**	**48**	**4**	**94% (3 yr)**	**83% (3 Yr)**
Beijing [113]	**43**	**50**	**10**	**95% (3 yr)**	**91% (3 Yr)**
Tohoku U [114]	**31**	**45**	**3**	**T1 = 78%**	**T1 = 72%**
				T2 = 40%	**T2 = 84%**
U Marburg [115]	40	30	1	81% (3 yr)	53% (3 Yr)
Sweden [116]	45	45	3	80% (3 yr)	55% (3 Yr)
Heidelberg [117]	42	19–30	1	68% (3 yr)	37.4% (3 yr)
UPMC [118]	100	20–60	1–3	75% (crude)	50% (2 Yr)
Tokyo [119]	59 (included mets)	30–34	1	78% (2 yr)	41% (2 YR)
Japan (multi-institution) [119]	257	18–75	1–22	BED >100 = 92%	71% (5 Yr)
				BED <100 = 43%	30% (5 Yr)

BED, biologically effective dose.

57.5 and 60 Gy in five fractions were 2, 2.7, 4.3, 5.7, and 7.2% respectively, all below protocol-specified thresholds. Other commonly used fractionations are 60 Gy in eight fractions at 7.5 Gy per fraction [56], and 70 Gy in 10 fractions at 7 Gy per fraction [57]. At ASTRO 2015, Park *et al.* presented an evaluation of 4950 SBRT-treated patients from the National Cancer Data Base, including stage cT1-2a NSCLC patients treated between 2004 and 2011. Of these patients, 2325 were treated with three fractions (mostly either 54 or 60 Gy total dose), and 2625 were treated with four to five fractions (mostly 48 or 50 Gy in four fractions or 50 Gy in five fractions). Propensity-matching demonstrated no significant survival differences between the groups [58].

As SBRT is increasingly being accepted as the standard of care approach for medically inoperable patients, the obvious next question is to assess its role in comparison to surgery for medically operable patients. RTOG1021/ACOPSOG Z4099 was a randomized Phase III study initiated to address outcomes of sublobar resection (± brachytherapy) versus SBRT in high-risk patients with stage I NSCLC. Targeting an ambitious 420 patients, the study closed after enrolling only 10 patients due to poor accrual rates. This was in part due to difficult randomization of patients to two varied treatment modalities. As a repeat attempt, the industry-funded Joint Lung Cancer Trialist's Coalition has initiated a multi-institutional Stablemates Trial evaluating the same two cohorts. However, this study follows a pre-randomization approach, with the randomization performed prior to consultation which is then offered to the patient during consultation. When comparing SBRT to lobar resection in patients with operable stage I NSCLC, a pooled analysis from two small randomized trials (STARS and ROSEL) demonstrated an improvement in overall survival at three years with the use of SBRT (95% versus 79%, p = 0.037) [59]. SBRT has been reported to have a better survival compared to conventionally fractionated radiotherapy in retrospective studies, population-based studies, and matched analyses, but no randomized trials have backed this assertion. Hallqvist *et al.* presented results of the Scandinavian SBRT group randomized trial, SPACE (Stereotactic Precision And Conventional radiotherapy Evaluation) at the IASLC World Conference on Lung Cancer in 2015 [60]. Both arms – SBRT and conventionally fractionated 3D – yielded equivalent survival results. The one-, two- and three-year overall survival rates were 85% versus 89%, 71% versus 72%, and 57% versus 59% for SBRT versus 3D radiotherapy, calling into question whether there is really something truly unique about SBRT.

Planning Parameters

A variety of dose constraints have been recognized as important in the treatment of lung tumors with SBRT. The planning techniques employed are designed to maximize dose within the target while creating a rapid dose fall-off outside the target. In order to achieve this, increased heterogeneity within the target is necessary (often prescribing the dose between the 60% and 90% isodose surface). A variety of parameters have been proposed to help limit toxicity and maximize local control. One such parameter involves reducing the volume of chest wall tissue peripheral to the lung receiving 30 Gy to less than 30 cm^3 in a three- to five-fraction regimen [61].

Given that treatment times can be quite extensive, an SBRT approach requires consistent and reproducible immobilization. There are many commercially available systems designed for this purpose. Some of the systems require fiducials on the surface for tracking motion, while others utilize imaging with KV or MVCT, or continuous orthogonal x-ray images. One particular technology utilizes intrathoracically embedded electromagnetic signal emitters which can track the tumor externally many times per second without exposing the patient to radiation from the imaging modalities [62].

With ablative doses of radiation that exceed the tolerances of all the normal tissue within the mediastinum and chest such as the heart, normal lung, diaphragm, brachial plexus, and tracheobronchial tree, it is necessary to pay particular attention to the motion associated with the tumor to minimize the dose to these normal critical structures. The motion envelope can vary substantially based on tumor location. It is not uncommon to see motion in excess of 2 cm or more for tumors located in the lower lobes of the lung, especially if diaphragmatic control is not employed. Superiorly located tumors, however, may show very little motion. The motion can be difficult to assess, and 4D CT or a slow CT typically covering the entire motion envelope of the tumor is highly recommended. With a fast spiral CT, multiple image sets are necessary in order to truly capture the entire tumor trajectory. This can be achieved with a formal 4D CT scan in which the images are coordinated with the patient's respiration. Further, PET/CT scans can also be incorporated, since the long duration of the scan automatically encodes motion. Assessing the appropriate PET-defined target in terms of the standardized uptake value (SUV) remains challenging.

Definition of the gross target volume (GTV) is typically performed using the lung windows of the planning CT scan. PET scans may be useful in patients that have significant atelectasis. MRI can be incorporated for patients that have chest wall tumors that are close to the brachial plexus. When applying SBRT, attention to margins is important. An internal target volume (ITV) representing the tumor motion envelope is delineated, using the techniques described above. Even though published CT-pathology correlative studies have sugested that a margin of 6–8 mm for clinical target volue (CTV) will have >90% probability of covering microscopic disease beyond the imaging-identified GTV, clinical practices and trials have typically incorporated 0–3 mm CTV margins with SBRT. The use of high-dose fractions allows considerable dose to delivered to these marginal zones which is felt to be adequate to cover microscopic disease. An additional planning target volume (PTV) margin is also incorporated to account for daily set-up errors. This can vary from institution to institution, but in some centers, where 4D CT is not utilized, the typical value is 5 mm in the axial plane and 10 mm in the cranio-caudal direction. If 4D CT is available, a 3–5-mm

margin is generally added for the PTV as motion has already been accounted for in the ITV contours. This approach is preferred, and individual institutions are encouraged to incorporate 4D-CT-based planning for SBRT. Breath-holding, tumor tracking using fiducials, and respiratory-gated approaches have also been described to minimize PTV margins.

To produce safe dose-distributions, multiple beam angles are usually needed (with eight to ten beams incorporated in the planning). The beams are typically all non-opposing beams and often non-coplanar, although with certain technologies far more beams are utilized and these tend to be coplanar. All beams need to be checked at the treatment machine or with appropriate machine software prior to plan approval to ensure that collisions with the patient are avoided. If fewer than 10 beams are used, no overlap should exist at the skin surface. For patients treated with arc-based technologies, a minimum of 340° should be utilized. For the Radiation Therapy Oncology Group (RTOG) protocols, the recommended prescription lines covering the PTV are 60–90%. The goal is to have 95% of the PTV covered by the prescription dose, and for 99% of the PTV to receive a minimum of 90% of the prescription dose. However, the Japanese Clinical Oncology Group protocols prescribe plan to the isocenter with a minimum dose to PTV around 85–95% of the isocenter [63,64].

The ablative effect occurs not only within the GTV itself but also in the surrounding tissues exposed to high doses, ultimately leading to surrounding fibrosis with or without distal atelectasis. Any dose greater than 105% of the prescription dose should occur primarily within the PTV, and not in the normal tissues outside of the PTV. The cumulative volume of all tissue outside of the PTV receiving >105% of the prescription dose should be no more than 15% of the size of the PTV volume. Ideally, the conformality index should be less than 1.2. This refers to the ratio of the volume of the prescription isodose line to the volume of the PTV. Other parameters for low-dose spillage include D2cm which refers to the dose to ≥2 cm from PTV, and theR50%, which is the ratio of volume of 50% prescription dose to the volume of PTV. With regards to organs at risk, a variety of dose limits have been proposed (Fig. 19.5a). The criteria utilized in the ACOSOG Z4099 study are listed in Table 19.6. This is based on a three-fraction regimen with a total prescription dose of 54 Gy.

Locally Advanced NSCLC

Locally advanced and metastatic NSCLC represents roughly 60–70% of lung cancers in the United States. Stage III lung cancer, accounting for slightly less than half of this group, represents a very heterogeneous group (see Table 19.1). The American College of Chest

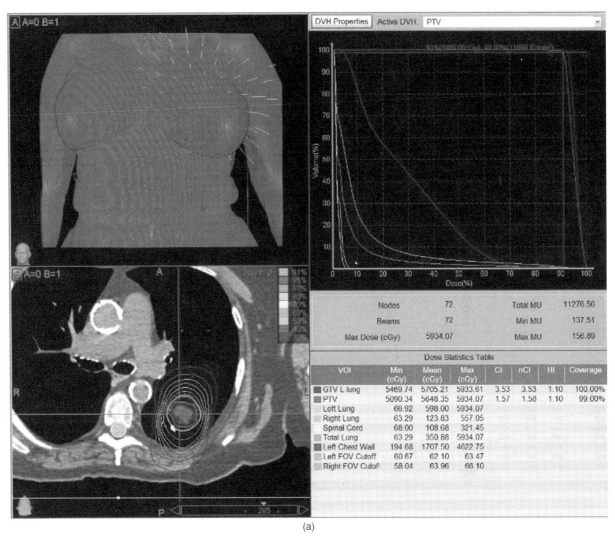

(a)

Figure 19.5 (a) SBRT patient with medically inoperable lung cancer. Note the rapid fall off of dose outside of the primary target. (b) A case example with locoregionally advanced NSCLC treated with IMRT technique to a dose of 66 Gy in 33 fractions, five fractions per week. Panel A: CT scan images in three planes showing target volumes and organs at risk. Panel B: Isodose distribution demonstrating highly conformal distribution of higher isodoses with relative spreading of lower isodoses. Panel C: Dose–volume histogram demonstrating a rapid fall-off of isodoses covering the target volume shown by curves on the right with significant sparing of normal tissues as represented by curves on the left. Illustration courtesy Dr George Cannon, University of Wisconsin. For a color version of this figure, see the color plate section.

Physicians (AACP) advocates treating patients with T3 N1 tumors in similar manner to those with Stage II tumors – that is, resection followed by adjuvant therapy. However, a prospective randomized trial has shown that there is no survival benefit with an *en-bloc* mediastinal sampling; furthermore, this trial failed to show any definitive increase in survival with mediastinal lymph node dissection (for right-sided lung tumors) [65,66].

In general, patients with resectable stage IIIA$_1$ and IIIA$_2$ lung cancers are treated in the manner described above – that is, resection followed by adjuvant therapy (Table 19.7). After completion of planned resection and systematic mediastinal lymph node sampling or dissection, patients would receive adjuvant chemotherapy.

Typically, this involves a platinum-based regimen and provides an approximate 5% improvement in overall survival [67]. Generally speaking, patients in this group only undergo adjuvant radiation therapy if there are multiple nodal stations involved, extracapsular extension, close or microscopically positive resection margins, or N2 disease.

For patients with Stage IIIA$_3$ NSCLC (potentially resectable), neoadjuvant therapy involving chemotherapy or chemoradiation may improve resectability with acceptable morbidity. This may allow for potentially improved overall survival versus chemoradiation. The randomized Intergroup trial 0139 showed an approximately 10% progression-free survival advantage with

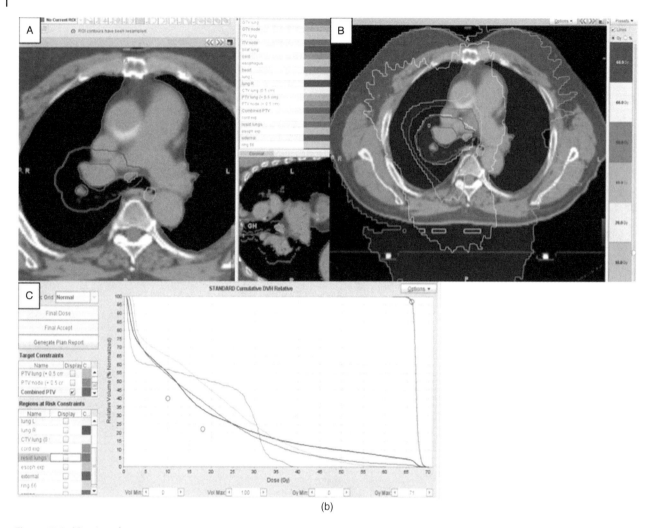

(b)

Figure 19.5 *(Continued)*

Table 19.6 Organs-at-risk table based on a 54 Gy in three-fraction SBRT regimen.

Serial tissue	Volume (ml)	Volume max (Gy)	Max point dose (Gy)	Endpoint ($\geq$ Grade 3)
Spinal cord and medulla	<0.35	18 Gy (6 Gy/fx)	21.9 Gy (7.3 Gy/fx)	Myelitis
	<1.2	12.3 Gy (4.1 Gy/fx)		
Esophagus	<5	17.7 Gy (5.9 Gy/fx)	25.2 Gy (8.4 Gy/fx)	Stenosis/fistula
Brachial plexus	<3	20.4 Gy (6.8 Gy/fx)	24 Gy (8 Gy/fx)	Neuropathy
Heart/pericardium	<15	24 Gy (8 Gy/fx)	30 Gy (10 Gy/fx)	Pericarditis
Great vessels	<10	39 Gy (13 Gy/fx)	45 Gy (15 Gy/fx)	Aneurysm
Trachea and large bronchus	<4	15 Gy (5 Gy/fx)	30 Gy (10 Gy/fx)	Stenosis/fistula
Rib	<1	28.8 Gy (9.6 Gy/fx)	36.9 Gy (12.3 Gy/fx)	Pain or fracture
Skin	<10	30 Gy (10 Gy/fx)	33 Gy (11 Gy/fx)	Ulceration
Stomach	<10	16.5 Gy (5.5 Gy/fx)	22.2 Gy (7.4 Gy/fx)	Ulceration/fistula
Colon	<20	24 Gy (8 Gy/fx)	28.2 Gy (9.4 Gy/fx)	Colitis/fistula

Parallel tissue	Critical volume (ml)	Critical volume dose max (Gy)	Endpoint (> Grade 3)
Lung (right and left)	1500	10.5 Gy (3.5 Gy/fx)	Basic lung function
Lung (right and left)	1000	11.4 Gy (3.8 Gy/fx)	Pneumonitis
Liver	700	17.1 Gy (5.7 Gy/fx)	Basic liver function
Renal cortex (right and left)	200	14.4 Gy (4.8 Gy/fx)	Basic renal function

Table 19.7 Subclassification of Stage III lung cancer.

Stage	Description
$IIIA_1$	Occult nodal metastases found on final pathologic examination of the resection specimen
$IIIA_2$	Incidental, resectable single nodal station metastases recognized intraoperatively
$IIIA_3$	Potentially resectable tumors with single or multiple station lymphadenopathy recognized by prethoractomy staging
$IIIA_4$	Unresectable with bulky or fixed multistation mediastinal disease

surgical intervention as part of multimodality therapy versus chemoradiotherapy alone for patients with pathologic N2 disease, but without increasing survival. The induction regimen included neoadjuvant radiotherapy (45 Gy) along with cisplatin (50 mg m^{-2} on days 1, 8, 29, and 36) and etoposide (50 mg m^{-2} on days 1–5, and 29–33). The control arm included an interrupted radiation dose of 61 Gy and two cycles of consolidation with cisplatin and etoposide. A total of 396 patients was randomized on this trial, and nearly 40% of patients converted down to N0 status. The primary endpoint of survival was not improved in the resection arm compared to patients not undergoing resection, when the entire cohort was analyzed. However, the median survival for patients converting to N0 status was 34.4 months, compared to 26.4 months for those with node-positive disease, and 7.9 months for those treated with induction therapy that were unable to undergo surgery ($p < 0.0001$) [68]. On subset analysis, those patients that underwent lobectomy had an improvement in survival versus those requiring a pneumonectomy (median survival of 33.6 versus 21.7 months).

One of the major controversies here is the definition of what is resectable, unresectable, or marginally resectable. As a general rule, subtotal surgical debulking is not recommended, though this is sometimes considered for patients requiring palliative therapy. The other controversy regards the choice of neoadjuvant chemotherapy versus chemoradiotherapy. In a recent NSCLC Meta-Analysis Collaborative Group, individual patient data meta-analysis of 15 randomized trials involving predominantly stage IB-IIIA NSCLC, the use of preoperative chemotherapy resulted in improved five-year survival from 40% to 45%, and a 13% reduction in relative risk for death ($p = 0.007$). The time to distant recurrence was also reduced with preoperative chemotherapy [69]. More recently, in an analysis of stage IIIA patients in the National Cancer Database (NCDB), no differences in survival were noted between preoperative chemotherapy versus preoperative chemoradiotherapy approaches, although the addition of radiation improved pathological nodal clearance and reduced the likelihood of adverse pathological features, including margins. No differences in postoperative mortality were seen [70]. Pless *et al.* reported the results of a European multi-national

23-center Phase III trial for stage III/N2 NSCLC conducted between 2001 and 2012, in which 232 patients were randomized to chemotherapy (three cycles of cisplatin + docetaxel), followed by three weeks of radiotherapy (44 Gy in 22 fractions, concomitant boost technique), followed 21–28 days later by surgery versus chemotherapy without radiotherapy, followed 21 days later by surgery. Postoperatively, there was a further randomization to radiotherapy or not for R1/2 resections only. In this study, radiotherapy did not add any benefit to induction chemotherapy followed by surgery when evaluating overall survival or event-free survival [71]. It should be noted that 16% of the patients in the neoadjuvant chemotherapy group were unable to start radiotherapy due to progression. Further objective responses at the end of all neoadjuvant therapy were in favor of the chemoradiotherapy group (61% versus 44%, $p < 0.05$). Thus, it might be prudent to offer combination chemoradiotherapy to patients where a surgical attempt is critically hinged on the extent of response to treatment. Also, it is unclear if use of concurrent chemoradiotherapy (over sequential as used in this study) and the use of higher-dose radiotherapy ($\sim$60 Gy) would maximize the benefit from chemoradiotherapy. Given the emerging and somewhat contradictory results regarding this issue, it is recommended that patients with locally advanced lung cancer should undergo multidisciplinary management for assessing the best possible treatment modality.

Patients with Stage $IIIA_4$ NSCLC are generally treated with definitive concurrent chemoradiotherapy only without resection, for those whose medical comorbidities will allow for it, or potentially sequential chemoradiotherapy or even radiation therapy alone for those who are unable to tolerate concurrent chemoradiotherapy. In the meta-analysis of concomitant versus sequential chemoradiotheapy in locally advanced NSCLC, the use of a concurrent regimen resulted in 4.5% absolute improvement in survival at five years, with 6% absolute benefit in locoregional control [72]. Distant disease control was not different between the two arms. As anticipated, the use of concurrent therapy resulted in an increased incidence of grade 3-4 esophagitis (18% versus 4%, $p < 0.001$).

For patients with unresectable disease with lymphadenopathy treated with radiation therapy or chemoradiotherapy, prognostic factors have been defined based on a recursive partitioning analysis of nine RTOG trials [73]. The most important favorable prognostic factor was Karnofsky Performance Score (KPS) ≥90. Other prognostic factors included age <70 years, non-large-cell histology, and an absence of malignant pleural effusion.

With regards to radiation technique, treatment fields and doses have changed substantially over the past two decades. Older techniques utilizing definitive radiation or definitive chemoradiation included elective nodal radiation involving bilateral supraclavicular, and mediastinal as well as bilateral hilar nodes. This technique significantly limited the ability to escalate dose. Modern clinical trials often treat only gross disease or limited lymph node stations, eliminating contralateral hilar and bilateral supraclavicular elective nodal coverage. RTOG 9311 showed less than 8% elective nodal failures in regions omitted from elective nodal treatment [74]. In a randomized controlled trial conducted by Yuan and colleagues, in which involved field radiation therapy (IFRT) was compared with elective nodal coverage, there was only a 7% rate of local failure in the IFRT [75]. Ironically, an improvement in overall survival was seen in the IFRT arm, likely related to a reduction in toxicity (radiation pneumonitis; 17% versus 29%, p = 0.044 and trends towards reduced esophagitis, myelosuppression and pericarditis), an improved local control in the IFRT arm (49% versus 41%), incidental coverage of elective nodes in the 40–50 Gy region anyway, and perhaps the use of PET-CT for creating targets that include hilar and mediastinal nodes that may not have been appreciated in previous studies when targets were delineated on CT alone. The ongoing clinical trials do not recommend elective nodal irradiation in appropriately staged patients. Another major advance in modern radiotherapy planning is the routine utilization of 3D planning which allows the generation of dose–volume histograms, and detailed analysis of these have established several important parameters that allow for risk-prediction for toxicities such as esophagitis and pneumonitis. Intensity-modulated radiotherapy (IMRT) is also being increasingly used to further reduce radiation dose to normal tissues, and to optimize dose to target volumes. The National Comprehensive Cancer Network (NCCN) provides reference guidelines for normal tissue constraints for conventionally fractionated, conformal radiotherapy techniques [76,77]. A case study of locoregionally advanced, non-metastatic lung cancer treated using tomotherapy-based IMRT is shown in Figure 19.5.

The optimal dose of radiation is also controversial for patients with unresectable, locally advanced, NSCLC. Originally, the dose of radiation alone was felt to be 60 Gy (versus 50 Gy in 25 fractions, 40 Gy in 20 fractions, and 40 y in 10 fractions split course) based on a landmark dose escalation trial conducted by Perez and colleagues [78]. Subsequently, RTOG 8311 compared

twice-daily treatment schedules with 69.6 Gy in 1.2-Gy twice-daily fractions as the optimal dose, and perhaps better than the standard 60 Gy in 30 fractions [79]. Through an intergroup effort, a three-arm prospective randomized study comparing radiation alone (60 Gy) with hyperfractionated x-ray therapy (XRT) (69.6 Gy) and induction chemotherapy followed by radiation (60 Gy) [80]. The median survival of the three arms were 11.6 months, 12.3 months, and 13.8 months, respectively; yielding induction chemotherapy followed by standard radiation as the standard. It was not until the completion of RTOG 9410 that additional clarity was realized with regards to twice-daily radiation, and conventional fractionated radiation with chemotherapy [81]. RTOG 9410 was a prospective randomized trial of 611 patients with unresected Stage II–III NSCLC, comparing two concurrent chemoradiation regimens to a standard sequential chemoradiation approach. Patients with a KPS ≥70 and weight loss ≤5% were eligible, and the arms of the study were as follows: (i) chemotherapy with cisplatin and vinblastine with standard radiation beginning on day 50; (ii) the same chemotherapy as arm 1, with concurrent standard radiation beginning on day 1; (iii) cisplatin 50 mg m^{-2} on days 1, 8, 29, and 36, and oral VP-16 (etoposide) 50 mg bid × 10 days on weeks 1, 2, 5, and 6, with concurrent hyperfractionated radiation beginning on day 1. Standard radiation consisted of 45 Gy in 25 fractions, followed by a boost of 18 Gy (nine fractions) for a total dose of 63 Gy. Hyperfractionated radiation consisted of 69.6 Gy (58 fractions each of 1.2 Gy, bid). The final results showed that concurrent once-daily radiation resulted in the best outcome (median survival 17 months) as opposed to sequential treatments (14.6 months) or concurrent hyperfractionated therapy (15.6 months).

Although RTOG 9410 did not show any improvement with hyperfractionation with concurrent chemotherapy versus standard fractionation, studies in the UK examining extreme hyperfractionation did show some benefit to the accelerated course of radiotherapy. In this effort, 536 patients were randomized 3:2 to continuous hyperfractionated accelerated radiotherapy (CHART) with 1.5 Gy thrice daily for 15 consecutive days to a total dose of 57 Gy, versus 60 Gy in 30 fractions (standard fractionation). This effort was made without concurrent chemotherapy. An improvement was noted in the two-year overall survival (29% versus 20%, p = 0.004) for CHART versus standard fractionation. The benefit was even more pronounced in squamous cell histologies (33% versus 20%, p = 0.0007). There was also a reduction in local control, regional failure, and distant failure with CHART, though this did come at the expense of more pronounced grade 3 dysphagia (19% versus 3%). It is unclear where the exact benefit to this regimen is, but it is postulated that this may be a result of relative dose intensification or perhaps reduction of

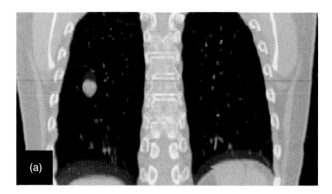 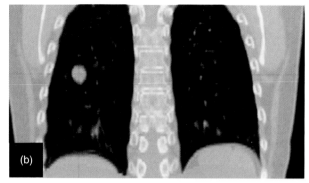

Figure 3.5 (a) Image at inhale and exhale showing different positions of the tumor and diaphragm. (b) After deformable image registration, the organs are aligned in 3D. Note after optimized DIR alignment, the vessels and airways show residual differences.

Figure 3.6 (a–d) Propagation of liver contour from manually contoured phase (panel b) to other phases. The arrows indicate imperfect registration at areas of high curvature.

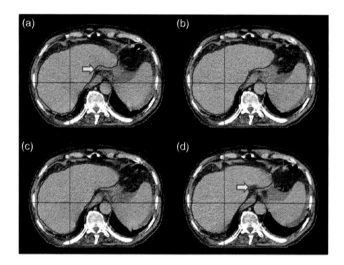

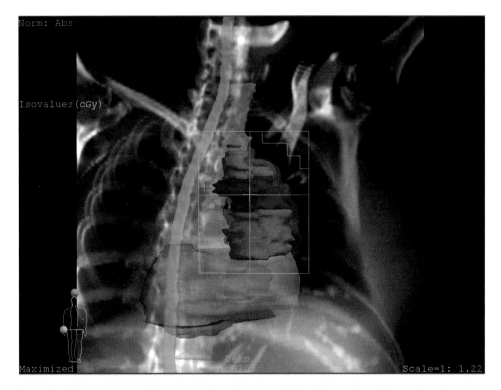

Figure 3.7 Beam's-eye view from a commercial treatment planning system. This right anterior oblique view shows separation of various CTVs of target (purple, red) and spinal cord (green). The lower heart is shown in gold.

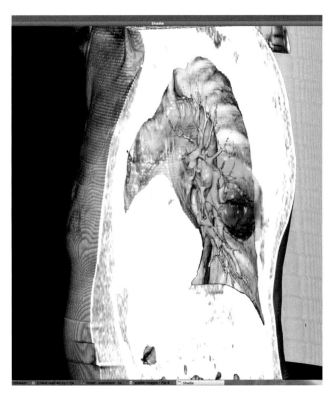

Figure 3.8 Volume rendering of a lung tumor. A cut plane is advanced from patient's left. The tumor, vessels and airways are visualized without image segmentation. The colors encode radiological pathlength variations from the skin surface to structures.

Figure 3.9 (a) Single-field dosimetry schematically indicating dose at point P is sum of primary dose from radiation source, and secondary scattered dose from point S. (b) Depth dose along the central axis. (c) Transverse profile at different depths show that the penumbra increases with depth.

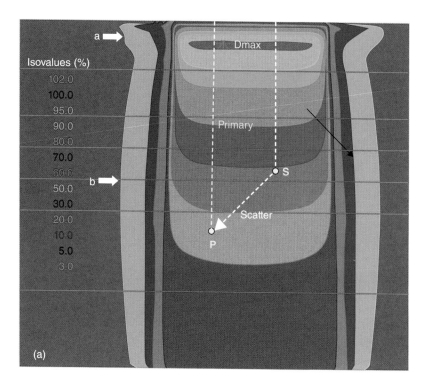

(a)

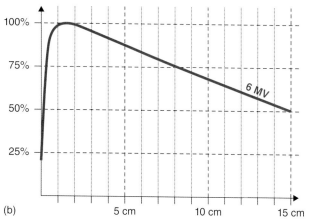

(b)

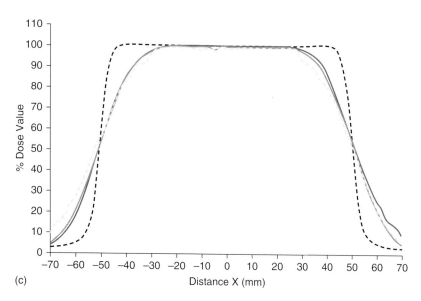

(c)

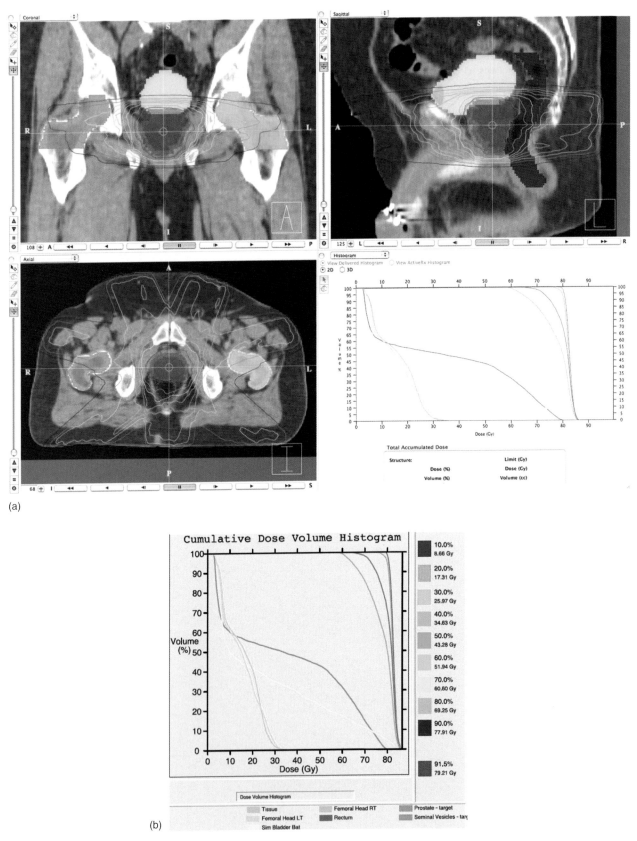

Figure 3.11 (a) Dose distribution in coronal, saggital and transverse planes. The target is red; OARs: bladder (yellow); femoral heads (light and dark blue). (b) Expanded view of the prostate plan cumulative DVH.

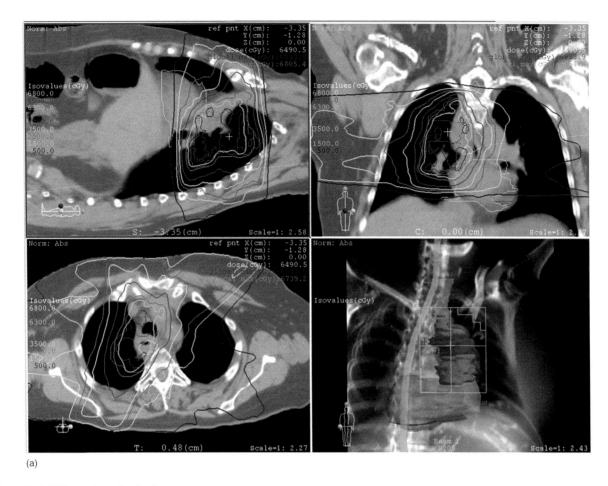

(a)

Figure 3.12 (a) Lung dose distributions in saggital, coronal and axial plane. A BEV view from the right anterior oblique field is also included. (b, c) Dose–volume histograms for lung example case (composite plan). The cumulative DVHs are color-coded to match the structure label in the legend (upper left-hand corner).

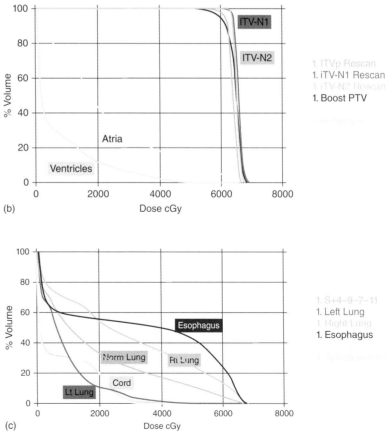

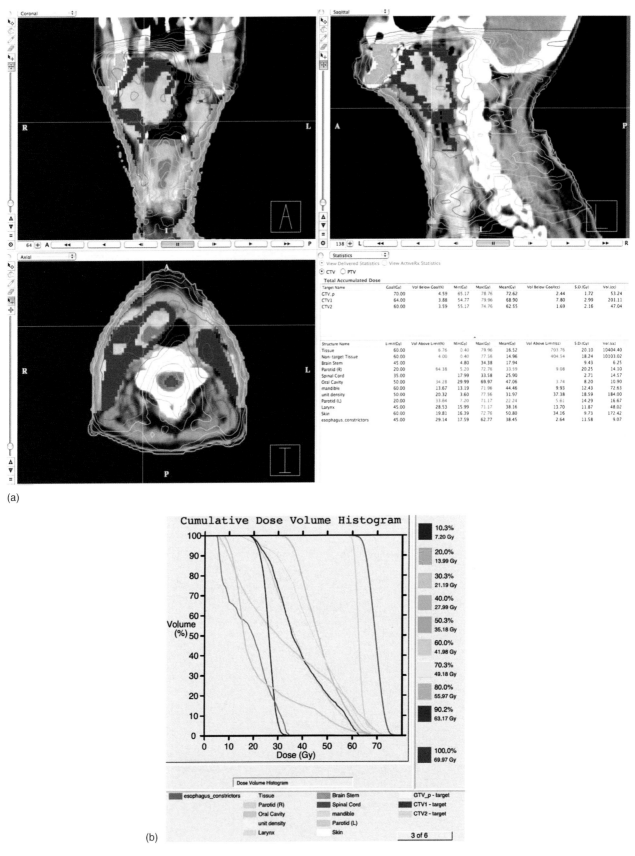

Figure 3.13 (a) Dose distribution for head and neck plan. Targets are shown in red/gold. OARs, the mandible is coded in blue. (b) Corresponding cumulative DVHs for targets and multiple OARs.

Figure 4.2 The gross tumor volume (GTV), clinical target volume (CTV) and internal target volume (ITV) to account for asymmetrical motion due to respiration (with the patient set-up in exhale breath-hold), and the planned target volume (PTV).

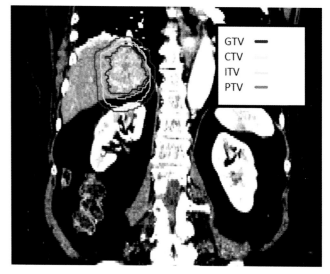

Figure 4.3 Overlay of planning CT scan and verification cone beam CT acquired during a course of radiation therapy for a posterior pharyngeal wall cancer. The gray color represents excellent alignment, whereas purple (reference CT) and green (CBCT) represents regions not well aligned due to deformation. Image registration was focused on the primary tumor and the cervical spine vertebral bodies adjacent to the tumor, as shown within a 'clipbox' (dotted line box). This region was registered to the planning CT dataset.

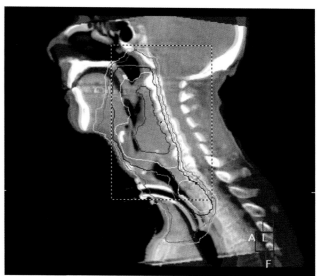

Figure 4.4 Stereotactic body radiotherapy, 33 Gy in six fractions, to treat a cholangiocarcinoma. (a,b) Images from the planning CT. The PTVs (primary tumor PTV = dark blue, liver metastasis PTV = light blue) and the liver (pink) are overlaid on the planning CT and the CBCT. (c,d) On day 1 of treatment, the CBCT showed an increase in gastric gas that resulted in deformation of the liver, as well as bringing the stomach in close proximity to the PTV of the primary tumor. Radiation was not delivered on this day and an anti-gas preparation was recommended for subsequent treatments.

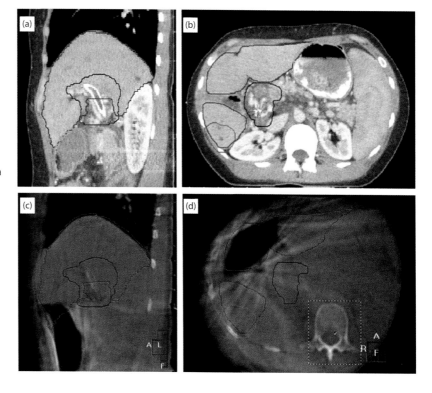

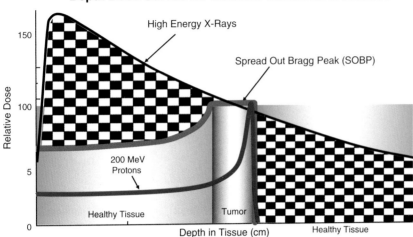

Depth Dose Curves for Different Treatment Modalities

High Energy X-Rays

Spread Out Bragg Peak (SOBP)

200 MeV Protons

Healthy Tissue

Tumor

Healthy Tissue

Relative Dose

Depth in Tissue (cm)

Figure 6.1 Depth dose curves for protons and photons. A single Bragg peak (red line) does not cover the target area, so several peaks are integrated together to form the spread-out Bragg peak (blue line). The checkered areas define where dose is deposited with photons, but is not delivered with protons.

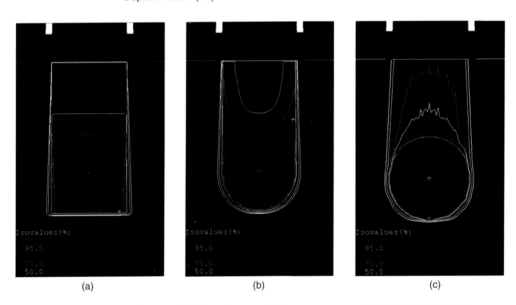

(a)   (b)   (c)

Figure 6.3 A sphere is treated with a single proton field from the top. (a) An uncompensated SOBP. (b) A SOBP with a range compensator providing improved distal conformality. Distal dose is displaced from the distal side to the proximal end when using the compensator. (c) A PBS beam; PBS allows for both distal and proximal shaping of the dose.

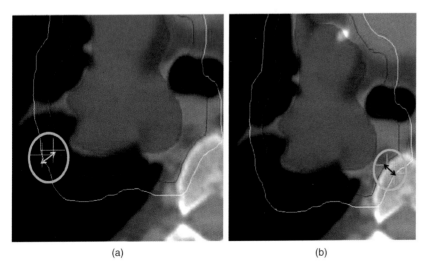

(a)   (b)

Figure 6.4 A GTV (red) and CTV (blue) are defined. The PTV (yellow) is generated by expanding the CTV by 0.5 cm. The physical expansion of 0.5 cm can be used to avoid geometric misses of the target. When addressing range uncertainty, expansions are dependent on the water equivalent thicknesses (WET), which can be very different depending on the beam angle. In panel (a), the physical distance of 0.5 mm is only 0.12 cm of WET due to the low density of the lung tissues. In panel (b) the WET is 0.57 cm, and is greater than the physical expansion of 0.5 cm due to the higher-density bone.

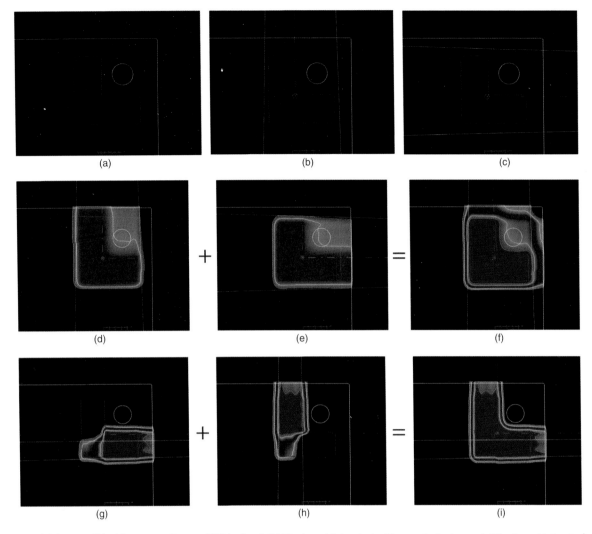

Figure 6.5 (a) A target (blue) is surrounding an OAR (yellow). (b) The target is treated with an anterior beam. (c) The target is treated with a lateral beam. (d–f) Single-field uniform dose (SFUD) optimized. Each proton field delivers a uniform dose to the target. SFUD plans are less sensitive to uncertainties. (g–i) Multi-field-optimized (MFO). Each individual field is optimized with dosimetric information of other fields. MFO allows for better sparing of OARs but is more sensitive to set-up and range uncertainties.

Figure 6.6 A typical CSI dose distribution using PBS delivery. The entire cranial and spinal axis for most children can be treated with two fields. Smooth intensity gradients are planned into the matchline regions to minimize sensitivities to misalignment.

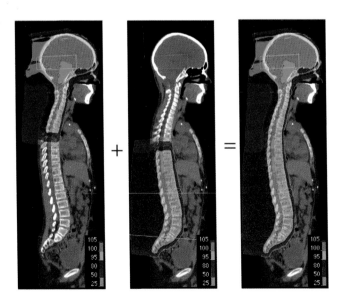

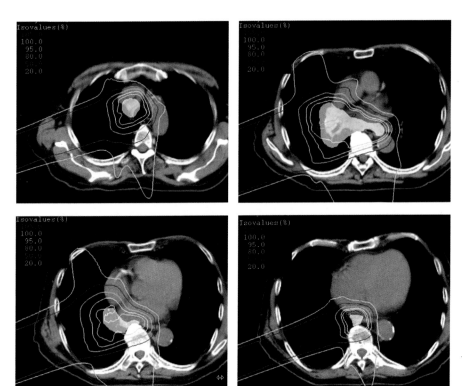

Figure 6.7 The dose distribution for a squamous cell carcinoma of the right hilum. Posterior oblique angles are used to keep the spinal cord below tolerance while sparing much of the heart and lungs.

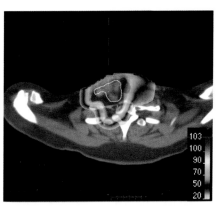
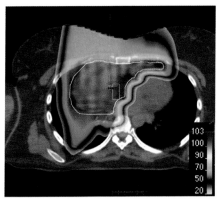
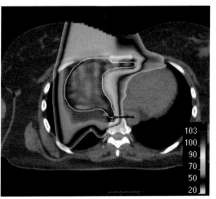
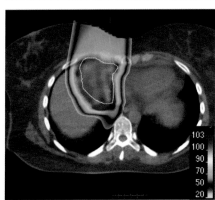

Figure 6.8 A PBS dose distribution for a 40-year-old female with Hodgkin's lymphoma. Protons were considered in this patient to minimize dose to the heart, lungs, and breast.

Figure 6.9 A PBS dose distribution for a left-sided breast with comprehensive nodal irradiation, including the internal mammary chain. This plan makes use of a single, *en-face* PBS field.

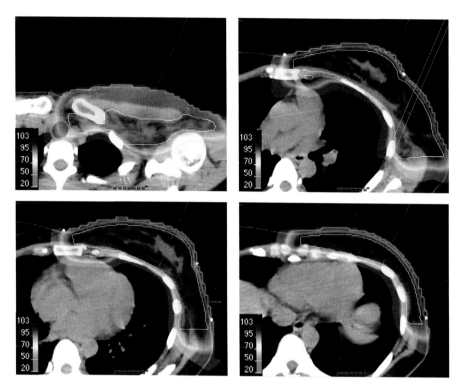

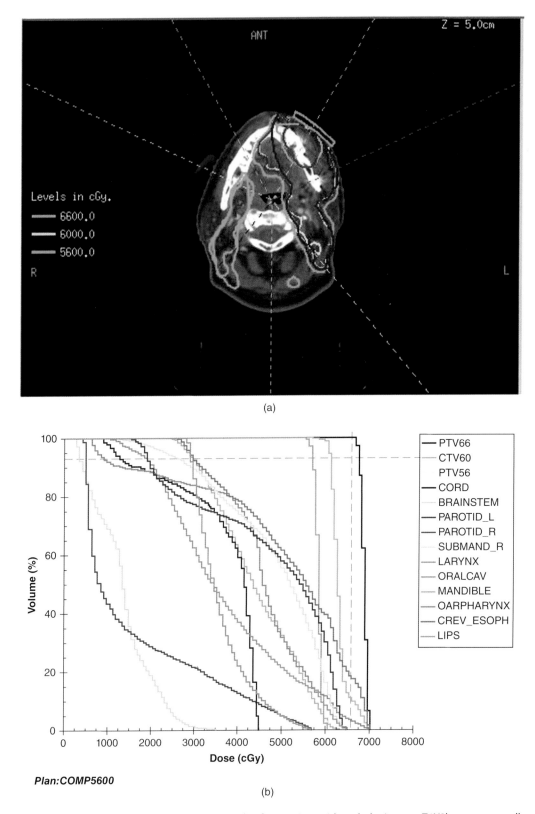

Figure 9.10 (A) Intensity-modulated radiation therapy (IMRT) plan for a patient with pathologic stage T4N2b squamous cell carcinoma of the gingiva shown in the axial plane. (B) Dose–volume histogram for the relevant structures. Note that the bolus is placed over the surgical scar.

Figure 9.11 Contours for a patient with unresectable T3N2b squamous cell carcinoma of the oral tongue treated with intensity-modulated radiation therapy (IMRT). The dose levels are as follows: red (inner line), gross tumor volume (GTV); red (outer line), planning target volume (PTV) 70 Gy; blue, PTV 70 Gy; yellow, PTV 59.4 Gy; green, PTV 54 Gy. Note the coverage of the base of tongue due to the risk of subclinical spread.

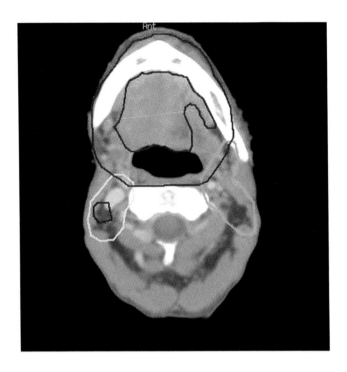

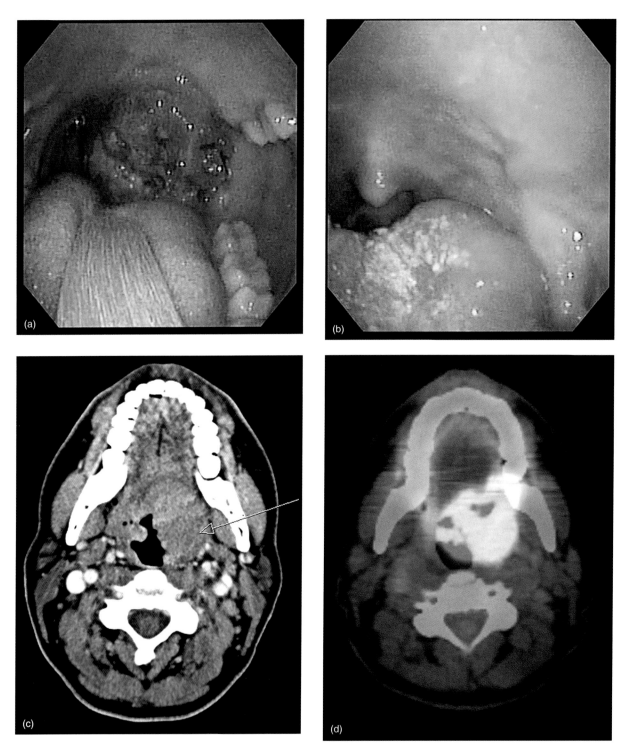

Figure 10.6 A patient with stage T4bN2bM0 left tonsillar cancer treated with an IMRT (Tomotherapy) technique with concurrent cisplatin. (a) Pretreatment. (b) At 3 months after treatment. (c) Pretreatment CT. (d) Pretreatment PET/CT. (e) 3 months post-treatment PET/CT showing resolution of abnormal FDG uptake. (f) IMRT (Tomotherapy) plan demonstrating the 70 Gy (red), 63 Gy (green), and 56 Gy (blue) dose regions.

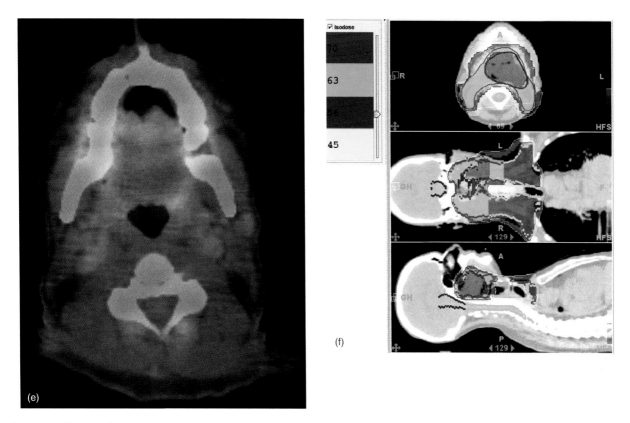

(e)

(f)

Figure 10.6 (*Continued*)

Figure 10.7 A patient with stage T1N2aM0 right tonsillar cancer status after trans-oral laser resection of the primary tumor and right neck dissection treated with postoperative IMRT (Tomotherapy) according to protocol RTOG 0920. (a) Preoperative CT demonstrating right Level II lymphadenopathy. (b) IMRT (Tomotherapy) plan showing the 66 Gy (red), 60 Gy (yellow), and 56 Gy (blue) dose regions.

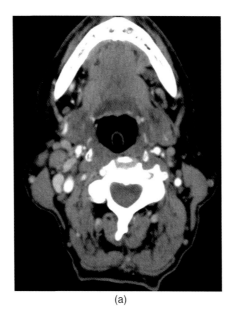

(a)

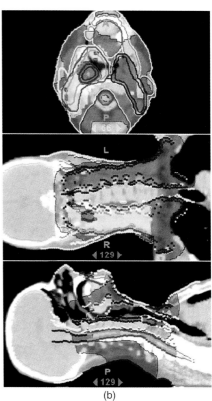

(b)

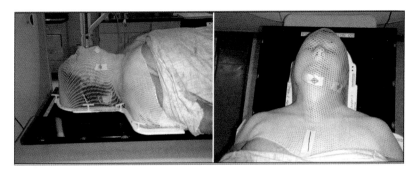

Figure 11.3 A thermoplastic mask for head and neck immobilization.

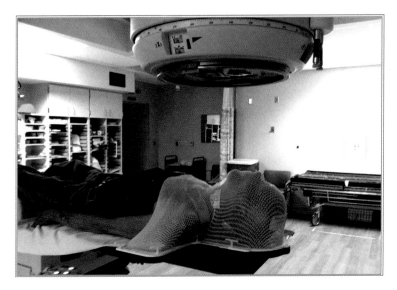

Figure 11.4 A patient in the treatment position fitted with an immobilization mask.

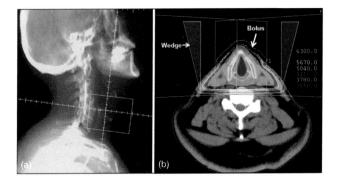

Figure 11.5 (a) Digitally reconstructed radiograph (DRR) showing a lateral field for a patient with a T1 laryngeal carcinoma. (b) Wedge pair and bolus are used to optimize dose distribution.

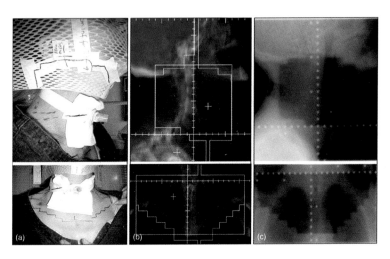

Figure 11.6 Three-field technique with upper neck opposed lateral fields (upper row) and lower neck anterior-posterior field (lower row). (a) Photographs for patient set-up. (b) Digitally reconstructed radiographs. (c) X-ray portals.

Figure 11.7 Target volume contouring, axial view, gross tumor volumes (GTV in red) including the primary tumor and gross lymph nodes, and clinical target volumes, CTV1 (light red), CTV2 (light green) and CTV3 (light blue). The spinal cord and esophagus are also delineated.

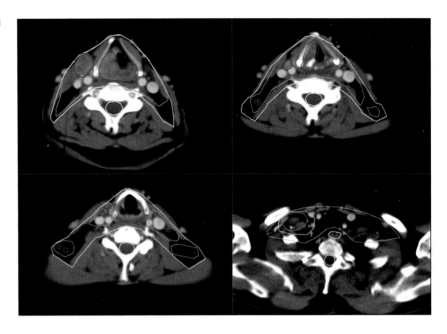

Figure 11.8 Target volume contouring, sagittal (a) and coronal (b) views. Parotids, oral cavity and spinal cord as well as the esophagus are also contoured.

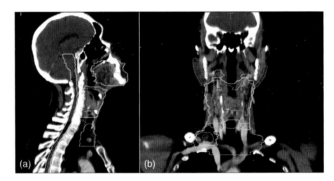

Figure 11.9 Reduction of the initial opposed lateral upper neck fields in order to be off the spinal cord after 45–46 Gy. (a) Photograph of the patient set-up. (b) Digitally reconstructed radiograph. (c) X-ray portal.

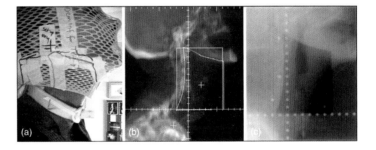

Figure 11.10 Final boost with three-dimensional (3D) technique. A right oblique field is showing. (a) Photograph of the patient set-up; (b) Digitally reconstructed radiograph. (c) X-ray portal.

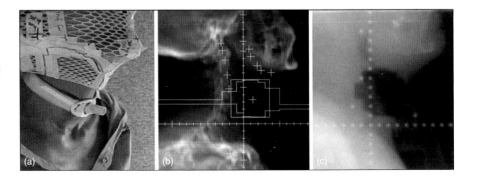

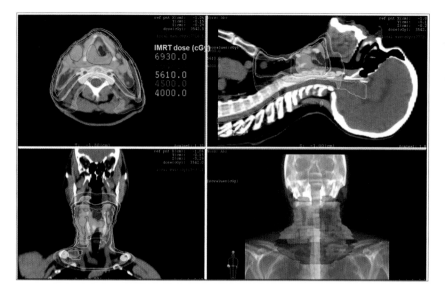

Figure 11.11 IMRT plan showing radiation dose distribution for a patient with a T3N2cM0 squamous cell carcinoma of the glottis. 6930 cGy (green) to the PTV1, 5940 cGy (blue) to the PTV2, and 5610 cGy (light green) to the PTV3 in 33 fractions.

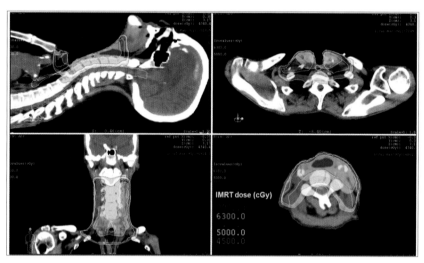

Figure 11.12 Postoperative IMRT plan showing radiation dose distribution for a patient with a T4N2bM0 Squamous cell carcinoma of the glottis after total laryngectomy and bilateral neck dissection. 6300 cGy (green) to the PTV1 and 5400 cGy (blue) to the PTV2 in 30 fractions. PTV3 was not needed in this case.

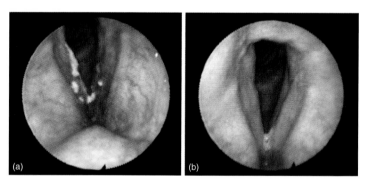

Figure 11.13 (a) A patient with CIS involving both true vocal cords. (b) Five months after radiation therapy of 63 Gy in 2.25 Gy per fraction.

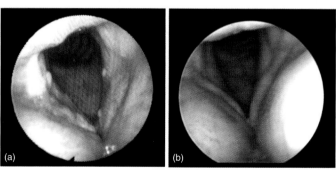

Figure 11.14 (a) A patient with a T1b squamous cell carcinoma arising from CIS involving both true vocal cords. (b) Six months after radiation therapy of 63 Gy in 2.25 Gy per fraction.

Figure 11.15 (a) A patient with a T2 squamous cell carcinoma involving right side true vocal cord and anterior commissure. (b) Five months after radiation therapy of 65.25 Gy in 2.25 Gy per fraction.

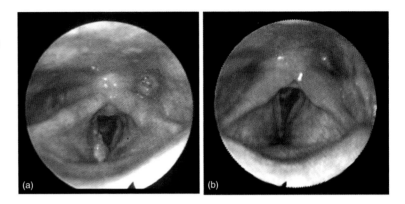

Figure 11.16 (a) A patient with a T1N0 squamous cell carcinoma in the epiglottis. (b) Three months after radiation therapy of 66 Gy in 2.2 Gy per fraction with concurrent chemotherapy.

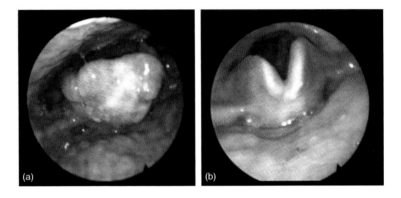

Figure 11.17 (a,b) A patient with a T3N2aM0 supraglottic squamous cell carcinoma. (a) Photograph. (b) Axial CT image. (c,d) At four months after concurrent cisplatin chemotherapy and IMRT to 69.3 Gy in 2.1 Gy per fraction. (c) Photograph. (d) Axial CT image.

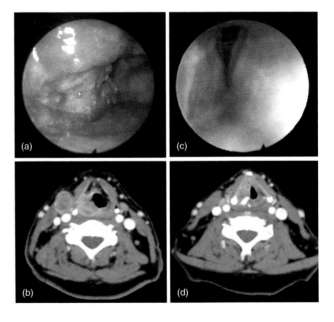

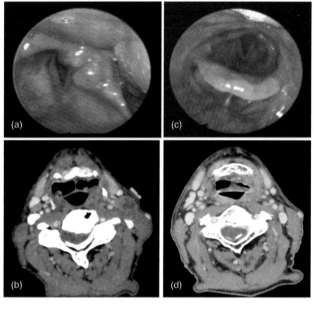

Figure 11.18 (a,b) A patient with a T3N2bM0 squamous cell carcinoma of the hypopharynx involving the left aryepiglottic fold and arytenoids. (a) Photograph. (b) Axial CT image. (c,d) At three months after concurrent chemotherapy and IMRT of 69.3 Gy in 2.1 Gy per fraction. (c) Photograph. (d) Axial CT image.

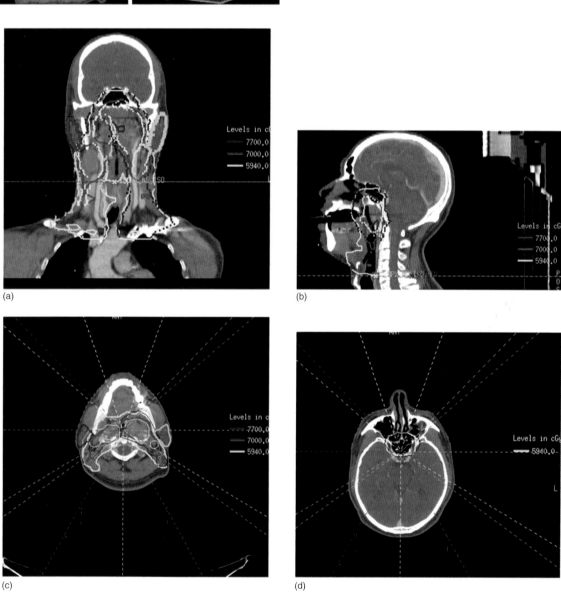

Figure 12.5 Intensity-modulated radiation therapy (IMRT) plan for a patient with T2N2 carcinoma of the nasopharyx displayed in the (A) coronal, (B) sagittal, and (C–E) axial planes. (F) Dose-volume histogram for the relevant structures.

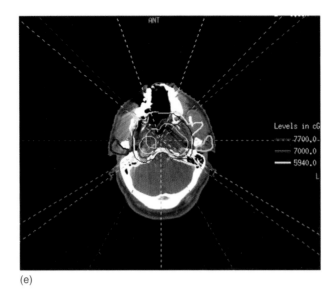

(e)

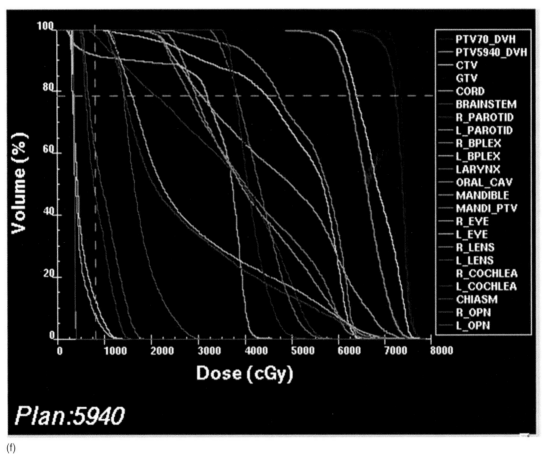

(f)

Figure 12.5 (*Continued*)

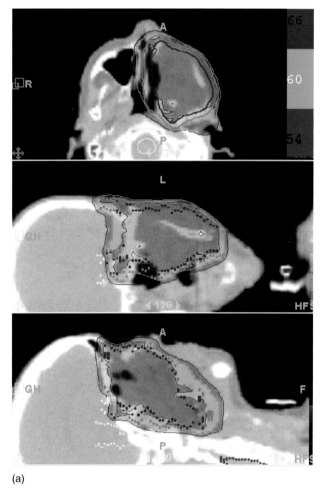

(a)

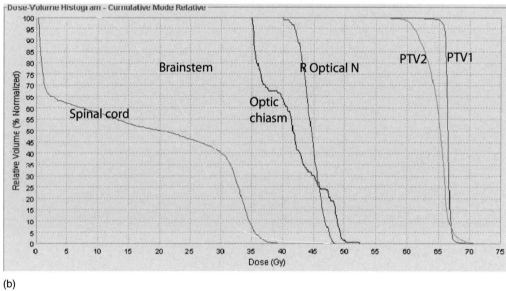

(b)

Figure 13.2 A patient with stage T4AN0 left maxillary sinus squamous cell carcinoma treated with postoperative radiotherapy. (a) Isodose distribution of the treatment plan. (b) Dose–volume histogram for the relevant structures.

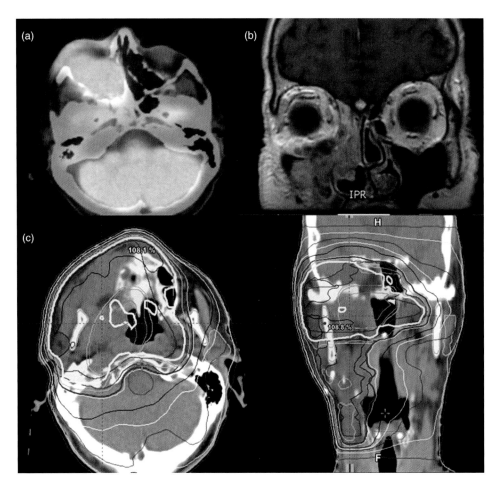

Figure 13.3 A patient with stage T4AN0 right maxillary sinus squamous cell carcinoma treated with postoperative radiotherapy. (a) Pre-operative PET scan showing FDG avid lesion in the right maxillary sinus involving the orbit and causing bone instruction. (b) Coronal MRI image showing disease in the right maxillary sinus with disruption of the floor of orbit. (c) Axial and coronal images of the planning CT scan showing the dose distribution. Green line, 66 Gy isodose; yellow line, 60 Gy isodose; blue line, 54 Gy isodose.

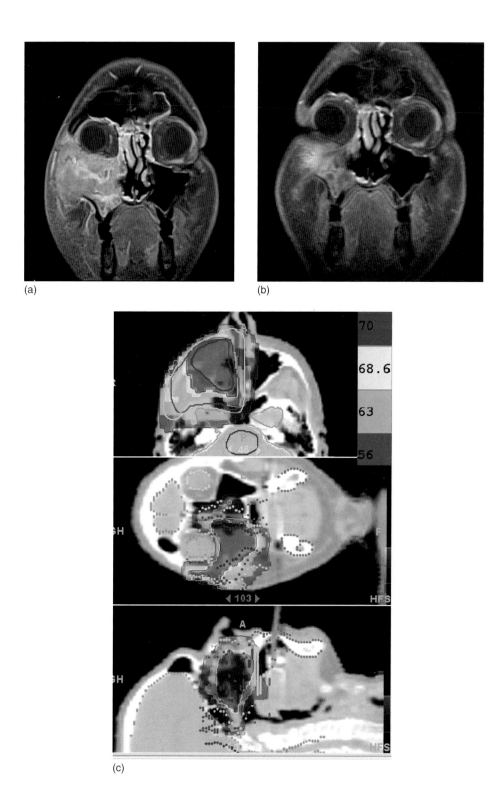

(a)

(b)

(c)

Figure 13.4 A patient with stage T4AN0 right maxillary sinus squamous cell carcinoma treated with induction chemotherapy followed by definitive concurrent chemoradiation. (a) MRI at diagnosis. (b) MRI after induction chemotherapy. (c) Isodose distribution of the treatment plan. Note that the postchemotherapy tumor volume was delivered to 70 Gy.

Figure 13.5 A patient with unresectable squamous cell carcinoma of sphenoid sinus and nasal cavity. (a) MRI at diagnosis. (b) IMRT plan to 50.4 Gy at 1.8 Gy per fraction. (c) MRI at one month after IMRT. (d) SBRT using Cyberknife for additional 18 Gy at 6 Gy per fraction. (e) MRI at three years after the initial treatment. Enhancement (arrow) was noted in the right temporal lobe suspicious for brain necrosis.

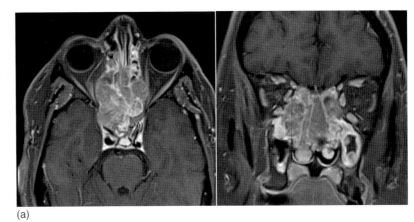

(a)

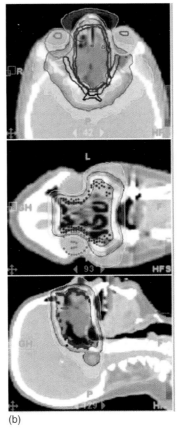

(b)

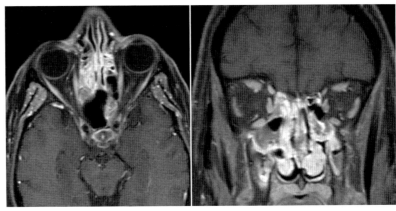

(c)

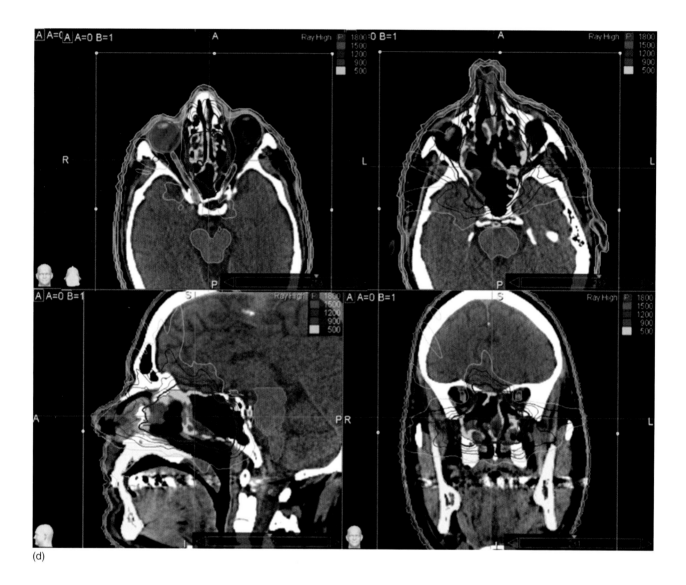

(d)

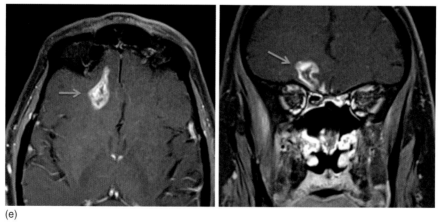

(e)

Figure 13.5 (*Continued*)

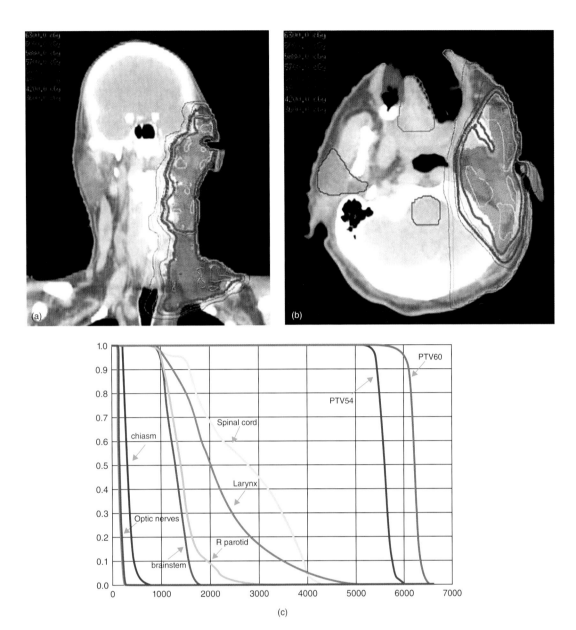

Figure 14.4 A 70-year-old male status post left-sided superficial parotidectomy and ipsilateral neck dissection for T2N1, high-grade mucoepidermoid carcinoma. The IMRT plan, shown in (a) coronal and (b) axial dimensions was designed to deliver a dose of 6000 cGy to the parotid bed and level II/III neck and 5400 cGy to the ipsilateral supraclavicular fossa, using a simultaneous-integrated boost technique. Visualized avoidance structures include the oral cavity (green), contralateral right parotid gland (light green), brainstem with margin (purple), and mandible (orange). (c) Dose–volume histogram illustrating the ability of IMRT to maximize dose to the 6000 cGy and 5400 cGy planning target volume (PTV) while minimizing dose to avoidance structures.

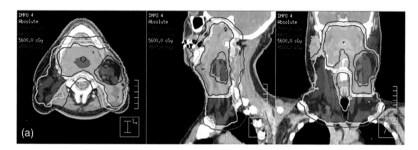

(a)

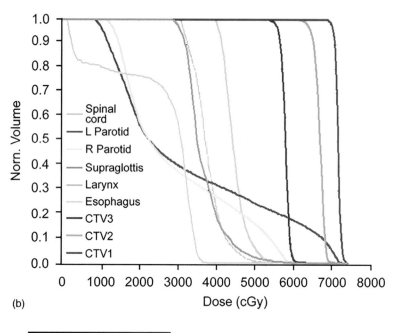

(b)

Figure 15.4 This patient received definitive IMRT with concurrent chemotherapy. (a) CTV1 included the lymphadenopathy with margin and was treated to 70 Gy. CTV2 included the nasopharynx, oropharynx and the high-risk lymphatic region, and was treated to 63 Gy. CTV3 was treated to 56 Gy. This was done with one plan using simultaneously integrated boost technique and delivered in 35 fractions. The segment of esophagus in the radiation field was also outlined as a dose-limiting structure. (b) Dose–volume histogram. Note acceptable doses to the parotids, larynx, and supraglottis. *Source:* Lu, Yao, and Tan 2009 [43]. Reproduced with permission of Elsevier. (c) Representative axial slices of the IMRT plan for this patient.

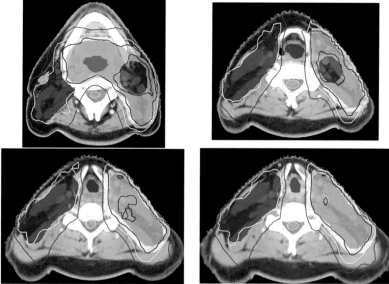

(c) **Red CTV1; Green CTV2; Blue CTV3**

Figure 15.5 This patient with bulky level II lymph node with extracapsular extension after neck dissection received postoperative IMRT with concurrent cisplatin. (a) CTV1 included the surgical bed, the high-risk lymphatic regions, the oropharynx and nasopharynx; CTV2 included the lower-risk cervical lymphatic regions. These were treated to 64 Gy (2 Gy per fraction) and 54.4 Gy (1.7 Gy per fraction) in 32 fractions in one plan using simultaneously integrated boost technique. The segment of esophagus in the radiation field was also outlined as a dose-limiting structure. (b) Dose–volume histogram. Note acceptable doses to the parotids, larynx, and supraglottis. *Source:* Lu, Yao, and Tan 2009 [43]. Reproduced with permission of Elsevier. (c) Representative axial slices of the IMRT plan for this patient.

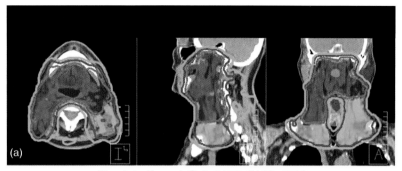

Absolute Dose (cGy): 6400 5440 4600

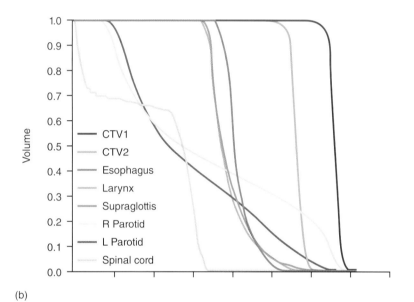

(b)

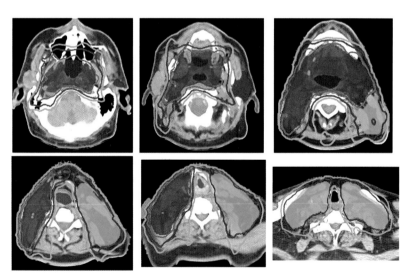

(c)   Red CTV1 and CTV2; Green CTV3

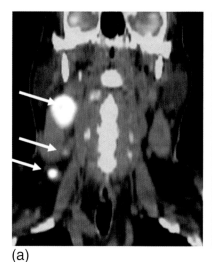

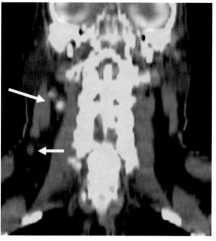

(a)

Figure 15.6 A patient with multiple lymphadenopathy at right level II to level IV. (a) FDG-PET scan of the patient. (b) IMRT plan. CTV1 included the all involved lymph nodes with margin and was treated to 70 Gy. CTV2 included the nasopharynx, oropharynx, ipsilateral larynx and hypopharynx, and the high-risk lymphatic region and was treated to 63 Gy. CTV3 was treated to 56 Gy. This was done with one plan using simultaneously integrated boost technique and delivered in 35 fractions. The segment of esophagus in the radiation field was also outlined as a dose-limiting structure. (c) Dose–volume histogram.

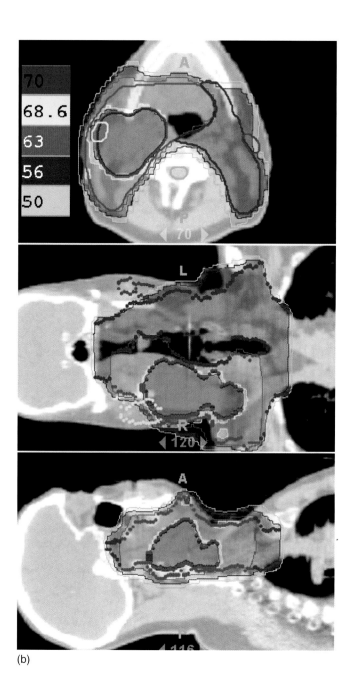

(b)

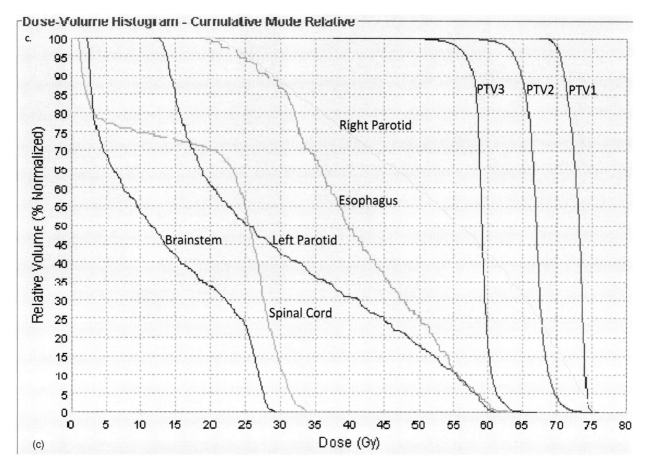

Dose-Volume Histogram - Cumulative Mode Relative

Right Parotid

Esophagus

Brainstem   Left Parotid

Spinal Cord

PTV3   PTV2   PTV1

Relative Volume (% Normalized)

Dose (Gy)

(c)

Figure 15.6 (*Continued*)

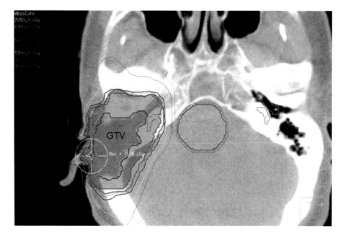

Figure 16.1 Intensity-modulated radiation therapy plan for a 75-year-old male who presented with a large squamous cell carcinoma involving the skin of the right temporal face. Notably, the patient had previously been treated to a dose of 70 Gy with cisplatin for squamous cell carcinoma of the oropharynx four years previously. He refused surgical resection for his new primary cancer and was treated with radiation to a dose of 66 Gy delivered to 95% of the planning target volume encompassing gross disease. Visible organs at risk on this axial section include the ipsilateral auditory structures (in the high-dose planning target volume), contralateral auditory structures, and brainstem. GTV, gross tumor volume.

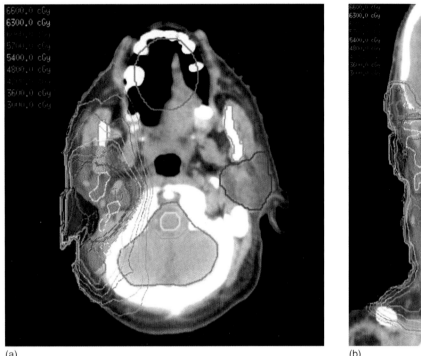
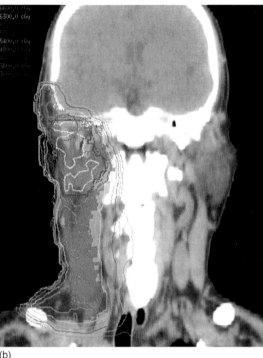

(a)

(b)

Figure 16.2 Intensity-modulated radiation therapy (IMRT) plan for a 55-year-old male who was status post gross total resection consisting of partial temporal bone resection and auriculectomy for squamous cell carcinoma of the external ear canal. The patient was subsequently treated to a total dose of 60 Gy to the tumor bed and 54 Gy to high-risk ipsilateral neck, respectively, using a simultaneous-integrated boost technique. Water bolus was employed to fill the surgical defect. (a) Visible organs at risk on this axial section include the oral cavity, spinal cord, brain, brainstem, and contralateral parotid gland. (b) Coronal view of the IMRT plan.

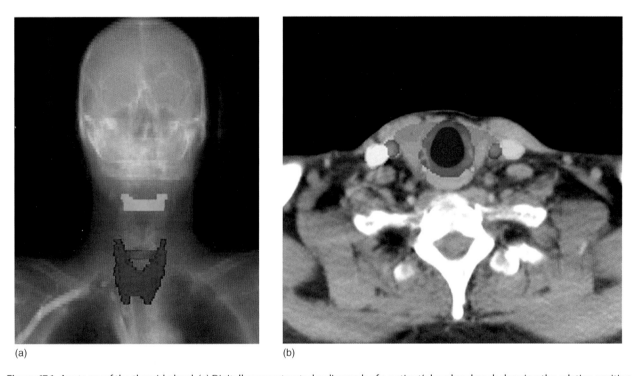

(a)

(b)

Figure 17.1 Anatomy of the thyroid gland. (a) Digitally reconstructed radiograph of a patient's head and neck showing the relative position of the thyroid gland (blue) to the hyoid bone (green) and bottom of the cricoid cartilage (purple). (b) Contrast-enhanced axial computed tomography (CT) slice at the level of the bottom of the cricoid cartilage (purple) showing the position of the thyroid gland (blue) relative to the esophagus (orange), carotid arteries (red), jugular vein (lavender) and the approximate position of the recurrent laryngeal nerves (yellow-green). *Source:* Halperin *et al.* 2013. Reproduced with permission of Wolters Kluwer Health.

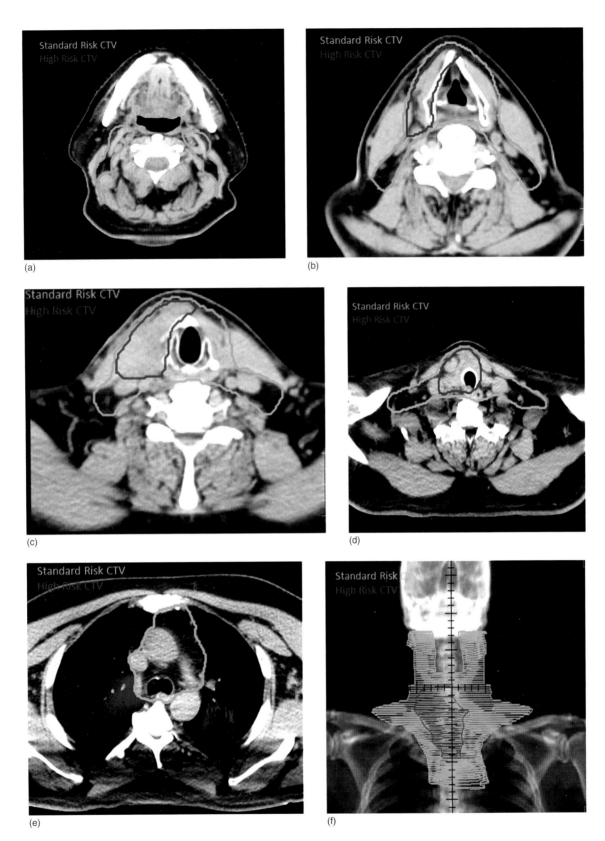

Figure 17.4 Intensity-modulated radiation therapy (IMRT) clinical target volume (CTV) contouring atlas for a patient with T2N0M0 insular thyroid carcinoma status-post total thyroidectomy and radioactive iodine (RAI). (a) Highest level of CTV for elective nodal irradiation where the posterior belly of the digastric muscle crosses the jugular vein. (b) CTV contours at the level of the thyroid notch. (c) CTV contours through the level of the cricoid cartilage. (d) CTV contours through the level of the first tracheal ring. (e) Lowest level of CTV contours covering the upper mediastinal lymph nodes at the level of the carina. (f) Digital reconstructed radiograph depicting the CTV volumes. Indications for external-beam radiation therapy (EBRT) were insular carcinoma (poorly differentiated) and positive margin.

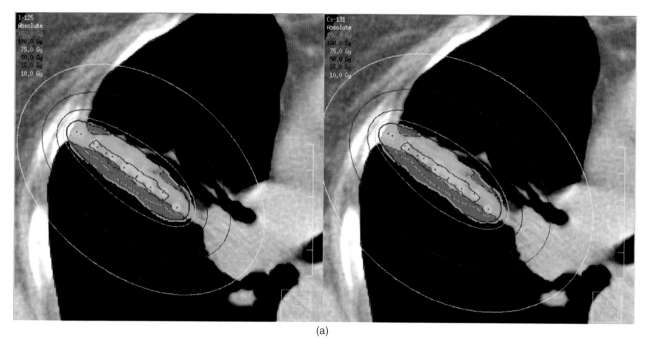

(a)

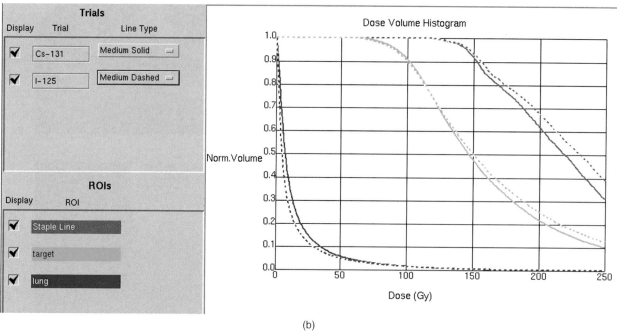

(b)

Figure 19.3 (a) Isodose lines for ^{125}I permanent implant on the left and [131]Cs permanent implant on the right. Very similar physical dose distributions are obtained. (b) Dose–volume histogram of the lung, target, and staple line for ^{125}I and [131]Cs permanent implants. Excellent coverage of the staple line is obtained with 100% of the staple line receiving the prescription dose. There is a over 90% coverage of the staple line plus 5 mm margin with both isotopes, yielding similar physical DVHs.

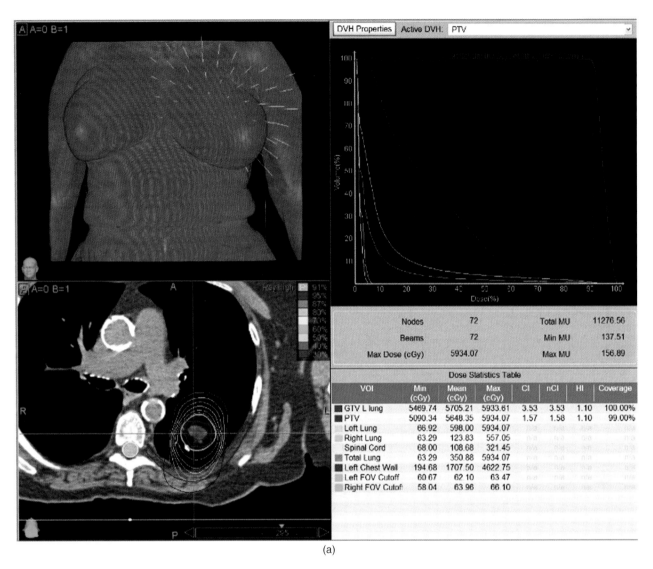

(a)

Figure 19.5 (a) SBRT patient with medically inoperable lung cancer. Note the rapid fall off of dose outside of the primary target. (b) A case example with locoregionally advanced NSCLC treated with IMRT technique to a dose of 66 Gy in 33 fractions, five fractions per week. Panel A: CT scan images in three planes showing target volumes and organs at risk. Panel B: Isodose distribution demonstrating highly conformal distribution of higher isodoses with relative spreading of lower isodoses. Panel C: Dose–volume histogram demonstrating a rapid fall-off of isodoses covering the target volume shown by curves on the right with significant sparing of normal tissues as represented by curves on the left. Illustration courtesy Dr George Cannon, University of Wisconsin.

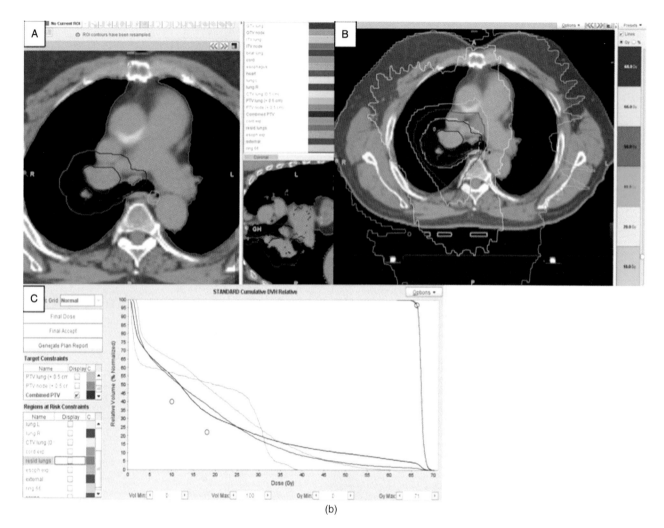

(b)

Figure 19.5 (*Continued*)

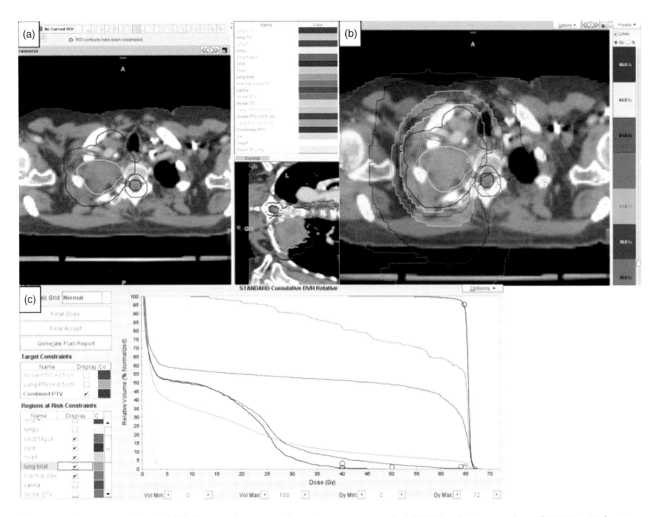

Figure 19.7 A case example with NSCLC presenting as superior sulcus tumor treated with IMRT technique to a dose of 64.8 Gy in 36 fractions, five fractions per week. Prescribed dose was limited by close proximity of target volume to spinal cord (purple). (a) CT scan images in three planes showing target volumes and organ at risks. (b) Isodose distribution demonstrating highly conformal distribution of higher isodoses with relative spreading of lower isodoses. (c) Dose–volume histogram demonstrating a rapid fall-off of isodoses covering the target volume shown by curves on the right with attempted sparing of normal tissues. Relatively high doses were delivered to the brachial plexus (green) and esophagus (pink) due to close proximity to target volumes. Illustration courtesy Dr George Cannon, University of Wisconsin.

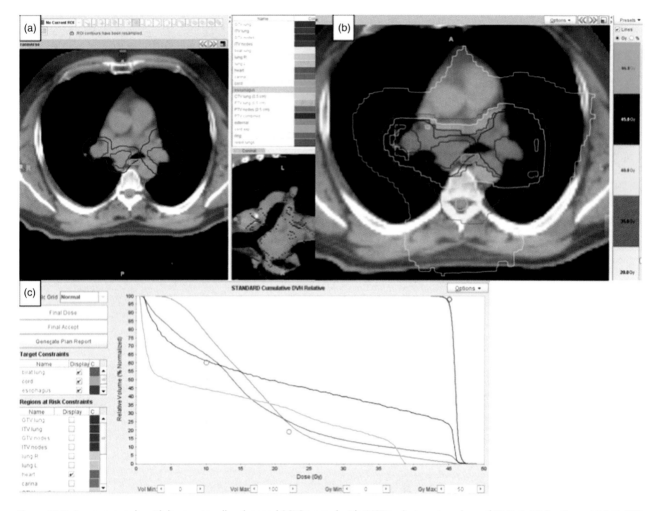

Figure 19.8 A case example with locoregionally advanced SCLC treated with IMRT technique to a dose of 45 Gy in 30 fractions at 1.5 Gy BID, 10 fractions per week as per the Turrisi regimen. (a) CT scan images in three planes showing target volumes and organs at risk. (b) Isodose distribution demonstrating highly conformal distribution of higher isodoses with relative spreading of lower isodoses. (c) Dose–volume histogram demonstrating a rapid fall-off of isodoses covering the target volume shown by curves on the right with significant sparing of normal tissues as represented by curves on the left. Illustration courtesy Dr George Cannon, University of Wisconsin.

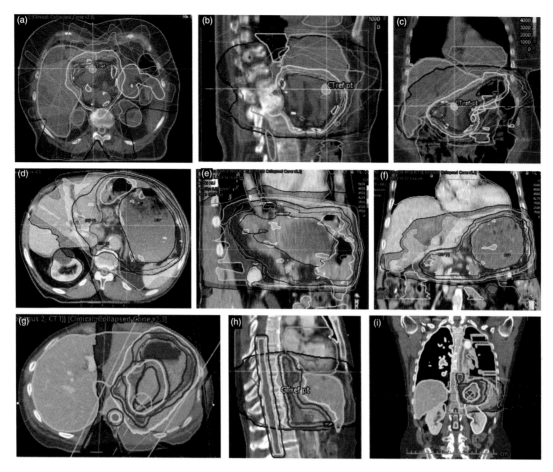

Figure 21.1 Representative postoperative (a–f) and neoadjuvant (g–j) radiation treatment plans for gastric cancer. Prescription dose of 45 Gy is shown in orange. (a–c) Adjuvant IMRT plan for a pT3N2 gastric body tumor following subtotal gastrectomy and D1+ lymphadenectomy, Roux-en-Y gastrojejunostomy and adjuvant chemotherapy. (d–f) Adjuvant IMRT plan for a pT4aN0 tumor in the lesser curvature following distal gastrectomy and D0 lymphadenectomy, Billroth II gastrojejunostomy and adjuvant chemotherapy. Note the larger field size due to large remnant and lack of surgical lymph node evaluation. (g–j) Neoadjuvant radiation plan for a T3N1 tumor in the GE junction. The primary tumor, outlined in red and marked by a blue X in circle, was given a boost of 5.4 Gy to a total dose of 50.4 Gy.

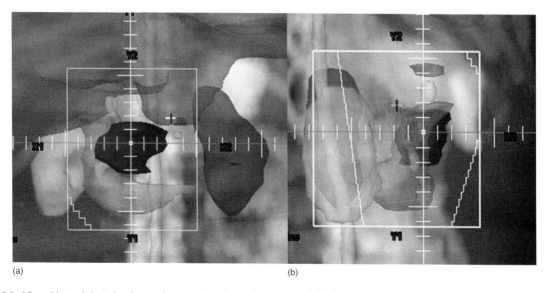

(a)   (b)

Figure 22.2 AP and lateral digital radiograph reconstructions of treatment fields for patient with pancreatic head cancer. (a) The antero-posterior/posteroanterior (AP/PA) field, which includes gross tumor (red), duodenal loop (pink) (plus approximately 50% of the right kidney (light green)), liver (brown) and nodal areas at risk (porta hepatis, orange; SMA, green; celiac-magenta). Most of the left kidney (blue) is excluded from the AP/PA field. (b) The right lateral field with an anterior margin beyond gross disease and a posterior margin behind front edge of vertebral body. The liver contour (brown) has been removed from lateral field for visualization of other structures.

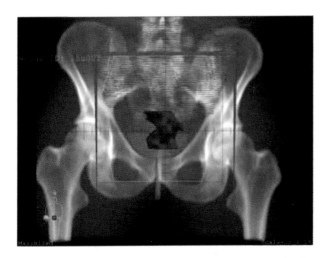

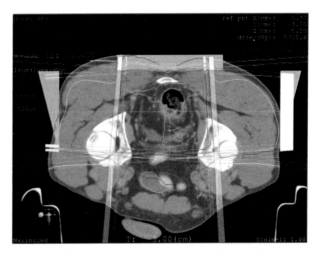

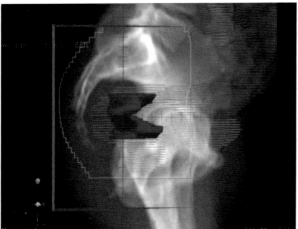

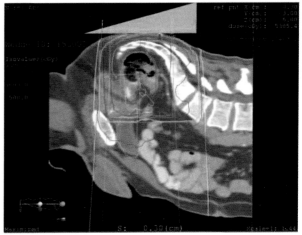

Figure 24.1 Standard radiation field for rectal cancer. Illustration courtesy of Theodore Hong.

Figure 24.2 Standard three-field radiation plan for rectal cancer. Illustration courtesy of Theodore Hong.

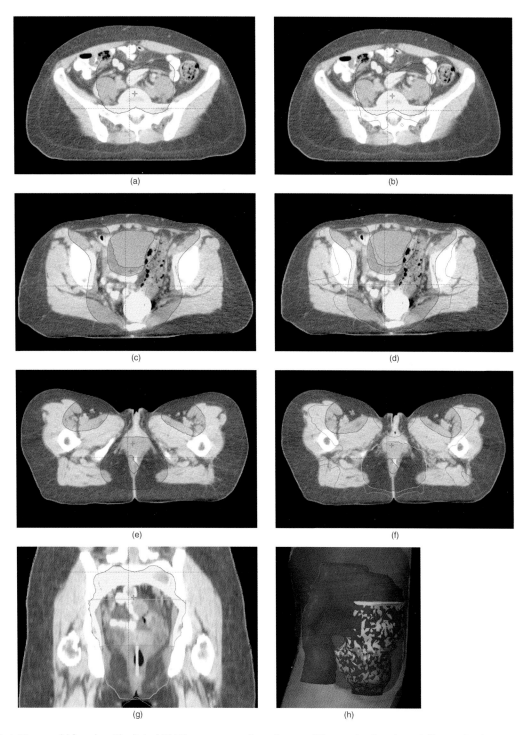

Figure 25.1 A 48-year-old female with clinical T2 N0 squamous cell carcinoma of the proximal anal canal. She received concurrent 5-FU and mitomycin-based chemoradiotherapy using IMRT techniques with serial PTV reductions. (a) Axial CT slice of the patient; the PTV 3060 is shown in red. (b) Corresponding image with the isodose line superimposed (pink line = 3060 cGy). (c) More inferior axial slice with PTV 3060 shown in red and bladder outlined in green. (d) Corresponding isodose lines. Note the relative sparing of the bladder anteriorly and femoral heads laterally. Pink isodose line = 3060 cGy; blue isodose line = 4500 cGy. (e) PTV 3060 shown more inferiorly. Note the centrally located GTV adjacent to the rectal tube. (f) The same image with relative isodoses superimposed from the IMRT plan. The patient was treated with a series of sequential PTV reductions. Note the relative sparing of the genitalia anteriorly and the proximal femora laterally. Pink isodose line = 3060 cGy; blue isodose line = 4500 cGy; yellow isodose line = 5400 cGy. (g) Sequential PTV reductions in the treatment of anal cancer. Red = PTV 3060; green = PTV 4500; blue = PTV 5400. (h) Lateral view of sequential PTVs. Red = PTV 3060; green = PTV 4500; blue = PTV 5400.

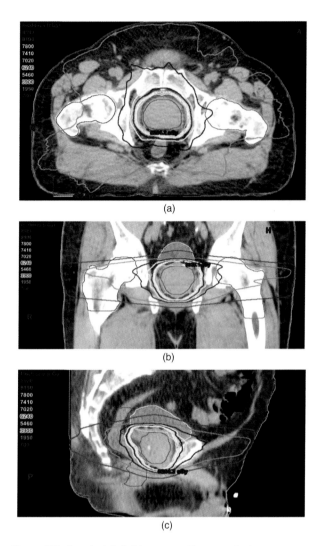

(a)

(b)

(c)

Figure 27.2 A typical definitive external beam radiotherapy isodose distribution using a VMAT plan to 78 Gy for an intermediate-risk prostate cancer patient. (a) Axial, (b) coronal, and (c) sagittal planes. The clinical target volume (CTV) is in red and the planning target volume (PTV) is in green.

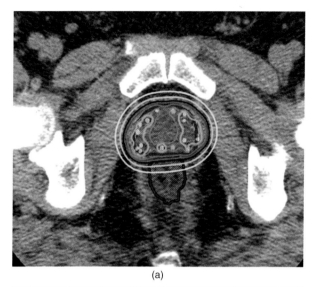

(a)

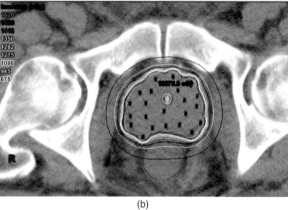

(b)

Figure 27.3 Typical isodose distributions for definitive prostate brachytherapy using (a) LDR and (b) HDR brachytherapy. The LDR plan uses iodine-125 and a modified peripheral loading, central-sparing technique. The HDR plan uses iridium-192 and dwell time/dwell position optimization after placement of the catheters.

Figure 27.4 (a–c) A typical post-prostatectomy radiotherapy isodose distribution using VMAT. The clinical target volume (CTV) is shown in red, and the planning target volume (PTV) in green. (a) Axial image. (b) Sagittal image. (c) Coronal image.

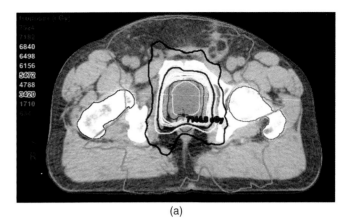

(a)

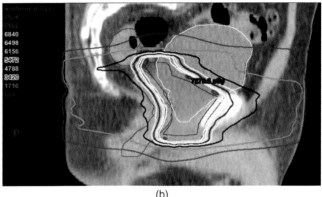

(b)

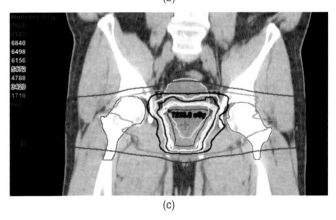

(c)

Figure 28.2 Staging and five-year survival for renal cell carcinoma. Figure modified from Cohen, H.T., McGovern, F.J. (2005) Survival statistics. *N. Engl. J. Med.*, **353**, 2477–2490. Modified with permission from The NCCN Clinical Practice Guidelines in Oncology for Kidney Cancer V.2.2012.

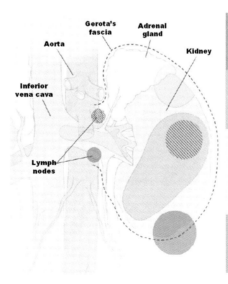

Stage I
Tumor ≤7 cm in greatest dimension and limited to kidney;
5-year survival, 96%

Stage II
Tumor >7 cm in greatest dimension and limited to kidney;
5-year survival, 82%

Stage III
Tumor extends into major veins or perinephric tissues but not into the ipsilateral adrenal gland and not beyond Gerota fascia **or** regional lymph nodes are involved;
5-year survival, 64%

Stage IV
Tumor beyond Gerota's fascia or distant metastasis;
5-year survival, 23%

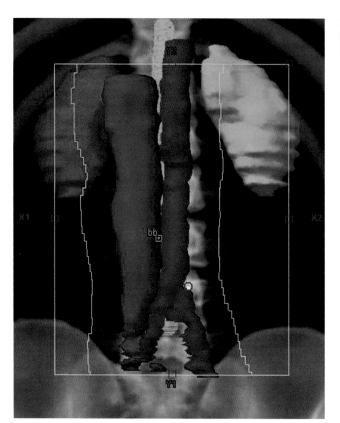

Figure 29.1 Standard para-aortic strip field. A standard para-aortic field for a CS I seminoma based on vascular anatomy. Illustration courtesy of Clair Beard, MD.

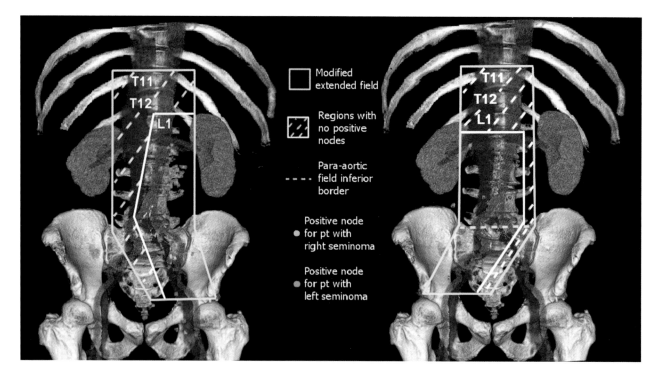

Figure 29.2 Dog-leg fields and nodal maps. The distribution of positive nodes in 90 stage IIA/B and recurrent stage I seminoma patients. Conventional and modified fields have been overlaid on the template [29].

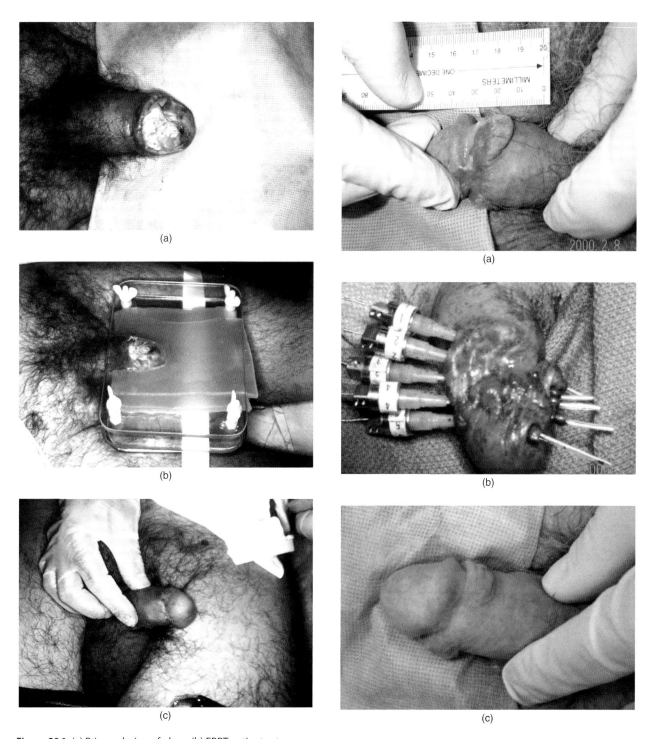

Figure 30.1 (a) Primary lesion of glans. (b) EBRT patient set-up with penis within a lucite 'sandwich'. The lucite acts as a bolus and additional bolus material is packed around the sides of the glans. A lead shield lies below to block the transmission to the testes. (c) One year post-EBRT. There is a well-healed, pale scar at the primary site.

Figure 30.2 (a) Primary lesion of the corona radiata. (b) Interstitial, single-plane brachytherapy with catheters placed perpendicular to the penile shaft. The patient is catheterized and care is taken to avoid the urethra. (c) One year post-brachytherapy.

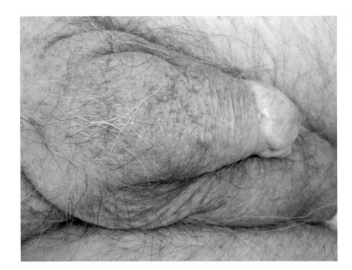

Figure 30.3 Post-treatment effects can include telangiectasia and penile swelling. The latter can result from the direct effect of radiation on the penile lymphatics or from irradiation of the inguinal lymph nodes.

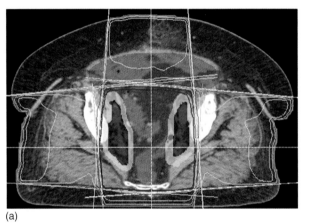

(a)

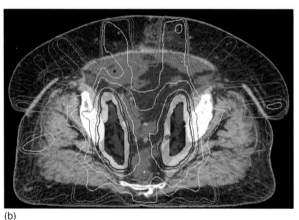

(b)

Figure 31.3 Standard three-dimensional conformal irradiation (a) requires treatment of small bowel (contoured in brown) which can be spared with IMRT (b).

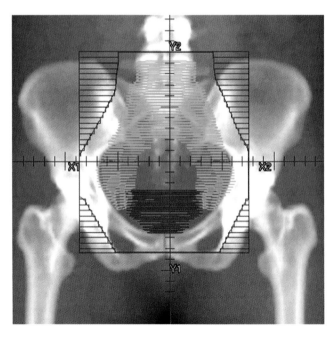

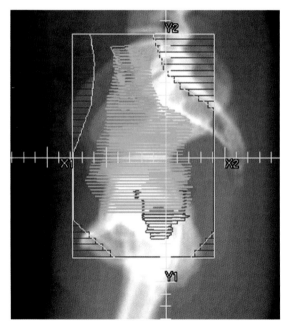

Figure 31.4 Examples of standard AP and lateral fields for pelvic radiation. Contours used for IMRT planning are shown as wireframe on the DRRs. The green contours represent the pelvic nodal CTV and the red volume is the vaginal CTV.

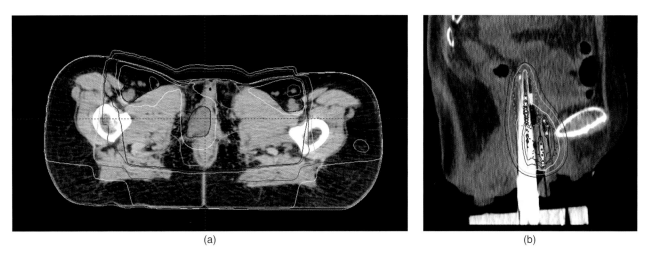

Figure 32.2 Dose distribution in a patient with vulvar cancer. Vaginal involvement was treated with IMRT (a) and interstitial brachytherapy (b). The external beam target volume included elective treatment of groin nodes with bolus covering the vulvar and groin areas. The interstitial brachytherapy boost dose is to the primary tumor, which involves the vagina.

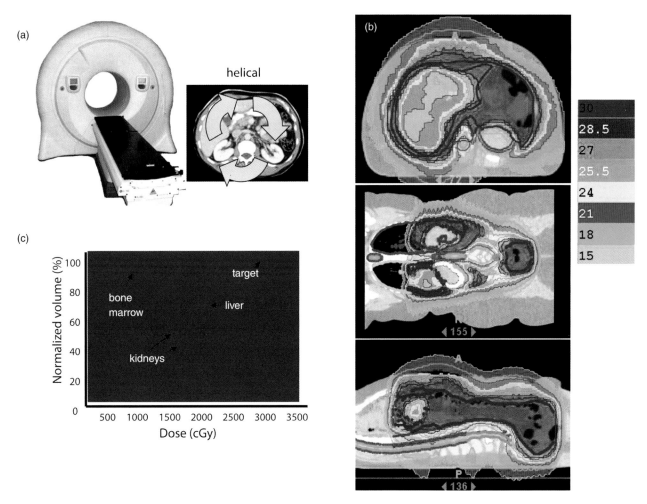

Figure 33.4 Helical tomotherapy for ovarian cancer. (a) Helical tomotherapy involves gradual passage through a circular bore with radiation delivered in helical arcs. (b) Avoidance structures (e.g., central liver parenchyma excluding 1 cm peripheral rim, central kidney excluding 1 cm peripheral rim) can be identified and prioritized for radiation dose exclusion. In this way, peritoneal surfaces are dosed by radiation, while underlying organ at-risk parenchyma are relatively spared from excessive radiation dose.

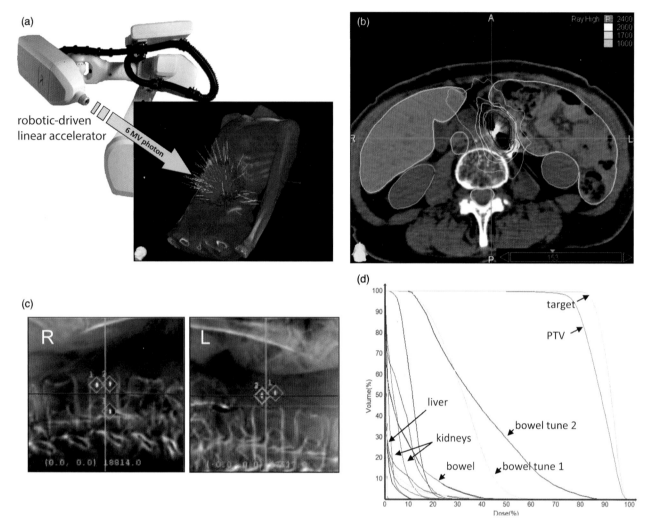

Figure 33.5 Stereotactic radiosurgery for ovarian cancer. (a) Depicted is a robotic stereotactic body radiosurgery system (Cyberknife®; Accuray, Sunnyvale, CA). The system allows for increased freedom in the number and in the angle of non-coplanar treatment beam trajectories (blue vectors) to focus high-dose radiation on localized area(s) of disease. (b) Robotic systems have submillimeter accuracy such that highly conformal radiation dose plans sparing normal tissues from excessive radiation dose per fraction can be achieved. Pictured is a radiosurgery plan for a para-aortic relapse of ovarian cancer with a gold fiducial placed within the target. (c) Orthogonal right (R) and left (L) fluoroscopic images taken by treatment room cameras allow on-board real-time tracking of implanted gold fiducials (green diamonds). (d) Dose–volume histograms indicate high percentage target coverage (red) while simultaneously distributing low radiation dose to critical organs (such as bowel, liver, and kidneys).

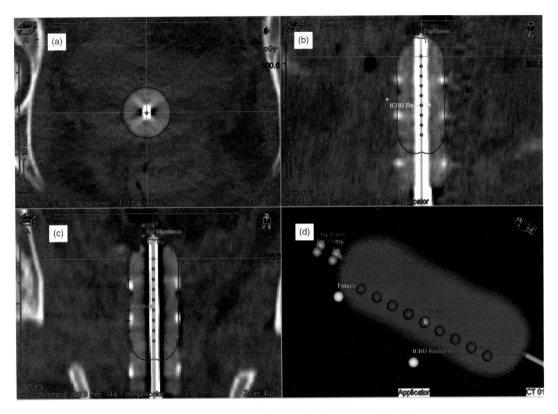

Figure 34.1 Endocavitary vaginal brachytherapy. (a–c) Three-field view of high-dose-rate 192-iridium endocavitary vaginal brachytherapy to deliver 3000 cGy in five divided fractions of 600 cGy radiation prescribed to the vaginal surface for a woman with vaginal intraepithelial neoplasia. (d) Optimization points along the vaginal surface (blue circles) and the vaginal apex (green circles) are depicted. The rectal International Commission on Radiation Units (ICRU) point is indicated (yellow circle). A fiducial (yellow circle) was placed in the right proximal vaginal apex pretherapy to ensure proper radiotherapy device placement during dosimetry planning.

Figure 34.2 Pelvic radiotherapy for vaginal cancer. (a,b) Anteroposterior and right lateral portal images for conventional four-field radiation are shown for treatment of the vagina and pelvic lymph nodes. (c,d) Anteroposterior and posteroanterior portal images are depicted for two-field radiation treatment of the vagina, pelvic lymph nodes, and inguinal lymph nodes. Care must be taken to ensure that inguinal nodes (occasionally lying 3 cm or deeper in groin tissue) are adequately covered by radiation dose. Supplemental electron or photon fields to boost radiation dose to the groins may be needed.

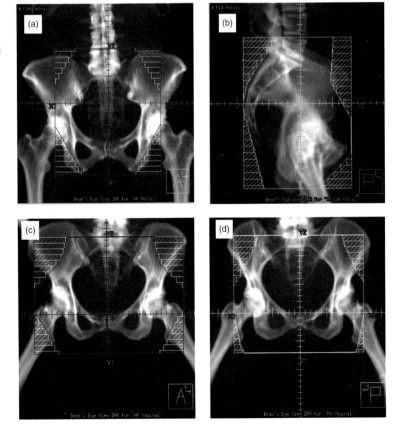

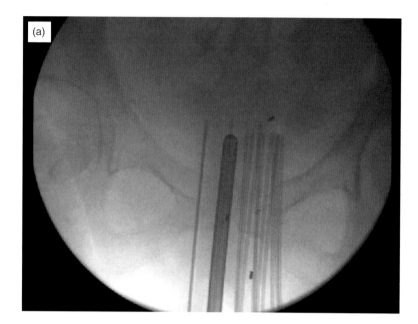
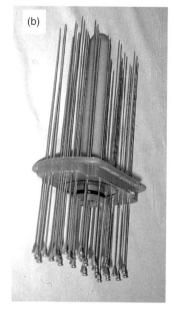
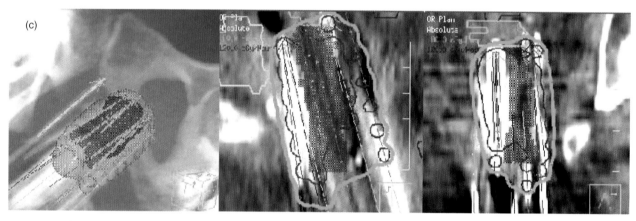

Figure 34.3 Vaginal interstitial brachytherapy. (a) Intraoperative anteroposterior radiograph of 192-iridium needle and 137-cesium tandem interstitial implant in a woman with stage II squamous cell carcinoma of the left lateral wall of the upper to mid-vagina having undergone pelvic radiation (4500 cGy). Four gold seed markers are implanted around the periphery of the disease to guide needle positioning. A central obturator with tandem for 137-cesium sources has been positioned in the vagina. Ten hollow interstitial needles for 192-iridium sources have been introduced percutaneously using a Syed–Neblett grid template (b, example of fully deployed template) according to preoperative CT/MRI planning. (c) Depicted is interstitial implant dosimetry of six 192-iridium sources 1 cm apart in 10 needles supplemented with five 137-cesium tandem sources to deliver 4000 cGy over 50 h (80 cGy h–1 isodose line, green outline).

Figure 35.2 Pelvic radiotherapy for cervical cancer. (a,b) Anteroposterior and right lateral portal images for conventional four-field radiation are shown for treatment of the uterine cervix and pelvic lymph nodes. (c,d) Anteroposterior and posteroanterior portal images are depicted for two-field parametrial boost sparing the central portion of the bladder and rectum. Dose to tumor not covered by these fields is made up with intracavitary brachytherapy.

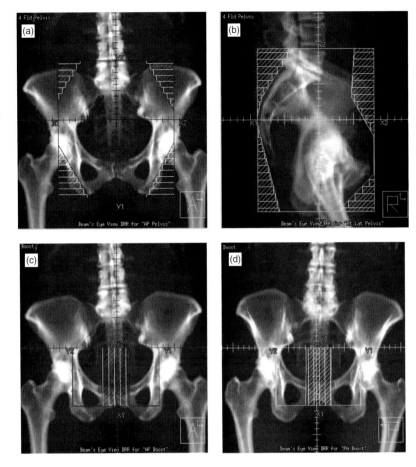

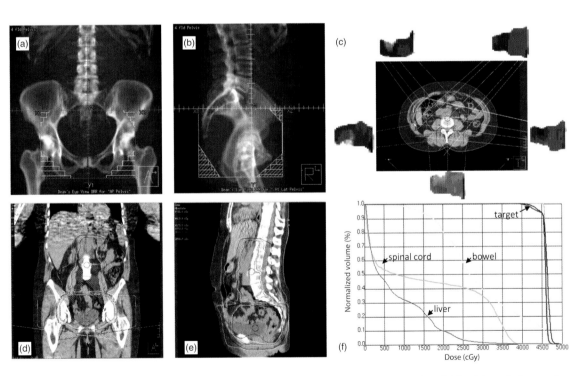

Figure 35.3 Extended field para-aortic intensity-modulated radiation therapy (IMRT) matched to four-field pelvic radiotherapy for cervical cancer. (a,b) Half-beam anteroposterior and right lateral portal images for four-field radiation are shown for treatment of the uterine cervix and pelvic lymph nodes. (c) A matched IMRT field is applied in five fields. Opening density matrices modeling the intensity of each control point are depicted for each beam. Coronal (d) and sagittal (e) dosimetry images for the composite pelvic plus IMRT para-aortic treatment fields. The heavy red contour identifies the 4500 cGy isodose line for which the daily prescription of 180 cGy was given for 25 divided fractions. (f) Dose–volume histogram plots for cancer targets and critical structures for this technique.

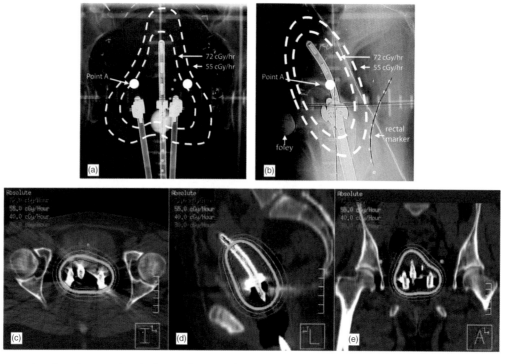

Figure 35.4 Intracavitary low-dose-rate brachytherapy for cervical cancer. (a,b) Anteroposterior and left lateral portal images are shown for a Henschke device low-dose-rate 137-cesium implant. Typical isodose contours are depicted with labeled dashed lines when five sources are loaded in the uterine tandem and one source is positioned in each ovoid colpostat. The point A prescription point is identified. (c–e) 3-D computed tomography dosimetry is shown for a low-dose-rate implant to deliver 4000 cGy, with a source not loaded in the first tandem position to spare bowel. Prescription point A (red circle) and point B (green circle) are shown for this implant dosing at a rate of 55 cGy h^{-1} (thick green line).

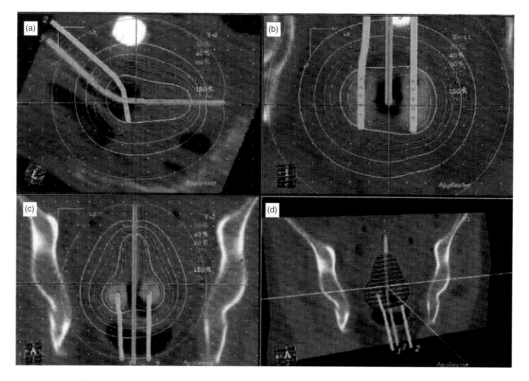

Figure 35.5 Intracavitary high-dose-rate brachytherapy for cervical cancer. (a–c) Cross-plane digital reconstructed radiographs obtained by computed tomography (CT)-based dosimetry planning are shown for a Henschke device high-dose-rate 192-iridium implant. Isodose contours are depicted after tailored dwell point dose calculations. (d) 3-D CT isodose contour (blue) for delivery of 600 cGy delivered for one of five fractions of brachytherapy.

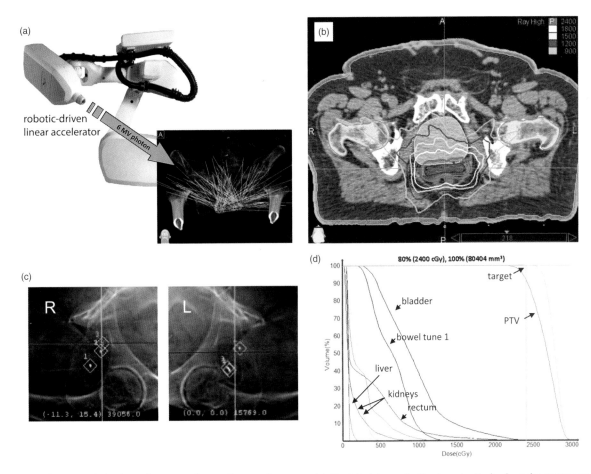

Figure 35.7 Stereotactic body radiosurgery for uterine cervix cancer. (a) Depicted is a robotic stereotactic body radiosurgery system (CyberKnife®; Accuray, Sunnyvale, CA). The robotic system increases freedom in the number and in the angle of non-coplanar treatment beam trajectories (blue vectors) to focus high-dose radiation on localized area(s) of disease. (b) Robotic systems have submillimeter accuracy such that highly conformal radiation dose plans sparing normal tissues from excessive radiation dose per fraction can be achieved. Pictured is a radiosurgery plan for a vaginal relapse of cervical cancer. (c) Orthogonal right (R) and left (L) fluoroscopic images taken by treatment room cameras allow on-board real-time tracking of implanted gold fiducials (green diamonds). (d) Dose–volume histograms indicate a high percentage of target coverage (light blue) while simultaneously distributing low radiation dose to critical organs (e.g., rectum, bladder, small bowel, liver, and kidneys).

Figure 36.2 Axial (upper panel) and sagittal (lower panel) circumferential homogeneous distribution of 100% isodose (yellow) at 3 mm in tissue with sparing of deep structures and avoidance of 125% isodose from skin in a refractory cutaneous T-cell lymphoma lesion.

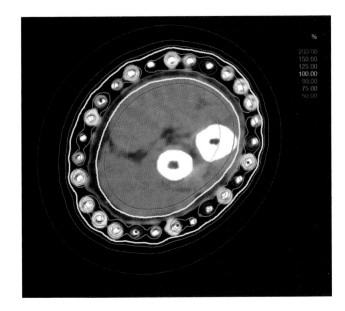

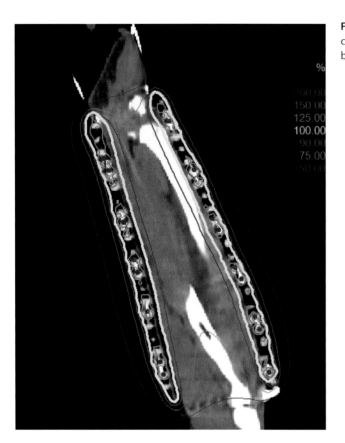

Figure 36.3 The Freiburg applicator with dummy wires in channels is tightly wrapped onto the clinical target with an elastic bandage.

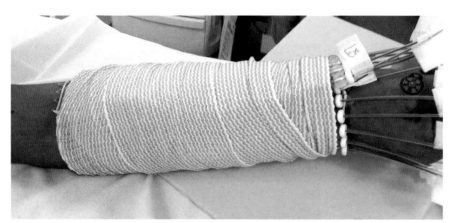

Figure 36.4 Freiburg applicator wrapped to the left forearm. The clinical target and margin are demarcated with radiopaque copper wire on the right forearm.

Figure 37.2 A mono-isocentric match with a half beam block approach, creating a perfect geometric match between the chest wall and the nodal field.

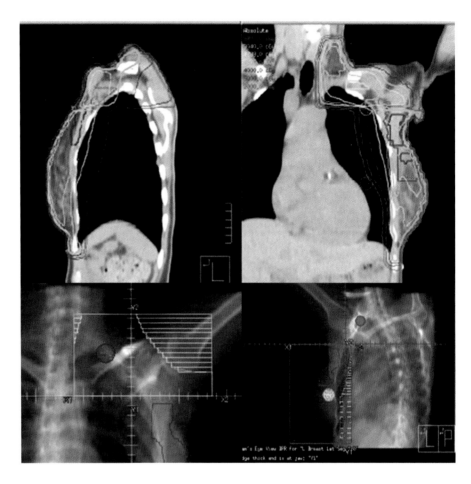

Figure 37.3 A nodal field encompassing the supraclavicular fossa and undissected axillary apex (defined on CT contour using clips).

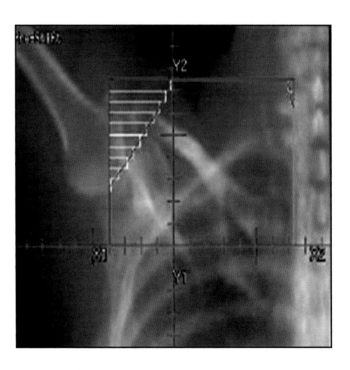

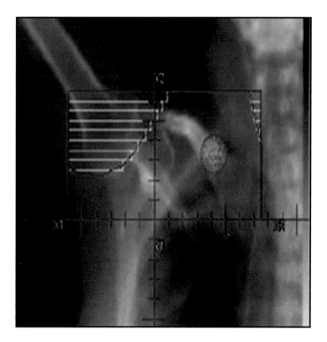

Figure 37.4 A nodal field encompassing the supraclavicular fossa and full axilla.

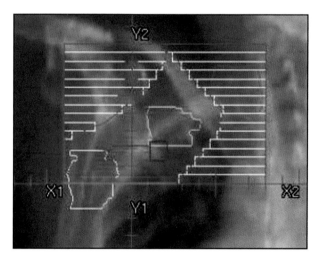

Figure 37.5 A posterior axillary boost (PAB) encompassing the lateral axilla for improved dosimetric coverage.

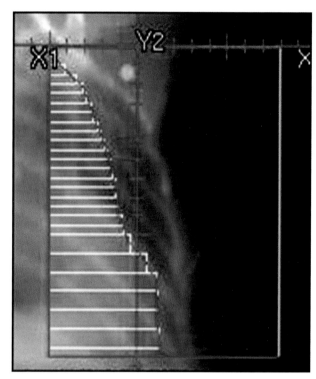

Figure 37.6 A partially-wide tangent (PWT) field encompassing the internal mammary nodes in the superior aspect of the field.

Figure 37.7 Post-mastectomy radiotherapy using a medial electron strip matched to a shallow photon tangent for chest wall coverage.

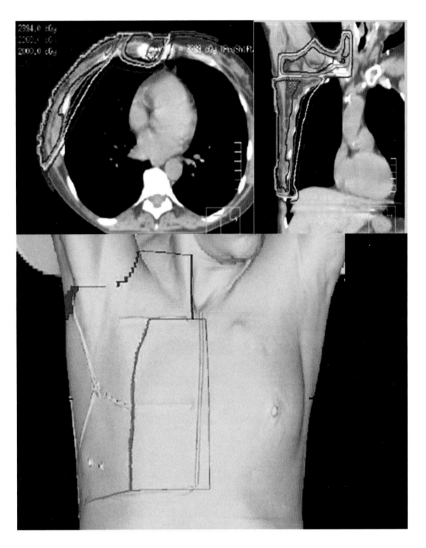

Figure 38.4 Clinical target volume (CTV; orange), planned target volume (PTV; cyan) expansions from gross tumor volume (GTV; yellow).

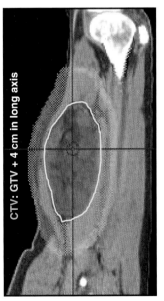

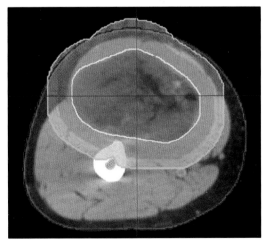

CTV: GTV + 1-1.5 cm in radial axis

CTV: GTV + 4 cm in long axis

PTV: CTV plus 1 cm margin in all directions

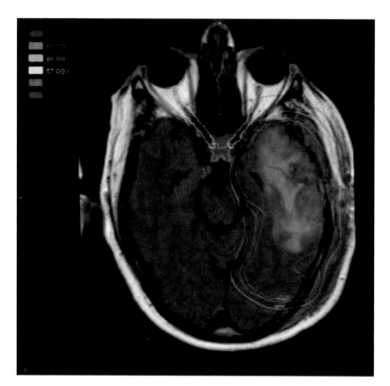

Figure 39.1 Case of a glioblastoma patient treated with IMRT using five fields prescribed to 60 Gy. The high-dose GTV is in red, CTV is in pink. The plan is overlayed on the fused FLAIR MRI image.

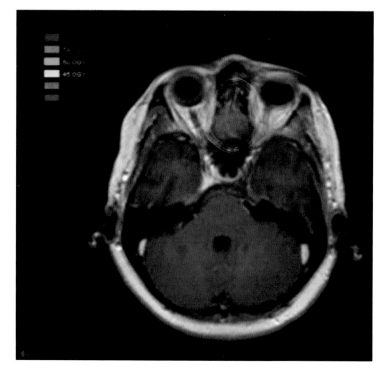

Figure 39.2 Case of a meningioma patient treated with fractionated proton therapy. The GTV is shown in red.

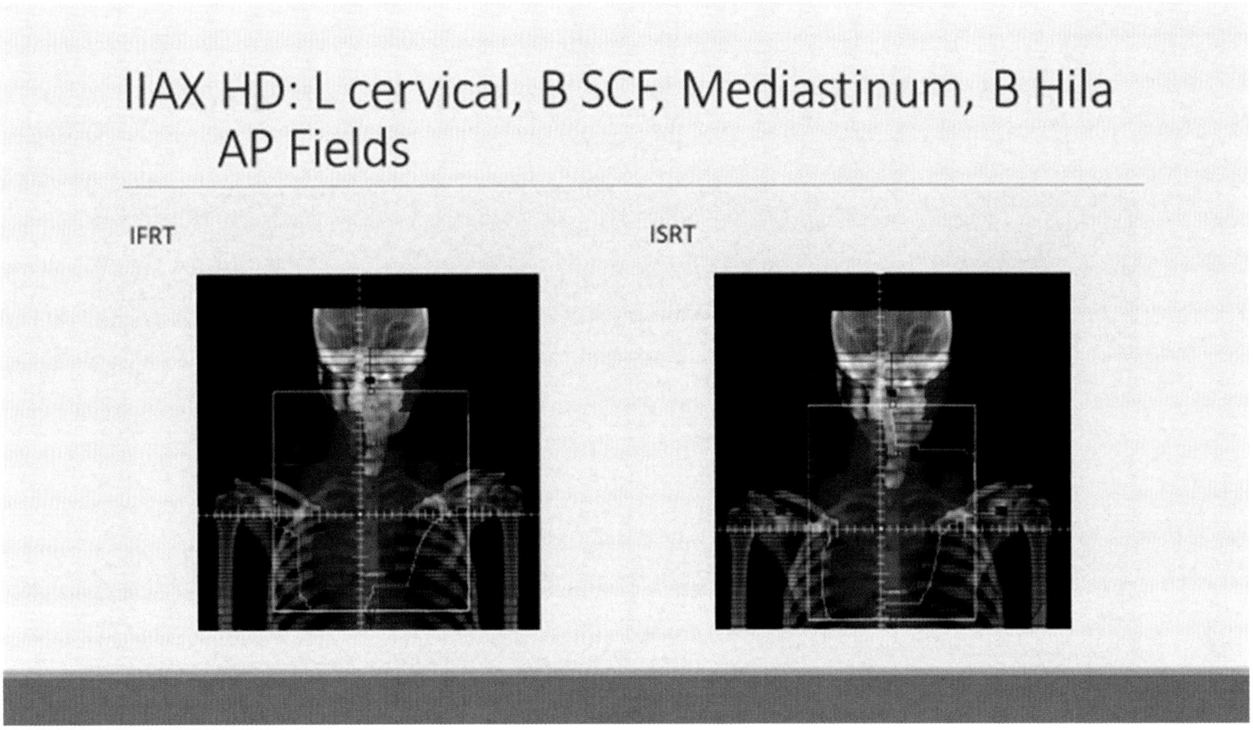

Figure 40.1 Stage IIAX nodular sclerosing Hodgkin's lymphoma. Left: IFRT (AP block). Right: ISRT (AP block).

Free breathing vs. Deep Inspiration Breath Hold
Lungs

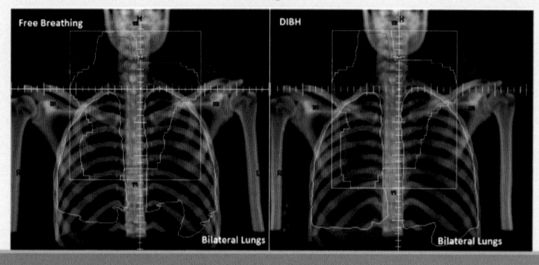

(a)

Free breathing vs. Deep Inspiration Breath Hold
Heart

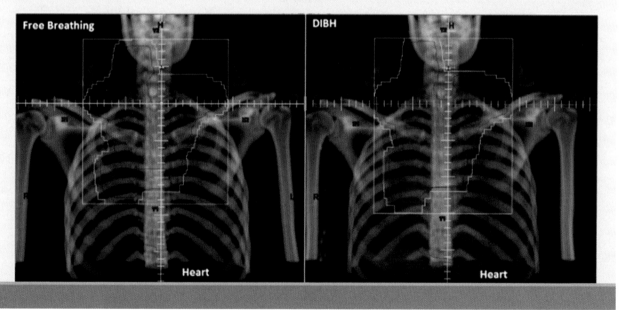

(b)

Figure 40.5 (a) Comparison of free-breathing versus deep-inspiration breath-hold. Pulmonary-sparing figure. (b) Comparison of free-breathing versus deep inspiration breath-hold. Cardiac sparing.

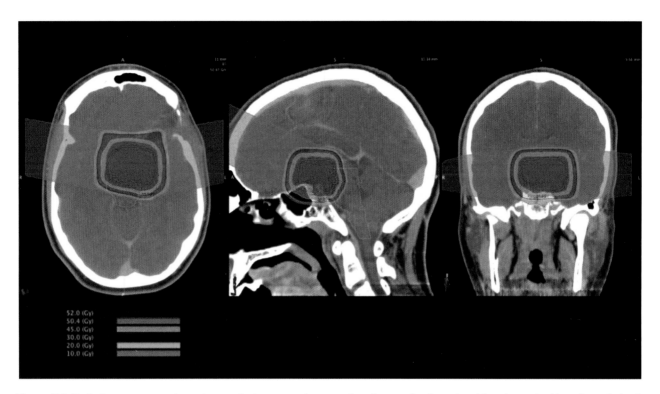

52.0 (Gy)
50.4 (Gy)
45.0 (Gy)
30.0 (Gy)
20.0 (Gy)
10.0 (Gy)

Figure 41.2 Radiation treatment plan using passively scattered protons for a low-grade glioma involving the optic chiasm/hypothalamic region.

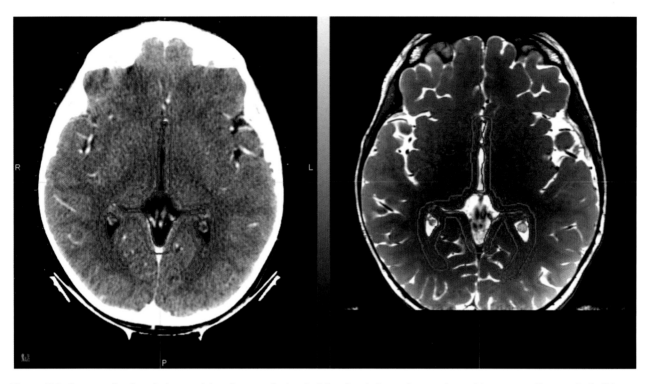

Figure 41.3 Contours for the whole-ventricle volume at the level of the pineal cistern for a patient with a germ-cell tumor. Left, CT scan. Right, T2 MRI.

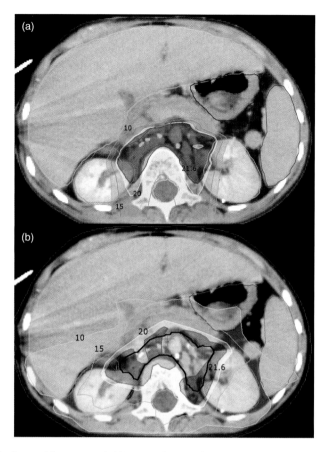

Figure 41.4 Treatment of paraspinal neuroblastoma with (a) scanned proton beam treatment and (b) IMRT (Individual isodose lines indicate dose in Gy).

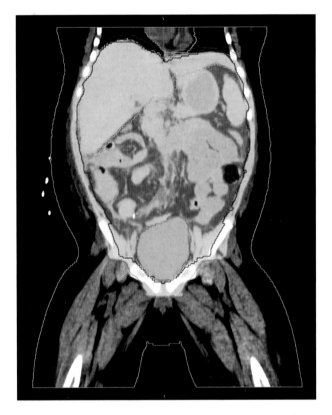

Figure 41.5 Whole-abdomen radiation therapy (WART) field for a patient with Wilms tumor. The field encompasses the entire peritoneal cavity with shielding of the femoral heads and heart.

total treatment time which avoids accelerated repopulation of resistant clonagens that often present during week 6 of treatment or beyond [82,83]. This concept of extreme hyperfractionation was further corroborated by the ECOG 2597 randomized trial of standard radiation versus HART after induction chemotherapy [84]. This was a Phase III prospective randomized trial where 119 patients received induction carboplatin and paclitaxel for two cycles, followed by either standard radiation to 64 Gy at 2 Gy per fraction (including elective nodal coverage) versus hyperfractionated accelerated radiotherapy (HART), with 1.5 Gy, 1.8 Gy, and 1.5 Gy given thrice daily for 12 treatment days (15 days overall) to a dose of 57.6 Gy (the middle fraction was treating gross disease only). Although the study closed early due to poor accrual, it did show a trend towards improved overall survival with HART (20.3 months versus 14.9 months). More grade 3 esophagitis, but less pneumonitis, was noted with the HART regimen. Although underpowered, the results were intriguing and set the stage for other types of accelerated radiation treatments for lung cancer.

Despite significant data suggesting a possible benefit to dose escalation (RTOG, University of Michigan, Memorial Sloan Kettering, UNC, Fudan University experience), recent data from RTOG 0617 has called into question the benefit of dose escalation with standard fractionation escalation [74,85–88]. In this study, 544 unresectable Stage IIIA and IIIB NSCLC patients were randomized to one of four arms: (i) high-dose (74 Gy) radiation with carboplatin, paclitaxel, and cetuximab; (ii) high-dose radiation with carboplatin and paclitaxel; (iii) standard dose radiation (60 Gy) with carboplatin, paclitaxel and cetuximab; and (iv) standard dose radiation with carboplatin and paclitaxel [89]. The target volume included the involved field only at 2 Gy per fraction utilizing 3D-CRT or IMRT. All patients received concurrent and adjuvant chemotherapy (carboplatin-paclitaxel). No survival advantage was achieved by using higher doses of radiation, or with the use of cetuximab. In fact, the median overall survival was lower in the 74 Gy arms (20.3 versus 28.7 months, p = 0.004). Comparison with the radiotherapy dose was closed early for the high-dose arms, and 60 Gy in standard fractionation was considered the standard of care. While there was no increase in grade 3 or higher toxic effects overall between the radiotherapy groups, the rates of severe esophagitis was increased (21% versus 7%, p < 0.0001). A higher number of treatment-related deaths, and more difficulty in completing concurrent chemotherapy, was noted in the high-dose arms. Post-hoc analyses are underway to better understand the negative outcomes in the high-dose arm. It is noted that the PTV coverage by the 95% and 100% isodose line was better in the 60-Gy groups (p < 0.001), which suggests that coverage of the target may have been compromised in the high-dose arm due to potential

biases of treating physicians unblended to the dose level. The authors performed a subgroup analysis by including only patients wherein 90% of PTV received at least 95% dose and the negative outcomes of the 74-Gy arm were persistent. However, it was also noted that a little less than one-fourth of the patients (470 of 2017) assigned to the high-dose arm received a radiation dose <74 Gy or no radiotherapy, as against 6.25% in the standard dose arm. Esophageal and heart doses were higher in the high-dose group. On multivariate analyses, all of these factors (maximum esophagitis grade, PTV, heart V5 and V30) were associated with predicting overall survival. A longer treatment duration and an unclear cause of death further confounded the true interpretation of these results. Hence, most experts in thoracic radiotherapy acknowledge that, despite the absence of clear level 1 evidence, there likely is a role for dose escalation, but the optimal schedule and patient population still needs to be defined. Alternate fractionation schedules with better attention to normal tissue dosimetry may potentially allow biological-dose escalation while limiting toxicity.

Mehta and colleagues at the University of Wisconsin described a new concept of dose escalation in NSCLC [90]. Given that NSCLC repopulation is rapid and the cell doubling time is less than four days, they proposed a dose per fraction escalation strategy which maintained the number of fractions at 25 treatments, but increased the dose per fraction to help maintain the same risk of pneumonitis, while increasing the local control (Figure 19.6). This model was later tested clinically in a Phase I dose

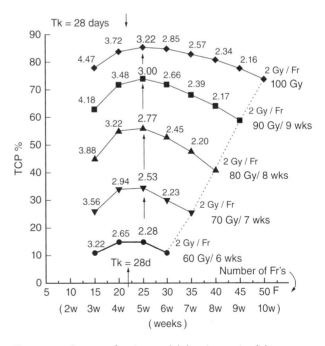

Figure 19.6 Dose per fraction model showing optimal dose escalation occurring at 25 fractions ranging from 2.28 Gy up to 3.22 Gy per fraction [65].

escalation model [91,92]. In this study, patients were placed in one of five dose bins to 25 fractions, with doses ranging from 2.28 Gy to 3.22 Gy per fraction. Normalized total dose (NTD) equivalents (assuming α/β ratio of 3 Gy) were between 60 and 110 Gy (with absolute non-corrected doses ranging from 57 to 85.5 Gy). The starting dose of each bin was determined by the relative normalized tissue mean dose modeled to cause <20% risk of grade 2 pneumonitis, and the NTD mean dose to esophagus <64 Gy. Initial toxicity results from 79 accrued patients showed no evidence of grade 3 acute pneumonitis or esophagitis. With 17 months median follow-up, six patients had late grade 4/5 toxicity that was felt to be related to therapy, primarily due to damage to central and perihilar structures, mainly at a dose ≥75 Gy. A maximum tolerated dose (MTD) was identified at 63.25 Gy (safety of 69.25 Gy could not be determined as only three patients were accrued at that dose level). Median and three-year overall survival was 16 months and 29%, respectively. More impressive was the fact that 44% of patients were stage IIIB and 27% stage IIIA. Of note, chemotherapy was not given during radiation (but could be done before or after).

As an alternate approach to reduce normal tissue irradiation while allowing dose-escalation, proton beam radiotherapy is currently under evaluation. This is especially relevant in reducing dose to the heart which, from the analysis of RTOG 0617 data, was a significant predictor of survival. In a retrospective review conducted at the M.D. Anderson Cancer Center, it was noted that use of proton beam therapy allow the safe delivery of a higher radiation dose, yet the incidence of severe radiation pneumonitis and esophagitis was lower [93]. These results were reproduced in a subsequent Phase II single-arm study from the same institution [94]. The dosimetric superiority of proton beam dose-distribution needs to be weighed against increased uncertainty with dose-deposition due to the lung–tissue interface further complicated by tumor motion. The ongoing RTOG 1308 study is comparing photon versus proton beam radiotherapy, with treatment planned to a total dose of 70 Gy (or 70 CGE).

For patients in the postoperative setting, adjuvant therapy is guided by pathological features. In the Lung Adjuvant Cisplatin Evaluation (LACE) meta-analysis, the use of adjuvant cisplatin-based chemotherapy resulted in a 5.4% absolute increase in five-year survival, with a 11% reduction in risk of death [95]. When analyzing by stage, benefit was mainly seen in stage II patients (HR 0.83; 95% CI, 0.73 to 0.95) and stage III patients (HR: 0.83; 95% CI, 0.72 to 0.94). The HR for stage IA patients was 1.40; 95% CI, 0.95 to 2.06, while for stage IB patients it was 0.93; 95% CI, 0.78 to 1.10 (both not statistically significant), raising concern for potential detriment in early-stage patients. Adjuvant chemotherapy is typically recommended for all

patients with node-positive disease, and is considered for high-risk patients (poorly differentiated tumors, lymphovascular invasion, sublobar surgery, tumor size >4 cm and visceral pleural involvement). The role of postoperative radiotherapy (PORT) continues to be an area of controversy, especially regarding benefit in non-N2 nodal group patients. The PORT meta-analysis, which primarily included trials conducted during the pre-conformal radiotherapy era, showed an overall detriment in survival with PORT [96] (7% at two years). On subgroup analysis, only patients with N2 disease did not have a negative effect. An analysis of Surveillance, Epidemiology, and End Results (SEER) Program database [97] showed a 7% improvement in five-year survival for pathological N2 group (20% versus 27%, p = 0.0036), with a detriment of 4% and 10% in five-year survival for pN1 and pN0 patients, respectively. Analysis of the Adjuvant Navelbine International Trialist Association (ANITA) data showed the benefit of PORT in patients with pN2 disease, irrespective of the use of chemotherapy or for patients with pN1 disease not receiving chemotherapy [98]. A recent report evaluating the use of modern technology demonstrated an improvement in survival with use of PORT only when patients were treated on linear accelerators [99]. The ongoing Lung Adjuvant radiotherapy (ART) study is a Phase III trial that will hopefully help to answer the question regarding the benefit of PORT in pN2 disease group patients with the use of modern radiation planning techniques (NCT00410683).

When delivering PORT (especially with N2 disease), elective nodal radiation is often employed. Since elective nodal irradiation is being eliminated from the definitive radiotherapy approaches for unresected patients, this underscores a dichotomy. For patients receiving definitive radiotherapy in the unresectable setting, local as well as distant failure is common. Efforts are made to intensify local radiation to gross disease as this is more difficult to control. Therefore, dose escalation to the gross disease is employed knowing that the likelihood of elective nodal recurrence is less than 10%. In the postoperative setting, however, all gross disease has been removed and the goals of therapy are to eradicate any microscopic foci that may be present within the mediastinum. The dose is typically significantly lower (50–54 Gy) compared to patients receiving definitive radiotherapy or chemotherapy alone (60–74 Gy).

Pancoast tumors represent a unique presentation of NSCLC that often is approached slightly differently from other types of NSCLC. This entity was characterized clinically by Pancoast in 1924, but was first described by Hare in 1838. Pancoast originally believed that these tumors arose embryologically from the 5th branchial cleft. These tumors are commonly referred to as 'superior sulcus tumors,' as this is the groove formed by the subclavian artery as it passes over the apex of the lung. A Pancoast tumor refers to any tumor located in the lung apex manifesting any of the associated clinical symptoms, including pain (generally along the innervation of the brachial plexus), Horner's syndrome, or weakness and atrophy of the intrinsic muscles of the ipsilateral hand. These tumors represent only about 3% of all primary lung cancers, and the majority of them (90% or higher) are non-small-cell lung in origin. Small-cell lung cancer makes up less than 5% of Pancoast tumors.

Single-modality therapy for Pancoast tumors has yielded poor results. The standard of care typically involves concurrent chemoradiotherapy followed by surgical resection based on the protocol SWOG 9416. In this intergroup study, 110 patients with T3-4 N0-1 NSCLC (Pancoast presentation) were treated with induction chemoradiotherapy using cisplatin and etoposide concurrently with 45 Gy in 25 fractions, with radiation directed to the tumor and ipsilateral supraclavicular fossa. Thoracotomy was performed within five weeks after induction therapy. Postoperatively, two additional cycles of cisplatin and etoposide were administered. This regimen was well tolerated, with over 95% of the patients completing induction therapy. At restaging, nine of the 110 patients had progressed. Eighty-eight patients proceeded to thoracotomy, with 93% of the resected patients achieving R0 resections. Some 36% of patients undergoing surgery were noted to have a complete pathologic response, and an additional 30% had minimal residual microscopic disease. The median survival of patients with an R0 resection was 94 months, with five-year overall survival 44% for all patients, and 54% for those with an R0 resection [100]. In a single-institution experience with higher radiation dose (mean 56.9 Gy)-based chemoradiotherapy, the pathologic complete response (pCR) rates were noted to be 40.5% with a 7.8 years median overall survival for these patients, suggesting a dose–response effect [101].

In situations where the disease is not considered surgically resectable, concurrent chemoradiotherapy is recommended. The prescribed radiation dose is, however, often limited by dose to critical normal structures such as spinal cord and brachial plexus (Figure 19.7). Very tight planning margins with the help of advanced image-guidance are highly important in such scenarios.

A relatively less common scenario for patients with locally advanced lung cancer is inability to receiving concurrent or sequential chemotherapy due to associated medical comorbidities. The Cancer and Leukemia Group B (CALGB) 8433 study, which evaluated the role of sequential chemoradiotheapy versus radiotherapy alone, had shown a median and five-year survival in the radiotherapy-alone cohort of 9.6 months and 6%, respectively [102]. This and other such trials in this era led to a general understanding that radiation alone is a non-curative treatment for locally advanced

lung cancer. However, these trials did not use modern staging and radiation treatment techniques. A more recent Phase III randomized Japanese Clinical Oncology Group (JCOG) 0301 study evaluating the role of low-dose carboplatin concurrent in elderly patients with locally advanced NSCLC, demonstrated a median survival of 16.9 months with a two-year survival of 35.1% in the radiotherapy-alone arm [103]. Such a treatment plan should be guided by patient's performance status and the extent of disease with the use of modern radiotherapy planning approaches to respect normal tissue dosimetry. The use of mild hypofractionation (2.5–3 Gy per fraction) could also be considered to limit treatment duration, while obtaining improved radiation response.

Limited Stage-Small-Cell Lung Cancer (LS-SCLC)

Role of Surgery

Combination chemotherapy with thoracic radiotherapy forms the backbone of therapy with a very limited role for surgical resection. During the early 1960s, the Medical Research Council of Great Britain conducted a Phase III trial that demonstrated the superiority of radiation therapy over surgery in patients with operable and resectable SCLC (long-term survival of 4% versus 0%) [104,105]. The role of surgery was evaluated further in an intergroup study of 328 patients with LS-SCLC who received combination chemotherapy (five cycles of cyclophosphamide, doxorubicin and vincristine), followed by randomization to surgery or no-surgery in responders [106]. Thoracic radiotherapy was delivered to both arms of the study. In the surgery arm, 83% patients were resectable, but the final survival curves were not different between the two arms.

Schreiber *et al.* analyzed LS-SCLC patients enrolled in the SEER registry from 1988 to 2002 [107]. Some 6% of patients (863 of 14 179) underwent surgical resection and demonstrated better survival both in localized (median 42 versus 15 months, p < 0.001) and regional disease (median 22 versus 12 months, p < 0.001) respectively. The best results were seen in patients undergoing lobectomy (median survival 65 months, five-year overall survival 53%). In the SEER registry dataset, the role of postoperative radiotherapy was evaluated in 241 patients. Similar to results in general with NSCLC, a trend towards inferior survival was noted in the entire cohort with the addition of radiotherapy (median survival 26 versus 31 months, p = 0.06). On subgroup analysis, positive outcomes with radiotherapy were restricted to patients with N2 disease (22 versus 16 months, p = 0.011), with non-significant differences in N0

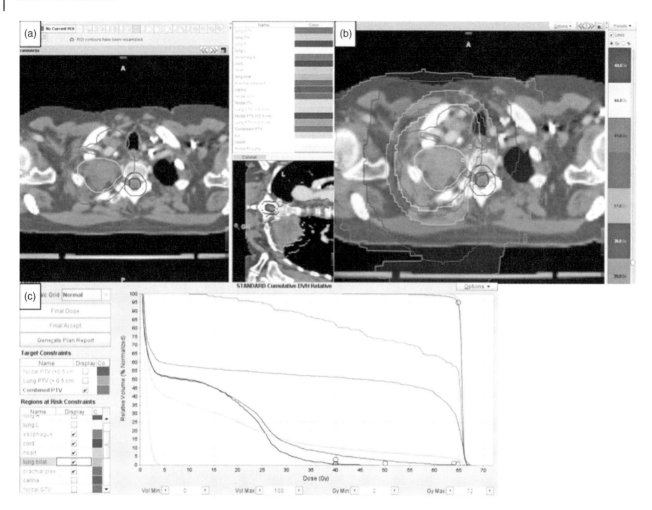

Figure 19.7 A case example with NSCLC presenting as superior sulcus tumor treated with IMRT technique to a dose of 64.8 Gy in 36 fractions, five fractions per week. Prescribed dose was limited by close proximity of target volume to spinal cord (purple). (a) CT scan images in three planes showing target volumes and organ at risks. (b) Isodose distribution demonstrating highly conformal distribution of higher isodoses with relative spreading of lower isodoses. (c) Dose–volume histogram demonstrating a rapid fall-off of isodoses covering the target volume shown by curves on the right with attempted sparing of normal tissues. Relatively high doses were delivered to the brachial plexus (green) and esophagus (pink) due to close proximity to target volumes. Illustration courtesy Dr George Cannon, University of Wisconsin. For a color version of this figure, see the color plate section.

(41 versus 40 months, p = 0.44) and N1 (22 versus 35 months, p = 0.179) patients. In a smaller SEER study focusing on patients with stage I SCLC, three- and five-year survival rates of 58.1% and 50.3% were observed with lobectomy alone (n = 205), compared to 64.9% and 57.1% respectively, with postoperative radiotherapy, although the differences were not statistically significant [108]. In a similar Japanese registry study, five-year survival rates for patients with clinical/pathological stage IA and IB were 58.8% (n = 161)/58.3% (n = 127) and 58.0% (n = 77)/60.2% (n = 79), respectively [109].

Role of Chemoradiotherapy

The advent of multidrug therapy during the late 1970s significantly improved median survival for patients with

LS-SCLC, from five to six months with thoracic radiotherapy alone to 10 to 14 months with chemoradiotherapy or chemotherapy alone [110,111]. Initial chemotherapy regimens included cyclophosphamide, etoposide, vincristine and doxorubicin, which were later replaced by platinum-based doublet regimens. The Cancer and Leukemia Group B (CALGB) randomized 426 patients to initial radiotherapy plus chemotherapy (18 months), delayed radiotherapy plus chemotherapy, or chemotherapy alone. Radiotherapy was delivered to a total dose of 50 Gy (40 Gy + 10 Gy boost to residual disease) and included the primary tumor, ipsilateral hilum, mediastinum and bilateral supraclavicular fields [112]. Prophylactic cranial irradiation (PCI) was used for all patients. Improved complete response (CR) rates, locoregional failure rate (20% versus 80%), failure-free survival (FFS) (20% versus 8%) and overall survival was seen in the two radiation arms. No significant differences were noted in the early versus delayed radiotherapy arms. The National Cancer Institute (NCI) performed a smaller trial with 96 LS-SCLC patients who were randomized to concurrent chemotherapy (48 weeks) with radiotherapy (40 Gy in 15 fractions with first cycle chemotherapy) or chemotherapy alone [113]. Again, improved CR rates (81%), intrathoracic control rates and overall survival (15 versus 11.6 months, p = 0.035) were noted with combination therapy at the cost of increased acute toxicity.

The Southwest Oncology Group (SWOG) evaluated the role of consolidation radiotherapy in patients achieving a CR to induction chemotherapy [114]. Radiotherapy was delivered as a split course (18 Gy in 10 fractions including supraclavicular fields, followed by 30 Gy in 12 fractions to reduced volumes), and was given to all patients who had a partial response (PR) or stable disease (SD) to induction chemotherapy, with randomization between treatment volumes (pre-induction versus post-induction). Reduced local recurrence rates (56% versus 90%) were seen with the addition of radiotherapy in patients with CR to induction chemotherapy, although this did not translate into survival improvement. Similarly, in patients with PR/SD to induction chemotherapy, no significant survival differences were noted between the pre- versus post-induction volumes.

Two meta-analyses have assessed the significance of consolidation radiotherapy in patients with LS-SCLC. Warde et al. reported the details of 11 randomized trials evaluating radiotherapy in combination with chemotherapy in patients with LS-SCLC [115]. The odds ratio (OR) benefit for two-year overall survival was 1.53 (95% CI 1.3-1.8, p < 0.001), with an absolute two-year survival benefit of 5.4%. From nine eligible studies, the OR for benefit in local control was estimated at 3.02 (p < 0.0001), with improvement in intrathoracic control by 25%. Interestingly, the addition of thoracic radiation also increased the OR for excess treatment-related deaths to 2.54 (p < 0.01). Pignon et al. conducted an individual patient data meta-analysis of 13 trials with 2140 patients [116]. Radiation therapy reduced the relative risk of death by 14% with an absolute $5.4 \pm 1.4\%$ overall survival benefit at three years. The same group also performed an indirect analysis on the impact of timing of radiotherapy, and found no significant differences between early versus late radiotherapy. The survival benefit was greatest for younger patients (age <55 years). Most of the chemotherapy regimens used in this era were cyclophosphamide- or doxorubicin-based.

Radiation Dose and Fractionation

Uncontrolled locoregional disease is still an important obstacle in SCLC. The radiation fractionation schemas have evolved from split-course, once-daily, low-dose regimens to accelerated hyperfractionation in an attempt to counteract tumor clonogen repopulation. The standard of care was set by a Phase III randomized intergroup study (INT 0096) reported by Turrisi et al. [12]. Concurrent cisplatin–etoposide doublet was delivered to 417 patients randomized to 45 Gy of thoracic radiotherapy administered either twice daily over a three-week period (1.5-Gy fractions) or once daily over a five-week period (1.8-Gy fractions). Radiotherapy was delivered along with first cycle of chemotherapy with no planned split. At a median follow-up of eight years, significant improvement in two-year (41% versus 47%) and five-year survival (16% versus 26%) (p = 0.04) were noted. This was at the cost of a significant increase in radiation esophagitis (11% versus 27%, p < 0.001). A case example of SCLC treated as per this regimen using an IMRT planning technique is shown in Figure 19.8. A critique of this trial is the use of what would now be considered a suboptimal dose in the once-daily fractionation arm. Attempts to deliver twice-daily radiation treatments with split course and delivered later in the course of chemotherapy, still resulted in significant toxicity while losing out on any positive impact on survival [117]. This highlights the importance of delivering radiotherapy as early as possible, to counteract tumor repopulation. The Radiation Therapy Oncology Group (RTOG) conducted a prospective Phase I, dose-escalation study (RTOG 97-12) with 64 patients receiving thoracic radiotherapy starting on day 1 of concurrent cisplatin-etoposide chemotherapy [118]. Radiotherapy was delivered with 1.8 Gy per fraction for the first four weeks, followed by a boost to the gross tumor volume with twice-daily fractions for the last 3, 5, 7, 9 or 11 days, reaching total doses of 50.4, 54.0, 57.6, 61.2, or 64.8 Gy, respectively. Radiotherapy was completed in five weeks for all arms. The maximally tolerated dose was determined to be 61.2 Gy, resulting in 82% 18-month survival compared to 25% survival at 50.4 Gy. This regimen was tested in the RTOG 0239 Phase II study, demonstrating median and two-year overall survivals of 19 months and 36.6% respectively, with 18% incidence of severe acute esophagitis, published results from which are awaited [119]. The CALGB performed a Phase II study, CALGB 39808, wherein thoracic radiotherapy (70 Gy in 35 fractions over seven weeks) was started concurrently with carboplatin–etoposide-based chemotherapy after two cycles of induction chemotherapy with paclitaxel and topotecan [120]. Radiation was delivered to the post-induction tumor volume and the pre-chemotherapy-involved nodal regions were included. Some 90% of patients proceeded to radiotherapy as per protocol, with a median overall survival of 22.4 months, but with one treatment-related fatality (fatal exsanguination at 64 Gy). Results from this trial compared favorably with those from the Intergroup study of Turrisi et al. Based on the results from these trials, and in the modern setting of improvements in

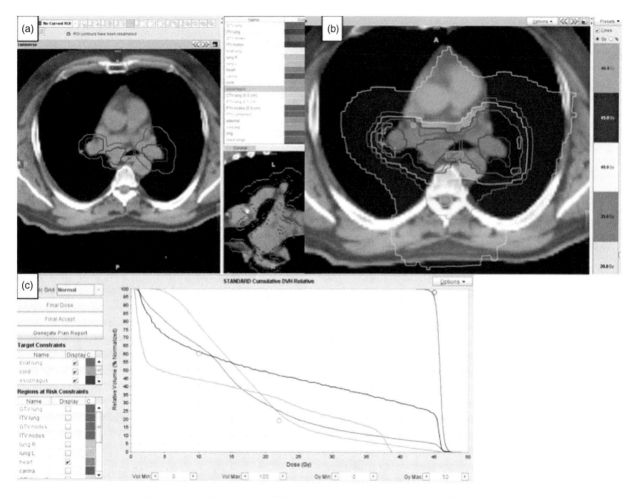

Figure 19.8 A case example with locoregionally advanced SCLC treated with IMRT technique to a dose of 45 Gy in 30 fractions at 1.5 Gy BID, 10 fractions per week as per the Turrisi regimen. (a) CT scan images in three planes showing target volumes and organs at risk. (b) Isodose distribution demonstrating highly conformal distribution of higher isodoses with relative spreading of lower isodoses. (c) Dose–volume histogram demonstrating a rapid fall-off of isodoses covering the target volume shown by curves on the right with significant sparing of normal tissues as represented by curves on the left. Illustration courtesy Dr George Cannon, University of Wisconsin. For a color version of this figure, see the color plate section.

radiation planning techniques which provide the ability to deliver more conformal radiotherapy, there is renewed interest in defining the optimal and safe dose and fractionation schedule for LS-SCLC. Two large clinical trials (CONVERT trial: NCT00433563 and CALGB 30610: NCT00632853) are further addressing the dose escalation question. The CALGB 30610 trial evaluated 70 Gy in 35 fractions versus 61.2 Gy concomitant boost approach in the first part of the study, and selected the 70 Gy arm for the final comparison with the standard of care 45 Gy twice-daily arm, which is ongoing. Initial results from the CONVERT trial wherein the experimental arm radiation dose was 66 Gy in 33 once daily fractions, were presented at the 2016 ASCO annual meeting. Among 547 patients with a median follow up of 45 months for those alive, there was no statistical significance in 2-yr (56% vs 51%) and median survival (30 m vs 25 m) between twice-daily vs. once-daily arms (p = 0.15) [121].

Timing of Radiotherapy and Chemotherapy

The timing decision regarding radiotherapy in conjunction with chemotherapy for LS-SCLC has been a topic of intense clinical evaluation and debate. Multiple Phase III randomized studies were performed which led to subsequent meta-analyses (Table 19.8). Three out of five meta-analyses, each with slightly different patient populations, have supported the early addition of radiotherapy (prior to starting the third cycle of chemotherapy).

Radiation Field Design

Radiation fields for LS-SCLC have been refined from 2D-based anatomical borders used in the Intergroup study to 3D-target volume-based designs used in the present

Table 19.8 Meta-analyses assessing timing of radiotherapy in relation to chemotherapy for definitive management of LS-SCLC.

Meta-analysis	No./Type of trials included	Trials included	No. of patients	Outcome	Subgroups
Huncharek et al., 2004	8/RCT	Jeremic et al.; Murray et al.; Perry et al.; Skarlos et al.; Takada et al.; Work et al.; Goto et al.; Lebeau et al.	1575 LS-SCLC, Early RT with 1st or 2nd cycle chemotherapy	ORp for 2-yr survival 1.60 (95% CI 1.3–2.0) – SS ORp for 3-yr survival 1.49 (95% CI 1.2–1.9) – SS Outcome: Survival favors early RT	ORp for 2-yr survival 1.81 for three trials using cisplatin–etoposide – SS Outcome: Survival favors early RT
Fried et al., 2004	7/RCT	Jeremic et al.; Murray et al.; Perry et al.; Skarlos et al.; Takada et al.; Work et al.; Gregor et al.	1524 LS-SCLC, Early RT within 9 weeks of 1st cycle of chemotherapy and before 3rd cycle.	RRs for 2-yr survival 1.17 (95% CI 1.02–1.35) – SS Outcome: Survival favors early RT	RRs for 2-yr survival 1.44 for trials using hyperfractionation RT and 1.30 for platinum-based chemotherapy – SS Outcome: Survival favors early RT
Spiro et al., 2006	8/RCT	Jeremic et al.; Murray et al.; Perry et al.; Skarlos et al.; Takada et al.; Work et al.; Gregor et al.; Spiro et al.	1849 LS-SCLC	RR for 2-yr survival 1.11 (95% CI 0.92–1.34) – NS	RR for 2-yr survival 1.35 for trials where early and later arms had similar percentage of patients receiving all chemotherapy – SS Outcome: Survival favors early RT
De Ruysscher et al., 2006	7/RCT	Jeremic et al.; Murray et al.; Perry et al.; Skarlos et al.; Takada et al.; Work et al.; James et al.	1514 LS-SCLC, Early RT within 30 days of start of chemotherapy	OR for 2–3 yr survival 0.84 (95% CI 0.56–1.28) – NS OS for 5-yr survival 0.80 (95% CI 0.47–1.38) – NS Outcome: Death	OR for 5-yr survival 0.64 for trials using platinum-based chemotherapy – SS OR for 5-yr survival 0.56 for trials with overall treatment time of RT <30 days – SS Outcome: Death favors early RT
De Ruysscher et al., 2006	4/RCT	Jeremic et al; Murray et al.; Takada et al.; Turrisi et al.	1056 LS-SCLC, Impact of start of any therapy until end of radiotherapy (SER)	RR for 5-yr survival 0.62; (95% CI 0.49–0.80) – SS	Each week of extension of the SER beyond the shortest SER resulted in an overall absolute decrease in the 5-year survival rate of 1.83%

ORp, Summary odds ratio; RCT, randomized control trial; RT, radiotherapy; SS; statistically significant.

generation clinical trials. In the Intergroup study, gross tumor, bilateral mediastinal and ipsilateral hilar lymph nodes were expanded by 1–1.5 cm to generate the block edge. Irradiation of the uninvolved supraclavicular fossa was not allowed. The inferior border was extended 5 cm below the carina or to include the ipsilateral hilar structures, whichever was lower. Oblique off-cord portals were used after 36 Gy to the spinal cord.

In a prospective study from the Netherlands, De Ruysscher et al. omitted elective nodal irradiation (ENI) in 27 patients with LS-SCLC that were staged with CT and treated as per the Turrisi et al. radiation regimen with concurrent carboplatin–etoposide [122]. Isolated nodal recurrence without distant disease was noted in 11% of patients, all in the supraclavicular fossa, which was not included even in the Intergroup 0096 trial. The same group then reported results of a prospective study in 60 patients with LS-SCLC for whom only the pretreatment PET identified primary tumor and mediastinal lymph nodes were irradiated [123]. Only two patients (3%) developed isolated nodal failure in the absence of distant disease with this approach, justifying the omission of ENI by incorporating PET scans into the radiation planning process. However, it is worth noting that an additional five patients (9%) had nodal failure in the presence of distant disease, and the cumulative 12% failure was similar to the 11% failure in the Netherlands study. The International Atomic Energy Agency (IAEA) consultant's meeting on ENI for SCLC could draw no firm conclusions from the available data, and clinical judgment was recommended [124]. Based on the above Phase II study, it was felt that PET staging might be employed to help with the decision, though again a firm recommendation was not feasible. In the RTOG 0239 protocol, 3D-conformal radiotherapy (3D-CRT) techniques were required. The clinical target volume (CTV) was defined as the gross target volume (GTV) plus a 1-cm margin. While ipsilateral supraclavicular irradiation was allowed when necessary for primary tumor coverage, contralateral hilar or supraclavicular treatment was not allowed. The inferior border was recommended to be 3 cm below the carina for upper and middle lobe tumors for the initial large fields, and 1 cm beyond the GTV for the boost fields. In the setting of gross subcarinal lymph node involvement, the CTV was defined as 1 cm beyond the nodal involvement for both the large and the boost fields. A 1.5-cm CTV expansion was recommended for any mediastinal lymph node. A planning target volume (PTV) of 0.5–1.5 cm was recommended based on tumor location and to account for daily set-up variations. No heterogeneity correction was allowed. As part of normal tissue constraints, 15 Gy to the contralateral whole lung, 36, 40, 45, and 50 Gy to the 100%, 50%, 10 cm and 5 cm of spinal cord, respectively, 45 Gy to whole esophagus with 10 cm of the esophagus receiving up to 60 Gy and 5 cm up to 65 Gy within the boost field was allowed. It was strongly recommended that the spinal cord should not be irradiated during the BID fractions.

In the post-induction setting, typical volumes are defined as the post-induction primary tumor volume and pre-induction involved nodal region. In the SWOG study (described previously), in patients with PR/SD to induction chemotherapy no significant survival differences were noted between radiotherapy to pre- versus post-induction volumes [114]. The CALGB 39808 trial defined the GTV as the post-induction residual tumor at both the primary and involved lymph node regions [120]. Ipsilateral hilar, mediastinal lymph node stations 3, 4, and 7 (e.g., precarinal, lower paratracheal, and subcarinal) and mediastinal lymph node stations 5 and 6 (e.g., aorta-pulmonary window and para-aortic) for left-sided tumors were included in the CTV. Boost fields were used after a tumor dose of 44 Gy, wherein the CTV included only the GTV and ipsilateral hilar lymph nodes. A 1-cm planning target volume was used. Treatment was prescribed to the isocenter and tissue heterogeneity corrections were not used. A spinal cord dose maximum dose of ≤50 Gy, a total lung V_{25} of ≤50% and heart $D_{100\%}$ ≤25 Gy was recommended. A recently reported interim analysis of a Phase III trial from China showed that

radiotherapy to the post-chemotherapy primary tumor volume (compared to the pre-chemotherapy volume) with no ENI did not significantly impact locoregional recurrence rates (31.6% versus 28.6%, p = 0.81) in patients with LS-SCLC [125]. Pre-chemotherapy nodal regions were treated in both arms. Less than 3% isolated out-of-field recurrences in the absence of distant metastases were noted in both arms, while the incidence of out-of-field recurrences in the presence of distant metastases was observed in 5.3% and 2.4% of cases. All out-of-field recurrences were in the non-irradiated ipsilateral supraclavicular fossa. Mediastinal N3 disease was the only factor predicting isolated nodal failure. FDG-PET/CT was employed in defining treatment volumes.

During recent years there has been increasing use of PET/CT-based volume definition in lung cancer. It helps in differentiating primary tumor from atelectasis, and also in detecting subclinical nodal/regional disease. Kamel *et al.* performed a retrospective review of the impact of FDG-PET in decision making for 42 patients with SCLC [126]. In 12 patients (29%) the findings from the PET scan changed the patient's management; five patients required a change in the radiation field and volume to encompass disease identified by PET scan. In another retrospective study, Van Loon *et al.* noted that the incorporation of PET would have resulted in a modification of radiation treatment fields in 24% of patients (*n* = 5), with both increases and decreases in volumes [127]. They subsequently performed a prospective study in 60 patients with LS-SCLC and found that PET led to changes in the irradiated involved nodal stations in nearly one-third of patients [123]. Some 5% of patients were noted to have positive supraclavicular disease on PET scanning that was reported as negative on CT scanning. In a small prospective study from Washington University, increased FDG uptake was noted in one-fourth of the patients with CT-negative nodes [128]. This resulted in an alteration in the radiation therapy plan in order to include these nodes in the high-dose volumes. Histological verification of increased uptake was not available for these studies. At this point, the impact of use of FDG-PET in the treatment algorithm for SCLC patients is still unclear [129]. The recently completed Phase III CONVERT trial (NCT00433563) is evaluating the optimal radiation dose-fractionation with the omission of ENI. At this point, the authors recommend incorporating PET-CT findings in radiation planning with treatment volumes limited to gross/FDG avid disease with appropriate CTV margins. Routine treatment of elective nodal regions beyond the involved site may not be needed. This will help minimize rates of radiation esophagitis, and also myelosuppression which in turn will help improve compliance to the full course of systemic therapy. For patients receiving prior chemotherapy, only post-induction volumes (circumferential extent) need to be targeted, though the entire pre-chemotherapy involved nodal region should be included in the CTV. While twice-daily fractionation to a total dose of 45 Gy continues to be the standard dose, once-daily fractionation to 60–70 Gy may be used in situation where twice-daily treatments are not feasible due to logistic reasons.

Extensive-Stage Small-Cell Lung Cancer (ES-SCLC)

The primary therapy for ES-SCLC is chemotherapy. Three meta-analyses have been performed to identify the most effective chemotherapy regime. Results from Pujol *et al.* and Mascaux *et al.* clearly supported the use of a cisplatin–etoposide doublet with improvements in survival and response rates [130,131]. A third analysis (Amarasena *et al.*) showed significantly higher rates of CR with platinum-based regimes but no significant differences in survival were noted [132]. The cisplatin–etoposide doublet remains the first-choice regimen, with cisplatin replaced by carboplatin in patients with poor performance status [11]. Irinotecan- and platinum-based combinations have also shown superior results than the cisplatin–etoposide doublet, as revealed in a fourth meta-analysis [133]. However, there is some concern that, due to epidemiological variations in the alleles that relate to irinotecan metabolism, toxicities may vary by race [10]. The addition of paclitaxel to the cisplatin–etoposide combination resulted in increased non-hematological toxicity and treatment-related mortality, without improvement in survival [134,135]. Therapy is usually given for four to six cycles, with anticipated CR rates of 20–25% and overall objective response rates of 80–90% [10,136]. Maintenance chemotherapy has not shown significant benefit as compared to salvage second-line therapy at progression [11]. In view of the exquisite chemosensitivity of this disease, there is usually a rapid response to therapy with the potential for significant symptom improvement.

The routine use of large-field radiotherapy in ES-SCLC has resulted in poor overall outcomes in view of the rapid development of disseminated metastatic disease. However, patients who achieve a CR to systemic chemotherapy have a much better survival and may benefit from the addition of consolidative radiotherapy to the primary and regional lymph nodes, as noted in a Phase III trial conducted by Jeremic *et al.* [136]. In this study, ES-SCLC patients received induction cisplatin–etoposide (PE) therapy. Patients achieving a CR of distant disease and PR or CR of thoracic disease underwent randomization to thoracic radiotherapy with concurrent low-dose carboplatin–etoposide (CE) or PE alone, both arms followed by PCI (25 Gy in 10 fractions). For patients obtaining a PR of distant disease, two additional cycles of PE were given followed by thoracic radiotherapy with concurrent CE. Radiotherapy was delivered using an accelerated regimen. Anteroposterior/posteroanterior fields were used to deliver 36 Gy in 24 fractions in 12 treatment days over 2.5 weeks, followed by oblique fields to give an additional 18 Gy in 12 fractions in six treatment days, thereby reaching a total dose of 54 Gy in 36 fractions, 1.5 Gy twice-daily. The use of thoracic radiotherapy after a CR/PR at primary and CR at distant disease improved median survival by six months (17 versus 11 months, p = 0.041) and five-year survival by 5.4% (9.1% versus 3.7%). For patients with CR at the primary and PR at distant disease sites, a two-year survival of 8.8% was reached when thoracic radiotherapy formed part of the regime. More recently, results from the Dutch randomized trial (CREST) [137] were published, in which the use of thoracic radiotherapy (30 Gy in 10 fractions) resulted in improved two-year survival (13% versus 3%, p = 0.004), with a reduced risk of thoracic progression and acceptable toxicity. The protocol recommended targeting post-chemotherapy volume including hilar/mediastinal nodal stations that were initially involved. Extra-thoracic sites were not treated, though all patients were recommended to receive PCI. On a planned susbset analysis, thoracic radiotherapy yielded maximum benefit in patients with residual intrathoracic disease (the predominant population in the trial); HR 0.81, 95% CI 0.66-1.00, p = 0.044, with no such benefit seen in patients without residual intrathoracic disease. The RTOG 0937 study (NCT01055197) was recently closed to accrual based on a planned interim analysis which revealed that the futility boundary for the primary end-point of overall survival had been crossed, with no improvement in overall survival expected with continued accrual and not because of toxicity. It should be noted that this study was different from the Dutch study in that it allowed the treatment of up to four extra-thoracic metastatic sites with residual disease and treatment to a higher dose of 45 Gy in 3 Gy per fraction (30–40 Gy in 10 fractions was also allowed). A late-breaking presentation at the 2015 Annual Meeting of American Society for Radiation Oncology (ASTRO), San Antonio noted a one-year survival of 60.1% (standard arm) versus 50.8% (experimental arm) (p = 0.21). While the progression rates were not different, time to progression favored the PCI + radiotherapy arm (p = 0.01). Furthermore, of the 39 patients accrued to the experimental arm, seven (18%) had grade 4/5 toxicity while none of the PCI patients had grade 4/5 toxicity. Final results from the study are awaited. The conflicting results between the CREST study and the RTOG 0937 study add fuel to the controversy regarding the role of extra-cranial radiotherapy for patients with ES-SCLC. A multidisciplinary discussion of risks/benefits is recommended. It is imperative for radiation oncologists to understand the potential toxicities with overzealous use of radiotherapy. Tight volumes targeting thoracic gross disease with limited margins may be considered, minimizing irradiation of the normal lung, esophagus, and vertebral marrow. Until further information from RTOG 0937 is available, the treatment of extra-thoracic metastatic sites may not be necessary, unless symptomatic. Finally, for those patients who do not achieve a significant response to chemotherapy, the palliative use of radiation to relieve symptoms of primary or metastatic disease may be considered.

Prophylactic Cranial Irradiation

The brain is one of the most common sites of metastatic disease in SCLC, with about 50–70% of patients developing brain metastases at some point during the natural history. 'Prophylactic' cranial irradiation (PCI) reduces the incidence of overt brain metastases by treating subclinical disease. Arriagada *et al.* randomized 294 patients in CR to PCI (24 Gy in eight 8 fractions, 12 days) or observation [138]. PCI reduced the cumulative incidence of brain as the first site of relapse from 45% to 19% (statistically significant). There was a 27% absolute reduction in the two-year rate of all brain metastases, with a non-significant 7.5% absolute improvement in survival (29% versus 21.5%, RR 0.83). No significant differences in neuropsychological results were seen between the two arms. Additional trials confirmed this observation, and led to a meta-analysis of individual patient data [139]. Almost 1000 patients with SCLC in complete remission were evaluated. PCI improved three-year survival by 5.4% (from 15.3% to 20.7%, p = 0.01) and reduced the incidence of brain metastasis (from 58.6% to 33.3%, p < 0.001). A dose–response relationship was noted with a trend toward superior results associated with early administration of PCI. An intergroup (PCI 99-01, EORTC 22003-08004, RTOG 0212, and IFCT 99-01) Phase III study randomized 720 LS-SCLC patients in CR to two doses of PCI (25 Gy in 10 fractions versus 36 Gy in 18 q.d. or 24 b.i.d. fractions) [140]. There was no significant difference in the two-year incidence of brain metastases between the two arms. The toxicities from PCI included fatigue (in 106 patients [30%] of the standard-dose group versus 121 patients [34%] in the higher-dose group), headache (85 [24%] versus 99 [28%]), and nausea or vomiting (80 [23%] versus 101 [28%]). A subsequent report confirmed no significant differences between the two groups in any of the 17 selected items evaluating quality of life, neurological and cognitive functions [141]. Mild decrements in time of communication deficit, weakness of legs, intellectual deficit and memory were seen with PCI (p < 0.005).

To evaluate role of PCI specifically in ES-SCLC, Slotman *et al.* randomized patients with any response to four to six cycles of chemotherapy to PCI starting four to six weeks after chemotherapy [142]. The cumulative risk of brain metastases was reduced from 40.4% to 14.6%, p < 0.001). There was a relative doubling of one-year survival (from 13.3% to 27.1%). Neither the chemotherapy regimen nor PCI dose was standardized in this study.

Seute *et al.* noted that for patients diagnosed with SCLC, the use of regular contrast-enhanced MRI of the brain instead of CT increased the prevalence of brain metastases from 10% to 24% [143]. In addition, the survival of patients detected with brain metastases during the MRI era was better than during the CT era, due to the detection of smaller and clinically asymptomatic cases. This, however, impacted the number of patients eligible for PCI. While the study by Slotman *et al.* did not require use of imaging for pre-treatment intracranial staging for asymptomatic patients, an interim analysis of a Japanese randomized study was presented at the 2014 American Society of Clinical Oncology (ASCO) meeting. In patients with any response to platinum doublet chemotherapy and negative brain MRI at baseline, the median overall survival was inferior in the PCI arm (10.1 versus 15.1 months, p = 0.09). However, even in MRI-staged patients, the use of PCI significantly reduced the incidence of subsequent diagnosis of brain metastases (32.4% versus 58%, p = 0.001). It was noted that the follow-up evaluation was more stringent than for the Slotman *et al.* study, with three-monthly imaging evaluations performed. A little over 80% of the patients in the no-PCI arm received radiotherapy at the time of manifestation of brain metastases. No increase in toxicities were noted, though there was a trend towards decreased use of third- and fourth-line systemic therapy in the PCI arm. The trial was closed early due to meeting futility boundaries. This study did raise questions regarding the benefit of PCI in the era of MRI staging, though it requires stringent follow-up MRI evaluation for the early detection of radiographic brain metastases. Further, in the setting of brain metastases, intracranial control has been shown to impact neurocognitive function and survival [144]. In a Phase III trial, the baseline Spitzer Quality of Life Index (SQLI) score was reduced by almost 30–40% in patients diagnosed to have brain metastases [145]. In addition, more than 90% patients may have changes in one or more neurocognitive domains, with up to 40% having changes in more than three domains [146]. These risks need to be discussed in detail with the patients, with PCI best avoided where compliance to follow-up is doubtful or, in younger, good performance status patients, in whom the likelihood of chronic neurotoxicity is lower [147]. When given, PCI should not be combined with concurrent chemotherapy. The ongoing NRG Oncology clinical trial CC003 (NCT02635009) is testing whole-brain radiation therapy with or without hippocampal avoidance in treating patients with limited-stage or extensive-stage SCLC.

The use of PCI among the NSCLC population has also been tested [148]. The randomized RTOG 0214 study was unfortunately closed early due to slow accrual [149]. No significant differences in one-year overall survival and disease-free survival were seen, though there was significant reduction in the incidence of detected brain metastases with the use of PCI (7.7% versus 18%, p = 0.004). At the Princess Margaret Hospital study (Toronto, Canada), no statistically significant differences

were seen in EORTC quality of life analyses, though a trend for reduction in patient-reported cognitive functioning was noted. Like the RTOG study, this study also closed early due to poor accrual (33% of planned accrual). At this point, PCI is not routinely used in the management of NSCLC.

References

1 Brady, L., Heilmann, H.P., Molls, M., Nieder, C. (2011) *Advances in Radiation Oncology in Lung Cancer*, 2nd edition (ed. B. Jeremic). Springer, Heidelberg.

2 Surmont, V., Aerts, J.G., Pouw, E., *et al.* (2009) Oral UFT, etoposide and leucovorin in recurrent non-small cell lung cancer: a non-randomized phase II study. *Lung Cancer*, **66** (3), 333–337.

3 Siegel, R., Miller, K., Jemal, A. (2017) Cancer Statistics 2017. *CA Cancer J. Clin.*, **67**, 7–30.

4 Aberle, D.R., Adams, A.M., Berg, C.D., *et al.* (2011) Reduced lung-cancer mortality with low-dose computed tomographic screening. *N. Engl. J. Med.*, **365** (5), 395–409.

5 National Cancer Institute (2012) Small Cell Lung Cancer Treatment PDQ Bethesda: National Cancer Institute 2012 [updated 1/20/2012; cited 2012 2/8/2012]. Available at: http://www.cancer.gov/cancertopics/pdq/treatment/small-cell-lung/healthprofessional.

6 Govindan, R., Page, N., Morgensztern, D., *et al.* (2006) Changing epidemiology of small-cell lung cancer in the United States over the last 30 years: analysis of the surveillance, epidemiologic, and end results database. *J. Clin. Oncol.*, **24** (28), 4539–4544.

7 Hoffmann, D., Hoffmann, I., El-Bayoumy, K. (2001) The less harmful cigarette: a controversial issue. A tribute to Ernst L. Wynder. *Chem. Res. Toxicol.*, **14** (7), 767–790.

8 Wynder, E.L., Muscat, J.E. (1995) The changing epidemiology of smoking and lung cancer histology. *Environ. Health Perspect.*, **103** (Suppl. 8), 143–148.

9 Kato, Y., Ferguson, T.B., Bennett, D.E., Burford, T.H. (1969) Oat cell carcinoma of the lung. A review of 138 cases. *Cancer*, **23** (3), 517–524.

10 van Meerbeeck, J.P., Fennell, D.A., De Ruysscher, D.K. (2011) Small-cell lung cancer. *Lancet*, **378** (9804), 1741–1755.

11 Sorensen, M., Pijls-Johannesma, M., Felip, E. (2010) Small-cell lung cancer: ESMO Clinical Practice Guidelines for diagnosis, treatment and follow-up. *Ann. Oncol.*, **21** (Suppl. 5), v120–v125.

12 Turrisi, A.T., 3rd, Kim, K., Blum, R., *et al.* (1999) Twice-daily compared with once-daily thoracic radiotherapy in limited small-cell lung cancer treated concurrently with cisplatin and etoposide. *N. Engl. J. Med.*, **340** (4), 265–271.

13 Takada, M., Fukuoka, M., Kawahara, M., *et al.* (2002) Phase III study of concurrent versus sequential thoracic radiotherapy in combination with cisplatin and etoposide for limited-stage small-cell lung cancer: results of the Japan Clinical Oncology Group Study 9104. *J. Clin. Oncol.*, **20** (14), 3054–3060.

14 Bayman, N.A., Sheikh, H., Kularatne, B., *et al.* (2009) Radiotherapy for small-cell lung cancer – Where are we heading? *Lung Cancer*, **63** (3), 307–314.

15 Gultekin, S.H., Rosenfeld, M.R., Voltz, R., Eichen, J., Posner, J.B., Dalmau, J. (2000) Paraneoplastic limbic encephalitis: neurological symptoms, immunological findings and tumour association in 50 patients. *Brain*, **123** (Pt 7), 1481–1494.

16 Gure, A.O., Stockert, E., Scanlan, M.J., *et al.* (2000) Serological identification of embryonic neural proteins as highly immunogenic tumor antigens in small cell lung cancer. *Proc. Natl Acad. Sci. USA*, **97** (8), 4198–4203.

17 Maddison, P., Lang, B. (2008) Paraneoplastic neurological autoimmunity and survival in small-cell lung cancer. *J. Neuroimmunol.*, **201–202**, 159–162.

18 Masters, G.A. (2010) *Clinical Presentation of Small Cell Lung Cancer*, 4th edition (eds H.I. Pass, D.P. Carbone, D.H. Johnson, J.D. Minna, G.V. Scagliotti, A.T. Turrisi). Lippincott Williams & Wilkins, Philadelphia, PA.

19 Clines, G.A. (2011) Mechanisms and treatment of hypercalcemia of malignancy. *Curr. Opin. Endocrinol. Diabetes Obes.*, **18** (6), 339–346.

20 Stovold, R., Blackhall, F., Meredith, S., Hou, J., Dive, C., White, A. (2012) Biomarkers for small cell lung cancer: Neuroendocrine, epithelial and circulating tumour cells. *Lung Cancer*, **76** (3), 263–268.

21 Hou, J.M., Greystoke, A., Lancashire, L., *et al.* (2009) Evaluation of circulating tumor cells and serological cell death biomarkers in small cell lung cancer patients undergoing chemotherapy. *Am. J. Pathol.*, **175** (2), 808–816.

22 Frisch, S.M., Francis, H. (1994) Disruption of epithelial cell-matrix interactions induces apoptosis. *J. Cell Biol.*, **124** (4), 619–626.

23 Muhm, J.R., Miller, W.E., Fontana, R.S., Sanderson, D.R., Uhlenhopp, M.A. (1983) Lung cancer detected during a screening program using four-month chest radiographs. *Radiology*, **148** (3), 609–615.

24 van Klaveren, R.J., Oudkerk, M., Prokop, M., *et al.* (2009) Management of lung nodules detected by volume CT scanning. *N. Engl. J. Med.*, **361** (23), 2221–2229.

25 Aoki, T., Tomoda, Y., Watanabe, H., *et al.* (2001) Peripheral lung adenocarcinoma: correlation of thin-section CT findings with histologic prognostic factors and survival. *Radiology*, **220** (3), 803–809.

26 Gu, P., Zhao, Y.Z., Jiang, L.Y., Zhang, W., Xin, Y., Han, B.H. (2009) Endobronchial ultrasound-guided transbronchial needle aspiration for staging of lung cancer: a systematic review and meta-analysis. *Eur. J. Cancer*, **45** (8), 1389–1396.

27 Amin, M.B. (2017) *AJCC Cancer Staging Manual*, 8th edition. Springer, New York.

28 Zelen, M. (1973) Keynote address on biostatistics and data retrieval. *Cancer Chemother. Rep.*, **4** (2), 31–42.

29 Stahel, R.A., Ginsberg, R., Havermann, K., *et al.* (1989) Staging and prognostic factors in small cell lung cancer: a consensus report. *Lung Cancer*, **5** (4-6), 119–126.

30 Shepherd, F.A., Crowley, J., Van Houtte, P., *et al.* (2007) The International Association for the Study of Lung Cancer lung cancer staging project: proposals regarding the clinical staging of small cell lung cancer in the forthcoming (seventh) edition of the tumor, node, metastasis classification for lung cancer. *J. Thorac. Oncol.*, **2** (12), 1067–1077.

31 Travis, W.D., Brambilla, E., Noguchi, M., *et al.*, American Thoracic Society (2011) International Association for the Study of Lung Cancer/American Thoracic Society/European Respiratory Society: international multidisciplinary classification of lung adenocarcinoma: executive summary. *Proc. Am. Thorac. Soc.*, **8** (5), 381–385.

32 Riely, G.J., Politi, K.A., Miller, V.A., Pao, W. (2006) Update on epidermal growth factor receptor mutations in non-small cell lung cancer. *Clin Cancer Res.*, **12** (24), 7232–7241.

33 Rudin, C.M., Avila-Tang, E., Harris, C.C., *et al.* (2009) Lung cancer in never smokers: molecular profiles and therapeutic implications. *Clin. Cancer Res.*, **15** (18), 5646–5661.

34 Franklin, W.F., Noguchi, M., Gonzalez, A. (2010) *Molecular and Cellular Pathology of Lung Cancer*, 4th edition (eds H.I. Pass, D.P. Carbone, D.H. Johnson, J.D. Minna, G.V. Scagliotti, A.T. Turrisi). Lippincott Williams & Wilkins, Philadelphia, PA.

35 McGarry, R.C., Song, G., des Rosiers, P., Timmerman, R. (2002) Observation-only management of early stage, medically inoperable lung cancer: poor outcome. *Chest*, **121** (4), 1155–1158.

36 Ginsberg, R.J., Rubinstein, L.V. (1995) Randomized trial of lobectomy versus limited resection for T1 N0 non-small cell lung cancer. Lung Cancer Study Group. *Ann. Thorac. Surg.*, **60** (3), 615–622; discussion 622–623.

37 Ginsberg, R.J., Rubinstein, L.V. and the Lung Cancer Study Group (1995) Randomized trial of lobectomy versus limited resection for T1 N0 non-small cell lung cancer. *Ann. Thorac. Surg.*, **60** (3), 615–622.

38 Swanson, S.J., Herndon, J.E., 2nd, D'Amico, T.A., *et al.* (2007) Video-assisted thoracic surgery lobectomy: report of CALGB 39802 – a prospective, multi-institution feasibility study. *J. Clin. Oncol.*, **25** (31), 4993–4997.

39 Darling, G.E., Allen, M.S., Decker, P.A., *et al.* (2011) Randomized trial of mediastinal lymph node sampling versus complete lymphadenectomy during pulmonary resection in the patient with N0 or N1 (less than hilar) non-small cell carcinoma: results of the American College of Surgery Oncology Group Z0030 Trial. *J. Thorac. Cardiovasc. Surg.*, **141** (3), 662–670.

40 Darling, G.E., Allen, M.S., Decker, P.A., *et al.* (2011) Number of lymph nodes harvested from a mediastinal lymphadenectomy: results of the randomized, prospective American College of Surgeons Oncology Group Z0030 trial. *Chest*, **139** (5), 1124–1129.

41 Schultz, S. (2011) Combination of Landmark Internal Radiation Therapy and da Vinci Robotics Represents Paradigm Shift in Early Stage Lung Cancer Treatment 2011 [11/12/2011]. Available at: http://www.business wire.com/news/home/20110712005558/en/IsoRay-Announces-Worlds-Cesium-131-Treatment-Lung-Cancer.

42 Thomas, S.R., Odau, H., Das, R.K., Bentzen, S.M., Patel, R.R., Khuntia, D. (eds) (2007) Feasibility of Cs-131 for intraoperative brachytherapy for patients undergoing sublobar resections for early stage nonsmall cell lung cancer (NSCLC): A dosimetric comparison with I-125 and Cs-131. American Brachytherapy Society, April 29–May 2, 2007, Chicago.

43 Santos, R., Colonias, A., Parda, D., *et al.* (2003) Comparison between sublobar resection and 125Iodine brachytherapy after sublobar resection in high-risk patients with Stage I non-small-cell lung cancer. *Surgery*, **134** (4), 691–697; discussion 697.

44 Fernando, H.C., Landreneau, R.J., Mandrekar, S.J., *et al.* (2011) The impact of adjuvant brachytherapy with sublobar resection on pulmonary function and dyspnea in high-risk patients with operable disease: preliminary results from the American College of Surgeons Oncology Group Z4032 trial. *J. Thorac. Cardiovasc Surg.*, **142** (3), 554–562.

45 Landreneau, J.P., Schuchert, M.J., Weyant, R., *et al.* (2014) Anatomic segmentectomy and brachytherapy mesh implantation for clinical stage I non-small cell lung cancer (NSCLC). *Surgery*, **155** (2), 340–346.

46 Gill, B.S., Clump, D.A., Burton, S.A., Christie, N.A., Schuchert, M.J., Heron, D.E. (2015) Salvage stereotactic body radiotherapy for locally recurrent non-small cell lung cancer after sublobar resection and i(125) vicryl mesh brachytherapy. *Front. Oncol.*, **5**, 109.

47 Wisnivesky, J.P., Bonomi, M., Henschke, C., Iannuzzi, M., McGinn, T. (2005) Radiation therapy for the treatment of unresected stage I-II non-small cell lung cancer. *Chest*, **128** (3), 1461–1467.

48 Timmerman, R., Papiez, L., McGarry, R., Likes, L., DesRosiers, C., Frost, S., Williams, M. (2003) Extracranial stereotactic radioablation: results of a phase I study in medically inoperable stage I non-small cell lung cancer. *Chest*, **124** (5), 1946–1955.

49 Uematsu, M., Shioda, A., Suda, A., Fukui, T., Ozeki, Y., Hama, Y., Wong, J.R., Kusano, S. (2001) Computed tomography-guided frameless stereotactic radiotherapy for stage I non-small cell lung cancer: a 5-year experience. *Int. J. Radiat. Oncol. Biol. Phys.*, **51** (3), 666–670.

50 Pan, H., Simpson, D.R., Mell, L.K., Mundt, A.J., Lawson, J.D. (2011) A survey of stereotactic body radiotherapy use in the United States. *Cancer*, **117** (19), 4566–4572.

51 Benedict, S.H., Yenice, K.M., Followill, D., *et al.* (2010) Stereotactic body radiation therapy: the report of AAPM Task Group 101. *Med. Phys.*, **37** (8), 4078–4101.

52 Soldberg, T.D., Balter, J.M., Benedict, S. (2011) Quality and safety considerations in stereotactic radiosurgery and stereotactic body radiation therapy executive summary. *Pract. Radiat. Oncol.*, **2** (1), 2–9.

53 Onishi, H., Araki, T., Shirato, H., *et al.* (2004) Stereotactic hypofractionated high-dose irradiation for stage I nonsmall cell lung carcinoma: clinical outcomes in 245 subjects in a Japanese multiinstitutional study. *Cancer*, **101** (7), 1623–1631.

54 Videtic, G.M., Hu, C., Singh, A.K., *et al.* (2015) A randomized Phase 2 study comparing 2 stereotactic body radiation therapy schedules for medically inoperable patients with Stage I peripheral non-small cell lung cancer: NRG Oncology RTOG 0915 (NCCTG N0927). *Int. J. Radiat. Oncol. Biol. Phys.*, **93** (4), 757–764.

55 Timmerman, R., McGarry, R., Yiannoutsos, C., *et al.* (2006) Excessive toxicity when treating central tumors in a phase II study of stereotactic body radiation therapy for medically inoperable early-stage lung cancer. *J. Clin. Oncol.*, **24** (30), 4833–4839.

56 Haasbeek, C.J., Lagerwaard, F.J., Slotman, B.J., Senan, S. (2011) Outcomes of stereotactic ablative radiotherapy for centrally located early-stage lung cancer. *J. Thorac. Oncol.*, **6** (12), 2036–2043.

57 Li, Q., Swanick, C.W., Allen, P.K., *et al.* (2014) Stereotactic ablative radiotherapy (SABR) using 70 Gy in 10 fractions for non-small cell lung cancer: exploration of clinical indications. *Radiother. Oncol.*, **112** (2), 256–261.

58 Park, H.S., Corso, C.D., Rutter, C.E., Kim, A.W., Yu, J.B., Husain, Z.A., Decker, R.H. (2015) Survival comparison of 3 versus 4-5 fractions for stereotactic body radiation therapy in Stage I non-small cell lung cancer. ASTRO 2015, 1st November 2015, San Antonio, p. s100.

59 Chang, J.Y., Senan, S., Paul, M.A., *et al.* (2015) Stereotactic ablative radiotherapy versus lobectomy for operable stage I non-small-cell lung cancer: a pooled analysis of two randomised trials. *Lancet Oncol.*, **16** (6), 630–637.

60 Hallvqist, A. (2015) The SPACE Study: A Randomized Phase II Trial Comparing SBRT and 3DCRT in Stage I NSCLC Patients; Final Analysis including HRQL. IASLC World Congress, 8th September 2015, Denver, CO.

61 Dunlap, N.E., Cai, J., Biedermann, G.B., *et al.* (2010) Chest wall volume receiving >30 Gy predicts risk of severe pain and/or rib fracture after lung stereotactic body radiotherapy. *Int. J. Radiat. Oncol. Biol. Phys.*, **76** (3), 796–801.

62 Balter, J.M., Wright, J.N., Newell, L.J., *et al.* (2005) Accuracy of a wireless localization system for radiotherapy. *Int. J. Radiat. Oncol. Biol. Phys.*, **61** (3), 933–937.

63 Onishi, H., Shirato, H., Nagata, Y., *et al.* (2011) Stereotactic body radiotherapy (SBRT) for operable stage I non-small-cell lung cancer: can SBRT be comparable to surgery? *Int. J. Radiat. Oncol. Biol. Phys.*, **81** (5), 1352–1358.

64 Nagata, Y., Hiraoka, M., Shibata, T., *et al.* (2015) Prospective trial of stereotactic body radiation therapy for both operable and inoperable T1N0M0 non-small cell lung cancer: Japan Clinical Oncology Group Study JCOG0403. *Int. J. Radiat. Oncol. Biol. Phys.*, **93** (5), 989–996.

65 Izbicki, J.R., Thetter, O., Habekost, M., *et al.* (1994) Radical systematic mediastinal lymphadenectomy in non-small cell lung cancer: a randomized controlled trial. *Br. J. Surg.*, **81** (2), 229–235.

66 Keller, S.M., Adak, S., Wagner, H., *et al.* (2000) A randomized trial of postoperative adjuvant therapy in patients with completely resected stage II or IIIA non-small-cell lung cancer. Eastern Cooperative Oncology Group. *N. Engl. J. Med.*, **343** (17), 1217–1222.

67 Berghmans, T., Paesmans, M., Meert, A.P., Mascaux, C., Lothaire, P., Lafitte, J.J., Sculier, J.P. (2005) Survival improvement in resectable non-small cell lung cancer with (neo)adjuvant chemotherapy: results of a meta-analysis of the literature. *Lung Cancer*, **49** (1), 13–23.

68 Albain, K.S., Swann, R.S., Rusch, V.W., *et al.* (2009) Radiotherapy plus chemotherapy with or without surgical resection for stage III non-small-cell lung cancer: a phase III randomised controlled trial. *Lancet*, **374** (9687), 379–386.

69 NSCLC Meta-analysis Collaborative Group (2014) Preoperative chemotherapy for non-small-cell lung cancer: a systematic review and meta-analysis of individual participant data. *Lancet*, **383** (9928), 1561–1571.

70 Sher, D.J., Fidler, M.J., Liptay, M.J., Koshy, M. (2015) Comparative effectiveness of neoadjuvant chemoradiotherapy versus chemotherapy alone followed by surgery for patients with stage IIIA non-small cell lung cancer. *Lung Cancer*, **88** (3), 267–274.

71 Pless, M., Stupp, R., Ris, H.B., *et al.* and Group SLCP (2015) Induction chemoradiation in stage IIIA/N2 non-small-cell lung cancer: a phase 3 randomised trial. *Lancet*, **386** (9998), 1049–1056.

72 Auperin, A., Le Pechoux, C., Rolland, E., *et al.* (2010) Meta-analysis of concomitant versus sequential radiochemotherapy in locally advanced non-small-cell lung cancer. *J. Clin. Oncol.*, **28** (13), 2181–2190.

73 Werner-Wasik, M., Scott, C., Cox, J.D., *et al.* (2000) Recursive partitioning analysis of 1999 Radiation Therapy Oncology Group (RTOG) patients with locally-advanced non-small-cell lung cancer (LA-NSCLC): identification of five groups with different survival. *Int. J. Radiat. Oncol. Biol. Phys.*, **48** (5), 1475–1482.

74 Bradley, J., Graham, M.V., Winter, K., *et al.* (2005) Toxicity and outcome results of RTOG 9311: a phase I-II dose-escalation study using three-dimensional conformal radiotherapy in patients with inoperable non-small-cell lung carcinoma. *Int. J. Radiat. Oncol. Biol. Phys.*, **61** (2), 318–328.

75 Yuan, S., Sun, X., Li, M., *et al.* (2007) A randomized study of involved-field irradiation versus elective nodal irradiation in combination with concurrent chemotherapy for inoperable stage III nonsmall cell lung cancer. *Am. J. Clin. Oncol.*, **30** (3), 239–244.

76 National Comprehensive Cancer Network. Non-small cell lung cancer 2012 [cited 2012]; 2.2012:[

77 National Comprehensive Cancer Network. Non-small cell lung cancer 2016 [1/19/2016]. Available at: http://www.nccn.org/professionals/physician゛gls/pdf/nscl.pdf.

78 Perez, C.A., Pajak, T.F., Rubin, P., *et al.* (1987) Long-term observations of the patterns of failure in patients with unresectable non-oat cell carcinoma of the lung treated with definitive radiotherapy. Report by the Radiation Therapy Oncology Group. *Cancer*, **59** (11), 1874–1881.

79 Cox, J.D., Pajak, T.F., Herskovic, A., Urtasun, R., Podolsky, W.J., Seydel, H.G. (1991) Five-year survival after hyperfractionated radiation therapy for non-small-cell carcinoma of the lung (NSCCL): results of RTOG protocol 81-08. *Am. J. Clin. Oncol.*, **14** (4), 280–284.

80 Sause, W.T., Scott, C., Taylor, S., *et al.* (1995) Radiation Therapy Oncology Group (RTOG) 88-08 and Eastern Cooperative Oncology Group (ECOG) 4588: preliminary results of a phase III trial in regionally advanced, unresectable non-small-cell lung cancer. *J. Natl Cancer Inst.*, **87** (3), 198–205.

81 Curran, W.J., Jr, Paulus, R., Langer, C.J., *et al.* (2011) Sequential vs. concurrent chemoradiation for stage III non-small cell lung cancer: randomized phase III trial RTOG 9410. *J. Natl Cancer Inst.*, **103** (19), 1452–1460.

82 Saunders, M., Dische, S., Barrett, A., Harvey, A., Griffiths, G., Palmar, M. (1999) Continuous, hyperfractionated, accelerated radiotherapy (CHART) versus conventional radiotherapy in non-small cell lung cancer: mature data from the randomised multicentre trial. CHART Steering committee. *Radiother. Oncol.*, **52** (2), 137–148.

83 Saunders, M., Dische, S., Barrett, A., Harvey, A., Gibson, D., Parmar, M. (1997) Continuous hyperfractionated accelerated radiotherapy (CHART) versus conventional radiotherapy in non-small-cell lung cancer: a randomised multicentre trial. CHART Steering Committee. *Lancet*, **350** (9072), 161–165.

84 Belani, C.P., Wang, W., Johnson, D.H., Wagner, H., Schiller, J., Veeder, M., Mehta, M. (2005) Phase III study of the Eastern Cooperative Oncology Group (ECOG 2597): induction chemotherapy followed by either standard thoracic radiotherapy or hyperfractionated accelerated radiotherapy for patients with unresectable stage IIIA and B non-small-cell lung cancer. *J. Clin. Oncol.*, **23** (16), 3760–3767.

85 Bradley, J.D., Moughan, J., Graham, M.V., *et al.* (2010) A phase I/II radiation dose escalation study with concurrent chemotherapy for patients with inoperable stages I to III non-small-cell lung cancer: phase I results of RTOG 0117. *Int. J. Radiat. Oncol. Biol. Phys.*, **77** (2), 367–372.

86 Rosenzweig, K.E., Sura, S., Jackson, A., Yorke, E. (2007) Involved-field radiation therapy for inoperable non small-cell lung cancer. *J. Clin. Oncol.*, **25** (35), 5557–5561.

87 Fried, D.B., Morris, D.E., Poole, C., *et al.* (2004) Systematic review evaluating the timing of thoracic radiation therapy in combined modality therapy for limited-stage small-cell lung cancer. *J. Clin. Oncol.*, **22** (23), 4837–4845.

88 Jeremic, B. (2011) *Advances in Radiation Oncology in Lung Cancer*, 2nd edition. Springer, New York.

89 Bradley, J.D., Paulus, R., Komaki, R., Masters, G., Blumenschein, G., Schild, S., Bogart, J., Hu, C., Forster, K., Magliocco, A., Kavadi, V., Garces, Y.I., Narayan, S., Iyengar, P., Robinson, C., Wynn, R.B., Koprowski, C., Meng, J., Beitler, J., Gaur, R., Curran, W., Jr, Choy, H. (2015) Standard-dose versus high-dose conformal radiotherapy with concurrent and consolidation carboplatin plus paclitaxel with or without cetuximab for patients with stage IIIA or IIIB non-small-cell lung cancer (RTOG 0617): a randomised, two-by-two factorial phase 3 study. *Lancet Oncol.*, **16** (2), 187–199.

90 Mehta, M., Scrimger, R., Mackie, R., Paliwal, B., Chappell, R., Fowler, J. (2001) A new approach to dose escalation in non-small-cell lung cancer. *Int. J. Radiat. Oncol. Biol. Phys.*, **49** (1), 23–33.

91 Adkison, J.B., Khuntia, D., Bentzen, S.M., *et al.* (2008) Dose escalated, hypofractionated radiotherapy using helical tomotherapy for inoperable non-small cell lung cancer: preliminary results of a risk-stratified phase I dose escalation study. *Technol. Cancer Res. Treat.*, **7** (6), 441–447.

92 Cannon, D.M., Mehta, M.P., Adkison, J.B., *et al.* (2013) Dose-limiting toxicity after hypofractionated dose-escalated radiotherapy in non-small-cell lung cancer. *J. Clin. Oncol.*, **31** (34), 4343–4348.

93 Sejpal, S., Komaki, R., Tsao, A., *et al.* (2011) Early findings on toxicity of proton beam therapy with concurrent chemotherapy for nonsmall cell lung cancer. *Cancer*, **117** (13), 3004–3013.

94 Chang, J.Y., Komaki, R., Lu, C., *et al.* (2011) Phase 2 study of high-dose proton therapy with concurrent chemotherapy for unresectable stage III nonsmall cell lung cancer. *Cancer*, **117** (20), 4707–4713.

95 Pignon, J.P., Tribodet, H., Scagliotti, G.V., *et al.*, Group LC (2008) Lung adjuvant cisplatin evaluation: a pooled analysis by the LACE Collaborative Group. *J. Clin. Oncol.*, **26** (21), 3552–3559.

96 PORT Meta-analysis Trialists Group (1998) Postoperative radiotherapy in non-small-cell lung cancer: systematic review and meta-analysis of individual patient data from nine randomised controlled trials. *Lancet*, **352** (9124), 257–263.

97 Lally, B.E., Zelterman, D., Colasanto, J.M., Haffty, B.G., Detterbeck, F.C., Wilson, L.D. (2006) Postoperative radiotherapy for stage II or III non-small-cell lung cancer using the surveillance, epidemiology, and end results database. *J. Clin. Oncol.*, **24** (19), 2998–3006.

98 Douillard, J.Y., Rosell, R., De Lena, M., Riggi, M., Hurteloup, P., Mahe, M.A., Adjuvant Navelbine International Trialist Association (2008) Impact of postoperative radiation therapy on survival in patients with complete resection and stage I, II, or IIIA non-small-cell lung cancer treated with adjuvant chemotherapy: the adjuvant Navelbine International Trialist Association (ANITA) Randomized Trial. *Int. J. Radiat. Oncol. Biol. Phys.*, **72** (3), 695–701.

99 Billiet, C., Decaluwe, H., Peeters, S., *et al.* (2014) Modern post-operative radiotherapy for stage III non-small cell lung cancer may improve local control and survival: a meta-analysis. *Radiother. Oncol.*, **110** (1), 3–8.

100 Rusch, V.W., Giroux, D.J., Kraut, M.J., *et al.* (2007) Induction chemoradiation and surgical resection for superior sulcus non-small-cell lung carcinomas: long-term results of Southwest Oncology Group Trial 9416 (Intergroup Trial 0160). *J. Clin. Oncol.*, **25** (3), 313–318.

101 Kwong, K.F., Edelman, M.J., Suntharalingam, M., *et al.* (2005) High-dose radiotherapy in trimodality treatment of Pancoast tumors results in high pathologic complete response rates and excellent long-term survival. *J. Thorac. Cardiovasc. Surg.*, **129** (6), 1250–1257.

102 Dillman, R.O., Herndon, J., Seagren, S.L., Eaton, W.L., Jr, Green, M.R. (1996) Improved survival in stage III non-small-cell lung cancer: seven-year follow-up of cancer and leukemia group B (CALGB) 8433 trial. *J. Natl Cancer Inst.*, **88** (17), 1210–1215.

103 Atagi, S., Kawahara, M., Yokoyama, A., *et al.*, Japan Clinical Oncology Group Lung Cancer Study Group (2012) Thoracic radiotherapy with or without daily low-dose carboplatin in elderly patients with non-small-cell lung cancer: a randomised, controlled, phase 3 trial by the Japan Clinical Oncology Group (JCOG0301). *Lancet Oncol.*, **13** (7), 671–678.

104 Scadding, J.G., *et al.* (1966) Comparative trial of surgery and radiotherapy for the primary treatment of small-celled or oat-celled carcinoma of the bronchus. First report to the Medical Research Council by the working-party on the evaluation of different methods of therapy in carcinoma of the bronchus. *Lancet*, **2** (7471), 979–986.

105 Fox, W., Scadding, J.G. (1973) Medical Research Council comparative trial of surgery and radiotherapy for primary treatment of small-celled or oat-celled carcinoma of bronchus. Ten-year follow-up. *Lancet*, **2** (7820), 63–65.

106 Lad, T., Piantadosi, S., Thomas, P., Payne, D., Ruckdeschel, J., Giaccone, G. (1994) A prospective randomized trial to determine the benefit of surgical resection of residual disease following response of small cell lung cancer to combination chemotherapy. *Chest*, **106** (6 Suppl.), 320S–323S.

107 Schreiber, D., Rineer, J., Weedon, J., *et al.* (2010) Survival outcomes with the use of surgery in limited-stage small cell lung cancer: should its role be re-evaluated? *Cancer*, **116** (5), 1350–1357.

108 Yu, J.B., Decker, R.H., Detterbeck, F.C., Wilson, L.D. (2010) Surveillance epidemiology and end results evaluation of the role of surgery for stage I small cell lung cancer. *J. Thorac. Oncol.*, **5** (2), 215–219.

109 Asamura, H., Goya, T., Koshiishi, Y., *et al.* (2008) A Japanese Lung Cancer Registry study: prognosis of 13,010 resected lung cancers. *J. Thorac. Oncol.*, **3** (1), 46–52.

110 Medical Research Council Lung Cancer Working Party (1979) Radiotherapy alone or with chemotherapy in the treatment of small-cell carcinoma of the lung. *Br. J. Cancer*, **40** (1), 1–10.

111 Livingston, R.B., Moore, T.N., Heilbrun, L., Bottomley, R., Lehane, D., Rivkin, S.E., Thigpen, T. (1978) Small-cell carcinoma of the lung: combined chemotherapy and radiation: a Southwest Oncology Group study. *Ann. Intern. Med.*, **88** (2), 194–199.

112 Perry, M.C., Eaton, W.L., Propert, K.J., *et al.* (1987) Chemotherapy with or without radiation therapy in limited small-cell carcinoma of the lung. *N. Engl. J. Med.*, **316** (15), 912–918.

113 Bunn, P.A., Jr, Lichter, A.S., Makuch, R.W., *et al.* (1987) Chemotherapy alone or chemotherapy with chest radiation therapy in limited stage small cell lung cancer. A prospective, randomized trial. *Ann. Intern. Med.*, **106** (5), 655–662.

114 Kies, M.S., Mira, J.G., Crowley, J.J., *et al.* (1987) Multimodal therapy for limited small-cell lung cancer: a randomized study of induction combination chemotherapy with or without thoracic radiation in complete responders; and with wide-field versus reduced-field radiation in partial responders: a Southwest Oncology Group Study. *J. Clin. Oncol.*, **5** (4), 592–600.

115 Warde, P., Payne, D. (1992) Does thoracic irradiation improve survival and local control in limited-stage small-cell carcinoma of the lung? A meta-analysis. *J. Clin. Oncol.*, **10** (6), 890–895.

116 Pignon, J.P., Arriagada, R., Ihde, D.C., *et al.* (1992) A meta-analysis of thoracic radiotherapy for small-cell lung cancer. *N. Engl. J. Med.*, **327** (23), 1618–1624.

117 Schild, S.E., Bonner, J.A., Shanahan, T.G., *et al.* (2004) Long-term results of a phase III trial comparing once-daily radiotherapy with twice-daily radiotherapy in limited-stage small-cell lung cancer. *Int. J. Radiat. Oncol. Biol. Phys.*, **59** (4), 943–951.

118 Komaki, R., Swann, R.S., Ettinger, D.S., *et al.* (2005) Phase I study of thoracic radiation dose escalation with concurrent chemotherapy for patients with limited small-cell lung cancer: Report of Radiation Therapy Oncology Group (RTOG) protocol 97-12. *Int. J. Radiat. Oncol. Biol. Phys.*, **62** (2), 342–350.

119 Komaki, R., Paulus, R., Ettinger, D.S., *et al.* (2012) Phase II study of accelerated high-dose radiotherapy with concurrent chemotherapy for patients with limited small-cell lung cancer: Radiation Therapy Oncology Group protocol 0239. *Int. J. Radiat. Oncol. Biol. Phys.*, **83** (4), e531–e536.

120 Bogart, J.A., Herndon, J.E., 2nd, Lyss, A.P., *et al.* (2004) 70 Gy thoracic radiotherapy is feasible concurrent with chemotherapy for limited-stage small-cell lung cancer: analysis of Cancer and Leukemia Group B study 39808. *Int. J. Radiat. Oncol. Biol. Phys.*, **59** (2), 460–468.

121 Faivre-Finn, C., Snee, M., Ashcroft, L., Appel, W., Barlesi, F., Bhatnagar, A., Bezjak, A., Cardenal, F., Fournel, P., Harden, S., Le Pechoux, C., McMenemin, R.M., Mohammed, N., O'Brien, M.E.R., Pantarotto, J.R., Surmont, V., Van Meerbeeck, J., Woll, P.J., Lorigan, P., Blackhall, F.H. (2016) CONVERT: An international randomised trial of concurrent chemo-radiotherapy (cCTRT) comparing twice-daily (BD) and once-daily (OD) radiotherapy schedules in patients with limited stage small cell lung cancer (LS-SCLC) and good performance status (PS). *J. Clin. Oncol.*, **34**, (suppl; abstr 8504).

122 De Ruysscher, D., Bremer, R.H., Koppe, F., *et al.* (2006) Omission of elective node irradiation on basis of CT-scans in patients with limited disease small cell lung cancer: a phase II trial. *Radiother. Oncol.*, **80** (3), 307–312.

123 van Loon, J., De Ruysscher, D., Wanders, R., *et al.* (2010) Selective nodal irradiation on basis of (18)FDG-PET scans in limited-disease small-cell lung cancer: a prospective study. *Int. J. Radiat. Oncol. Biol. Phys.*, **77** (2), 329–336.

124 Videtic, G.M., Belderbos, J.S., Spring Kong, F.M., Kepka, L., Martel, M.K., Jeremic, B. (2008) Report from the International Atomic Energy Agency (IAEA) consultants' meeting on elective nodal irradiation in lung cancer: small-cell lung cancer (SCLC). *Int. J. Radiat. Oncol. Biol. Phys.*, **72** (2), 327–334.

125 Hu, X., Bao, Y., Zhang, L., *et al.* (2012) Omitting elective nodal irradiation and irradiating postinduction versus preinduction chemotherapy tumor extent for limited-stage small cell lung cancer: interim analysis of a prospective randomized noninferiority trial. *Cancer*, **118** (1), 278–287.

126 Kamel, E.M., Zwahlen, D., Wyss, M.T., Stumpe, K.D., von Schulthess, G.K., Steinert, H.C. (2003) Whole-body (18)F-FDG PET improves the

management of patients with small cell lung cancer. *J. Nucl. Med.*, **44** (12), 1911–1917.

127 van Loon, J., Offermann, C., Bosmans, G., *et al.* (2008) 18FDG-PET based radiation planning of mediastinal lymph nodes in limited disease small cell lung cancer changes radiotherapy fields: a planning study. *Radiother. Oncol.*, **87** (1), 49–54.

128 Bradley, J.D., Dehdashti, F., Mintun, M.A., Govindan, R., Trinkaus, K., Siegel, B.A. (2004) Positron emission tomography in limited-stage small-cell lung cancer: a prospective study. *J. Clin. Oncol.*, **22** (16), 3248–3254.

129 Thomson, D., Hulse, P., Lorigan, P., Faivre-Finn, C. (2011) The role of positron emission tomography in management of small cell lung cancer. *Lung Cancer*, **73** (2), 121–126.

130 Pujol, J.L., Carestia, L., Daures, J.P. (2000) Is there a case for cisplatin in the treatment of small-cell lung cancer? A meta-analysis of randomized trials of a cisplatin-containing regimen versus a regimen without this alkylating agent. *Br. J. Cancer*, **83** (1), 8–15.

131 Mascaux, C., Paesmans, M., Berghmans, T., *et al.* (2000) A systematic review of the role of etoposide and cisplatin in the chemotherapy of small cell lung cancer with methodology assessment and meta-analysis. *Lung Cancer*, **30** (1), 23–36.

132 Amarasena, I.U., Walters, J.A., Wood-Baker, R., Fong, K. (2008) Platinum versus non-platinum chemotherapy regimens for small cell lung cancer. *Cochrane Database Syst. Rev.* 2008 (4): CD006849.

133 Shao, N., Jin, S., Zhu, W. (2012) An updated meta-analysis of randomized controlled trials comparing irinotecan/platinum with etoposide/platinum in patients with previously untreated extensive-stage small cell lung cancer. *J. Thorac. Oncol.*, **7** (2), 470–472.

134 Niell, H.B., Herndon, J.E., 2nd, Miller, A.A., *et al.* (2005) Randomized phase III intergroup trial of etoposide and cisplatin with or without paclitaxel and granulocyte colony-stimulating factor in patients with extensive-stage small-cell lung cancer: Cancer and Leukemia Group B Trial 9732. *J. Clin. Oncol.*, **23** (16), 3752–3759.

135 Mavroudis, D., Papadakis, E., Veslemes, M., *et al.* (2001) A multicenter randomized clinical trial comparing paclitaxel-cisplatin-etoposide versus cisplatin-etoposide as first-line treatment in patients with small-cell lung cancer. *Ann. Oncol.*, **12** (4), 463–470.

136 Jeremic, B., Shibamoto, Y., Nikolic, N., *et al.* (1991) Role of radiation therapy in the combined-modality treatment of patients with extensive disease small-cell lung cancer: A randomized study. *J. Clin. Oncol.*, **17** (7), 2092–2099.

137 Slotman, B.J., van Tinteren, H., Praag, J.O., *et al.* (2015) Use of thoracic radiotherapy for extensive stage small-cell lung cancer: a phase 3 randomised controlled trial. *Lancet*, **385** (9962), 36–42.

138 Arriagada, R., Le Chevalier, T., Borie, F., *et al.* (1995) Prophylactic cranial irradiation for patients with small-cell lung cancer in complete remission. *J. Natl Cancer Inst.*, **87** (3), 183–190.

139 Auperin, A., Arriagada, R., Pignon, J.P., *et al.* (1999) Prophylactic cranial irradiation for patients with small-cell lung cancer in complete remission. Prophylactic Cranial Irradiation Overview Collaborative Group. *N. Engl. J. Med.*, **341** (7), 476–484.

140 Le Pechoux, C., Dunant, A., Senan, S., *et al.* (2009) Standard-dose versus higher-dose prophylactic cranial irradiation (PCI) in patients with limited-stage small-cell lung cancer in complete remission after chemotherapy and thoracic radiotherapy (PCI 99-01, EORTC 22003-08004, RTOG 0212, and IFCT 99-01): a randomised clinical trial. *Lancet Oncol.*, **10** (5), 467–474.

141 Le Pechoux, C., Laplanche, A., Faivre-Finn, C., *et al.*, Prophylactic Cranial Irradiation Collaborative Group (2011) Clinical neurological outcome and quality of life among patients with limited small-cell cancer treated with two different doses of prophylactic cranial irradiation in the intergroup phase III trial (PCI99-01, EORTC 22003-08004, RTOG 0212 and IFCT 99-01). *Ann. Oncol.*, **22** (5), 1154–1163.

142 Slotman, B., Faivre-Finn, C., Kramer, G., *et al.* (2007) Prophylactic cranial irradiation in extensive small-cell lung cancer. *N. Engl. J. Med.*, **357** (7), 664–672.

143 Seute, T., Leffers, P., ten Velde, G.P., Twijnstra, A. (2008) Detection of brain metastases from small cell lung cancer: consequences of changing imaging techniques (CT versus MRI). *Cancer*, **112** (8), 1827–1834.

144 Li, J., Bentzen, S.M., Renschler, M., Mehta, M.P. (2007) Regression after whole-brain radiation therapy for brain metastases correlates with survival and improved neurocognitive function. *J. Clin. Oncol.*, **25** (10), 1260–1266.

145 Scott, C., Suh, J., Stea, B., Nabid, A., Hackman, J. (2007) Improved survival, quality of life, and quality-adjusted survival in breast cancer patients treated with efaproxiral (Efaproxyn) plus whole-brain radiation therapy for brain metastases. *Am. J. Clin. Oncol.*, **30** (6), 580–587.

146 Meyers, C.A., Smith, J.A., Bezjak, A., *et al.* (2004) Neurocognitive function and progression in patients with brain metastases treated with whole-brain radiation and motexafin gadolinium: results of a randomized phase III trial. *J. Clin. Oncol.*, **22** (1), 157–165.

147 Wolfson, A.H., Bae, K., Komaki, R., *et al.* (2011) Primary analysis of a phase II randomized trial Radiation Therapy Oncology Group (RTOG) 0212: impact of different total doses and schedules of prophylactic cranial irradiation on chronic neurotoxicity and quality of life for patients with limited-disease small-cell lung cancer. *Int. J. Radiat. Oncol. Biol. Phys.*, **81** (1), 77–84.

148 Lester, J.F., MacBeth, F.R., Coles, B. (2005) Prophylactic cranial irradiation for preventing brain metastases in patients undergoing radical treatment for non-small-cell lung cancer: a Cochrane Review. *Int. J. Radiat. Oncol. Biol. Phys.*, **63** (3), 690–694.

149 Gore, E.M., Bae, K., Wong, S.J., *et al.* (2011) Phase III comparison of prophylactic cranial irradiation versus observation in patients with locally advanced non-small-cell lung cancer: primary analysis of radiation therapy oncology group study RTOG 0214. *J. Clin. Oncol.*, **29** (3), 272–278.

20

Carcinoma of the Esophagus

Grace J. Kim and Mohan Suntharalingam

Introduction

Despite remarkable advances having been made in the diagnosis and management of cancer over the past century, esophageal cancer continues to pose a significant therapeutic challenge. In 2017, the American Cancer Society estimates that a total of 16 940 new cases of esophageal cancer would be identified in the United States, and 15 690 resultant deaths [1]. The high mortality rate relative to the number of newly diagnosed cases is indicative of the aggressive nature of this disease. The majority of patients present with locally advanced disease, and up to 40% of patients have metastatic disease at presentation [2]. The understanding that there is a high chance of both local and systemic failure in patients presenting with locally advanced disease has led to the development of combined-modality treatment strategies that have attempted to deal with these competing risks. In this chapter, attention will be focused on the work-up and management of esophageal cancer and its treatment with either definitive chemoradiotherapy or trimodality therapy. Novel esophageal cancer treatment strategies such as intensity-modulated radiation therapy (IMRT) and biologic therapy will also be reviewed.

Etiology

Etiologic factors and predisposing conditions for esophageal cancer vary depending on histology. For squamous cell cancers of the esophagus, risk factors include alcohol and tobacco use, radiation, Plummer–Vinson syndrome, and occupational exposures including asbestos and perchoroethylene. Squamous cell carcinoma had previously accounted for more than 90% of all esophageal cancers; however, lower esophageal adenocarcinomas in the setting of Barrett esophagus

have increased in incidence during recent years and now represent more than 50% of all patients [3–6]. Between 1975 and 2004, Surveillance, Epidemiology and End Results Program (SEER) data analysis reported that the incidence of adenocarcinoma in the United States had increased by 335% and 463% among white women and men, respectively, while the incidence of squamous cell carcinoma had declined in the population regardless of race or gender. Clear reasons for the increase in adenocarcinoma are unknown but are thought to be largely due to increases in obesity and reflux. It should be noted that obesity has been found to be a risk factor independent of reflux [7,8].

Presentation

Esophageal cancer presents as a fungating, ulcerative, or infiltrative tumor. The most common gross appearance of the tumor is a combination of these features, with fungating, ulcerated intraluminal tumor infiltrating the esophageal wall and causing concentric narrowing of the central esophageal lumen. Submucosal spread of this tumor can be quite extensive, and skip metastasis along the submucosal lymphatics has been found as far as 8 cm from the site of the gross tumor [9]. The absence of a serosal covering of the esophagus is another significant factor for early radial extension of the tumor into surrounding structures. Over 50% of patients present with locally advanced or metastatic disease.

Several updates have been made in the staging system reflecting the evolving understanding of esophageal cancer (Figure 20.1). Histology has been incorporated into the staging system where squamous cell and adenocarcinomas are divided into separate stage groupings reflecting their different biologies and outcomes [7, 10]. Location has also been incorporated into staging where

Clinical Radiation Oncology: Indications, Techniques, and Results, Third Edition. Edited by William Small Jr.
© 2017 John Wiley & Sons, Inc. Published 2017 by John Wiley & Sons, Inc.

T-stage:

T1 – invades lamina propria, muscular mucosae, or submucosa

T1a – invades lamina propria or muscular mucosae

T1b – invades submucosa

T2 – invades mucularis propria

T3 – invades adventitia

T4 – invades adjacent structures

T4a – resectable tumor invading pleura, pericardium, or diaphragm

T4b – unresectable tumor invading other adjacent structures, such as aorta, vertebral body, trachea, etc.

N-stage:

Regional lymph nodes "extend from periesophageal cervical nodes to celiac nodes."

N0 – no lymph node metastases

N1 – metastasis in 1-2 regional nodes

N2 – metastasis in 3-6 regional nodes

N3 – metastasis in 7 or more nodes

M-stage:

M0 – no distant metastasis

M1 – distant metastasis

Squamous
- IA – Any location: T1a N0 and Grade 1 (or Grade unknown)
- IB – Any location: T1a N0 and Grade 2-3, T1b N0 and Grade 1-3 (or Grade Unknown)
- IB – Any location: T2 N0 and Grade 1
- IIA – Upper or middle tumor: T3 N0 and Grade 1

- IIA – Lower tumor/X: T3 N0 and Any Grade
- IIA – Any location: T2 N0 and Grade 1, Grade 2-3 (or Grade unkown)
- IIB – Upper or middle tumor: T2-3 N0 and Grade 2-3
- IIB – Any location: T1 N1, or T3 N0, Grade Unknown

The stages below are the same for squamous + adeno:
- IIIA – Any location: T1 N2, T2 N1
- IIIB – Any location: T2 N2, T3 N1-2, T4a N0-1
- IVA – Any location: T4a N2, T4b, N0-2, Any T N3
- IV – M1

Adenocarcinoma
- IA – T1a N0 and Grade 1 (or Grade unknown)
- IB – T1a N0 and Grade 2, T1b N0 and Grade 1-2 (or GX)
- IC – T1 N0 and Grade 3, T2 N0 and Grade 1-2
- IIA – T2 N0 and Grade 3 (or Grade unknown)
- IIB – T3 N0, T1 N1

The stages below are the same for squamous + adeno:
- IIIA – T1 N2, T2 N1
- IIIB – T2 N2, T3 N1-2, T4a N0-1
- IVA – T4a N2, T4b, N0-2, Any T N3
- IVB – M1

Figure 20.1 Tumor staging. Reprinted with permission from: Amin, M.B., *et al.* (eds) (2017) Esophagus and Esophagogastric Junction, in *AJCC Cancer Staging Manual*, 8th edition. Springer, New York, pp. 185–202.

upper- or mid-esophageal tumors are staged higher than anatomically lower tumors. In addition, N-staging has been updated from an emphasis on location of involved lymph node chains to the number of involved lymph nodes. Previously, involvement of celiac and supraclavicular nodes was classified as M1 disease, but these have now been redefined as regional nodes [11, 12].

Anatomic Considerations

The esophagus is generally divided into three anatomic regions [13]. The cervical esophagus extends from the cricopharyngeal sphincter at the pharyngoesophageal junction, down to the level of the thoracic inlet, approximately 18 cm from the upper incisor teeth. The middle third extends from the thoracic inlet to a point 10 cm above the gastroesophageal junction, a point usually at the level of the eighth thoracic vertebra and approximately 31 cm from the upper incisors. In the upper two-thirds region, the esophagus is in immediate contact with the tracheobronchus, aorta, the azygous vein, and the vertebral column. The lower third of the esophagus extends from a point 10 cm above the gastroesophageal junction to the cardiac orifice of the stomach, a point approximately 40 cm from the upper incisors. The distal thoracic esophagus is also in close contact with the pericardium of the left atrium, the inferior vena cava, and the descending aorta. Squamous cell carcinomas are often found in the upper to middle third of the esophagus, while adenocarcinomas are commonly found in the distal esophagus.

Work-Up

Currently, upper gastrointestinal endoscopy is the chief modality used to identify tumor presence and location with respect to the incisors or esophagogastric junction. For patients with esophageal cancer involving the upper two-thirds of the esophagus, bronchoscopy may also be performed at the physician's discretion at the time of esophagoscopy to evaluate the trachea or tracheobronchi for tumor invasion.

Computed tomography (CT) is used to rule out metastatic disease and to evaluate the periesophageal area for enlarged lymph nodes. Locoregional assessment of esophageal tumor involvement however is not adequate with CT. Endoscopic ultrasound (EUS) is the most reliable in assessing the tumor's depth of invasion, and involvement of the surrounding normal tissue and regional lymph nodes [14–16]. EUS was shown to be 82% accurate in determining transmural extension (T3 or T4), and 85.5% accurate in detecting mediastinal nodal disease [17,18]. However, for superficial T1 lesions its accuracy drops to 67% [19]. In general, EUS is better than CT, positron emission tomography (PET) or magnetic resonance imaging (MRI) for local staging [20]. An additional benefit of EUS is that abnormal appearing nodes also can be biopsied during the procedure.

For the evaluation of distant disease, PET imaging is the most sensitive [21]. Flamen *et al.* reported PET/CT to be more accurate at detecting stage IV disease than the combination of CT and EUS (82% versus 64%), with a higher specificity for regional and distant lymph node involvement (98% versus 90%). When PET staging was added to CT and EUS, 22% of patients also had a significant change in stage: 15% were upstaged to stage IV disease, while 7% were downstaged to a stage in which curative therapy became appropriate [22].

PET scanning also aids in identifying the extent of the primary tumor. The degree of standardized uptake value (SUV) of the primary tumor has also been found to be prognostic, as a high SUV portends a worse survival [23]. PET can also be useful in identifying involved lymph nodes, but EUS staging is still considered to be more accurate [22].

In many institutions, PET is also used to re-stage patients after induction chemoradiation therapy. In a retrospective review of potential trimodality candidates, PET-CT identified the appearance of metastatic disease in 8% after completion of neoadjuvant therapy. These authors also reported that the pathologic response was unpredictable using PET-CT [24]. However, other retrospective series have reported that PET-CT may have a significant predictive benefit with the potential to detect which patients may need salvage surgery versus those patients that may avoid surgery. The use of PET after neoadjuvant therapy to determine prognosis, or as an

indication for surgery, still needs to be validated. The Phase II MUNICON study evaluated PET-CT response as a guide for administering continued chemotherapy in locally advanced esophageal and gastroesophageal junction adenocarcinomas. Using PET-CT, 110 evaluable patients were assessed for metabolic response after two weeks of induction chemotherapy. Subsequently, 49% of patients had a metabolic response and were designated to receive chemotherapy for another 10 weeks before undergoing resection. Those that did not respond to chemotherapy immediately went for resection. In responders, the median overall survival had not been reached at a follow-up time of 2.3 years, but the median overall survival in non-responders was 25.8 months. Median event-free survivals between the responders and non-responders were 29.7 months and 14.1 months, respectively [25]. The results of this and other trials have led to the currently accruing CALGB 80803 trial, which will use PET-CT scanning SUV after induction chemotherapy to determine subsequent chemotherapy administered during radiation.

Indication for Radiation Therapy in Multimodality Therapy for Carcinoma of the Esophagus

The role of radiation therapy in the management of esophageal cancer can be categorized as follows: (i) concurrent chemoradiotherapy for locally advanced and/or medically inoperable esophageal cancer; (ii) radiation therapy in combination with multi-drug chemotherapy as preoperative therapy for marginally resectable or resectable esophageal cancer; and (iii) palliative radiation therapy for obstructive symptoms.

Early reports of single modality therapy for esophageal cancer yielded disappointing results, with long-term survival achieved in less than 10% of patients [26,27]. Earlam *et al.* performed two separate meta-analyses examining both surgery-alone and radiation-alone trials for esophageal cancer. Surgery-alone trials revealed a five-year overall survival of 12%, while radiation-alone trials yielded equally disappointing results with a five-year overall survival rate of 6%. The patterns of failure in patients treated with radiation therapy alone have consistently shown poor local control as well as distant failure rates of up to 66%, even when patients were treated with doses greater than 50 Gy [28]. The addition of chemotherapy to radiation therapy was, therefore, a logical next step in the evolution of therapy for esophageal carcinoma.

Some of the first reports of combined modality therapy were led by Fujimake *et al.*, who described increased pathologic response rates of up to almost 70% with the addition of bleomycin to radiation [29]. Herskovic and colleagues at Wayne State University reported results

Table 20.1 Single-institution results for definitive chemoradiation therapy in patients with esophageal cancer.

Trial/Reference	No. of patients	Radiation dose (Gy)	Chemotherapeutic agents	Median survival (months)	2-Year survival (%)
Herskovic *et al.* [30]	39	30.0	Cisplatin, 5-FU	9.8	20
	22	50.0	Cisplatin, 5-FU	19.5	36
Coia *et al.* [31]	30	60.0	Cisplatin, Mitomycin C	18.0	47
Keane *et al.* [66]	20	22.5–25.0	5-FU, Mitomycin C	–	12
	15	45.0–50.0		–	48
John *et al.* [67]	30	41.4–50.4	Cisplatin, 5-FU, Mitomycin C	11.0	29

5-FU, 5-fluorouracil.

from 39 patients who received definitive chemoradiation therapy with or without surgery, with a radiation therapy dose of 30 Gy and concurrent cisplatin and 5-fluorouracil (5-FU). Because the initial two-year survival was 20%, the radiation dose was increased to 50 Gy in an additional 22 patients and two-year survivals were subsequently increased to 36% [30].

Coia *et al.* from the Fox Chase Cancer Center reported a Phase II study of 57 stage I–II patients who were treated definitively with concurrent chemoradiation, and 33 stage III and IV patients who were treated palliatively. Definitive treatment consisted of a radiation therapy dose to 60 Gy with continuous infusion of 5-FU (days 1-4) during weeks 1 and 2, and mitomycin C ($10\,mg\,m^{-2}$) on day 2. For these stage I and II patients, the median survival was 18 months and the three- and five-year overall survivals were 29% and 18%, respectively. Moderate and severe acute toxicity rates approached 56%, which was deemed acceptable [31]. Other initial Phase II experiences of combined modality therapy with platinum chemotherapy and radiation are listed in Table 20.1.

The standard of care for definitive esophageal cancer treatment was defined by a Phase III trial performed by the Radiation Therapy Oncology Group. The RTOG 85-01 study involved a randomization between concurrent combination of chemotherapy (four cycles of 5-FU, 1000 mg m^2, continuous 24-h intravenous infusion for the first four days of weeks 1, 5, 8, and 11, and cisplatin 75 mg m^{-2} on the first day of each cycle) and radiation therapy (50 Gy in 2-Gy fractions), or with radiation therapy (64 Gy, 2-Gy fractions) alone for patients with carcinoma of the thoracic esophagus. A total of 202 patients was enrolled in the study, and after a planned interim analysis the study met stopping rules and was closed early. Squamous cell cancer accounted for 90% of all patients. The five-year median survival in the radiation-alone arm was 9.3 months versus 14.1 months in those treated with chemoradiation therapy. The five-year overall survival was accordingly 0% in the single-modality arm versus 26% for the combined modality arm. Improvements in local control and distant

failure with chemoradiation were met with increased acute toxicity with severe toxicity rates (44% versus 20%); late toxicity was similar in both arms [30]. Other randomized trials also revealed increased acute toxicity with the addition of chemotherapy, with esophagitis and hematologic toxicity as the most substantial side effects. To date, four major randomized Phase III studies have been conducted (see Table 20.2) comparing definitive chemoradiation with radiation therapy alone, all showing a benefit to combined modality therapy.

Despite the survival benefit with chemoradiation therapy, local control still remained in the 50–70% range. As a result, the Intergroup trial 0123 was designed to examine the role of radiation dose escalation with concurrent chemotherapy [32]. Because of the acute toxicity identified in the RTOG 85-01 trial, dose and field size adjustments were made in an attempt to offset expected increases in toxicity that might be seen with dose escalation. In RTOG 85-01, the daily radiation dose was 2.0 Gy and field size was the entire esophagus to 30 Gy, with a smaller boost to 20 Gy to a field size with a 5 cm superior and inferior margin [32]. In the Intergroup trial, the dose was 1.8 Gy per day and the field size was 5 cm superior and inferior to the tumor and 2 cm radially. In total, 236 patients were accrued, and after a planned interim analysis the study was closed after the high-dose arm was found unlikely to have a statistical benefit with a median survival of 13 months in the high-dose arm and 18 months in the low-dose arm, with similar local controls in each arm (56% versus 52%, respectively). There was also higher grade V toxicity in the high-dose arm (11 versus 2 deaths). It is important to note that seven deaths in the high-dose arm occurred in patients who had received less than 50 Gy [32].

Definitive Chemoradiation versus Trimodality Therapy

In efforts to improve local control, adding surgery to chemoradiation has been investigated in two randomized trials. Bedenne *et al.* randomized patients who had

Table 20.2 Results from randomized trials evaluating radiation therapy alone versus chemoradiotherapy in patients with esophageal cancer.

Trial/Reference	No. of patients	Radiation dose (Gy)	Chemotherapeutic agents	2-Year survival (%)
Araujo *et al.* [68]	28	50.0	None	22
	31	50.0	5-FU, Mitomycin C	38
Smith *et al.* [69]	62	40.0	None	12*
	65	40.0	5-FU, Mitomycin C	27*
Wobbes *et al.* [70]	111	40.0*	None	15*
	110	40.0*	Cisplatin	20*
		*split course		
Cooper *et al.* [71]	62	64.0	None	0*^
	61	50.0	Cisplatin, 5-FU	26*^
				^3-year survival

*Statistically significant.
FU, 5-fluorouracil.

potentially resectable esophageal cancer to chemoradiation alone or trimodality therapy. For this, 455 patients were enrolled and all received two cycles of cisplatin and 5-FU concurrently, with a total radiation dose of 46 Gy. Some 89% of the patients had squamous cell histology. Patients with at least a partial response were then randomized to surgical resection or an additional three cycles of chemotherapy and 20 Gy. Overall survival (36% versus 40%) and local control (34% versus 40%) were not significantly different between both arms. The three-month mortality was significantly greater in the trimodality arm (9.3% versus 0.8%; p = 0.002) [33]. However, in a 2008 update of the trial, non-randomized patients who were non-responders were found to have a survival benefit with surgical resection [34].

Similarly, Stahl and colleagues published the details of a Phase III randomized trial of 172 patients with T3 or T4 and N0 or N1 squamous cell carcinomas staged by CT and EUS. After randomization, all patients underwent induction chemotherapy with three cycles of 5-FU, leucovorin, etoposide, and cisplatin. Patients randomized to the trimodality arm then received concurrent chemoradiotherapy (cisplatin, etoposide, and 40 Gy) followed by surgery, while patients assigned to the definitive chemoradiotherapy arm received the same chemotherapy with >65 Gy. The three-year overall survival was not statistically different between those patients who underwent definitive chemoradiation and those with trimodality therapy (20% versus 28%). The two-year progression-free survival was significantly better in the trimodality arm (64% versus 40%), but treatment-related mortality was also significantly higher in the surgical group. On multivariate analysis, several prognostic factors were evaluated, though only tumor response after induction chemotherapy proved to be statistically significant. Although an improvement in local control was

observed in the trimodality therapy arm, the high postoperative mortality rate counteracted any potential gain in survival associated with the addition of surgery [35].

The results of these two Phase III randomized trials comparing trimodality therapy to definitive chemoradiation are strikingly similar in their outcomes. In both trials, the addition of surgery to chemoradiation therapy was associated with an increased treatment-related toxicity, which ultimately compromised overall survival. Further investigation is warranted in delineating factors associated with increased risk of mortality after surgery, and in the identification of suitable patient populations for trimodality therapy, which may yield more favorable results. Because all patients on the Stahl trial, and 89% on the Bedenne trial, had a squamous cell histology, definitive conclusions from these two randomized trials may be limited. Ultimately, both studies reinforced definitive chemoradiation therapy as the standard of care in the management of locally advanced esophageal cancer. For squamous cell carcinoma of the esophagus, pathologic response rates appear to be higher than adenocarcinoma [36], so in the case of a pathologic complete response a potentially morbid surgery for additional local control may be avoided.

Several randomized trials have also been conducted to examine the benefit of adding chemoradiation followed by surgery compared to surgery alone (Table 20.3). Walsh *et al.* compared preoperative chemoradiotherapy and surgery with surgery alone in 113 patients with esophageal adenocarcinoma. The preoperative therapy included two cycles of chemotherapy during weeks 1 and 6 (5-FU 15 mg kg^{-1} daily for five days, and cisplatin 75 mg m^{-2} on day 7 of each cycle) and concurrent radiotherapy (40 Gy in 15 fractions in three weeks). The median survival time was 16 months for the multimodality therapy, compared to 11 months for surgery alone. The

Table 20.3 Trimodality versus surgery-alone trials.

Trial	No. of patients	Radiation dose (Gy)	Chemotherapeutic agents	3-Year survival (%)
Bosset *et al.* [72]	139	None	None	37
	143	37	Cisplatin	38
Urba *et al.* [38]	50	None	None	16
	50	45	5-FU, Cisplatin, Vincristine	30
Burmeister *et al.* [73]	128	None	None	33
	128	35	Cisplatin, 5-FU	36
Mariette *et al.* (only	98	None	None	43.8 months
Stage I and II patients	97	45	Cisplatin, 5-FU	31.8 months
included in this trial) [74]				
Walsh *et al.* [37]	58	None	None	6*
	50	40	Cisplatin, 5-FU	32*
Tepper *et al.* [39]	26	None	None	20*
	30	50.4	Cisplatin, 5-FU	65*
Shapiro *et al.* [40]	162	None	None	48*
	158	41.4	Carboplatin, Paclitaxel	59*

*Statistically significant.

survival rates at one, two and three years were 52%, 37%, and 32%, respectively, for patients treated with a multimodality regimen, compared to 44%, 26%, and 6% for those assigned to surgery alone, with the survival advantage favoring multimodality therapy (p = 0.01) [37].

Urba *et al.* also reported a randomized study in which the combination of preoperative chemoradiotherapy and surgery was compared with surgery alone. The preoperative therapy consisted of an intensive course of chemotherapy (cisplatin 20 mg m^{-2} on days 1–5 and 17–21; vinblastine 1 mg m^{-2} on days 1–4 and 17–20; 5-FU 300 mg^{-2} on days 1–21) and radiotherapy (45 Gy in fractions of 1.5 Gy, twice daily for three weeks). Surgery was performed on day 42. Fifty patients were randomized to each arm. Adenocarcinoma accounted for 75% of all patients. The median survival time and three-year survival rate were 16.9 months and 30%, respectively, for the combined therapy group, compared to 17.6 months and 16%, respectively, for the surgery-alone group (p = 0.15). Local-regional recurrence as the first site of failure was noted in 39% of patients treated with surgery alone, compared to 19% of patients in the combined-therapy group (p = 0.039). Pathologic complete response was associated with improved survival (p = 0.006) [38].

Tepper *et al.* randomized esophageal and gastroesophageal junction tumors to either surgery alone or trimodality therapy with cisplatin 100 mg m^{-2} and 5-FU 1000 mg m^{-2} per day for 4 days during weeks 1 and 5, with concurrent radiation therapy 50.4 Gy in 1.8-Gy daily fractions. The trial was closed due to poor accrual, and ultimately 30 patients were assigned to the trimodality arm and 26 underwent surgery alone. The five-year survival was in favor of trimodality therapy, with 39% versus 16% and a median survival of 4.48 years versus 1.79 years (p = 0.002) [39].

More recently, the Phase III CROSS trial enrolled 364 esophageal trimodality candidates, with patients randomized to either surgery alone or chemoradiation followed by surgery. Chemoradiation consisted of weekly carboplatin and paclitaxel with 41.4 Gy of radiation therapy. Surgery was scheduled within six weeks of neoadjuvant therapy completion. Some 92.3% of the chemoradiotherapy arm were able to have R0 resections, in contrast to 67% of those in the surgery-alone arm. The three-year survival was improved with the addition of chemoradiation (59% versus 48%; p = 0.011). Post-treatment toxicity rates were similar in both groups [40].

Radiation Therapy Technique

Radiotherapeutic factors important in the achievement of therapeutic goals include a clear definition of target volume, optimal radiation dose and fractionation schedules, and proper radiation portal arrangements to secure adequate dose distribution within the target volume while the surrounding normal tissues are protected.

Target Volume

The target volume consists of the clinical target volume (CTV) and gross tumor volume (GTV). The use of esophagogastroduodenoscopy (EGD), EUS, CT and

PET/CT can aid in delineating the GTV. The CTV often includes 4 cm proximal and distal and 1 cm radially beyond the gross tumor. Depending on the esophagus region involved, respective regional nodal groups should be covered. For cervical esophageal lesions (10–15 cm from incisors), supraclavicular regions should be covered; mid-esophageal (>15–30 cm from incisors): paraesophageal nodes; and distal esophageal lesions (>30 cm from incisors), celiac nodes. The planning target volume (PTV) can be created by adding a 1- to 2-cm margin around the CTV.

Optimal Dose and Fractionation Schedules

Several different fractionation schedules have similar biologic effects on normal and neoplastic tissues. Recent advances in radiation biology indicate that, for the same total dose, the late reaction of the intrathoracic normal tissue can be reduced if small daily fractions (i.e., 1.8–2.0 Gy instead of 2.5–3.0 Gy) are used [41, 42].

In preoperative chemoradiotherapy for resectable carcinoma of the esophagus, a total dose of 45–50.4 Gy administered at 1.8-Gy daily fractions, five days a week, has been the standard regimen [43]. In the setting of trimodality therapy, the CROSS trial used 41.4 Gy with carboplatin and paclitaxel chemotherapy [44], and if there is any difficulty in reaching normal tissue constraints then using a lower radiation dose is reasonable. Altered fractionation schedules such as accelerated schedule (45 Gy in 30 fractions in three weeks using a 1.5-Gy per fraction, twice-daily treatment schedule) and a hybrid schedule of twice-daily radiation treatment during chemotherapy cycles and once-daily treatment between the chemotherapy cycles (58.5Gy in 34 fractions in five weeks) have been also been tested for tolerance, tumor response, and survival.

Patients judged incurable because of their poor general condition or the presence of distant metastases can be treated with speedy fractionation schedules. A total dose of 40–45 Gy at 2.2–2.5 Gy daily fractions, five days a week, is a reasonable schedule for palliation of dysphagia.

New Trends

Targeted Therapies

The discovery of growth factors, cell-surface receptors, and their resultant signaling cascades, has led to a greater understanding of tumorigenesis. Dysregulation of angiogenesis, inflammation, cell cycle control, growth, and cell migration are all essential components of neoplastic transformation which involve growth factors and cell-surface receptors. A new class of systemic therapy specifically targeting cellular growth protein receptors and downstream signaling pathways has shown promising results in improving the therapeutic ratio of oncologic treatment.

The epidermal growth factor receptor (EGFR, ErbB-1) is a member of the ErbB family of receptor tyrosine kinases. These receptors combine an extracellular ligand-binding domain with an intracellular tyrosine kinase which, upon activation, initiates cell signaling cascades. Activation of these receptors in cancer cells results in several downstream effects, including autocrine stimulation, mutation, and/or overexpression. Approximately 90% of esophageal carcinomas have been shown to overexpress EGFR, which has been correlated with a poor prognosis in several studies [45–48]. As a result, several molecular targeting strategies have been developed, and these include antibodies to the extracellular ligand-binding domain or small-molecule inhibitors blocking the receptor tyrosine kinase activity. Several targeted agents and their mechanisms of action are listed in Table 20.4.

Cetuximab, a monoclonal (IgG1) antibody against the extracellular domain of EGFR, has been studied in conjunction with radiation therapy. Pre-clinical studies have suggested a synergistic effect with the addition of cetuximab to radiation therapy in head and neck squamous-cell carcinoma lines [49]. Proposed mechanisms of radiosensitization include: induction of G1 cell-cycle arrest; inhibition of cellular proliferation; promotion of radiation-induced apoptosis; inhibition of radiation-induced damage repair; and inhibition of tumor angiogenesis.

Recently, a Phase III randomized study of radiation therapy versus radiation therapy and cetuximab in patients with locally advanced head and neck cancer demonstrated a local control and overall survival benefit with the addition of cetuximab. Notably, there was no increase in treatment-related toxicity in patients who received cetuximab [50]. While cetuximab and radiation therapy has been shown to be tolerable and efficacious, the addition of chemotherapy to this treatment strategy remains investigational.

Two Phase II studies incorporating cetuximab with chemoradiation, in esophageal carcinoma, have recently been reported but with conflicting results. In the first study 50.4 Gy was administered in 28 fractions of radiation therapy and concurrent weekly cisplatin 30 mg m^{-2}, irinotecan 65 mg m^{-2}, and cetuximab 250 mg on weeks 1, 2, 4, and 5, followed by surgery four to eight weeks after completion of radiotherapy. When compared to similar studies in patients undergoing trimodality therapy, the addition of cetuximab resulted in a lower complete response rate and higher overall toxicity [51]. Conversely, investigators from the Brown University Oncology Group and the University of Maryland

Table 20.4 Selected targeted biologic agents.

Agent	Target	Mechanism of action
Cetuximab	EGFR	Antibody to the extracellular domain which prevents ligand binding and subsequent activation of the receptor.
Erlotinib	EGFR	Small-molecule tyrosine kinase inhibitor which prevents kinase activity from initiating downstream signaling cascade.
Trastuzumab	HER-2	Antibody to the extracellular domain which prevents ligand binding and subsequent activation of the receptor.
Laptinib	EGFR/HER-2	Small-molecule tyrosine kinase inhibitor which prevents kinase activity from initiating downstream signaling cascade.
Bevacizumab	VEGF	Antibody to the VEGF ligand which prevents its binding to and activation of the VEGFR.
Sorafenib	PDGFR/VEGFR/Flt-3/c-Kit/Raf	Small-molecule tyrosine kinase inhibitor which prevents kinase activity from initiating downstream signaling cascade.

EGFR, epidermal growth factor receptor; PDGFR, platelet-derived growth factor receptor; VEGF, vascular endothelial growth factor; VEGFR, vascular endothelial growth factor receptor.

Greenebaum Cancer Center found an endoscopic complete response rate of 65% and acceptable toxicity in a Phase II trial of cetuximab, carboplatin, paclitaxel, and 50.4 Gy of radiation therapy [52]. Ultimately, the role of cetuximab in combination with definitive chemoradiotherapy was evaluated in a Phase III trial run by the RTOG, where preliminary findings found no survival or local control benefit with the addition of cetuximab [53].

HER-2 (ErbB2), another member of the ErbB receptor family, has also been shown in several studies to be overexpressed in esophageal carcinoma lines [54–56]. HER-2 overexpression has been linked to increased tumor invasiveness, lymph node metastasis, and chemoresistance. Trastuzumab is a humanized IgG1 antibody against the HER-2 receptor. There appear to be multiple mechanisms through which the antibody exerts its effect, including: G1 cell-cycle arrest; downregulation of the HER-2 receptor; disruption of downstream signaling cascades; suppression of angiogenesis; and promotion of apoptosis. Safran and associates recently reported the details of a Phase I/II trial of locally advanced adenocarcinoma treated with trastuzumab, paclitaxel, cisplatin, and radiation therapy in patients with HER-2 overexpression. Some 33% of screened patients overexpressed HER-2, as assessed by immunohistochemistry. The median survival for the cohort was 18 months, with 42% of patients alive at two years [58]. In addition, the randomized Phase III ToGA trial tested the benefit of adding trastuzumab to standard chemotherapy in advanced gastric or gastroesophageal junction cancer. Trastuzumab increased the median survival to 13.8 months versus 11.1 months (p = 0.0046) for those that received chemotherapy alone [58]. These findings, therefore, warrant further investigation in patients with HER-2 overexpression and are currently being investigated in RTOG 10-10. In this current trimodality trial, Her-2-positive esophageal cancer patients will be randomized between Arm 1 (chemoradiation with trastuzumab) and Arm 2 (chemoradiation alone). All patients then are to undergo surgical resection. Patients in arm 1 are to receive 13 more cycles after surgery.

Vascular endothelial growth factor (VEGF) is a family of potent endothelial growth factors which have been extensively investigated in cancer therapy. VEGF has been shown to be involved in the regulation of vascular permeability and proliferation and also has apoptotic effects. Bevacizumab, an antibody against VEGF, has been shown to have radiosensitizing effects in preclinical studies with esophageal cancer lines [59]. As a result, ongoing trials incorporating bevacizumab into chemoradiation regimens are being evaluated in Phase II trials. However, in light of recent reports of increased associated tracheoesophageal fistula formation in other disease sites, the use of bevacizumab may be limited.

Intensity-Modulated Radiotherapy (IMRT)

IMRT has been found invaluable in the treatment of cancers such as prostate and head and neck, in allowing dose escalation while limiting the radiation dose to surrounding normal tissues. IMRT has also been shown to be useful in the treatment of esophageal cancers, with the potential to reduce lung and heart doses, as demonstrated in several dosimetric studies. In an M.D. Anderson study, the dose-volume of normal lung was reduced in distal esophageal cancers with IMRT with mean absolute improvements of 10% for V_{10}, 5% for V_{20}, and 2.5 Gy for Mean Lung Dose over 3D conformal radiation [60]. Wu and Nutting both showed IMRT planning to be superior to 3D planning in terms of dose-sparing of the lung and spinal cord, homogeneity, and dose conformity [61, 62]. In addition, IMRT may be useful in treating the cervical esophagus because of the anatomical challenge of the upper esophageal location [63]. Likewise, in the cervical esophagus, Fu *et al.* showed that IMRT reduced V_{20} and V_{30} lung volumes [64]. La *et al.* at Stanford, used IMRT either as a definitive or a preoperative therapy and found it to be effective and well-tolerated, with an actuarial two-year local control of 64% and two-year disease-free and overall survival rates of 38% and 35%, respectively [65]. Additional studies are required to confirm whether IMRT provides a definite benefit over 3D conformal radiation therapy.

Conclusions

Over the past 50 years, the management of locally advanced esophageal cancer has evolved from single-modality therapy to a combined-modality approach. The addition of chemotherapy to radiation therapy has led to a dramatic increase in overall survival when compared to radiation alone; however, five-year survival rates of 20–25% leave room for improvement. Increases in distant failure seen over the past 20 years are likely the result of improved local control, and therefore newer strategies should address this changing pattern of failure. The addition of surgery to chemoradiation continues to remain controversial and, ultimately, further investigation is warranted to identify subgroups of patients who are most likely to benefit from this aggressive approach. Recent advances in understanding the molecular biology of cancer have led to the development of targeted systemic therapy. As biologic agents are integrated into chemoradiation regimens, comparisons to standard cisplatin and 5-FU must be performed in Phase III trials. As the present understanding of the biology of esophageal carcinoma improves, better patient-specific therapies will surely lead to improved long-term survival.

References

1 Siegel, R.L., Miller, K.D., Jemal, A. (2017) Cancer statistics, 2017. *CA Cancer J. Clin.*, **67** (1), 7–30.

2 Jemal, A., Siegel, R., Ward, E., Murray, T., Xu, J., Smigal, C., *et al.* (2006) Cancer statistics, 2006. *CA Cancer J. Clin.*, **56** (2), 106–130.

3 Naef, A.P., Savary, M., Ozzello, L. (1975) Columnar-lined lower esophagus: an acquired lesion with malignant predisposition. Report on 140 cases of Barrett's esophagus with 12 adenocarcinomas. *J. Thorac. Cardiovasc. Surg.*, **70** (5), 826–835.

4 Poleynard, G.D., Marty, A.T., Birnbaum, W.B., Nelson, L.E., O'Reilly, R.R. (1977) Adenocarcinoma in the columnar-lined (Barrett) esophagus. Case report and review of the literature. *Arch. Surg.*, **112** (8), 997–1000.

5 Cameron, A.J., Ott, B.J., Payne, W.S. (1985) The incidence of adenocarcinoma in columnar-lined (Barrett's) esophagus. *N. Engl. J. Med.*, **313** (14), 857–859.

6 Blot, W.J., Devesa, S.S., Fraumeni, J.F., Jr. (1993) Continuing climb in rates of esophageal adenocarcinoma: an update. *JAMA*, **270** (11), 1320.

7 Brown, L.M., Devesa, S.S. (2002) Epidemiologic trends in esophageal and gastric cancer in the United States. *Surg. Oncol. Clin. North Am.*, **11** (2), 235–256.

8 Brown, L.M., Devesa, S.S., Chow, W.H. (2008) Incidence of adenocarcinoma of the esophagus among white Americans by sex, stage, and age. *J. Natl Cancer Inst.*, **100** (16), 1184–1187.

9 Goodner, J.T., Miller, T.P., Pack, G.T., Watson, W.L. (1956) Torek esophagectomy; the case against segmental resection for esophageal cancer. *J. Thorac. Surg.*, **32** (3), 347–359.

10 Rizk, N.P., Venkatraman, E., Bains, M.S., *et al.* (2007) American Joint Committee on Cancer staging system does not accurately predict survival in patients receiving multimodality therapy for esophageal adenocarcinoma. *J. Clin. Oncol.*, **25** (5), 507–512.

11 Rizk, N., Venkatraman, E., Park, B., *et al.* (2006) The prognostic importance of the number of involved lymph nodes in esophageal cancer: implications for revisions of the American Joint Committee on Cancer staging system. *J. Thorac. Cardiovasc. Surg.*, **132** (6), 1374–1381.

12 Peyre, C.G., Hagen, J.A., DeMeester, S.R., *et al.* (2008) Predicting systemic disease in patients with esophageal cancer after esophagectomy: a multinational study on the significance of the number of involved lymph nodes. *Ann. Surg.*, **248** (6), 979–985.

13 Edge, S.B., Byrd, D.R., Compton, C.C., Fritz, A.G., Greene, F.L., Trotti, A. (2002) *AJCC Cancer Staging Manual*. Springer.

14 Leichman, L., Herskovic, A., Leichman, C.G., *et al.* (1987) Nonoperative therapy for squamous-cell cancer of the esophagus. *J. Clin. Oncol.*, **5** (3), 365–370.

15 Leichman, L., Steiger, Z., Seydel, H.G., *et al.* (1984) Preoperative chemotherapy and radiation therapy for patients with cancer of the esophagus: a potentially curative approach. *J. Clin. Oncol.*, **2** (2), 75–79.

16 Douple, E.B., Richmond, R.C. (1982) Enhancement of the potentiation of radiotherapy by platinum drugs in a

mouse tumor. *Int. J. Radiat. Oncol. Biol. Phys.*, **8** (3-4), 501–503.

17 Natsugoe, S., Yoshinaka, H., Morinaga, T., *et al.* (1996) Ultrasonographic detection of lymph-node metastases in superficial carcinoma of the esophagus. *Endoscopy*, **28** (8), 674–679.

18 Hiele, M., De Leyn, P., Schurmans, P., *et al.* (1997) Relation between endoscopic ultrasound findings and outcome of patients with tumors of the esophagus or esophagogastric junction. *Gastrointest. Endosc.*, **45** (5), 381–386.

19 Young, P.E., Gentry, A.B., Acosta, R.D., Greenwald, B.D., Riddle, M. (2010) Endoscopic ultrasound does not accurately stage early adenocarcinoma or high-grade dysplasia of the esophagus. *Clin. Gastroenterol. Hepatol.*, **8** (12), 1037–1041.

20 van Vliet, E.P., Heijenbrok-Kal, M.H., Hunink, M.G., Kuipers, E.J., Siersema, P.D. (2008) Staging investigations for oesophageal cancer: a meta-analysis. *Br. J. Cancer*, **98** (3), 547–557.

21 Flanagan, F.L., Dehdashti, F., Siegel, B.A., *et al.* (1997) Staging of esophageal cancer with 18F-fluorodeoxyglucose positron emission tomography. *Am. J. Roentgenol.*, **168** (2), 417–424.

22 Flamen, P., Lerut, A., Van Cutsem, E., *et al.* (2000) Utility of positron emission tomography for the staging of patients with potentially operable esophageal carcinoma. *J. Clin. Oncol.*, **18** (18), 3202–3210.

23 Pan, L., Gu, P., Huang, G., Xue, H., Wu, S. (2009) Prognostic significance of SUV on PET/CT in patients with esophageal cancer: a systematic review and meta-analysis. *Eur. J. Gastroenterol. Hepatol.*, **21** (9), 1008–1015.

24 Bruzzi, J.F., Swisher, S.G., Truong, M.T., *et al.* (2007) Detection of interval distant metastases: clinical utility of integrated CT-PET imaging in patients with esophageal carcinoma after neoadjuvant therapy. *Cancer*, **109** (1), 125–134.

25 Lordick, F., Ott, K., Krause, B.J., *et al.* (2007) PET to assess early metabolic response and to guide treatment of adenocarcinoma of the oesophagogastric junction: the MUNICON phase II trial. *Lancet Oncol.*, **8** (9), 797–805.

26 Adams, W., Phemister, D. (1933) Carcinoma of the lower thoracic esophagus: report of successful resection and esophagogastrostomy. *J. Thorac. Surg.*, **7**, 621–632.

27 Torek, F. (1913) The first successful case of resection of the thoracic portion of the oesophagus for carcinoma. *Surg. Gynecol.*, **16**, 614–617.

28 Aisner, J., Forastiere, A., Aroney, R. (1983) Patterns of recurrence for cancer of the lung and esophagus, in *Cancer Treatment Symposia: Proceedings of the Workshop on Patterns of Failure After Cancer Treatment*, Vol. **2** (ed. R.E. Wittes), US Department of Health and Human Services, Washington, DC.

29 Fujimake, M., Soga, J., Kawaguchi, M., Maeda, M., Sasaki, K. (1975) Role of preoperative administration of bleomycin and radiation in the treatment of esophageal cancer. *Jpn. J. Surg.*, **5** (1), 48–55.

30 Herskovic, A., Martz, K., al-Sarraf, M., *et al.* (1992) Combined chemotherapy and radiotherapy compared with radiotherapy alone in patients with cancer of the esophagus. *N. Engl. J. Med.*, **326** (24), 1593–1598.

31 Coia, L.R., Engstrom, P.F., Paul, A.R., Stafford, P.M., Hanks, G.E. (1991) Long-term results of infusional 5-FU, mitomycin-C and radiation as primary management of esophageal carcinoma. *Int. J. Radiat. Oncol. Biol. Phys.*, **20** (1), 29–36.

32 Minsky, B.D., Pajak, T.F., Ginsberg, R.J., *et al.* (2002) INT 0123 (Radiation Therapy Oncology Group 94-05) phase III trial of combined-modality therapy for esophageal cancer: high-dose versus standard-dose radiation therapy. *J. Clin. Oncol.*, **20** (5), 1167–1174.

33 Bedenne, L., Michel, P., Bouche, O., *et al.* (2007) Chemoradiation followed by surgery compared with chemoradiation alone in squamous cancer of the esophagus: FFCD 9102. *J. Clin. Oncol.*, **25** (10), 1160–1168.

34 Jouve, J., Michel, P., Mariette, C., *et al.* (2008) Outcome of the nonrandomized patients in the FFCD 9102 trial: Chemoradiation followed by surgery compared with chemoradiation alone in squamous cancer of the esophagus. *J. Clin. Oncol.*, **26** (20s), 4555.

35 Stahl, M., Stuschke, M., Lehmann, N., *et al.* (2005) Chemoradiation with and without surgery in patients with locally advanced squamous cell carcinoma of the esophagus. *J. Clin. Oncol.*, **23** (10), 2310–2317.

36 Cheedella, N.K., Suzuki, A., Fau-Xiao, L., *et al.* (2013) Association between clinical complete response and pathological complete response after preoperative chemoradiation in patients with gastroesophageal cancer: analysis in a large cohort. *Ann. Oncol.*, **24** (5), 1262–1266.

37 Walsh, T.N., Noonan, N., Hollywood, D., Kelly, A., Keeling, N., Hennessy, T.P. (1996) A comparison of multimodal therapy and surgery for esophageal adenocarcinoma. *N. Engl. J. Med.*, **335** (7), 462–467.

38 Urba, S.G., Orringer, M.B., Turrisi, A., Iannettoni, M., Forastiere, A., Strawderman, M. (2001) Randomized trial of preoperative chemoradiation versus surgery alone in patients with locoregional esophageal carcinoma. *J. Clin. Oncol.*, **19** (2), 305–313.

39 Tepper, J., Krasna, M.J., Niedzwiecki, D., *et al.* (2008) Phase III trial of trimodality therapy with cisplatin, fluorouracil, radiotherapy, and surgery compared with surgery alone for esophageal cancer: CALGB 9781. *J. Clin. Oncol.*, **26** (7), 1086–1092.

40 Shapiro, J., van Lanschot, J.J., Hulshof, M.C., *et al.* and the CROSS study group (2015) Neoadjuvant

chemoradiotherapy plus surgery versus surgery alone for oesophageal or junctional cancer (CROSS): long-term results of a randomised controlled trial. *Lancet Oncol.*, **16** (9), 1090–1098.

41 Thames, H.D., Jr, Peters, L.J., Withers, H.R., Fletcher, G.H. (1983) Accelerated fractionation vs hyperfractionation: rationales for several treatments per day. *Int. J. Radiat. Oncol. Biol. Phys.*, **9** (2), 127–138.

42 Withers, H.R. (1985) Biologic basis for altered fractionation schemes. *Cancer*, **55** (9 Suppl.), 2086–2095.

43 Forastiere, A.A., Heitmiller, R.F., Lee, D.J., *et al.* (1997) Intensive chemoradiation followed by esophagectomy for squamous cell and adenocarcinoma of the esophagus. *Cancer J. Sci. Am.*, **3** (3), 144–152.

44 van Hagen, P., Hulshof Mc Fau, van Lanschot, J.J.B., *et al.* (2012) Preoperative chemoradiotherapy for esophageal or junctional cancer. *N. Engl. J. Med.*, **366** (22), 2074–2084.

45 Kitagawa, Y., Ueda, M., Ando, N., Ozawa, S., Shimizu, N., Kitajima, M. (1996) Further evidence for prognostic significance of epidermal growth factor receptor gene amplification in patients with esophageal squamous cell carcinoma. *Clin. Cancer Res.*, **2** (5), 909–914.

46 Ozawa, S., Ueda, M., Ando, N., Shimizu, N., Abe, O. (1989) Prognostic significance of epidermal growth factor receptor in esophageal squamous cell carcinomas. *Cancer*, **63** (11), 2169–2173.

47 Itakura, Y., Sasano, H., Shiga, C., *et al.* (1994) Epidermal growth factor receptor overexpression in esophageal carcinoma. An immunohistochemical study correlated with clinicopathologic findings and DNA amplification. *Cancer*, **74** (3), 795–804.

48 Yoshida, K., Kuniyasu, H., Yasui, W., Kitadai, Y., Toge, T., Tahara, E. (1993) Expression of growth factors and their receptors in human esophageal carcinomas: regulation of expression by epidermal growth factor and transforming growth factor alpha. *J. Cancer Res. Clin. Oncol.*, **119**, 401–407.

49 Gibson, M.K., Abraham, S.C., Wu, T.T., *et al.* (2003) Epidermal growth factor receptor, p53 mutation, and pathological response predict survival in patients with locally advanced esophageal cancer treated with preoperative chemoradiotherapy. *Clin. Cancer Res.*, **9** (17), 6461–6468.

50 Bonner, J.A., Harari, P.M., Giralt, J., *et al.* (2006) Radiotherapy plus cetuximab for squamous-cell carcinoma of the head and neck. *N. Engl. J. Med.*, **354** (6), 567–578.

51 Enzinger, P.C., Yock, T., Suh, W., *et al.* (2006) Phase II cisplatin, irinotecan, cetuximab and concurrent radiation therapy followed by surgery for locally advanced esophageal cancer. *J. Clin. Oncol.*, **24** (18s), 4064.

52 Suntharalingam, M., Dipetrillo, T., Akerman, P., *et al.* (2006) Cetuximab, paclitaxel, carboplatin, and radiation for esophageal and gastric cancer. *J. Clin. Oncol.*, **24** (18S), 4029.

53 Suntharalingam, M., Winter, K., Ilson, D., *et al.* (2014) The initial report of local control on RTOG 0436: A Phase 3 trial evaluating the addition of cetuximab to paclitaxel, cisplatin, and radiation for patients with esophageal cancer treated without surgery. *Int. J. Radiat. Oncol. Biol. Phys.*, **90**, S3.

54 al-Kasspooles, M., Moore, J.H., Orringer, M.B., Beer, D.G. (1993) Amplification and over-expression of the EGFR and erbB-2 genes in human esophageal adenocarcinomas. *Int. J. Cancer*, **54** (2), 213–219.

55 Dahlberg, P.S., Jacobson, B.A., Dahal, G., *et al.* (2004) ERBB2 amplifications in esophageal adenocarcinoma. *Ann. Thorac. Surg.*, **78** (5), 1790–1800.

56 Shiga, K., Shiga, C., Sasano, H., *et al.* Expression of c-erbB-2 in human esophageal carcinoma cells: overexpression correlated with gene amplification or with GATA-3 transcription factor expression. *Anticancer Res.*, **13** (5A), 1293–1301.

57 Safran, H., DiPetrillo, T., Nadeem, A., *et al.* (2004) Trastuzumab, paclitaxel, cisplatin, and radiation for adenocarcinoma of the esophagus: a phase I study. *Cancer Invest.*, **22** (5), 670–677.

58 Bang, Y.J., Van Cutsem, E., Feyereislova, A., *et al.* (2010) Trastuzumab in combination with chemotherapy versus chemotherapy alone for treatment of HER2-positive advanced gastric or gastro-oesophageal junction cancer (ToGA): a phase 3, open-label, randomised controlled trial. *Lancet*, **376** (9742), 687–697.

59 Gorski, D.H., Beckett, M.A., Jaskowiak, N.T., *et al.* (1999) Blockage of the vascular endothelial growth factor stress response increases the antitumor effects of ionizing radiation. *Cancer Res.*, **59** (14), 3374–3378.

60 Chandra, A., Guerrero, T.M., Liu, H.H., *et al.* (2005) Feasibility of using intensity-modulated radiotherapy to improve lung sparing in treatment planning for distal esophageal cancer. *Radiother. Oncol.*, **77** (3), 247–253.

61 Nutting, C.M., Bedford, J.L., Cosgrove, V.P., Tait, D.M., Dearnaley, D.P., Webb, S. (2002) Intensity-modulated radiotherapy reduces lung irradiation in patients with carcinoma of the oesophagus. *Front. Radiat. Ther. Oncol.*, **37**, 128–131.

62 Wu, V.W., Sham, J.S., Kwong, D.L. (2004) Inverse planning in three-dimensional conformal and intensity-modulated radiotherapy of mid-thoracic oesophageal cancer. *Br. J. Radiol.*, **77** (919), 568–572.

63 Wang, S.L., Liao, Z., Liu, H., *et al.* (2006) Intensity-modulated radiation therapy with concurrent chemotherapy for locally advanced cervical and upper thoracic esophageal cancer. *World J. Gastroenterol.*, **12** (34), 5501–5508.

64 Fu, W.H., Wang, L.H., Zhou, Z.M., Dai, J.R., Hu, Y.M., Zhao, L.J. (2004) Comparison of conformal and intensity-modulated techniques for simultaneous integrated boost radiotherapy of upper esophageal carcinoma. *World J. Gastroenterol.*, **10** (8), 1098–1102.

65 La, T.H., Minn, A.Y., Su, Z., *et al.* (2010) Multimodality treatment with intensity modulated radiation therapy for esophageal cancer. *Dis. Esoph.*, **23** (4), 300–388.

66 Keane, T.J., Harwood, A.R., Elhakim, T., *et al.* (1985) Radical radiation therapy with 5-fluorouracil infusion and mitomycin C for oesophageal squamous carcinoma. *Radiother. Oncol.*, **4** (3), 205–210.

67 John, M.J., Flam, M.S., Mowry, P.A., *et al.* Radiotherapy alone and chemoradiation for nonmetastatic esophageal carcinoma. A critical review of chemoradiation. *Cancer*, **63** (12), 2397–2403.

68 Araujo, C.M., Souhami, L., Gil, R.A., *et al.* (1991) A randomized trial comparing radiation therapy versus concomitant radiation therapy and chemotherapy in carcinoma of the thoracic esophagus. *Cancer*, **67** (9), 2258–2261.

69 Smith, T.J., Ryan, L.M., Douglass, H.O., Jr, *et al.* (1998) Combined chemoradiotherapy vs. radiotherapy alone for early stage squamous cell carcinoma of the esophagus: a study of the Eastern Cooperative Oncology Group. *Int. J. Radiat. Oncol. Biol. Phys.*, **42** (2), 269–276.

70 Wobbes, T., Baron, B., Paillot, B., *et al.* (2001) Prospective randomised study of split-course radiotherapy versus cisplatin plus split-course radiotherapy in inoperable squamous cell carcinoma of the oesophagus. *Eur. J. Cancer*, **37** (4), 470–477.

71 Cooper, J.S., Guo, M.D., Herskovic, A., *et al.* (1999) Chemoradiotherapy of locally advanced esophageal cancer: long-term follow-up of a prospective randomized trial (RTOG 85-01). Radiation Therapy Oncology Group. *JAMA*, **281** (17), 1623–1627.

72 Bosset, J.F., Gignoux, M., Triboulet, J.P., *et al.* (1997) Chemoradiotherapy followed by surgery compared with surgery alone in squamous-cell cancer of the esophagus. *N. Engl. J. Med.*, **337** (3), 161–167.

73 Burmeister, B.H., Smithers, B.M., Gebski, V., *et al.* (2005) Surgery alone versus chemoradiotherapy followed by surgery for resectable cancer of the oesophagus: a randomised controlled phase III trial. *Lancet Oncol.*, **6** (9), 659–668.

74 Mariette, C., Dahan, L., Mornex, F., *et al.* (2014) Surgery alone versus chemoradiotherapy followed by surgery for stage I and II esophageal cancer: final analysis of randomized controlled phase III trial FFCD 9901. *J. Clin. Oncol.*, **32** (23), 2416–2422.

Section 4

Gastrointestinal Malignancies

Section Editor: Christopher G. Willett

21

Gastric Cancer

Joanna Y. Chin and Theodore S. Hong

Introduction

Although the incidence of gastric cancer is declining in the United States, with an estimated 28 000 new cases in 2017, the worldwide annual incidence is as much as tenfold higher in some countries in Asia, Eastern Europe, and South America [1–3]. Worldwide, developing countries account for more than 70% of cases, and incidence rates are about twice as high in men than in women. Gastric cancer was the third leading cause of cancer deaths worldwide in 2012. While surgical treatment alone is adequate in patients who present with early-stage disease, the majority present with locally advanced disease or with metastatic disease, for whom overall survival at five years is 30% and 4.5%, respectively [1]. Therefore, adjuvant treatment for gastric cancer remains an important area of study and improvement.

Clinical Presentation and Diagnostic Evaluation

Common symptoms at diagnosis are weight loss and persistent epigastric pain; other symptoms include nausea, anorexia, early satiety, melena and/or dysphagia, with the latter more common in tumors at the gastroesophageal (GE) junction. Early-stage gastric cancers can be asymptomatic but these only represent 10–20% of cases at diagnosis in the United States. Early satiety can result from gastric outlet obstruction or an aggressive form of diffuse-type gastric cancer in which the stomach loses distensibility, termed 'linitus plastica.' Approximately 25% of patients have a history of gastric ulcer. Other risk factors include *Helicobacter pylori* gastric infection, increased age, male gender, diets low in fruits and vegetables, diets high in salted, smoked or preserved

foods, chronic atropic gastritis, intestinal metaplasia, pernicious anemia, gastric adenomatous polyps, family history of gastric cancer, and cigarette smoking [4]. Advanced disease can present with a palpable abdominal mass, and a full lymph node assessment includes the left supraclavicular region (Virchow's node), the periumbilicus (Sister Mary Joseph's node), and the left axilla (Irish node).

Esophagoduodenoscopy with biopsy is typically used to determine tumor location and size, and to obtain tissue for diagnosis. Endoscopic ultrasound is useful in determining the depth of invasion and therefore helpful for staging. Chest, abdominal and pelvis computed tomography (CT) imaging is used to assess distant metastases in the liver, peritoneal surfaces, and distant lymph nodes. Less commonly, metastatic disease can involve the ovaries (Krukenberg's tumor), central nervous system, bone, lung, or soft tissue. Suspicious visceral lesions warrant a biopsy. While positron emission tomography–computed tomography (PET-CT) can be helpful to evaluate for distant disease, most diffuse-type gastric cancers are not fluoro-2-deoxyglucose (FDG)-avid, and PET-CT is only 50% sensitive in detecting peritoneal carcinomatosis [5]. Therefore, PET-CT is not yet routinely used in gastric cancer staging.

At some institutions, a preoperative laparoscopy is used to assess the peritoneum, surface of the liver and local-regional lymph nodes, particularly as preoperative assessment of nodal involvement and of peritoneal metastases by non-invasive methods can be challenging [6]. A peritoneal cytology sample may also be obtained during preoperative laparoscopy to select patients who may benefit from neoadjuvant therapy (e.g., in the case of occult positive peritoneal washings). Intraperitoneal metastases have been identified at the time of exploratory laparotomy or open surgery in 20–30% of patients with negative CT, arguing for the routine use of exploratory

Clinical Radiation Oncology: Indications, Techniques, and Results, Third Edition. Edited by William Small Jr.
© 2017 John Wiley & Sons, Inc. Published 2017 by John Wiley & Sons, Inc.

laparotomy to identify patients who would not benefit from surgery [6, 7].

Anatomy

The stomach consists of the cardia, the fundus, the gastric body (divided into the lesser and greater curvatures), and the pyloric antrum. The regional lymph nodes at risk for involvement depend on the location of the primary tumor. Regional nodes for tumors located along the greater curvature include greater curvature, greater omental, gastroduodenal, gastroepiploic, prepyloric antrum, and pancreaticoduodenal nodes. For tumors along the lesser curvature, these include lesser curvature, lesser omental, left gastric, cardioesophageal, common hepatic, celiac and hepatoduodenal nodes. The pancreatic and splenic area (pancreaticolienal, peripancreatic, splenic) are at risk for both greater and lesser curvature tumors. Hepatoduodenal, retropancreatic, portal, mesenteric, and para-aortic node involvement is classified as distant metastases.

Since the 1990s, there has been a shift in the location of gastric tumors, with an increasing number arising near the GE junction and proximal stomach, compared with the body and antrum of the stomach [1]. In surgical series, GE junction tumors are associated with a less favorable outcome compared with tumors arising in the distal stomach. Several studies have examined histologic, environmental and genetic factors as contributory to this trend towards the GE junction, but the data are inconclusive. It is essential that future trials be precise regarding the inclusion of GE junction tumors for appropriate comparisons. Notably, the current AJCC staging system clarifies that tumors arising within 5 cm of the GE junction, whereas the 8th edition of the AJCC staging system proposes the boundary between esophagus and stomach to be at 2 cm are classified as esophageal tumors [8].

Histology

The Lauren classification divides gastric cancers into two main histologic variants: the intestinal and diffuse types. The former type demonstrates defined glandular structures, while the latter type shows submucosal spread of infiltrative cells [9]. The intestinal type of gastric cancer accounts for approximately 70–80%, is more common in males, is more prevalent in high-risk populations, and is likely linked to environmental factors. The diffuse type is associated with a younger age at diagnosis, and portends a worse prognosis than the intestinal type.

A small proportion of gastric cancers (<10%) are hereditary [9], and 3–5% are associated with inherited cancer predisposition syndrome such as Lynch syndrome, Peutz–Jeghers syndrome, familial adenomatous polyposis, hereditary breast and ovarian cancers and Li–Fraumeni syndrome. An entity known as hereditary diffuse gastric cancer (HDGC) is associated with a young age of onset and diffuse-type histology. Some 50% of HDGC cases are attributable to an underlying genetic defect of *CDH-1* (E-cadherin gene), and having the defect is associated with a 40–60% lifetime risk of gastric cancer [10]. HER2 receptor overexpression and amplification of the encoding *ERBB2* gene has been found in between 7% and 34% of gastric cancers, but there are conflicting data whether overexpression is correlated with clinical outcome [11–18a]. Compellingly, the addition of a HER2-targeting agent, trastuzumab, to chemotherapy for advanced gastric cancer demonstrates a survival advantage in the ToGA trial [19]. However, in the final update of the randomized phase III ARTIST trial, which compared chemoradiation to chemotherapy alone for resected gastric cancer (discussed below), no difference in disease-free survival was associated with HER2 overexpression [20]. Other molecular targets currently under investigation in gastric cancer include EGFR overexpression, angiogenesis pathway targets such as vascular endothelial growth factor receptors (VEGFA, VEGFR) [20a], fibroblast growth factor receptors (FGFRs), hepatocyte growth factor receptors (HGFR and the tyrosine receptor kinase MET), and the mammalian target of rapamycin (mTOR).

Finally, the Cancer Genome Atlas molecularly characterized gastric adenocarcinoma, based on 25 frequently mutated genes, resulting in four main types: Epstein–Barr virus-associated; microsatellite unstable (hypermutated); genomically stable tumors; and tumors with chromosomal instability [21]. This characterization will not only provide important clues as to etiology and pathogenesis, but will also facilitate molecular stratification in clinical trial design of targeted therapeutics. For example, the current SWOG 1201 trial is using expression levels of a protein involved in nucleotide excision repair, excision repair cross-complementation group 1 (ERCC1), to stratify response to different chemotherapy regimens in advanced gastric cancer.

Staging

The most commonly used classification system is the TNM system, developed by the AJCC/UICC, which is based on depth of invasion for the T stage and number of regional involved nodes for the N stage. Notably, tumor size and location of involved lymph nodes is not reported in the staging system. The T stage corresponds to the staging systems for esophageal and rectal cancers. The N category is defined by the number of regional lymph nodes involved. The 8th edition of the AJCC staging system now includes clinical prognostic stage groups, in addition to pathological staging. However, the new staging system has been criticized for upstaging 60% of patients without a correlated change in prognosis [22, 23]. For example, stage IIA cancers according to the AJCC 7th edition includes pT3pN0, pT2pN1 and pT1bpN2 tumors, which have median survival times of 35.8 months, 21.9 months, and 16.0 months, respectively, in a retrospective analysis of patients treated in one institution [22]. Furthermore, some investigators propose the use of the N-ratio (number of lymph nodes involved as a proportion of those examined) to highlight the importance of extensive lymph node dissections (discussed below) in accurate staging [24, 25].

Management

Surgical resection of the primary gastric tumor is the cornerstone of curative treatment for gastric cancer. At experienced centers, curative intent requires an R0 resection accompanied by an extended lymphadenectomy (see next section) and omentectomy. The extent of surgery is dependent on the location of the primary tumor. Total gastrectomy is not always required, particularly for distal lesions, where subtotal resections have similar survival results and fewer morbidities [26, 27]. For subtotal gastrectomies for intestinal-type histologies, intragastric margins of 5 cm are recommended; larger margins may be needed for diffuse-type disease [28]. For tumors arising in the proximal third or in the body of the stomach, a total gastrectomy is typically performed, often with a splenectomy, as tumors in this location can metastasize to the splenic hilum. Subtotal proximal gastrectomies often lead to reflux, and thus are not preferred.

Extent of Lymph Node Dissection

In addition to removal of the primary gastric tumor with adequate margins, increasing evidence supports a more extensive lymph node dissection than has been performed historically, with improved survival outcome. In a surgical series of gastrectomies at MSKCC between 1985 and 1999, Karpeh *et al.* [29] found that examining 15 or more lymph nodes was associated with a higher five-year overall survival in stage II patients (54%), compared with a 30% five-year overall survival in patients having less than 15 lymph nodes examined. It was believed that increasing lymph node dissection allowed for more appropriate and adequate staging.

Furthermore, a comparison of surgical series performed in Japan and in Europe/US demonstrated superior five-year survival and operative mortality rates in Japan. Although patients in the Japanese series tended to present at an earlier stage than in Europe/US, this was

true even when patients were stage-matched. This was partly attributed to increased experience of Japanese surgeons with the surgery from higher gastric cancer incidence rates in Japan. The improved survival, however, was also attributed to the routine use of D2 lymph node dissection, versus D1 node dissection, with gastrectomy in Japan. A so-called D1 dissection involves only removal of the peri-gastric, that is, directly attached and greater and lesser omental, lymph nodes. A D2 level dissection includes a D1 dissection, and also removes the lymph nodes of the celiac trunk and the nodes that track along the portal, splenic, and celiac arteries.

Extended node dissection requires increased surgical expertise, and the more extensive surgery required in a D2 node dissection has confounded trials comparing overall survival following gastrectomy with a D1 or D2 node dissection. In the Phase III multicenter Dutch Gastric Cancer Trial, 711 patients undergoing a complete gastric primary resection were also randomized to receive either a D1 or D2 lymph node dissection [30–32]. The study arms, however, were not well-matched in that more patients in the arm undergoing a D2 dissection also received a splenectomy (37% versus 11% of patients receiving a D1 dissection) and a pancreatic tail resection (30% versus 3%), procedures that by themselves are more intensive and associated with increased morbidity and mortality. Indeed, the rate of complications was higher in the group of patients receiving a D2 dissection (43% versus 25%, p = 0.001), and had an increased rate of postoperative mortality (10% versus 4%, p = 0.004). Not surprisingly, the 15-year overall survival was not significantly different between the two study groups, nor did age, pathologic stage, lymph node involvement, nor extent of primary resection have an effect on overall survival rates. Recurrence rates in the 15-year update, however, were higher in the group of patients receiving a D1 lymph node resection (49% versus 40%). Similarly, a meta-analysis of 2044 patients from eight randomized trials failed to demonstrate a survival benefit for D2 dissections, which were associated with a higher rate of postoperative complications [33].

Improvements in surgical technique and training, and referral to specialized surgical centers for improved quality control, have reduced the rates of spleen and pancreas removal when D2 dissections are performed. The Italian Gastric Cancer Study Group showed that when a select group of highly trained surgeons is used, gastrectomy with D2 lymph node dissections are associated with the same postoperative complication and mortality rates as gastrectomies performed with D1 node dissection [34]. This equivalence of morbidity and operative mortality between patients receiving a D1 lymphadenectomy and a D2 lymphadenectomy was also demonstrated in a subsequent randomized Phase III trial by the same group. Furthermore, there was no difference in five-year overall survival between patients who had a D1 versus D2 dissection (i.e., 66.5% versus 64.2%), both of which are considerably higher than historical Western studies. On subgroup analyses, D2 lymphadenectomy appeared to benefit patients with pT2-4 disease and positive lymph nodes [35]. Although this suggests that D2 dissections may be preferred in locally advanced disease, extended lymphadenectomy is still not routine practice in the US and Europe.

Adjuvant Chemoradiation

The high rates of locoregional recurrence following surgery alone speaks to the importance of adjuvant therapy in overall gastric cancer management (Table 21.1). Both adjuvant chemotherapy and adjuvant chemoradiation have been studied. MacDonald *et al.* [36] randomized patients following primary tumor resection to observation or adjuvant 5-FU chemotherapy and chemoradiation in the Intergroup 0116 trial [36, 37]. After one cycle of 5-FU chemotherapy, radiation to 45 Gy was given to the surgical tumor bed with a 2 cm margin to the resection and to regional lymph nodes, with 5-FU radiosensitizer given during radiation. One month following radiation, patients received an additional two cycles of 5-FU chemotherapy, for a total of three cycles of adjuvant chemotherapy. The three-year overall survival was improved in the group of patients receiving surgery with adjuvant chemotherapy and chemoradiation, compared to those who had surgery alone (50% versus 41%). The benefit of chemoradiation continued to be seen with more than 10 years of follow-up (HR 1.32, 95% CI 1.10–1.60, p = 0.0046). Median survival time and recurrence-free survival was also increased (35 months versus 27 months, and 27 months versus 19 months, respectively) in patients receiving adjuvant chemotherapy and chemoradiation. One major criticism of this study, however, is that over half (54%) of the patients had a D0 resection, defined as any lymph node removal less than a D1. As discussed previously, adequate lymph node dissection is thought to be a major prognostic factor for survival after surgery, and adjuvant chemotherapy and chemoradiation in this study may be compensating for substandard surgery.

The question of chemoradiation compensating for suboptimal lymph node excision was studied in a retrospective analysis of patients enrolled in Phase I/II trials modeled after the adjuvant chemotherapy and chemoradiation regimen used in the MacDonald study [38]. Among this group of patients, 27% had a D0 dissection,

Table 21.1 Table of major clinical trials of adjuvant therapy following gastrectomy for gastric cancer.

Trial	Adjuvant treatment arms	No. of patients	Overall survival	Other clinical endpoints	Comments
Intergroup 0116 Macdonald *et al.* 2001 1991–1998	5-FU + RT vs. none	556	50% vs. 41% (p = 0.005) at 3 years	Relapse-free survival 48% vs. 31% (p > .001) at 3 years	84% of patients had node-positive disease; 54% had less than complete dissection of N1-level nodes
ARTIST Lee *et al.* 2012 2004–2008	Capecitabine/cisplatin + RT vs. capecitabine/cisplatin	458	–	Disease-free survival 78.2% vs. 74.2% (p = 0.0862) at 3 years	In subgroup analysis of LN+ pts (*n* = 396), DFS improved in arm with RT (77.5% vs. 72.3% in cape/cis – alone arm, p = 0.0365)
MAGIC Cunningham *et al.* 2006 1994–2002	Epirubicin/cisplatin/ 5-FU perioperatively vs. none	503	36.3% vs 23.0% (p = 0.009) at 5 years	Progression-free survival 30% vs. 18% (p > 0.001) at 5 years	Included esophageal and GE junction tumors; 41.6% of patients in perioperative chemotherapy arm did not complete chemotherapy
ACTS-GC Sasako *et al.* 2011 2001–2004	S-1 vs. none	1059	71.7% vs 61.1% (HR 0.669, 95% CI 0.540 to 0.828) at 5 years	Recurrence free survival 65.4% vs. 53.1% (HR 0.653, 95% CI 0.537–0.793) at 5 years	OS in surgery alone group improved compared to other trials; benefit of S-1 adjuvant therapy more significant in stage II patients
CLASSIC Bang *et al.* 2012 2006–2009	capecitabine/oxaliplatin vs. none	1035	83% vs. 78% (p = 0.0493) at 3 years	Disease-free survival 74% vs. 59% (HR 0.56, 95% CI 0.44 to 0.72) at 3 years	OS in surgery-alone group improved compared to other trials

39% D1, and 25% D2. These patients, who received post-operative adjuvant chemoradiation, were compared with patients enrolled in the Dutch Gastric Cancer Trial, who received radical gastrectomy with a D1 or D2 dissection (i.e., surgery alone). This retrospective analysis showed that postoperative chemoradiation led to a reduction in local recurrence (5% versus 17% at two years), while regional or distant recurrence rates were not different between the two groups. Notably, the difference in local recurrence rates was magnified in patients who had chemoradiation following a D1 dissection (2% versus 18% at two years), while there was no advantage of chemoradiation following a D2 dissection. This suggests that chemoradiation is particularly important in the management of postoperative patients receiving a D1 rather than a D2 dissection.

More recently, the results of the Phase III ARTIST trial looked at the benefit of adding chemoradiation to adjuvant chemotherapy, and this study required a radical primary resection with a D2 lymph node dissection to ensure an adequate surgery in all patients. This trial randomized 458 patients, following surgery, to either six cycles of capecitabine and cisplatin, or to four total cycles of the same adjuvant chemotherapy sandwiching a five-week course of chemoradiation [20, 39]. Radiation was to 45 Gy to the tumor bed and regional lymph nodes, and capecitabine 825 mg m^{-2} twice daily was used as the radiosensitizer. In this study, no significant difference was seen in five-year overall survival between the two study arms (75% in the adjuvant chemotherapy and chemoradiation arm versus 73% in the adjuvant chemotherapy-alone arm; HR 1.13, 95% CI 0.775–1.647, p = 0.5272). However, in a subgroup analysis of patients with positive lymph nodes, which includes 84.6% of patients in the adjuvant chemotherapy arm and 88.3% of those in the adjuvant chemotherapy and chemoradiation arm, disease-free survival at three years was improved with chemoradiation (76% versus 72%, p = 0.04). This suggested that patients with more extensive local-regional disease at time of surgery benefitted from additional local therapy with chemoradiation. In fact, locoregional relapse was more frequent in the chemotherapy-alone arm (13% versus 7%, p = 0.0033), while there was no difference in distant metastases rate in the two arms (27% versus 24%, p = 0.5568). The applicability of the ARTIST trial to patients in the U.S. and Europe is cautioned, however, as 60% of their study population had stage IB or II disease, and 60% had diffuse-type gastric cancer. The relatively high proportion of early-stage disease and of diffuse-type histology, may in part account for the apparent lack of benefit of chemoradiation in the ARTIST trial.

Both the Intergroup 0116 trial and the ARTIST trial discussed above used adjuvant chemotherapy in both arms, with the addition of chemoradiation in one of the study arms. Two other trials are studying chemotherapy agents in the setting of adjuvant chemoradiation. The CALGB 80101 trial compared two different chemotherapy regimens that are commonly used (5-FU/leucovorin versus epirubicin, cisplatin, and continuous-infusion 5-FU (ECF)), and patients in both adjuvant chemotherapy arms also received adjuvant chemoradiation. No overall survival or disease-free survival advantage was seen, with a three-year overall survival of 50% in the 5-FU arm and 52% in the ECF arm (HR, 1.03; 95% CI, 0.80–1.34; p = 0.80) [40]. The Dutch CRITICS trial is also comparing adjuvant ECX (epirubicin, cis/oxaliplatin, and capecitabine) chemotherapy with adjuvant chemoradiation to 45 Gy with concurrent cisplatin/capecitabine. Both groups will receive neoadjuvant ECX and gastrectomy with D1+ dissection [41]. This study will help to address the question of systemic versus local therapy following surgical resection, and to perhaps minimize toxicity of adjuvant treatment by identifying the critical components of an effective chemotherapy regimen.

Perioperative and Adjuvant Chemotherapy

Several major randomized trials show a benefit to the use of perioperative or adjuvant chemotherapy alone following surgical resection. These trials have used various chemotherapy regimens. In the MAGIC trial, 503 patients were randomized to surgery alone, or to three cycles of ECF chemotherapy before and after surgery for a total of six cycles of perioperative chemotherapy [42]. The chemotherapy regimen used was epirubicin, cisplatin, and 5-FU. With a median follow-up of four years, the addition of perioperative chemotherapy improved overall survival and progression-free survival (three-year survival was 36.3% versus 23% in the group of patients receiving surgery alone). Of note, this study included tumors in the lower esophagus (14%) and in the esophagogastric junction (12%), which may be biologically distinct from gastric tumors. In addition, only 41% of patients in the perioperative chemotherapy arm actually completed chemotherapy, though treatment-related toxicity was not different among the two arms. Nevertheless, patients in the perioperative chemotherapy arm had lower T-stage disease (51.7% T1-2 versus 36.8% in the surgery-alone arm) and lower N-stage disease (84.1% 0-6 lymph nodes involved versus 70.5%) at the time of surgery, suggesting that neoadjuvant treatment may be useful for tumor downstaging, though no patients had a pathologic complete response after three cycles of preoperative chemotherapy.

More recently, two large Asian trials were reported which studied the role of adjuvant 5-FU-based chemotherapy following complete primary resection and D2 lymph node dissection. The ACTS-GC trial in Japan used a one-year course of adjuvant S-1, an oral form of fluoropyrimidine with improved bioavailability, following surgery [43]. Compared with patients undergoing surgical resection alone, patients receiving surgery with adjuvant S-1 had an improved five-year overall survival (71.7% versus 61.1% with surgery alone), and a decreased number of relapses (25.1% versus 35.5%). Similarly, the CLASSIC trial investigators demonstrated improved disease-free survival with the use of adjuvant capecitabine/oxaliplatin compared with surgery alone (68% at five years versus 53% with surgery alone, p < 0.0001), and improved overall survival at five years with the use of adjuvant chemotherapy (78% versus 69%, p = 0.0015) [44,45]. Treatment-related toxicity, however, was increased in the adjuvant chemotherapy arm, and only one-third of patients in this arm received the eight cycles of chemotherapy as planned. It is important to note that the overall survival rates of the patients receiving surgery alone in these two studies are higher than similar arms in European or US-based trials. This again emphasizes that biology, surgical expertise, and earlier tumor stage are still important factors that distinguish Asian from Western studies of gastric cancer.

The question of what adjuvant chemotherapy to use, whether as systemic therapy or as a radiosensitizer, is an area of active study. The venous access and continuous infusion required of 5-FU treatment makes oral capecitabine attractive as an alternative. Similarly, oxaliplatin has been used in place of the standard platinum agent, cisplatin, due to the higher renal toxicity profile of cisplatin. With these adjustments in mind, the REAL 2 trial enrolled 1002 patients in a 2× 2 design, comparing epirubicin/cisplatin with 5-FU or capecitabine, or epirubicin/oxaliplatin with 5-FU or capecitabine, in patients with previously untreated advanced gastric cancer [46]. Their results demonstrated that capecitabine is not inferior to 5-FU in terms of overall and progression-free survival, and that oxaliplatin is not inferior to cisplatin. Interestingly, in a secondary analysis, at one-year the overall survival was 46.8% in patients receiving EOX (epirubicin/oxaliplatin/capecitabine) versus 37.7% in those receiving ECF (p = 0.02), and median survival time was improved by almost two months in the EOX arm. This suggests that a more convenient, possibly safer and efficacious chemotherapy regimen may be possible for adjuvant use, which would be expected to increase adherence to the regimen. Though not directly used in the adjuvant chemoradiation setting, the results also suggest that capecitabine may be an effective radiosensitizer in place of the current standard continuous infusion 5-FU. Furthermore, the addition of a taxane or anthracycline is being addressed in ongoing trials, including the Dutch Phase II/III study comparing 5-FU, oxaliplatin and docetaxel (FLOT) with ECF in the adjuvant setting (ClinicalTrials.gov NCT01216644).

Finally, the effect of neoadjuvant treatment on outcome is complicated by the mixed inclusion of gastric,

gastroesophageal junction, and esophageal cancers in the various randomized studies. A meta-analysis of neoadjuvant treatment (chemotherapy or chemoradiation) suggests an advantage to neoadjuvant chemotherapy when all sites are pooled; however, the benefit is more modest when restricted to patients with gastric cancer compared with esophageal cancer patients [47]. A meta-analysis of 12 randomized trials of neoadjuvant chemotherapy suggested an absolute survival benefit of 12% for the addition of chemotherapy prior to surgery [48]. The question of which neoadjuvant treatment is more effective – that is, chemotherapy or chemoradiation – is currently being studied in the Australian Phase II/III TOPGEAR trial (Trial of Preoperative Therapy for Gastric and Esophagogastric Junction Adenocarcinoma). Patients will receive either preoperative ECF or ECX (epirubicin/cisplatin/capecitabine), or preoperative chemoradiation to 45 Gy with concurrent CI 5-FU or capecitabine. Both pathological complete response and overall survival are endpoints of the study.

Radiation Therapy Techniques

Radiation for gastric cancer is typically in the post-surgical setting to the tumor bed and associated lymph nodes. The resultant radiation volume can be large, particularly for gastroesophageal junction tumors, and adequate coverage while respecting neighboring organ constraints typically requires IMRT or 3D conformal radiation at the present authors' institution. Tumors arising near the esophagogastric junction are particularly associated with large CTVs in order to cover the esophagogastric anastomosis, which is typically within the thoracic cavity.

Preoperative and postoperative imaging, as well as endoscopic reports to determine radial and longitudinal involvement, are used to define the CTV. Intravenous and oral contrast during simulation are often helpful for treatment planning. 4D-CT is occasionally helpful for proximal tumors to account for organ motion. For gastroesophageal junction tumors, 4–5 cm of proximal normal esophagus is included in the CTV. For evidence of nodal involvement, any remaining stomach is also included in the CTV. The inclusion of lymph nodes is dependent on the location of the primary tumor. For gastroesophageal junction tumors, perigastric, periesophageal and celiac lymph nodes are included. These three lymph node fields are also covered for gastric cardia lesions, as well as the splenic, pancreaticoduodenal and porta hepatis lymph nodes. For gastric body lesions, perigastric, celiac, splenic, suprapancreatic, pancreaticoduodenal and porta hepatis nodes are included. The same lymph node regions are covered for gastric antrum and pyloric lesions, except the splenic region is excluded. PTV expansion is typically 0.5-1 cm. An adjuvant dose of 45–50.4 Gy in 1.8-Gy

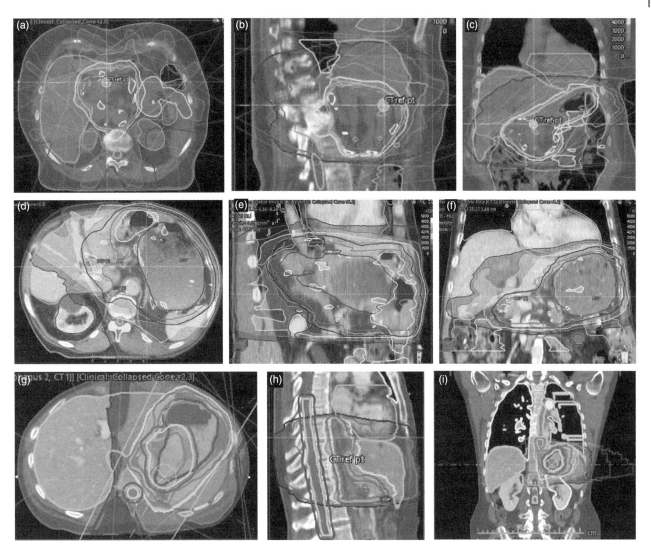

Figure 21.1 Representative postoperative (a–f) and neoadjuvant (g–i) radiation treatment plans for gastric cancer. Prescription dose of 45 Gy is shown in orange. (a–c) Adjuvant IMRT plan for a pT3N2 gastric body tumor following subtotal gastrectomy and D1+ lymphadenectomy, Roux-en-Y gastrojejunostomy and adjuvant chemotherapy. (d–f) Adjuvant IMRT plan for a pT4aN0 tumor in the lesser curvature following distal gastrectomy and D0 lymphadenectomy, Billroth II gastrojejunostomy and adjuvant chemotherapy. Note the larger field size due to large remnant and lack of surgical lymph node evaluation. (g–i) Neoadjuvant radiation plan for a T3N1 tumor in the GE junction. The primary tumor, outlined in red and marked by a blue X in circle, was given a boost of 5.4 Gy to a total dose of 50.4 Gy. For a color version of this figure, see the color plate section.

fractions is typically used. Representative treatment plans for various scenarios in gastric cancer radiation are shown in Figure 21.1; these highlight the customization of field design based on tumor location, the extent of surgery and operative findings, and whether treatment is delivered in the preoperative or postoperative setting.

Conclusions

The treatment of gastric cancer remains a worldwide challenge. Considerable scientific and clinical studies have been conducted to refine the use of adjuvant systemic and local therapy, to define the benefit of radiation, to optimize its sequencing, and to select effective chemotherapy regimens. Treatment patterns continue to differ based on geography, and this may also reflect different inherent biology, pathogenesis, and stage at presentation. It is paramount that patients are discussed in a multidisciplinary setting to personalize treatment selection upfront. At the present authors' institution, perioperative chemotherapy is generally recommended due to the potential for tumor downstaging, the concern for inability to tolerate postoperative treatment, and the apparent benefit in reducing distant recurrence risk as observed in the MAGIC trial. Typically, neoadjuvant chemoradiation is favored for gastroesophageal junction tumors, as per the CROSS trial. Adjuvant chemoradiation is given to those patients with T2 or larger primary tumors, or with N+ disease who have not had neoadjuvant treatment. Currently ongoing studies, such as the Dutch CRITICS and TOPGEAR trials, will likely have a significant impact on the use of chemoradiation and selection of systemic agents, and their results are eagerly awaited.

References

1 Howlader, N., Noone, A.M., Krapcho, M., *et al.* (eds) (2015) SEER Cancer Statistics Review, 1975–2012, National Cancer Institute, Bethesda, MD. Available at: http://seer.cancer.gov/csr/1975_2012/, based on November 2014 SEER data submission, posted to the SEER web site, April 2015.

2 Ferlay, J., Soerjomataram, I., Ervik, M., *et al.* GLOBOCAN 2012 v1.0, Cancer Incidence and Mortality Worldwide: IARC CancerBase No. 11 [Internet]. Lyon, France: International Agency for Research on Cancer; 2013. Available at: http://globocan.iarc.fr, accessed on 5/8/2015.

3 Siegel, R., Miller, K., Jemal, A. (2017) Cancer Statistics 2017. *CA Cancer J. Clin.*, **67**, 7–30.

4 Buas, M.F., Vaughan, T.L. (2013) Epidemiology and risk factors for gastroesophageal junction tumors: understanding the rising incidence of this disease. *Semin. Radiat. Oncol.*, **23** (1), 3–9.

5 Yoshioka, T., Yamaguchi, K, Kubota, K., *et al.* (2003) Evaluation of 18F-FDG PET in patients with advanced, metastatic, or recurrent gastric cancer. *J. Nucl. Med.*, **44** (5), 690–699.

6 Sarela, A.I., Lefkowitz, R., Brennan, M.F., Karpeh, M.S. (2006) Selection of patients with gastric adenocarcinoma for laparoscopic staging. *Am. J. Surg.*, **191** (1), 134–138.

7 Power, D.G., Schattner, M.A., Gerdes, H., *et al.* (2009) Endoscopic ultrasound can improve the selection for laparoscopy in patients with localized gastric cancer. *J. Am. Coll. Surg.*, **208** (2), 173–178.

8 AJCC (2017) Stomach, in *AJCC Cancer Staging Manual*, 8th edition (ed M.B. Amin), Springer, New York, pp. 203–213.

9 Stoffel, E.M. (2015) Screening in GI cancers: The role of genetics. *J. Clin. Oncol.*, **33**, 1721–1728.

10 Fitzgerald, R.C., Hardwick, R., Huntsman, D., *et al.* (2010) Hereditary diffuse gastric cancer: updated consensus guidelines for clinical management and directions for future research. *J. Med. Genet.*, **47** (7), 436–444.

11 Gravalos, C., Jimeno, A. (2008) HER2 in gastric cancer: a new prognostic factor and a novel therapeutic target. *Ann. Oncol.*, **19** (9), 1523–1529.

12 Hofmann, M., Stoss, O., Shi, D., *et al.* (2008) Assessment of a HER2 scoring system for gastric cancer: results from a validation study. *Histopathology*, **52** (7), 797–805.

13 Tanner, M., Hollmen, M., Junttila, T.T., *et al.* (2005) Amplification of HER-2 in gastric carcinoma: association with Topoisomerase IIalpha gene amplification, intestinal type, poor prognosis and sensitivity to trastuzumab. *Ann. Oncol.*, **16** (2), 273–278.

14 Bar-Sela, G., Hershkovitz, D., Haim, N., *et al.* (2013) The incidence and prognostic value of HER2 overexpression and cyclin D1 expression in patients with gastric or gastroesophageal junction adenocarcinoma in Israel. *Oncol. Lett.*, **5** (2), 559–563.

15 Barros-Silva, J.D., Leitao, D., Afonso, L., *et al.* (2009) Association of ERBB2 gene status with histopathological parameters and disease-specific survival in gastric carcinoma patients. *Br. J. Cancer*, **100** (3), 487–493.

16 Gordon, M.A., Gundacker, H.M., Benedetti, J., *et al.* (2013) Assessment of HER2 gene amplification in adenocarcinomas of the stomach or gastroesophageal junction in the INT-0116/SWOG9008 clinical trial. *Ann. Oncol.*, **24** (7), 1754–1761.

17 Grabsch, H., Sivakumar, S., Gray, S., Gabbert, H.E., Muller, W. (2010) HER2 expression in gastric cancer: Rare, heterogeneous and of no prognostic value – conclusions from 924 cases of two independent series. *Cell Oncol.*, **32** (1-2), 57–65.

18 Okines, A.F., Thompson, L.C., Cunningham, D., *et al.* (2013) Effect of HER2 on prognosis and benefit from peri-operative chemotherapy in early oesophago-gastric adenocarcinoma in the MAGIC trial. *Ann. Oncol.*, **24** (5), 1253–1261.

18a Aizawa, M., Nagatsuma, A.K., Kitada, K., Kuwata, T., Fujii, S., Kinoshita, T., Ochiai, A. (2014) Evaluation of HER2-based biology in 1,006 cases of gastric cancer in a Japanese population. *Gastric Cancer*, **17** (1), 34–42.

19 Bang, Y.J., Van Cutsem, E., Feyereislova, A., *et al.*, and ToGA Trial Investigators (2010) Trastuzumab in combination with chemotherapy versus chemotherapy alone for treatment of HER2-positive advanced gastric or gastro-oesophageal junction cancer (ToGA): a phase 3, open-label, randomised controlled trial. *Lancet*, **376** (9742), 687–697.

20 Park, S.H., Sohn, T.S., Lee, J., *et al.* (2015) Phase III trial to compare adjuvant chemotherapy with capecitabine and cisplatin versus concurrent chemoradiotherapy in gastric cancer: Final Report of

the Adjuvant Chemoradiotherapy in Stomach Tumors Trial, Including Survival and Subset Analyses. *J. Clin. Oncol.*, **33**, 3130–3136.

20a Fuchs, C.S., Tomasek, J., Yong, C.J., *et al.* and the REGARD Trial Investigators (2014) Ramucirumab monotherapy for previously treated advanced gastric or gastro-oesophageal junction adenocarcinoma (REGARD): an international, randomised, multicentre, placebo-controlled, phase 3 trial. *Lancet*, **383** (9911), 31–39.

21 Cancer Genome Atlas Research (2014) Comprehensive molecular characterization of gastric adenocarcinoma. *Nature*, **513** (7517), 202–209.

22 Warneke, V.S., Behrens, H.M., Hartmann, J.T., *et al.* (2011) Cohort study based on the seventh edition of the TNM classification for gastric cancer: proposal of a new staging system. *J. Clin. Oncol.*, **29** (17), 2364–2371.

23 Rocken, C., Behrens, H.M. (2015) Validating the prognostic and discriminating value of the TNM-classification for gastric cancer – a critical appraisal. *Eur. J. Cancer*, **51** (5), 577–586.

24 Marchet, A., Mocellin, S., Ambrosi, A., *et al.* and Italian Research Group for Gastric Cancer (2008) The prognostic value of N-ratio in patients with gastric cancer: validation in a large, multicenter series. *Eur. J. Surg. Oncol.*, **34** (2), 159–165.

25 Kutlu, O.C., Watchell, M., Dissanaike, S. (2015) Metastatic lymph node ratio successfully predicts prognosis in western gastric cancer patients. *Surg. Oncol.*, **24**, 84–88.

26 Gouzi, J.L., Huguier, M., Fagniez, P.L., *et al.* (1999) Total versus subtotal gastrectomy for adenocarcinoma of the gastric antrum. A French prospective controlled study. *Ann. Surg.*, **209** (2), 162–166.

27 Bozzetti, F., Marubini, E., Bonfanti, G., Miceli, R., Piano, C., Gennari, L. (1999) Subtotal versus total gastrectomy for gastric cancer: five-year survival rates in a multicenter randomized Italian trial. Italian Gastrointestinal Tumor Study Group. *Ann. Surg.*, **230** (2), 170–178.

28 Schwarz, R.E. (2015) Current status of management of malignant disease: current management of gastric cancer. *J. Gastrointest. Surg.*, **19** (4), 782–788.

29 Karpeh, M.S., Leon, L., Klimstra, D., Brennan, M.F. (2000) Lymph node staging in gastric cancer: is location more important than number? An analysis of 1,038 patients. *Ann. Surg.*, **232** (3), 362–371.

30 Bonenkamp, J.J., Sasako, M., Hermans, J., *et al.* and the Dutch Gastric Cancer Group (1999) Extended lymph-node dissection for gastric cancer. *N. Engl. J. Med.*, **340**, 908–914.

31 Hartgrink, H.H., van de Helde, C.J., Putter, H., *et al.* (2004) Extended lymph node dissection for gastric cancer: who may benefit? Final results of the randomized Dutch Gastric Cancer Group trial. *J. Clin. Oncol.*, **22**, 2069–2077.

32 Songun, I., Putter, H., Meershoek-Klein Kranenbarg, E., Sasako, M., van de Helde, J.H. (2010) Surgical treatment of gastric cancer: 15-year follow-up results of the randomized nationwide D1D2 trial. *Lancet*, **ii**, 439–449.

33 Jiang, L., Yang, K.H., Chen, Y., Guan, Q.L., Zhao, P., Tian, J.H., Wang, Q. (2014) Systematic review and meta-analysis of the effectiveness and safety of extended lymphadenectomy in patients with resectable gastric cancer. *Br. J. Surg.*, **101** (6), 595–604.

34 Degiuli, M., Sasako, M., Ponti, A., Calvo, F. (2004) Survival results of a multicenter phase II study to evaluate D2 gastrectomy for gastric cancer. *Br. J. Cancer*, **90** (9), 1727–1732.

35 Degiuli, M., Sasako, M., Ponti, A., *et al.* and Italian Gastric Cancer Study Group (2014) Randomized clinical trial comparing survival after D1 or D2 gastrectomy for gastric cancer. *Br. J. Surg.*, **101** (2), 23–31.

36 Macdonald, J.S., Smalley, S.R., Benedetti, J., *et al.* (2001) Chemoradiotherapy after surgery compared with surgery alone for adenocarcinoma of the stomach or gastroesophageal junction. *N. Engl. J. Med.*, **345** (10), 725–730.

37 Smalley, S.R., Benedetti, J.K., Haller, D.G., *et al.* (2012) Updated analysis of SWOG-directed intergroup study 0116: a phase III trial of adjuvant radiochemotherapy versus observation after curative gastric cancer resection. *J. Clin. Oncol.*, **30** (19), 2327–2333.

38 Dikken, J.L., Jansen, E.P.M., Cats, A., *et al.* (2010) Impact of the extent of surgery and postoperative chemoradiotherapy on recurrence patterns in gastric cancer. *J. Clin. Oncol.*, **28**, 2430–2436.

39 Lee, J., Lim, D.H., Kim, S., *et al.* (2011) Phase III trial comparing capecitabine plus cisplatin versus capecitabine radiotherapy in completely resected gastric cancer with D2 lymph node dissection: the ARTIST trial. *J. Clin. Oncol.*, **30**, 268–273.

40 Fuchs, C.S., Tepper, J.E., Niedzwiecki, D., *et al.* (2011) Postoperative adjuvant chemoradiation for gastric or gastroesophageal junction (GEJ) adenocarcinoma using epirubicin, cisplatin, and infusional (CI) 5-FU (ECF) before and after CI 5-FU and radiotherapy (CRT) compared with bolus 5-FU/LV before and after CRT: Intergroup trial CALGB 80101. Oral Abstract Session, 2011 ASCO Annual Meeting. *J. Clin. Oncol.*, **29** (Suppl.; abstract 4003).

41 Dikken, J.L., van Sandick, J.W., Maurits Swellengrebel, H.A., *et al.* (2011) Neo-adjuvant chemotherapy followed by surgery and chemotherapy or by surgery and chemoradiotherapy for patients with resectable gastric cancer (CRITICS). *BMC Cancer*, **11**, 329.

42 Cunningham, D., Allum, W.H., Stenning, S.P., *et al.* (2006) Perioperative chemotherapy versus surgery alone for resectable gastroesophageal cancer. *N. Engl. J. Med.*, **355** (1), 11–20.

43 Sasako, M., Sakuramoto, S., Katai, H., *et al.* (2011) Five-year outcomes of a randomized phase III trial comparing adjuvant chemotherapy with S-1 versus surgery alone in stage II or stage III gastric cancer. *J. Clin. Oncol.*, **29**, 4387–4393.

44 Bang, Y.J., Kim, Y.W., Yang, H.K., *et al.* (2012) Adjuvant capecitabine and oxaliplatin for gastric cancer after D2 gastrectomy (CLASSIC): a phase 3 open-label, randomized controlled trial. *Lancet*, **379**, 315–321.

45 Noh, S.H., Park, S.R., Yang H.K., *et al.* (2014) Adjuvant capecitabine plus oxaliplatin for gastric cancer after D2 gastrectomy (CLASSIC): 5-year follow-up of an open-label, randomised phase 3 trial. *Lancet Oncol.*, **15**, 1389–1396.

46 Cunningham, D., Starling, N., Rao, S., *et al.* (2008) Capecitabine and oxaliplatin for advanced esophogastric cancer. *N. Engl. J. Med.*, **358**, 36–46.

47 Ronellenfitsch, U., Schwarzbach, M., Hofheinz, R., *et al.* (2013) Preoperative chemo(radio)therapy versus primary surgery for gastroesophageal adenocarcinoma: systematic review with meta-analysis combining individual patient and aggregate data. *Eur. J. Cancer*, **49** (15), 3149–3158.

48 Jiang, L., Yang, K.H., Guan, Q.L., Chen, Y., Zhao, P., Tian, J.H. (2015) Survival benefit of neoadjuvant chemotherapy for resectable cancer of the gastric and gastroesophageal junction: a meta-analysis. *J. Clin. Gastroenterol.*, **49** (5), 387–394.

22

Pancreatic Cancer

Manisha Palta, Christopher G. Willett and Brian G. Czito

Introduction

Pancreatic cancer is the fourth leading cause of cancer-related death in the United States, where it accounts for approximately 43 000 deaths each year [1]. At present, surgery offers the only means of cure but, unfortunately, only 10–20% of patients present with tumors amenable to resection. Even among patients who present with localized disease, the five-year overall survival (OS) rate is approximately 20% and median survival ranges from approximately 13 to 20 months [2]. Contemporary survival rates have reported improved results, particularly in patients with complete surgical resection (R0) and node-negative (N0) disease [3–5]. Patients who present with locally advanced and unresectable pancreatic cancer have a median survival of approximately nine to 16 months, with rare long-term survival. Nearly 60% of patients present with metastatic disease, which carries a shorter median survival of less than a year [6].

Evaluation

During recent years, significant advances have been achieved in the imaging and staging of pancreatic cancer [7]. Currently, the principal diagnostic tools are helical computed tomography (CT) scanning, endoscopic ultrasound (EUS), and laparoscopy. Magnetic resonance imaging (MRI) and positron emission tomography (PET) are emerging imaging techniques in the evaluation of pancreatic malignancies. These tools have facilitated characterization of the primary tumor (resectable/borderline resectable versus unresectable), as well as the identification of metastatic disease, so patients can be appropriately and reliably triaged to operative and non-operative therapies.

The most commonly used staging and diagnostic examination tool is abdominal CT scanning. Newer generation, multidetector, high-speed helical CT performed with timed contrast enhancement and thin-section imaging allows high-resolution, motion-free images of the pancreas and its surrounding structures to be obtained at varying phases of enhancement. This allows for adequate imaging of the primary tumor and its proximity to adjacent vessels, as well as the assessment of metastatic deposits in other intra-abdominal organs such as the liver [8]. Over 90% of patients deemed unresectable due to vascular involvement by CT are truly inoperable at time of surgery [9]. CT staging is limited, however, in the detection of nodal involvement and peritoneal disease. Pathologic confirmation of malignancy is a necessary step prior to initiating therapy for patients with pancreatic cancer; CT can be utilized to facilitate fine-needle aspiration (FNA).

Another tool for staging and diagnosis is EUS. In this procedure, an endoscope with an ultrasound transducer at its tip is passed into the stomach and duodenum, where it provides high-resolution images of the pancreas and surrounding vessels. EUS may also be performed in conjunction with endoscopic retrograde cholangiopancreatography (ERCP). This combined diagnostic approach allows for staging, therapeutic stenting of the common bile duct when indicated, and retrieval of tumor cells by FNA without exposing the peritoneum to potential tumor seeding, as may occur with CT-guided biopsies. The sensitivity for EUS is at least comparable to that of CT, with tumor detection reported as high as 97% [10]. An advantage of EUS over CT is ability to detect small lesions that might not be well visualized on cross-sectional imaging [11]. Caution must be applied, however, as the interpretation of EUS is highly operator-dependent [10, 12].

As current imaging techniques cannot visualize small (1–2 mm) liver and peritoneal implants, staging laparoscopy has been used preoperatively to exclude intraperitoneal metastases. A recent meta-analysis showed that the adoption of staging laparoscopy and laparoscopic ultrasound can detect otherwise occult disease, preventing up to 50% of patients from undergoing unnecessary laparotomy [13]. Patients with locally advanced disease and involved peritoneal washings or positive peritoneal biopsies have the same prognosis as those with metastatic disease; these patients are more appropriately treated with systemic therapies [14].

Advances in MRI, including high-resolution imaging, faster acquisition time, 3D reconstruction, functional imaging and magnetic resonance cholangiopancreatography (MRCP), have led to an improved ability of MRI to diagnose and stage pancreatic cancer [8]. This modality can be used in patients with poor renal function to assess the primary tumor and determine resectability, although some studies suggest that MRI is not as sensitive as EUS or CT in tumor detection [15]. A potential advantage of MRI is the identification of small foci of hepatic metastatic disease that are difficult to appreciate by CT, or to further characterize ill-defined lesions seen on CT [16].

Initial studies showed that PET has a higher sensitivity, specificity, and accuracy than CT in diagnosing pancreatic carcinomas [17–19]. More recent studies have compared integrated PET-CT with PET or CT alone in pancreatic cancers, and have demonstrated a higher sensitivity for malignancy detection with PET-CT [17]. PET may also be a useful adjunct in the identification of benign versus malignant lesions and presence of metastatic disease. Although PET-CT may be useful in initial diagnosis, its role in determining resectability has been questioned as co-registration is often performed with lesser-resolution CT images and areas of high metabolism can obscure peripancreatic planes [20].

Despite the number of imaging modalities available for the assessment of pancreatic malignancies, all imaging modalities are inadequate to stage lymph node involvement, and further advances may improve the ability to diagnose, stage, and appropriately select patients for further therapies.

Therapy for Resectable Disease

Following surgical resection alone of pancreatic cancer, local recurrence rates range from 50% to 90% and distant recurrence rates from 40% to 90%, most commonly to the liver and/or peritoneum [21–27]. This provides rationale for adjuvant therapy including radiation therapy (RT), chemotherapy, and combined radiation and chemotherapy (CRT), which have been employed in an effort to improve patient outcomes. Despite multiple randomized trials, a definitive role for adjuvant radiation therapy for resected pancreatic cancer has not been established.

Early Adjuvant Therapy Trials

An early randomized control trial for resectable pancreatic cancer, designed by the Gastrointestinal Tumor Study Group (GITSG), laid the foundation for the adoption of CRT in the United States (Table 22.1). In this study, 43 patients were enrolled to evaluate the outcomes of surgery alone compared to CRT. All patients

Table 22.1 Randomized trials of adjuvant therapy.

Trial/Reference	Year	No. of patients	Treatment arms	DFS months	Median months	OS
GITSG [30]	1985	43	Observation	9	11	2 yr 15%
			5-FU CRT then 5FU	11	20	2 yr 42%
EORTC [31,32]	1999	114	Observation	–	19.2	5 yr 22%
			5-FU CRT	–	21.6	5 yr 25%
ESPAC-1 [35]	2004	289	No CT vs. CT	–	15.5 vs 20.1	5 yr 8 vs 21%
			No CRT vs. CRT	–	17.9 vs 15.9	5 yr 20 vs 10%
CONKO [37]	2007	368	Observation	6.9	20.2	5 yr 9%
			Gem	13.4	22.8	5 yr 21%
RTOG 9704 [113]	2008	388	5-FU, 5-FU CRT, 5-FU	–	17.2	5 yr 18%
			Gem, 5-FU CRT, Gem	–	20.5	5 yr 22%
ESPAC-3 [39]	2010	1088	5-FU	14.1	23	2 yr 48%
			Gem	14.3	23.6	2 yr 49%

CRT, chemoradiotherapy; CT, chemotherapy; 5-FU, 5-Fluorouracil; Gem, gemcitabine.

underwent curative resection of pancreatic adenocarcinoma without evidence of intraperitoneal disease. Split-course RT was administered to a total dose of 40 Gy with a two-week treatment break. Chemotherapy consisted of bolus infusion 5-flourouracil (5-FU) (500 mg/m^2) during the first three days of each RT course, and weekly thereafter for a planned course of two years or until disease progression. At interim analysis, an improvement in median disease-free survival (DFS) and OS with CRT was observed: 11 months versus 9 months, and 20 months versus 11 months, respectively. The two-year OS was 42% in the CRT group versus 15% in the surgery-alone arm [28]. An additional 30 patients were later enrolled to receive adjuvant CRT. These patients confirmed the survival outcomes seen in the original trial, with median survival of 18 months and a two-year survival of 46% [29].

The GITSG trial closed prematurely following the enrollment of 43 of an intended 100 patients due to slow accrual over the eight-year enrollment period. The RT approach in this trial, by contemporary standards, was considered low dose and antiquated due to the split-course technique and large treatment fields encompassing the entire pancreas/pancreatic bed and celiac, pancreaticosplenic, peripancreatic, and retroperitoneal regional lymph nodes [30]. Additionally, the inclusion of both CRT and adjuvant chemotherapy after surgery alone evaluated two treatment variables, making it difficult to discern the true effect of either treatment alone. In the CRT arm there were issues of compliance, with 32% of patients assigned to CRT receiving inappropriate radiation, and 25% of patients failing to initiate treatment within 10 weeks post-surgery, the protocol-specified time limit. Only 9% of patients completed the planned two-year maintenance chemotherapy course. In addition, survival in the control arm was low compared to historical controls. Despite these caveats and the inability to reach the desired patient accrual, the GITSG trial demonstrated a benefit to CRT and became standard adjuvant therapy, particularly in the United States.

In Europe, the use of adjuvant CRT underwent further assessment by the European Organization for Research and Treatment of Cancer (EORTC), who designed a trial to confirm the findings of the original GITSG study. A total of 218 patients with resected pancreas (*n* = 114) or non-pancreas periampullary tumors (*n* = 104) were randomly assigned to surgery and adjuvant CRT or surgery alone. RT, as in the GITSG trial, was delivered split course to 40 Gy with a two-week treatment break. Chemotherapy was delivered by continuous infusion (25 mg kg^{-1} for the first five days of each RT course) without further adjuvant therapy [31]. Long-term follow-up of the EORTC trial demonstrated no difference in five-year OS with CRT use: 25% (CRT) versus 22% (surgery alone). Post hoc analysis of the pancreatic head lesions failed to demonstrate a benefit with CRT, with a median OS of 1.3 years (CRT) versus one year (surgery alone) [32].

This trial has been criticized for its heterogeneous patient population, including patients with both pancreatic and periampullary primary tumors. Periampullary carcinomas have a significantly better prognosis compared to pancreatic cancer; the two entities thus represent truly different diseases and this potentially dilutes any evidence of benefit for adjuvant CRT [33]. Similar to the GITSG trial, older RT techniques of split course and low total dose were used. Additionally, more than 20% of patients in the CRT arm did not receive the intended treatment due to postoperative complications and/or patient refusal. Although a small subset, patients undergoing non-curative resection were still eligible for enrollment. The discordant results of the EORTC and GITSG trials have led some investigators to attribute the OS benefit seen in the GITSG trial to be a function of adjuvant chemotherapy administration rather than RT.

An additional European trial conducted by the European Study Group for Pancreatic Cancer (ESPAC) aimed to further answer the question of appropriate adjuvant therapy for 'macroscopically' resected pancreatic cancer patients. ESPAC-1 enrolled 541 patients with pancreatic adenocarcinoma undergoing surgery to receive CRT, chemotherapy, CRT followed by chemotherapy, or no further treatment. Although planned as a 2 × 2 randomization design, only 285 patients were randomized to one of the above treatment arms. The remainder were, as per patient or physician preference, randomized for CRT (versus not) or chemotherapy (versus not) in an attempts to enhance patient accrual. RT was delivered in similar fashion as the GITSG and EORTC trials, with split-course treatment to 40 Gy, and bolus 5-FU (425 mg/m^2) chemotherapy was administered with leucovorin (LV; 20 mg/m^2). On initial analysis, outcomes from all three cohorts (2 × 2 factorial, chemotherapy versus no chemotherapy and CRT versus no CRT) were analyzed collectively, specifically evaluating patients receiving CRT versus no CRT and chemotherapy versus no chemotherapy. No difference in survival was seen in patients receiving CRT compared to patients who did not receive CRT. In the chemotherapy arm, however, a 35% reduction in death was seen in the group receiving chemotherapy compared to no chemotherapy, with a median survival of 19.7 months versus 14 months [34]. Long-term results of only those patients randomized in the 2 × 2 schema were subsequently reported. This analysis suggested a survival detriment in patients receiving CRT, with a five-year OS of 10% (CRT) versus 20% (no CRT). However, an improvement in OS continued to be seen in patients receiving chemotherapy at five years: 21% (chemotherapy) versus 8% (no chemotherapy) [35].

This complex trial design has the potential for bias as patients and/or physicians could select randomization for one treatment variable. As in the aforementioned trials, the RT technique used is, by contemporary standards, considered outdated with split-course and low total dose. No details of RT delivery or central quality assurance for RT, surgery, or pathology were available. Similarly, many treatment violations occurred as only 62% of patients received full CRT treatment and 42% of patients in the chemotherapy arms completed the predefined regimen. Although many have attempted to draw conclusions from the updated publication, the 2×2 cohort of the study was not powered to detect OS differences. Patients receiving CRT in the ESPAC trial experienced poorer survival outcomes compared to other reported CRT series, and patients who had received prior chemotherapy and/or radiation therapy were still eligible for enrollment. Despite these critiques, it has been speculated that the detriment seen in the CRT group may be due to delayed systemic therapy administration.

Another common critique of the early trials of adjuvant therapy is the lack of restaging after surgical resection and prior to the initiation of adjuvant therapy to evaluate presence of persistent or metastatic disease. The time between initial staging and commencement of adjuvant treatment can be as long as three to four months, during which time a significant minority of patients would be expected to develop radiographically apparent metastases. Without interval restaging, these patients may inappropriately receive CRT. Although these three trials, each fraught with its own flaws, created the foundation for adjuvant treatment approaches of resectable pancreatic cancer, there continues to be little consensus regarding the 'most appropriate' treatment. A relative dichotomy in adjuvant treatment approaches for resectable pancreatic cancer has emerged between the US and parts of Europe, with adjuvant CRT frequently implemented in the US and adjuvant chemotherapy alone in parts of Europe.

Adjuvant Gemcitabine-Based Therapy Trials

In parts of Europe, the EORTC and ESPAC-1 trials were felt to provide sufficient evidence to exclude the routine use of adjuvant CRT in favor of adjuvant chemotherapy alone. The Charite Onkologie (CONKO) trial from Germany randomized 368 patients with R0 or R1 resection to six cycles (with one cycle generally consisting of three weekly infusions followed by one week off) of adjuvant gemcitabine (1000 mg/m^2) versus observation. Patients with cancer antigen 19-9 (CA19-9) or carcinoembryonic antigen (CEA) levels greater than 2.5-fold the upper limits of normal were excluded. Low rates of grade 3–4 toxicities were seen with gemcitabine, the majority consisting of hematologic toxicities. The primary study endpoint of DFS was significantly improved to 14.2 months (gemcitabine) versus 7.5 months (surgery alone). This improvement was sustained in both R0 and R1 subgroups [36]. At the initial publication there was no difference in OS,

but with a longer follow-up median survival and five-year OS were both improved in patients receiving gemcitabine (23 months versus 20 months, and 21% versus 9%, respectively) [37]. This well-conceived and implemented trial established gemcitabine as the adjuvant chemotherapy of choice. These findings were supported by a smaller randomized study from Japan, again demonstrating a DFS benefit of gemcitabine compared to surgery alone [38].

At the same time the CONKO trial was enrolling patients, ESPAC-3 – the largest randomized control trial in pancreatic cancer to date – enrolled 1088 patients with pancreatic adenocarcinoma undergoing R0 or R1 resection. Patients were randomized to six cycles of adjuvant gemcitabine (three weekly infusions at 1000 mg/m^2) or six cycles of bolus 5-FU/LV (5-FU 425 mg/m^2; LV 20 mg/m^2). Patients receiving 5FU/LV experienced significantly higher rates of grade 3–4 gastrointestinal toxicity (stomatitis and diarrhea), whereas those receiving gemcitabine experienced significantly higher rates of grade 3–4 hematologic toxicity. At median follow-up of 34.2 months, there was no difference in the primary endpoint of OS between the two groups. Given the favorable toxicity profile, gemcitabine alone is considered the standard adjuvant treatment in patients with resectable pancreatic cancer throughout many parts of Europe [39]. The focus of future European adjuvant therapies for resectable pancreatic cancer has centered on finding the ideal combination of systemic agents. The ongoing ESPAC-4 is accruing patients with resected pancreatic cancer for randomization to gemcitabine alone versus gemcitabine/capecitabine.

As opposed to parts of Europe where the focus of adjuvant therapy has centered on chemotherapy, adjuvant CRT continues to be commonly utilized in the US. The Radiation Therapy Oncology Group (RTOG) 9704 conducted a randomized trial comparing adjuvant 5-FU-based versus gemcitabine-based chemotherapy integrated with CRT. A total of 451 patients with resected pancreatic adenocarcinoma were randomized to receive continuous-infusion 5-FU (250 mg/m^2 per day) or gemcitabine (1000 mg/m^2 weekly for three weeks) prior to CRT, and for 12 weeks after CRT. In both groups, CRT consisted of 50.4 Gy delivered with continuous-infusion 5-FU (250 mg/m^2 per day) throughout treatment. Prospective quality assurance of all RT plans was required. This trial was powered to demonstrate a survival benefit for the entire cohort and the subgroup of patients with pancreatic head lesions. On initial analysis of the pancreatic head subgroup, a non-significant trend toward improved median and three-year OS was seen in the gemcitabine arm: 20.5 months versus 16.9 months, and 31% versus 22%, respectively. However, a higher incidence of grade 3 or higher hematologic toxicity was also seen in the gemcitabine group, with no significant differences seen in severe non-hematologic toxicities [40]. An update of this trial reported median and five-year OS rates in patients with pancreatic head tumors of 20.5 months and 22% with gemcitabine versus 17.2 months and 18% with 5-FU. On multivariate analysis, in the subgroup of patients with pancreatic head lesions who received gemcitabine, there was a nonsignificant trend toward improved OS (p = 0.08) [41].

A secondary endpoint of RTOG 9704 was to assess the ability of post-resection CA 19-9 to predict survival. In a cohort of 385 patients, when CA 19-9 was analyzed as a dichotomized variable (<180 versus ≥180, ≤90 versus >90 U ml^{-1}), there was a significant survival difference favoring patients with CA 19-9 less than 180 U ml^{-1}. This corresponded to a 72% risk reduction in death [42]. Follow-up analysis showed that patients with pancreatic head tumors treated with gemcitabine with a CA 19-9 serum level of <90 U ml^{-1} and as per protocol RT, had favorable survival compared to that seen in the CONKO trial (median survival and five-year rate of 24 months and 34% versus 22 months and 21%, respectively) [42a].

As opposed to previously described randomized trials evaluating the role of adjuvant radiation therapy, a major strength of the RTOG study was the rigorous, centralized quality control of RT techniques and delivery. Modern techniques with three or four field beam arrangements were used. A recent analysis demonstrated that patients treated as per study guidelines had a significant survival advantage, indicating the importance of centralized review and treatment technique in this disease [43].

In this study, 28% of patients experienced local recurrence as first site of relapse, which was considerably lower than previously discussed randomized trials (including CONKO) and historical series implementing chemotherapy alone approaches. Distant failure, however, remained high at 73% as a first site of relapse. These high rates of distant failure and need for more effective systemic therapy, as well as controversy surrounding the role of CRT in resected patients, led to the design of the current, multinational RTOG 0848/EORTC trial.

The current RTOG 0848/EORTC trial randomizes patients with resected pancreatic head adenocarcinoma (stratified based on CA 19-9, nodal and margin status) to gemcitabine alone or gemcitabine combined with erlotinib for five cycles. The trial was recently amended to remove the first randomization to gemcitabine or gemcitabine/erlotinib. If no progression is seen on restaging following completion of systemic therapy, patients are then randomized to receive an additional cycle (total six cycles) of previously administered chemotherapy and no further treatment versus CRT (50.4 Gy) using modern techniques/central RT quality assurance, with concurrent capecitabine or 5-FU (Figure 22.1). This trial seeks to answer two primary questions: (i) the role of the small-molecule EGFR inhibitor, erlotinib, in the adjuvant therapy of pancreatic cancer; and (ii) the role of CRT in the era of modern chemotherapy, particularly in patients who do not experience early disease progression. This is the only contemporary randomized clinical trial currently evaluating the role of CRT in the adjuvant setting.

Single-Institution/Large Retrospective Experiences

In addition to the above-randomized studies, several large, single-institution series have suggested a benefit of adjuvant CRT. A review of the Mayo Clinic experience reported the outcomes of 472 patients who underwent

Figure 22.1 RTOG 0848/EORTC trial schema. *Source:* Palta 2011. Reproduced with permission of UBM Media LLC.

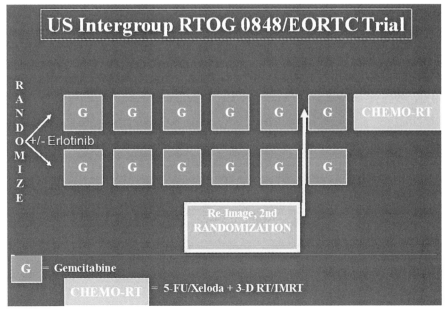

R0 resection between 1975 and 2005. Despite more adverse prognostic features in patients receiving CRT (higher histological grade and lymph node involvement rates), median, two-year and five-year OS were significantly improved in the CRT cohort: 25.2 months versus 19.2 months, 50% versus 39%, and 28% versus 17%, respectively [44]. A similar series from Johns Hopkins compared 908 patients who underwent pancreaticoduodenectomy between 1993 and 2005 and received surgery alone or CRT. Patients receiving CRT experienced a significant improvement in median, two-year and five-year OS: 21.2 months versus 14.4 months, 43.9% versus 31.9%, and 20.1% versus 15.4%, respectively [45]. A pooled retrospective analysis of nearly 1100 patients from both institutions demonstrated similar results in favor of adjuvant CRT [46]. Despite inherent biases of non-randomized, retrospective trials, these data, along with patterns of failure data in the above-randomized studies, suggest that there are patient subgroups that stand to benefit from the addition of CRT to surgical resection.

Data with the highest survival after adjuvant therapy for pancreatic cancer come from a Phase II trial conducted at the Virginia Mason Clinic. Some 43 of a planned enrollment of 53 patients were treated with CRT to 50 Gy with 5-FU (200 mg/m^2 per day) continuous infusion, weekly cisplatin (30 mg/m^2), and interferon-α (3 × 10^6 units) subcutaneously every other day. After completion of CRT, patients received further adjuvant 5-FU (200 mg/m^2 per day) continuous infusion [47]. The two- and five-year OS were 64% and 55%, respectively. Median survival was not reached at time of initial publication. With these encouraging data came significant toxicity, as 70% of patients experienced grade 3 or higher toxicities and 42% required hospitalization. The American College of Surgeons Oncology Group (ACOSOG) subsequently opened a multicenter, Phase II trial evaluating the Virginia Mason adjuvant regimen. Although survival outcomes were promising (median survival 25 months), the trial closed early after accrual of 89 patients due to high toxicity rates; 95% of patients experienced grade 3 or higher toxicity, and 50% failed to complete the entire treatment protocol [48].

Neoadjuvant Chemoradiotherapy

In other gastrointestinal malignancies (i.e., rectum, esophagus), the use of neoadjuvant CRT has become standard practice. Given the potential for significant delays in delivery of adjuvant therapy in one-third or more of patients following surgical resection and modest survival gains associated with adjuvant therapy, the delivery of neoadjuvant therapy offers a potentially attractive alternative [49]. Potential advantages of preoperative therapy include an undisrupted tumor vasculature,

allowing for improved delivery of chemotherapy and radiosensitizing oxygenation [50, 51]. Downstaging may occur, potentially allowing more advanced lesions to be resected as well as sterilization of operative region, reducing the risk of spread during surgical manipulation. Preoperative treatment avoids delay in adjuvant therapy delivery due to postoperative recovery and, importantly, avoids potentially morbid radical resection in patients with rapidly progressive disease. This is important for the minority of patients who will develop clinically apparent metastatic disease during the course of neoadjuvant therapy [52–54]. Finally, neoadjuvant CRT has also been associated with a reduction in the incidence of pancreatic leak, as well as leak-associated morbidity and mortality [50].

Unlike with adjuvant therapy, no Phase III randomized trials of neoadjuvant CRT have been performed, and the vast majority of data derives from single- and multi-institution Phase II and retrospective studies (Table 22.2). At M.D. Anderson Cancer Center, multiple trials of neoadjuvant 5-FU-based CRT have been performed. The earliest trial treated 28 patients with continuous-infusion 5-FU (300 mg/m^2 per day) and concurrent external beam radiotherapy (EBRT) to 50.4 Gy over 5.5 weeks. Patients who underwent surgical resection also received intraoperative radiation therapy (IORT). Some 25% of patients had evidence of metastatic disease on preoperative restaging, while 15% had metastatic disease that was found on laparoscopy. For those patients who underwent surgery, median survival was 18 months and 41% achieved pathologic partial response to therapy. However, 33% of patients treated on this study required hospitalization for gastrointestinal toxicity from therapy [55]. In an effort to minimize hospitalization, this group subsequently focused on rapid-fractionation EBRT. In this case, a prospective trial of 35 patients treated with EBRT to 30 Gy (3 Gy per fraction for 10 fractions) with concurrent continuous-infusion 5-FU (300 mg/m^2 per day) found grade 3 nausea and vomiting in only 9% of patients, with no grade 4 toxicities. Of these patients, 27 underwent surgery and 20 underwent resection and IORT to 10–15 Gy. Locoregional recurrence occurred in only two of the 20 resected patients. Median survival for patients who underwent surgery was 25 months, with a three-year survival rate of 23% [56].

Trials of neoadjuvant CRT with paclitaxel as radiosensitizer have been conducted. In an M.D. Anderson study, 35 patients received weekly paclitaxel (60 mg/m^2) with concurrent EBRT to 30 Gy. Among patients, 80% underwent resection, with 21% of pathology specimens showing >50% tumor necrosis. The three-year survival for patients who underwent preoperative therapy and resection was 28%. Hospitalization was required in 11% of patients for toxicity, primarily nausea and vomiting. These preliminary data show an increased toxicity

Table 22.2 Trials of neoadjuvant therapy for resectable disease.

Trial/Reference	Year	No. of patients	Treatment arms	Complete resection	Survival (entire cohort) Median OS	Survival (resected patients) Median OS
Pisters *et al.* [56]	1998	35	5-FU CRT (30 Gy) + IORT	20 (57%)	–	25 mo, 3 yr 23%
Hoffman *et al.* [114]	1998	53	MMC/5-FU CRT (50.4 Gy)	24 (45%)	9.7 mo	15.7 mo, 2 yr 27%
Pisters *et al.* [57]	2002	37	Paclitaxel CRT (30 Gy) + IORT	20 (54%)	12 mo, 3yr 14%	19 mo, 3yr 28%
Evans *et al.* [59]	2008	86	Gem CRT (30 Gy)	64 (74%)	22.7 mo, 5yr 27%	34 mo, 5 yr 36%
Varadhachary *et al.* [60]	2008	90	Gem/CDDP CT, Gem CRT (30 Gy)	52 (58%)	17.4 mo	31 mo
Le Scodan *et al.* [58]	2009	41	Gem/CDDP CRT (50 Gy)	26 (63%)	9.4 mo	12 mo 2yr 32%
Talamonti *et al.* [61]	2006	20	Gem CRT (36Gy)	16 (80%)	26 mo	
Small *et al.* [62]	2008	41	Gem CRT (36 Gy)	1 yr 73%	2 yr 61%	
Golcher *et al.* [63]	2015	73	Surgery / Gem/CDDP CRT (50–54 Gy) + Surgery	48% / 52%	14.4 mo / 17.4 mo	18.9 mo / 25 mo

5-FU, 5-Flourouracil; CDDP, cisplatin; CRT, chemoradiotherapy; CT, chemotherapy; Gem, gemcitabine; IORT, intraoperative radiotherapy; MMC, mitomycin-C; mo, months; OS, overall survival.

without a significant improvement in histological response rate or survival [57].

The French SFRO-FFCD 9704 trial incorporated further radiosensitizing chemotherapy with radiation therapy. Here, 41 patients received CRT to 50 Gy with 5-FU (300 mg/m^2 per day) and two cycles of CDDP (20 mg/m^2) followed by surgical resection in patients without progression. Some 63% of patients underwent curative surgery, with 80% obtaining an R0 resection and 50% of specimens showing a major histological response. In patients who underwent curative surgery, the median survival was 11.7 months with 32% two-year OS [58].

The evolution of CRT in the neoadjuvant setting appears to parallel advances made with adjuvant therapy and transition to gemcitabine-containing regimens. In 2008, two published Phase II studies from the M.D. Anderson Cancer Center evaluated the use of gemcitabine as part of a neoadjuvant regimen. One trial enrolled 86 patients with radiographically resectable adenocarcinoma of the pancreatic head/uncinate. Patients received weekly gemcitabine (400 mg/m^2) with 30 Gy RT over two weeks. After re-staging four to six weeks post-CRT, 73 patients (85%) underwent surgery, with 64 (74%) undergoing successful resection. The median survival in resected versus unresected patients was 34 months versus 7 months, with corresponding five-year OS rates of

36% and 0%, respectively. Among patients undergoing pancreaticoduodenectomy, only 11% failed locally, with distant failure accounting for the major cause of mortality [59].

Given the high incidence of distant disease development, a simultaneously conducted Phase II trial incorporated cisplatin (CDDP) and gemcitabine prior to initiation of CRT with gemcitabine. Induction chemotherapy consisted of CDDP (30 mg/m^2) and gemcitabine (750 mg/m^2) every two weeks for four cycles, followed by four weekly infusions of gemcitabine (400 mg/m^2) with 30 Gy RT. Sixty-two patients (78%) underwent surgery and 52 (66%) had successful resection. The median survival for patients undergoing surgery was 31 months versus 10.5 months in the unresected patients [60].

In addition to data from M.D. Anderson there are a number of small, multi-institutional studies evaluating a neoadjuvant approach to potentially resectable pancreatic cancer. One study of 20 patients delivered three cycles of gemcitabine (1000 mg/m^2) with concurrent radiation during cycle 2 (36 Gy in 2.4-Gy fractions). Seventeen patients (85%) underwent surgical resection, with R0 resection in 94% [61]. In a second study 39 of 41 enrolled patients with non-metastatic pancreatic cancer also used full-dose gemcitabine with 3D-CRT radiation of 36 Gy in 2.4-Gy fractions delivered with cycle 2. Seventeen patients underwent surgery, and this regimen was well tolerated [62].

A multi-institutional randomized Phase II study from Germany published results on 73 patients with resectable pancreatic cancer randomized to upfront surgery or neoadjuvant chemoradiation (gemcitabine/CDDP 50.4–55.8 Gy) followed by surgical resection. Surgical resection was performed in 23 patients (upfront surgery) and 19 patients (CRT arm), with R0 resection in 48% and 52%, respectively. Postoperative complications were similar in both groups, and the median survival for all patients was not statistically significant: 14.4 months in the upfront surgery arm and 17.4 months in upfront CRT arm [63]. This trial was closed prematurely as a larger Phase III study comparing these arms was commenced.

A review of the Surveillance, Epidemiology, and End Results (SEER) database also supports the use of neoadjuvant treatment. This analysis included 3885 patient treated for resectable pancreatic cancer: 70 patients (2%) received neoadjuvant RT, 1478 (38%) adjuvant RT, and 2337 (60%) surgery alone. Given that the SEER database does not provide information on the administration of CT, this variable could not be assessed. The median OS was 23 months in patients receiving neoadjuvant RT, 17 months with adjuvant RT, and 12 months in the surgery-alone cohort [64].

Despite the potential advantages and encouraging results using a neoadjuvant CRT approach, no randomized trial results exist comparing neoadjuvant to adjuvant therapy, and its role continues to be investigational. In addition to the previously mentioned Phase III European trial, another multi-institutional European trial is evaluating adjuvant gemcitabine versus neoadjuvant gemcitabine/oxaliplatin (no radiation) plus adjuvant gemcitabine in resectable pancreatic cancer patients [65].

Borderline Resectable Disease

As surgery of the primary tumor remains the only potentially curative treatment for pancreatic cancer, neoadjuvant therapy has also been evaluated to assess its ability to convert locally unresectable pancreatic cancer to resectable disease. Although the definition of borderline resectable disease is contentious, the NCCN definition is accepted by many institutions (Table 22.3). Although variable, approximately 30% or more of patients with borderline resectable disease become resectable after neoadjuvant therapy [66, 67]. Similarly, there appears to be higher rates of local control, R0 resection, and N0 disease in this patient subset after neoadjuvant therapy [68–71].

A number of single-institution retrospective studies have evaluated this patient subset. The earliest study from M.D. Anderson assessed 160 patients with borderline

resectable disease. Patients received 50.4 Gy in 28 fractions or 30 Gy in 10 fractions with concurrent 5-FU, paclitaxel, gemcitabine, or capecitabine at radiosensitizing doses. Among patients, 41% underwent pancreatectomy with margin-negative resection in 94%. Median survival in the 66 patients who completed preoperative therapy and surgery was 44 months, comparable to patients with initially resectable disease [69].

A review from Fox Chase evaluated 109 patients who underwent resection of pancreatic adenocarcinoma with varying involvement of the portal vein and/or superior mesenteric vein as determined by CT. Patients received 5-FU- or gemcitabine-based CRT. Median survival in the 74 patients who received preoperative therapy was 23 months, compared to 15 months in the cohort undergoing upfront surgery. Preoperative CRT was associated with higher rate of R0 resection and N0 disease [70].

A smaller series from the University of Virginia reviewed the outcome of 40 patients with borderline resectable disease. Patients received 50.4 Gy in 28 fractions or 50 Gy in 20 fractions, with concurrent capecitabine. Among these patients, 46% underwent surgery, with 75% undergoing an R0 resection. Patients undergoing surgery after neoadjuvant treatment had similar median survival rates as those undergoing upfront surgery [71].

The ECOG initiated a randomized Phase II study of two neoadjuvant gemcitabine-containing regimens in patients with potentially resectable cancer. Patients received 50.4 Gy EBRT with weekly gemcitabine (500 mg/m^2) or induction chemotherapy with gemcitabine (175 mg/m^2), CDDP (20 mg/m^2), 5-FU (600 mg/m^2) prior to CRT with 5-FU (225 mg/m^2). All patients received adjuvant gemcitabine (1000 mg/m^2). This trial – the only randomized trial of borderline resectable pancreatic cancer – closed early due to poor accrual, with only 21 patients enrolled [72]. Whether a neoadjuvant approach is superior to upfront surgery in patients with borderline resectable pancreatic cancer is not established, and further studies will need to be conducted to clarify its role.

Therapy for Locally Advanced Disease

Approximately 30% of patients fall within the category of locally advanced carcinoma of the pancreas, composing a group with an intermediate prognosis between resectable and metastatic. These patients have pancreatic tumors which are defined as surgically unresectable (Table 22.3), but have no evidence of distant metastases. Of note, advances in surgical technique may allow for the resection of selected patients with tumors involving the superior mesenteric vein (SMV), depending on the extent of involvement [73,74]. Combined treatment with

Table 22.3 Criteria defining resectability status.

Resectability Status	Arterial	Venous
Resectable	No arterial tumor contact (celiac axis [CA], superior mesenteric artery [SMA], or common hepatic artery [CHA]).	No tumor contact with the superior mesenteric vein (SMV) or portal vein (PV) or ≤180° contact without vein contour irregularity
Borderline Resectable	Pancreatic head/uncinate process: • Solid tumor contact with CHA without extension to celiac axis or hepatic artery bifurcation allowing for safe and complete resection and reconstruction. • Solid tumor contact with the SMA of ≤180° • Presence of variant arterial anatomy (ex: accessory right hepatic artery, replaced right hepatic artery, replaced CHA and the origin of replaced or accessory artery) and the presence and degree of tumor contact should be noted if present as it may affect surgical planning. Pancreatic body/tail: • Solid tumor contact with the CA of ≤180° • Solid tumor contact with the CA of ≤180° without involvement of the aorta and with intact and uninvolved gastroduodenal artery [some members prefer this criteria to be in the unresectable category].	• Solid tumor contact with the SMV or PV of >180°, contact of ≤180° with contour irregularity of the vein or thrombosis of the vein but with suitable vessel proximal and distal to the site of involvement allowing for safe and complete resection and vein reconstruction. • Solid tumor contact with the inferior vena cava (IVC)
Unresectable	• Distant metastasis (including non-regional lymph node metastasis) Head/uncinate process: • Solid tumor contact with SMA >180° • Solid tumor contact with the CA >180° • Solid tumor contact with the first jejunal SMA branch Body and tail: • Solid tumor contact of >180° with the SMA or CA • Solid tumor contact with the CA and aortic involvement	Head/uncinate process: • Unreconstructible SMV/PV due to tumor involvement or occlusion (can be due to tumor or bland thrombus) • Contact with most proximal draining jejunal branch into SMV Body and tail: • Unreconstructible SMV/PV due to tumor involvement or occlusion (can be due to tumor or bland thrombus)

From NCCN (National Comprehensive Cancer Network), version 2.2016.

radiation and chemotherapy increases median survival for patients with locally advanced cancers to approximately nine to 14 months, but rarely results in long-term survival. The radiation-based therapeutic options for patients with locally advanced pancreatic cancer include CRT with 5-FU chemotherapy, IORT and, more recently, RT with novel chemotherapeutic and targeted agents. In evaluating the results of these various therapies, it is useful to remember that a median survival of three to six months has been reported for this subset of patients undergoing palliative gastric or biliary bypass only [75].

Prospective Trials

Prospective trials have evaluated the role of RT versus CRT, variations in CRT regimens, and CRT versus chemotherapy alone. With conflicting results, there is little consensus as to the most appropriate management of locally advanced patients, and most are considered reasonable options. Most trials of conventional RT for locally advanced pancreatic cancer have been shown to improve survival when combined with 5-FU compared to RT alone or chemotherapy alone (Table 22.4). Mayo Clinic investigators undertook an early randomized trial during the 1960s in which 64 patients with locally unresectable, non-metastatic stomach, large-bowel and pancreas adenocarcinoma received 35–40 Gy RT with concurrent 5-FU versus the same RT schedule plus placebo. A significant survival advantage was seen for patients receiving CRT versus RT alone (10.4 months versus 6.3 months) [76].

The GITSG followed with a similar study comparing RT alone to CRT with concurrent and maintenance 5-FU. A total of 194 eligible patients with surgically confirmed unresectable and non-metastatic pancreatic adenocarcinoma were randomized to receive 60 Gy split-course RT alone, 40 Gy split-course RT with two to three cycles of concurrent bolus 5-FU chemotherapy (500 mg/m^2), or 60 Gy split-course RT using a similar chemotherapy regimen. Patients in the latter groups received two years of

Table 22.4 Prospective randomized trials for locally advanced, unresectable pancreatic cancer.

Series/Reference	No. of patients	Median survival (months)	Local failure (%)	1-Year (%)	18-Month (est. %)
EBRT versus CRT					
Mayo Clinic [76]					
EBRT (35–40 Gy/3–4 weeks) alone	32	6.3	NA	6	6
EBRT (35–40 Gy/3–4 weeks) + 5-FU	32	10.4	NA	22	13
GITSG [77]					
EBRT (60 Gy/10 weeks) alone	25	5.3	24	10	5
EBRT (40 Gy/6 weeks) + 5-FU	83	9.7	26	35	20
EBRT (60 Gy/10 weeks) + 5-FU	86	9.3	27	46	20
ECOG [78]					
EBRT (59.4 Gy) alone	49	7.1	NA	NA	NA
EBRT (59.5 Gy) + 5-FU/MMC	55	8.4	NA	NA	NA
Variations in CRT Regimen					
GITSG [79]					
EBRT (60 Gy/10 weeks) + 5-FU	73	8.5	58 (first site)	33	15
EBRT (40 Gy/4 weeks) + doxorubicin	70	7.6	51 (first site)	27	17
Taipei [80]					
EBRT (50.4-61.2 Gy) +5-FU	16	6.7	56	31	0 (2 year)
EBRT (50.4-61.2 Gy) + Gemcitabine	18	14.5	34	56	15 (2 year)
CRT versus Chemotherapy					
GITSG [81,115]					
EBRT (54 Gy/6 weeks) + 5-FU and SMF	22	9.7	45 (first site)	41	18
SMF alone	21	7.4	48 (first site)	19	0
ECOG [82]					
EBRT (40 Gy/4 weeks) + 5-FU	47	8.3	32	26	11
5-FU alone	44	8.2	32	32	21
FFCD/SFRO [83]					
EBRT (60 Gy) +5-FU/CDDP	59	8.6	NA	32	NA
Gemcitabine alone	60	13	NA	53	NA
ECOG [84]					
EBRT (50.4 Gy)+ Gemcitabine	34	11.1	12 (first site)	50	29
Gemcitabine alone	37	9.2	30 (first site)	32	11

EBRT, external-beam radiation therapy; CRT, chemoradiation; NA, not available; 5-FU, 5-flurouracil; GITSG, Gastrointestinal Tumor Study Group; ECOG, Eastern Cooperative Oncology Group;; MMC, mitomycin-C; SMF, streptozocin, mitomycin-C, and 5-flurouracil; FFCD/SFRO, Fédération Francophone de Cancérologie Digestive/Société Francophone de Radiothérapie Oncologique.

maintenance 5-FU after RT completion. The RT-alone arm was closed early as a result of an inferior survival. The one-year OS in the two combined modality therapy arms was 38% and 36%, respectively, versus 11% in the EBRT-alone arm [77].

The ECOG 8282 study randomized 114 patients to EBRT alone (59.4 Gy) with or without continuous-infusion 5-FU (1000 mg/m^2 per day) on days 2–5 and 28–31, and MMC (10 mg/m^2) on day 2. There was no difference in response rates, DFS or OS with the addition of concurrent chemotherapy. Higher rates of toxicity, primarily hematologic, where noted in the CRT group [78].

Further studies sought to determine a more efficacious CRT regimen. A second GITSG trial randomized 157 eligible patients with unresectable disease to 60 Gy split-course RT with concurrent and maintenance 5-FU (as in the prior GITSG trial) or 40 Gy continuous-course radia-

tion with weekly, concurrent doxorubicin chemotherapy (10 mg/m^2), followed by maintenance doxorubicin and 5-FU. A significant increase in treatment-related toxicity was seen in the doxorubicin arm, but no survival difference was observed between the two groups (median survival 37 versus 33 weeks). No clinical benefit was seen in substituting doxorubicin for 5-FU [79].

As studies emerged demonstrating significant survival advantages with gemcitabine-based chemotherapy in the metastatic setting, this strategy was incorporated into the locally advanced setting with radiation therapy. A trial from Taiwan randomized 34 patients to EBRT (50.4–61.2 Gy) with concurrent 5-FU (500 mg/m^2/d for 3 days repeated every 2 weeks for 6 weeks) or gemcitabine (600 mg/m^2/wk for 6 weeks). Patients received maintenance gemcitabine (1000 mg/m^2) at the completion of CRT. The median OS and time to progression were prolonged in the gemcitabine arm: 14.5 months and 7.1 months (gemcitabine) versus 6.7 months and 2.7 months (5-FU). There were no observed differences in grade 3–4 toxicity or hospitalization days between the two arms. Study criticisms include the small number of patients and relatively poor outcomes in the 5-FU arm compared to historical controls [80].

A number of trials have compared CRT with chemotherapy alone. A follow-up GITSG trial compared chemotherapy alone to CRT, again in surgically confirmed unresectable tumors. For this, 43 patients were randomized to receive combination streptozocin, mitomycin-C and 5-FU (SMF) chemotherapy or 54 Gy RT with two cycles of concurrent bolus 5-FU chemotherapy, followed by adjuvant SMF chemotherapy. The CRT arm demonstrated a significant survival advantage over the chemotherapy alone arm (one-year survival 41% versus 19%) [81].

In contrast to the results of the prior studies, the Eastern Cooperative Oncology Group (ECOG) reported no benefit to CRT versus chemotherapy only. In this study, 191 patients with unresectable, non-metastatic pancreatic or gastric adenocarcinoma were randomized to receive either 5-FU chemotherapy alone (600 mg/m^2) or 40 Gy EBRT with concurrent bolus 5-FU in week one (600 mg/m^2) followed by maintenance chemotherapy. Patients with locally recurrent disease, as well as those undergoing surgery with residual disease, were eligible for this trial. In the 91 analyzable pancreatic patients, no survival difference was observed between the two groups (median survival 8.2 versus 8.3 months) [82].

The Fédération Francophone de Cancérologie Digestive/Société Francophone de Radiothérapie Oncologique (FFCD/SFRO) trial randomized 119 patients to CRT consisting of 60 Gy EBRT with continuous-infusion 5-FU (300 mg/m^2 per day) on days 1–5 for six weeks, and intermittent CDDP (20 mg/m^2 per day) on days 1–5 for weeks 1 and 5 with maintenance gemcitabine (1000 mg/m^2) versus gemcitabine alone (1000 mg/m^2). Survival was inferior in the CRT arm at 8.6 months compared to 13 months with gemcitabine alone. Higher grade 3–4 toxicity rates were observed in the CRT arm during treatment (36% versus 22%) and maintenance (32% versus 18%) chemotherapy phases. This trial closed early due to poor accrual. Criticisms included an inferior survival in the CRT arm, which was similar to early GITSG trials, despite the use of continuous-infusion chemotherapy and modern EBRT technique, as well as excess toxicity associated with the chosen CRT regimen [83].

The ECOG also published results from a randomized trial of CRT (50.4 Gy with concurrent gemcitabine: 600 mg/m^2 per week for weeks 1–5) versus gemcitabine alone (1000 mg/m^2 per week). The trial closed early due to poor accrual. Analysis of the 74 patients randomized demonstrated no difference in progression-free survival;

however, a survival benefit was seen in the CRT arm: 11.1 versus 9.2 months. This benefit came at the expense of higher grade 4–5 toxicity rates in the CRT arm (mainly hematologic), but with no difference in the long-term quality of life [84].

At present, there is no consensus regarding the appropriate management of locally advanced patients. A meta-analysis of locally advanced patients demonstrated a survival benefit for CRT versus EBRT, but no such benefit was seen for CRT with adjuvant chemotherapy versus chemotherapy alone. Many consider upfront chemotherapy alone with subsequent response assessment and directed CRT in responders to facilitate selection of patients most likely to benefit from CRT [85]. The French Groupe Cooperateur Multidisciplinaire en Oncologie (GERCOR) conducted a randomized multicenter Phase III study in patients with locally advanced adenocarcinoma of the pancreas, evaluating gemcitabine with or without the EGFR inhibitor erlotinib, with further randomization to chemoradiotherapy versus additional chemotherapy alone in patients who do not progress. Preliminary results indicate no difference in overall survival in patients receiving chemotherapy alone or chemoradiation; however, in patients with no evidence of progression after four months of systemic gemcitabine, there is an improvement in local tumor control and longer interval to additional treatment in patients receiving chemoradiation [85a].

Many patients with locally advanced disease present with local symptoms (pain, obstruction, bleeding), in which case RT can potentially offer more prompt and durable palliation. At present, CRT (with continuous-infusion 5-FU/capecitabine or gemcitabine) or gemcitabine-based chemotherapy alone are considered reasonable options in patients with locally advanced disease.

Radiation Dose Escalation

Given poor local control results achieved with CRT, attempts have been made to evaluate whether increasing doses of RT may improve outcomes through IORT, intensity-modulated radiation therapy (IMRT), or stereotactic body radiotherapy (SBRT).

IORT is an alternative method to deliver higher radiation doses. This technique allows for the administration of a single high dose of radiotherapy, with the advantage of enabling healthy tissues to be displaced and shielded from radiation. IORT has been utilized postoperatively and in the treatment of locally advanced disease. Institutional reports and a randomized trial have shown that resection followed by IORT yields lower rates of locoregional recurrence, though no significant difference in survival has been seen [86–89]. IORT has also been evaluated in patients with unresectable disease [90, 91]. A study from investigators at Massachusetts General Hospital reported the results of 150 patients with unresectable pancreatic cancer treated with IORT, EBRT, and chemotherapy. Although the study spanned nearly 25 years, it demonstrated that long-term survival is possible for patients with unresectable pancreatic cancer. Furthermore, the study showed that postoperative and late treatment-related toxicity rates were acceptable [91]. A lower incidence of local failure in most series, and improved median survival in some, have been reported with these techniques when compared with conventional external beam irradiation, but it is uncertain whether this is due to treatment superiority or case selection [92].

Advances in radiation technique and delivery, such as IMRT and SBRT, also enable dose escalation and potential sparing of normal tissues. IMRT is a technique that breaks up a typical radiation treatment field into smaller 'beamlets.' It is implemented either as dynamic IMRT (where collimating leaves move in and out of the radiation beam path during treatment) or as 'step and shoot' IMRT (where leaves change the field shape while beam delivery is off). The cumulative effect is that the prescription dose conforms around delineated target volumes, significantly reducing doses to adjacent normal tissues. This technology has increasingly been used in a number of gastrointestinal malignancies, including pancreatic cancer. Early clinical data support both the feasibility of this technique and its potential for reducing acute gastrointestinal toxicity [93–95]. An analysis from the University of Maryland evaluated 46 patients treated with IMRT and concurrent 5-FU-based chemotherapy. Acute toxicities in these patients were compared with those in a control group enrolled in RTOG 9704 who received conventional 3D treatment. There was a statistically significant reduction in acute grade 3–4 gastrointestinal toxicity in patients who received radiotherapy via IMRT compared to those who received 3D conformal radiotherapy [95]. IMRT can also result in a significant reduction of dose to normal structures, including the liver, kidneys, stomach, and small bowel [94]. This may allow alternate novel systemic agents to be administered with radiotherapy [93].

Another radiation technique being investigated in the treatment of pancreatic cancers is SBRT, which involves the delivery of high dose-per-fraction radiation treatments over a small number of fractions (generally one to five treatments), utilizing techniques that permit very highly conformal dose delivery of EBRT. The postulated advantage of SBRT is potentially improving local control through the delivery of ablative doses of radiation, while minimizing associated side effects. Few institutions have published experiences utilizing this technique, and the data are largely in the setting of locally advanced disease [96, 97]. A recent Phase II multi-institutional study evaluated 49 patients with locally advanced pancreatic cancer receiving gemcitabine (1000 mg/m^2) followed by a one-week break and SBRT (33 Gy in five fractions). Rates of acute and late (the primary endpoint) grade ≥2 gastritis, fistula, enteritis, or ulcer toxicities were 2% and 11%, respectively. The median overall survival was 13.9 months. Freedom from local disease progression at one year was 78%. Four patients (8%) underwent margin-negative and lymph node-negative surgical resections [98].

The role of SBRT in the treatment of pancreatic cancer continues to be a topic of prospective study. However, the minimal gain with dose escalation and high rates of local and distant failures achieved begs for further improvements in both local and systemic therapies.

Chemoradiation for Metastatic Disease and Effects on Quality of Life

Despite the potential survival benefits for patients receiving CRT, these gains are modest. With the exception of resectable disease, nearly all patients will ultimately succumb to their disease. In spite of this, CRT can achieve significant palliative benefit. Pain, anorexia, fatigue and cachexia are relatively common symptoms, which significantly impact on the patient's quality of life. Using RT alone or CRT, approximately 35–65% of patients will experience pain resolution and some improvement in wasting and obstructive symptoms [79,99,100]. Definite, but less dramatic, improvements in performance status and anorexia may also be observed [99, 100]. Palliation from therapy can take many weeks for maximal effect and alternative treatments, such as biliary and duodenal stents, and may provide more rapid relief of obstructive symptoms. Given the high mortality rate associated with pancreatic cancer, quality of life should be an endpoint in trial design for these patients.

Radiation Techniques

After resection, antero-posterior (AP)/postero-anterior (PA) and lateral fields are frequently designed on the basis of preoperative CT primary tumor volumes, preoperative duodenal location, operative clip placement, and postoperative CT nodal volumes (RTOG contouring atlas accessible at RTOG.org). The anterior border is determined by vascular or nodal boundaries (porta hepatis, superior mesenteric, and celiac), as demonstrated on CT as well as preoperative tumor location.

The patient is placed in a supine position for simulation and treatment. Until the mid-1990s conventional simulation was the standard for radiotherapy treatment planning in pancreatic malignancies. During conventional simulation an initial set of AP/PA and cross-table lateral films is obtained after the injection of renal contrast medium to identify operative clips and renal position relative to the field isocenter. Additional films can be obtained with contrast medium in the stomach and duodenal loop in unresected patients.

3D-CRT represented a major paradigm shift in radiation oncology treatment planning, with better visualization of internal organs and target delineation. CT-based treatment planning permits the construction of normal tissue dose–volume histograms and the generation of treatment plans that optimize radiation dose delivery to tumor while sparing critical normal tissues. Despite this advancement, the intent of treatment remains the same. Multiple field, fractionated, external-beam techniques utilizing high-energy photons deliver 45–50 Gy in 1.8-Gy fractions to the tumor bed, unresected or residual tumor, and lymph node-bearing areas at risk. After 45–50.4 Gy, a boost field can be designed to include unresected or gross residual disease, as defined by CT scans and clips, while excluding most of the stomach and small bowel.

For pancreatic head lesions, the primary draining lymph nodes at risk are the pancreaticoduodenal, suprapancreatic, celiac and porta hepatic nodes, and these are often covered. Approximately two-thirds of the left kidney must be excluded from the AP/PA field since the right kidney is often in the field owing to duodenal inclusion. The entire duodenal loop with margin is generally included, as pancreatic head lesions may invade the medial wall of the duodenum and place the entire circumference and pancreaticoduodenal nodal basins at risk. The superior field extent is often at the middle or upper portion of the T11 vertebral body for adequate margins on the celiac vessels (T12, L1) and the inferior limit at the level L2–3 to include the superior mesenteric lymph nodes and third portion of the duodenum. With lateral fields, the anterior field margin is 1.5–2.0 cm beyond gross disease. The posterior margin is often 1.5 cm behind the anterior portion of the vertebral body to allow adequate margins on para-aortic nodes, which are at risk with posterior tumor extension in head or body lesions. The lateral contribution usually is limited to 15–18 Gy, since a moderate volume of kidney or liver may be in the irradiated volume. If a biliary stent has been placed to alleviate obstruction, the stent should be included with coverage of the common bile duct and any tumor that may have tracked superiorly (Figure 22.2). For patients with locally advanced pancreatic cancer, many clinicians advocate for treatment of gross tumor volume (GTV) alone (with an appropriate margin) and no elective nodal radiation.

For body and tail lesions, it may be necessary to increase the superior and left borders to allow adequate coverage of the primary tumor as well as lateral suprapancreatic, splenic artery, and splenic hilar nodes. Unfortunately, this also increases the volume of the left kidney in the field, and a reduction in the right kidney volume

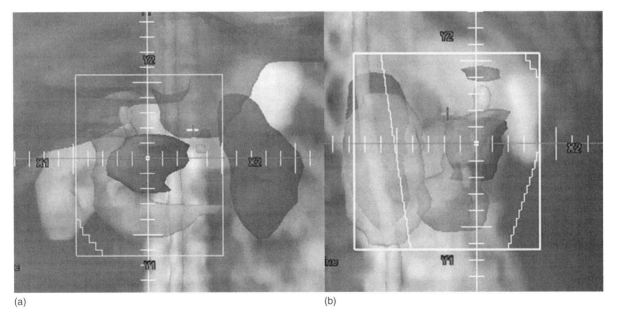

(a) (b)

Figure 22.2 AP and lateral digital radiograph reconstructions of treatment fields for patient with pancreatic head cancer. (a) The antero-posterior/posteroanterior (AP/PA) field, which includes gross tumor (red), duodenal loop (pink) (plus approximately 50% of the right kidney (light green)), liver (brown) and nodal areas at risk (porta hepatis, orange; SMA, green, celiac-magenta). Most of the left kidney (blue) is excluded from the AP/PA field. (b) The right lateral field with an anterior margin beyond gross disease and a posterior margin behind front edge of vertebral body. The liver contour (brown) has been removed from lateral field for visualization of other structures. For a color version of this figure, see the color plate section.

being treated is accomplished by omission of the entirety of the C-loop, as duodenal involvement by tumors in these locations is uncommon. With customized multi-leaf collimator (MLC) blocking it is usually possible to cover the pancreaticoduodenal and porta hepatis nodes adequately.

4D-CT simulation or fluoroscopic evaluation of target motion are important given the potential pancreatic motion with respiration, with breath-hold techniques sometimes implemented to control for such. With more conformal radiotherapy techniques, instructions on empty stomach for simulation and treatment should be given.

Future Directions/Targeted Therapies

In the metastatic setting, two recent randomized trials have demonstrated survival benefit with newer chemotherapy combinations. There is much room for improvement in the diagnosis and treatment of pancreatic cancer. Screening of high-risk individuals may allow for the detection of disease in earlier disease states by means of novel imaging methods or assessment of serum biomarkers [101, 102]. As the biological basis of cancer is better understood, the successful use of cancer-specific targeted therapies in other cancers supports the need to identify new targets and better predictors of response to therapy in pancreatic cancer.

There is evidence of additive or synergistic effects for several targeted agents (such as antibodies against epidermal growth factor receptor [EGFR] and vascular endothelial factor receptor [VEGF]) with both chemotherapy and radiation therapy, making these approaches especially promising. These targeted agents have been studied most extensively in the metastatic setting prior to evaluation in locally advanced and resectable disease. Currently, the only targeted agent that has shown a modest statistically significant survival benefit in the metastatic setting compared to chemotherapy alone is erlotinib, an anti-EGFR tyrosine kinase inhibitor. However, the survival benefit with addition of erlotinib is small, with median survival increased from 5.9 to 6.2 months and one-year survival improvement from 17% to 24% [103]. The clinical significance of this difference has been questioned by investigators and treating physicians.

Another EGFR/HER-1 inhibitor, cetuximab, initially showed promising Phase II results in the metastatic setting. Efficacy was initially seen with the combination of cetuximab and EBRT in the treatment of locally advanced squamous cell carcinoma of the head and neck, and this was subsequently tested in a Phase III trial [104]. However, in pancreatic cancer, a Phase III randomized study of gemcitabine plus cetuximab versus gemcitabine

plus placebo (Southwest Oncology Group S0205) as first-line therapy in locally advanced, unresectable, or metastatic disease enrolled over 700 patients from the US and Canada. No survival improvement was seen with the addition of cetuximab to gemcitabine (6.3 months gemcitabine plus cetuximab versus 5.9 months gemcitabine alone). Even amongst patients tested for EGFR expression (90% specimens proved positive for expression), no benefit to cetuximab was seen in this patient subgroup [105]. An additional Phase II study evaluated the efficacy and safety of multi-agent chemotherapy in combination with cetuximab. Here, 69 patients with locally advanced pancreatic cancer received cetuximab, gemcitabine, and oxaliplatin followed by cetuximab, capecitabine and radiotherapy. Diagnostic cytology specimens were stained for Smad4 (Dpc4) expression. The median overall survival was 19.2 months, and the pattern of failure for patients with Smad4 (Dpc4) expression was primarily local, rather than distant, disease failure [106]. The addition of EGFR inhibitors in localized disease is currently being evaluated in Phase I and II trials.

VEGF inhibitors bind to receptors involved in tumor growth via angiogenesis pathways. Preclinical data have shown that the inhibition of VEGF has radiosensitizing effects. Initially promising results in the metastatic setting, however, have ultimately not shown benefit from the addition of an anti-VEGF antibody to chemotherapy. A Phase II trial of the combination of gemcitabine and bevacizumab in 52 treated patients with advanced pancreatic cancer showed a response rate of 21%, a median progression-free survival of 5.4 months, and median OS of 8.8 months [107]. In response to these positive results, a Phase III randomized study of gemcitabine plus bevacizumab versus placebo (CALGB 80303) was initiated, but no significant difference was observed in OS or PFS [108]. Bevacizumab has also been evaluated in combination with radiotherapy. An initial Phase I study of radiotherapy, capecitabine, and bevacizumab led to incorporation in the Phase II setting in patients with locally advanced pancreatic cancer (RTOG 0411) [109]. In this case, 82 patients were treated with radiotherapy to the gross tumor, capecitabine (825 mg/m^2), and bevacizumab (5 mg/kg^1 on days 1, 15, 29), followed by adjuvant gemcitabine (1000 mg/m^2). The median and one-year survival rates were 11.9 months and 47%, respectively. These results were similar to those in prior RTOG trials of locally advanced pancreatic cancer [110]. An additional Phase II trial assessed the efficacy of full-dose gemcitabine (1000 mg/m^2), bevacizumab (10 mg/kg^1) and radiotherapy to 36 Gy (in 2.4-Gy fractions) with maintenance gemcitabine and bevacizumab in patients with unresected tumors, with no evidence of disease progression. The median progression-free survival and OS were 9.9 and 11.8 months, respectively

[111]. Therefore, the incorporation of bevacizumab with radiotherapy has not led to profound improvements in treatment outcomes compared to 5-FU-based CRT.

Although improvements with targeted agents have been modest, other pathways are being evaluated. Pancreatic cells deficient in BRCA repair pathways are sensitive to poly ADP-ribose polymerase (PARP) inhibitors. PARP inhibitors have been evaluated in ovarian and breast cancer, with response rates of 40%; clinical trials of PARP inhibitors in the treatment of pancreatic cancer are underway [6]. Other therapeutic agents under evaluation include hedgehog pathway inhibitors, multi-kinase inhibitors (sorafenib), and agents targeting v-src sarcoma (SRC), γ-secretase, stem-cell factor receptor (c-kit), secreted protein acidic and rich in cysteine (SPARC), mitogen-activated protein kinase (MEK), mesothelin, RAS, prostate stem cell antigen (PSCA), tumor necrosis factor-alpha (TNF-α), Mucin-1, mammalian target of rapamycin (mTOR), tumor necrosis factor superfamily member 10 (TNFSF10), and type 1 insulin-like growth factor receptor (IGF1) [6, 112].

Conclusions

Older adjuvant trials evaluating the outcomes of CRT, chemotherapy and surgery alone in resected pancreatic cancer patients are fraught with flaws. Despite this, adjuvant chemotherapy alone has evolved and remains the standard of care in adjuvant treatment of resectable pancreatic cancer throughout much of Europe. In the US, the role of CRT continues to be redefined in the era of modern chemotherapeutics. The currently active RTOG 0848/EORTC study will help to not only further clarify the role of adjuvant CRT, but also to assess to utility of small-molecule EGFR therapy in the treatment of this disease. The use of neoadjuvant CRT in resectable patients offers potential advantages as well as promising local control and survival results based on institutional data, although randomized trials are lacking. Modest improvements in median survival have been attained for patients with locally advanced tumors. Prospective trials have evaluated the role of RT versus CRT, variations in CRT regimens, and CRT versus chemotherapy alone. With conflicting results, there is little consensus as to the appropriate management of locally advanced patients, and most are considered reasonable options. Despite advances in many aspects of oncologic evaluation and management, including preoperative evaluation (e.g., EUS, CT), surgical techniques, perioperative care, systemic therapy and radiotherapy, the five-year OS rate for patients with resectable pancreatic remains approximately 20%, and long-term survival for locally advanced disease is rare. Further advances in systemic therapies, the study of optimal sequencing of therapies, the earlier detection of disease and the development of new therapeutic options are urgently needed in the treatment of this formidable disease.

References

1 Siegel, R., Miller, K., Jemal, A. (2017) Cancer statistics, 2017. *CA Cancer J. Clin.*, **67**, 7–30.

2 Geer, R.J., Brennan, M.F. (1993) Prognostic indicators for survival after resection of pancreatic adenocarcinoma. *Am. J. Surg.*, **165**, 68–72; discussion 73.

3 Yeo, C.J., Cameron, J.L., Lillemoe, K.D., *et al.* (1995) Pancreaticoduodenectomy for cancer of the head of the pancreas. 201 patients. *Ann. Surg.*, **221**, 721–731; discussion 731–733.

4 Wagner, M., Redaelli, C., Lietz, M., Seiler, C.A., Friess, H., Buchler, M.W. (2004) Curative resection is the single most important factor determining outcome in patients with pancreatic adenocarcinoma. *Br. J. Surg.*, **91**, 586–594.

5 Lim, J.E., Chien, M.W., Earle, C.C. (2003) Prognostic factors following curative resection for pancreatic adenocarcinoma: a population-based, linked database analysis of 396 patients. *Ann. Surg.*, **237**, 74–85.

6 Vincent, A., Herman, J., Schulick, R., Hruban, R.H., Goggins, M. (2011) Pancreatic cancer. *Lancet*, **378**, 607–620.

7 Willett, C.G., Czito, B.G., Bendell, J.C., Ryan, D.P. (2005) Locally advanced pancreatic cancer. *J. Clin. Oncol.*, **23**, 4538–4544.

8 Kinney, T. (2010) Evidence-based imaging of pancreatic malignancies. *Surg. Clin. North Am.*, **90**, 235–249.

9 Karmazanovsky, G., Fedorov, V., Kubyshkin, V., Kotchatkov, A. (2005) Pancreatic head cancer: accuracy of CT in determination of resectability. *Abdom. Imag.*, **30**, 488–500.

10 Hunt, G.C., Faigel, D.O. (2002) Assessment of EUS for diagnosing, staging, and determining resectability of pancreatic cancer: a review. *Gastroint. Endosc.*, **55**, 232–237.

11 Rosch, T., Lorenz, R., Braig, C., *et al.* (1991) Endoscopic ultrasound in pancreatic tumor diagnosis. *Gastroint. Endosc.*, **37**, 347–352.

12 Meyenberger, C., Huch Boni, R.A., Bertschinger, P., Zala, G.F., Klotz, H.P., Krestin, G.P. (1995) Endoscopic ultrasound and endorectal magnetic resonance imaging: a prospective, comparative study for

preoperative staging and follow-up of rectal cancer. *Endoscopy*, **27**, 469–479.

13 Hariharan, D., Constantinides, V.A., Froeling, F.E., Tekkis, P.P., Kocher, H.M. (2010) The role of laparoscopy and laparoscopic ultrasound in the preoperative staging of pancreatico-biliary cancers – A meta-analysis. *Eur. J. Surg. Oncol.*, **36**, 941–948.

14 Fernandez-del Castillo, C., Rattner, D.W., Warshaw, A.L. (1995) Further experience with laparoscopy and peritoneal cytology in the staging of pancreatic cancer. *Br. J. Surg.*, **82**, 1127–1129.

15 Bipat, S., Phoa, S.S., van Delden, O.M., *et al.* (2005) Ultrasonography, computed tomography and magnetic resonance imaging for diagnosis and determining resectability of pancreatic adenocarcinoma: a meta-analysis. *J. Comput. Assist. Tomogr.*, **29**, 438–445.

16 Sica, G.T., Ji, H., Ros, P.R. (2002) Computed tomography and magnetic resonance imaging of hepatic metastases. *Clin. Liver Dis.*, **6**, 165–179, vii.

17 Lemke, A.J., Niehues, S.M., Hosten, N., *et al.* (2004) Retrospective digital image fusion of multidetector CT and 18F-FDG PET: clinical value in pancreatic lesions – a prospective study with 104 patients. *J. Nucl. Med.*, **45**, 1279–1286.

18 Sachelarie, I., Kerr, K., Ghesani, M., Blum, R.H. (2005) Integrated PET-CT: evidence-based review of oncology indications. *Oncology*, **19**, 481–490; discussion 490–492, 495–496.

19 Rose, D.M., Delbeke, D., Beauchamp, R.D., *et al.* (1999) 18Fluorodeoxyglucose-positron emission tomography in the management of patients with suspected pancreatic cancer. *Ann. Surg.*, **229**, 729–737; discussion 737–738.

20 Grassetto, G., Rubello, D. (2011) Role of FDG-PET/CT in diagnosis, staging, response to treatment, and prognosis of pancreatic cancer. *Am. J. Clin. Oncol.*, **34**, 111–114.

21 Raut, C.P., Tseng, J.F., Sun, C.C., *et al.* (2007) Impact of resection status on pattern of failure and survival after pancreaticoduodenectomy for pancreatic adenocarcinoma. *Ann. Surg.*, **246**, 52–60.

22 Willett, C.G., Lewandrowski, K., Warshaw, A.L., Efird, J., Compton, C.C. (1993) Resection margins in carcinoma of the head of the pancreas. Implications for radiation therapy. *Ann. Surg.*, **217**, 144–148.

23 Tepper, J., Nardi, G., Suit, H. (1976) Carcinoma of the pancreas: review of MGH experience from 1963 to 1973. Analysis of surgical failure and implications for radiation therapy. *Cancer*, **37**, 1519–1524.

24 Griffin, J.F., Smalley, S.R., Jewell, W., *et al.* (1990) Patterns of failure after curative resection of pancreatic carcinoma. *Cancer*, **66**, 56–61.

25 Ozaki, H. (1992) Improvement of pancreatic cancer treatment from the Japanese experience in the 1980s. *Int. J. Pancreatol.*, **12**, 5–9.

26 Westerdahl, J., Andren-Sandberg, A., Ihse, I. (1993) Recurrence of exocrine pancreatic cancer – local or hepatic? *Hepato-gastroenterology*, **40**, 384–387.

27 Allema, J.H., Reinders, M.E., van Gulik, T.M., *et al.* (1995) Prognostic factors for survival after pancreaticoduodenectomy for patients with carcinoma of the pancreatic head region. *Cancer*, **75**, 2069–2076.

28 Kalser, M.H., Ellenberg, S.S. (1985) Pancreatic cancer. Adjuvant combined radiation and chemotherapy following curative resection. *Arch. Surg.*, **120**, 899–903.

29 Gastrointestinal Tumor Study Group (1987) Further evidence of effective adjuvant combined radiation and chemotherapy following curative resection of pancreatic cancer. *Cancer*, **59**, 2006–2010.

30 Kalser, M.H., Barkin, J., MacIntyre, J.M. (1985) Pancreatic cancer. Assessment of prognosis by clinical presentation. *Cancer*, **56**, 397–402.

31 Klinkenbijl, J.H., Jeekel, J., Sahmoud, T., *et al.* (1999) Adjuvant radiotherapy and 5-fluorouracil after curative resection of cancer of the pancreas and periampullary region: phase III trial of the EORTC gastrointestinal tract cancer cooperative group. *Ann. Surg.*, **230**, 776–782; discussion 782–784.

32 Smeenk, H.G., van Eijck, C.H., Hop, W.C., *et al.* (2007) Long-term survival and metastatic pattern of pancreatic and periampullary cancer after adjuvant chemoradiation or observation: long-term results of EORTC trial 40891. *Ann. Surg.*, **246**, 734–740.

33 Mehta, V.K., Fisher, G.A., Ford, J.M., *et al.* (2001) Adjuvant chemoradiotherapy for "unfavorable" carcinoma of the ampulla of Vater. *Arch. Surg.*, **136**, 65–69.

34 Neoptolemos, J.P., Dunn, J.A., Stocken, D.D., *et al.* (2001) Adjuvant chemoradiotherapy and chemotherapy in resectable pancreatic cancer: a randomised controlled trial. *Lancet*, **358**, 1576–1585.

35 Neoptolemos, J.P., Stocken, D.D., Friess, H., *et al.* (2004) A randomized trial of chemoradiotherapy and chemotherapy after resection of pancreatic cancer. *N. Engl. J. Med.*, **350**, 1200–1210.

36 Oettle, H., Post, S., Neuhaus, P., *et al.* (2007) Adjuvant chemotherapy with gemcitabine vs observation in patients undergoing curative-intent resection of pancreatic cancer: a randomized controlled trial. *JAMA*, **297**, 267–277.

37 Oettle, H., Neuhaus, P., Hochous, A. *et al.* (2013) CONKO-001: Adjuvant chemotherapy with gemcitabine and long-term outcomes among patients with resected pancreatic cancer. *JAMA*, **310**, 1473–1481.

38 Ueno, H., Kosuge, T., Matsuyama, Y., *et al.* (2009) A randomised phase III trial comparing gemcitabine with surgery-only in patients with resected pancreatic cancer: Japanese Study Group of Adjuvant Therapy for Pancreatic Cancer. *Br. J. Cancer*, **101**, 908–915.

39 Neoptolemos, J.P., Stocken, D.D., Bassi, C., *et al.* (2010) Adjuvant chemotherapy with fluorouracil plus folinic acid vs gemcitabine following pancreatic cancer resection: a randomized controlled trial. *JAMA*, **304**, 1073–1081.

40 Regine, W.F., Winter, K.A., Abrams, R.A., *et al.* (2008) Fluorouracil vs gemcitabine chemotherapy before and after fluorouracil-based chemoradiation following resection of pancreatic adenocarcinoma: a randomized controlled trial. *JAMA*, **299**, 1019–1026.

41 Regine, W.F., Winter, K.A., Abrams, R., *et al.* (2011) Fluorouracil-based chemoradiation with either gemcitabine or fluorouracil chemotherapy after resection of pancreatic adenocarcinoma: 5-year analysis of the U.S. Intergroup/RTOG 9704 Phase III Trial. *Ann. Surg. Oncol.*, **18**, 1319–1326.

42 Berger, A.C., Garcia, M., Jr, Hoffman, J.P., *et al.* (2008) Postresection CA 19-9 predicts overall survival in patients with pancreatic cancer treated with adjuvant chemoradiation: a prospective validation by RTOG 9704. *J. Clin. Oncol.*, **26**, 5918–5922.

42a Berger, A.C., Winter, K., Hoffman, J.P., *et al.* (2012) Five year results of US intergroup/RTOG 9704 with postoperative CA 19-9 ≤90 U/mL and comparison to the CONKO-001 trial. *Int. J. Radiat. Oncol. Biol. Phys.*, **84**, e291–e297.

43 Abrams, R.A., Winter, K.A., Regine, W.F., *et al.* (2012) Failure to adhere to protocol specified radiation therapy guidelines was associated with decreased survival in RTOG 9704-A Phase III trial of adjuvant chemotherapy and chemoradiotherapy for patients with resected adenocarcinoma of the pancreas. *Int. J. Radiat. Oncol. Biol. Phys.*, **82** (2), 809–816.

44 Corsini, M.M., Miller, R.C., Haddock, M.G., *et al.* (2008) Adjuvant radiotherapy and chemotherapy for pancreatic carcinoma: the Mayo Clinic experience (1975–2005). *J. Clin. Oncol.*, **26**, 3511–3516.

45 Herman, J.M., Swartz, M.J., Hsu, C.C., *et al.* (2008) Analysis of fluorouracil-based adjuvant chemotherapy and radiation after pancreaticoduodenectomy for ductal adenocarcinoma of the pancreas: results of a large, prospectively collected database at the Johns Hopkins Hospital. *J. Clin. Oncol.*, **26**, 3503–3510.

46 Hsu, C.C., Herman, J.M., Corsini, M.M., *et al.* (2010) Adjuvant chemoradiation for pancreatic adenocarcinoma: the Johns Hopkins Hospital–Mayo Clinic collaborative study. *Ann. Surg. Oncol.*, **17**, 981–990.

47 Picozzi, V.J., Kozarek, R.A., Traverso, L.W. (2003) Interferon-based adjuvant chemoradiation therapy after pancreaticoduodenectomy for pancreatic adenocarcinoma. *Am. J. Surg.*, **185**, 476–480.

48 Picozzi, V.J., Abrams, R.A., Decker, P.A., *et al.* (2011) Multicenter phase II trial of adjuvant therapy for resected pancreatic cancer using cisplatin, 5-fluorouracil, and interferon-alfa-2b-based chemoradiation: ACOSOG Trial Z05031. *Ann. Oncol.*, **22**, 348–354.

49 Aloia, T.A., Lee, J.E., Vauthey, J.N., *et al.* (2007) Delayed recovery after pancreaticoduodenectomy: a major factor impairing the delivery of adjuvant therapy? *J. Am. Coll. Surg.*, **204**, 347–355.

50 Cheng, T.Y., Sheth, K., White, R.R., *et al.* (2006) Effect of neoadjuvant chemoradiation on operative mortality and morbidity for pancreaticoduodenectomy. *Ann. Surg. Oncol.*, **13**, 66–74.

51 White, R.R., Tyler, D.S. (2004) Neoadjuvant therapy for pancreatic cancer: the Duke experience. *Surg. Oncol. Clin. North Am.*, **13**, 675–684, ix–x.

52 Evans, D.B., Pisters, P.W., Lee, J.E., *et al.* (1998) Preoperative chemoradiation strategies for localized adenocarcinoma of the pancreas. *J. Hepatobiliary Pancreatic Surg.*, **5**, 242–250.

53 Raut, C.P., Evans, D.B., Crane, C.H., Pisters, P.W., Wolff, R.A. (2004) Neoadjuvant therapy for resectable pancreatic cancer. *Surg. Oncol. Clin. North Am.*, **13**, 639–661, ix.

54 Wayne, J.D., Abdalla, E.K., Wolff, R.A., Crane, C.H., Pisters, P.W., Evans, D.B. (2002) Localized adenocarcinoma of the pancreas: the rationale for preoperative chemoradiation. *Oncologist*, **7**, 34–45.

55 Evans, D.B., Rich, T.A., Byrd, D.R., *et al.* (1992) Preoperative chemoradiation and pancreaticoduodenectomy for adenocarcinoma of the pancreas. *Arch. Surg.*, **127**, 1335–1339.

56 Pisters, P.W., Abbruzzese, J.L., Janjan, N.A., *et al.* (1998) Rapid-fractionation preoperative chemoradiation, pancreaticoduodenectomy, and intraoperative radiation therapy for resectable pancreatic adenocarcinoma. *J. Clin. Oncol.*, **16**, 3843–3850.

57 Pisters, P.W., Wolff, R.A., Janjan, N.A., *et al.* (2002) Preoperative paclitaxel and concurrent rapid-fractionation radiation for resectable pancreatic adenocarcinoma: toxicities, histologic response rates, and event-free outcome. *J. Clin. Oncol.*, **20**, 2537–2544.

58 Le Scodan, R., Mornex, F., Girard, N., *et al.* (2009) Preoperative chemoradiation in potentially resectable pancreatic adenocarcinoma: feasibility, treatment effect evaluation and prognostic factors, analysis of the SFRO-FFCD 9704 trial and literature review. *Ann. Oncol.*, **20**, 1387–1396.

59 Evans, D.B., Varadhachary, G.R., Crane, C.H., *et al.* (2008) Preoperative gemcitabine-based chemoradiation for patients with resectable adenocarcinoma of the pancreatic head. *J. Clin. Oncol.*, **26**, 3496–3502.

60 Varadhachary, G.R., Wolff, R.A., Crane, C.H., *et al.* (2008) Preoperative gemcitabine and cisplatin followed by gemcitabine-based chemoradiation for resectable adenocarcinoma of the pancreatic head. *J. Clin. Oncol.*, **26**, 3487–3495.

61 Talamonti, M.S., Small, W., Jr, Mulcahy, M.F., *et al.* (2006) A multi-institutional phase II trial of preoperative full-dose gemcitabine and concurrent radiation for patients with potentially resectable pancreatic carcinoma. *Ann. Surg. Oncol.*, **13**, 150–158.

62 Small, W., Berlin, J., Freedman, G.M., *et al.* (2008) Full-dose gemcitabine with concurrent radiation therapy in patients with nonmetastatic pancreatic cancer: A multicenter phase II trial. *J. Clin. Oncol.*, **26**, 942–947.

63 Golcher, H., Brunner, T.B., Witzigmann, H., *et al.* (2015) Neoadjuvant chemoradiation therapy with gemcitabine/cisplatin and surgery versus immediate surgery in resectable pancreatic cancer. *Strahlenther. Onkol.*, **191**, 7–16.

64 Stessin, A.M., Meyer, J.E., Sherr, D.L. (2008) Neoadjuvant radiation is associated with improved survival in patients with resectable pancreatic cancer: an analysis of data from the surveillance, epidemiology, and end results (SEER) registry. *Int. J. Radiat. Oncol. Biol. Phys.*, **72**, 1128–1133.

65 Heinrich, S., Pestalozzi, B., Lesurtel, M., *et al.* (2011) Adjuvant gemcitabine versus NEOadjuvant gemcitabine/oxaliplatin plus adjuvant gemcitabine in resectable pancreatic cancer: a randomized multicenter phase III study (NEOPAC study). *BMC Cancer*, **11**, 346.

66 Gillen, S., Schuster, T., Meyer Zum Buschenfelde, C., Friess, H., Kleeff, J. (2010) Preoperative/neoadjuvant therapy in pancreatic cancer: a systematic review and meta-analysis of response and resection percentages. *PLoS Med.*, **7**, e1000267.

67 Massucco, P., Capussotti, L., Magnino, A., *et al.* (2006) Pancreatic resections after chemoradiotherapy for locally advanced ductal adenocarcinoma: analysis of perioperative outcome and survival. *Ann. Surg. Oncol.*, **13**, 1201–1208.

68 Greer, S.E., Pipas, J.M., Sutton, J.E., *et al.* (2008) Effect of neoadjuvant therapy on local recurrence after resection of pancreatic adenocarcinoma. *J. Am. Coll. Surg.*, **206**, 451–457.

69 Katz, M.H., Pisters, P.W., Evans, D.B., *et al.* (2008) Borderline resectable pancreatic cancer: the importance of this emerging stage of disease. *J. Am. Coll. Surg.*, **206**, 833–846; discussion 846–848.

70 Chun, Y.S., Milestone, B.N., Watson, J.C., *et al.* (2010) Defining venous involvement in borderline resectable pancreatic cancer. *Ann. Surg. Oncol.*, **17**, 2832–2838.

71 Stokes, J.B., Nolan, N.J., Stelow, E.B., *et al.* (2011) Preoperative capecitabine and concurrent radiation for borderline resectable pancreatic cancer. *Ann. Surg. Oncol.*, **18**, 619–627.

72 Landry, J., Catalano, P.J., Staley, C., *et al.* (2010) Randomized phase II study of gemcitabine plus radiotherapy versus gemcitabine, 5-fluorouracil, and cisplatin followed by radiotherapy and 5-fluorouracil for patients with locally advanced, potentially resectable pancreatic adenocarcinoma. *J. Surg. Oncol.*, **101**, 587–592.

73 Tseng, J.F., Tamm, E.P., Lee, J.E., Pisters, P.W., Evans, D.B. (2006) Venous resection in pancreatic cancer surgery. *Best Pract. Res. Clin. Gastroenterol.*, **20**, 349–364.

74 Leach, S.D., Lee, J.E., Charnsangavej, C., *et al.* (1998) Survival following pancreaticoduodenectomy with resection of the superior mesenteric-portal vein confluence for adenocarcinoma of the pancreatic head. *Br. J. Surg.*, **85**, 611–617.

75 Gunderson, L.L., Haddock, M.G., Burch, P., Nagorney, D., Foo, M.L., Todoroki, T. (1999) Future role of radiotherapy as a component of treatment in biliopancreatic cancers. *Ann. Oncol.*, **10** (Suppl. 4), 291–295.

76 Moertel, C.G., Childs, D.S., Jr, Reitemeier, R.J., Colby, M.Y., Jr, Holbrook, M.A. (1969) Combined 5-fluorouracil and supervoltage radiation therapy of locally unresectable gastrointestinal cancer. *Lancet*, **2**, 865–867.

77 Moertel, C.G., Frytak, S., Hahn, R.G., *et al.* (1981) Therapy of locally unresectable pancreatic carcinoma: a randomized comparison of high dose (6000 rads) radiation alone, moderate dose radiation (4000 rads + 5-fluorouracil), and high dose radiation + 5-fluorouracil: The Gastrointestinal Tumor Study Group. *Cancer*, **48**, 1705–1710.

78 Cohen, S.J., Dobelbower, R., Jr, Lipsitz, S., *et al.* (2005) A randomized phase III study of radiotherapy alone or with 5-fluorouracil and mitomycin-C in patients with locally advanced adenocarcinoma of the pancreas: Eastern Cooperative Oncology Group study E8282. *Int. J. Radiat. Oncol. Biol. Phys.*, **62**, 1345–1350.

79 Gastrointestinal Tumor Study Group (1985) Radiation therapy combined with adriamycin or 5-fluorouracil for the treatment of locally unresectable pancreatic carcinoma. *Cancer*, **56**, 2563–2568.

80 Li, C.P., Chao, Y., Chi, K.H., *et al.* (2003) Concurrent chemoradiotherapy treatment of locally advanced pancreatic cancer: gemcitabine versus 5-fluorouracil, a randomized controlled study. *Int. J. Radiat. Oncol. Biol. Phys.*, **57**, 98–104.

81 Gastrointestinal Tumor Study Group (1988) Treatment of locally unresectable carcinoma of the pancreas: comparison of combined-modality therapy (chemotherapy plus radiotherapy) to chemotherapy alone. *J. Natl Cancer Inst.*, **80**, 751–755.

82 Klaassen, D.J., MacIntyre, J.M., Catton, G.E., Engstrom, P.F., Moertel, C.G. (1985) Treatment of locally unresectable cancer of the stomach and pancreas: a randomized comparison of 5-fluorouracil alone with radiation plus concurrent and maintenance 5-fluorouracil–an Eastern Cooperative Oncology Group study. *J. Clin. Oncol.*, **3**, 373–378.

83 Chauffert, B., Mornex, F., Bonnetain, F., *et al.* (2008) Phase III trial comparing intensive induction chemoradiotherapy (60 Gy, infusional 5-FU and intermittent cisplatin) followed by maintenance gemcitabine with gemcitabine alone for locally advanced unresectable pancreatic cancer. Definitive results of the 2000-01 FFCD/SFRO study. *Ann. Oncol.*, **19**, 1592–1599.

84 Loehrer, P.J., Sr, Feng, Y., Cardenes, H., *et al.* (2011) Gemcitabine alone versus gemcitabine plus radiotherapy in patients with locally advanced pancreatic cancer: an eastern cooperative oncology group trial. *J. Clin. Oncol.*, **29**, 4105–4112.

85 Huguet, F., Andre, T., Hammel, P., *et al.* (2007) Impact of chemoradiotherapy after disease control with chemotherapy in locally advanced pancreatic adenocarcinoma in GERCOR phase II and III studies. *J. Clin. Oncol.*, **25**, 326–331.

85a Huguet, F., Hammel, P., Vernerey, D., *et al.* (2014) Impact of chemoradiotherapy (CRT) on local control and time without treatment in patients with locally advanced pancreatic cancer (LAPC) included in the international phase III LAP 07 study. *J. Clin. Oncol.*, **32** (5S), abstract number 4001.

86 Hiraoka, T., Watanabe, E., Mochinaga, M., *et al.* (1984) Intraoperative irradiation combined with radical resection for cancer of the head of the pancreas. *World J. Surg.*, **8**, 766–771.

87 Sindelar, W.F., Kinsella, T.J. (1999) Studies of intraoperative radiotherapy in carcinoma of the pancreas. *Ann. Oncol.*, **10** (Suppl. 4), 226–230.

88 Showalter, T.N., Rao, A.S., Rani Anne, P., *et al.* (2009) Does intraoperative radiation therapy improve local tumor control in patients undergoing pancreaticoduodenectomy for pancreatic adenocarcinoma? A propensity score analysis. *Ann. Surg. Oncol.*, **16**, 2116–2122.

89 Ogawa, K., Karasawa, K., Ito, Y., *et al.* Intraoperative radiotherapy for resected pancreatic cancer: a multi-institutional retrospective analysis of 210 patients. *Int. J. Radiat. Oncol. Biol. Phys.*, **77**, 734–742.

90 Ogawa, K., Karasawa, K., Ito, Y., *et al.* Intraoperative radiotherapy for unresectable pancreatic cancer: a multi-institutional retrospective analysis of 144 patients. *Int. J. Radiat. Oncol. Biol. Phys.*, **80**, 111–118.

91 Willett, C.G., Del Castillo, C.F., Shih, H.A., *et al.* (2005) Long-term results of intraoperative electron beam irradiation (IOERT) for patients with unresectable pancreatic cancer. *Ann. Surg.*, **241**, 295–299.

92 Roldan, G.E., Gunderson, L.L., Nagorney, D.M., *et al.* (1988) External beam versus intraoperative and external beam irradiation for locally advanced pancreatic cancer. *Cancer*, **61**, 1110–1116.

93 Ben-Josef, E., Shields, A.F., Vaishampayan, U., *et al.* (2004) Intensity-modulated radiotherapy (IMRT) and concurrent capecitabine for pancreatic cancer. *Int. J. Radiat. Oncol. Biol. Phys.*, **59**, 454–459.

94 Milano, M.T., Chmura, S.J., Garofalo, M.C., *et al.* (2004) Intensity-modulated radiotherapy in treatment of pancreatic and bile duct malignancies: toxicity and clinical outcome. *Int. J. Radiat. Oncol. Biol. Phys.*, **59**, 445–453.

95 Yovino, S., Poppe, M., Jabbour, S., *et al.* (2011) Intensity-modulated radiation therapy significantly improves acute gastrointestinal toxicity in pancreatic and ampullary cancers. *Int. J. Radiat. Oncol. Biol. Phys.*, **79**, 158–162.

96 Rwigema, J.C., Parikh, S.D., Heron, D.E., *et al.* (2011) Stereotactic body radiotherapy in the treatment of advanced adenocarcinoma of the pancreas. *Am. J. Clin. Oncol.*, **34**, 63–69.

97 Chang, D.T., Schellenberg, D., Shen, J., *et al.* (2009) Stereotactic radiotherapy for unresectable adenocarcinoma of the pancreas. *Cancer*, **115**, 665–672.

98 Herman, J.M., Chang, D.T., Goodman, K.A., *et al.* (2015) Phase 2 multi-institutional trial evaluating gemcitabine and stereotactic body radiotherapy for patients with locally advanced unresectable pancreatic adenocarcinoma. *Cancer*, **121**, 1128–1137.

99 Haslam, J.B., Cavanaugh, P.J., Stroup, S.L. (1973) Radiation therapy in the treatment of irresectable adenocarcinoma of the pancreas. *Cancer*, **32**, 1341–1345.

100 Dobelbower, R.R., Jr, Borgelt, B.B., Strubler, K.A., Kutcher, G.J., Suntharalingam, N. (1980) Precision radiotherapy for cancer of the pancreas: technique and results. *Int. J. Radiat. Oncol. Biol. Phys.*, **6**, 1127–1133.

101 Larghi, A., Verna, E.C., Lecca, P.G., Costamagna, G. (2009) Screening for pancreatic cancer in high-risk individuals: a call for endoscopic ultrasound. *Clin. Cancer Res.*, **15**, 1907–1914.

102 Greenhalf, W., Grocock, C., Harcus, M., Neoptolemos, J. (2009) Screening of high-risk families for pancreatic cancer. *Pancreatology*, **9**, 215–222.

103 Moore, M.J., Goldstein, D., Hamm, J., *et al.* (2007) Erlotinib plus gemcitabine compared with gemcitabine alone in patients with advanced

pancreatic cancer: a phase III trial of the National Cancer Institute of Canada Clinical Trials Group. *J. Clin. Oncol.*, **25**, 1960–1966.

104 Bonner, J.A., Harari, P.M., Giralt, J., *et al.* (2010) Radiotherapy plus cetuximab for locoregionally advanced head and neck cancer: 5-year survival data from a phase 3 randomised trial, and relation between cetuximab-induced rash and survival. *Lancet Oncol.*, **11**, 21–28.

105 Philip, P.A., Benedetti, J., Corless, C.L., *et al.* (2010) Phase III study comparing gemcitabine plus cetuximab versus gemcitabine in patients with advanced pancreatic adenocarcinoma: Southwest Oncology Group-directed intergroup trial S0205. *J. Clin. Oncol.*, **28**, 3605–3610.

106 Crane, C.H., Varadhachary, G.R., Yordy, J.S., *et al.* (2011) Phase II trial of cetuximab, gemcitabine, and oxaliplatin followed by chemoradiation with cetuximab for locally advanced (T4) pancreatic adenocarcinoma: correlation of Smad4(Dpc4) immunostaining with pattern of disease progression. *J. Clin. Oncol.*, **29**, 3037–3043.

107 Kindler, H.L., Friberg, G., Singh, D.A., *et al.* (2005) Phase II trial of bevacizumab plus gemcitabine in patients with advanced pancreatic cancer. *J. Clin. Oncol.*, **23**, 8033–8040.

108 Kindler, H.L., Niedzwiecki, D., Hollis, D., *et al.* (2010) Gemcitabine plus bevacizumab compared with gemcitabine plus placebo in patients with advanced pancreatic cancer: phase III trial of the Cancer and Leukemia Group B (CALGB 80303). *J. Clin. Oncol.*, **28**, 3617–3622.

109 Crane, C.H., Ellis, L.M., Abbruzzese, J.L., *et al.* (2006) Phase I trial evaluating the safety of bevacizumab with concurrent radiotherapy and capecitabine in locally advanced pancreatic cancer. *J. Clin. Oncol.*, **24**, 1145–1151.

110 Crane, C.H., Winter, K., Regine, W.F., *et al.* (2009) Phase II study of bevacizumab with concurrent capecitabine and radiation followed by maintenance gemcitabine and bevacizumab for locally advanced pancreatic cancer: Radiation Therapy Oncology Group RTOG 0411. *J. Clin. Oncol.*, **27**, 4096–4102.

111 Small, W., Jr, Mulcahy, M.F., Rademaker, A., *et al.* (2011) Phase II trial of full-dose gemcitabine and bevacizumab in combination with attenuated three-dimensional conformal radiotherapy in patients with localized pancreatic cancer. *Int. J. Radiat. Oncol. Biol. Phys.*, **80**, 476–482.

112 Hidalgo, M. (2010) Pancreatic cancer. *N. Engl. J. Med.*, **362**, 1605–1617.

113 Regine, W.F. (2009) Five-year results of the Phase III Intergroup Trial (RTOG 97-04) of adjuvant pre- and postchemoradiation (CRT) 5-FU vs. gemcitabine (G) for resected pancreatic adenocarcinoma: Implications for Future International Trial Design. *Int. J. Radiat. Oncol. Biol. Phys.*, **75**, S55–S56.

114 Hoffman, J.P., Lipsitz, S., Pisansky, T., Weese, J.L., Solin, L., Benson, A.B., 3rd (1998) Phase II trial of preoperative radiation therapy and chemotherapy for patients with localized, resectable adenocarcinoma of the pancreas: an Eastern Cooperative Oncology Group Study. *J. Clin. Oncol.*, **16**, 317–323.

115 The Gastrointestinal Tumor Study Group (1986) Phase II studies of drug combinations in advanced pancreatic carcinoma: fluorouracil plus doxorubicin plus mitomycin C and two regimens of streptozotocin plus mitomycin C plus fluorouracil. *J. Clin. Oncol.*, **4**, 1794–1798.

23

Colon Cancer

Jennifer Y. Wo

Introduction

With an estimated incidence of 1.2 million cases worldwide each year, colorectal cancer is the third most commonly diagnosed cancer in males and the second most common in females [1]. In the United States, approximately 135 400 new cases of colorectal cancer are diagnosed each year, and 50 300 colorectal cancer-related deaths [2]. Although surgical resection remains the mainstay curative therapy, the five-year overall survival (OS) for patients with stage II and stage III colon cancer can range from 30% to 70% [3]. As a result, the benefit of adjuvant therapy has been extensively investigated to decrease the risk of disease recurrence after potentially curative resection.

During the 1970s, studies examining the outcome and patterns of failure of patients undergoing resection of colon and rectal cancer identified subsets of patients at risk for local and/or systemic recurrence (classically by anatomic stage). These investigations determined the frequency and anatomic location of recurrence, and served as the basis for the development of adjuvant and neoadjuvant therapies. During the 1970s and 1980s, treatment strategies utilizing external-beam irradiation, 5-fluorouracil (5-FU)-based chemotherapy, and combinations of these treatments were under way, with the goal of eradicating micrometastases, thereby maximizing the disease-free survival (DFS) and OS. These initial studies pointed to the possible benefits of these therapies, and subsequently, numerous multi-institutional randomized prospective trials have assessed and demonstrated their efficacy. For patients with resected high-risk colon cancer, these studies have established the value of adjuvant chemotherapy. Currently, adjuvant chemotherapy has been clearly demonstrated to benefit patients with stage III (node-positive) disease [4–6]. In contrast, the benefit of adjuvant chemotherapy remains controversial in patients with stage II disease and, based on current published data, the National Comprehensive Cancer Network (NCCN) guidelines have not recommended the routine use of adjuvant chemotherapy for stage II colon cancer [7]. Regarding the role of postoperative radiation therapy in completely resected colon cancer, although there are retrospective single-institutional series supporting adjuvant irradiation in combination with 5-FU-based chemotherapy for patients with locally advanced colon cancer, the only randomized prospective trial published to date failed to demonstrate a benefit with the addition of adjuvant radiation therapy. The rationale for the use of radiation therapy and 5-FU-based chemotherapy in the treatment of colon cancer is reviewed in this chapter. Previously established Duke's staging classification and the most recent updated AJCC 2017 Staging System for Colon Cancer are summarized in Table 23.1.

The Role of Adjuvant Chemotherapy

Prospective randomized trials have established the value of adjuvant chemotherapy for patients with resected high-risk colon cancer. For more than a decade, adjuvant 5-FU and leucovorin was considered the standard adjuvant therapy for stage III colon cancer after three major clinical trials had demonstrated a statistically significant improvement in survival among patients treated with 5-FU/leucovorin compared to patients receiving no adjuvant therapy or levamisole alone [8–10]. More recently, the benefit of adding oxaliplatin to 5-FU and leucovorin has been established in patients with resected colon cancer [5,6]. In 2004, Andre *et al.* published the results of the MOSAIC trial, which randomly assigned 2246 patients with resected stage II or III colon cancer to receive either the de Gramont regimen of 5-FU/

Table 23.1 Staging classification system of colon cancer.

Primary Tumor (T Category)

Tis	Carcinoma *in situ*; intraepithelial or invasion of lamina propria
T1	Tumor invades submucosa
T2	Tumor invades muscularis propria
T3	Tumor invades through the muscularis propria into pericolorectal tissues
T4a	Tumor penetrates to the surface of the visceral peritoneum
T4b	Tumor directly invades or is adherent to other organs or structures

Regional Lymph Nodes (N Category)

N0	No regional lymph node metastases
N1	1–3 lymph nodes involved
N1a	1 lymph node involved
N1b	2–3 lymph nodes involved
N1c	No positive lymph nodes, but tumor deposits in the subserosa, mesentery, or nonperitonealized pericolic, or perirectal/mesorectal tissues
N2	4 or more regional lymph nodes involved
N2a	4–6 regional lymph nodes involved
N2b	7 regional lymph nodes involved

Distant Metastasis (M)

M0	No distant metastases
M1	Distant metastases
M1a	Metastasis confined to one organ or site
M1b	Metastasis in more than one organ/site or the peritoneum
M1c	Metastasis to the peritoneal surface alone or with other site or organ metastases

AJCC Stage	TNM	Dukes classification	Modified Astler–Coller
I	T1N0	A	A
	T2N0		B1
IIA	T3N0	B	B2
IIB	T4aN0		B2
IIC	T4bN0		B3
IIIA	T1-2N1, N1c	C	C1
	T1N2a		C1
IIIB	T3-T4aN1, N1c		C2
	T2-T3, N2a		C1/C2
	T1-T2, N2b		C1
IIIC	T4aN2a		C2
	T3-T4a,N2b		C2
	T4b,N1-2		C3
IVA	M1a	–	–
IVB	M1b	–	–
IVC	M1c	–	–

leucovorin (LV 200 mg m^{-2} over 2 h, followed by bolus 5-FU 400 mg m^{-2}, followed by a 22-h continuous-infusion of 5-FU 600 mg m^{-2} given every two weeks) with or without oxaliplatin [5]. With a median follow-up of 82 months, the addition of oxaliplatin (FOLFOX4 regimen) yielded a significant benefit in five-year DFS (73% versus 67%, HR 0.80, p = 0.003). Additionally, six-year OS rates were improved from 76% to 78.5% (HR 0.84, p = 0.046) with the addition of oxaliplatin. When stratified by stage, there was only a statistically significant improvement in six-year OS among stage III patients (73% versus 69%, HR 0.80, p = 0.02), but not stage II patients. The principal toxicity associated with the addition of oxaliplatin was grade 3 neuropathy, which resolved in the majority of patients. Among patients receiving oxaliplatin, the rate of grade 3 peripheral sensory neuropathy was only 1.3% at 12 months after the completion of treatment [11].

Within the United States, NSABP C-07 was launched to similarly address the role of oxaliplatin in the adjuvant setting [6]. In total, 2409 patients with stage II or III resected colon cancer were randomized to receive either bolus 5-FU/leucovorin (5-FU 500 mg m^{-2}, leucovorin 500 mg m^{-2} both weekly for six weeks for an eight-week cycle) with or without oxaliplatin given every two weeks. With a median follow-up of eight years, among all patients the addition of oxaliplatin (FLOX) improved five-year DFS (69% versus 64%, HR 0.82, p = 0.002), and yielded a non-significant trend towards improved five-year OS (80% versus 78%, HR 0.88, p = 0.08). In an unplanned subset analysis, oxaliplatin appeared to confer a survival benefit among patients aged <70 years, though no positive effect was seen in patients aged >70 years [12]. As seen in the MOSAIC study, there was a higher incidence of neurosensory toxicity and diarrhea that occurred among patients treated with oxaliplatin-containing regimens. Comparison of the toxicity profile reported in the MOSAIC trial (FOLFOX4 regimen) with that reported in NSABP C-07 (FLOX) suggested higher rates of grade 3 and 4 diarrhea associated with the FLOX regimen (38% versus 10%). Based on the positive results of these two studies and the improved toxicity profile with infusional 5-FU compared to bolus weekly 5-FU, the FOLFOX regimen has been established as the standard regimen for adjuvant systemic therapy of completely resected stage III colon cancer.

Capecitabine

More recently, the possibility of substituting capecitabine, an orally active fluoropyridimine, has been evaluated in the adjuvant setting for colon cancer. Study NO16968 randomly assigned 1886 patients to receive either capecitabine plus oxaliplatin (XELOX) or bolus 5-FU and folinic acid (FA) as adjuvant therapy for patients with stage III colon cancer. After 57 months of follow-up, XELOX was found to confer an improvement in DFS compared to 5-FU and FA (three-year DFS 71% versus 67%, HR 0.80, p = 0.0045). Although there was a trend towards improved OS favoring XELOX, the difference was not significant (five-year OS: 78% versus 74%, HR 0.87, p = 0.15) [13].

Moreover, the X-ACT study (Xeloda in Adjuvant Colon Cancer Therapy) study sought to compare the efficacy and safety of capecitabine versus bolus 5-FU/leucovorin as adjuvant therapy for stage III colon cancer. This international, multicenter, prospective Phase III study randomized 1987 patients to receive either 24 weeks of capecitabine 1250 mg m^{-2} twice daily for days 1–14 every three weeks, or 5-FU/leucovorin. With a median follow-up of 6.9 years, capecitabine was found to be at least equivalent to 5-FU/leucovorin with respect to DFS (HR 0.88) and OS (HR 0.86). Additionally, pre-planned multivariate analyses showed that capecitabine yielded statistically significant beneficial effects on DFS (P = 0.021) and OS (P = 0.020). Capecitabine was also associated with significantly fewer grade 3 and 4 adverse

events (p < 0.01) requiring fewer hospital admissions [14]. Thus, the X-ACT study suggested that capecitabine offered at least equivalent clinical benefit, with a potentially improved toxicity profile, and was a possibly more cost-effective therapeutic option for patients with stage III colon cancer in the adjuvant setting [14].

Irinotecan

In the metastatic setting, the addition of irinotecan has been shown to improve median survival and response rate compared to 5-FU and leukovorin alone [15]. However, randomized studies evaluating the role of irinotecan in the adjuvant setting have not confirmed a benefit. Study CALGB 89803 randomly assigned 1264 patients to receive either standard weekly bolus 5-FU plus leucovorin, or weekly bolus irinotecan plus 5-FU plus leucovorin. With a median follow-up of 4.8 years, there were no differences in either DFS or OS between the two treatment arms. Febrile neutropenia and neutropenia were significantly higher for patients receiving irinotecan, and significantly more patients died secondary to treatment-related events in the irinotecan arm (2.8% versus 1.0%, p = 0.008) [16]. Subsequently, the PETACC-3 trial similarly confirmed the lack of benefit with the addition of irinotecan to short-term infusion 5-FU and leucovorin. After randomization of 2094 patients with stage III disease, there was no significant improvements were seen in five-year DFS or OS with the addition of irinotecan [17]. Based on these results, it is important to recognize that advances in the metastatic setting do not necessarily translate into the adjuvant setting, and should be evaluated in randomized, prospective studies [16].

Targeted Therapies

Bevacizumab
Bevacizumab (Avastin®) is a humanized monoclonal antibody directed against vascular endothelial growth factor (VEGF), which has been shown to improve survival in the metastatic setting in combination with 5-FU-based regimens [18]. Recently, the NSABP sought to assess the safety and efficacy of bevacizumab in the adjuvant setting. Study NSABP C-08 randomized 2672 patients with stage II/III colon cancer to receive FOLFOX with or without bevacizumab for six months, with bevacizumab continued as monotherapy for an additional six months [19,20]. After a median follow-up of 35.6 months, there was no improvement in three-year DFS (HR 0.89, p = 0.15) in stage II/III colon cancer. Additionally, bevacizumab was associated with significantly higher rates of hypertension, wound complications, pain, proteinuria, and neuropathy [19]. Running concurrent with NSABP C-08, the AVANT trial, which closed to accrual in 2007, also sought to address the role of bevacizumab in the setting of either FOLFOX or XELOX. Preliminary results

presented in 2011 confirmed the lack of benefit of bevacizumab to either FOLFOX or XELOX regimens in the adjuvant setting [21]. Based on these results, there does not appear to be a role for bevacizumab in the adjuvant setting.

Cetuximab

Cetuximab is a human/mouse chimeric monoclonal antibody directed against the epidermal growth factor receptor (EGFR) which has been extensively evaluated in metastatic colon cancer. To date, there has been one randomized prospective, phase III study which addressed the role of cetuximab in the adjuvant setting. The NO147 trial randomized 2418 patients (1760 K-ras wild-type, 658 K-ras mutants) with resected stage III colon cancer to receive either FOLFOX with or without cetuximab. After interim analysis, the study was closed prematurely when the preliminary results suggested that there was no benefit of cetuximab to any subgroups of patients [22,23]. Hence, at the present time cetuximab does not appear to have a role in the adjuvant setting.

The Role of Adjuvant Radiation Therapy

Due to the documented efficacy of adjuvant chemotherapy and the perception among many oncologists that colon cancer, in contrast to rectal cancer, is much more likely to recur systemically than locally, the role of postoperative radiation therapy is less well-established in the adjuvant setting for colon cancer. The potential indications for postoperative irradiation in patients with colon cancer stem from examinations of the patterns of failure after resection [24,25]. For colon cancer, both the stage of the primary tumor and the location are important. For lesions in the ascending and descending colon – which is considered to be anatomically immobile bowel – invasion into the retroperitoneum may limit a wide surgical resection. As a result of compromised radial resection margins, the risk of local failure may be considerably higher. Unless there is invasion into an adjacent organ, local failure is rare for tumors in the sigmoid colon and transverse colon (mobile bowel), since a wide resection margin is usually achievable regardless of the extent of invasion into the mesentery. For tumors that arise in the cecum, flexures, or proximal or distal ends of the sigmoid colon, the risk of local failure may be variable depending on the amount of mesentery and the ability to obtain a satisfactory circumferential margin. For any colon tumor adherent to adjacent structures (with and without lymph node involvement), local failure rates can exceed 30%. In summary, local failure may be a consideration for large-bowel tumors, where there are anatomic constraints of radial resection margins, and for tumors invading adjacent structures.

Reports on the use of adjuvant postoperative radiation therapy to the tumor bed without chemotherapy for colon cancer are limited to single-institution retrospective analyses [26–28]. These retrospective studies suggest that failure rates in the operative bed are potentially reduced in patients receiving radiation therapy compared to historical controls. In 1993, Willett *et al.* published details of their experience at Massachusetts General Hospital evaluating the role of postoperative radiation therapy for high-risk, completely resected colon cancer. In total, 171 patients with high-risk colon cancer treated between 1976 and 1989 – including patients with stage B3 and C3 disease, patients with stage C2 disease except middle sigmoid and transverse colon cancer, and selected patients with stage B2 disease with 'tight' margins – were reviewed. These all received postoperative radiation therapy via a high-energy linear accelerator by parallel opposed fields or multifield techniques to irradiate the tumor bed with approximately 3–5 cm margins to a total dose of 45 Gy in 1.8-Gy fractions, followed by a boost to 50.4 Gy. Additional treatment above 50.4 Gy was attempted in patients with stage B3 and C3 disease only if the small bowel could be displaced from the field. Of the 171 patients, 53 were treated with adjuvant chemotherapy, usually 5-FU as intravenous bolus for three consecutive days (500 mg m^{-2} per day) during the first and last weeks of radiation therapy. These 171 patients were compared with 395 patients in the Massachusetts General Hospital series with similarly staged tumors who underwent surgery alone during the period between 1970 and 1977. The five-year actuarial local control and recurrence-free survival rates for patients undergoing postoperative radiation therapy compared to surgery alone (by stage) are listed in Table 23.2. Among patients with stage B3 and C3 tumors, postoperative radiation therapy resulted in a statistically significant improved local control, with rates of local control of 93% versus 72% for B3 tumors, and 69% versus 47% for C3 tumors. Patients with stage B3 and C3 disease receiving postoperative radiotherapy experienced 16% and 15% improvements, respectively, in DFS compared to surgery alone. In contrast, there was no improvement seen among patients with stage B2 and C2 treated with postoperative radiotherapy. However, this result may be confounded by treatment bias, with patients at greater risk of margin positivity more likely to receive postoperative radiation therapy [26]. The authors concluded that patients with T4 tumors, tumors with abscess/fistula formation, or margin-positive resections may benefit from postoperative irradiation.

Other studies have demonstrated improved local control in irradiated patients with high-risk colon cancer [27,28]. The results of postoperative radiotherapy at the Mayo Clinic for 103 patients with locally advanced colon cancers were analyzed. More than 90% of these patients

Table 23.2 The MGH Experience: Five-year actuarial local control and recurrence-free survival after adjuvant radiation therapy versus surgery alone according to stage.

Stage	Surgery + Radiation			Surgery Alone		
	No. of patients	Local control (%)	Recurrence-free survival (%)	No. of patients	Local control (%)	Recurrence-free survival (%)
B2	23	91	72	163	90	78
B3	54	93	79	83	69	63
C2	55	70	47	100	64	48
C3	39	72	53	49	47	38

had modified Astler–Coller stage B3 and C3 lesions. With a median follow-up of 5.8 years, the five-year actuarial local failure rate was 10% for patients with no residual disease, 54% for those with microscopic residual disease, and 79% for those with gross residual disease (p < 0.001) [27]. The five-year actuarial survival rate was 66% for patients with no residual disease, 47% for those with microscopic residual disease, and 23% for those with gross residual disease (p = 0.0009) [27].

In 1996, the University of Florida also published their experience of 78 patients with locally advanced, completely resected colon cancer treated with postoperative radiotherapy [28]. This study reported a local control rate of 88%, similar to the 90% reported by the Mayo Clinic in patients with completely resected tumors. In addition, a significant relationship between the radiation dose delivered and the rate of local control was found. The five-year local control was 96% for those who had received 50–55 Gy, compared to 76% for those who had received less than 50 Gy (p = 0.0095).

Few data are available evaluating the combined effect of 5-FU and irradiation in colon cancer. In the MGH adjuvant series, 53 patients received three days of bolus 5-FU (500 mg m^{-2} per day) for three consecutive days during the first and last weeks of irradiation. Local control and recurrence-free survival rates for the adjuvantly treated patients based on 5-FU administration during radiation therapy are listed in Table 23.3. Although no statistically significant differences in local control or

recurrence-free survival were observed based on the addition of 5-FU, there was a trend towards improved local control in patients receiving 5-FU. Interestingly, the incidence of acute enteritis in patients receiving irradiation and 5-FU was 16%, versus 4% in patients undergoing irradiation only. No differences in late bowel complications were observed following 5-FU administration [26]. This higher incidence of acute enteritis is consistent with other reports of combined 5-FU and irradiation in rectal cancer. The current policy at MGH for patients receiving postoperative irradiation for colon cancer is to utilize continuous-infusion 5-FU (225 mg m^{-2} per 24 h) or capecitabine 825 mg m^{-2} twice daily five days per week, throughout the irradiation.

To date, only one prospective randomized controlled trial, the US Intergroup INT 0130, has been conducted in an attempt to definitively assess the merits of postoperative radiation therapy for high-risk colon cancer. Although the initial target accrual was 700 patients, the study closed early due to poor accrual. In total, 222 patients with completely resected colon cancer with high-risk features, defined as either: (i) tumor adherence to or invasion of surrounding structures; or (ii) tumor in the ascending/descending colon with penetration through the colon wall with involvement of regional lymph nodes (T3,N1-2), were enrolled between 1992 and 1996. All patients received adjuvant levamisole and 5-FU with or without adjuvant radiation therapy. Patients received 45 Gy at 1.8 Gy per fraction over five weeks,

Table 23.3 Five-year actuarial local control and recurrence-free survival of adjuvantly irradiated patients based on 5-FU administration.

Stage	Without 5-FU			With 5-FU		
	No. of patients	Local control (%)	Recurrence-free survival (%)	No. of patients	Local control (%)	Recurrence-free survival (%)
B2	16	87	69	7	100	80
B3	37	94	78	16	100	83
C2	41	69	48	14	70	43
C3	24	67	53	15	79	52

Table 23.4 Summary of results from Intergroup 0130.

Parameter	Chemotherapy alone	Chemoradiation	P-value
5-year DFS	52%	51%	0.85
5-year OS	62%	58%	0.60
Acute grade 3+ toxicity	42	54	0.04

DFS, disease-free survival; OS, overall survival.

with an optional 5.4 Gy boost. With a median follow-up of 6.6 years, there were no significant differences in five-year OS (62% versus 58%, p >0.5 for chemotherapy alone and chemoradiation, respectively) or five-year DFS (51% for both groups, p >0.5). There were 18 local recurrences within each study arm. As expected, chemoradiation was associated with increased grade 3+ toxicity (54% versus 42%, p = 0.04). Due to limitations of the study, the results should be interpreted with caution. First, the poor study accrual limited the study power to detect potentially clinically significant differences in outcomes. Second, only a minority of patients had placement of surgical clips to guide the design of radiation therapy treatment fields. Third, computed tomography (CT) imaging was not required for patient follow-up, which limited the ability to detect local recurrences. The results of the study are summarized in Table 23.4 [29].

The Role of Hepatic or Whole-Abdomen Irradiation

Because of the high incidence of hepatic metastases and peritoneal failures developing in patients with advanced-stage colon cancer, there have been clinical investigations of the efficacy of adjuvant hepatic irradiation as well as whole-abdomen radiation therapy. However, only one randomized prospective trial has been reported, namely the Phase III trial of adjuvant hepatic irradiation reported by the Gastrointestinal Tumor Study Group [30]. In this study, 300 patients with completely resected transmural or node-positive colon carcinoma were randomized between two treatment arms: (i) observation; or (ii) 5-FU and 21 Gy to the liver (1.5 Gy per fraction for 14 treatments). The 5-FU was given as an intravenous bolus during the first three days of radiation therapy, as well as maintenance treatment. No statistical difference in survival, recurrence-free survival, or liver recurrence was seen between the control patients and the treatment patients.

Several investigators have reported the results and toxicity of whole-abdomen irradiation as an adjuvant treatment for patients at high risk for hepatic and peritoneal

failure [31–33], but none of these studies had concurrent controls. Wong *et al.* reported their experience at Princess Margaret Hospital of 30 patients receiving whole-abdomen irradiation of 14–25 Gy over three to five weeks, with or without local tumor boost [31]. The five-year actuarial survival was 55%. For patients without regional nodal involvement, the survival was 72%, compared with 41% for those with nodal involvement. After treatment, four patients had failure in the peritoneum and 12 had hepatic and extra-abdominal failure. Brenner *et al.* described 21 patients with Duke C colon cancer who received whole-abdomen irradiation to 20–30 Gy in three weeks to areas at high risk, with concurrent weekly 350 mg m^{-2} doses of 5-FU given intravenously [32]. Those patients who underwent radiation therapy were compared with a matched control group who underwent surgery alone, and a statistically significant improvement in the disease-free survival was noted (55% versus 12%, respectively).

In 1995, the results were described of a Phase I/II Southwest Oncology Group study (SWOG 8572) utilizing 30 Gy of whole-abdomen irradiation (given 1 Gy per fraction daily) and an additional 16 Gy tumor boost with continuous infusional 5-FU (200 mg m^{-2} per 24 h) for 41 patients with T3 N1-2 colon cancer [33]. In view of the early intolerance, the protocol was amended to insert a one-week break from external beam irradiation and 5-FU. The five-year actuarial DFS and OS for all 41 patients were 58% and 67%, respectively. For the 19 patients with four or fewer positive nodes, both the five-year OS and DFS rate were 61%. For the 20 patients with more than four involved nodes, the five-year actuarial DFS and OS rates with chemoradiation were 55% and 74%, respectively. This was higher than the DFS and OS results of 35% and 39% reported in the 5-FU and levamisole intergroup trial.

Estes *et al.* [34] compared patterns of relapse for MAC C2 patients in SWOG 8591 (arms of surgery alone or surgery plus 5-FU/levamisole), SWOG 8572 (whole-abdomen irradiation plus tumor bed irradiation and 5-FU infusion), and the surgery-alone arm from the Willett MGH analysis. In SWOG 8591, although lung relapse was decreased from 34% to 21% with the addition of 5-FU/levamisole to surgical resection, the chemotherapy adjuvant had no impact on the rate of locoregional relapse (surgery alone 20%, 5-FU/levamisole 27%), which is equivalent to the 32% incidence alone in the MGH analysis. Patients who received chemoradiation (whole-abdomen irradiation and tumor bed irradiation with infusion of 5-FU) in SWOG 8572 had only a 12% tumor bed nodal relapse rate, along with a reduction in liver and peritoneal relapse rates (liver relapse rate of 22% with chemoradiation versus 54% and 57% in the two arms of SWOG 8591; peritoneal relapse rates of 15% in SWOG 8572 versus 37% and 40% in SWOG 8591).

Techniques of Irradiation of Colon Cancer

As is true in the treatment of rectal cancer, great care must be taken in the postoperative treatment of adenocarcinoma of the colon. Field arrangements will vary to a great degree depending on the exact site of the primary tumor and the areas thought to be at high risk for local recurrence. Although recommendations of specific fields cannot be made, some general suggestions are possible.

Attempts should be made to treat the primary tumor site with a 4–5 cm margin proximally and distally, and a 3–4 cm margin medially and laterally, to provide adequate coverage of the local tumor spread. Generally, the lymph nodes in the mesentery beyond the margins of the surgical resection are not treated. At times, there may be a need to treat lymph nodes draining from adjacent structures that are involved by tumor, such as the para-aortic nodes with deep retroperitoneal involvement. The surgeon can usually obtain good mesenteric nodal margins with standard lymph node dissection. In rare instances, it may be appropriate to treat proximally located lymph nodes in the surgical resection. However, the long-term survival benefit from this treatment is likely to be minimal.

It may be helpful to treat patients in the right or left decubitus position. When patients are treated with one side up, often much of the small bowel will fall by gravity away from the radiation field. The total radiation dose should be adjusted to the amount of small bowel included within the field.

It is often found that part or all of one kidney may be in the radiation field. In general, the finding has been accepted that the irradiation of a large portion of one kidney results in long-term lack of function in that kidney. Nonetheless, these patients may always be treated if their other kidney functions well, and their blood urea nitrogen and creatinine values are within normal limits. Renal scan to confirm functionality of the contralateral kidney may be useful. An evaluation of long-term effects of renal irradiation performed at the MGH has shown minimal long-term clinical sequelae from unilateral renal irradiation.

For colon cancer, a dose of 45 Gy is delivered to a larger, elective field, as described above, in 1.8-Gy daily fractions. At this point, an attempt is made to design a boost that will optimally exclude the small bowel from the radiation field, with the small bowel dose limited to 50 Gy. The exact dose delivered to the boost area may vary according to stage, degree of resection, and location of the tumor. All patients should receive concurrent 5-FU-based chemotherapy during radiation treatment. Although relevant data are currently unavailable, intraoperative radiation therapy for T4, margin-positive, or recurrent cancers may be appropriate.

Conclusions

The role of adjuvant radiation therapy in resected colon cancer remains poorly defined. Although several single-institution retrospective series have suggested a potential benefit with adjuvant radiation therapy, the only randomized study to date addressing this issue was underpowered to detect a difference, and failed to demonstrate an improvement in DFS or OS. There may be a subgroup of patients with 30% or more greater risk of local recurrence, particularly those with T4 disease or positive margins, in whom postoperative radiation therapy may be considered. However, based on existing data, treatment recommendations should be made on a case-by-case basis. A thorough discussion regarding the risks, benefits and potential side effects of radiation therapy should be discussed in detail with the patient. At the present author's institution, adjuvant chemoradiation is considered for patients with positive or close margins after surgical resection and/or for tumors with adherence to structures or organs for which wide surgical margins cannot be achieved.

References

1 Jemal, A., Bray, F., Center, M.M., Ferlay, J., Ward, E., Forman, D. (2011) Global cancer statistics. *CA Cancer J. Clin.*, **61** (2), 69–90.

2 Siegel, R., Miller, K., Jemal, A. (2017) Cancer Statistics 2017. *CA Cancer J. Clin.*, **67**, 7–30.

3 Amin, M.B. (ed) (2017) *American Joint Committee on Cancer (AJCC) Cancer Staging Manual*, 8th edition. Springer, New York.

4 Wolmark, N., Rockette, H., Fisher, B., *et al.* (1993) The benefit of leucovorin-modulated fluorouracil as postoperative adjuvant therapy for primary colon cancer: results from National Surgical Adjuvant Breast and Bowel Project protocol C-03. *J. Clin. Oncol.*, **11** (10), 1879–1887.

5 Andre, T., Boni, C., Mounedji-Boudiaf, L., *et al.* (2004) Oxaliplatin, fluorouracil, and leucovorin as adjuvant treatment for colon cancer. *N. Engl. J. Med.*, **350** (23), 2343–2351.

6 Kuebler, J.P., Wieand, H.S., O'Connell, M.J., *et al.* (2007) Oxaliplatin combined with weekly bolus fluorouracil and leucovorin as surgical adjuvant chemotherapy for stage II and III colon cancer: results from NSABP C-07. *J. Clin. Oncol.*, **25** (16), 2198–2204.

7 www.nccn.org

8 Moertel, C.G., Fleming, T.R., Macdonald, J.S., *et al.* (1990) Levamisole and fluorouracil for adjuvant therapy of resected colon carcinoma. *N. Engl. J. Med.*, **322** (6), 352–358.

9 International Multicentre Pooled Analysis of Colon Cancer Trials (IMPACT) Investigators (1995) Efficacy of adjuvant fluorouracil and folinic acid in colon cancer. *Lancet*, **345** (8955), 939–944.

10 O'Connell, M.J., Mailliard, J.A., Kahn, M.J., *et al.* (1997) Controlled trial of fluorouracil and low-dose leucovorin given for 6 months as postoperative adjuvant therapy for colon cancer. *J. Clin. Oncol.*, **15** (1), 246–250.

11 Andre, T., Boni, C., Navarro, M., *et al.* (2009) Improved overall survival with oxaliplatin, fluorouracil, and leucovorin as adjuvant treatment in stage II or III colon cancer in the MOSAIC trial. *J. Clin. Oncol.*, **27** (19), 3109–3116.

12 Yothers, G., O'Connell, M.J., Allegra, C.J., *et al.* (2011) Oxaliplatin as adjuvant therapy for colon cancer: Updated results of NSABP C-07 trial, including survival and subset analyses. *J. Clin. Oncol.*, **29** (28), 3768–3774.

13 Haller, D.G., Tabernero, J., Maroun, J., *et al.* (2011) Capecitabine plus oxaliplatin compared with fluorouracil and folinic acid as adjuvant therapy for stage III colon cancer. *J. Clin. Oncol.*, **29** (11), 1465–1471.

14 Twelves, C., Scheithauer, W., McKendrick, J., *et al.* (2012) Capecitabine versus 5-fluorouracil/folinic acid as adjuvant therapy for stage III colon cancer: final results from the X-ACT trial with analysis by age and preliminary evidence of a pharmacodynamic marker of efficacy. *Ann. Oncol.*, **23** (5), 1190–1197.

15 Saltz, L.B., Cox, J.V., Blanke, C., *et al.* (2000) Irinotecan plus fluorouracil and leucovorin for metastatic colorectal cancer. Irinotecan Study Group. *N. Engl. J. Med.*, **343** (13), 905–914.

16 Saltz, L.B., Niedzwiecki, D., Hollis, D., *et al.* (2007) Irinotecan fluorouracil plus leucovorin is not superior to fluorouracil plus leucovorin alone as adjuvant treatment for stage III colon cancer: results of CALGB 89803. *J. Clin. Oncol.*, **25** (23), 3456–3461.

17 Van Cutsem, E., Labianca, R., Bodoky, G., *et al.* (2009) Randomized phase III trial comparing biweekly infusional fluorouracil/leucovorin alone or with irinotecan in the adjuvant treatment of stage III colon cancer: PETACC-3. *J. Clin. Oncol.*, **27** (19), 3117–3125.

18 Hurwitz, H., Fehrenbacher, L., Novotny, W., *et al.* (2004) Bevacizumab plus irinotecan, fluorouracil, and leucovorin for metastatic colorectal cancer. *N. Engl. J. Med.*, **350** (23), 2335–2342.

19 Allegra, C.J., Yothers, G., O'Connell, M.J., *et al.* (2009) Initial safety report of NSABP C-08: A randomized phase III study of modified FOLFOX6 with or without bevacizumab for the adjuvant treatment of patients with stage II or III colon cancer. *J. Clin. Oncol.*, **27** (20), 3385–3390.

20 Allegra, C.J., Yothers, G., O'Connell, M.J., *et al.* (2011) Phase III trial assessing bevacizumab in stages II and III carcinoma of the colon: results of NSABP protocol C-08. *J. Clin. Oncol.*, **29** (1), 11–16.

21 De Gramont, A., van Cutsem, E., Tabernero, J., *et al.* (2011) AVANT: Results from a randomized, three-arm multinational phase III study to investigate bevacizumab with either XELOX or FOLFOX 4 versus FOLFOX alone as adjuvant treatment for colon cancer. Paper presented at GI ASCO GI Cancers Symposium, 20–22 January 2011, San Francisco, California.

22 Alberts, S.R., Sargent, D.J., Smyrk, T.C., *et al.* (2010) Adjuvant mFOLFOX6 with and without cetuximab (Cmab) in KRAS wild-type (WT) patients with resected stage III colon cancer: Results from NCCTG Intergroup Phase III Trial N0147.2010. *J. Clin. Oncol.* (Suppl.), abstract CRA3507.

23 Goldberg, R.M., Sargent, D.J., Thibodeau, S.N., *et al.* (2010) Adjuvant mFOLFOX6 plus or minus cetuximab in patients with KRAS-mutant resected stage III colon cancer: NCCTG Intergroup Phase III Trial N0147. *J. Clin. Oncol.* (Suppl.), abstract CRA3507.

24 Willett, C.G., Tepper, J.E., Cohen, A.M., Orlow, E., Welch, C.E. (1984) Failure patterns following curative resection of colonic carcinoma. *Ann. Surg.*, **200** (6), 685–690.

25 Gunderson, L.L., Sosin, H., Levitt, S. (1985) Extrapelvic colon – areas of failure in a reoperation series: implications for adjuvant therapy. *Int. J. Radiat. Oncol. Biol. Phys.*, **11** (4), 731–741.

26 Willett, C.G., Fung, C.Y., Kaufman, D.S., Efird, J., Shellito, P.C. (1993) Postoperative radiation therapy for high-risk colon carcinoma. *J. Clin. Oncol.*, **11** (6), 1112–1117.

27 Schild, S.E., Gunderson, L.L., Haddock, M.G., Wong, W.W., Nelson, H. (1997) The treatment of locally advanced colon cancer. *Int. J. Radiat. Oncol. Biol. Phys.*, **37** (1), 51–58.

28 Amos, E.H., Mendenhall, W.M., McCarty, P.J., *et al.* (1996) Postoperative radiotherapy for locally advanced colon cancer. *Ann. Surg. Oncol.*, **3** (5), 431–436.

29 Martenson, J.A., Jr, Willett, C.G., Sargent, D.J., *et al.* (2004) Phase III study of adjuvant chemotherapy and radiation therapy compared with chemotherapy alone in the surgical adjuvant treatment of colon cancer: results of intergroup protocol 0130. *J. Clin. Oncol.*, **22** (16), 3277–3283.

30 The Gastrointestinal Tumor Study Group (1991) Adjuvant therapy with hepatic irradiation plus fluorouracil in colon carcinoma. *Int. J. Radiat. Oncol. Biol. Phys.*, **21** (5), 1151–1156.

31 Wong, C.S., Harwood, A.R., Cummings, B.J., Keane, T.J., Thomas, G.M., Rider, W.D. (1984) Total abdominal

irradiation for cancer of the colon. *Radiother. Oncol.*, **2** (3), 209–214.

32 Brenner, H.J., Bibi, C., Chaitchik, S. (1983) Adjuvant therapy for Dukes C adenocarcinoma of colon. *Int. J. Radiat. Oncol. Biol. Phys.*, **9** (12), 1789–1792.

33 Fabian, C., Giri, S., Estes, N., *et al.* (1995) Adjuvant continuous infusion 5-FU, whole-abdominal radiation, and tumor bed boost in high-risk stage III colon carcinoma: a Southwest Oncology Group Pilot study. *Int. J. Radiat. Oncol. Biol. Phys.*, **32** (2), 457–464.

34 Estes, N.C., Giri, S., Fabian, C. (1996) Patterns of recurrence for advanced colon cancer modified by whole abdominal radiation and chemotherapy. *Am. Surg.*, **62** (7), 546–549; discussion 549–550.

24

Rectal Cancer

Jennifer Y. Wo

Introduction

Carcinoma of the rectum is a heterogeneous disease. At one end of the clinical spectrum, a small number of patients who present with superficially invasive favorable cancers may be served by limited procedures, such as local excision or endocavitary irradiation. The great majority of patients with rectal cancer, however, present with mobile, but more deeply invasive tumors that require definitive surgical resection with either low anterior resection or abdominoperineal resection. At the other and less-favorable end of the clinical spectrum, a subset of patients present with locally advanced, unresectable tumors that are adherent or fixed to adjoining structures such as the sacrum, pelvic sidewalls, prostate or bladder. Relevant clinical issues in the three presentations of: (i) favorable; (ii) mobile, resectable; and (iii) locally advanced unresectable rectal cancer are reviewed in this chapter.

Favorable Rectal Cancer

Since the introduction of abdominoperineal resection by Miles, this surgical approach with removal of the tumor and its adjacent tissues has offered a high probability of local control and survival. Despite its merits, however, abdominoperineal resection has profound drawbacks, notably a loss of anorectal function, with a permanent colostomy and a high incidence of sexual and genitourinary dysfunction. To overcome these limitations, an array of surgical procedures has been developed, ranging from full-thickness wide local excisions to complex resections with reconstruction. In appropriately staged patients, these operations appear to offer not only comparable rates of local control as the abdominoperineal resection, but also and importantly, to preserve sphincter integrity. With continued experience, selection

criteria and the role of radiation therapy and chemotherapy have become more clearly defined.

One obvious consideration in the selection of patients for sphincter preservation is tumor location within the rectum. Patients with tumors in the upper rectum have long been well managed by a sphincter-preserving anastomosis. With the advent of the end-to-end anastomosis stapling instrument, tumors of the mid-rectum, even in a narrow pelvis, become amenable to treatment by low anterior resection and preservation of the anal sphincter. Although with the lower anastomoses there is a real incidence of sexual dysfunction and less than perfect anorectal function, the avoidance of a permanent colostomy is perceived by the patient as an extremely fortunate situation. In contrast to tumors of the upper and middle rectum, the management of distal rectal cancer continues to pose a major challenge to the surgeon and the oncologist. An important consideration in the treatment selection of patients with low rectal cancer is the local extent of the primary tumor.

For small lesions in the distal rectum, there has been interest in local excision procedures as an alternative to abdominoperineal resection. The most commonly practiced local surgical management option is transanal tumor excision, which can be accomplished either via a conventional transanal excision (TAE) technique or via an operating microscope with transanal endoscopic microsurgery (TEM). Other potential approaches include the posterior parasacral approach (Kraske) first described in 1885, or the posterior trans-sphincteric approach of Mason, first described in the 1900s and later re-introduced in the 1970s.

Clinical and Radiographic Evidence

The usual criteria for rectal cancers suitable for full-thickness wide local excision are as follows: mobile,

Clinical Radiation Oncology: Indications, Techniques, and Results, Third Edition. Edited by William Small Jr.
© 2017 John Wiley & Sons, Inc. Published 2017 by John Wiley & Sons, Inc.

tumor size <4 cm, location 8 cm or less from the anal verge, well- or moderately-well differentiated histology, comprising <40% of the rectal circumference, without ulceration, no evidence of lymphovascular invasion, and no suspicion of perirectal lymph nodes [1]. With this approach, an attempt is being made to select patients with tumors confined to the rectal wall where there is a low probability of lymph node metastases.

Although impressive advances have been made in the radiographic imaging of rectal cancer, digital rectal examination by an experienced practitioner is one of the most reliable (and inexpensive!) methods of determining the depth of penetration of the primary tumor. The accuracy rate of staging the primary tumor by digital rectal examination has been reported to be approximately 80% [2]. Because lymph nodes are seen only microscopically in a high percentage of cases, it is not surprising that digital examination is insensitive at identifying metastatic perirectal nodal involvement.

In addition to digital examination, endoscopic ultrasonography (EUS) has been used as a staging tool in assessing local tumor extent as well as lymph node involvement. A recent meta-analysis reported a sensitivity and specificity for EUS in the determination of perirectal tissue invasion of 90% and 75%, respectively. To achieve high accuracy rates (≥90%), this examination must be performed by experienced operators. In a study from University of Minnesota, the accuracy rates rose from 59% during the early phase of the study to 88% in the latter phase [3]. In assessing perirectal lymph node involvement, EUS has been generally less helpful, with reported sensitivity and specificity of 67% and 78%, respectively [4]. With these caveats, EUS is generally acknowledged to be complementary to digital examination in staging, and more accurate than axial computed tomography (CT) and pelvic magnetic resonance imaging (MRI) for the determination of local tumor invasion [4], although the increasing use of newer MRI techniques may yield improved accuracy in tumor staging [5].

Compared to EUS, obtaining a pelvic MRI provides several potential advantages, including a larger field of view compared to EUS, less operator and technique dependence, and the ability to thoroughly evaluate stenotic tumors [3,6]. Additionally, in general, MRI scans provide improved accuracy in the assessment of perirectal lymph node involvement compared to endorectal ultrasound based on both evaluation of the size and contour of lymph nodes, with reported accuracy rates of up to 95% [7]. More recently, a prospective multicenter European MERCURY study showed that high-resolution MRI is the best technique for predicting mesorectal fascial involvement at the time of resection [8]. However, similar to EUS, the evaluation of MRI is both dependent on the technical aspects of imaging and image interpretation. Therefore, at the present time both EUS and high-resolution MRI are acceptable radiographic methods of assessing preoperative tumor and nodal stage.

Surgical and Pathological Evaluation

The two most commonly practiced local excisional approaches include conventional TAE and TEM. For a conventional TAE, patients are placed under general anesthesia in either the prone jackknife position (for anterior and lateral lesions), or the dorsal lithotomy position (for posterior lesions). The aim of the TAE is to completely excise the tumor with a full-thickness specimen, which can be confirmed by visualization of the mesorectal fat after excision. All surgical margins should include at least 1 cm of normal tissue circumferentially. The pathologist should use an inked margin to carefully define the narrowest margin in fresh tissues and on slides. Alternatively, TEM is a minimally invasive technique developed to overcome some of the technical limitations of TAE. By incorporating carbon dioxide insufflations and a lighted rectoscope, TEM can be used to access tumors within the upper rectum and is performed with a magnified view of the tumor. However, obtaining a full-thickness excision of a high anterior lesion is associated with a risk of intraperitoneal perforation, and therefore should be approached with caution [9,10]. Neither of these procedures aims to remove nodal tissue in the mesorectum. In contrast, total mesorectal excision (TME) involves sharp dissection of the avascular plane between the visceral covering of the mesorectum and the parietal fascia of the pelvis. A TME surgically removes the primary tumor, draining lymphatic tissue, and any other involved pelvic structures in an *en bloc* fashion and provides the best clearance of proximal, distal, and radial margins. To date, there are no prospective randomized clinical trials comparing wide local excision with TAE or TEM compared to radical resection. Numerous retrospective multi-institutional cohort studies, however, have suggested that local excision yields inferior local control compared to radical resection, although it is unclear whether this translates into an overall survival decrement [11–14]. Fulguration or electrocoagulation is not recommended: these procedures are associated with a high likelihood of residual disease after the procedure and inadequate pathologic analysis.

A critical limitation of wide local excision procedures is the inability to sample or resect perirectal lymphatics. The incidence of perirectal lymph node metastases progressively rises as the tumor penetrates from submucosa through muscularis propria to fat [15, 16]. Lymph node metastases have been reported in 5–12% of T1 lesions, in 10–35% of T2 lesions, and in up to 70% of T3 lesions [1, 15–17]. In addition to the T stage, histologic grade and vascular involvement are independent predictors of

Table 24.1 Risk of perirectal lymph nodes by primary tumor histopathology.

Low-risk: Well-differentiated histology Submucosa or inner muscularis propria invasion	<10%
Intermediate-risk: Moderately well-differentiated histology Muscularis propria invasion	10–20%
High-risk Poorly differentiated histology Muscularis propria or perirectal fat invasion Lymphatic or venous vessel invasion	>30%

lymph node metastasis. One analysis reported a 29% to 50% risk of perirectal nodal metastasis for patients with T1 and T2 tumors showing poorly differentiated histology or lymphatic/blood vessel involvement [16]. The incidence of perirectal nodal metastases by T stage, and histologic features of the primary tumor, are summarized in Table 24.1

Because many patients with pathologically high-risk T1 and T2 tumors have perirectal lymph node metastases, local excision procedures alone would be inadequate. Studies examining the outcome of patients undergoing local excision show a clear association of local failure to the risk of perirectal nodal metastases as assessed by primary tumor histopathology. In a study from Erlangen, patients with 'low-risk' tumors had less has a 10% local failure, whereas patients with 'high-risk' tumors had a greater than 30% local failure [18]. To improve the outcome of these patients, treatment programs of postoperative pelvic irradiation with concurrent 5-fluorouracil (5-FU) after local excision of 'high-risk' tumors have been investigated.

Post Local Excision Treatment Recommendations and Results

Treatment recommendations should be guided by the surgical and pathological finding of the full-thickness wide local excision. For patients with small tumors invading the mucosa and the submucosa, a full-thickness wide local excision, which includes the entire muscularis propria and perirectal fat in the pathologic specimen, may potentially suffice. Among pathologic T1 tumors without adverse pathologic features, the risk of local failure or having positive lymph nodes may be less than 10%, and patients may be able to forego adjuvant radiation therapy. However, in the presence of adverse pathologic features such as larger tumor size, lymphovascular invasion or high grade, the risk of local recurrence and/or positive lymph nodes can be much higher [17, 19]. For this subset of patients, radical surgical resection or postoperative therapy should be considered. Several single-institution retrospective series (see Table 24.2) suggest that local control rates after wide local excision and postoperative radiation may range from 73% to 92% [20–25]. Although salvage after local failure is possible with an abdominoperineal resection (APR), most series report that little more than half of the patients are successfully salvaged [20–23].

In tumors that are somewhat larger, or in which there is deeper invasion of the tumor into the rectal wall, several studies have suggested that postoperative radiation therapy with concurrent 5-FU-based chemotherapy may improve outcomes. Single-institution studies reporting on the results of postoperative irradiation for these patients indicate excellent local control and survival rates. A series published from M.D. Anderson Cancer Center reported a local control rate of 93% among 15 patients with T2 tumors treated by local excision with postoperative chemoradiation [26]. Similar results were reported by Massachusetts General Hospital, where all 11 patients with T2 tumors treated by local excision and adjuvant chemoradiation have maintained local control [27]. The only prospective data comes from the CALGB 8984 trial, which enrolled 51 T2 patients treated with transanal excision followed by postoperative chemoradiation (54 Gy in 30 fractions with concurrent 5-FU). The 10-year actuarial local recurrence was 18%, with a 10-year overall survival (OS) of 66% [28]. Although postoperative chemoradiation may benefit some patients with

Table 24.2 Summary of published series of wide local excision and postoperative radiotherapy.

Institution/Reference	No. of patients	Follow-up (months)	Local control (%)	Sphincter preservation (%)	Successful salvage rates with APR
Massachusetts General Hospital [21]	47	51	90	NA	56
Memorial Sloan Kettering [22]	39	41	73	87	62.5
M.D. Anderson [25]	46	36	92	NA	NA
Fox Chase [20]	21	56	91	NA	75
University of Florida [144]	67	65	86	85	80

NA, not available.

high-risk T1 or T2 tumors, the predominant site of disease failure is still local despite the addition of radiation therapy. To date, however, there are no published randomized studies comparing this approach to radical surgical resection with respect to local control and long term outcomes. Thus, whether these outcomes are comparable to those reported for radical surgery remains controversial.

For patients with tumors invading the perirectal fat (T3), radical surgical resection is recommended because of the risk of tumor cut-through and inadequate lymph node removal by local excision procedures. The experience of local excision with postoperative chemoradiation is limited, and the available data suggest higher local failure rates. Three of the 15 patients (20%) with T3 tumors from M.D. Anderson experienced local failure following local excision and postoperative chemoradiation [26]. In a study from Massachusetts General Hospital, three of four patients (75%) with T3 tumors developed local recurrence after local excision and postoperative irradiation [27]. Unless there is a medical contraindication or patient refusal, for all patients with T3 tumors, it is strongly advised that radical resection be undertaken.

Currently, very few published data are available regarding the effectiveness of preoperative radiotherapy with or without adjuvant chemotherapy followed by wide local excision for patients who desire sphincter-preservation. To minimize the risk of local recurrence, both accurate preoperative radiographic assessment to optimally select for patients with adequate tumor down-staging and thorough intraoperative resection margins to confirm successful resection of the lesion is required. Due to difficulties in selecting appropriate candidates for wide local excision alone after preoperative therapy, most of the published series with preoperative radiotherapy limit the use of wide local excision to highly selected patients, including those with clinically T3 tumors that are either medically inoperable or who refuse surgery [29, 30]. A recent study by Schell *et al.* reported that only 15% of patients treated with preoperative chemoradiotherapy that demonstrated significant tumor down-staging went on to receive transanal excision of the primary tumor [29]. In addition to tumor down-staging however, the degree of local tumor invasion and primary tumor size may be predictive of the rate of local recurrence after wide local excision alone [30].

Although some surgeons have recommended local excision alone without lymphadenectomy when preoperative chemoradiotherapy yields significant tumor regression [29, 31, 32], some studies have demonstrated up to a 10% risk of lymph node positivity among patients with complete pathologic response of the primary tumor [33]. Additionally, although current guidelines state that a minimum of 12 lymph nodes should be retrieved for accurate staging [34], treatment with preoperative

chemoradiotherapy may decrease the number of retrievable lymph nodes [35]. As a result, definitive surgical resection with TME with thorough lymph node dissections is still recommended as standard treatment, regardless of treatment response.

Recently, a prospective study of 70 patients with T2N0 low-grade, rectal tumors (<6 cm from anal verge, <3 cm in size) treated with preoperative chemoradiotherapy randomized patients to TEM or TME. With a median follow-up of 84 months, the authors reported low rates of local failure after both TEM (5.7%) and TME (2.8%) [36]. However, this study is limited due to the small number of patients, leading to the potential for unbalanced patient and tumor characteristics in the two surgical arms. Additionally, a prospective Phase II clinical trial sponsored by the American College of Surgeons Oncology Group (ACOSOG Z6041) enrolled 90 patients with T2 rectal cancer defined by pretreatment EUS or pelvic MRI. All patients were treated with neoadjuvant radiation, capecitabine, and oxaliplatin followed by wide local excision. The preliminary results revealed that 81% of patients completed the course of neoadjuvant chemoradiation, with a complete pathologic complete response rate in 44% [37]. Future prospective studies may help to elucidate clinical prognostic factors that select for patients at minimal risk of local failure after wide local excision. Additionally, larger, multi-institutional randomized studies should be performed to assess the role of TEM in the treatment of T2N0 patients.

An alternative, non-standard approach for the treatment of early rectal cancers is intracavitary radiation therapy. First described by Papillon, contact x-ray therapy and interstitial brachytherapy have been described as potentially curative, non-surgical treatment techniques. In a review of 312 cases, Papillon reported a five-year local failure rate of 4.5% [37a]. More recently, high-dose rate brachytherapy has been evaluated as a potential non-surgical treatment technique, but at the present time this approach should be considered investigational.

Summary

Local excision and postoperative chemoradiation appear to offer the potential for satisfactory local control and survival but, importantly, sphincter preservation for selected patients with distal rectal cancer. For patients with favorable histology T1 rectal cancer, local excision alone may suffice. To date, however, there are no published randomized studies comparing this approach to radical surgical resection with respect to local control and long-term outcomes. Although postoperative chemoradiation may benefit some patients with high-risk T1 or T2 tumors, the predominant site of disease failure is still local despite the addition of radiation therapy. Thus, whether these outcomes are comparable to those reported for radical surgery remains controversial. At the present time, wide local excision should only be performed as part of a clinical trial, or if the patient is medically unfit or refuses definitive surgical resection.

Although postoperative chemoradiation may benefit some patients with high-risk T1 or T2 tumors, to date there are no published randomized studies comparing this approach to radical surgical resection. Because of the predominance of local failure among patients with high-risk T1 or T2, despite the addition of radiation therapy, radical resection is favored at Massachusetts General Hospital. However, for patients who refuse radical resection, postoperative irradiation and chemotherapy should be strongly considered following local excision procedures for patients with unfavorable histology T1 or all T2 lesions. The data for T3 tumors with this approach is limited; however, results from single-institution studies suggest unacceptably high local failure rates. Radical resection is strongly advised.

Mobile Rectal Cancers

The role and sequencing of radiation therapy in the management of mobile T3-4, or node-positive tumors has gradually evolved over the past few decades. Although surgery remains the mainstay of curative therapy for rectal cancer, the addition of radiation therapy has been shown to decrease the risk of locoregional recurrence, an event which can be associated with significant morbidity and decreased quality of life [38–40]. Numerous randomized controlled trials have been successfully completed and have addressed multiple different issues with respect to radiation therapy, including: (i) the optimal sequencing of radiation therapy, with comparison of preoperative versus postoperative radiation therapy; (ii) the optimal fractionation scheme for radiation therapy, with comparison of short-course preoperative radiation therapy to standard fractionation preoperative radiation therapy; and (iii) the potential role of chemotherapy given in combination with radiation therapy. A thorough overview of the published literature that has established radiation therapy as the standard of care as it exists today is provided in the flowing sections.

Postoperative Radiotherapy for Mobile Rectal Cancer

Prior to 1990, locally advanced rectal cancer in the US was treated with surgery with or without the addition of adjuvant radiation therapy depending on pathologic tumor characteristics, based on a heterogeneous series of non-randomized published reports [41–43]. As a result, in 1977, the National Surgical Adjuvant Breast and Bowel Project (NSABP) launched the NSABP R-01 trial to define the role of postoperative adjuvant chemotherapy and radiation for locally advanced rectal cancer. In total, 555 patients with stage II or III rectal cancer were randomized to receive either no further therapy, postoperative adjuvant chemotherapy with a combination of semustine, vincristine, and 5-FU, or postoperative radiation therapy. With a mean follow-up of 64 months, treatment with postoperative radiation therapy was associated with lower rates of local recurrence (LRR) (five-year 24.5% versus 16.3%, p = 0.06), without a significant improvement in disease-free survival (DFS) or overall survival (OS), compared to surgery alone [44]. In contrast, postoperative chemotherapy conferred an improvement in DFS (five-year 42% versus 30%, p = 0.006) and OS (five-year 53% versus 43%, p = 0.05), compared to surgery alone.

While NSABP R-01 explored the benefit for postoperative chemotherapy and postoperative radiation therapy alone, several other prospective randomized trials sought to evaluate the potential benefit of postoperative concurrent chemoradiation over chemotherapy or radiation therapy alone. One of the earliest studies to evaluate the role of combined postoperative chemoradiotherapy was the Gastrointestinal Study Group (GITSG) Protocol 7175, which randomly assigned 227 patients with stage II/III rectal cancer to one of four treatment arms after surgical resection: (i) no further therapy; (ii) chemotherapy alone with bolus 5-FU and methyl-CCNU; (iii) postoperative radiation therapy alone; or (iv) chemoradiation with concurrent 5-FU followed by adjuvant 5-FU/methyl-CCNU. With an initial target accrual of 520 patients, the study was terminated early due to a significant benefit seen for patients treated with concurrent chemoradiation. With a median follow-up of 80 months, postoperative chemoradiation decreased rates of recurrence compared to surgery alone (33% versus 55%, p <0.009). There was a trend towards improved OS at seven years with chemoradiation compared to surgery alone (56% versus 36%, p <0.07), which with longer follow-up has become significant. The benefit of chemoradiation was attributed both to radiation therapy reducing rates of local failures (16% versus 25%, p = 0.06) and chemotherapy reducing rates of distant metastases (20% versus 30%, p = 0.06). Thus, GITSG 71-75 demonstrated an OS benefit among patients receiving postoperative chemoradiation. This study, however, has been criticized for being underpowered to detect a significant benefit among patients treated with either radiation or chemotherapy alone, and for unequal randomization between the treatment arms [40].

The North Central Cancer Treatment Group (NCCTG) 79-47-51 study also sought to establish the additional benefit of concurrent postoperative chemoradiation. This study randomized 204 patients with T3–4 or node-positive rectal cancer to either:

(i) adjuvant radiation therapy alone (50.4 Gy); or (ii) concurrent chemoradiation with bolus 5-FU followed by adjuvant 5-FU/semustine (methyl-CCNU). With a median follow-up of seven years, combined postoperative chemoradiation demonstrated a significant 34% relative reduction in disease recurrence at five years (p = 0.002), a 36% relative reduction in cancer-related death (p = 0.07), and a 29% relative reduction in the risk of overall death (p = 0.025) compared to postoperative radiation therapy alone [45]. On the basis of the results from NCCTG 79-47-51 and GITSG 7175, in 1990 the consensus statement by the US National Institutes for Health recommended postoperative chemoradiotherapy as the standard treatment for all patients with completely resected stage II or III rectal cancer [40, 45, 46].

Although GITSG 7175 demonstrated that postoperative concurrent chemoradiation improved OS compared to surgery alone, and NCCTG 79-47-51 demonstrated superiority of concurrent chemoradiation over radiation therapy alone, neither study was designed to assess the additional benefit of radiation therapy to chemotherapy alone. Therefore, in order to further address the role of the combined modality therapy over chemotherapy alone, from 1987 to 1992, the NSABP R-02 study randomized 694 patients with Duke's B or C rectal carcinoma to either: (i) postoperative adjuvant chemotherapy alone with a 5-FU-based regimen; or (ii) postoperative chemoradiation with concurrent bolus 5-FU. With a mean follow-up of 93 months, the addition of postoperative radiotherapy failed to improve DFS (p = 0.90) or OS (p = 0.89), but resulted in an improvement in five-year LRRs from 13% to 8% (p = 0.02) compared to chemotherapy alone [47].

The majority of these early chemotherapy regimens included methyl-CCNU, a known risk factor for acute non-lymphocytic leukemia. The estimated risk of delayed acute leukemia in patients receiving multiple doses of methyl-CCNU over 12–18 months is 2.3 cases per 1000 persons per year (14 cases of leukemia in 2067 patients given methyl-CCNU; six-year cumulative risk of developing leukemia is 4%). Importantly, two subsequent postoperative trials from the GITSG and NCCTG have shown that methyl-CCNU does not produce an additive benefit to irradiation plus 5-FU [48, 49]. Thus, methyl-CCNU is no longer utilized in the adjuvant chemotherapy regimens in colorectal cancer.

All of the published prospective, randomized trials to date evaluating treatment with postoperative radiation therapy for locally advanced rectal cancer are summarized in Table 24.3. In summary, only postoperative chemotherapy alone [44] and postoperative chemoradiotherapy [40] have both been demonstrated to improve OS compared to surgery alone. Postoperative radiation therapy appears to decrease the risk of local recurrence compared to surgery alone [44] or

postoperative chemotherapy alone [40, 47], without a significant impact on DFS or OS [40, 44, 45, 47]. Despite this, a reduction in local recurrence is considered by many to be a meaningful endpoint, as the development of locoregional recurrence can often be associated with significant morbidity and decrement of quality of life.

Although the 1990 US National Institutes for Health consensus statement recommended postoperative chemoradiation for all patients with pathologic T3 and above or node-positive disease [46], several retrospective studies have attempted to identify subsets of patients in whom postoperative therapy could be excluded. Several single-institution retrospective series have suggested that subsets of patients with pT3N0 disease may not require adjuvant radiation therapy [50, 51]. Moreover, a recent pooled analysis of five Phase III cooperative group studies found that patients with pT1-2N1 and pT3N0 disease may have an 'intermediate' risk of recurrence with five-year LRRs of 7% and 9%, respectively [52]. Among these 'intermediate'-risk patients, five-year OS rates were similar when comparing adjuvant chemotherapy alone to tri-modality combinations, suggesting perhaps that tri-modality postoperative chemoradiation may not be necessary for all patients with T1-2N1 and T3N0 lesions. However, the pooled analysis also found that for patients with T3N0 lesions treated without radiation therapy, the rate of DFS was 69%, with a five-year actuarial rate of local recurrence of 11%. Based on these findings, and in conjunction with significant patient and treatment heterogeneity seen across the different trials included in the analysis, it is difficult to draw any definitive conclusions regarding in which patient subsets radiation can safely excluded [52]. Currently, postoperative radiation therapy is generally recommended for all patients found with pathologic T3–T4 and node-positive disease. Future prospective and retrospective studies will hopefully further aid in the identification of patient subsets at minimal risk of local recurrence, in whom adjuvant radiation therapy can be safely avoided.

Preoperative Radiotherapy for Locally Advanced Rectal Cancer

Over the past decade, preoperative therapy either with radiation alone or combined modality therapy has slowly gained acceptance as the standard of care. Several distinct advantages of preoperative radiotherapy have emerged in comparison to postoperative radiotherapy. Proponents of preoperative radiotherapy argue that it allows for clearer tumor definition, potential tumor down-staging, increased resectability rates, improvement in sphincter preservation rates, decreased operative tumor seeding, less normal tissue irradiation

Table 24.3 Summary of Phase III data of postoperative radiotherapy.

Trial/ Reference	No. of patients	Stage	Study arms	RT Dose/fx	Chemo	5-year local failure (%)	p-value	5-year DFS (%)	p-value	5-year OS (%)	p-value
\multicolumn{12}{c}{**Postoperative Radiotherapy versus Surgery Alone**}
GITSG 7175 [40]	227	II/III	Surgery	N	N	24	NA	34	<0.01	36	0.07
			Post-op. C	N	5-FU/ Semustine	27		30		46	
			Post-op. RT	40–48 Gy	N	20		27		44	
			Post-op. CRT	40–44 Gy	Bolus 5-FU/Semustine	11		26		56	
NSABP R-01 [44]	555	II/III	Surgery	N	N	25§	0.06*	~30	0.4*	~43	0.7*
			Post-op. RT	46.8 Gy/26 fx	N	16§		~33		~42	
			Post-op. C	N	MOF	22§	NS	~42	<0.01*	~53	0.05*
NSABP R-02 [47]	694	II/III	Post-op. C	N	MOF or 5FU/LV	8 (5)	0.02	~55	0.90	~65	0.89
			Post-op. CRT	50.4 Gy/28 fx	Bolus 5-FU	13 (5)		~55		~65	
NCCTG 794751 [45]	204	II/III	Post-op. RT	45–50.4 Gy	N	25	0.04	37	0.002	48	0.03
			Post-op. CRT	45–50.4 Gy	Bolus 5-FU	13		59		58	

N, not applicable; NA, not available.
C, Chemotherapy; RT, Radiation therapy; CRT, Chemoradiotherapy; MOF, 5-FU, Semustine, Vincristine; LV, Leukovorin.
DFS, disease-free survival; OS, overall survival.
§Crude rates; *Compared to surgery alone; ~Estimated from Kaplan-Meier curve.

leading to lower long-term treatment-related toxicity, and the ability to test the efficacy of novel systemic agents and radiation.

However, there are several disadvantages of preoperative radiotherapy. A major disadvantage of preoperative chemoradiotherapy is the potential risk of overtreatment among patients with early-stage, node-negative or undetected metastatic disease in whom radiation therapy may not indicated. Preoperative chemoradiotherapy results in significant nodal down-staging, and patients with initially positive nodes may develop a pathological complete response within the lymph nodes. Due to difficulties in discerning patients with upfront node-negative disease from patients with upfront node-positive

disease that converted to pathologic node negative status after preoperative chemoradiotherapy, all patients treated with preoperative chemoradiotherapy are usually committed to four to six months of adjuvant chemotherapy. A recent study which used CT and transrectal ultrasound to clinically stage patients preoperatively found that 18% of patients were overstaged, and thus would receive preoperative therapy unnecessarily [53]. Additionally, preoperative chemoradiotherapy may increase surgical morbidity and confer loss of prognostic information of nodal involvement at initial presentation. The advantages and disadvantages of postoperative versus preoperative radiotherapy are summarized in Table 24.4.

Table 24.4 Theoretical advantages of preoperative versus postoperative radiotherapy (RT).

	Advantages of preoperative RT	Advantages of postoperative RT
Tumor definition	Improved	Worse
Volume of normal tissue irradiated	Less	More
Tumor/nodal down-staging	Potentially Yes	No
Surgical resectability	Improved	Unchanged
Sphincter preservation	Improved	Unchanged
Ability to test novel agents	Better	Worse
Potential to overtreat patients	Yes	No
Have prognostic nodal information	No	Yes
Dependent on radiographic staging	Yes	No

Due to the numerous potential advantages of preoperative radiotherapy, several large multi-institutional studies have sought to determine if there is a role for preoperative radiation therapy in the treatment of rectal cancer. A summary of the results of prospective randomized trials evaluating the role of preoperative radiotherapy is provided in Table 24.5. Within these studies, two predominant radiation fractionation schemes have emerged, including a standard fractionation radiotherapy

course typically consisting of 45–50.4 Gy in 25–28 fractions typically given with concurrent chemotherapy [53, 54], and a hypofractionated 'short' preoperative radiotherapy course consisting of 25 Gy in five fractions [38, 54–56] given without chemotherapy. To date, two prospective randomized controlled studies have compared these two regimens with respect to rates of sphincter preservation and local control [54, 57]. Additionally, two recently published randomized,

Table 24.5 Summary of Phase III data of preoperative radiotherapy.

Trial/ Reference	No. of patients	Stage	Study arms	RT dose/Fx	Chemo with RT?	5-year local failure (%)	p-value	5-year DFS (%)	p-value	5-year OS (%)	p-value
\multicolumn{12}{c}{**Preoperative Short-Course Radiotherapy versus Surgery Alone**}
Swedish* Trial [38]	1168	Resectable	Surgery			26	<0.01	NA	NA	30	0.008
			Pre-op. RT	25 Gy/5 fx	N	9		NA		38	
Dutch CKVO Trial [39]	1861	Resectable	Surgery			10.9	<0.01	NA	NA	63.5	0.90
			Pre-op. RT	25 Gy/5fx	N	5.6		NA		64.2	
Stockholm I [145]§	849	Resectable	Surgery			28	<0.01	72	NS	69	NS
			Preop. RT	25 Gy/5fx	N	14		70		70	
\multicolumn{12}{c}{**Preoperative Standard Fractionation Radiotherapy versus Preoperative Chemoradiotherapy**}
FFCD 9203 [65]	733	T3-4	Pre-op. RT	45 Gy/25 fx	N	16.5	<0.05	55.5	NA	67.9	0.68
			Pre-op. CRT	45 Gy/25 fx	Bolus 5-FU	8.1		59.4		67.4	
EORTC 22921 [69]	1011	T3-4	Pre-op. RT	45 Gy/25 fx		17.1	<0.01	54.4	0.52	64.8	0.43
			Pre-op. RT S→CT	45 Gy/25 fx		9.6					
			Pre-op. CRT	45 Gy/25 fx	Bolus 5-FU	8.7		56.1		65.8	
			Pre-op. CRT→S→CT	45 Gy/25 fx	Bolus 5-FU	7.6					
\multicolumn{12}{c}{**Preoperative Standard Chemoradiotherapy versus Postoperative Standard Chemoradiotherapy**}
Uppsala Trial [78]	471	Resectable	Pre-op. RT	25.5 Gy/5 fx	N	14.3	0.02	NA	NA	NA	0.42
			Post-op. RT	60 Gy/30 fx	N	26.8		NA		NA	
German Rectal Trial [53]	823	cT3-4, N+	Pre-op. CRT	50.4 Gy/28 fx	CI 5-FU	6	0.006	68	0.32	76	0.80
			Post-op. CRT	55.8 Gy/31 fx	CI 5-FU	13		65		74	
NSABP R-03 [58]	267	cT3-4, N+	Pre-op. CRT	50.4 Gy/28 fx	CI 5-FU	10.7	0.69	64.7	0.01	74.5	0.065
			Post-op. CRT	50.4 Gy/28 fx	CI 5-FU	10.7		53.4		65.6	

*13 year follow-up; §Crude rates with median follow-up of 107 months.
Other abbreviations as Table 24.3

Phase III studies in the era of TME have compared the efficacy of preoperative versus postoperative chemoradiotherapy with respect to local control and DFS, and have established preoperative chemoradiotherapy as the current standard of care [53, 58]. Moreover, a recent meta-analysis of 14 randomized controlled trials comparing preoperative radiotherapy plus surgery with surgery alone found an improvement in five-year overall mortality rate (OR 0.84, p = 0.03), cancer-related mortality rate (OR 0.71, p <0.001), and LRR (OR 0.49, p <0.001), without any observed reduction in rate of distant metastases (OR 0.93, p = 0.54) [59]. The major randomized Phase III studies that have defined the integral role of preoperative radiation therapy as it exists today in the management of locally advanced rectal cancer are reviewed in the following section.

Preoperative Standard Fractionation Radiotherapy and the Role of Chemotherapy

During the early 1990s, although postoperative adjuvant chemoradiation was the recommended standard of care in the US [46], many European countries sought to examine the potential role for preoperative radiation with or without chemotherapy in the treatment of locally advanced, resectable tumors [60,61]. Concurrent chemoradiotherapy had proven to improve outcomes in other disease sites [62–64], and thus several European cooperative groups launched randomized controlled trials to evaluate whether there was a potential additional benefit of concurrent chemotherapy in the setting of locally advanced rectal cancer.

In 1993, the Federation Francophone de Cancerologie Digestive (FFCD) 9203 randomized 733 patients with palpable T3/T4 tumors of the mid to lower rectum to receive 45 Gy preoperative radiotherapy given alone or in conjunction with 5-FU 350 mg m^{-2} for five days with leukovorin 20 mg m^{-2} during the first and fifth weeks, with all patients receiving an additional four cycles of adjuvant chemotherapy with the same regimen [65]. TME within 3–10 weeks was recommended, although no specific training or monitoring of this type of surgery was performed. With overall survival as the primary study endpoint and a median follow-up of 81 months, no significant difference in five-year OS was seen between the two groups. However, the five-year incidence of local recurrence was significantly lower with preoperative chemoradiotherapy compared to preoperative radiation alone (8.1% versus 16.5%, p <0.05), with a relative risk of local recurrence of 0.5 (95% CI, 0.31–0.80) in patients treated with chemoradiotherapy.

In an unplanned post-randomization subgroup analysis, chemoradiotherapy was found to offer a significant local control benefit, even amongst patients treated in more recent years, which was felt to be a surrogate for treatment with TME surgery.

The complete pathologic rate was also significantly higher in patients treated with chemoradiotherapy (11.4% versus 3.6%, p <0.05), although there was no difference in sphincter preservation rates. As expected, grade 3 or 4 toxicity was more frequent in patients treated with chemoradiotherapy (14.6% versus 2.7%, p <0.05). Thus, the authors concluded that despite a moderate increase in acute toxicity and no impact on OS, preoperative chemoradiotherapy improved local control and therefore should be considered for all patients with locally advanced rectal cancer. Although this study was limited by a suboptimal chemotherapy regimen with delivery of bolus 5-FU [66, 67], a lack of surgical standardization with TME surgery [68], and a lack of standardization for pathologic analysis of the surgical specimen, the findings helped cement the role of concurrent chemotherapy for preoperative radiation therapy.

Similar to the FFCD 9203 study, the European Organization for Research and Treatment of Cancer (EORTC) Radiotherapy Group initiated a study to determine the addition of chemotherapy to preoperative radiotherapy and the use of postoperative chemotherapy in the treatment of rectal cancer [69]. In total, EORTC 22921 randomized 1011 patients with resectable T3 or T4N0 rectal cancer by 2 × 2 randomization to receive either: (i) preoperative radiotherapy alone; (ii) preoperative chemoradiotherapy alone; (iii) preoperative radiotherapy and postoperative chemotherapy; or (iv) preoperative chemoradiotherapy and postoperative chemotherapy. Radiation therapy consisted of 45 Gy in 25 fractions, and chemotherapy included two, five-day preoperative courses of bolus 5-FU and leucovorin (5FU 350 mg m^{-2} per day; leukovorin 20 mg m^{-2} per day) during the first and fifth weeks of radiotherapy, and four additional courses of the same regimen given postoperatively. With respect to surgical technique, after 1999 all patients were recommended to undergo TME [69].

With a primary study endpoint of OS, at a median follow-up of 5.4 years, there was no significant difference in OS between the groups that received chemotherapy preoperatively or postoperatively (p = 0.12). However, patients that received chemotherapy either preoperatively or postoperatively were found with significantly lower rates of local recurrence compared to those who did not receive chemotherapy (p = 0.002). Specifically, the five-year cumulative incidence rates of local recurrence were 8.7%, 9.6%, and 7.6% respectively for patients treated with chemotherapy preoperatively, postoperatively, or both, compared to 17.1% among patients treated with radiotherapy alone. The rate of

17.1% local failure in patients treated with preoperative radiotherapy alone is much higher than that in other studies, and is mostly likely inadequate surgical resection with only 35% of patients undergoing TME [69]. Interestingly, the cumulative incidence of distant metastases did not differ significantly according to the preoperative or the postoperative treatment (p = 0.14, p = 0.62, respectively). A subsequent exploratory subset analysis suggested that only patients with ypT0-2 (pathologic stage after neoadjuvant therapy) seemed to benefit from adjuvant chemotherapy (p = 0.011) with respect to improved DFS and OS. Additionally, no difference was seen in rates of sphincter preservation (50.5% versus 52.8%, p = 0.47). However, patients treated with preoperative chemoradiotherapy had less advanced pathological tumor staging, less advanced pathological nodal staging, fewer examined nodes, and less-frequent lymphatic, venous, and perineural invasion compared to patients treated with preoperative radiotherapy alone [69].

Therefore, similar to the findings of FFCD 9203, this study also showed that the addition of chemotherapy to preoperative radiation therapy yielded no improvement in overall survival, but improved tumor down-staging and local control compared to preoperative radiation therapy alone [65]. The results of the study also suggested that chemotherapy administered at any time, conferred a significant benefit with respect to local control, but not distant metastases.

Moreover, a recent meta-analysis of four randomized trials evaluating the benefit of concurrent chemotherapy in addition to neoadjuvant radiotherapy found that preoperative chemotherapy increased the likelihood of a complete pathologic response (95% CI associated with OR, 2.52–5.27, p <0.001) and improved local control (95% CI associated with OR 0.39–0.72, p <0.001), without a significant impact on sphincter preservation (95% CI associated with OR 0.92–1.31, p = 0.29), DFS (95% CI associated with OR 0.92–1.34, P = 0.27) or OS (95% CI associated with OR 0.79–1.14, P = 0.58). Not surprisingly, the addition of preoperative chemoradiotherapy was associated with an increased risk of grade 3 or 4 toxicity (95% CI associated with OR 1.68–10, p-0.002), without a difference observed on postoperative morbidity or mortality [70].

A major issue at present in the adjuvant therapy of rectal cancer is how to optimize the proven combination of radiation and 5-FU. If there is a combined modality effect of radiation therapy and 5-FU, it is logical to try to use both modalities optimally. Both, the use of the 5-FU as a long-term continuous infusion (225 mg m^{-2} per day) and 5-FU combined with leucovorin have been shown to produce higher response rates in patients with metastatic disease than the use of conventional bolus 5-FU. The GI Intergroup has run a study testing the value of continuous-infusion 5-FU given with radiation therapy compared with bolus 5-FU during radiation therapy [49]. Both groups of patients also received pre- and post-irradiation 5-FU. The results showed a reduction in distant metastases with improved relapse-free and OS for patients treated with continuous infusion.

In summary, in contrast to postoperative chemotherapy, which has been demonstrated to improve overall survival [44], no studies have yet demonstrated that chemotherapy improves survival in the setting of preoperative radiation therapy. As a result, the recommendation for preoperative chemotherapy remains an extrapolation from the studies from postoperative radiation therapy [40, 44] and the German Rectal Study (see below) [53], which includes outback chemotherapy.

Preoperative versus Postoperative Standard Fractionation Chemoradiotherapy

To date, three randomized, controlled trials of standard fractionation preoperative versus postoperative chemoradiotherapy have been performed for clinically resectable rectal cancer. All studies enrolled patients with T3–4 disease, and treated with conventional doses and techniques of radiation therapy combined with 5-FU-based chemotherapy, and required surgeons to perform preoperative clinical assessments and to declare the type of operation required. Unfortunately, the two studies performed in the US (RTOG 9401/INT 0147, NSABP R-03) were closed due to poor target accrual. Details of the German Rectal Study (CAO/ARO/AIO 94) and the NSABP R-03 have both been recently published, and available results of these studies are reviewed below.

Between 1995 and 2002, the German Rectal Cancer Study Group enrolled 823 patients on a Phase III trial (CAO/ARO/AIO-94 trial) comparing conventionally fractionated preoperative radiotherapy given with concurrent 5-FU chemotherapy ($n = 421$) with the same treatment given postoperatively ($n = 402$) in patients with clinically staged T3/T4 or node-positive rectal cancer. All patients received underwent EUS to determine T/N stage, and CT of the abdomen/pelvis to evaluate for distant metastases. Preoperative radiotherapy was prescribed to the primary tumor and pelvic lymph nodes, with a total of 50.4 Gy delivered over 28 days, while postoperative radiotherapy included an additional boost of 5.4 Gy. Concurrent continuous-infusion 5-FU was given over five days at a dose of 1000 mg m^{-2} per day during the first and fifth weeks of radiotherapy, and all patients received an four additional cycles of adjuvant 5-FU (500 mg m^{-2} per day) were given. Prior to randomization, surgeons reported whether sphincter-preservation was possible, and all patients underwent TME. Surgery was performed within six weeks after the completion of chemoradiation [53].

After a median follow-up of 134 months, patients treated with preoperative chemoradiation had a decreased 10-year cumulative incidence of pelvic relapse compared to those in the postoperative treatment group (10-year local failure (LF) 7.1% versus 10.1%, p = 0.048). Despite the improvement in local relapse, there was no significant difference with respect to DFS (10-year 68.1% versus 67.8%, p = 0.65) or OS (5-year 59.6% versus 59.9%, p = 0.85) between the two groups. Additionally, preoperative radiotherapy was significantly associated with tumor down-staging (p <0.001), yielding an 8% pathologic complete response rate and a 15% absolute reduction in lymph node involvement (25% versus 40%).

Among 194 patients for which abdominoperineal resection (APR) was deemed necessary by surgeons at presentation, those who received preoperative chemoradiation were twice as likely to undergo sphincter-preserving surgery (39% versus 19%). However, the absolute rate of APR in the two cohorts was not significantly different. With respect to postoperative morbidity, there was no significant difference in postoperative mortality, postoperative complication rates, or anastomotic leak rates. However, patients treated preoperatively had lower rates of acute Grade 3/4 toxicities (27% versus 40%, p = 0.001) and chronic Grade 3/4 toxicities (14% versus 24%, p = 0.01), especially with respect to acute and chronic diarrhea and development of anastomotic strictures.

Given the improvements in local failure and sphincter-preservation rates, and the decrease in acute and late toxicity, this study demonstrated the superiority of preoperative chemoradiotherapy over postoperative chemoradiotherapy for patients with clinical T3 or greater or node-positive rectal cancer. Of note, 18% of patients randomized to receive postoperative chemoradiotherapy were found with pathologic stage I disease at the time of surgery; these represented the patients that would be overtreated in the era of standard preoperative chemoradiation. Although improvements in pretreatment assessment of tumor and nodal staging may help to decrease these overtreatment rates, at present, neither MRI of the pelvis, CT of the abdomen/pelvis, or transrectal ultrasound can accurately identify patients with node-positive disease [71].

While the German Rectal Study was accruing in Europe, the NSABP R-03 study was launched in the US [58]. The study sought to compare preoperative versus postoperative chemoradiotherapy with the primary study endpoints of DFS and OS. Although the study initially targeted an enrollment of 900 patients, it was closed early due to poor patient accrual. Between 1993 and 1999, a total of 256 patients with T3/T4 or node-positive rectal cancer were randomly assigned to receive either preoperative chemoradiotherapy ($n = 123$) or postoperative chemoradiotherapy ($n = 131$). Patients randomized to the neoadjuvant treatment arm received one cycle of chemotherapy consisting of 5-FU (500 mg m^{-2} weekly for six weeks) and leucovorin, followed by chemoradiotherapy with concurrent 5-FU 325 mg m^{-2} for five days and leucovorin. The pelvis received 45 Gy in 25 fractions to isocenter with a four-field box technique, followed by a 5.4 Gy boost to a restricted volume. Patients randomized to the postoperative treatment arm received the same regimen, and all received an additional four cycles of adjuvant 5-FU-based chemotherapy.

With a median follow-up of 8.4 years, patients treated with preoperative compared to postoperative chemoradiotherapy demonstrated an improved five-year DFS (64.7% versus 53.4%, p = 0.011), and a trend towards improved five-year OS (74.5% versus 65.6%, p = 0.065). Some 15% of patients treated with preoperative chemoradiotherapy had pathologic-complete responses, and none of these patients has subsequently developed local recurrences. Preoperative chemoradiation was also significantly associated with lower rates of pathologic lymph node involvement (pN0: 66.7% versus 52.5%, p = 0.04) due to nodal down-staging.

Interestingly, however, in contrast to the results of the German Rectal Cancer Study, there was also no difference with respect to locoregional recurrence between the two treatment arms (10.7% versus 10.7%, p = 0.69) or rates of sphincter preservation (47.8% versus 39.2%, p = 0.227) [53, 58]. Thus, the authors concluded that preoperative chemoradiation, compared to postoperative chemoradiation, significantly improved DFS with a trend towards improved OS. One of the main limitations of this study was the small number of patients, which limited the statistical power to detect differences between treatment arms with respect to locoregional recurrence. Additionally, not all patients in NSABP R-03 underwent TME, which is now considered the surgical standard of care for locally advanced rectal cancers.

A recent collaborative meta-analysis of 22 randomized trials including 8507 patients evaluated the efficacy of preoperative radiotherapy and postoperative radiotherapy compared to surgery alone. Consistent with results seen in the individual randomized controlled trials, radiation therapy was not associated with a significant improvement in OS. However, the yearly risk of local recurrence was significantly reduced by 46% with preoperative radiotherapy (p = 0.0001), and significantly reduced by 37% with postoperative radiotherapy (p = 0.002) [72]. Consistent with the studies discussed above, the largest reductions for local recurrence were found in studies of preoperative radiotherapy when biologically effective doses of 30 Gy or more were prescribed.

In summary, preoperative chemoradiation has been shown to yield lower rates of local failure, decreased acute and late treatment-related toxicity, higher rates of sphincter preservation, and improved DFS compared to postoperative chemoradiation [53, 58]. As a result, the current standard of care for locally advanced rectal cancer is treatment with preoperative chemoradiation to 45–50.4 Gy over five to six weeks given concurrently with continuous-infusion 5-FU, with TME performed at four to seven weeks after completion of neoadjuvant therapy, followed by an additional four months of postoperative 5-FU-based chemotherapy.

Preoperative Short-Course Radiotherapy

To date, several large randomized studies have investigated the long-term efficacy of preoperative short-course radiotherapy and demonstrated a reduction of local recurrence compared to surgery alone [38,39]. The Swedish Rectal Cancer Trial was the one of the first randomized studies to evaluate the efficacy of this fractionation schema, which randomized 908 with stage I–III patients between 1987 and 1990 to curative surgery alone ($n = 454$) or preoperative radiotherapy (25 Gy in five fractions; $n = 454$) followed by curative surgery within one week of completion of radiation [55]. With a median follow-up of 13 years, compared to surgery alone, preoperative radiotherapy significantly decreased rates of local recurrence (9% versus 26%, p <0.001) and increased rates of cancer-specific survival (72% versus 62%, p = 0.03) and OS (38% versus 30%, p = 0.008) [38]. However, there were no significant differences with respect to rates of distant failure between the irradiated and non-irradiated arms. With respect to treatment-related toxicities, although there was an increased risk of hospitalization after preoperative short-course radiotherapy during the initial six months after surgery (RR 1.64, 95% CI 1.21–2.22), there was no difference in hospitalization rates between treatment arms after six months. Among irradiated patients, however, there were increased hospitalization rates for bowel obstruction (RR: 1.88, p = 0.02), abdominal pain (RR 1.92, p = 0.01), and nausea (RR 4.04, p = 0.03) [73]. Generalizability of these results is limited by outdated, non-conformal radiation treatment fields which may have yielded higher rates of postoperative morbidity.

To date, this study is the only one to demonstrate an OS benefit with preoperative radiation therapy, though numerous factors likely contributed to this positive finding. First, the treatment arms were imbalanced with respect to stage, with a higher percentage of stage I randomized to surgery and radiation than to surgery alone. Second, the study was performed in the era before standardization of TME as the oncologic surgical procedure of choice, and thus the reported rates of local recurrence are much higher than those reported in subsequent trials [39,53,58]. As a result, preoperative radiation therapy may have compensated for inadequate oncologic surgery, thus, contributing to the marked reduction in the risk

of local recurrence and potential OS benefit seen after radiotherapy.

With increasing recognition that sharp, precise dissection of the entire mesorectum with TME reduced the risk of local recurrence in the absence of radiotherapy, the Dutch Colorectal Cancer Group performed a prospective, multicenter randomized trial evaluating the role of preoperative short-course radiotherapy in combination with standardized TME. For this, between 1996 and 1999 a total of 861 patients with resectable rectal cancer were randomized to preoperative radiotherapy (5 Gy × five 5 fractions; $n = 924$) followed by TME, or to TME alone ($n = 937$). The trial mandated standardization of techniques and quality control measures to ensure consistency of radiotherapy, surgical, and pathologic techniques [56]. With a median follow-up of six years, there was a significant improvement in local recurrence rates among patients treated with preoperative radiation compared to surgery alone (5-year 5.6% versus 10.9%, p <0.001), with a relative risk reduction of 49%. There was no significant difference in OS (5-year 64.2% versus 63.5%, p = 0.90) or distant metastases (5-year 25.8% versus 28.3%, p = 0.39) [39]. On multivariate analysis, treatment with surgery alone (HR 2.18, p < 0.001), tumors <10 cm from the anal verge (p = 0.03), higher TNM stage (p < 0.001), and the presence of a positive circumferential margin (HR 2.16, p < 0.001) were associated with increased rates of local recurrence [39]. Patients treated with preoperative radiotherapy had slightly increased blood loss (1000 versus 900 ml, p < 0.001) and increased perineal complications (26% versus 18%, p = 0.05) compared to patients treated with TME alone, with no other significant differences with respect to postoperative complications [74]. Thus, even in the setting of TME, the authors concluded that short-term preoperative radiotherapy reduced the risk of local recurrence. However, in contrast to the results of the Swedish trial, there was no significant difference in overall mortality among patients with resectable rectal cancer. Moreover, the low recurrence rate of 10.9% at five years in the surgery-alone arm confirmed the improvement in local control in the era of TME compared to 15–45% rates of local recurrence in studies of conventional, non-standardized surgery [75–77].

Although the Swedish trial [38] and the Dutch trial [39] each revealed that preoperative short-course radiotherapy improved outcomes compared to surgery alone, these studies did not address its efficacy compared to postoperative treatment. Between 1980 and 1985, the Uppsala study randomized 471 patients with resectable rectal cancer to receive either preoperative short-course radiotherapy (25.5 Gy in five fractions) or split-course, standard fractionation, postoperative radiotherapy (60 Gy in 30 fractions) [78]. With a mean follow-up of six years, the preoperative radiotherapy arm was associated with a significantly lower rate of local recurrence (13% versus 21%, p = 0.02), without a significant improvement in OS (43% versus 37%) [78] or treatment-related toxicities [79]. Although this study had numerous limitations, including outdated radiation and surgical techniques and a lack of concurrent chemotherapy in the postoperative treatment arm, the data obtained suggested that preoperative radiation therapy improved outcomes over postoperative radiotherapy.

More recently, the MRC CR07/NCIC-CTG C016 study compared the role of short-course preoperative radiotherapy to selective postoperative standard fractionation chemotherapy. After the findings of improved OS with preoperative short-course radiotherapy in the Swedish study had been published [55], the standard of care in most of the United Kingdom was considered to be preoperative short-course radiotherapy. However, the question of whether selective postoperative chemoradiotherapy would be equivalent to preoperative radiotherapy had not been addressed. The MRC CR07/NCIC-CTG C016 randomized 1350 patients with clinically operative adenocarcinoma of the rectum less than 15 cm from the anal verge to preoperative radiotherapy (25 Gy in five fractions) ($n = 674$) or selective postoperative chemoradiation for positive circumferential margins with standard fractionation chemoradiotherapy to 45 Gy in 28 fractions given concurrently with 5-FU ($n = 676$) [80]. As per the study guidelines, patients with negative circumferential margins were not to receive any postoperative chemoradiotherapy. Adjuvant chemotherapy was based on local institutional policy according to circumferential margin and lymph node status.

In total, 88% patients randomized to the selective postoperative radiotherapy arm had negative circumferential margins, and only 12% ($n = 77$) had positive circumferential margins. With a median follow-up of four years, the five-year local recurrence was significantly improved with preoperative radiotherapy (5% versus 17%, p < 0.001) compared to postoperative radiotherapy. Preoperative radiotherapy offered a relative risk reduction of 61% in local recurrence (HR 0.39, 95% CI 0.27–0.58, p < 0.0001) and a three-year absolute risk reduction of 6.2% (95% CI 5.3–7.1). Additionally, preoperative radiotherapy was found to confer a relative improvement in DFS of 24% (HR 0.76, 95% CI 0.62–0.94, p = 0.013) and an absolute difference at three years of 6.0% (95% CI 5.3–6.8). However, there was no difference in OS between the two groups [80]. Of note, the proportion of patients with pathologically assessed stage III disease was equivalent in both groups, suggesting the lack of significant downstaging effect from preoperative radiotherapy [80].

There were several limitations to this study. Most notably, although 93% of surgeons reported that TME was achieved, there was no formal surgical training of TME at participating centers. Moreover, in contrast to most studies of preoperative or postoperative radiation therapy that include only locally advanced rectal cancer, this study included stage I patients, thereby decreasing the statistical power to detect meaningful differences among higher-risk patients [80]. Lastly, because the study allowed local institutions to decide whether to administer adjuvant chemotherapy, there was significant heterogeneity with respect to administration of adjuvant chemotherapy, making the final results difficult to interpret [80].

Although the efficacy of preoperative short-course radiotherapy has been shown as an effective treatment in reducing the risk of local recurrence, there has been hesitation about adopting this radiation fractionation schema as the standard due to concerns of increased long-term toxicity of high fractional doses. Doses higher than the standard 1.8–2.0 Gy per fraction, such as 5.0 Gy per fraction administered in preoperative 'short'-course radiotherapy, may lower the therapeutic ratio, particularly with respect to late normal tissue complications. Additionally, preoperative short-course radiation treatment not been shown to result in tumor down-staging, which may explain why short-term preoperative radiotherapy has not been found to improve sphincter preservation. For this reason, preoperative short-course radiotherapy has not been routinely recommended for patients with locally advanced rectal cancer with the goal of sphincter preservation. However, for older patients or patients with significant medical comorbidities that have limited life expectancies, in which long-term treatment-related toxicities are of less concern, preoperative short-course radiotherapy offers the benefit of a shortened treatment course and should be considered.

Preoperative Short-Course Radiotherapy versus Preoperative Standard Fractionation Chemoradiotherapy

To date, there are two published Phase III randomized controlled trial that have sought to compare preoperative short-course radiotherapy with preoperative conventionally fractionated chemoradiation [54]. The Polish rectal study accrued 316 patients between 1999 and 2002, and randomized patients to receive either preoperative radiotherapy to 25 Gy in five fractions, or preoperative radiotherapy to 50.4 Gy in 28 fractions with concurrent 5-FU and leucovorin followed by surgery four to six weeks later. In contrast to other rectal cancer studies [53, 58], the primary endpoint of this study was the rate of sphincter preservation; therefore, surgeons were recommended to make a decision on the type of surgical resection based on tumor status after completion of preoperative therapy. Preoperative standard fractionation chemoradiotherapy resulted in significantly higher rates of clinical complete response rates (13% versus 2%, p < 0.001) and pathologic complete response rates (16% versus 1%, p < 0.001), with lower rates of positive circumferential margins (4% versus 13%, p = 0.017). Additionally, tumor size on average was 1.9 cm smaller among patients treated with preoperative chemoradiotherapy (p < 0.001). However, despite significantly higher tumor down-staging with standard fractionation preoperative chemoradiation, there was no difference in rates of sphincter preservation (61% versus 58%, respectively, p = 0.57).

The Polish study has been heavily criticized due to the subjectivity in surgeons' decisions regarding sphincter preservation and reliance on pre-treatment tumor volumes. This criticism is highlighted by the fact that 28% of patients (5/18) underwent APR despite achieving a clinically complete response after preoperative chemoradiotherapy. The study has also been criticized for a lack of standardization regarding clinical staging work-up, leading up to approximately 40% of patients being overstaged, and a lack of standardization of surgical technique with TME. Moreover, there was lack of central review of surgical technique, pathologic processing, and radiation techniques. Lastly, the outcomes of the Polish study were underpowered for local control and survival, and short follow-up and non-standardized patient evaluation precluded a thorough assessment of treatment-related toxicities [54].

More recently, the Trans-Tasman Radiation Oncology Group Trial 01.04 study randomized 326 patients with cT3N0-2 rectal cancer to receive either preoperative short-course or long-course (50.4 Gy in 1.8 Gy per fraction with continuous-infusion 5-FU 225 mg m^{-2}). Six monthly courses of 5-FU 425 mg m^{-2} and folinic acid (20 mg m^{-2}) administered daily for five days were commenced four to six weeks after surgery. With a median follow-up of 5.9 years, the three-year LRRs were 7.5% for short-course and 4.4% for long-course (p = 0.24). There was no significant difference in five-year rates of distant recurrence (27% versus 30%, p = 0.92), OS (74% versus 70%, p = 0.62), or grade 3 or 4 toxicity (5.8% versus 8.2%, p = 0.53) for short-course and long-course, respectively [57].

Role of Preoperative Radiation Therapy in Sphincter Preservation

For distal rectal tumors in close proximity to the dentate line, preoperative radiotherapy may yield tumor down-staging, and thus, allow for the possibility of conversion from a planned APR to a sphincter-preserving low anterior resection. For tumors with direct extension into the anal sphincter, however, sphincter preservation is unlikely even in the setting of a complete clinical response. Several Phase II studies have reported surgical conversion rates from an APR to sphincter preservation in between 30% and 89% patients initially believed

to require an APR after chemoradiation [82–85]. However, these published results were all single-institution studies from highly specialized centers, and thus it is unclear whether these results are generalizable to community practice.

As discussed, with respect to timing of surgery, a longer interval between the completion of preoperative therapy and surgery may increase the chance for tumor regression, and thus potentially, sphincter preservation [86, 87]. Consequently, standard fractionation preoperative radiotherapy is recommended when sphincter preservation is a goal of therapy, with surgery performed four to seven weeks after completion of preoperative therapy. A delay in surgery allows for both healing from any acute radiation-induced toxicity and maximal tumor response. Although the only Phase III randomized study comparing short-course and standard fractionation radiotherapy failed to find a difference in rates of sphincter preservation, it did identify a significant improvement in tumor down-staging with standard fractionation. However, as discussed above, the study has been highly criticized for the surgeons' subjectivity in decisions regarding sphincter preservation [54].

Tumor Response to Preoperative Chemoradiation: Pathologic Assessment and Prognostic Significance

With preoperative chemoradiation becoming the standard of care [53, 58], it has become increasingly important to assess the effect of tumor down-staging and its potential implications in predicting long-term outcomes. Numerous studies have demonstrated that preoperative chemotherapy and radiotherapy may alter pathologic T and N categories by reducing the depth of tumor invasion and causing complete disappearance of the malignant cells within the rectal wall and surrounding perirectal lymph nodes [53, 65]. Although down-staging can be clinically assessed by preoperative staging techniques of EUS, CT scans or MRI, they are have limited sensitivity and specificity in determination of pathologic T and N categories [88]. Alternatively, treatment response can be assessed by a thorough pathologic review of surgical specimens to determine the presence of histologic changes, including cytoplasmic alteration and stromal fibrosis [89–91].

By analyzing patients treated with preoperative chemoradiotherapy on the German Rectal Study, Rodel and colleagues established the importance of tumor regression as a significant prognostic factor [33, 53]. In this exploratory analysis, tumor regression grading (TRG) was performed on surgical specimens of 385 patients treated with preoperative chemoradiation. Tumor regression of the primary tumor was determined by the amount of viable tumor versus the amount of fibrosis, with grading as follows: Grade 0, no regression;

Grade 1, minor regression (fibrosis in ≤25% of tumor mass); Grade 2, moderate regression (obvious fibrosis of 26–50% of the tumor mass); Grade 3, good regression (>50% tumor regression); or Grade 4, total regression, no viable tumor cells, only fibrotic mass [90].

On pathologic review, 10.4% and 8.3% of patients were found with TRG 4 and TRG 0, respectively. When compared to TRG 4, patients with TRG 2/TRG 3 and with TRG 0/TRG 1 had significantly worse five-year DFS rates of 86%, 75%, and 63%, respectively (p = 0.006). No pretreatment factors significantly predicted TRG in this study, however, pretreatment tumor size has been implicated as a possible predictor for pathologic complete response after preoperative chemoradiotherapy in other studies [92,93]. Additionally, a higher TRG was significantly associated with a lower risk of post-treatment positive lymph nodes (p < 0.001) and higher R0 resection rates (p = 0.012). Due to the small number of events, TRG was not associated with increased rates of local failure, however, none of the patients with TRG 4 experienced a local recurrence, compared to 4% and 6% among patients with TRG 2+3 and 0+1, respectively (p = 0.33). In contrast, TRG was found to be significantly correlated with DFS and metastases-free survival. On multivariate analysis, the pathologic T category and nodal status after chemoradiotherapy were the most important prognostic factors for DFS. Thus, a higher grade of tumor regression has been demonstrated to predict for improved DFS after preoperative chemoradiotherapy [33].

Additionally, several studies have suggested that pathologic stage after preoperative chemoradiotherapy is a significant prognostic factor in the determination of OS [94, 95]. The degree of tumor regression has been associated with treatment-related factors, including overall doses to radiation [54], the use of concurrent chemotherapy [65, 69], and the time interval between preoperative treatment and surgery [54]. As discussed above, the Polish study demonstrated higher rates of clinical and pathologic complete response in patients treated with preoperative standard fractionation chemoradiotherapy compared to preoperative short-course radiotherapy [54]. Additionally, the results of FFCD 9203 highlighted the effect of concurrent chemotherapy with higher rates of pathologic complete response (11.4% versus 3.6%, p < 0.05) among patients treated with preoperative chemoradiotherapy compared to preoperative standard fractionation radiotherapy alone [65]. Likewise, the EORTC 22921 showed patients treated with preoperative chemoradiotherapy had less-advanced pathological tumor staging and less-advanced pathological nodal staging, compared to patients treated with preoperative standard fractionation radiotherapy alone [69].

With respect to timing of surgery, because rectal cancer typically regresses slowly, a longer interval between completion of preoperative therapy and surgery may increase the chance for tumor regression, and thus potentially, sphincter preservation [86,87]. Most notably, the issue of optimal timing of completion of preoperative radiotherapy and surgical resection was addressed in the Lyon R90-01 study [96]. This study randomized 201 patients, all of which received preoperative 39 Gy in 13 fractions, to either undergo surgical resection within two weeks (short interval, SI, group) or within six to eight weeks (long interval, LI, group). A longer interval between preoperative radiotherapy and surgery yielded significantly higher rates of clinical tumor response (53.1% in SI versus 71.7% in LI, p = 0.007) and pathologic down-staging (10.3% in SI versus 26% in LI, p = 0.005). With a median follow-up of 33 months, however, improved tumor response did not translate into improved rates of treatment morbidity, local control, or short-term overall survival. Although there was a slight trend in improved rates of sphincter preservation with the LI group (76% versus 68%, p = 0.27), the difference was not significant [96].

Why would tumor regression after preoperative chemoradiotherapy be associated with improved prognosis? One hypothesis is that greater tumor regression after preoperative chemoradiotherapy may be a surrogate for smaller tumor size and pathologic stage at presentation [92, 93]. A second hypothesis is that the extent of tumor regression is a surrogate for how responsive the tumor is either to 5-FU chemotherapy or radiation. The underlying assumption of this hypothesis is that patients with treatment-responsive tumors will ultimately fare better than patients with treatment-resistant tumors.

Locally Advanced, Unresectable Rectal Cancer

Within the group of patients categorized as having 'locally advanced' rectal cancer, there is also variability in disease extent with no uniform definition of resectability. Depending on the series, a locally advanced lesion can range from a tethered or marginally resectable tumor to a fixed cancer with direction invasion of adjacent organs or structures. The definition will also depend on whether the assessment of resectability is made clinically or at the time of surgery. In some cases, tumors thought to be unresectable at the time of clinical or radiographic examination may be more mobile when the patient is examined under anesthesia. With these caveats, a good working definition of a locally advanced, unresectable tumor is "…a tumor that cannot be resected without leaving microscopic or gross residual disease in the local site because of tumor adherence or fixation to that site." Since these patients do poorly with surgery alone, treatment programs of irradiation, chemotherapy and surgery have evolved to improve their outcome. For patients who present with metastatic disease, systemic therapy remains the standard of care, and radiation therapy is typically reserved for symptom palliation. For patients with oligometastatic disease deemed to have surgical resectable disease for curative intent, patients should be referred to a multidisciplinary clinic for consideration of preoperative pelvic radiation therapy.

External Beam Irradiation

In the past, the management of locally advanced, unresectable rectal cancer had been variable. Some patients had incomplete surgical resections alone, while others had radiation alone or surgery combined with postoperative or preoperative irradiation. The results of high-dose external beam irradiation as a primary curative treatment have been unsatisfactory, with local failure rates of at least 90% or greater and five-year survivals of less than 10%. Wang and Schulz reported that, of 58 patients with recurrent, inoperable, or residual rectosigmoid carcinoma treated with 35–50 Gy in four to five weeks, six patients survived five years disease-free [97]. O'Connell *et al.* noted that 37 of 44 patients with locally unresectable or recurrent rectal cancer treated with 50 Gy in a split-course fashion over seven weeks with and without adjuvant immunotherapy had progression of disease [98]. Of 31 patients assessable for sites of initial tumor progression, 17 had local progression only, 11 had concurrent local progression and distant metastases only, and three developed only distant metastases. Brierley *et al.* reported that of 77 patients with clinically fixed tumors who were treated with 50 Gy in 20 fractions over four years, local control was 3% and survival was 4%. Unless the patient is not a candidate for surgery, external beam irradiation has no role as definitive treatment [99].

External Beam and Surgery

Combinations of external beam irradiation and surgical resection have been used to improve local control and survival. Radiation therapy after subtotal resection gives better local control and survival in patients treated for residual microscopic disease than to patients treated with gross residual disease. Allee *et al.* reported the results of 31 patients with residual microscopic cancer treated with 45 Gy followed by additional radiation therapy to as much as 60–70 Gy if the small bowel could be moved from the irradiation field [100]. Local control rates and five-year DFS rates were 70% and 45%, respectively. In contrast, these figures were 43% and 11% for 25 patients treated for gross residual disease. A possible dose–response correlation was seen in patients with microscopic residual disease; the risk of local failure was 11% (1/9) with doses of 60 Gy or greater versus 40% (8/20) if the boost dose

was less than 60 Gy. There was no clear dose–response relationship in patients with gross disease. In 17 patients receiving external beam irradiation after subtotal resection, Schild *et al.* observed that local control was achieved in three of 10 patients (30%) with microscopic residual cancer, and in one of seven (14%) with gross residual cancer [101]. Four of the 17 patients (24%) have remained disease free for more than five years. Ghossein *et al.* treated patients to 46 Gy in 1.8-Gy fractions followed by a field reduction to the area of persistent disease which received 60 Gy [102]. For patients treated with microscopic disease, the incidence of local failure and survival was 16% and 84%, whereas for patients with gross disease these figures were 50% and 39%, respectively.

For patients presenting with locally advanced, unresectable disease, high-dose preoperative irradiation (45–50 Gy) has been used to reduce tumor size and facilitate resection. Emami *et al.* reported that the rate of resectability of 28 patients after full-dose preoperative irradiation was 50% [103]. Dosoretz *et al.* described 25 patients (57%) with unresectable tumors in the rectum or rectosigmoid treated with 40–52 Gy preoperative radiation therapy [104]. Sixteen of the 25 patients underwent potentially curative resection, and the six-year survival was 26% (with three postoperative deaths). Total pelvic failure after curative resection was 39% (five of 13 patients). Mendenhall *et al.* reviewed 23 patients with locally advanced, unresectable carcinoma who received 35–60 Gy of preoperative irradiation [105]. Eleven patients were able to undergo complete resection with a five-year absolute survival of 18% and a local failure of 55%. Of 20 patients with unresectable rectal cancer undergoing 43–55.8 Gy preoperative irradiation reported by Whiting *et al.*, 13 patients (65%) underwent resection with curative intent. Three of 13 (23%) subsequently developed a local failure with a five-year survival of 40% [106].

One randomized prospective study has been conducted examining the merits of preoperative irradiation in patients with locally advanced, unresectable rectal cancer. Under the auspices of the Northwest rectal cancer Group (Manchester, United Kingdom), 284 patients with tethered or fixed rectal cancer were entered into a prospective randomized trial between 1982 and 1986 to assess the effects of preoperative irradiation given one week before surgery [107]. Of these patients, 141 were allowed to undergo surgical treatment alone, and 143 were allocated to receive 20 Gy in four fractions. This study showed a highly significant reduction in local recurrences in the irradiated group (12.8%) versus the surgery-alone group (36.5%). Although there was no significant difference in either OS or cancer-related mortality between the two treatment groups, subset analysis of the patients who underwent curative surgery alone revealed a significant reduction in overall mortality of 53.3% for patients allocated to surgery alone compared to 44.9% for patients allocated to preoperative radiotherapy.

In summary, following full-dose preoperative irradiation, most series report that half to two-thirds of patients will be converted to a resectable status. However, despite a complete resection and negative margins, the local failure rate depending on the degree of tumor fixation varies from 23% to 55%.

Preoperative Chemoradiotherapy and Surgery

With the landmark results of the German Rectal Study Group and NSABP R-03 establishing preoperative chemoradiation as the standard of care in patients with T3–4, node-positive rectal cancer, these results have similarly solidified the benefit of preoperative chemoradiation in locally advanced, unresectable rectal cancer. Moreover, the superiority of preoperative chemoradiation over preoperative radiation therapy alone was demonstrated in a randomized Phase III study of unresectable primary or locally recurrent rectal cancer. In total, 207 patients were randomly assigned to either receive radiation therapy (50 Gy) with or without bolus 5-FU and leucovorin chemotherapy. The addition of chemotherapy yielded a significantly higher R0 rate (84% versus 68%, p = 0.009), and improved five-year local control (82% versus 67%, p = 0.03), DFS (63% versus 44%, p = 0.003), and disease-specific survival (72% versus 55%, p = 0.02) [108]. Not surprisingly, chemotherapy was associated with increased rates of acute toxicity (29% versus 6%, p = 0.03), but no difference in late toxicity.

Intraoperative Electron Beam Radiation Therapy

Despite full-dose preoperative irradiation and complete resection of locally advanced, initially unresectable rectal cancer, local failures can occur in at least one-third of patients. These local failure rates are even higher in patients undergoing subtotal resection. Intraoperative electron beam radiation therapy (IOERT) has been used in combination with preoperative irradiation (with and without 5-FU) and surgical resection when there is gross residual cancer, position or close resection margins, or simply tumor adherence. IOERT is an intensive radiation therapy modality that delivers a single concentrated dose of radiation to the open surgical cavity with electrons at the time of surgical resection. IOERT allows for direct targeting of the radiation to the tumor bed, while sparing normal surrounding tissues. IOERT requires close coordination of the surgical team and the radiation oncologist in order to define all high-risk areas, as well as supplemental shielding within the walls of the operating rooms for radiation safety protection. Although most IOERT treatments in rectal cancer are given through the abdomen, occasionally a perineal port is used to treat low-lying tumors of the coccyx, or distal pelvic side wall. IOERT has been used in conjunction with preoperative chemoradiation and surgery if there is gross residual disease or tumor adherence to the pelvic sidewall [109–112].

At MGH, all patients with locally advanced rectal cancer receive full-dose preoperative irradiation with infusion 5-FU (225 mg m^{-2} per day, five days per week, throughout irradiation). Surgical exploration is undertaken four to six weeks later. At surgery, the abdomen is carefully evaluated for liver and peritoneal metastases. If metastases are found, intraoperative irradiation is not performed and treatment ends with surgical resection or IOERT alone. If no metastases are found, the patients undergo abdominoperineal resection, low anterior resection, or pelvic exenteration, depending on the extent and location of the tumor. Attempts are made to resect as much disease as possible, even if some gross residual disease remains. The surgical specimen and tumor bed are examined pathologically to define areas of possible residual disease, microscopic positive margins, or gross residual tumor. It is critical to define all high-risk areas accurately, to determine the optimal position for the IOERT field. If no tumor adherence and adequate soft-tissue radial margins are present (>1 cm), IOERT is usually not used. Patients with residual cancer or with positive or minimal margins (<5 mm) radial soft-tissue margins are evaluated for IOERT.

The areas of highest risk for local tumor recurrence are defined by the surgeon and radiation oncologist. To direct the IOERT, cones are used with internal diameters ranging from 4 to 8 cm. Some have beveled ends, enabling good apposition of the cone to sloping surfaces in the pelvis. Cone size is selected to cover fully the high-risk area generally on the sacrum or the pelvic sidewall. These cones allow the geometry of the cone to fit the specific situation of tumor versus normal tissue. The cone must abut the site being treated, which can be difficult if the high-risk area is located in an anatomically confined region such as the pelvis. Further, the angle of the edge of the cone should optimally be placed flat against the body surface to maximize dose homogeneity. It is important that the applicator be placed so that the tumor is fully covered, that no sensitive normal tissues be included in the beam, and that no fluid build-up occurs in the treatment area. During treatment, suction tubes are positioned to minimize fluid build-up. If necessary, lead sheets can be cut out to block sensitive normal tissues that cannot be removed from the path of the beam: retraction and packing are often necessary to move normal tissues. Most IOERT treatments in rectal cancer are given through the abdomen, but a perineal port is occasionally used to treat a very low-lying tumor involving the coccyx, distal pelvic sidewall, or portions of the prostate and bladder when an exenteration is not performed.

Typical doses of radiation delivered intraoperatively are in the range of 10 to 20 Gy, with the lower doses being given for minimal residual disease and the higher doses for gross residual disease after resection. For patients undergoing complete resection with negative margins, the IOERT dose is usually 10–12.5 Gy, whereas for patients undergoing subtotal resection with microscopic residual the dose is 12.5–15 Gy. For patients with macroscopic tumor after resection, the dose is 17.5–20 Gy. Typical electron energies used are 9–15 MeV, depending on the thickness of the residual tumor. The dose is quoted at the 90% isodose.

Recent studies have shown that IOERT is highly effective at reducing the risk of local failure, particularly for T4 [111] or locally recurrent tumors. Nakfoor *et al.* reported details of the MGH experience of 73 patients with locally advanced rectal cancer treated with preoperative chemoradiation, followed by surgical resection and IOERT [113]. The authors reported five-year actuarial rates of local control and disease-specific survival of 89% and 63% for patients treated with R0 resection. However, the rates of five-year local control and disease-specific survival were considerably lower at 57% and 14%, respectively, for patients with R2 resection. Some 11% of patients developed IOERT-related complications, with two patients developing osteoradionecrosis of the sacrum requiring surgical intervention.

The Mayo Clinic has also reported on their long-standing experience of treating 146 patients with a combination of preoperative radiation with surgery and IOERT. They reported a five-year local recurrence-free survival of 85%, and five-year DFS of 43%. Additionally, they reported an 8% rate of perioperative complications and a 53% rate of long-term complications, most commonly peripheral neuropathy (19%), bowel obstruction (14%) and ureteral obstruction (12%) [114].

Krempien *et al.* recently reported on the long-term experience at University of Heidelberg of 210 patients with locally advanced rectal cancer treated with TME, IOERT, and preoperative or postoperative chemotherapy. With a median follow-up of 61 months, the patients experienced a five-year actuarial overall survival of 69%, disease-free survival of 66%, and local control rate of 93%. Acute complications and late complications of grade 3 or more were seen in 17% and 13% of patients, respectively [115]. A subsequent patterns of failure study reported from the same group found that among 243 patients treated with IOERT after TME and external beam radiation therapy (EBRT) (87%), seven infield recurrences were seen in the presacral space. The remaining local relapses were located in the retrovesical/retroprostatic space ($n = 5$), anastomotic site ($n = 2$), sacral promontory ($n = 1$), ileocecal region ($n = 1$) and perineal ($n = 1$). Rates of acute and long-term toxicity have been reported to range from 8% to 53%, and most commonly include

peripheral neuropathy, bowel obstruction, and ureteral obstruction [113, 114].

High-dose rate-intraoperative radiation therapy (HDR-IORT) may also be a potentially safe and feasible treatment modality. A published series from Memorial Sloan Kettering Cancer Center reported the results of 66 patients treated with HDR-IORT. With a median follow-up of 17.5 months, they reported a two-year local control rate of 81%. The authors noted a significant complication rate of 38%, the majority with manageable to complete recovery.

Thus, multimodality treatment with TME and IOERT boost in combination with preoperative or postoperative chemoradiation is feasible and results in excellent long-term local control rates in patients with intermediate to high-risk locally advanced rectal cancer.

Role of Chemotherapy Alone

Although the current treatment paradigm for stage II–III rectal cancer centers around neoadjuvant chemoradiation followed by surgery and postoperative chemotherapy, concerns have been raised regarding the long-term side effects of pelvic irradiation in the setting of improved surgical techniques and chemotherapy options. To evaluate the feasibility of omitting radiation therapy, the Memorial-Sloan Kettering Cancer Center investigators conducted a pilot feasibility of preoperative 5-FU/leucovorin/oxaliplatin (FOLFOX) and bevacizumab without concurrent radiation in patients with stage II–III rectal cancer. The primary endpoint was the R0 resection rate. All 29 patients who completed preoperative chemotherapy had R0 resections, and 27% (8/29) had a pathologic complete response (pCR). With a short follow-up, there were no patients with a LR and three distant recurrences, all pulmonary. This prompted the Preoperative Radiation Or Selective Preoperative Radiation and Evaluation before Chemotherapy and Total Mesorectal Excision (PROSPECT) trial, the aim of which is to reduce the delivery of pelvic radiation in those patients who may not benefit from such. There are two preoperative arms of this Phase II/III trial for patients prior to TME: neoadjuvant FOLFOX (oxaliplatin, leucovorin, and 5-FU) with selective use of chemoradiation (5-FU and radiation) versus standard fractionation preoperative chemoradiation with 5-FU. The primary endpoints of the study are R0 resection rate, DFS, and time to local recurrence.

Radiation Techniques

In designing radiation treatment fields, the goal is to encompass regions at risk for local regional recurrence after treatment with surgery alone. For locally advanced tumors, sites of relapse may include the anastomotic site, pelvic sidewall, presacral space, or the pelvic lymph nodes [116, 117]. In patients requiring an APR, the perineum is at a higher risk of recurrence and coverage should be considered [117]. Typically, whole pelvic fields have been used to cover the primary tumor/surgical bed and the primary at risk lymph nodes. A RTOG consensus panel contouring atlas for elective clinical target volumes for rectal cancer has been recently published.

Traditionally, patients are treated in the prone position and radiation fields have been designed as a three-field approach with two lateral fields, and a single posterior-anterior (PA) field or as a four-field approach with either paired posterior obliques or the addition of an anterior-posterior (AP) field. The advantage of the three-field approach is that it allows for a greater sparing of anterior pelvic structures, including the small bowel and bladder. For locally aggressive tumors with anterior extension, however, the addition of an AP field may be necessary for adequate dose coverage of the tumor. For the AP/PA fields, the typical radiation field borders are as follows: superior field edge – sacral promontory (L5/S1 junction); inferior field edge – bottom of the obturator foramen after low anterior resection or includes the perineal scar after APR; lateral field edges – 1–2 cm beyond the widest part of the pelvic brim. To treat the entire presacral space with adequate margins and full dose, the lateral fields are designed so that the posterior border encompasses the entire sacrum with a 1 cm margin posterior to the sacrum. Anteriorly, the fields are designed to encompass the original tumor with at least a 2 cm margin. Blocks can often be used to spare a portion of the femoral neck on the lateral fields.

With conventionally fractionated radiation therapy, the doses most commonly prescribed are in the range of 45 to 50.4 Gy to the whole pelvis in 25–28 fractions, followed by an additional boost of 5.4 Gy in three fractions to the primary tumor and mesorectum. During the 5.5-week course of irradiation, patients receive a continuous infusion of 5-FU (225 mg m^{-2} per day) for five days per week, or capecitabine 825 mg m^{-2} given twice daily. Based on the final results of NSABP R-04, 5-FU and capecitabine yield equivalent outcomes.

3D-conformal radiation therapy (3D-CRT) planning has become the standard of care for the treatment of rectal cancer, which allows for CT-based localization of target and normal tissue structures. Additionally, based on 3D reconstructions of CT images taken during treatment planning, a dose–volume histogram (DVH) can be generated, summarizing 3D dose distributions to the planning target volume and normal tissue structures in a graphical, user friendly, 2D format.

Patients can be treated with a full bladder, in order to push some of the small intestine out of the radiation field. Great effort should be made to minimize the dose to the

small bowel to 45 Gy, with a particular attention paid to ensuring that no small bowel is within the boost fields. For patients treated in the postoperative setting, it may be helpful to have the surgeon (at the time of the initial surgical procedure) try to move the small intestine out of the pelvis. This can best be accomplished by reperitonealizing the pelvic floor, but when this is not possible it is helpful to have a loop of omentum swung to cover the pelvic floor, or to have the uterus retroverted to accomplish the same purpose. Some centers have considered the use of prostheses or artificial mesh, but these are still being investigated. This is most important when treating patients after an abdominoperineal resection, since after a low anterior resection the remaining rectum and colon prevent some small bowel from being immobilized deep in the pelvis. Examples of a standard field arrangement in the treatment of rectal cancer are shown in Figures 24.1 and 24.2. Additionally, bolus should be placed on the perineal scar in the postoperative APR setting, to ensure that full dose will be delivered to the scar in this region. If

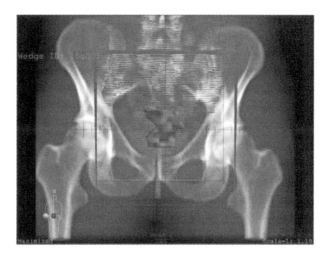

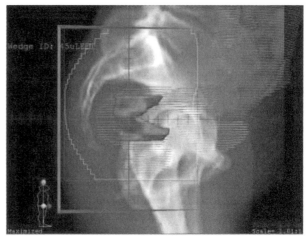

Figure 24.1 Standard radiation fields for rectal cancer. Illustration courtesy of Theodore Hong. For a color version of this figure, see the color plate section.

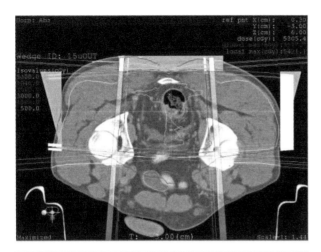

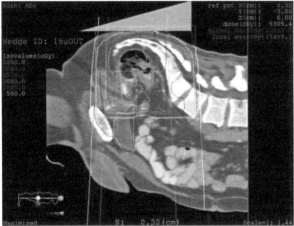

Figure 24.2 Standard three-field radiation plan for rectal cancer. Illustration courtesy of Theodore Hong. For a color version of this figure, see the color plate section.

the reaction becomes marked, the bolus can be removed. Generally, perineal reactions have not produced major symptoms.

Novel Radiation Techniques and Radiosensitizing Agents

With the emergence of technologic advancements into the field of radiation therapy, there has been growing interest in maximizing dose to the tumor and minimizing dose to the normal tissue structures. Intensity-modulated radiation therapy (IMRT) is a novel technique based on the concept of inverse planning and computer-controlled radiation deposition, allowing for normal tissue avoidance. Dosimetric comparison studies of IMRT and 3D-CRT have suggested a reduction in small bowel volume receiving 45 Gy by 63% for IMRT [118]. A Phase II RTOG study, RTOG 0822, which seeks to evaluate the role of capecitabine and oxaliplatin in conjunction with

IMRT, has recently completed accrual and final results are pending at this time.

Additionally, with the ability to create multiple targets and multiple avoidance structures, IMRT enables radiation treatment delivery with greater precision and minimizes treatment-related morbidity, making dose escalation with a consequent improvement in local control feasible at certain disease sites [119]. Similarly, the question of dose escalation has been explored with IMRT. A recent Phase I study evaluated the safety of preoperative hypofractionated radiotherapy using IMRT and an incorporated boost with concurrent capecitabine in patients with locally advanced rectal cancer [120]. Photon IMRT and an incorporated boost, via a radiation treatment technique called 'dose-painting,' were used to treat the whole pelvis to 45 Gy and the gross tumor volume plus 2 cm to 55 Gy in 25 treatments. Eight patients completed radiotherapy at the initial study dose level of 55 Gy, but the study was discontinued due to excessive grade 3 toxicity (38%). Additionally, all patients went on to definitive surgical resection, and no patient had a pathological complete response [120]. Thus, at the present time conventional radiotherapy has remained the standard of care, and further studies will hopefully help to elucidate whether IMRT offers either improved clinical outcomes or decreased treatment-related toxicities compared to conventional radiotherapy.

Recent studies have attempted to identify new chemotherapeutic and biologically targeted agents that can be used in conjunction with radiation therapy to improve upon current preoperative chemoradiotherapy regimens. The potential efficacy of capecitabine [121, 122], oxaliplatin [123], irinotecan [124], cetuximab [125], and bevacizumab [126] have been extrapolated from the adjuvant and metastatic setting, and are currently being investigated in conjunction with preoperative radiation therapy. With studies demonstrating equivalent efficacy of 5-FU and capecitabine (an orally active prodrug of 5-FU), there has been increasing interest in incorporating this agent into preoperative regimens [127]. A recent Phase II randomized study, RTOG 02-47, sought to evaluate the potential efficacy of concurrent preoperative chemoradiation with capecitabine with either irinotecan or oxaliplatin. However, due to unexpectedly high rates of grade 3 and 4 toxicities, this study has been temporarily closed to accrual. The Phase III ACCORD 12/0405-Prodige 2 trial of T3–4 M0 rectal cancer recently failed to demonstrate an additional benefit of oxaliplatin to concurrent capecitabine and preoperative radiation, and was associated with increased acute grade 3 and 4 toxicity (10.9% versus 25.4%, p < 0.001) [128]. The results of this study support the preliminary findings of a recent Studio Terapia Adjuvante Retto (STAR-01) trial of 747 patients with T3–4 rectal tumors comparing preoperative chemoradiation with concurrent continuous-infusion 5-FU with or without oxaliplatin. Among the two arms, there were similar rates of APR, pathologic complete response, pathologic node positivity or T3 disease, and margin positivity. However, grade 3 to 4 adverse events during preoperative treatment were more frequent with oxaliplatin plus 5-FU and radiation than with radiation and 5-FU alone (24% versus 8% of treated patients; P < .0001) [129]. Given these findings, there does not appear to be a role for the addition of oxaliplatin to the course of preoperative chemoradiation at this time.

Additional strategies have included the incorporation of biologically targeted agents, such as bevacizumab and cetuximab, and are currently undergoing investigation. Recent studies in the metastatic setting have evaluated the efficacy of cetuximab and have clearly demonstrated a benefit restricted to patients with KRAS wild-type disease [125]. On-going Phase I/II studies are evaluating the efficacy of cetuximab in the preoperative setting given in combination with concurrent chemoradiation. Willett *et al.* recently published the results of a Phase II prospective study evaluating the efficacy of neoadjuvant bevacizumab with standard chemoradiotherapy in locally advanced rectal cancer. For this, 32 patients were enrolled and treated with a preoperative course of bevacizumab (5 or 10 mg kg^{-1}) on day 1 of each cycle, 5-FU infusion (225 mg m^{-2} per day) during cycles 2 and 4, and radiation therapy to 50.4 Gy in 28 fractions. With this preoperative regimen, the authors reported a 100% five-year actuarial local control and OS. In all patients, histologic examination demonstrated either no cancer or varying numbers of scattered cancer cells in a bed of fibrosis at the primary site [130]. The results of this single-arm study are encouraging, and should be evaluated in larger, Phase III studies to determine whether any of these novel agents will offer an advantage compared to the current standard 5-FU-based concurrent chemoradiation regimens.

Gastrointestinal Toxicity of Radiation Therapy

Pelvic irradiation may result in the development of acute and late treatment-related toxicities. The severity and likelihood of experiencing adverse radiation toxicities depend on the total radiation dose delivered, the fractional dose of radiation prescribed, and the total volume of normal tissues irradiated. For a given total dose, the higher dose per fraction may result in a greater risk of acute and late normal tissue toxicity. Acute radiation-related side effects are cumulative over the course of radiation therapy, occur during or shortly after completion of radiation therapy, and may include fatigue, dysuria,

urinary frequency, cramping and diarrhea, and rarely, nausea. In contrast, late effects may develop months to years after completion of radiation, and can include sexual dysfunction [131], long-term bowel and bladder impairment [132–134], significant perineal wound healing delays after APR [74], and increased risk of secondary malignancies [135].

Numerous patient- and treatment-related factors have been found to increase the risk of developing acute and late radiation toxicity. For example, a history of prior abdominal or pelvic surgery has been associated with an increased risk of developing small bowel obstructions in patients treated with more than 50 Gy to the pelvis [136], and can lead to adhesions which limit intestinal displacement [137, 138]. Additionally, patients with coexisting collagen vascular disease or inflammatory bowel disease may be at higher risk for development of acute and long-term radiation side effects [139–141]. For patients with inflammatory bowel treated with abdominopelvic irradiation, one study reported a 45% overall crude rate of severe toxicity, with 21% of patients developing acute toxicity requiring a treatment break; however, toxicity was significantly lower for patients treated with more modern and specialized radiation techniques [140]. Lastly, patients receiving concurrent therapy with chemotherapy or biologically targeted agents may be at increased risk for radiation toxicity. Several recent Phase I/II studies have demonstrated increased gastrointestinal toxicity with the integration of agents including oxaliplatin and irinotecan to a 5-FU-based chemoradiation regimen [128, 142].

Improvements in imaging and computer planning systems have allowed for more precise radiation treatment planning and delivery and, consequently, decreased dose to normal tissue structures. Many radiation treatment techniques have recently been adopted to minimize doses and volumes of normal tissue receiving radiation. These techniques have included employing multiple radiation fields to avoid significant dose inhomogeneity, and use of a 'belly board' with the patient in the prone position or treatment of the patient with their bladder full in order to optimize physical displacement of the small bowel [143].

Conclusion

Although surgery remains the mainstay of curative treatment for rectal cancer, the addition of adjuvant radiation, given either preoperatively or postoperatively, has been shown to decrease the risk of local failure. Two recently published Phase III trials comparing preoperative to postoperative chemoradiotherapy have demonstrated the superiority of preoperative treatment with respect to local control, acute and late treatment-related toxicity, sphincter preservation, and DFS compared to postoperative chemoradiation. As a result, the current standard of care for locally advanced rectal cancer is treatment with a preoperative 5-FU-based chemotherapy regimen with concurrent radiation to 45–50.4 Gy over five to six weeks, with TME four to seven weeks after completion of neoadjuvant therapy, followed by an additional four months of postoperative 5-FU-based chemotherapy. Preoperative short-course radiotherapy has been demonstrated as an effective treatment in reducing the risk of local recurrence; however, there has been hesitation in adopting this regimen due to concerns

of increased long-term toxicity of high fractional doses. For older patients, or patients with significant medical comorbidities that have limited life expectancies, in which long-term treatment-related toxicities are of less concern, preoperative short-course radiotherapy offers the benefit of a shortened treatment course and should be considered. Lastly, technologic advancements with radiation therapy planning and the delivery and incorporation of novel radiosensitizing agents are currently being evaluated with the goal of improving tumor dose coverage and sparing radiation dose to normal tissue structures.

References

1 Billingham, R.P. (1992) Conservative treatment of rectal cancer. Extending the indications. *Cancer*, **70** (5 Suppl.), 1355–1363.

2 Nicholls, R.J., Mason, A.Y., Morson, B.C., Dixon, A.K., Fry, I.K. (1982) The clinical staging of rectal cancer. *Br. J. Surg.*, **69** (7), 404–409.

3 Orrom, W.J., Wong, W.D., Rothenberger, D.A., Jensen, L.L., Goldberg, S.M. (1990) Endorectal ultrasound in the preoperative staging of rectal tumors. A learning experience. *Dis. Colon Rectum*, **33** (8), 654–659.

4 Bipat, S., Glas, A.S., Slors, F.J., Zwinderman, A.H., Bossuyt, P.M., Stoker, J. (2004) Rectal cancer: local staging and assessment of lymph node involvement with endoluminal US, CT, and MR imaging – a meta-analysis. *Radiology*, **232** (3), 773–783.

5 Lahaye, M.J., Engelen, S.M., Nelemans, P.J., *et al.* (2005) Imaging for predicting the risk factors – the circumferential resection margin and nodal disease – of local recurrence in rectal cancer: a meta-analysis. *Semin. Ultrasound CT MR*, **26** (4), 259–268.

6 Ng, A.K., Recht, A., Busse, P.M. (1997) Sphincter preservation therapy for distal rectal carcinoma: a review. *Cancer*, **79** (4), 671–683.

7 Brown, G., Richards, C.J., Bourne, M.W., *et al.* (2003) Morphologic predictors of lymph node status in rectal cancer with use of high-spatial-resolution MR imaging with histopathologic comparison. *Radiology*, **227** (2), 371–377.

8 MERCURY Study Group (2006) Diagnostic accuracy of preoperative magnetic resonance imaging in predicting curative resection of rectal cancer: prospective observational study. *Br. Med. J.*, **333** (7572), 779.

9 Touzios, J., Ludwig, K.A. (2008) Local management of rectal neoplasia. *Clin. Colon Rectal Surg.*, **21** (4), 291–299.

10 Tytherleigh, M.G., Warren, B.F., Mortensen, N.J. (2008) Management of early rectal cancer. *Br. J. Surg.*, **95** (4), 409–423.

11 You, Y.N., Baxter, N.N., Stewart, A., Nelson, H. (2007) Is the increasing rate of local excision for stage I rectal cancer in the United States justified?: a nationwide cohort study from the National Cancer Database. *Ann. Surg.*, **245** (5), 726–733.

12 Ptok, H., Marusch, F., Meyer, F., *et al.* (2007) Oncological outcome of local vs radical resection of low-risk pT1 rectal cancer. *Arch. Surg.*, **142** (7), 649–655; discussion 656.

13 Endreseth, B.H., Myrvold, H.E., Romundstad, P., Hestvik, U.E., Bjerkeset, T., Wibe, A. (2005) Transanal excision vs. major surgery for T1 rectal cancer. *Dis. Colon Rectum*, **48** (7), 1380–1388.

14 Folkesson, J., Johansson, R., Pahlman, L., Gunnarsson, U. (2007) Population-based study of local surgery for rectal cancer. *Br. J. Surg.*, **94** (11), 1421–1426.

15 Minsky, B.D., Rich, T., Recht, A., Harvey, W., Mies, C. (1989) Selection criteria for local excision with or without adjuvant radiation therapy for rectal cancer. *Cancer*, **63** (7), 1421–1429.

16 Brodsky, J.T., Richard, G.K., Cohen, A.M., Minsky, B.D. (1992) Variables correlated with the risk of lymph node metastasis in early rectal cancer. *Cancer*, **69** (2), 322–326.

17 Willett, C.G., Tepper, J.E., Donnelly, S., *et al.* (1989) Patterns of failure following local excision and local excision and postoperative radiation therapy for invasive rectal adenocarcinoma. *J. Clin. Oncol.*, **7** (8), 1003–1008.

18 Gall, F., Hermanek, P. (1992) Update of the German experience with local excision of rectal cancer. *Surg. Oncol. Clin. North Am.*, **1**, 99–109.

19 Minsky, B.D., Mies, C., Rich, T.A., Recht, A. (1989) Lymphatic vessel invasion is an independent prognostic factor for survival in colorectal cancer. *Int. J. Radiat. Oncol. Biol. Phys.*, **17** (2), 311–318.

20 Fortunato, L., Ahmad, N.R., Yeung, R.S., *et al.* (1995) Long-term follow-up of local excision and radiation

therapy for invasive rectal cancer. *Dis. Colon Rectum*, **38** (11), 1193–1199.

21 Chakravarti, A., Compton, C.C., Shellito, P.C., *et al.* (1999) Long-term follow-up of patients with rectal cancer managed by local excision with and without adjuvant irradiation. *Ann. Surg.*, **230** (1), 49–54.

22 Wagman, R., Minsky, B.D., Cohen, A.M., Saltz, L., Paty, P.B., Guillem, J.G. (1999) Conservative management of rectal cancer with local excision and postoperative adjuvant therapy. *Int. J. Radiat. Oncol. Biol. Phys.*, **44** (4), 841–846.

23 Vauthey, J.N., Marsh, R.W., Zlotecki, R.A., *et al.* (1999) Recent advances in the treatment and outcome of locally advanced rectal cancer. *Ann. Surg.*, **229** (5), 745–752; discussion 752–754.

24 Steele, G.D., Jr, Herndon, J.E., Bleday, R., *et al.* (1999) Sphincter-sparing treatment for distal rectal adenocarcinoma. *Ann. Surg. Oncol.*, **6** (5), 433–441.

25 Bleday, R., Breen, E., Jessup, J.M., Burgess, A., Sentovich, S.M., Steele, G., Jr (1997) Prospective evaluation of local excision for small rectal cancers. *Dis. Colon Rectum*, **40** (4), 388–392.

26 Ota, D.M., Skibber, J., Rich, T.A., *et al.* (1992) MD Anderson Cancer Center experience with local excision and multimodality therapy for rectal cancer. *Surg. Oncol. Clin. North Am.*, **1**, 147–152.

27 Wood, W.C. (1992) Update of the Massachusetts General Hospital experience of combined local excision and radiotherapy for rectal cancer. *Surg. Oncol. Clin. North Am.*, **1**, 131–136.

28 Greenberg, J.A., Shibata, D., Herndon, J.E., 2nd, Steele, G.D., Jr, Mayer, R., Bleday, R. (2008) Local excision of distal rectal cancer: an update of cancer and leukemia group B 8984. *Dis. Colon Rectum*, **51** (8), 1185–1191; discussion 1191–1194.

29 Schell, S.R., Zlotecki, R.A., Mendenhall, W.M., Marsh, R.W., Vauthey, J.N., Copeland, E.M., 3rd (2002) Transanal excision of locally advanced rectal cancers downstaged using neoadjuvant chemoradiotherapy. *J. Am. Coll. Surg.*, **194** (5), 584–590; discussion 590–591.

30 Mohiuddin, M., Marks, G., Bannon, J. (1994) High-dose preoperative radiation and full thickness local excision: a new option for selected T3 distal rectal cancers. *Int. J. Radiat. Oncol. Biol. Phys.*, **30** (4), 845–849.

31 Kim, C.J., Yeatman, T.J., Coppola, D., *et al.* Local excision of T2 and T3 rectal cancers after downstaging chemoradiation. *Ann. Surg.*, **234** (3), 352–358; discussion 358–359.

32 Bonnen, M., Crane, C., Vauthey, J.N., *et al.* (2004) Long-term results using local excision after preoperative chemoradiation among selected T3 rectal cancer patients. *Int. J. Radiat. Oncol. Biol. Phys.*, **60** (4), 1098–1105.

33 Rodel, C., Martus, P., Papadoupolos, T., *et al.* (2005) Prognostic significance of tumor regression after preoperative chemoradiotherapy for rectal cancer. *J. Clin. Oncol.*, **23** (34), 8688–8696.

34 Stocchi, L., Nelson, H., Sargent, D.J., *et al.* (2001) Impact of surgical and pathologic variables in rectal cancer: a United States community and cooperative group report. *J. Clin. Oncol.*, **19** (18), 3895–3902.

35 Turner, R.R., Nora, D.T., Trocha, S.D., Bilchik, A.J. (2003) Colorectal carcinoma nodal staging. Frequency and nature of cytokeratin-positive cells in sentinel and nonsentinel lymph nodes. *Arch. Pathol. Lab. Med.*, **127** (6), 673–679.

36 Lezoche, G., Baldarelli, M., Guerrieri, M., *et al.* (2008) A prospective randomized study with a 5-year minimum follow-up evaluation of transanal endoscopic microsurgery versus laparoscopic total mesorectal excision after neoadjuvant therapy. *Surg. Endosc.*, **22** (2), 352–358.

37 Garcia-Aguilar, J., Shi, Q., Thomas, C.R., *et al.* (2010) Pathologic complete response to neoadjuvant chemoradiation of uT2N0 rectal cancer treated by local excision. *J. Clin. Oncol.* (Suppl.), abstract 3510.

37a Papillon, J., Berard, P. (1992) Endocavitary irradiation in the conservative treatment of adenocarcinoma of the low rectum. *World J. Surg.*, **16** (3), 451–457.

38 Folkesson, J., Birgisson, H., Pahlman, L., Cedermark, B., Glimelius, B., Gunnarsson, U. (2005) Swedish Rectal Cancer Trial: long lasting benefits from radiotherapy on survival and local recurrence rate. *J. Clin. Oncol.*, **23** (24), 5644–5650.

39 Peeters, K.C., Marijnen, C.A., Nagtegaal, I.D., *et al.* (2007) The TME trial after a median follow-up of 6 years: increased local control but no survival benefit in irradiated patients with resectable rectal carcinoma. *Ann. Surg.*, **246** (5), 693–701.

40 Gastrointestinal Tumor Study Group (1985) Prolongation of the disease-free interval in surgically treated rectal carcinoma. *N. Engl. J. Med.*, **312** (23), 1465–1472.

41 Withers, H.R., Romsdahl, M.M. (1977) Post-operative radiotherapy for adenocarcinoma of the rectum and rectosigmoid. *Int. J. Radiat. Oncol. Biol. Phys.*, **2** (11-12), 1069–1074.

42 Turner, S.S., Vieira, E.F., Ager, P.J., *et al.* (1977) Elective postoperative radiotherapy for locally advanced colorectal cancer. A preliminary report. *Cancer*, **40** (1), 105–108.

43 Hoskins, R.B., Gunderson, L.L., Dosoretz, D.E., *et al.* (1985) Adjuvant postoperative radiotherapy in carcinoma of the rectum and rectosigmoid. *Cancer*, **55** (1), 61–71.

44 Fisher, B., Wolmark, N., Rockette, H., *et al.* (1988) Postoperative adjuvant chemotherapy or radiation

therapy for rectal cancer: results from NSABP protocol R-01. *J. Natl Cancer Inst.*, **80** (1), 21–29.

45 Krook, J.E., Moertel, C.G., Gunderson, L.L., *et al.* (1991) Effective surgical adjuvant therapy for high-risk rectal carcinoma. *N. Engl. J. Med.*, **324** (11), 709–715.

46 NIH Consensus Conference (1990) Adjuvant therapy for patients with colon and rectal cancer. *JAMA*, **264** (11), 1444–1450.

47 Wolmark, N., Wieand, H.S., Hyams, D.M., *et al.* (2000) Randomized trial of postoperative adjuvant chemotherapy with or without radiotherapy for carcinoma of the rectum: National Surgical Adjuvant Breast and Bowel Project Protocol R-02. *J. Natl Cancer Inst.*, **92** (5), 388–396.

48 Gastrointestinal Tumor Study Group (1992) Radiation therapy and fluorouracil with or without semustine for the treatment of patients with surgical adjuvant adenocarcinoma of the rectum. *J. Clin. Oncol.*, **10** (4), 549–557.

49 O'Connell, M.J., Martenson, J.A., Wieand, H.S., *et al.* (1994) Improving adjuvant therapy for rectal cancer by combining protracted-infusion fluorouracil with radiation therapy after curative surgery. *N. Engl. J. Med.*, **331** (8), 502–507.

50 Willett, C.G., Badizadegan, K., Ancukiewicz, M., Shellito, P.C. (1999) Prognostic factors in stage T3N0 rectal cancer: do all patients require postoperative pelvic irradiation and chemotherapy? *Dis. Colon Rectum*, **42** (2), 167–173.

51 Merchant, N.B., Guillem, J.G., Paty, P.B., *et al.* (1999) T3N0 rectal cancer: results following sharp mesorectal excision and no adjuvant therapy. *J. Gastrointest. Surg.*, **3** (6), 642–647.

52 Gunderson, L.L., Sargent, D.J., Tepper, J.E., *et al.* (2004) Impact of T and N stage and treatment on survival and relapse in adjuvant rectal cancer: a pooled analysis. *J. Clin. Oncol.*, **22** (10), 1785–1796.

53 Sauer, R., Becker, H., Hohenberger, W., *et al.* (2004) Preoperative versus postoperative chemoradiotherapy for rectal cancer. *N. Engl. J. Med.*, **351** (17), 1731–1740.

54 Bujko, K., Nowacki, M.P., Nasierowska-Guttmejer, A., *et al.* (2004) Sphincter preservation following preoperative radiotherapy for rectal cancer: report of a randomised trial comparing short-term radiotherapy vs. conventionally fractionated radiochemotherapy. *Radiother. Oncol.*, **72** (1), 15–24.

55 Anonymous (1997) Improved survival with preoperative radiotherapy in resectable rectal cancer. Swedish Rectal Cancer Trial. *N. Engl. J. Med.*, **336** (14), 980–987.

56 Kapiteijn, E., Marijnen, C.A., Nagtegaal, I.D., *et al.* (2001) Preoperative radiotherapy combined with total mesorectal excision for resectable rectal cancer. *N. Engl. J. Med.*, **345** (9), 638–646.

57 Ngan, S.Y., Burmeister, B., Fisher, R.J., *et al.* (2012) Randomized trial of short-course radiotherapy versus long-course chemoradiation comparing rates of local recurrence in patients with T3 rectal cancer: Trans-Tasman Radiation Oncology Group Trial 01.04. *J. Clin. Oncol.*, **30** (31), 3827–3832.

58 Roh, M.S., Colangelo, L.H., O'Connell, M.J., *et al.* (2009) Preoperative multimodality therapy improves disease-free survival in patients with carcinoma of the rectum: NSABP R-03. *J. Clin. Oncol.*, **27** (31), 5124–5130.

59 Camma, C., Giunta, M., Fiorica, F., Pagliaro, L., Craxi, A., Cottone, M. (2000) Preoperative radiotherapy for resectable rectal cancer: A meta-analysis. *JAMA*, **284** (8), 1008–1015.

60 Gerard, A., Buyse, M., Nordlinger, B., *et al.* (1988) Preoperative radiotherapy as adjuvant treatment in rectal cancer. Final results of a randomized study of the European Organization for Research and Treatment of Cancer (EORTC). *Ann. Surg.*, **208** (5), 606–614.

61 Pahlman, L., Glimelius, B. (1990) Radiotherapy additional to surgery in the management of primary rectal carcinoma. *Acta Chir. Scand.*, **156** (6-7), 475–485.

62 UKCCCR Anal Cancer Trial Working Party. UK Co-ordinating Committee on Cancer Research (1996) Epidermoid anal cancer: results from the UKCCCR randomised trial of radiotherapy alone versus radiotherapy, 5-fluorouracil, and mitomycin. *Lancet*, **348** (9034), 1049–1054.

63 Bartelink, H., Roelofsen, F., Eschwege, F., *et al.* (1997) Concomitant radiotherapy and chemotherapy is superior to radiotherapy alone in the treatment of locally advanced anal cancer: results of a phase III randomized trial of the European Organization for Research and Treatment of Cancer Radiotherapy and Gastrointestinal Cooperative Groups. *J. Clin. Oncol.*, **15** (5), 2040–2049.

64 Morris, M., Eifel, P.J., Lu, J., *et al.* (1999) Pelvic radiation with concurrent chemotherapy compared with pelvic and para-aortic radiation for high-risk cervical cancer. *N. Engl. J. Med.*, **340** (15), 1137–1143.

65 Gerard, J.P., Conroy, T., Bonnetain, F., *et al.* (2006) Preoperative radiotherapy with or without concurrent fluorouracil and leucovorin in T3-4 rectal cancers: results of FFCD 9203. *J. Clin. Oncol.*, **24** (28), 4620–4625.

66 O'Connell, M.J., Mailliard, J.A., Kahn, M.J., *et al.* (1997) Controlled trial of fluorouracil and low-dose leucovorin given for 6 months as postoperative adjuvant therapy for colon cancer. *J. Clin. Oncol.*, **15** (1), 246–250.

67 James, R.D., Donaldson, D., Gray, R., Northover, J.M., Stenning, S.P., Taylor, I. (2003) Randomized clinical

trial of adjuvant radiotherapy and 5-fluorouracil infusion in colorectal cancer (AXIS). *Br. J. Surg.*, **90** (10), 1200–1212.

68 Heald, R.J., Moran, B.J., Ryall, R.D., Sexton, R., MacFarlane, J.K. (1998) Rectal cancer: the Basingstoke experience of total mesorectal excision, 1978-1997. *Arch. Surg.*, **133** (8), 894–899.

69 Bosset, J.F., Collette, L., Calais, G., *et al.* (2006) Chemotherapy with preoperative radiotherapy in rectal cancer. *N. Engl. J. Med.*, **355** (11), 1114–1123.

70 Ceelen, W.P., Van Nieuwenhove, Y., Fierens, K. (2009) Preoperative chemoradiation versus radiation alone for stage II and III resectable rectal cancer. *Cochrane Database Syst. Rev.*, **2009**(1):CD006041.

71 Kim, J.H., Beets, G.L., Kim, M.J., Kessels, A.G., Beets-Tan, R.G. (2004) High-resolution MR imaging for nodal staging in rectal cancer: are there any criteria in addition to the size? *Eur. J. Radiol.*, **52** (1), 78–83.

72 Colorectal Cancer Collaborative Group (2001) Adjuvant radiotherapy for rectal cancer: a systematic overview of 8,507 patients from 22 randomised trials. *Lancet*, **358** (9290), 1291–1304.

73 Birgisson, H., Pahlman, L., Gunnarsson, U., Glimelius, B. (2005) Adverse effects of preoperative radiation therapy for rectal cancer: long-term follow-up of the Swedish Rectal Cancer Trial. *J. Clin. Oncol.*, **23** (34), 8697–8705.

74 Marijnen, C.A., Kapiteijn, E., van de Velde, C.J., *et al.* (2002) Acute side effects and complications after short-term preoperative radiotherapy combined with total mesorectal excision in primary rectal cancer: report of a multicenter randomized trial. *J. Clin. Oncol.*, **20** (3), 817–825.

75 Harnsberger, J.R., Vernava, V.M., Longo, W.E. (1994) Radical abdominopelvic lymphadenectomy: historic perspective and current role in the surgical management of rectal cancer. *Dis. Colon Rectum*, **37**, 73–87.

76 Phillips, R.K., Hittinger, R., Blesovsky, L., Fry, J.S., Fielding, L.P. (1984) Local recurrence following 'curative' surgery for large bowel cancer: I. The overall picture. *Br. J. Surg.*, **71** (1), 12–16.

77 Kapiteijn, E., Marijnen, C.A., Colenbrander, A.C., *et al.* (1998) Local recurrence in patients with rectal cancer diagnosed between 1988 and 1992: a population-based study in the west Netherlands. *Eur. J. Surg. Oncol.*, **24** (6), 528–535.

78 Pahlman, L., Glimelius, B. (1990) Pre- or postoperative radiotherapy in rectal and rectosigmoid carcinoma. Report from a randomized multicenter trial. *Ann. Surg.*, **211** (2), 187–195.

79 Frykholm, G.J., Glimelius, B., Pahlman, L. (1993) Preoperative or postoperative irradiation in adenocarcinoma of the rectum: final treatment results

of a randomized trial and an evaluation of late secondary effects. *Dis. Colon Rectum*, **36** (6), 564–572.

80 Sebag-Montefiore, D., Stephens, R.J., Steele, R., *et al.* (2009) Preoperative radiotherapy versus selective postoperative chemoradiotherapy in patients with rectal cancer (MRC CR07 and NCIC-CTG C016): a multicentre, randomised trial. *Lancet*, **373** (9666), 811–820.

81 Bujko, K., Nowacki, M.P., Nasierowska-Guttmejer, A., Michalski, W., Bebenek, M., Kryj, M. (2006) Long-term results of a randomized trial comparing preoperative short-course radiotherapy with preoperative conventionally fractionated chemoradiation for rectal cancer. *Br. J. Surg.*, **93** (10), 1215–1223.

82 Grann, A., Feng, C., Wong, D., *et al.* (2001) Preoperative combined modality therapy for clinically resectable uT3 rectal adenocarcinoma. *Int. J. Radiat. Oncol. Biol. Phys.*, **49** (4), 987–995.

83 Bozzetti, F., Baratti, D., Andreola, S., *et al.* (1999) Preoperative radiation therapy for patients with T2-T3 carcinoma of the middle-to-lower rectum. *Cancer*, **86** (3), 398–404.

84 Mehta, V.K., Poen, J., Ford, J., *et al.* (2001) Radiotherapy, concomitant protracted-venous-infusion 5-fluorouracil, and surgery for ultrasound-staged T3 or T4 rectal cancer. *Dis. Colon Rectum*, **44** (1), 52–58.

85 Wagman, R., Minsky, B.D., Cohen, A.M., Guillem, J.G., Paty, P.P. (1998) Sphincter preservation in rectal cancer with preoperative radiation therapy and coloanal anastomosis: long term follow-up. *Int. J. Radiat. Oncol. Biol. Phys.*, **42** (1), 51–57.

86 Marijnen, C.A., Nagtegaal, I.D., Klein Kranenbarg, E., *et al.* (2001) No downstaging after short-term preoperative radiotherapy in rectal cancer patients. *J. Clin. Oncol.*, **19** (7), 1976–1984.

87 Graf, W., Dahlberg, M., Osman, M.M., Holmberg, L., Pahlman, L., Glimelius, B. (1997) Short-term preoperative radiotherapy results in down-staging of rectal cancer: a study of 1316 patients. *Radiother. Oncol.*, **43** (2), 133–137.

88 Kwok, H., Bissett, I.P., Hill, G.L. (2000) Preoperative staging of rectal cancer. *Int. J. Colorectal Dis.*, **15** (1), 9–20.

89 Shia, J., Guillem, J.G., Moore, H.G., *et al.* (2004) Patterns of morphologic alteration in residual rectal carcinoma following preoperative chemoradiation and their association with long-term outcome. *Am. J. Surg. Pathol.*, **28** (2), 215–223.

90 Dworak, O., Keilholz, L., Hoffmann, A. (1997) Pathological features of rectal cancer after preoperative radiochemotherapy. *Int. J. Colorectal Dis.*, **12** (1), 19–23.

91 Wheeler, J.M., Warren, B.F., Mortensen, N.J., *et al.* (2002) Quantification of histologic regression of rectal cancer after irradiation: a proposal for a modified staging system. *Dis. Colon Rectum*, **45** (8), 1051–1056.

92 Janjan, N.A., Khoo, V.S., Abbruzzese, J., *et al.* (1999) Tumor downstaging and sphincter preservation with preoperative chemoradiation in locally advanced rectal cancer: the M. D. Anderson Cancer Center experience. *Int. J. Radiat. Oncol. Biol. Phys.*, **44** (5), 1027–1038.

93 Willett, C.G., Warland, G., Coen, J., Shellito, P.C., Compton, C.C. (1995) Rectal cancer: the influence of tumor proliferation on response to preoperative irradiation. *Int. J. Radiat. Oncol. Biol. Phys.*, **32** (1), 57–61.

94 Quah, H.M., Chou, J.F., Gonen, M., *et al.* (2008) Pathologic stage is most prognostic of disease-free survival in locally advanced rectal cancer patients after preoperative chemoradiation. *Cancer*, **113** (1), 57–64.

95 Ruo, L., Tickoo, S., Klimstra, D.S., *et al.* (2002) Long-term prognostic significance of extent of rectal cancer response to preoperative radiation and chemotherapy. *Ann. Surg.*, **236** (1), 75–81.

96 Francois, Y., Nemoz, C.J., Baulieux, J., *et al.* (1999) Influence of the interval between preoperative radiation therapy and surgery on downstaging and on the rate of sphincter-sparing surgery for rectal cancer: the Lyon R90-01 randomized trial. *J. Clin. Oncol.*, **17** (8), 2396.

97 Wang, C.C., Schulz, M.D. (1962) The role of radiation therapy in the management of carcinoma of the sigmoid, rectosigmoid, and rectum. *Radiology*, **79**, 1–5.

98 O'Connell, M.J., Childs, D.S., Moertel, C.G., *et al.* (1982) A prospective controlled evaluation of combined pelvic radiotherapy and methanol extraction residue of BCG (MER) for locally unresectable or recurrent rectal carcinoma. *Int. J. Radiat. Oncol. Biol. Phys.*, **8** (7), 1115–1119.

99 Brierley, J.D., Cummings, B.J., Wong, C.S., *et al.* 91995) Adenocarcinoma of the rectum treated by radical external radiation therapy. *Int. J. Radiat. Oncol. Biol. Phys.*, **31** (2), 255–259.

100 Allee, P.E., Tepper, J.E., Gunderson, L.L., Munzenrider, J.E. (1989) Postoperative radiation therapy for incompletely resected colorectal carcinoma. *Int. J. Radiat. Oncol. Biol. Phys.*, **17** (6), 1171–1176.

101 Schild, S.E., Martenson, J.A., Jr, Gunderson, L.L., Dozois, R.R. (1989) Long-term survival and patterns of failure after postoperative radiation therapy for subtotally resected rectal adenocarcinoma. *Int. J. Radiat. Oncol. Biol. Phys.*, **16** (2), 459–463.

102 Ghossein, N.A., Samala, E.C., Alpert, S., *et al.* (1981) Elective postoperative radiotherapy after incomplete resection of colorectal cancer. *Dis. Colon Rectum*, **24** (4), 252–256.

103 Emami, B., Pilepich, M., Willett, C., Munzenrider, J.E., Miller, H.H. (1982) Effect of preoperative irradiation on resectability of colorectal carcinomas. *Int. J. Radiat. Oncol. Biol. Phys.*, **8** (8), 1295–1299.

104 Dosoretz, D.E., Gunderson, L.L., Hedberg, S., *et al.* (1983) Preoperative irradiation for unresectable rectal and rectosigmoid carcinomas. *Cancer*, **52** (5), 814–818.

105 Mendenhall, W.M., Million, R.R., Bland, K.I., Pfaff, W.W., Copeland, E.M., 3rd (1987) Initially unresectable rectal adenocarcinoma treated with preoperative irradiation and surgery. *Ann. Surg.*, **205** (1), 41–44.

106 Whiting, J.F., Howes, A., Osteen, R.T. (1993) Preoperative irradiation for unresectable carcinoma of the rectum. *Surg. Gynecol. Obstet.*, **176** (3), 203–207.

107 Marsh, P.J., James, R.D., Schofield, P.F. (1994) Adjuvant preoperative radiotherapy for locally advanced rectal carcinoma. Results of a prospective, randomized trial. *Dis. Colon Rectum*, **37** (12), 1205–1214.

108 Braendengen, M., Tveit, K.M., Berglund, A., *et al.* (2008) Randomized phase III study comparing preoperative radiotherapy with chemoradiotherapy in nonresectable rectal cancer. *J. Clin. Oncol.*, **26** (22), 3687–3694.

109 Valentini, V., Coco, C., Rizzo, G., *et al.* (2009) Outcomes of clinical T4M0 extra-peritoneal rectal cancer treated with preoperative radiochemotherapy and surgery: a prospective evaluation of a single institutional experience. *Surgery*, **145** (5), 486–494.

110 Kim, H.K., Jessup, J.M., Beard, C.J., *et al.* (1997) Locally advanced rectal carcinoma: pelvic control and morbidity following preoperative radiation therapy, resection, and intraoperative radiation therapy. *Int. J. Radiat. Oncol. Biol. Phys.*, **38** (4), 777–783.

111 Roeder, F., Treiber, M., Oertel, S., *et al.* (2007) Patterns of failure and local control after intraoperative electron boost radiotherapy to the presacral space in combination with total mesorectal excision in patients with locally advanced rectal cancer. *Int. J. Radiat. Oncol. Biol. Phys.*, **67** (5), 1381–1388.

112 Kusters, M., Holman, F.A., Martijn, H., *et al.* (2009) Patterns of local recurrence in locally advanced rectal cancer after intra-operative radiotherapy containing multimodality treatment. *Radiother. Oncol.*, **92** (2), 221–225.

113 Nakfoor, B.M., Willett, C.G., Shellito, P.C., Kaufman, D.S., Daly, W.J. (1998) The impact of 5-fluorouracil and intraoperative electron beam radiation therapy on the outcome of patients with locally advanced primary rectal and rectosigmoid cancer. *Ann. Surg.*, **228** (2), 194–200.

114 Mathis, K.L., Nelson, H., Pemberton, J.H., Haddock, M.G., Gunderson, L.L. (2008) Unresectable colorectal cancer can be cured with multimodality therapy. *Ann. Surg.*, **248** (4), 592–598.

115 Krempien, R., Roeder, F., Oertel, S., *et al.* (2006) Long-term results of intraoperative presacral electron boost radiotherapy (IOERT) in combination with total mesorectal excision (TME) and chemoradiation in patients with locally advanced rectal cancer. *Int. J. Radiat. Oncol. Biol. Phys.*, **66** (4), 1143–1151.

116 Gunderson, L.L., Sosin, H. (1974) Areas of failure found at reoperation (second or symptomatic look) following 'curative surgery' for adenocarcinoma of the rectum. Clinicopathologic correlation and implications for adjuvant therapy. *Cancer*, **34** (4), 1278–1292.

117 Hruby, G., Barton, M., Miles, S., Carroll, S., Nasser, E., Stevens, G. (2003) Sites of local recurrence after surgery, with or without chemotherapy, for rectal cancer: implications for radiotherapy field design. *Int. J. Radiat. Oncol. Biol. Phys.*, **55** (1), 138–143.

118 Guerrero Urbano, M.T., Henrys, A.J., Adams, E.J., *et al.* (2006) Intensity-modulated radiotherapy in patients with locally advanced rectal cancer reduces volume of bowel treated to high dose levels. *Int. J. Radiat. Oncol. Biol. Phys.*, **65** (3), 907–916.

119 Zietman, A.L., DeSilvio, M.L., Slater, J.D., *et al.* (2005) Comparison of conventional-dose vs high-dose conformal radiation therapy in clinically localized adenocarcinoma of the prostate: a randomized controlled trial. *JAMA*, **294** (10), 1233–1239.

120 Freedman, G.M., Meropol, N.J., Sigurdson, E.R., *et al.* (2007) Phase I trial of preoperative hypofractionated intensity-modulated radiotherapy with incorporated boost and oral capecitabine in locally advanced rectal cancer. *Int. J. Radiat. Oncol. Biol. Phys.*, **67** (5), 1389–1393.

121 Twelves, C., Wong, A., Nowacki, M.P., *et al.* (2005) Capecitabine as adjuvant treatment for stage III colon cancer. *N. Engl. J. Med.*, **352** (26), 2696–2704.

122 Twelves, C., Gollins, S., Grieve, R., Samuel, L. (2006) A randomised cross-over trial comparing patient preference for oral capecitabine and 5-fluorouracil/leucovorin regimens in patients with advanced colorectal cancer. *Ann. Oncol.*, **17** (2), 239–245.

123 Andre, T., Boni, C., Mounedji-Boudiaf, L., *et al.* (2004) Oxaliplatin, fluorouracil, and leucovorin as adjuvant treatment for colon cancer. *N. Engl. J. Med.*, **350** (23), 2343–2351.

124 Saltz, L.B., Cox, J.V., Blanke, C., *et al.* (2000) Irinotecan plus fluorouracil and leucovorin for metastatic colorectal cancer. Irinotecan Study Group. *N. Engl. J. Med.*, **343** (13), 905–914.

125 Van Cutsem, E., Kohne, C.H., Hitre, E., *et al.* (2009) Cetuximab and chemotherapy as initial treatment for metastatic colorectal cancer. *N. Engl. J. Med.*, **360** (14), 1408–1417.

126 Hurwitz, H., Fehrenbacher, L., Novotny, W., *et al.* (2004) Bevacizumab plus irinotecan, fluorouracil, and leucovorin for metastatic colorectal cancer. *N. Engl. J. Med.*, **350** (23), 2335–2342.

127 Das, P., Lin, E.H., Bhatia, S., *et al.* (2006) Preoperative chemoradiotherapy with capecitabine versus protracted infusion 5-fluorouracil for rectal cancer: a matched-pair analysis. *Int. J. Radiat. Oncol. Biol. Phys.*, **66** (5), 1378–1383.

128 Gerard, J.P., Azria, D., Gourgou-Bourgade, S., *et al.* (2010) Comparison of two neoadjuvant chemoradiotherapy regimens for locally advanced rectal cancer: results of the phase III trial ACCORD 12/0405-Prodige 2. *J. Clin. Oncol.*, **28** (10), 1638–1644.

129 Aschele, C., Cionini, L., Lonardi, S., *et al.* (2011) Primary tumor response to preoperative chemoradiation with or without oxaliplatin in locally advanced rectal cancer: pathologic results of the STAR-01 randomized phase III trial. *J. Clin. Oncol.*, **29** (20), 2773–2780.

130 Willett, C.G., Duda, D.G., di Tomaso, E., *et al.* (2009) Efficacy, safety, and biomarkers of neoadjuvant bevacizumab, radiation therapy, and fluorouracil in rectal cancer: a multidisciplinary phase II study. *J. Clin. Oncol.*, **27** (18), 3020–3026.

131 Marijnen, C.A., van de Velde, C.J., Putter, H., *et al.* (2005) Impact of short-term preoperative radiotherapy on health-related quality of life and sexual functioning in primary rectal cancer: report of a multicenter randomized trial. *J. Clin. Oncol.*, **23** (9), 1847–1858.

132 Peeters, K.C., van de Velde, C.J., Leer, J.W., *et al.* (2005) Late side effects of short-course preoperative radiotherapy combined with total mesorectal excision for rectal cancer: increased bowel dysfunction in irradiated patients – a Dutch colorectal cancer group study. *J. Clin. Oncol.*, **23** (25), 6199–6206.

133 Kollmorgen, C.F., Meagher, A.P., Wolff, B.G., Pemberton, J.H., Martenson, J.A., Illstrup, D.M. (1994) The long-term effect of adjuvant postoperative chemoradiotherapy for rectal carcinoma on bowel function. *Ann. Surg.*, **220** (5), 676–682.

134 Dahlberg, M., Glimelius, B., Graf, W., Pahlman, L. (1998) Preoperative irradiation affects functional results after surgery for rectal cancer: results from a randomized study. *Dis. Colon Rectum*, **41** (5), 543–549; discussion 549–551.

135 Birgisson, H., Pahlman, L., Gunnarsson, U., Glimelius, B. (2005) Occurrence of second cancers in patients

treated with radiotherapy for rectal cancer. *J. Clin. Oncol.*, **23** (25), 6126–6131.

136 Letschert, J.G., Lebesque, J.V., Aleman, B.M., *et al.* (1994) The volume effect in radiation-related late small bowel complications: results of a clinical study of the EORTC Radiotherapy Cooperative Group in patients treated for rectal carcinoma. *Radiother. Oncol.*, **32** (2), 116–123.

137 Green, N. (1983) The avoidance of small intestine injury in gynecologic cancer. *Int. J. Radiat. Oncol. Biol. Phys.*, **9** (9), 1385–1390.

138 Eifel, P.J., Levenback, C., Wharton, J.T., Oswald, M.J. (1995) Time course and incidence of late complications in patients treated with radiation therapy for FIGO stage IB carcinoma of the uterine cervix. *Int. J. Radiat. Oncol. Biol. Phys.*, **32** (5), 1289–1300.

139 Song, D.Y., Lawrie, W.T., Abrams, R.A., *et al.* (2001) Acute and late radiotherapy toxicity in patients with inflammatory bowel disease. *Int. J. Radiat. Oncol. Biol. Phys.*, **51** (2), 455–459.

140 Willett, C.G., Ooi, C.J., Zietman, A.L., *et al.* (2000)Acute and late toxicity of patients with inflammatory bowel disease undergoing irradiation for abdominal and pelvic neoplasms. *Int. J. Radiat. Oncol. Biol. Phys.*, **46** (4), 995–998.

141 Lin, A., Abu-Isa, E., Griffith, K.A., Ben-Josef, E. (2008) Toxicity of radiotherapy in patients with collagen vascular disease. *Cancer*, **113** (3), 648–653.

142 Aschele, A., Pinto, C., Cordio, S., *et al.* (2009) Preoperative fluorouracil (FU)-based chemoradiation with and without weekly oxaliplatin in locally advanced rectal cancer: pathologic response analysis of the Studio Terapia Adiuvante Retto (STAR)-01 randomized phase III trial. *J. Clin. Oncol.*, **27** (170 Suppl.), abstract CRA4008.

143 Gallagher, M.J., Brereton, H.D., Rostock, R.A., *et al.* (1986) A prospective study of treatment techniques to minimize the volume of pelvic small bowel with reduction of acute and late effects associated with pelvic irradiation. *Int. J. Radiat. Oncol. Biol. Phys.*, **12** (9), 1565–1573.

144 Mendenhall, W.M., Morris, C.G., Rout, W.R., *et al.* (2001) Local excision and postoperative radiation therapy for rectal adenocarcinoma. *Int. J. Cancer*, **96** (Suppl.), 89–96.

145 Cedermark, B., Johansson, H., Rutqvist, L.E., Wilking, N. (1995) The Stockholm I trial of preoperative short term radiotherapy in operable rectal carcinoma. A prospective randomized trial. Stockholm Colorectal Cancer Study Group. *Cancer*, **75** (9), 2269–2275.

25

Anal Cancer

Brian G. Czito, Manisha Palta and Christopher G. Willett

Anatomy, Histology, and Epidemiology

The anal canal extends from the anorectal ring (the palpable muscle bundle formed by the junction of the puborectalis, distal longitudinal bowel, upper internal sphincter and deep external sphincter musculature) distally to the anal verge (the mucocutaneous junction). The skin radiating 5 cm out from the anal verge is often called the *anal margin*, a term which has also been applied to the distal anal canal, creating confusion in the literature. Although the canal spans only 4–5 cm in most people, it is a heterogeneous structure, arbitrarily divided by the dentate line near its mid aspect. The dentate line is not a true 'line' *per se* but an endoscopically visible zone of epithelial transition, where the anal glands empty into the lumen of the canal. Above the dentate line, transitional epithelium evolves into the glandular rectal mucosa superiorly.

A variety of malignancies arise within the anal canal; these can be divided into squamous and non-squamous tumors. Squamous cell tumors are the most common cell type. Histologic descriptions such as basaloid/cloacogenic/junctional (tumors arising in the transitional mucosa of the proximal canal described above) are not clinically relevant distinctions and thus not included in the current World Health Organization (WHO) classification system for anal cancer. Tumors arising in this area are considered squamous cell tumors (generally non-keratinizing), whereas tumors below the dentate line are often keratinizing squamous cell carcinomas. Non-squamous cell tumors are rare and include adenocarcinomas, melanomas, lymphomas, and sarcomas. A suspected anal adenocarcinoma is often an extension from a distal rectal adenocarcinoma. True adenocarcinomas of the anal canal have a different clinical biology than squamous cell carcinoma and usually are managed similar to rectal adenocarcinomas. Ultimately, tumor location within the anal canal is not as important as histological subtype. Anatomically, lymphatic and vascular drainage above the dentate line is to the superior and middle rectal veins and lymphatics, ultimately flowing into the periaortic/portal system. In contrast, lymphatics of the distal canal generally flow to inguinofemoral vasculature and nodal basins, ultimately draining systemically. There are extensive interconnections of lymphatics within the anal canal allowing for 'cross-drainage'.

Squamous cell anal canal tumors are uncommon, with approximately 8200 new cases annually in the United States [1], though the incidence has increased steadily in recent years. Epidemiological investigations have identified risk factors associated with development of squamous cell anal tumors. An increased number of sexual partners has been associated with a higher risk of developing anal cancer. In a large case-control series, an increasing number of sexual partners was associated with development of anal cancer in both women and men (odds ratio of 4.5 for women and 2.5 for men with ≥10 sexual partners) [2]. Studies have also demonstrated that a history of anal condyloma and receptive anal intercourse in women was associated with a higher risk of developing anal cancer [3]. Similarly, a prior history of cervical and genital malignancies has also been found to be associated with a higher risk of anal cancer [4,5]. These data strongly suggest the role of a sexually transmitted factor in anal cancer carcinogenesis. A clear association between viral infection with certain subtypes of human papillomavirus (HPV) and the development of preinvasive and invasive squamous cell anal DNA has been delineated [2,6,7]. As with cervical cancer, there are certain subtypes of HPV (primarily HPV-16/18) commonly found in the cells of malignant lesions. The relationship between high-risk HPV subtype infection and subsequent malignant cellular transformation is well studied in squamous cell carcinomas of the uterine cervix, and women with cervical cancer are also at increased risk of developing squamous cell anal cancer compared to the

Clinical Radiation Oncology: Indications, Techniques, and Results, Third Edition. Edited by William Small Jr.
© 2017 John Wiley & Sons, Inc. Published 2017 by John Wiley & Sons, Inc.

general population [4]. HPV infection can lead to a progression from preinvasive (anal intraepithelial neoplasia; AIN) to frankly invasive tumors [8].

Other independent risk factors include non-HIV-related chronic immunosuppression and cigarette smoking [9–11]. Patients receiving immunosuppressive therapy following renal transplantation are at increased risk of developing anal cancer. In one study, there was an approximately 100-fold increased risk of developing anogenital cancer in patients who were recipients of kidney transplants. In another series, patients receiving chronic steroid therapy for the amelioration of autoimmune effects were also found to be predisposed to HPV-associated anogenital tumor formation. Immunosuppression may prevent effective immune responses to HPV and also hinder anti-tumor immunity. Cigarette smoking is also associated with the development of anal cancer [12]. The risk of anal cancer appears to be higher with an increased pack–year history of smoking. The etiologic association of smoking to anal cancer is unclear, but it may act as a co-carcinogen with HPV infection [13].

The association between HIV and the development of anal cancer is controversial. HIV may facilitate the development of anal cancer in HPV-positive patients [8,14]. In one series, patients who were HPV-positive and simultaneously HIV-positive had a higher risk of developing AIN and anal cancer compared to those who were HIV-negative. In a separate analysis, patients with low CD4+ T-cell counts were more likely to demonstrate progression from AIN to invasive disease.

Diagnosis

Histologic confirmation of malignancy by tissue biopsy is required prior to any therapy. Staging involves categorizing the local extent of primary and nodal disease as well as an assessment of distant metastases. Digital and endoscopic examinations of the anus and rectum, in addition to palpation of the inguinal region, is necessary to delineate the extent of gross tumor. Positron emission tomography-computed tomography (PET-CT) is now also routinely integrated into the staging algorithm for these patients [15–17]. In one series, PET-CT had a higher sensitivity than conventional imaging (CT and/or magnetic resonance imaging; MRI) in detecting regional lymph node metastases (89% versus 62%), although for practical reasons not all nodes could be biopsied for a true measure of sensitivity and specificity. Additionally, PET imaging results in a modification of planned radiation therapy fields in 13% of patients and should be included in staging [17]. Of note, HIV-positive patients may have falsely positive fluorodeoxyglucose (FDG)-avid lymph nodes. Biopsy may be necessary in these situations to determine whether or not there is true nodal involvement. The role of PET-CT is discussed further below.

Historical Treatment of Squamous Cell Carcinoma of the Anal Canal

Historically, the treatment for localized squamous cell carcinoma of the anal canal entailed abdominoperineal resection (APR), leading to removal of the anorectum and creation of a permanent colostomy. APR results in high rates of urinary/sexual dysfunction, wound morbidity and additional perioperative morbidity and mortality. Studies on the management of anal cancer with APR alone have reported five-year survival rates of 30% to 71%, with local regional recurrence rates in between 19% and 60% of patients. A series from the Mayo Clinic showed that local recurrence following APR occurred in approximately 30% of patients [18].

Because of the inferior results achieved with APR, Nigro (a surgeon from Wayne State University) and coinvestigators treated three patients with preoperative radiation therapy (30 Gy) concurrently with continuous infusional 5-fluorouracil (5-FU) and mitomycin, followed by APR. The surgical specimens of two patients showed no evidence of residual disease, whereas a third patient refused surgery and remained disease-free [19]. Later experience from this group and others confirmed high rates of clinical and pathologic complete response using preoperative chemoradiotherapy and surgery [20–24]. These results led to further trials evaluating radiation therapy alone or combined chemoradiotherapy as 'definitive', nonsurgical therapy.

Current Treatment of Anal Canal Squamous Cell Carcinoma

The contemporary treatment of anal cancer is founded on the results of multiple randomized trials. Because high rates of local control and disease-free survival could be achieved with radiation therapy alone, the role of chemotherapy in the 'definitive' management of this disease was less clear. To address this, the United Kingdom Coordinating Committee on Cancer Research (UKC-CCR) Anal Canal Trial Working Party performed the ACT I study, randomizing 585 patients with anal cancer to receive either 45 Gy of radiation therapy alone or with concurrent chemotherapy (continuous infusion 5-FU weeks 1 and 5 and mitomycin week 1). Patients with a good clinical response following a six-week break received a 'boost' dose of radiation therapy, while poor responders underwent salvage surgery [25]. Local control was significantly enhanced in the combined modality therapy group (64% versus 41%, p < 0.0001), with a significant improvement in anal cancer-related mortality (28% versus 39%, p = 0.02) in concurrently treated patients. However, the three-year overall survival was not different between the arms (65% versus 58%, p = 0.25). The authors concluded that patients with squamous cell carcinoma of the anal canal can be treated with radiation therapy, 5-FU and mitomycin, with surgery reserved for salvage. After a 13-year follow-up, no differences were reported in long-term morbidity rates, although an excess in non-anal cancer deaths was seen in the chemoradiotherapy group during the first ten years following treatment (cardiovascular, treatment-related, pulmonary disease and second malignancies). Locoregional failure rates remained significantly lower in patients treated with chemoradiotherapy (25% absolute difference at 12 years), with a corresponding improvement in relapse-free survival (12% absolute at 12 years). Although not statistically significant, an absolute improvement in 12-year survival of 5.6% was seen in the combined modality cohort [25a].

Similarly, a study by the European Organization for Research and Treatment of Cancer (EORTC) randomized 110 patients to radiation therapy alone (45 Gy) followed by a 'boost' radiation dose (dose depending on response) versus the same regimen plus 5-FU in weeks 1 and 5 and mitomycin in week 1. As in the ACT I study, patients undergoing combined modality therapy had a significant improvement in local control, colostomy-free and progression-free survival rates. No significant survival difference was seen between the groups (three-year survival 72% versus 65%, p = 0.17) [26].

A third randomized trial from the United States conducted by the Radiation Therapy Oncology Group (RTOG) and Eastern Cooperative Oncology Group (ECOG) evaluated the role of mitomycin in this treatment regimen. Mitomycin has potentially severe toxicities, including thrombocytopenia, leucopenia, pulmonary toxicity, nephrotoxicity and hemolytic-uremic syndrome. A total of 310 patients was randomized to receive radiation therapy (45–50.4 Gy) with infusional 5-FU in week 1 versus the same regimen with an infusion of mitomycin in weeks 1 and 5. Patients with biopsy-proven residual disease following combined therapy were eligible to receive additional pelvic radiation therapy (9 Gy) with 5-FU and cisplatin chemotherapy. The four-year colostomy-free and disease-free survival rates were significantly higher in patients receiving 5-FU/mitomycin compared to 5-FU alone. No difference in overall survival was observed between the treatment arms. Grade 4/5 toxicities (primarily related to neutropenia and sepsis) were significantly higher in patients receiving mitomycin. Of 24 patients with positive post-treatment biopsy, half were rendered disease-free by 'salvage' chemoradiotherapy [27]. These results were confirmed after a five-year follow-up [27a].

An important caveat to these trials is that there may be a long period of tumor regression for anal malignancies after chemoradiotherapy (up to one year). There are reports noting that many patients with biopsy-positive disease following combined modality therapy will experience long-term disease-free survival with no additional therapy. Historically, in the absence of overt disease progression, it is generally recommended that patients should not be biopsied for at least three months following treatment completion. In the recent ACT II study (see below), mandated time-points for clinical tumor response occurred at 11 and 18 weeks, and by CT imaging at 24 weeks. Preliminary trial results showed that an assessment of complete response at 11 weeks was able to discriminate between patients achieving (versus not) clinical complete response for progression-free survival (PFS) and overall survival (OS) [27b]. Hazard ratios indicate that assessment at 26 weeks significantly predicts outcome, and is an appropriate tumor assessment time point. This is supported by the fact that only 83 of 265 patients not achieving a clinical response at week 11 ultimately experienced progression/persistent disease.

In comparing anal cancer trials, it is important to recognize that the dose of mitomycin has not been standardized. The aforementioned RTOG/ECOG trial used a dose of 10 mg/m^2 in weeks 1 and 5, while European trials have used a single 12–15 mg m^2 dose of mitomycin on day 1. Retrospective studies have failed to demonstrate that two doses are more effective in terms of clinical outcome than a single dose, although two doses are associated with significant increases in acute hematologic and skin toxicity [27c].

In summary, the results of these randomized trials showed that combined modality therapy with radiation therapy, 5-FU and mitomycin results in long-term disease-free survival and sphincter preservation in the majority of patients with anal cancer and superior outcomes relative to radiation therapy alone or radiation therapy combined with 5-FU alone, albeit at the expense of higher treatment-related morbidity.

Given the significant toxicities associated with mitomycin and the role of cisplatin-based chemoradiotherapy in squamous cell carcinoma of other sites (head and neck, esophageal and cervical cancers), there has been interest in substituting cisplatin for mitomycin in the combined modality treatment of anal cancer. Phase I and II trials from the United States and Europe using this strategy have reported high rates of local control and disease-free survival, with acceptable toxicity. Based on these data, RTOG investigators initiated the 98-11 trial, randomizing 682 patients to receive radiation therapy (45–59 Gy) with continuous-infusion 5-FU and bolus mitomycin in weeks 1 and 5, or a regimen of continuous-infusion 5-FU and bolus cisplatin in weeks 1, 5, 9, and 13, with radiation (45–59 Gy) starting in week 9 (i.e., a 'neoadjuvant' chemotherapy-alone approach). The rate of Grade 3+ hematologic toxicity was higher in patients receiving mitomycin (61% versus 42%, p < 0.001). On initial report, no significant difference was seen in the five-year disease-free survival (60% versus 54%, p = 0.17), overall survival (75% versus 70%, P = 0.10) or local-regional relapse (25% versus 33%, p = 0.07) rates. However, the five-year colostomy rate was 10% in patients receiving mitomycin compared to 19% in the cisplatin arm (p = 0.02) [28–30]. An update of these results, however, demonstrated a significant improvement in disease-free survival (67.7% versus 57.6%, p = 0.005), overall survival (78.2% versus 70.5%, p = 0.02), and colostomy-free survival (71.8% versus 64.9%, p = 0.05) in favor of mitomycin-based chemoradiotherapy [31].

A Phase III trial conducted by the UKCCR (the ACT II study) more directly compared cisplatin to mitomycin with radiation therapy [32]. In this largest of anal cancer randomized studies, 950 patients were randomized to the same radiotherapy regimen (50.4 Gy in 1.8-Gy fractions) with either concurrent 5-FU and cisplatin versus 5-FU and mitomycin, followed by a second randomization to receive two cycles of adjuvant 5-FU/cisplatin or no further therapy following the completion of chemoradiation. Grade 3-4 acute non-hematologic toxicity rates were similar (60% versus 65%, p = 0.17) between arms, but grade 3 and higher hematologic toxicity rates were higher in the mitomycin group (25% versus 13%, p < 0.001). Complete clinical response at six months (the trial primary endpoint) was not significantly different between the two groups. At a median follow up of 5.1 years, clinical complete response at 26 weeks was 91% in the mitomycin group compared to 90% in the cisplatin group, while the three-year colostomy rate was similar between the two groups (14% mitomycin versus 11% cisplatin). Additionally, the use of maintenance therapy in this trial showed no benefit, with three-year recurrence-free survival of 75% in both arms with similar overall survival rates between the maintenance compared to the non-maintenance groups (85% versus 84%). The authors concluded that, given similar efficacy and toxic effects, fewer cycles of chemotherapy, fewer non-chemotherapy drugs, less time in the chemotherapy suite, less expense, and no risk of neuropathy compared with cisplatin, mitomycin given concurrently with 5-FU and radiation therapy should remain the standard in the treatment of anal cancer, and that there is no role for maintenance chemotherapy following definitive chemoradiotherapy.

In summary, the results of published randomized trials to date show that the standard of care for anal cancer remains radiation therapy combined with 5-FU and mitomycin. A summary of randomized studies is presented in Tables 25.1 and 25.2. As discussed in later sections, recent technologic advances in radiation therapy,

as well as interest in examining less toxic but more active chemotherapy regimens, are currently directing future treatment approaches of this disease.

Perianal Skin Tumors

Tumors arising from the perianal skin may be managed as skin tumors. Treatment options for squamous cell tumors of the perianal skin include local excision with or without adjuvant radiation, or radiation therapy with or without chemotherapy. Chapet *et al.* reviewed their experience of 26 patients with tumors of the perianal skin (five patients also had involvement of the anal canal). Of the tumors identified, 21 were ≤5 cm in diameter. Fourteen patients were treated with definitive radiation (with or without chemotherapy) and 12 with radiation after initial local excision. The initial crude local control rate was 61.4% (16/26), but after salvage surgical treatment this increased to 80.8%. The five-year cause-specific survival was 88.3% [33]. Khanfir *et al.* reported similar results in their experience with 45 patients, 29 of whom underwent local excision followed by postoperative radiation therapy. The five-year local-regional control was 78%, and five-year disease-free survival 86% [34]. Balamucki *et al.* updated the University of Florida experience of definitive radiotherapy and chemoradiotherapy for squamous cell tumors of the perianal skin by treating 26 patients, two of whom developed local recurrence of disease and two of whom developed regional nodal recurrence. The ten-year cause-specific survival was 92%. Of note, two patients with clinically node-negative disease who did not receive prophylactic inguinal nodal irradiation developed groin recurrences [35].

Although small perianal skin tumors without adverse histologic features may be treated with local excision alone or radiation-alone based approaches, the authors' general approach to larger lesions and/or tumors with adverse histologic features (i.e., factors increasing the likelihood of lymphatic spread) is to treat with combination chemoradiotherapy, similar to tumors of the anal canal.

Imaging

The introduction of PET and subsequent PET-CT has improved the staging and treatment of patients with anal cancer. PET-detected nodal metastases occurred in 17–24% of patients judged to have clinically uninvolved lymph nodes by CT [15,16]. In the absence of PET, these sites would usually receive 'subclinical' doses of radiation therapy (as compared to higher doses used to treat gross disease), thus leading to underdosage and potentially predisposing patients to pelvic failure. In a recent series of patients with anorectal cancer

Table 25.1 Summary of randomized Phase III clinical trials of chemoradiotherapy for anal cancer.

Study/Reference	Treatment arms*	Local regional failure**	Relapse-free survival**	Colostomy-free survival**	Overall survival**
UKCCCR/ACT I [25a]	1) Radiation versus 2) Radiation + 5-FU + MMC	1) 57% 2) 32%	1) 34% 2) 47%	1) 37% 2) 47%	1) 53% 2) 58% P = NS
EORTC [26]	1) Radiation versus 2) Radiation + 5-FU + MMC	1) 50% 2) 32%	Estimated improvement of 18% in disease-free survival	1) 40% 2) 72%	1) 54% 2) 58% P = 0.17
RTOG/ECOG [27, 27a]	1) Radiation + 5-FU versus 2) Radiation + 5-FU + MMC	1) 34% 2) 16%	1) 51% 2) 73% (disease-free survival at 4 years)	1) 59% 2) 71% (at 4 years)	1) 71% 2) 78% (at 4 years) P = NS
RTOG 98-11 [31]	1) Radiation + 5-FU + MMC versus 2) Cisplatin + 5-FU → Radiation + 5-FU + Cisplatin	1) 20% 2) 26% P = 0.09	1) 68% 2) 58% (disease-free survival at 5 years)	1) 12% 2) 17% (Cumulative incidence of colostomy) P = 0.08	1) 78% 2) 71% (at 5 years)
UKCCCR/ ACT II [32]	1) Radiation + 5-FU + MMC versus 2) Radiation + 5-FU + Cisplatin Versus 3) Radiation + 5-FU + MMC→ Cisplatin/5FU 4) Radiation + 5-FU + Cisplatin→ Cisplatin/5FU	NS	69% MMC 69% CisP P = 0.63 70% maintenance 69% no maintenance P = 0.7	1) 75% 2) 72% 3) 73% 4) 75% P = NS (at 3 years)	1) 86% 2) 84% 3) 82% 4) 83% P = NS (at 3 years)
ACCORD 3 [48]	1) 5-FU + cisplatin → RT + 5-FU + cisplatin versus 2) 5-FU + cisplatin →high-dose RT + 5-FU + cisplatin versus 3) Same as 1) but without induction therapy versus 4) Same as 2) but without induction therapy	1) 28% 2) 12% 3) 16% 4) 22% P = NS	1) 64% 2) 78% 3) 67% 4) 62% P = NS (tumor-free survival at 5 years)	1) 70% 2) 82% 3) 77% 4) 73% P = NS	No difference when analyzed by induction chemotherapy or high-dose boost delivery

*Details of treatment arms noted in text.
**p-values significant for comparisons unless otherwise noted.
RT, radiotherapy.

Table 25.2 Summary of conclusions from selected randomized trials in anal cancer.

Trial (Reference)	Tested therapies	Results
UKCCCR [25,25a] EORTC [26]	1) RT versus 2) RT + 5-FU + MMC	Addition of chemotherapy to radiation therapy improves local disease control, relapse-free and colostomy-free survival.
RTOG/ECOG [27, 27a]	1) RT + 5-FU versus 2) RT + 5-FU + MMC	Although associated with more toxicity, addition of MMC improves local disease control, relapse-free and colostomy-free survival.
RTOG 98-11 [31]	1) Cisplatin/5-FU followed by RT + 5-FU + cisplatin versus 2) RT + 5-FU + MMC	Induction cisplatin/5-FU associated with lower overall, disease-free and colostomy-free survival.
ACT II [32]	1) RT + 5-FU + MMC versus 2) RT + 5-FU + cisplatin Additional randomization to no further therapy or maintenance 5-FU and cisplatin	Results show equivalent regimens with respect to disease control; differing toxicities. No benefit to maintenance chemotherapy.
ACCORD 03 [48]	1) 5-FU + cisplatin followed by RT + 5-FU + cisplatin versus 2) 5-FU + cisplatin followed by high-dose RT + 5-FU + cisplatin versus 3) Same as 1) but without induction therapy versus 4) Same as 2) but without induction therapy	Induction chemotherapy and higher radiation dose do not improve disease-related outcomes.
EORTC 22011-40014 (closed prematurely) [47]	RT + MMC + 5-FU versus RT + MCC + cisplatin	Higher response rates in the MMC-cisplatin treated patients albeit with lower compliance rates.

MMC, mitomycin-C; RT, radiation therapy.

undergoing PET-CT-based radiation planning, one-fourth of patients had PET-detected metastases resulting in a change in overall patient management and modification of radiation volumes [36]. Similarly, a report from Hamburg evaluating pre-therapy PET staging in anal cancer patients revealed that radiotherapy fields were changed in 23% of patients undergoing contrasted PET-CT versus CT or PET scanning alone [37]. Another report from the Curie Hospital evaluating the role of PET-CT scanning showed that 36% of patients had a change in stage as a result of contrast-enhanced PET/CT compared to either study alone, suggesting a complementary role of both imaging modalities [38]. Therefore, it is the present authors' practice to obtain contrast enhanced PET-CT scans for patients with anal cancer as part of their initial staging evaluation.

In assessing response to therapy, Curie Hospital investigators also showed that the sensitivity and specificity of PET in detecting persistent or recurrent disease was 93% and 81%, respectively, impacting management in 20% of patients [38]. Other studies have also suggested that patients achieving less than a complete metabolic response following combined modality therapy may experience inferior disease-related outcomes [39,40]. The role of PET in this disease remains an active area of investigation.

Time Factors and Novel Chemotherapeutic Approaches

As discussed previously, the results of the RTOG 98-11 trial have not supported the use of 'induction' chemotherapy, possibly due to the protracted duration of treatment. In many cancers the overall duration of treatment influences clinical outcomes. In anal cancer, a Phase II dose-escalation trial conducted by the RTOG mandating a two-week treatment break showed inferior outcomes compared to historical controls [41]. Similarly, other institutional experiences have reported that patients with prolonged treatment duration were more likely to suffer disease failure [42]. An analysis of two randomized

RTOG trials showed a significant association between overall treatment duration and colostomy failure, local failure, regional failure and time-to-failure rates. On multivariate analysis, a significant association with local failure and statistical trend toward an association with colostomy failure and overall treatment duration were seen. The authors concluded that prolonged treatment time may have a detrimental effect on local failure and colostomy rate in anal cancer patients [43]. The inferior results with induction chemotherapy may be due to the development of a tumor clonogen 'accelerated repopulation', which occurs as treatments progress, and the role of neoadjuvant chemotherapy in upregulating pathways that confer radioresistance remains unknown [44–46].

As opposed to the previously discussed RTOG and ACT II trials that evaluated cisplatin as a potential substitute for mitomycin, cisplatin has also been studied as an alternative to 5-FU, maintaining mitomycin in the treatment regimen. The EORTC closed (prematurely) a randomized Phase II/III trial (EORTC 22001/400014) comparing mitomycin plus weekly cisplatin given concurrently with radiation therapy versus mitomycin and continuous infusion 5-FU during the entire radiation course given concurrently with radiation therapy. The initial radiation course consisted of 36 Gy delivered over four weeks, followed by a two-week break, followed by an additional 23.4 Gy given over 2.5 weeks, with concurrent chemotherapy delivered during both radiation sessions [47]. The Phase II trial results reported increased high-grade hematologic toxicity rates in the mitomycin + cisplatin group, with impaired treatment compliance. However, overall response rates (at eight weeks following therapy completion) were higher in patients treated with mitomycin + cisplatin. In an even more intensive chemotherapeutic regimen, a United Kingdom Act II pilot study suggested that the use of triple-drug combination of mitomycin, 5-FU and cisplatin was poorly tolerated and associated with significant morbidity, prohibiting this regimen to be taken into a subsequent randomized Phase III trial [47a].

In the French Federation Nationale des Centres de Lutte Contre le Cancer ACCORD 03 trial [48], patients were randomized to one of four following study arms:

1) Neoadjuvant 5-FU and cisplatin alone followed by combined therapy with 5-FU and cisplatin (radiation dose 45 Gy). Patients then underwent a scheduled treatment break followed by additional radiation to a dose of 15 Gy delivered as a boost.
2) As in arm '1' with a boost dose of 20–25 Gy depending on the initial response.
3) As in arm '1' but without a neoadjuvant chemotherapy component.
4) As in arm '2' but without a neoadjuvant chemotherapy component.

The results of this study showed that at a median follow-up of 50 months, the five-year colostomy-free survival (CFS) rates were 69.6%, 82.4%, 77.1%, and 72.7%, respectively. The five-year CFS was 76.5% versus 75.0% (P = 0.37) for groups 1 and 2 versus groups 3 and 4, respectively (i.e., neoadjuvant chemotherapy versus not), and 73.7% versus 77.8% in groups 1 and 3 versus groups 2 and 4 (i.e., standard radiation dose boost versus high-dose boost (P = 0.067). The authors concluded that neither neoadjuvant chemotherapy nor high-dose boost improved CFS rates, although there was a trend towards an improved CFS in the high-dose boost group. Hence, they recommended arm 2 for further investigation (see Tables 25.1 and 25.2).

Several clinical trials have been conducted examining other agents beyond 5-FU, cisplatin and mitomycin. In a Phase II trial from the United Kingdom, capecitabine, an oral 5-FU prodrug, was combined with mitomycin in 31 anal cancer patients. Of these patients, 18 completed treatment as planned with low rates of high-grade diarrhea and neutropenia. At one month, 24 patients had achieved a complete clinical response, and at a median follow-up of 14 months three local regional relapses had occurred. The authors concluded that capecitabine, mitomycin and radiation therapy is well tolerated in anal carcinoma patients, and should be studied in future national Phase III studies in anal cancer [49]. Investigators from the MD Anderson Hospital conducted a Phase II study of capecitabine and oxaliplatin combined with radiation therapy in patients with stage II–III anal cancer. The radiation dose was prescribed based on the T-stage of the tumor. Capecitabine was delivered twice daily on weekdays, and oxaliplatin was (initially) given weekly. When five of 11 patients developed high-grade diarrhea, the protocol was modified to eliminate chemotherapy during weeks 3 and 6. Among the nine patients enrolled in the modified protocol, one patient developed grade 3 diarrhea. At a median follow-up of 19 months there were no local recurrences, and one patient experienced distant failure of disease [50].

The French Federation Nationale des Centres de Lutte Contre le Cancer also conducted a multi-institutional Phase II study of chemoradiotherapy (65 Gy + cisplatin + 5-FU) combined with cetuximab in patients with locally advanced anal cancer. A preliminary report of this trial detailed trial suspension due to a high number of serious adverse events following treatment of the initial patient cohort. This prompted a 5-FU/cisplatin dose reduction and the implementation of intensity-modulated radiotherapy (IMRT) techniques. Despite this, an additional cohort of patients experienced significant toxicities that included neutropenia, diarrhea, fatigue, rash and thrombocytopenia, with three patients experiencing severe long-term toxicity including radionecrosis and colostomy placement for fistula formation. The study was later closed due to high rates of toxicity and insufficient efficacy [51]. The AIDS Associated Malignancies Clinical Trials Consortium is conducting a Phase II trial combining cisplatin, 5-FU and the anti-epidermal growth factor receptor monoclonal antibody cetuximab with radiation therapy in HIV-positive patients with anal cancer. Similarly, the ECOG is also conducting a Phase II trial using a similar regimen in non-HIV patients. Preliminary safety and efficacy results were presented in immunocompetent (ECOG 3205, *n* = 28) and HIV+ (AMC045, *n* = 45) patients with non-metastatic squamous cell carcinoma of the anal canal [51a]. The PFS and overall survival rates at two years were 80% and 89% for HIV-positive patients, compared to 92% and 93%, respectively for HIV-negative patients. The Grupo Espanol Multidisciplinario del cancer Digestivo in Spain is conducting a Phase II trial to assess the efficacy and safety of chemoradiation with 5-FU, mitomycin and the anti-epidermal growth factor receptor monoclonal antibody panitumumab. Similarly, a Phase II trial from Switzerland is recruiting patients to evaluate the outcomes and toxicities of panitumumab/capecitabine/mitomycin-C with concurrent IMRT. The results of these and other studies may further refine the optimal chemotherapy regimen, toxicities and sequencing in the treatment of this disease, particularly for more advanced lesions.

Radiation Therapy

Although the addition of chemotherapy increases acute toxicity, radiotherapy contributes to significant acute and late toxicities. Dermatologic, hematologic, genitourinary and gastrointestinal toxicities are often experienced by patients during a course of chemoradiotherapy due to the irradiation of a significant amount of perianal and genital skin, bone, pelvic bone marrow, bladder, and bowel. Severe acute toxicity results in treatment breaks, leading to a protracted treatment course and potentially compromising chemoradiotherapy antitumor efficacy [41,42]. As noted above, an analysis of the two randomized RTOG trials confirmed that shorter, more intense radiation courses were associated with a reduction in colostomy rates [43].

Radiation therapy in early studies was based on 2-dimensional (2D)-based planning, where known anatomic (bony) landmarks guide field design using orthogonal x-ray images. Since the late 1980s, however, conformal (CT-guided or three-dimensional; 3D) radiotherapy-based treatments have allowed the radiation oncologist to identify normal as well as target structures on axial CT images, facilitating improved treatment accuracy and delivery. These techniques use 'uniform' fields for radiation therapy delivery, inclusive of a significant amount of perianal/genital skin, pelvic

bone/bone marrow, bladder and bowel. Beginning in the late 1990s, IMRT was introduced and involves the 3D identification of normal pelvic organs as well as target structures, including the primary disease and draining lymph nodes. In 3D-based planning the physician designs treatment fields based on a 'beams-eye view' of the target volumes and normal structures (i.e., fields are designed as if one were inside the machine looking into the patient). In IMRT-based planning, strict radiation dose constraints to normal organs are established, doses prescribed to different target volumes, and computer software 'inverse planning' algorithms are used to design unconventional treatment fields which would not otherwise be possible with standard planning methods. Importantly, IMRT involves the partitioning of a given radiation field into multiple smaller fields, which can occur in the form of dynamic IMRT (in which collimating 'leaves' or blocks move across an active radiation field using highly specific leaf sequences) or 'step-and-shoot' IMRT (in which leaves sculpt the field shape while the beam is off). The end result of these approaches is that the intensity of the radiation beam for any one field varies. Similarly, the approach of volumetric-modulated arc therapy (VMAT) involves a technique that implements intensity-modulated techniques in the setting of continuous gantry rotation. When these IMRT fields are summed, the cumulative effect is a radiation dose-distribution that closely conforms the radiation dose around the target volumes while significantly reducing the dose to surrounding normal tissues. An example of IMRT-based treatment in a case of anal cancer is shown in Figure 25.1. The advantage of IMRT techniques is the reduction in normal tissue irradiation and thereby also in chronic radiation-related toxicities.

Clinical studies of IMRT-based therapy of anal cancer have reported a significant reduction in acute treatment-related toxicity (primarily bowel- and skin-related) with similar disease-related outcomes versus historical controls using 2D and 3D planning [52,53]. RTOG investigators completed a prospective, Phase II study (RTOG 0529) combining 5-FU, mitomycin and IMRT-based radiotherapy. Of note is that this trial (as opposed to some reported series) used a 'dose-painting' approach whereby the primary/elective nodal planning target volumes (PTVs) as well as involved lymph nodes received differing radiation doses (synchronously) using differing doses per fraction, based on absolute size. The primary goal of this study was to determine the feasibility of this approach in a cooperative group setting, as well as to determine treatment-related toxicity and preliminary disease-related outcomes in these patients. In comparing toxicity outcomes to patients treated in the RTOG 9811 study (described previously), where conventional radiation planning was used, rates of ≥Grade 3 dermatologic toxicity were superior in the IMRT study (23% versus

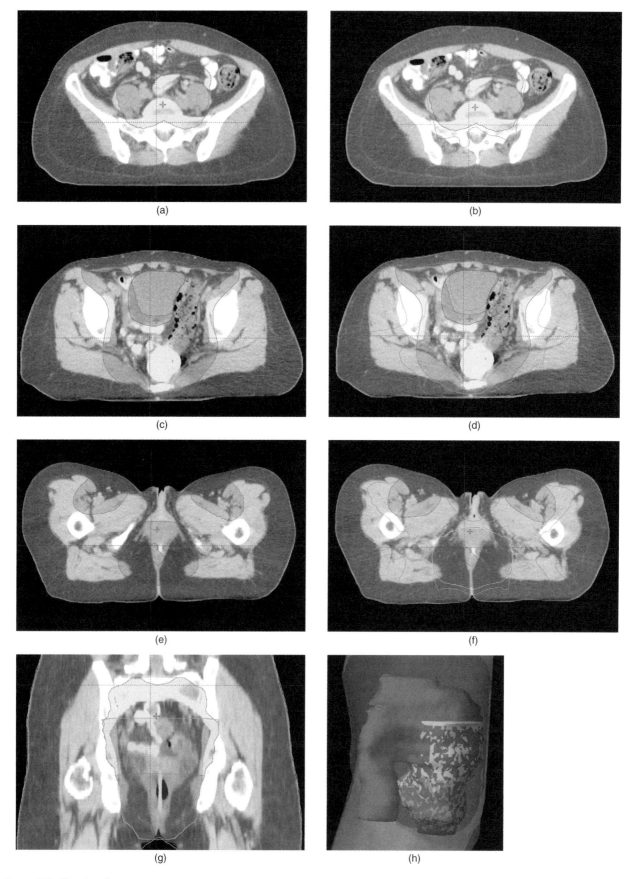

Figure 25.1 (*Continued*)

49%, p <0.001), as were rates of ≥grade 3 gastrointestinal and genitourinary toxicity (21% versus 37%, p = 0.0052). Although 77% of patients experienced ≥Grade 2 gastrointestinal/genitourinary adverse events, there was a significant reduction in ≥Grade 2 hematologic, ≥Grade 3 gastrointestinal, and ≥Grade 3 dermatologic toxicity relative to the mitomycin-containing arm of RTOG 98-11. The authors concluded that although the primary endpoint of reduction of ≥Grade 2 combined acute gastrointestinal/genitourinary adverse events was not met, significant toxicity sparing could be achieved [54]. A disease outcomes update of this study showed that this approach also yielded similar two-year disease-related outcomes compared to RTOG 9811 [55, 55a].

One of the most challenging aspects of treating patients with IMRT is the accurate definition of target volumes. With IMRT, there are very precise and conformal high-dose regions enveloping target volumes with a steep dose gradient. If a target/desired treatment volume is not accurately defined, there is risk of underdosing disease resulting in clinical failure [56]. Knowledge of patterns of failure and routes of spread are important. Along these lines, real-time quality assurance was performed in RTOG 0529, and a secondary endpoint was whether or not IMRT could be performed in a broader, multi-institutional setting. On an initial pretreatment review, 81% of patients in this trial required replanning using a dose-painting IMRT approach. This illustrates the challenge of implementing this new and complex planning technique in a cooperative group setting, and the importance of knowledge of target design using these advanced technologies in this often-curable malignancy.

Radiation Therapy Planning

Although many techniques have been described in the treatment of anal cancer, the present authors' general approach in the treatment of squamous cell carcinoma of the anal canal and perianal skin is to use IMRT. Patients are generally instructed to arrive for CT simulation with 'bladder-full', as well as during treatment. Alternatively, patients can undergo simulation with both full and empty bladder with subsequent scan fusion. Patients are usually immobilized in the supine position in a customized immobilization device, although some advocate prone positioning on a false tabletop to facilitate small-bowel sparing, frequently using a 'frog leg' position bilaterally as permitted by the CT bore diameter. Any palpable lymphadenopathy is demarcated using radio-opaque markers, as is any disease extending outside of the anal verge that may be visible on physical examination. Additionally, a marker is placed at the anal verge and a rectal tube inserted with instillation of anorectal contrast. Alternatively, patients can undergo simulation with and without rectal contrast with subsequent scan fusion. Similarly, intravenous contrast is administered, preferably during the arterial phase of the CT scan. Based on reviews of the patient's pre-simulation imaging studies, if there is a concern of potential underdosing of the inguinal lymph node basins, bolus may be placed over the inguinal regions at the time of CT scanning (in some patients this may be unnecessary using IMRT techniques). Although bolus material can be considered for disease extending onto the perianal skin, the above immobilization technique frequently facilitates 'self-bolus' such that additional bolus in the perianal region may not be necessary. In males, the genitalia are positioned midline at simulation and treatment. A radio-opaque vaginal cylinder may be used at simulation in female patients, although these devices may displace the posterior vaginal wall and immediately adjacent anal canal, thereby altering the normal anatomy in this region. Alternatively, smaller radio-opaque markers may be used to minimize such displacement. A report from the M.D. Anderson investigators evaluated placement of a vaginal dilator at simulation, and treatment showed that the dilator tended to be inserted more inferiorly during treatment than simulation, although this did not compromise tumor coverage and could potentially allow for improved genital sparing [56a]. The CT scan is usually performed using 2.5- to 5-mm slice intervals.

Once images are downloaded into the treatment planning system, normal organs are outlined including femoral heads, genitalia, large and small bowel, and bladder. A gross tumor volume (GTV) is defined, based on physical examination, endoscopy and imaging studies. This would include the primary sites of disease as well as

Figure 25.1 A 48-year-old female with clinical T2 N0 squamous cell carcinoma of the proximal anal canal. She received concurrent 5-FU and mitomycin-based chemoradiotherapy using IMRT techniques with serial PTV reductions. (a) Axial CT slice of the patient; the PTV 3060 is shown in red. (b) Corresponding image with the isodose line superimposed (pink line = 3060 cGy). (c) More inferior axial slice with PTV 3060 shown in red and bladder outlined in green. (d) Corresponding isodose lines. Note the relative sparing of the bladder anteriorly and femoral heads laterally. Pink isodose line = 3060 cGy; blue isodose line = 4500 cGy. (e) PTV 3060 shown more inferiorly. Note the centrally located GTV adjacent to the rectal tube. (f) The same image with relative isodoses superimposed from the IMRT plan. The patient was treated with a series of sequential PTV reductions. Note the relative sparing of the genitalia anteriorly and the proximal femora laterally. Pink isodose line = 3060 cGy; blue isodose line = 4500 cGy; yellow isodose line = 5400 cGy. (g) Sequential PTV reductions in the treatment of anal cancer. Red = PTV 3060; green = PTV 4500; blue = PTV 5400. (h) Lateral view of sequential PTVs. Red = PTV 3060; green = PTV 4500; blue = PTV 5400. For a color version of this figure, see the color plate section.

locoregional nodal involvement by physical examination, imaging, and biopsy. Subsequently, a clinical target volume (CTV) can be constructed, encompassing the GTV volume(s) as well as regions thought to be at high risk for harboring occult, micrometastatic disease. In anal cancer, this would include the mesorectal and presacral space nodal basins, as well as internal (obturator) and external iliac regions, extending out into the inguinofemoral basins. Subsequently, a planning target volume (PTV) is created, encompassing the CTV and accounting for uncertainties in patient position, physiologic variation in organ location, and so forth. It should be noted that the PTV volumes are individualized on a case-by-case basis depending on the extent of disease, individual patient anatomy, proximity of target to adjacent normal tissues, imaging frequency, and so forth. It should again be emphasized that target definition using this technique is of paramount importance. These volumes should be made as conformal as reasonably possible by reproducible positioning of patients with immobilization devices as above, as well as the frequent use of image-guidance technology (KV imaging, cone beam CT) to ascertain patient alignment immediately prior to treatments. In addition, there may be select situations in which extensive disease involvement/target uncertainty may prevent the dose-distribution advantages seen with IMRT.

Although a variety of techniques exists, the present authors' preferred technique includes the creation of an initial PTV encompassing the aforementioned targets/nodal basins, extending up to approximately the L5/S1 level. Subsequently, a second PTV is created, which generally involves only nodal basins in the 'true' pelvis (below the inferior sacroiliac joint). This, however, is dependent on the extent of nodal involvement. In clinically node-negative patients, the authors generally treat the initial PTV to a dose of 30.6 Gy, although others have treated these volumes to a dose of 45 Gy. Thereafter, a reduced PTV is treated to a total dose of 45 Gy, usually exclusive of inguinofemoral nodal basins

in patients without evidence of nodal metastases. Finally, a third PTV (encompassing areas of gross disease alone with margin) is treated to a total dose of 54 Gy.

Following the completion of volume delineation, strict dose constraints and prescription doses are defined and IMRT-treatment planning carried out. During this process, it is important that normal tissue tolerances be respected, including small and large bowel, femoral heads, genitalia, and bladder. During planning the necessity of inguinal (and sometimes perianal) bolus is determined on a case-by-case basis. Although a 'fixed gantry' IMRT technique is frequently implemented, in selected situations volumetric arc therapy may be used in the interest of decreasing treatment time, assuming equivalence to static-field therapy. Once planning is completed, analysis of adequacy of target coverage, normal tissue doses (including dose–volume histogram analysis) and dose heterogeneity is carried out. Once a satisfactory plan is generated, the patient initiates radiation with the simultaneous delivery of 5-FU and mitomycin-based chemotherapy. As above, it is imperative that patients undergo accurate daily treatment set-up, including the use of image guidance.

In addition to the above, close monitoring of the patient's clinical status during treatments in conjunction with the treating medical oncologist is paramount given the significant treatment-related toxicities encountered with the use of combined modality therapy in this disease. Patients have basic blood counts evaluated on at least a weekly basis. Additionally, close monitoring for symptoms related to decreased blood counts as well as skin, urinary and gastrointestinal tract irritation should be performed. Symptoms should be addressed promptly with aggressive treatment/supportive measures of side effects implemented, including the use of dietary modifications, analgesics, appropriate skin care, hydration, and chemotherapy-dose modification. It is the present authors' general policy to try to avoid treatment breaks where possible and to complete the treatment in a continuous fashion.

References

1 Siegel, R., Miller, K., Jemal, A. (2017) Cancer Statistics 2017. *CA Cancer J. Clin.*, **67**, 7–30.

2 Frisch, M., Glimelius, B., van den Brule, A.J., *et al.* (1997) Sexually transmitted infection as a cause of anal cancer. *N. Engl. J. Med.*, **337**, 1350–1358.

3 Daling, J.R., Weiss, N.S., Hislop, T.G., *et al.* (1987) Sexual practices, sexually transmitted diseases, and the incidence of anal cancer. *N. Engl. J. Med.*, **317**, 973–977.

4 Melbye, M., Sprogel, P. (1991) Aetiological parallel between anal cancer and cervical cancer. *Lancet*, **338**, 657–659.

5 Rabkin, C.S., Biggar, R.J., Melbye, M., Curtis, R.E. (1992) Second primary cancers following anal and cervical carcinoma: evidence of shared etiologic factors. *Am. J. Epidemiol.*, **136**, 54–58.

6 Bjorge, T., Engeland, A., Luostarinen, T., *et al.* (2002) Human papillomavirus infection as a risk factor for anal and perianal skin cancer in a prospective study. *Br. J. Cancer*, **87**, 61–64.

7 Daling, J.R., Madeleine, M.M., Johnson, L.G., *et al.* (2004) Human papillomavirus, smoking, and sexual practices in the etiology of anal cancer. *Cancer*, **101**, 270–280.

8 Palefsky, J.M., Holly, E.A., Ralston, M.L., Jay, N. (1998) Prevalence and risk factors for human papillomavirus infection of the anal canal in human immunodeficiency virus (HIV)-positive and HIV-negative homosexual men. *J. Infect. Dis.*, **177**, 361–367.

9 Penn, I. (1986) Cancers of the anogenital region in renal transplant recipients. Analysis of 65 cases. *Cancer*, **58**, 611–616.

10 Arends, M.J., Benton, E.C., McLaren, K.M., *et al.* (1997) Renal allograft recipients with high susceptibility to cutaneous malignancy have an increased prevalence of human papillomavirus DNA in skin tumours and a greater risk of anogenital malignancy. *Br. J. Cancer*, **75**, 722–728.

11 Sillman, F.H., Sedlis, A. (1991) Anogenital papillomavirus infection and neoplasia in immunodeficient women: an update. *Dermatol. Clin.*, **9**, 353–369.

12 Holly, E.A., Whittemore, A.S., Aston, D.A., *et al.* (1989) Anal cancer incidence: genital warts, anal fissure or fistula, hemorrhoids, and smoking. *J. Natl Cancer Inst.*, **81**, 1726–1731.

13 Sood, A.K. (1991) Cigarette smoking and cervical cancer: meta-analysis and critical review of recent studies. *Am. J. Prev. Med.*, **7**, 208–213.

14 Sobhani, I., Vuagnat, A., Walker, F., *et al.* (2001) Prevalence of high-grade dysplasia and cancer in the anal canal in human papillomavirus-infected individuals. *Gastroenterology*, **120**, 857–866.

15 Trautmann, T.G., Zuger, J.H. (2005) Positron emission tomography for pretreatment staging and posttreatment evaluation in cancer of the anal canal. *Mol. Imaging Biol.*, **7**, 309–313.

16 Cotter, S.E., Grigsby, P.W., Siegel, B.A., *et al.* (2006) FDG-PET/CT in the evaluation of anal carcinoma. *Int. J. Radiat. Oncol. Biol. Phys.*, **65**, 720–725.

17 Winton, E., Heriot, A.G., Ng, M., *et al.* (2009) The impact of 18-fluorodeoxyglucose positron emission tomography on the staging, management and outcome of anal cancer. *Br. J. Cancer*, **100**, 693–700.

18 Boman, B.M., Moertel, C.G., O'Connell, M.J., *et al.* (1984) Carcinoma of the anal canal. A clinical and pathologic study of 188 cases. *Cancer*, **54**, 114–125.

19 Nigro, N.D., Vaitkevicius, V.K., Considine, B., Jr (1974) Combined therapy for cancer of the anal canal: a preliminary report. *Dis. Colon Rectum*, **17**, 354–356.

20 Buroker, T.R., Nigro, N., Bradley, G., *et al.* (1977) Combined therapy for cancer of the anal canal: a follow-up report. *Dis. Colon Rectum*, **20**, 677–678.

21 Michaelson, R.A., Magill, G.B., Quan, S.H., *et al.* (1983) Preoperative chemotherapy and radiation therapy in the management of anal epidermoid carcinoma. *Cancer*, **51**, 390–395.

22 Nigro, N.D., Seydel, H.G., Considine, B., *et al.* (1983) Combined preoperative radiation and chemotherapy for squamous cell carcinoma of the anal canal. *Cancer*, **51**, 1826–1829.

23 Leichman, L., Nigro, N., Vaitkevicius, V.K., *et al.* (1985) Cancer of the anal canal. Model for preoperative adjuvant combined modality therapy. *Am. J. Med.*, **78**, 211–215.

24 Meeker, W.R., Jr, Sickle-Santanello, B.J., Philpott, G., *et al.* (1986) Combined chemotherapy, radiation, and surgery for epithelial cancer of the anal canal. *Cancer*, **57**, 525–529.

25 UK Co-ordinating Committee on Cancer Research (1996) Epidermoid anal cancer: results from the UKCCCR randomised trial of radiotherapy alone versus radiotherapy, 5-fluorouracil, and mitomycin. UKCCCR Anal Cancer Trial Working Party. *Lancet*, **348**, 1049–1054.

25a Northover, J., Glynne-Jones, R., Sebag-Montefiore, D., *et al.* (2010) Chemoradiation for the treatment of epidermoid anal cancer: 13-year follow-up of the first randomised UKCCCR Anal Cancer Trial (ACT I). *Br. J. Cancer*, **103**, 1123–1128.

26 Bartelink, H., Roelofsen, F., Eschwege, F., *et al.* (1997) Concomitant radiotherapy and chemotherapy is superior to radiotherapy alone in the treatment of locally advanced anal cancer: results of a phase III randomized trial of the European Organization for Research and Treatment of Cancer Radiotherapy and Gastrointestinal Cooperative Groups. *J. Clin. Oncol.*, **15**, 2040–2049.

27 Flam, M., John, M., Pajak, T.F., *et al.* (1996) Role of mitomycin in combination with fluorouracil and radiotherapy, and of salvage chemoradiation in the definitive nonsurgical treatment of epidermoid carcinoma of the anal canal: results of a phase III randomized intergroup study. *J. Clin. Oncol.*, **14**, 2527–2539.

27a John, M., Flam, M., Berkley, B., *et al.* (1998) Five year results and analyses of a phase III randomised RTOG/ECOG chemoradiation protocol for anal cancer. *Proc. Am. Soc. Clin. Oncol.*, **17**, abstract 989.

27b Glynne-Jones, R., James, R., Meadows, H., *et al.* (2012) Optimum time to assess complete clinical response (CR) following chemoradiation (CRT) using mitomycin (MMC) or cisplatin (CisP), with or without maintenance CisP/5FU in squamous cell carcinoma of the anus: Results of ACT II. *J. Clin. Oncol.*, **30** (Suppl.), abstract 4004.

27c Yeung, R., McConnell, Y., Roxin, G., *et al.* (2012) One versus 2 cycles of mitomycin C in concurrent chemoradiation for treatment of anal canal carcinoma: an analysis of outcomes and toxicity. *Int. J. Radiat. Oncol. Biol. Phys.*, **84** (3S), S351, abstract 2355.

28 Ajani, J.A., Winter, K.A., Gunderson, L.L., *et al.* (2008) Fluorouracil, mitomycin, and radiotherapy vs

fluorouracil, cisplatin, and radiotherapy for carcinoma of the anal canal: a randomized controlled trial. *JAMA*, **299**, 1914–1921.

29 Ajani, J.A., Winter, K.A., Gunderson, L.L., *et al.* (2006) Intergroup RTOG 98-11: a phase III randomized study of 5-fluorouracil (5-FU), mitomycin, and radiotherapy versus 5-fluorouracil, cisplatin and radiotherapy in carcinoma of the anal canal. *J. Clin. Oncol.*, **24**, 180s.

30 Gunderson, L.L., Winter, K.A., Ajani, J.A., *et al.* (2006) Intergroup RTOG 9811 phase III comparison of chemoradiation with 5-FU and mitomycin vs 5-FU and cisplatin for anal canal carcinoma: impact of disease-free, overall and colostomy-free survival. *Int. J. Radiat. Oncol. Biol. Phys.*, **66**, S24 (abstract).

31 Gunderson, L.L., Winter, K.A., Ajani, J.A., *et al.* (2012) Long-term update of U.S. GI Intergroup RTOG 98-11 phase III trial for anal carcinoma: Comparison of concurrent chemoradiation with 5FU mitomycin versus 5FU cisplatin for disease free and overall survival. *J. Clin. Oncol.*, **30** (35), 4344–4351.

32 James, R.D., Glynne-Jones, R., Meadows, H.M., *et al.* (2013) Mitomycin or cisplatin chemoradiation with or without maintenance chemotherapy for treatment of squamous-cell carcinoma of the anus (ACT II): a randomised, phase 3, open-label, 2 × 2 factorial trial. *Lancet Oncol.*, **14** (6), 516-524.

33 Chapet, O., Gerard, J.P., Mornex, F., *et al.* (2007) Prognostic factors of squamous cell carcinoma of the anal margin treated by radiotherapy: the Lyon experience. *Int. J. Colorectal Dis.*, **22**, 191–199.

34 Khanfir, K., Ozsahin, M., Bieri, S., *et al.* (2008) Patterns of failure and outcome in patients with carcinoma of the anal margin. *Ann. Surg. Oncol.*, **15**, 1092–1098.

35 Balamucki, C.J., Zlotecki, R.A., Rout, W.R., *et al.* (2011) Squamous cell carcinoma of the anal margin: the university of Florida experience. *Am. J. Clin. Oncol.*, **34**, 406–410.

36 Anderson, C., Koshy, M., Staley, C., *et al.* (2007) PET-CT fusion in radiation management of patients with anorectal tumors. *Int. J. Radiat. Oncol. Biol. Phys.*, **69**, 155–162.

37 Bannas, P., Weber, C., Adam, G., *et al.* (2011) Contrast-enhanced [(18)F]fluorodeoxyglucose-positron emission tomography/computed tomography for staging and radiotherapy planning in patients with anal cancer. *Int. J. Radiat. Oncol. Biol. Phys.*, **81** (2), 445–451.

38 Vercellino, L., Montravers, F., de Parades, V., *et al.* (2011) Impact of FDG PET/CT in the staging and the follow-up of anal carcinoma. *Int. J. Colorectal Dis.*, **26**, 201–210.

39 Schwarz, J.K., Siegel, B.A., Dehdashti, F., *et al.* (2008) Tumor response and survival predicted by post-therapy FDG-PET/CT in anal cancer. *Int. J. Radiat. Oncol. Biol. Phys.*, **71**, 180–186.

40 Day, F.L., Link, E., Ngan, S., *et al.* (2011) FDG-PET metabolic response predicts outcomes in anal cancer managed with chemoradiotherapy. *Br. J. Cancer*, **105** (4), 498–504.

41 John, M., Pajak, T., Flam, M., *et al.* (1996) Dose escalation in chemoradiation for anal cancer: preliminary results of RTOG 92-08. *Cancer J. Sci. Am.*, **2**, 205–211.

42 Roohipour, R., Patil, S., Goodman, K.A., *et al.* (2008) Squamous-cell carcinoma of the anal canal: predictors of treatment outcome. *Dis. Colon Rectum*, **51**, 147–153.

43 Ben-Josef, E., Moughan, J., Ajani, J.A., *et al.* (2010) Impact of overall treatment time on survival and local control in patients with anal cancer: a pooled data analysis of Radiation Therapy Oncology Group trials 87-04 and 98-11. *J. Clin. Oncol.*, **28**, 5061–5066.

44 Glynne-Jones, R., Hoskin, P. (2007) Neoadjuvant cisplatin chemotherapy before chemoradiation: a flawed paradigm? *J. Clin. Oncol.*, **25**, 5281–5286.

45 De Ruysscher, D., Pijls-Johannesma, M., Bentzen, S.M., *et al.* (2006) Time between the first day of chemotherapy and the last day of chest radiation is the most important predictor of survival in limited-disease small-cell lung cancer. *J. Clin. Oncol.*, **24**, 1057–1063.

46 Brade, A.M., Tannock, I.F. (2006) Scheduling of radiation and chemotherapy for limited-stage small-cell lung cancer: repopulation as a cause of treatment failure? *J. Clin. Oncol.*, **24**, 1020–1022.

47 Matzinger, O., Roelofsen, F., Mineur, L., *et al.* (2009) Mitomycin C with continuous fluorouracil or with cisplatin in combination with radiotherapy for locally advanced anal cancer (European Organisation for Research and Treatment of Cancer phase II study 22011-40014). *Eur. J. Cancer*, **45**, 2782–2791.

47a Sebag-Montefiore, D., Meadows, H.M., Cunningham, D., *et al.* (2012) Three cytotoxic drugs combined with pelvic radiation and as maintenance chemotherapy for patients with squamous cell carcinoma of the anus (SCCA): long-term follow-up of a phase II pilot study using 5-fluorouracil, mitomycin C and cisplatin. *Radiother. Oncol.*, **104** (2), 155–160.

48 Peiffert, D., Tournier-Rangeard, L., Gérard, J.P., *et al.* (2012) Induction chemotherapy and dose intensification of the radiation boost in locally advanced anal canal carcinoma: Final analysis of the randomized UNICANCER ACCORD 03 Trial. *J. Clin. Oncol.*, **30** (16), 1941–1948.

49 Glynne-Jones, R., Meadows, H., Wan, S., *et al.* (2008) EXTRA – a multicenter phase II study of chemoradiation using a 5 day per week oral regimen of capecitabine and intravenous mitomycin C in anal cancer. *Int. J. Radiat. Oncol. Biol. Phys.*, **72**, 119–126.

50 Eng, C., Chang, G., Das, P., *et al.* (2009) Phase II study of capecitabine and oxaliplatin with concurrent

radiation therapy (XELOX-XRT) for squamous cell carcinoma of the anal canal. *J. Clin. Oncol.*, **15** (Suppl.), abstract 4116.

51 Deutsch, E., Lemanski, C., Paris, E., *et al.* (2011) Cetuximab plus radiochemotherapy in locally advanced anal cancer: Interim results of the French multicenter phase II trial ACCORD16. *J. Clin. Oncol.*, **29** (Suppl.), abstract 4098.

51a Garg, M., Lee, J.Y., Kachnic, L., *et al.* (2012) Phase II trials of cetuximab (CX) plus cisplatin (CDDP), 5-fluorouracil (5-FU) and radiation (RT) in immunocompetent (ECOG 3205) and HIV-positive (AMC045) patients with squamous cell carcinoma of the anal canal (SCAC): Safety and preliminary efficacy results. *J. Clin. Oncol.*, **30** (Suppl.), abstract 4030.

52 Salama, J.K., Mell, L.K., Schomas, D.A., *et al.* (2007) Concurrent chemotherapy and intensity-modulated radiation therapy for anal canal cancer patients: a multicenter experience. *J. Clin. Oncol.*, **25**, 4581–4586.

53 Pepek, J.M., Willett, C.G., Wu, Q.J., *et al.* (2010) Intensity-modulated radiation therapy for anal malignancies: a preliminary toxicity and disease outcomes analysis. *Int. J. Radiat. Oncol. Biol. Phys.*, **78**, 1413–1419.

54 Kachnic, L.A., Tsai, H.K., Coen, J.J., *et al.* (2012) Dose-painted intensity-modulated radiation therapy for anal cancer: a multi-institutional report of acute toxicity and response to therapy. *Int. J. Radiat. Oncol. Biol. Phys.*, **82** (1), 153–158.

55 Kachnic, L., Winter, K.A., Myerson, R., *et al.* (2011) Two-year outcomes of RTOG 0529: A phase II evaluation of dose-painted IMRT in combination with 5-fluorouracil and mitomycin-C for the reduction of acute morbidity in carcinoma of the anal canal. *J. Clin. Oncol.*, **29** (Suppl.), abstract 368.

55a Kachnic, L., Winter, K.A., Myerson, R., *et al.* (2013) RTOG 0529: a phase 2 evaluation of dose-painted intensity modulated radiation therapy in combination with 5-fluorouracil and mitomycin-C for the reduction of acute morbidity in carcinoma of the anal canal. *Int. J. Radiat. Oncol. Biol. Phys.*, **82** (1), 153–158.

56 Wright, J.L., Patil, S.M., Temple, L.K., *et al.* (2010) Squamous cell carcinoma of the anal canal: patterns and predictors of failure and implications for intensity-modulated radiation treatment planning. *Int. J. Radiat. Oncol. Biol. Phys.*, **86** (1), 27-33.

56a Briere, T., Crane, C., Beddar, S., *et al.* (2012) Reproducibility and genital sparing with vaginal dilator used for female anal cancer patients. *Radiother. Oncol.*, **104**, 161–166.

Section 5

Genitourinary Malignancies

Section Editor: Jason A. Efstathiou

26

Bladder Cancer

Phillip J. Gray, William U. Shipley and Jason A. Efstathiou

Incidence and Pathology

Bladder cancer is the fourth most common cancer among men, and 11th among women in the United States, with 79 000 new cases and 17 000 deaths expected to occur in both sexes in 2017 [1]. The incidence of bladder cancer increases with age, and peaks in the seventh decade of life with less than 1% of bladder cancer cases occurring in patients aged under 40 years. The incidence rate among black men is 50% of that in whites; however, the disease often presents at a more advanced stage. Males are affected more than threefold as frequently as females, and this ratio approaches 4:1 in whites. Outside of the US, rates of bladder cancer vary dramatically, with the highest rates occurring in North America and Western Europe. Bladder cancer remains a relatively rare disease in Eastern Europe and Asia, though rates are increasing in most countries [2]. Exposure to toxins such as aniline dyes, nitrites, acrolein, aromatic amines, coal and arsenic have all been associated with an increased risk of bladder cancer, though the most common and important factor remains exposure to cigarette smoke [3–5]. Bladder cancer can be thought of as a wide spectrum of diseases which can roughly be placed into three major categories: non-muscle-invasive; muscle-invasive; and metastatic. The clinical behavior and standard treatment approach varies significantly between these categories and are described in detail in the following sections.

In the US over 90% of bladder cancers are urothelial cell carcinomas (also known as transitional cell carcinoma). Squamous cell carcinoma is the next most common pathologic entity, accounting for about 6% of cases in the US but over 70% of cases in Egypt due to infection with the parasite *Schistosoma haematobium* [6]. Other less-common entities include adenocarcinoma, small-cell carcinoma, giant-cell carcinoma, and lymphoepithe-lioma [7–9]. Macroscopically, urothelial cell carcinomas demonstrate a papillary growth pattern approximately 80% of the time. Solid tumors, which comprise the remaining 20%, are more likely to be high-grade and invasive of the muscularis propria. Tumor grade is an important predictor of clinical behavior in non-muscle-invasive disease, and is typically graded on a three-point scale according to the degree of mitoses, nuclear abnormalities, and cellular atypia. For muscle-invasive disease, however, almost all tumors are high-grade and thus the primary pathologic predictor of tumor aggressiveness is the depth of muscle invasion or invasion beyond the bladder wall. The presence of carcinoma *in situ* (CIS) in isolation is rare and accounts for less than 2% of cases. However, the presence of CIS adjacent to or involving sites distant from invasive lesions occurs in more than half of cases [10]. Travel through draining lymphatics is a common pathway for metastatic spread. First-echelon nodal basins include the perivesical nodes as well as the external and internal iliac chains. Common iliac, para-aortic and paracaval lymph nodes comprise the second echelon. Spread by direct extension into the pelvic side wall, prostate, vagina or rectum is also common. Hematogenous dissemination is most frequently seen in the form of lung and skeletal metastases.

Clinical Evaluation

Painless episodic hematuria is the presenting clinical manifestation in over 80% of patients with bladder cancer. Dysuria, stranguria (pain with straining to urinate), urinary frequency or bladder outlet obstruction should also prompt a thorough evaluation. The initial patient work-up should include voided urine analysis, urinary cytology, and office cystoscopy with biopsy [11]. Number, size, shape and location of tumors should be recorded, as

Clinical Radiation Oncology: Indications, Techniques, and Results, Third Edition. Edited by William Small Jr.
© 2017 John Wiley & Sons, Inc. Published 2017 by John Wiley & Sons, Inc.

well as the presence of any areas suspicious for involvement by CIS. Once a diagnosis of bladder cancer is made, additional work-up should include pelvic computed tomography (CT) and analysis of the upper tract collecting system by ultrasound, CT or magnetic resonance imaging (MRI) techniques. For patients with documented muscle-invasive disease, the work-up should also include chest radiography and a bone scan in the setting of elevated alkaline phosphatase or clinical symptoms.

Endoscopic evaluation and management forms the backbone of the initial treatment for bladder cancer. This should include a bimanual examination which fully characterizes the size and mobility of any palpable lesions in the bladder. Cystoscopy with biopsy of all suspicious areas followed by resection of all visible tumor (if possible) should be performed. This resection should include the muscularis propria, especially if the lamina propria is affected or the tumor is high-grade. If muscle is not seen on the biopsy specimen there should be a strong consideration for repeat resection due to the high risk of residual tumor being present [12, 13]. Upon completion of the endoscopic procedure, a careful diagram should be made showing the location of resected tumors, visibly residual disease, and the results of a second bimanual examination after transurethral resection of the bladder tumor (TURBT). An example of such a diagram for a male patient is shown in Figure 26.1.

The staging of bladder cancer focuses on the depth of tumor invasion, which was classically shown to correlate with the risk of regional lymph node involvement and distant metastases [14]. The TNM (tumor, node metastasis) system last updated by the AJCC in 2017 is shown in Table 26.1 [15].

In clinical practice, however, the depth of invasion based on endoscopic evaluation correlates with that seen on full pathologic analysis at the time of cystectomy in less than 50% of cases [16–18]. It is almost impossible to distinguish superficial versus deep muscle invasion based on TURBT alone. Furthermore, T3 disease is almost never detected at the time of TURBT. An older staging system developed by the Union Internationale Contre Cancer (UICC) is still sometimes used. In this system, patients with minimal residual induration after TURBT are staged as T2, and those with palpable residual induration or a mass are staged as T3 [19].

Treatment Selection

Non-Muscle-Invasive Bladder Cancer

Non-muscle invasive bladder cancers (NMIBCs) of clinical stage Ta, T1 or Tis comprise 70–80% of all newly diagnosed bladder cancer cases. These tumors are usually treated successfully by a variety of conservative (bladder-sparing) techniques. Recurrence after TURBT is common, however, and occurs in 50–70% of patients depending on the tumor grade, size, multifocality and presence of CIS [20–22]. Intravesical therapy is often added based on risk of tumor recurrence or progression which can be calculated with various nomograms [23, 24]. Bacillus Calmette–Guérin is the most common and most effective intravesical agent used for treatment, and has been shown to be superior to several chemotherapy regimens in head-to-head trials [25–27]. A single postoperative instillation of a chemotherapeutic agent (most commonly mitomycin C) is also commonly used and appears to improve the risk of relapse but not progression-free survival [28].

The role of definitive external beam radiotherapy (EBRT) in the treatment of patients with non-invasive bladder cancer is unclear, but is not likely to be beneficial in the majority of patients. Indeed, a multi-institution randomized trial of patients with T1G3 tumors treated with radiotherapy alone showed no benefit over conservative therapy, though in this trial there was no requirement for an up-front aggressive TURBT [29]. This particular subgroup is at high risk for progression to muscle-invasive disease despite appropriate surveillance and intravesical therapy [21]. Typically, for treatment refractory patients, cystectomy is recommended as second-line therapy [30]. However, in a recent study from Erlangen, Germany, a 10-year disease-specific survival rate of over 70% was reported using an approach combining chemotherapy and radiation for patients with high-risk T1 tumors [31]. Retrospective data for patients with T1 tumors failing intravesical therapy is also promising, with a combined modality approach showing similar disease-specific survival rates [32]. Currently, the RTOG is enrolling patients with a history of T1 disease who have failed intravesical therapy on a Phase II trial of combined chemoradiotherapy [33]. The use of interstitial radiation implants also appears effective. A recent publication from the Netherlands using a combination of TURBT, EBRT (3×3.5 Gy or 10×2 Gy) and interstitial radiotherapy in patients with T1G3 disease resulted in a 70% local control rate and a 10-year disease-specific survival rate of 66% [34].

Muscle-Invasive Tumors

Between 20% and 25% of bladder cancers invade the muscularis propria at the time of diagnosis. The most common treatment offered for muscle-invasive bladder cancer (MIBC) remains surgical in the form of radical cystoprostatectomy in men and an anterior exenteration (removal of the bladder, urethra, ventral vaginal wall and uterus) in women. Although this approach remains the standard at many centers unequipped with full multidisciplinary cancer services, organ-preserving

Figure 26.1 Template map for documenting extent of transurethral resection of bladder tumors. For a color version of this figure, see the color plate section.

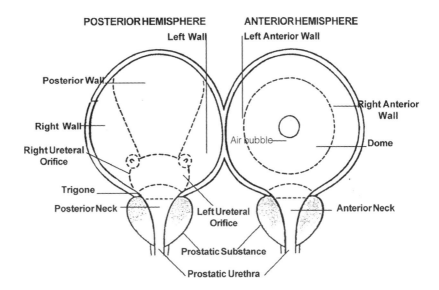

A. **TUMOR LOCATION** <u>**BEFORE TURB.**</u>

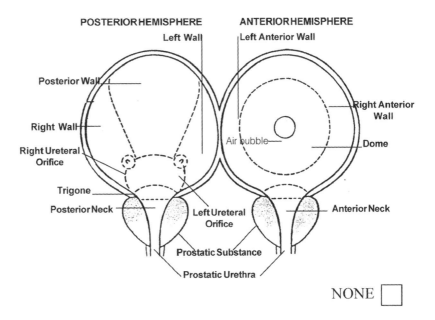

B. <u>**POST-TURB**</u>: IF MACROSCOPIC TUMOR REMAINS AT END OF PROCEDURE, INDICATE ITS LOCATION. IF NOT, CHECK "NONE."

techniques using multiple modality therapy including TURBT, chemotherapy and radiation are emerging as viable alternatives in selected patients. The ultimate goal of any therapy for MIBC should be to maximize post-treatment quality of life while maintaining maximal disease control. Unfortunately, randomized data comparing modern bladder-sparing techniques and radical cystectomy are lacking, and the only randomized controlled trial designed and opened in the UK was closed due to poor accrual [35]. As such, clinicians are left with only retrospective comparisons of these different

modalities. Such comparisons can be problematic for several reasons. First, approximately 5–10% of patients are excluded from cystectomy series because of discovery, at the time of surgery, of previously unidentified extravesicular tumor or lymph node metastases that preclude curative surgical resection. Second, despite advanced imaging, clinical staging still greatly underestimates the extent of disease found at the time of surgery, making comparisons of clinical and pathologic stage extremely difficult [16–18]. Finally, cystectomy patients tend to be younger and in better health than those treated

Table 26.1 Staging of bladder cancer.

Primary Tumor (T)

Ta - non-invasive papillary carcinoma

Tis - carcinoma in situ, 'flat tumor'

T1 - invades subepithelial connective tissue

T2 - invades muscularis propria

T2a - invades superficial muscle (inner half)

T2b - invades deep muscle (outer half)

T3 - invades perivesical tissue

T3a – microscopically

T3b - macroscopically (extravesical mass)

T4 - invades other organs

T4a - invades prostatic stroma, uterus, vagina

T4b - invades pelvic wall, abdominal wall

Regional Lymph Nodes (N)

Nx - Regional lymph nodes cannot be assessed

N0 – none

N1 - single LN metastasis in the true pelvis (below common iliac)

N2 - multiple LN metastases in the true pelvis (below common iliac)

N3 - metastases to the common iliac LNs

Distant Metastases (M)

Mx - Distant metastases cannot be assessed

M0 - No distant metastases

M1 - Distant metastases

M1a - Distant metastasis limited to lymph nodes beyond the common iliacs

M1b - Non-lymph node distant metastases

Source: AJCC Cancer Staging Manual, Eighth Edition (2017), Springer, New York, Inc.

with radiotherapy-based approaches. Despite these limitations, a comparison of modern surgical and chemoradiotherapy cohorts exhibit very similar overall survival outcomes and are listed in Table 26.2.

Surgical Approach

Following radical cystectomy, urinary flow through the ureters must be diverted. The most common and simple technique used to accomplish this is formation of a non-continent ileal conduit. In this procedure, urine flows from the ureters into a segment of isolated ileum to the skin surface, where it is collected from the stoma in an externally worn bag. More complicated continent diversions can be created in the form of an orthotopic neobladder or an abdominal pouch. During these procedures a segment of bowel is formed into a spherical form and connected to a continent catheterizable stoma in the case of a pouch, or to the patient's own urethra in the case of a neobladder. Complications associated with all ileumbased conduits include hyperchloremic metabolic acidosis, risk of sepsis, renal deterioration, and nutrient malabsorption. Such complications appear more commonly in continent diversions compared to non-continent diversions [43]. Relative contraindications of continent diversion include advanced age, intercurrent illness, impaired renal function, inability to prolong surgery by up to 2 h, hydroureter, and inflammatory bowel diseases.

In some patients, radical cystectomy may be considered to carry too much morbidity due to advanced age, poor performance status, or co-morbid disease. As an alternative, a partial cystectomy may be considered in some situations. This procedure requires a solitary lesion located in a region of the bladder that allows for complete excision with a 2-cm margin. Adequate residual bladder tissue must remain after resection to allow for a reasonable bladder capacity. Contraindications to partial cystectomy include multifocality, tumors involving the trigone or bladder neck and those associated with extensive CIS. As such, less than 5% of patients with MIBC undergo partial cystectomy [76]. Furthermore, local recurrence rates exceed 75% in some series [44].

Due to a high rate of occult distant metastases present at the time of cystectomy, which become clinically relevant one to three years following surgery, both the use of adjuvant and neoadjuvant chemotherapy with cystectomy has attracted great attention. Multiple randomized controlled trials of combination neoadjuvant chemotherapy and cystectomy have since been performed, and selected trials are summarized in Table 26.3.

Table 26.2 Large studies of patients treated with radical cystectomy or chemoradiotherapy for muscle-invasive bladder cancer.

Study/Reference	Stage	No. of patients	Accrual period	Median follow-up	5-year OS	10-year OS
Cystectomy						
USC [36]	pT2-4a	633	1971–2001	14.3 years	48%	32%
MSKCC [37]	pT2-4a	300	1990–1993	5.4 years	45%	–
SWOG [38]	cT2-4a	317	1987–1998	8.7 years	49%	34%
Chemo-Radiotherapy						
Erlangen [39]	cT2-4	326	1982–2000	5.0 years	45%	29%
MGH [40]	cT2-4a	348	1986–2006	7.7 years	52%	35%
BC2001 [41]	cT2-4a	182	2001–2008	5.8 years	48%	–
RTOG [42]	cT2-4a	468	1988–2007	4.3 years	57%	36%

Table 26.3 Recent studies of neoadjuvant chemotherapy use in bladder cancer.

Study group/ Reference	Chemotherapy regimen	Patients	Benefit to neoadjuvant therapy
SWOG [38]	MVAC	307	Yes
BA06 [45]	CMV	976	Yes
Italy (Guone) [46]	MVAC	206	No
Italy (GISTV) [47]	MVEC	171	No
Nordic 2 [48]	MC	317	No

C, cisplatin; M, methotrexate; V, vinblastine; A, doxorubicin; E, epirubicin.

The use of adjuvant rather than neoadjuvant chemotherapy has certain theoretical advantages, the greatest of which is providing risk-adapted therapy based on findings at the time of cystectomy. A meta-analysis of 491 patients treated on six adjuvant chemotherapy trials using cisplatin-based chemotherapy has recently been performed [49]. This study found insufficient evidence on which to base reliable treatment decisions for recommendation of adjuvant chemotherapy following cystectomy. Despite this, other studies have identified a survival benefit for patients who receive adjuvant chemotherapy [50]. Many centers favor the use of adjuvant gemcitabine and cisplatin (GC) given its similar efficacy to MVAC (methotrexate, vinblastine, doxorubicin, cisplatin) with an improved toxicity profile, but it has not been rigorously studied in the adjuvant setting [51].

Adjuvant Radiotherapy

If pathologic analysis at the time of cystectomy reveals extensive extravesicular disease or grossly positive margins, a significant risk for pelvic recurrence exists [52]. A recent review of 105 patients treated with radical cystectomy in Canada found an overall two-year actuarial pelvic failure rate of 51% for patients with pT3–T4 disease [53]. Postoperative radiotherapy has been evaluated in a randomized fashion in only a single trial that was performed by the National Cancer Institute of Egypt and randomized 236 patients with T3–T4 tumors to postoperative thrice-daily radiotherapy (37.5 Gy at 1.25 Gy per fraction), standard radiotherapy (50 Gy at 2 Gy per fraction), or observation. The five-year local control rates were 87% and 93% in the radiotherapy arms, respectively, versus 50 % in the observation arm. It is important to note, however, that 68% of the patients in this trial had squamous histology. Given the high associated morbidity, adjuvant therapy should be used selectively with careful attention paid to field size to reduce dose to the small bowel. A recent retrospective study identified pT3 disease or higher as the major predictive factor for pelvic nodal failure, while the only predictor for failure in the cystectomy bed was the presence of positive surgical margins [54]. NRG Oncology will be opening a randomized Phase II trial of adjuvant IMRT for pT3/T4 urothelial cell carcinoma in the near future.

Radiotherapy Alone Compared to Cystectomy

There are four reported randomized Phase III trials of cystectomy with preoperative radiotherapy versus EBRT with cystectomy reserved for salvage in patients with persistent or recurrent bladder cancer. All of these trials were conducted before the availability of cisplatin. These trials are summarized in Table 26.4.

Of these trials, only the one from M.D. Anderson showed a statistically significant survival advantage to immediate cystectomy. It is important to note that this trial included only patients with bulky T3 tumors that were unlikely to be cured with radiotherapy alone. The other three trials described showed no significant survival difference between the two arms. Despite these mixed results these trials are primarily of historic interest as their control and survival rates are somewhat lower than in contemporary cystectomy and multimodality bladder-sparing therapy series.

Table 26.4 Randomized Phase III trials of cystectomy with preoperative radiotherapy versus primary radiotherapy with cystectomy reserved for salvage.

Study/Reference	No. of patients	Period	5-year survival (%)	
			RT + RC	RT + salvage RC
M.D. Anderson [55]	67	1964–1970	46	22
Denmark [56]	183	1970–1977	29	23
Royal Marsden [57]	189	1965–1976	40	28
NBCG	72	1983–1986	27	40

RC, radical cystectomy; RT, radiotherapy.

Bladder-Preserving Approaches with Combined Modality Therapy

Multimodality organ-sparing therapy has become the standard of care for many common malignancies, including carcinoma of the uterine cervix, carcinoma of the anal canal, carcinomas of the head and neck region, and limb sarcomas. In many of these sites a combination of chemotherapy and radiation has been found to be the most beneficial, allowing the patient to be spared the morbidity of more radical surgery. In the case of anal cancer, adoption of the Nigro regimen and a move away from extirpative surgery occurred in the absence of Phase III data [58].

In the case of bladder cancer, chemotherapy as monotherapy achieves a clinical complete response only in 25–37% of patients, and typically only in the setting of lower-stage and smaller tumors (<5 cm) [59–64]. The two-year survival rate in patients treated with chemotherapy alone is approximately 30%. Even in patients who respond, chemotherapy spares the bladder in only 10–20% of cases. Chemotherapy alone is therefore considered inadequate treatment for patients eligible for more definitive therapies.

In appropriately selected patients, bladder-preserving treatment with transurethral resection of tumor, radiation therapy and concurrent chemotherapy offers a probability of long-term cure and overall survival comparable to cystectomy-based approaches (40–60% at five years) in patients of similar clinical stage, age, and comorbidities. In addition, these selective bladder-preserving approaches allow approximately 80% of the long-term survivors to retain normally functioning bladders [65–71]. The rationale for combining chemotherapy and radiation is two-fold. First, certain cytotoxic agents such as cisplatin, 5-fluorouracil (5-FU) and gemcitabine are potent radiosensitizers, thus increasing cell kill in response to a given dose of radiation synergistically. Second, as previously stated, approximately 50% of patients with MIBC harbor occult metastatic disease at the time of diagnosis. Thus, treatment of the primary tumor alone with radical surgery or radiation therapy would be insufficient for this group of patients.

Over the past few decades the Massachusetts General Hospital and the Radiation Therapy Oncology Group have conducted multiple Phase II and III protocols investigating concurrent chemoradiotherapy with or without neoadjuvant or adjuvant chemotherapy. Simultaneously, centers in Erlangen, Germany and Paris, France have evaluated concurrent chemoradiotherapy alone. Chemotherapy agents typically used include platinum and 5-FU combination regimens. A recent study from the University of Michigan also investigated the use of very low-dose gemcitabine (33 mg m^{-2}) with very encouraging preliminary results [72]. A summary of trials with long-term follow-up comprising 1398 patients is provided in Table 26.5.

Recently, a pooled analysis of the 468 patients treated on RTOG trials 8802, 8903, 9506, 9706, 9906, and 0233 has been performed [42]. Of those patients treated, 60.6% had T2 tumors, 29.1% T3a, 6.2% T3b, and 3.9% T4. Complete pathologic response to combined modality therapy

Table 26.5 Studies of bladder-sparing chemoradiotherapy for bladder cancer.

Series	Year	Therapy	No. of patients	5-year overall survival	5-year intact bladder survival
RTOG 8512	1993	EBRT+Cisplatin	42	52	42
RTOG 8802	1996	TURBT, MCV, EBRT+Cisplatin	91	51	44 (4 years)
RTOG 8903	1998	TURBT ± MCV, EBRT+Cisplatin	123	49	38
U. Paris	1997	TURBT, 5-FU, EBRT+Cisplatin	120	63	NR
U. Erlangen	2002	TURBT, EBRT, cisplatin/ carboplatin, 5-FU	415	50	42
RTOG 9506	2000	TURBT, EBRT+Cisplatin/5-FU	34	83% (3y)	83% (3 years)
RTOG 9706	2003	TURBT, EBRT+Cisplatin, MCV	52	61% (3y)	48% (3 years)
RTOG 9906	2008	TURBT, EBRT+Taxol/Cisplatin, Gemcitabine	80	56	47
RTOG 0233	2010	TURBT, EBRT+Taxol/Cisplatin/5FU, Gemcitabine	93	73 (4y)	69 (4 years)
MGH	2012	TURBT ± MCV, EBRT+Cisplatin ± 5FU/Taxol	348	52	45

RTOG, Radiation Therapy Oncology Group; EBRT, external beam radiation therapy; MCV, methotrexate, cisplatin, vinblastine; TURBT, transurethral resection of bladder tumor; 5-FU, 5-fluorouracil; NR, not reported; MGH, Massachusetts General Hospital.

was observed in 72% of patients. With a median follow-up of 4.3 years, the five-year overall survival rate was 57% and the five-year disease-specific survival (DFS) rate was 71%. It is important to note that in this combined analysis 94% of patients had urothelial cell histology. For those patients treated on protocol with variant histology the five-year overall survival (OS) rate was 41% and the five-year DFS rate was 66%. The role for combined modality therapy in the treatment of variant histology bladder cancer is a subject of ongoing investigation.

Similarly, the Massachusetts General Hospital recently updated their long-term experience of bladder-sparing therapy for 348 patients [40]. In this study, 123 of the patients received neoadjuvant chemotherapy. Among patients. 54% had T2 tumors while 38% had T3 and the remainder T4. Some 72% of patients achieved a complete response to induction chemoradiotherapy (78% for those with T2 tumors). At a median follow-up of 7.7 years, the five- and ten-year OS rates were 52% and 35%, respectively, while the five- and ten-year DFS rates were 64% and 59%, respectively. On a univariate Cox regression analysis of factors associated with reduced OS, the clinical stage, completeness of TURBT, hydronephrosis and induction response were all significant predictive factors. On multivariate analysis, only clinical stage and induction response remained significant predictive factors for OS. Despite this, hydronephrosis remains an important factor considered in the discussion of treatment options, as described in the following section. A nomogram now exists to aid clinicians with determining likely response and survival rates in such patients [73].

The use of cisplatin has been a common thread among most of the prospective trials of bladder-sparing therapy in the US. While cisplatin's radiosensitizing ability has been clearly demonstrated in multiple disease sites, it can be a difficult regimen for older patients or those with poor performance status. Additionally, the use of cisplatin requires adequate renal function in order to be used safely. A research group in the UK recently reported their experience using an alternative regimen consisting of 5-FU and mitomycin-C (MMC) concurrently with radiotherapy [41]. In study BC2001, patients were randomized in a 2 × 2 fashion to chemoradiotherapy or radiotherapy alone, and also to standard volume or reduced volume radiotherapy. The radiation dose was 64 Gy in 32 fractions or 55 Gy in 20 fractions. By April 2008, the study had accrued 458 patients, 360 of whom were randomized, while 182 received combined modality therapy. No difference in local recurrence or survival was seen between the arms testing different radiation treatment volumes. At a median follow-up of 69.9 months, the use of chemotherapy significantly improved local recurrence-free survival at two years (67% versus 54%). A significant OS benefit was not seen at five years (48% for combined modality therapy versus 35% for radiation alone). The implications of this study are twofold. First, this is one of only two randomized studies to show the superiority of combined modality therapy over radiotherapy alone (the second being an NCIC study using concurrent cisplatin) [74]. Second, the combination of 5-FU and MMC was well tolerated even by those with poor renal function and poor performance status. Indeed, the median age in BC2001 was much higher than that in the NCIC trial (72 years versus 65 years). As such, this regimen may allow for more inclusive trials of combined modality therapy in the future.

Conclusions

For patients with MIBC, bladder-preserving combined modality therapy in appropriately selected patients (based primarily on the response of the tumor to induction therapy) offers rates of long-term cure and survival comparable to those in patients undergoing immediate cystectomy. Bladder-preserving therapy is not considered suitable for patients with advanced tumors, especially those with tumor-related hydronephrosis. Some 20–30% of patients cured of their MIBC will go on to develop a new NMIBC. Such superficial tumors typically respond well to a combination of TURBT and intravesical therapy. All patients undergoing therapy for non-muscle invasive or muscle-invasive tumors require close urologic surveillance. Bladder-preserving combined modality therapy is not likely to increase the risk of distant metastases if non-responders receive a prompt salvage cystectomy. Bladder-preserving therapy also usually results in a normally functioning bladder without severe urgency, incontinence, or recurrent hematuria. For those patients that do require salvage cystectomy, however, a recent review of the MGH experience indicates that the morbidity associated with such procedures appears low [75]. The ideal candidate for bladder preservation is one with a clinical stage T2 tumor not associated with ureteral obstruction in whom a visibly complete TURBT can be performed. The delivery of multimodality therapy for bladder cancer requires careful cooperation between urologists, medical oncologists and radiation oncologists who are familiar with these techniques. Unfortunately, the utilization of trimodality therapy in the US remains quite low, with many – particularly elderly – patients being offered no definitive therapy [76]. Hence, further education regarding the potential of this therapy among care providers in the US is needed.

Radiotherapy Techniques

Pending validation of the data from the BC2001 trial, the standard approach to radiation delivery in the US involves including the first echelon draining lymphatics while sparing as much normal tissue as possible. This approach requires the use of a modern linear accelerator capable of delivering high-energy photons (10–25 MV) or intensity-modulated radiation therapy (IMRT). The classical treatment program includes the combination of a small pelvic field that includes the aforementioned lymph nodes, the entire bladder and tumor volume, as well as the prostatic urethra which is treated to a dose adequate to control microscopic disease (40–50 Gy using conventional fractionation). The bladder tumor volume is subsequently boosted to raise its total dose to 64–70 Gy, again using conventional fractionation. These treatment volumes are designed at the time of simulation using data from a CT scan of the pelvis, but also with careful reference to the bladder map created at the time of cystoscopy and bimanual examination. Before simulation the patient should be asked to void, at which time the bladder can be scanned or catheterized to check the post-void residual. If desired, 20–30 ml of dilute contrast and air may be introduced into the bladder to aid with planning, but the bladder should not contain more liquid than the patient's measured post-void residual as it is desirable to treat the patient with their bladder as empty as possible so as to minimize day-to-day organ mobility. Contrast in the rectum is not usually necessary, but a rectal tube without contrast may be helpful for anatomic identification. The rectum should be as empty as possible for simulation; an enema may be given prior to simulation to accomplish this. It is vital that the patient be instructed to void his or her bladder before each treatment to ensure proper daily set-up.

The Small Pelvic Field

The clinical target volume (CTV) includes the bladder, the total bladder tumor volume, the proximal urethra (in the male, the entire prostatic urethra) and the lymph nodes immediately adjacent to the bladder such as the distal hypogastric, external iliac, and obturator groups. The field borders for these small pelvic fields extend in the cranial–caudal dimension from the lower pole of the obturator foramen to the mid-sacrum (the anterior aspect of the S2–S3 junction). The field should extend 1.5 cm lateral to the bony margin of the pelvis at its widest point. These fields should have shaped inferior lateral blocks to shield the medial border of the femoral heads. An example of this field is shown in Figure 26.2.

For the lateral fields, the field border should be 2 cm anterior to the most anterior portion of the bladder mucosa, as seen on CT imaging. The field should also extend 2 cm posterior to the most posterior portion of the bladder tumor identified on CT images or information obtained from cystoscopic resection records. The lateral

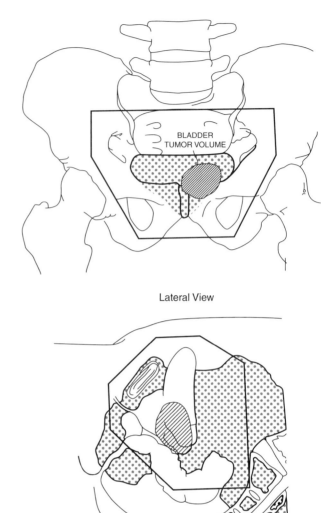

Lateral View

Figure 26.2 Example of a small pelvic field for treatment of bladder cancer.

fields should be shaped inferiorly with corner blocks to shield tissue outside the pubic symphysis anteriorly and to block the entire anal canal posteriorly. Superiorly, the lateral fields should have anterior blocks to exclude any portion of the bowel that lies anterior to the external iliac lymph node groups. Wedges or subfields should be considered for lateral fields if the transverse contour has significant slope or irregularity. Weighting of the AP-PA and lateral fields will depend on the technique chosen for the boost treatment to the bladder tumor volume. Critical structures include the femoral heads, which should not receive more than 45 Gy, and the rectum, which should not receive more than 55 Gy to 50% of its volume (as defined from the anus to the rectosigmoid flexure). If paired lateral fields can be used for the boost it is generally prudent to give one-third of the planned dose to the lateral fields, and the remaining two-thirds to the

AP-PA fields. The use of high-energy photons (>6 MV) to the lateral fields is often useful for reducing hotspots and improving dose conformality. Some anatomic variations may require special adjustments, such as in the case of women with vaginal prolapse where the bladder may extend below the lower border of the obturator foramen. Bladder diverticuli should also be included as part of the target volume. Radiation is typically delivered via the described three-dimensional conformal approach. Currently, more advanced techniques, such as IMRT are gaining favor among many providers. IMRT may be particularly helpful in patients with total hip replacements, which may complicate dose delivery through the lateral fields, and those with a significant amount of small bowel found in the pelvis. Given the high conformality of IMRT, special attention must be paid so that adequate CTV and PTV margins are placed around critical structures such as the bladder and the bladder tumor volume to account for variability in set-up and bladder filling. Ideally, the patient should be treated with image guidance including cone beam CT if available.

Boost Fields to the Bladder Tumor Volume

Boost volumes include the entire bladder mucosa, a defined bladder tumor volume with a 2-cm margin, or a combination of both. The design of the boost volume is derived both from anatomic CT data and from information obtained from the cystoscopy map, selective mucosal biopsies, and the bimanual examination. As with the small pelvis volume, it is vital that the patient void prior to each treatment. The CTV should include the gross tumor volume with a 1.5-cm margin. An additional 0.5 cm should be added to make a total of 2 cm from the border of the defined GTV to block edge. Conformal shielding of the surrounding tissue can be achieved by the use of multi-leaf collimators or custom-cut blocks. The majority of bladder tumors involve the trigone and/or posterior bladder wall. As such, the optimal field arrangement for the GTV of these tumors utilizes opposed lateral fields with beam energies of 10 MV or higher. If high-energy photons are not available, boost techniques may be delivered by employing a multi-field approach to minimize hotspots and dose to the femoral heads. The usual boost dose is 14.4–18.0 Gy in 1.8–2 Gy daily fractions with concurrent chemotherapy. If twice-daily radiotherapy is employed, the total dose to the bladder should between 64 and 65 Gy.

Current Radiation Treatment Policies

A flowchart for the evaluation and treatment of patients with non-metastatic MIBC with selective bladder-sparing therapy is shown in Figure 26.3.

Special Presentations

Patients Presenting with Symptomatic Pelvic Recurrences Following Radical Cystectomy

Isolated urethral recurrence following radical cystectomy can be approached with hope of cure by radiation therapy, though most centers have had limited success in curing patients with pelvic wall recurrences [77]. Patients with urethral recurrences after radical cystectomy with urinary diversion by ileal conduit may be treated with EBRT to a dose of 65–70 Gy, preferably with concurrent cisplatin or another radiosensitizing agent. This can be safely delivered using the standard 3D conformal techniques described previously, or IMRT. For those patients with pelvic sidewall recurrences and pain, a course of concurrent cisplatin and EBRT to a dose likely to be tolerated by the intestines (generally 50–56 Gy), the ileal loop, and its stoma is the standard approach. This should then be followed by multi-agent systemic chemotherapy.

Patients Presenting with MIBC and Hydronephrosis

For patients with tumor-associated hydronephrosis and clinically modest-size operable tumors, an immediate radical cystectomy is recommended, with consideration given to adjuvant chemotherapy or radiotherapy after the pathologic extent of disease has been fully defined. Pelvic radiotherapy is typically offered only in the face of positive surgical margins. In such a case, the recommended treatment would be to a dose of 40–45 Gy with concurrent cisplatin using conventional daily fractionation. This should then be followed by multi-agent systemic chemotherapy given the high likelihood of occult metastatic disease in such a presentation. For patients presenting with hydronephrosis and a locally advanced tumor of questionable resectability, a course of concurrent chemoradiotherapy could be offered following percutaneous upper-tract decompression. Provided that the patient's medical comorbidities do not preclude resection, he or she could then proceed on to radical cystectomy after restaging.

Patients with Biopsy-Confirmed Evidence of Local Nodal Metastases

For this subgroup of patients, three of four cycles of systemic multi-agent chemotherapy are recommended, followed by re-evaluation with full-body CT imaging and cystoscopy. If a good response to initial chemotherapy was seen and no development of distant metastases was found on restaging, a course of concurrent chemoradiotherapy to the bladder and involved nodal regions could be offered. Nodal target volumes and the entire bladder volume should be treated to a dose of 45–50 Gy followed by a boost to the primary bladder tumor to a dose of 65–70 Gy.

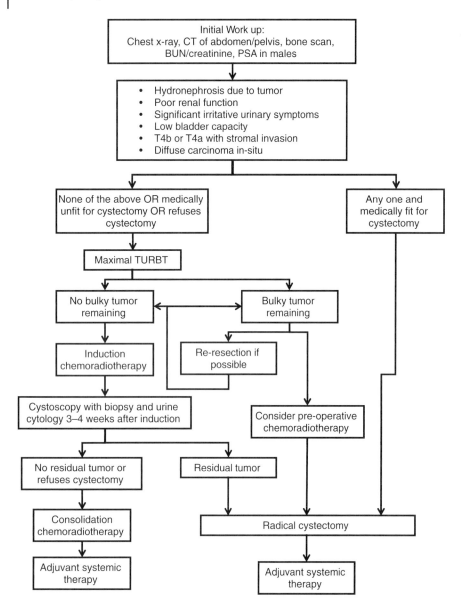

Figure 26.3 Flowchart of work-up and treatment of patients with muscle-invasive bladder cancer.

Patients Found to Have a Positive Margin Following Partial Cystectomy

Assuming an adequate bladder capacity, a pT2–T3 tumor, and adequate restaging studies, such a patient could be treated with concurrent chemoradiotherapy. If the pelvic lymph nodes were sampled and found to be negative, 45 Gy may be delivered to a target volume that is restricted to the entire bladder and abdominal incision. An additional boost dose of 20 Gy could then be delivered to the section of the residual bladder felt to be at highest risk of harboring microscopic residual disease.

Palliation of Bleeding from a Primary Bladder Tumor or Bladder Metastasis

Patients with severe bleeding will often have three-way irrigation catheters present at the time of presentation.

For patients with known metastatic disease elsewhere, a standard palliative approach of 30 Gy in 10 fractions is usually reasonable to stop bleeding. An alternative would be to offer 21 Gy in three fractions, delivered on alternating days. This regimen was found to be equivalent in effectiveness and toxicity to longer courses in a small randomized trial in Australia [78]. In the absence of clinical metastases, but in a patient with poor performance status, a hybrid regimen such as 50 Gy in 25 fractions with low-dose chemotherapy such as paclitaxel may afford a more durable response.

Interstitial Brachytherapy

Brachytherapy remains a common treatment technique for prostate, gynecologic, and other cancers in the US;

however, its use in bladder cancer is primarily limited to specialist centers throughout Europe. Appropriate candidates for brachytherapy include those with a solitary urothelial cell carcinoma with a diameter <5 cm, stage T1G3 to T3a. Early experience revealed clearly that urothelial cell carcinoma may be surgically seeded either into the wound or into the peritoneal cavity. This can be easily overcome by relatively low doses of preoperative EBRT [79]. Typical preoperative courses include 8.5 Gy × one fraction, 3.5 Gy × three fractions, or 5 Gy × two fractions. Reported local control rates at expert centers are between 70% and 90%, with similar disease-free survival rates and a high rate of bladder preservation. Toxicity rates are usually low, although some data exist that suggest the use of fractionated high-dose rate techniques may result in higher complication rates than low-dose rate techniques [80]. However, in the absence of any prospective randomized trials comparing the results and toxicities of brachytherapy to that of full-dose EBRT with or without chemotherapy, it is not possible to conclude whether brachytherapy approaches offer any specific advantages.

References

1 Siegel, R.L., Miller, K.D., Jemal, A. (2017) Cancer statistics, 2017. *CA Cancer J. Clin.*, **67** (1), 7–30.

2 Curado, M.P., Edwards, B., Shin, H.R., *et al.* (2007) *Cancer Incidence Five Continents*, vol. IX. IARC Scientific Publications, No. 160, IARC, Lyon.

3 Kaufman, D.S., Shipley, W.U., Feldman, A.S. (2009) Bladder cancer. *Lancet*, **374** (9685), 239–249.

4 Lamm, S.H., Engel, A., Penn, C.A., Chen, R., Feinleib, M. (2006) Arsenic cancer risk confounder in southwest Taiwan data set. *Environ. Health Perspect.*, **114** (7), 1077–1082.

5 Messing, E.M. (2004) Urothelial tumors of the urinary tract, in *Campbell's Urology*, 8th edition (eds P.C. Walsh, A.B. Retik, E.D. Vaughan, A.J. Wein), Saunders, Philadelphia.

6 Fried, B., Reddy, A., Mayer, D. (2011) Helminths in human carcinogenesis. *Cancer Lett.*, **305** (2), 239–249.

7 Montironi, R., Lopez-Beltran, A. (2005) The 2004 WHO classification of bladder tumors: a summary and commentary. *Int. J. Surg. Pathol.*, **13** (2), 143–153.

8 Young, R.H. (2000) Pathology of carcinomas of the urinary bladder, in *Comprehensive Textbook of Genitourinary Oncology*, 2nd edition (eds N.J. Vogelzang, P.T. Scardino, W.U. Shipley, D.S. Coffey), Lippincott Williams & Wilkins, Philadelphia.

9 Eble, J.N., Sauter, G., Epstein, J.I., Sesterhenn, I.A. (2004) Pathology and genetics of tumors of the urinary system and male genital organs, in *World Health Organization Classification of Tumors*. IARC Press, Lyon.

10 Farrow, G.M. (1992) Pathology of carcinoma in situ of the urinary bladder and related lesions. *J. Cell. Biochem. Suppl.*, **161**, 39–43.

11 Harving, N., Wolf, H., Melsen, F. (1988) Positive urinary cytology after tumor resection: an indicator for concomitant carcinoma in situ. *J. Urol.*, **140** (3), 495–497.

12 Herr, H.W., Donat, S.M., Dalbagni, G. (2007) Can restaging transurethral resection of T1 bladder cancer select patients for immediate cystectomy? *J. Urol.*, **177** (1), 75–79; discussion 79.

13 Schwaibold, H.E., Sivalingam, S., May, F., Hartung, R. (2006) The value of a second transurethral resection for T1 bladder cancer. *Br. J. Urol. Int.*, **97** (6), 1199–1201.

14 Jewett, H.J., Strong, G.H. (1946) Infiltrating carcinoma of the bladder; relation of depth of penetration of the bladder wall to incidence of local extension and metastases. *J. Urol.*, **55**, 366–372.

15 Amin, M.B. (2017) *AJCC Cancer Staging Manual*, 8th edition. Springer, New York.

16 Svatek, R.S., Shariat, S.F., Novara, G., *et al.* (2011) Discrepancy between clinical and pathological stage: external validation of the impact on prognosis in an international radical cystectomy cohort. *Br. J. Urol. Int.*, **107** (6), 898–904.

17 Turker, P., Bostrom, P.J., Wroclawski, M.L., *et al.* (2012) Upstaging of urothelial cancer at the time of radical cystectomy: factors associated with upstaging and its effect on outcome. *Br. J. Urol. Int.*, **110** (6), 804–811.

18 Gray, P.J., Lin, C.C., Jemal, A., *et al.* (2014) Clinical-pathologic stage discrepancy in bladder cancer patients treated with radical cystectomy: results from the national cancer data base. *Int. J. Radiat. Oncol. Biol. Phys.*, **88** (5), 1048–1056.

19 Union Internationale Contre Cancer (UICC) (1978) *TNM classification of malignant tumors*. UICC, Geneva.

20 Herr, H.W. (2000) Tumor progression and survival of patients with high grade, noninvasive papillary (TaG3) bladder tumors: 15-year outcome. *J. Urol.*, **163** (1), 60–61; discussion 61–62.

21 Heney, N.M., Ahmed, S., Flanagan, M.J., *et al.* (1983) Superficial bladder cancer: progression and recurrence. *J. Urol.*, **130** (6), 1083–1086.

22 Althausen, A.F., Prout, G.R., Jr, Daly, J.J. (1976) Non-invasive papillary carcinoma of the bladder

associated with carcinoma in situ. *J. Urol.*, **116** (5), 575–580.

23 Sylvester, R.J., van der Meijden, A.P., Oosterlinck, W., *et al.* (2006) Predicting recurrence and progression in individual patients with stage Ta T1 bladder cancer using EORTC risk tables: a combined analysis of 2596 patients from seven EORTC trials. *Eur. Urol.*, **49** (3), 466–475; discussion 475–477.

24 Shariat, S.F., Zippe, C., Ludecke, G., *et al.* (2005) Nomograms including nuclear matrix protein 22 for prediction of disease recurrence and progression in patients with Ta, T1 or CIS transitional cell carcinoma of the bladder. *J. Urol.*, **173** (5), 1518–1525.

25 Bohle, A., Jocham, D., Bock, P.R. (2003) Intravesical bacillus Calmette-Guerin versus mitomycin C for superficial bladder cancer: a formal meta-analysis of comparative studies on recurrence and toxicity. *J. Urol.*, **169** (1), 90–95.

26 Sylvester, R.J., van der Meijden, A., Lamm, D.L. (2002) Intravesical bacillus Calmette-Guerin reduces the risk of progression in patients with superficial bladder cancer: a meta-analysis of the published results of randomized clinical trials. *J. Urol.*, **168** (5), 1964–1970.

27 Lamm, D.L., Blumenstein, B.A., Crawford, E.D., *et al.* (1991) A randomized trial of intravesical doxorubicin and immunotherapy with bacille Calmette-Guerin for transitional-cell carcinoma of the bladder. *N. Engl. J. Med.*, **325** (17), 1205–1209.

28 Sylvester, R.J., Oosterlinck, W., van der Meijden, A.P. (2004) A single immediate postoperative instillation of chemotherapy decreases the risk of recurrence in patients with stage Ta T1 bladder cancer: a meta-analysis of published results of randomized clinical trials. *J. Urol.*, **171** (6 Pt 1), 2186–2190, quiz 2435.

29 Harland, S.J., Kynaston, H., Grigor, K., *et al.* (2007) A randomized trial of radical radiotherapy for the management of pT1G3 NXM0 transitional cell carcinoma of the bladder. *J. Urol.*, **178** (3 Pt 1), 807–813; discussion 813.

30 Bianco, F.J., Jr, Justa, D., Grignon, D.J., Sakr, W.A., Pontes, J.E., Wood, D.P., Jr (2004) Management of clinical T1 bladder transitional cell carcinoma by radical cystectomy. *Urol. Oncol.*, **22** (4), 290–294.

31 Weiss, C., Wolze, C., Engehausen, D.G., *et al.* (2006) Radiochemotherapy after transurethral resection for high-risk T1 bladder cancer: an alternative to intravesical therapy or early cystectomy? *J. Clin. Oncol.*, **24** (15), 2318–2324.

32 Wo, J.Y., Shipley, W.U., Dahl, D.M., *et al.* (2009) The results of concurrent chemo-radiotherapy for recurrence after treatment with bacillus Calmette-Guerin for non-muscle-invasive bladder

cancer: is immediate cystectomy always necessary? *Br. J. Urol. Int.*, **104** (2), 179–183.

33 Gray, P.J., Shipley, W.U., Efstathiou, J.A. (2013) T1 high-grade bladder cancer recurring after BCG therapy: a curative alternative to radical cystectomy exists. *Oncology (Williston Park)*, **27** (9), 873, 921.

34 Blank, L.E., Koedooder, K., van Os, R., van de Kar, M., van der Veen, J.H., Koning, C.C. (2007) Results of bladder-conserving treatment, consisting of brachytherapy combined with limited surgery and external beam radiotherapy, for patients with solitary T1-T3 bladder tumors less than 5 cm in diameter. *Int. J. Radiat. Oncol. Biol. Phys.*, **69** (2), 454–458.

35 Huddart, R.A., Hall, E., Lewis, R., Birtl, *et al.* (2011) Life and death of spare (selective bladder preservation against radical excision): reflections on why the spare trial closed. *Br. J. Urol. Int.*, **106** (6), 753–755.

36 Yu, R.J., Stein, J.P., Cai, J., Miranda, G., Groshen, S., Skinner, D.G. (2006) Superficial (pT2a) and deep (pT2b) muscle invasion in pathological staging of bladder cancer following radical cystectomy. *J. Urol.*, **176** (2), 493–498; discussion 498–499.

37 Dalbagni, G., Genega, E., Hashibe, M., *et al.* (2001) Cystectomy for bladder cancer: a contemporary series. *J. Urol.*, **165** (4), 1111–1116.

38 Grossman, H.B., Natale, R.B., Tangen, C.M., *et al.* (2003) Neoadjuvant chemotherapy plus cystectomy compared with cystectomy alone for locally advanced bladder cancer. *N. Engl. J. Med.*, **349** (9), 859–866.

39 Rodel, C., Grabenbauer, G.G., Kuhn, R., *et al.* (2002) Combined-modality treatment and selective organ preservation in invasive bladder cancer: long-term results. *J. Clin. Oncol.*, **20** (14), 3061–3071.

40 Efstathiou, J.A., Spiegel, D.Y., Shipley, W.U., *et al.* (2012) Long-term outcomes of selective bladder preservation by combined-modality therapy for invasive bladder cancer: The MGH experience. *Eur. Urol.*, **61** (4), 705–711.

41 James, N.D., Hussain, S.A., Hall, E., *et al.* (2012) Radiotherapy with or without chemotherapy in muscle-invasive bladder cancer. *N. Engl. J. Med.*, **366** (16), 1477–1488.

42 Mak, R.H., Hunt, D., Shipley, W.U., *et al.* (2014) Long-term outcomes in patients with muscle-invasive bladder cancer after selective bladder-preserving combined-modality therapy: a pooled analysis of Radiation Therapy Oncology Group protocols 8802, 8903, 9506, 9706, 9906, and 0233. *J. Clin. Oncol.*, **32** (34), 3801–3809.

43 Tanrikut, C., McDougal, W.S. (2005) Metabolic implications and electrolyte disturbances, in *Urinary Diversion: Scientific Foundation in Clinical Practice*, 2nd edition (eds K.J. Kreder, A. Stone), Isis Media Medical, Oxford.

44 Sweeney, P., Kursh, E.D., Resnick, M.I. (1992) Partial cystectomy. *Urol. Clin. North Am.*, **19** (4), 701–711.

45 International Collaboration of Trialists, Medical Research Council Advanced Bladder Cancer Working Party, European Organisation for Research and Treatment of Cancer Genito-Urinary Tract Cancer Group, *et al.* (2011) International Phase III trial assessing neoadjuvant cisplatin, methotrexate, and vinblastine chemotherapy for muscle-invasive bladder cancer: long-term results of the BA06 30894 trial. *J. Clin. Oncol.*, **29** (16), 2171–2177.

46 Bassi, P., Pagano, F., Pappagallo, G. (1998) Neo-adjuvant M-VAC of invasive bladder cancer: The GUONE multicenter phase III trial. *Eur. Urol.*, **33** (Suppl.1), 142.

47 GISTV (Italian Bladder Cancer Study Group) (1996) Neoadjuvant treatment for locally advanced bladder cancer: a randomized prospective clinical trial. *J. Chemother.*, **8** (Suppl. 4), 345–346.

48 Sherif, A., Rintala, E., Mestad, O., *et al.* (2002) Neoadjuvant cisplatin-methotrexate chemotherapy for invasive bladder cancer – Nordic cystectomy trial 2. *Scand. J. Urol. Nephrol.*, **36** (6), 419–425.

49 Advanced Bladder Cancer (ABC) Meta-analysis Collaboration (2005) Adjuvant chemotherapy in invasive bladder cancer: a systematic review and meta-analysis of individual patient data. *Eur. Urol.*, **48** (2), 189–199; discussion 199–201.

50 Ruggeri, E.M., Giannarelli, D., Bria, E., *et al.* (2006) Adjuvant chemotherapy in muscle-invasive bladder carcinoma: a pooled analysis from phase III studies. *Cancer*, **106** (4), 783–788.

51 von der Maase, H., Hansen, S.W., Roberts, J.T., *et al.* (2000) Gemcitabine and cisplatin versus methotrexate, vinblastine, doxorubicin, and cisplatin in advanced or metastatic bladder cancer: results of a large, randomized, multinational, multicenter, phase III study. *J. Clin. Oncol.*, **18** (17), 3068–3077.

52 Herr, H.W., Faulkner, J.R., Grossman, H.B., *et al.* (2004) Surgical factors influence bladder cancer outcomes: a cooperative group report. *J. Clin. Oncol.*, **22** (14), 2781–2789.

53 Eapen, L. (2012) Substantial pelvic recurrence (PR) rates after contemporary radical cystectomy (RC) for pT3/4 N0-2 transitional bladder cancer (TBC): A multi-institutional Canadian study. American Urologic Association Annual Meeting, 2012, Atlanta, GA.

54 Baumann, B.C., Guzzo, T., Vaughn, D., *et al.* (2011) Bladder cancer patterns of pelvic failure: implications for adjuvant radiation therapy. *Int. J. Radiat. Oncol. Biol. Phys.*, **81** (2), S72–S73.

55 Miller, L.S. (1977) Bladder cancer: superiority of preoperative irradiation and cystectomy in clinical stages B2 and C. *Cancer*, **39** (2 Suppl.), 973–980.

56 Sell, A., Jakobsen, A., Nerstrom, B., Sorensen, B.L., Steven, K., Barlebo, H. (1991) Treatment of advanced bladder cancer category T2 T3 and T4a. A randomized multicenter study of preoperative irradiation and cystectomy versus radical irradiation and early salvage cystectomy for residual tumor. DAVECA protocol 8201. Danish Vesical Cancer Group. Scand. *J. Urol. Nephrol. Suppl.*, **138**, 193–201.

57 Horwich, A., Pendlebury, S., Dearnaley, D.P. (1995) Organ conservation in bladder cancer. *Eur. J. Cancer*, **31**, S208–S209.

58 Nigro, N.D., Vaitkevicius, V.K., Considine, B., Jr (1974) Combined therapy for cancer of the anal canal: a preliminary report. *Dis. Colon Rectum*, **17** (3), 354–356.

59 Angulo, J.C., Sanchez-Chapado, M., Lopez, J.I., Flores, N. (1996) Primary cisplatin, methotrexate and vinblastine aiming at bladder preservation in invasive bladder cancer: multivariate analysis on prognostic factors. *J. Urol.*, **155** (6), 1897–1902.

60 Sternberg, C.N., Arena, M.G., Calabresi, F., *et al.* (1993) Neoadjuvant M-VAC (methotrexate, vinblastine, doxorubicin, and cisplatin) for infiltrating transitional cell carcinoma of the bladder. *Cancer*, **72** (6), 1975–1982.

61 Splinter, T.A., Pavone-Macaluso, M., Jacqmin, D., *et al.* (1992) A European Organization for Research and Treatment of Cancer – Genitourinary Group phase 2 study of chemotherapy in stage T3-4N0-XM0 transitional cell cancer of the bladder: evaluation of clinical response. *J. Urol.*, **148** (6), 1793–1796.

62 Roberts, J.T., Fossa, S.D., Richards, B., *et al.* (1991) Results of Medical Research Council phase II study of low dose cisplatin and methotrexate in the primary treatment of locally advanced (T3 and T4) transitional cell carcinoma of the bladder. *Br. J. Urol.*, **68** (2), 162–168.

63 Farah, R., Chodak, G.W., Vogelzang, N.J., *et al.* (1991) Curative radiotherapy following chemotherapy for invasive bladder carcinoma (a preliminary report). *Int. J. Radiat. Oncol. Biol. Phys.*, **20** (3), 413–417.

64 Dreicer, R., Messing, E.M., Loehrer, P.J., Trump, D.L. (1990) Perioperative methotrexate, vinblastine, doxorubicin and cisplatin (M-VAC) for poor risk transitional cell carcinoma of the bladder: an Eastern Cooperative Oncology Group pilot study. *J. Urol.*, **144** (5), 1123–1126; discussion 1126–1127.

65 Efstathiou, J.A., Bae, K., Shipley, W.U., *et al.* (2009) Late pelvic toxicity after bladder-sparing therapy in patients with invasive bladder cancer: RTOG 89-03, 95-06, 97-06, 99-06. *J. Clin. Oncol.*, **27** (25), 4055–4061.

66 Shipley, W.U., Prout, G.R., Jr, Einstein, A.B., *et al.* (1987) Treatment of invasive bladder cancer by cisplatin and radiation in patients unsuited for surgery. *JAMA*, **258** (7), 931–935.

67 Weiss, C., Engehausen, D.G., Krause, F.S., *et al.* (2007) Radiochemotherapy with cisplatin and 5-fluorouracil after transurethral surgery in patients with bladder cancer. *Int. J. Radiat. Oncol. Biol. Phys.*, **68** (4), 1072–1080.

68 Zietman, A.L., Sacco, D., Skowronski, U., *et al.* (2003) Organ conservation in invasive bladder cancer by transurethral resection, chemotherapy and radiation: results of a urodynamic and quality of life study on long-term survivors. *J. Urol.*, **170** (5), 1772–1776.

69 Kachnic, L.A., Kaufman, D.S., Heney, N.M., *et al.* (1997) Bladder preservation by combined modality therapy for invasive bladder cancer. *J. Clin. Oncol.*, **15** (3), 1022–1029.

70 Dunst, J., Sauer, R., Schrott, K.M., Kuhn, R., Wittekind, C., Altendorf-Hofmann, A. (1994) Organ-sparing treatment of advanced bladder cancer: a 10-year experience. *Int. J. Radiat. Oncol. Biol. Phys.*, **30** (2), 261–266.

71 Tester, W., Porter, A., Asbell, S., *et al.* (1993) Combined modality program with possible organ preservation for invasive bladder carcinoma: results of RTOG protocol 85-12. *Int. J. Radiat. Oncol. Biol. Phys.*, **25** (5), 783–790.

72 Kent, E., Sandler, H., Montie, J., *et al.* (2004) Combined-modality therapy with gemcitabine and radiotherapy as a bladder preservation strategy: results of a phase I trial. *J. Clin. Oncol.*, **22** (13), 2540–2545.

73 Coen, J.J., Paly, J.J., Niemierko, A., *et al.* (2013) Nomograms predicting response to therapy and outcomes after bladder-preserving trimodality therapy for muscle-invasive bladder cancer. *Int. J. Radiat. Oncol. Biol. Phys.*, **86** (2), 311–316.

74 Coppin, C.M., Gospodarowicz, M.K., James, K., *et al.* (1996) Improved local control of invasive bladder cancer by concurrent cisplatin and preoperative or definitive radiation. The National Cancer Institute of Canada Clinical Trials Group. *J. Clin. Oncol.*, **14** (11), 2901–2907.

75 Eswara, J.R., Efstathiou, J.A., Heney, N.M., *et al.* (2012) Complications and long-term results of salvage cystectomy after failed bladder sparing therapy for muscle invasive bladder cancer. *J. Urol.*, **187** (2), 463–468.

76 Gray, P.J., Fedewa, S.A., Shipley, W.U., *et al.* (2013) Use of potentially curative therapies for muscle-invasive bladder cancer in the United States: results from the National Cancer Data Base. *Eur. Urol.*, **63** (5), 823–829.

77 Dhar, N.B., Jones, J.S., Reuther, A.M., *et al.* (2008) Presentation, location and overall survival of pelvic recurrence after radical cystectomy for transitional cell carcinoma of the bladder. *Br. J. Urol. Int.*, **101** (8), 969–972.

78 Duchesne, G.M., Bolger, J.J., Griffiths, G.O., *et al.* (2000) A randomized trial of hypofractionated schedules of palliative radiotherapy in the management of bladder carcinoma: results of medical research council trial BA09. *Int. J. Radiat. Oncol. Biol. Phys.*, **47** (2), 379–388.

79 van der Werf-Messing, B. (1969) Carcinoma of the bladder treated by suprapubic radium implants. The value of additional external irradiation. *Eur. J. Cancer*, **5** (3), 277–285.

80 Pos, F.J., Horenblas, S., Lebesque, J., *et al.* (2004) Low-dose-rate brachytherapy is superior to high-dose-rate brachytherapy for bladder cancer. *Int. J. Radiat. Oncol. Biol. Phys.*, **59** (3), 696–705.

27

Prostate Cancer

Abhishek A. Solanki, Rebecca I. Hartman, Phillip J. Gray, Brent S. Rose, Jonathan J. Paly, Kent W. Mouw and Jason A. Efstathiou

Introduction

Prostate carcinoma is the most common form of non-skin cancer and the second most frequent cause of cancer deaths among males in the United States [1]. The estimated lifetime risk of developing prostate cancer for an American male is as high as one in seven [2]. In 2017, there will be an estimated 161 360 new diagnoses of prostate cancer and the disease will claim 26 730 lives [1].

Prostate-specific antigen (PSA) screening for prostate cancer, initiated during the late 1980s, led to an initial rise in incidence rates that has since declined by 4.3% each year on average over the past decade [2–4]. As important as PSA screening was when it was initiated, the U.S. Preventive Services Task Force's 2012 recommendation to discontinue PSA screening due to concerns of over-diagnosis and overtreatment may also drastically change the landscape of prostate cancer in the future.

While not all men need radical treatment, the majority elect for definitive management [5]. Radiation therapy is a mainstay of prostate cancer treatment, and treatment of the disease comprises a large proportion of the average radiation oncologist's workload. Innovations in the ability to use advanced radiotherapy techniques such as image-guided radiotherapy (IGRT), intensity-modulated radiotherapy (IMRT) and proton therapy, have led to an increase in the accuracy and complexity of treatments, but at increased cost. Additionally, based on the natural history of indolent prostate cancer, many men may not need treatment in their lifetime, and thus the risk of toxicities to impact a man's quality of life is of utmost importance.

These considerations are made more difficult to navigate due to relatively limited randomized data comparing the different treatment modalities. Added to these complexities is increased media coverage of the disease and patient advocacy groups promoting increased investigation into improving patient outcomes and limiting toxicity.

There are few disease states with as much controversy surrounding the benefits/harms of screening, concerns for overtreatment, and societal economic costs of treatment as prostate cancer. In this chapter, the key elements of the diagnosis, multidisciplinary management, radiotherapeutic techniques, and radiotherapy disease control and toxicity outcomes of men with prostate cancer in the modern era are discussed.

Epidemiology

The incidence of prostate cancer in the United States and globally has been intertwined with the use of PSA screening. The PSA test was first approved by the FDA in 1986 to monitor for biochemical recurrence after radical prostatectomy or external beam radiotherapy (EBRT) for men with a known diagnosis of prostate cancer. However, it was commonly used for screening which led to the peak incidence of prostate cancer in 1992. The PSA test and digital rectal examination (DRE) were approved for screening by the FDA in 1994, and since then the incidence of prostate cancer has declined but held relatively steady.

Prostate cancer is primarily a disease of the developed world, with the highest incidence rates in Australia/New Zealand, North America, and Europe, while Asia and Africa have the lowest rates [6]. These differences may be due to a combination of factors, including genetic susceptibility, environmental risk factors, or artifacts from variations in cancer registration and screening [7]. Japanese males who migrate to the US have a higher incidence of the disease, suggesting an environmental role for disease

Clinical Radiation Oncology: Indications, Techniques, and Results, Third Edition. Edited by William Small Jr.
© 2017 John Wiley & Sons, Inc. Published 2017 by John Wiley & Sons, Inc.

development [8]. Race is an important factor in the development and course of prostate cancer. African-American males have a higher incidence, frequency of advanced stage of disease at presentation, frequency of adverse pathologic features, and mortality than their white counterparts [2, 9]. The etiology of this difference, whether due to biology or access to care, including treatment and screening, remains unknown.

Age remains the most important risk factor, and prostate cancer has the strongest relationship with age of any cancer. The disease is rarely diagnosed in men aged under 50 years, and over 85% of men diagnosed are older than 65 years [7]. Autopsy series have shown that by the fifth decade of life, 50% of men have occult prostate cancer, and this rate exceeds 75% for men aged 85 years and older [10]. Interestingly, there is little variation among the incidences of latent prostate cancer throughout the world, although the incidence of clinically diagnosed disease varies significantly [11]. This finding suggests that the key difference among various countries is the incidence of progression from occult to clinically significant disease.

Approximately 10–15% of prostate cancer cases may be familial in nature [12]. First-degree relatives of men with prostate cancer have a twofold higher risk of developing prostate cancer themselves compared to the general population [13]. With additional affected first-degree relatives, the risk of prostate cancer is further increased [14]. Genome-wide association studies have provided evidence of a strong genetic component in the development of prostate cancer [15]. In addition, the *BRCA* gene has a known impact on disease incidence, and men with mutations in this tumor suppressor gene have an increased risk of developing prostate cancer, especially at a younger age [16].

Determining lifestyle risk factors for prostate cancer has proven difficult. In contrast to many other cancers, smoking, alcohol and sexually transmitted infections have no clear association with prostate cancer development [17, 18], although tobacco use has been associated with more aggressive prostate cancer [19]. Associations with some dietary factors have been noted, however. A high-fat diet has been associated with increased prostate cancer incidence, while soy and coffee may be protective [20, 21]. A decreased level of vitamin D has been suggested as a risk factor, but studies examining this relationship have provided conflicting results [22, 23]. The Selenium and Vitamin E Cancer Prevention Trial (SELECT) found no decreased incidence of prostate cancer with selenium or vitamin E supplementation [24]. The consumption of lycopene, an anti-oxidant found in tomatoes, has also been associated with a decreased disease risk, but study results have been mixed and an evidenced-based review found insufficient evidence for this association [25, 26]. Obesity has also been linked to prostate

cancer incidence [27], and may also be associated with cancer aggressiveness [28–30]. Endogenous sex hormones are not associated with incidence, while exogenous testosterone supplementation is controversial [31, 32].

Pharmacologic exposures have also been explored to find risk factors for prostate cancer, but the results have been conflicting [33]. Multiple studies have shown that the use of HMG-CoA reductase inhibitors ('statins') may decrease the overall incidence of prostate cancer, as well as decrease the incidence of aggressive prostate cancer, and statin-users may have less advanced prostate cancer [34, 35]. Antihypertensive use has also been associated with a decreased incidence of prostate cancer, as has as aspirin use [36, 37].

Thus, the development of clinically significant prostate cancer is complex. It is likely due to a combination of factors that are responsible for transforming the occult microscopic foci of prostate cancer commonly seen with aging into clinically significant disease.

Anatomy

The current understanding of prostatic anatomy has permitted considerable improvements in both surgical and radiotherapy-based treatments for the disease. The prostate is typically 20–30 ml in volume, but prostate size varies widely and increases with age. McNeal originally described the prostate as divided into three zones: peripheral, central, and transition [38]. The transition zone is the smallest zone and wraps around the mid-prostatic urethra. The enlargement of this zone that typically occurs with aging explains the bladder outflow symptoms of benign prostatic hyperplasia (BPH). The central zone, which contains the ejaculatory ducts, is a cone-shaped area located posterior to the transition zone. The largest zone in a normal prostate is the peripheral zone, which surrounds the transition and central zones, except anteriorly where the peripheral zone is incomplete. The peripheral zone is the most common site of prostatic carcinoma, with approximately 80% of prostate cancers arising from this zone. When the central zone is involved, it often is due to direct extension of malignancy that initially arose in the peripheral zone. Rarely, tumors can arise from the transition zone and can grow very large without extending beyond the prostate due to the internal location of this zone. Surrounding the prostate is a fibromuscular band that forms an ill-defined capsule that is incomplete anteriorly [39].

The prostate's nerve supply consists of bilateral neurovascular bundles, including autonomic nerves controlling erectile function, that course along the posterolateral edge of the prostate. The internal iliac artery provides the primary blood supply, and venous blood drains directly into the prostatic plexus, which drains into the internal iliac vein. The lymphatic drainage of the prostate includes a periprostatic network that drains to the internal and external iliac, obturator, and presacral nodes.

An understanding of the imaging anatomy of the prostate and prostate cancer is critical for clinicians. On ultrasound, the peripheral zone and central zones are typically a gray color, while the transition zone is usually more hypoechoic (darker), than these two regions. When present, a large median lobe can be visualized protruding into the bladder. On computed tomography (CT) scanning, the prostate can be visualized relatively well, though the anterior border, apex and base can be difficult to identify.

Ultimately, magnetic resonance imaging (MRI) allows for the most detailed demarcation of the borders of each of the prostatic zones and the prostatic capsule. The T2 sequence is usually the most useful for evaluating prostate anatomy. The peripheral zone is usually T2 hyperintense (brighter), while the transition zone is more heterogeneous-appearing due to the presence of BPH nodules. The central zone is often more hypointense (darker). The seminal vesicles are commonly T2-hyperintense, and can be described as appearing tubular. An example of the MRI of a patient with prostate cancer with the several pertinent anatomic structures identified is shown in Figure 27.1.

Knowledge of this anatomy has facilitated the use of directed biopsies with transrectal ultrasound (TRUS) guidance. It is also used in low-dose rate (LDR) brachytherapy seed implantation and high-dose rate (HDR) brachytherapy catheter implantation to adjust the distribution of the radiation dose across the prostate gland.

Histology

The diagnosis of prostatic carcinoma hinges upon both architectural and cytologic criteria. The characteristic adenomatous hyperplasia common with advanced age can be distinguished easily from cancer. However, prostatic intraepithelial neoplasia (PIN) cannot be distinguished as easily. PIN exhibits atypical cellular proliferation cytologically, but maintains the normal acinar structure. High-grade PIN is a premalignant lesion that is associated with extant or future prostate cancer, although an optimal rebiopsy strategy has yet to be defined [40]. In contrast, low-grade PIN lacks clinical significance and does not require rebiopsy. In fact, some PIN lesions may regress or remain unchanged [41]. As a result, PIN should be recognized as distinct from carcinoma *in-situ*.

More than 95% of prostatic cancers are adenocarcinomas; the remainder are comprised of sarcomatoid, basaloid, adenoid cystic, carcinoid, and small-cell

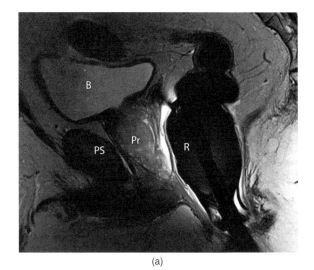

(a)

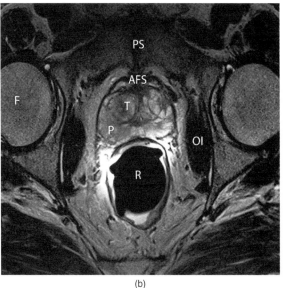

(b)

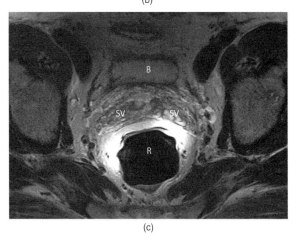

(c)

Figure 27.1 T2-weighted MRI images of the prostate. (a) Sagittal image of the prostate. (b, c) Axial images at two levels. Note that an endorectal coil was used in this study and is visible in the images. Pr, prostate; PS, pubic symphysis; B, bladder; R, rectum; F, femur; AFS, anterior fibromuscular stroma; OI, obturator internus; T, transitional zone; P, peripheral zone.

histologies. Although rare, the recognition of these categories is important because they may not respond to androgen deprivation. In addition, small-cell carcinomas may also be associated with paraneoplastic syndromes.

The Gleason histologic grading system was created in 1966 by Donald Gleason [42], and continues to be the most widely accepted grading system. The primary or dominant pattern of differentiation is assigned a score from 1 to 5, based largely on glandular architectural features. The second most commonly encountered pattern also receives a grade, and the two are summed to yield a value between 6 and 10 for men with prostate cancer. It is standard to report both individual scores rather than the sum as, for example, a 3+4 tumor has a better prognosis than a 4+3 tumor [43]. Numerous studies have demonstrated the clinical utility of the Gleason score in prognosis, and there is a stepwise increase in prostate cancer mortality with increases in Gleason score [44]. The Gleason system has evolved over time [42], with the highest Gleason score in a biopsy, irrespective of the percentage involvement, now also playing a role in patient management [44]. Some studies have described worse outcomes for patients with any degree of Gleason pattern 5, often referred to as tertiary grade 5 [45].

Gleason scores from biopsies correlate exactly with subsequent whole-gland pathologic scores in approximately 50% of cases, and within one unit in nearly 90% of cases [46]. Errors are significantly more likely to be due to undergrading rather than overgrading [46]. Critiques of the Gleason system include its omission of cytologic features and lack of robust interobserver reproducibility [44]. In addition, the Gleason system fails to address the heterogeneity of Gleason 7 tumors, a commonly reported score. There has been a recent initiative to create Gleason score groups based on differences in survival outcomes, particularly to address this difference between 3+4 and 4+3 tumors, and those with 8 and 9–10 tumors, but this has not yet become standard [47]. Additionally, molecular markers are presently being examined to further refine this group in order to guide cancer treatment and help refine selection of patients for active surveillance. Several commercial tests are available, but the optimal use in routine clinical practice has not been elucidated [48]. The Decipher® genomic classifier is a 22-gene expression profile that has been validated to be predictive of early distant metastases after radical prostatectomy (RP) and for metastases after post-operative radiotherapy, and may be more specific than standard clinical features [49–51].

The local spread of carcinoma beyond the prostate most frequently occurs along nerves and lymphatics. As a result, extracapsular extension is most commonly found around the neurovascular bundles and at the apex, where they enter and exit the prostate [20]. A pathologic review of RP specimens suggested that ≥90% of extracapsular extension is ≤5 mm from the capsule [52]. Direct extension into the seminal vesicles occurs along the ejaculatory ducts; alternatively, a tumor may embolize or metastasize to the seminal vesicles through blood vessels. Based on pathological analyses of specimens from patients undergoing RP, the length of seminal vesicle involvement is within 1 cm in ≥90% of patients overall. Looking specifically at the group of patients with pathologic seminal vesicle involvement, however, approximately 90% of patients have a length of involvement is actually within 2 cm [53].

Screening and Prevention

Prostate cancer survival is highly dependent on the extent of disease at the time of diagnosis. Men with early-stage localized disease confined to the prostate have five-year disease-specific survival rates approaching 100%, compared to only 28.7% for those with metastatic disease [54]. This survival difference and the disease's very high prevalence have prompted screening efforts using two tools, namely DRE and serum PSA, which are typically combined in practice.

The DRE is targeted at the peripheral zone of the prostate. Abnormal findings on DRE consistent with prostate cancer include asymmetry, nodules, and induration. Based on a meta-analysis, the sensitivity, specificity and positive predictive value of DRE alone are 53%, 84%, and 18%, respectively [55]. Cancers discovered using DRE alone (as were most cancers prior to the PSA era) are typically locally advanced or already metastatic [56].

In contrast, PSA testing allows for prostate cancer to be diagnosed prior to the development of palpable disease. The PSA is a glycoprotein produced by both benign and malignant prostate cells, which has serine protease activity and is involved in lysis of the seminal coagulum. The normal range for men has historically been defined between 0 and 4.0 ng ml^{-1}, although it is lower in young men and rises with age. PSA testing using this cut-off has a reported sensitivity of 20%, a specificity of 91%, and a positive predictive value of 30% [57]. False elevations in PSA can be caused by ejaculation, BPH, prostatitis, or prostatic trauma. PSA levels may also be inappropriately low in those with poorly differentiated cancers or with 5α-reductase inhibitor use (ca. 50% reduction with dutasteride or finasteride use).

Attempts have been made to refine the use of screening for PSA. Typically, PSA levels increase with age, and as a result age-specific ranges for PSA have been generated. The PSA density is the ratio of PSA to gland volume measured by TRUS, and thus takes into account BPH. The PSA density has not, however, been shown to have clear use either in lowering biopsy rates or in ascertaining prognosis. PSA is present in the bloodstream both free and complexed with extracellular protease inhibitors. Cancer, as opposed to BPH, is more likely when the free PSA represents less than 25% of the total [58]. In addition, a greater annual PSA velocity (increase in PSA level in one year) appears more commonly associated with cancer than benign conditions, though some studies have found that the PSA velocity offers minimal if any additional clinical value over PSA level alone for screening [59,60]. This finding is likely due to the lability of PSA levels. The Prostate Cancer Antigen 3 (PCA3) score, based on the ratio of PCA3 mRNA to PSA mRNA, is more specific to prostate cancer than PSA, although its clinical use in addition to PSA is unclear [61]. Research is presently being conducted on novel biomarkers to supplement PSA testing.

Currently, PSA screening remains one of the most controversial aspects of prostate cancer diagnosis and management. Two large randomized trials – the Prostate, Lung, Colorectal, and Ovarian (PLCO) Screening Trial in the US, and the European Randomized Study of Screening for Prostate Cancer (ERSPC) in Europe – randomized patients to a scheduled screening regimen or usual care [62,63]. Several criticisms were raised against these trials, particularly of the PLCO trial, in which a high percentage of patients in both arms had a screening PSA prior to enrolling in the study, and also PSA contamination of the control group. Both trials suggested that screening increases cancer detection, but there was no cancer-specific mortality reduction in the PLCO trial, and in the ERSPC trial the absolute benefit was 1.07 per 1000 men screened. The number needed to screen in order to prevent one death is thus estimated to be 1000. However, the Goteberg subset of the ERSPC trial included younger men, more frequent testing, a lower PSA threshold for biopsy, and a longer follow-up, and found that the number needed to screen may be as low as 243 [64]. Based on the findings of these randomized trials, the United States Preventative Service Task Force found insufficient evidence to recommend screening for average risk patients in their 2012 recommendation [65]. Conversely, the American Cancer Society recommended that men who are aged 50 years and have at least a 10-year life expectancy individually discuss the risks and benefits with their physicians of whether to initiate screening, while the National Comprehensive Cancer Network (NCCN) recommended discussing the risks and benefits for men aged 45–75 years and repeating the PSA and DRE based on the results and age of the patients [57,66].

Prostate cancer prevention has been studied using 5α-reductase inhibitors, which inhibit the conversion of testosterone to dihydrotestosterone, the most active androgen in the prostate. The rationale for this is that 5α-reductase leads to prostate growth via the conversion of testosterone to dihydrotestosterone, and therefore inhibiting this pathway may inhibit prostate cancer growth. The Prostate Cancer Prevention (PCPT) trial and the Reduction by Dutasteride of Prostate Cancer Events (REDUCE) trials tested the prevention of prostate cancer by finasteride and dutasteride, respectively [67–69]. There appeared to be an approximately 25–33% reduction in prostate cancer incidence, primarily in low-grade disease. The PCPT trial suggested an increased frequency of high-grade disease, though this may have been explained by decreased prostate gland size [70]. Based on these trials, there is no clear prostate cancer-specific mortality or overall survival benefit with these agents, and thus the benefit must be weighed against the risks related to the side effects. Selenium and vitamin E have also been proposed as chemopreventive agents, but the SELECT randomized trial did not provide evidence of any clinically significant effects [42].

Presentation and Diagnosis

With the widespread use of PSA screening, prostate cancer is usually asymptomatic at the time of diagnosis. Since 1990, there has been a progressive increase in the proportion of men who have low-risk disease, with almost 80% presenting without any findings on DRE, while two-thirds have a PSA level of 2-4 [71].

Nevertheless, a history should be obtained, including current genitourinary, bowel, and sexual function symptoms using validated metrics such as the American Urology Association International Prostate Symptom Score (IPSS), the Expanded Prostate Cancer Index Composite (EPIC) quality of life instrument, or International Index of Erectile Function-5 (IIEF-5). The presence of obstructive or irritative voiding symptoms such as hesitancy, intermittency, incomplete emptying, urgency, frequency, nocturia, and a dwindling urinary stream are much less common and, if present, are often due to BPH or bladder disorders. Uncommon presentations with symptoms such as hematuria and perineal pain are very worrisome, and may signify invasion of the bladder neck or the external sphincter. Despite widespread PSA screening throughout the US, men may still present with late-stage disease and the associated symptomatology of metastatic disease, including bone pain and unexplained fatigue. An elevated PSA or a positive DRE should prompt a referral for a biopsy to confirm the diagnosis. The aforementioned late-stage clinical symptoms are also indications for biopsy and radiographic imaging. The most recent NCCN guidelines recommend consideration of biopsy when the PSA is >3 ng ml^{-1} [66].

Biopsy is most commonly performed under TRUS guidance, and 12 cores are typically sampled throughout the gland. It is difficult to biopsy the anterior aspect of the gland via TRUS biopsy, and thus cancers arising from this region may be difficult to diagnose.

The role of multiparametric MRI to help decide whether a biopsy is indicated, and to help target biopsies in the diagnosis of prostate cancer, is evolving. The PI-RADS score – a score ranging from 1 to 5 given to lesions seen on prostate MRI and used to quantify the radiographic suspicion for prostate cancer – is being integrated into the evaluation of prostate MRI [72]. The PI-RADS score is increasingly being used to help identify biopsy target lesions and suspicious areas for prostate cancer. A prospective cohort study of patients undergoing multiparametric MRI with targeted biopsies and standard sextant biopsies found that targeted biopsies could identify 13% additional clinically relevant prostate cancers, while omitting biopsy in patients with a PI-RADS score of 1 or 2 would reduce the men requiring biopsy by approximately one-third [73]. Another series found that MRI-guided biopsies can detect more high-risk prostate cancers [74]. However, a randomized trial conducted in Finland showed no benefit in finding clinically significant cancers using MRI prior to biopsy [75]. MRI and ultrasound fusion to help guide biopsies may better identify and target higher-grade and clinically significant disease compared to standard ultrasound-guided sextant biopsy, and is being used at many institutions [74]. However, at the present time the standard remains sextant biopsy. Nonetheless, with growing experience and a better risk stratification of target lesions, MRI will likely play an increasingly important role in the initial diagnosis and work-up of prostate cancer.

Staging/Risk Stratification

The most widely accepted staging system is the tumor, node, and metastasis (TNM) system of the American Joint Committee on Cancer (Table 27.1). Key changes featured in the most recent update from 2017 include the removal of the subclassification of pT2a,b and c to just pT2, as these have not clearly been associated with outcomes. Additionally, a recommendation was made that the Gleason grade group should be reported, and Stage II and II were further subdivided into IIA-c and IIA (Tables 27.2, 27.3). Studies have shown that the inclusion of these two characteristics improves the prognostic ability of the anatomic stages [43]. Other prognostic factors, including the percentage of positive cores on biopsy and perineural invasion, are not included in the anatomic staging system, but may be prognostically relevant [76, 77]. The NCCN guidelines also propose categories stratified by recurrence risk (Table 27.4) [78]. Patients are treated based on whether they fall within the low-risk, intermediate-risk, or high-risk group, although there remains considerable heterogeneity within the risk groups, particularly the intermediate-risk and high-risk groups [76, 79, 80].

Key features of the local extent of disease, including extracapsular extension and seminal vesicle involvement, are difficult to determine by DRE, biopsy specimens, or standard imaging techniques. Non-palpable prostate cancer is difficult to identify on ultrasound, but when visible it is usually hypoechoic. Prostate cancer is usually not visible on CT, unless there is gross extension outside of the prostate into adjacent tissues. Some have found multiparametric MRI to provide incremental benefit in defining these features. Multiparametric MRI, which includes diffusion-weight imaging, dynamic contrast-enhancement imaging, and sometimes spectroscopy, can help improve the ability to identify high-grade disease [81]. An endorectal coil was historically used to help identify prostate cancer location, as well as to evaluate for extracapsular extension or seminal vesicle involvement. However, with advanced and high-quality MRI scans it may not be necessary and consequently many institutions have moved away from using the endorectal coil for patient comfort. Prostate cancer is typically hypointense on T2-weighted MRI, contrasting it from the high signal of the peripheral zone. Blurring of the prostatic capsule can be suggestive of extracapsular extension, while a hypointense appearance of the base of the seminal vesicles can suggest involvement with disease [82]. The normal prostate takes up contrast similar to prostate cancer, and therefore contrast-enhanced T1 MRI is less useful.

The need for additional imaging to search for nodal or distant metastases is determined by the T stage of the tumor, the PSA level, and the Gleason score. The NCCN guidelines recommend the following staging work-up for nodal or distant metastases: A bone scan is indicated to evaluate for metastases for T3 and T4 tumors, T1 tumors with PSA > 20, T2 tumors with PSA > 10, Gleason score > 7, as well as for all patients with clinical symptoms [78]. In addition, a pelvic CT scan or MRI to evaluate for nodal spread is indicated for T3 or T4 tumors, and T1–T2 tumors with nomogram indicated the probability of lymph node involvement as >10% [78]. It is unlikely that imaging for lower-risk tumors that do not meet either the aforementioned criteria will yield useful information. In one study, fewer than 1 in 120 bone scans performed on patients with a serum PSA below 20 ng ml^{-1} were found to be positive, and over 70% of those who tested positive had known symptoms of metastatic disease [83].

Despite the best efforts being made to stage prostate cancer with accuracy, prostatectomy series have shown that more than 10% of clinical T1–T2 patients actually have pathologic T3 or T4 disease [84]. The likelihood of extraprostatic extension or seminal vesicle involvement, designated pathologic T3 disease, is well-predicted by the judicious use of anatomic stage, serum PSA, and Gleason score. Several nomograms have been created to predict the risk of adverse pathologic features [85, 86].

Table 27.1 TNM stage definitions.

Clinical (cT)		
TX		Primary tumor cannot be assessed
T0		No evidence of primary tumor
T1		Clinically inapparent tumor neither palpable nor visible by imaging
	T1a	Tumor incidental histologic finding in 5% or less of tissue resected
	T1b	Tumor incidental histologic finding in more than 5% of tissue resected
	T1c	Tumor identified by needle biopsy (e.g., for elevated PSA)
T2		Tumor confined within prostate
	T2a	Tumor involves one-half of one lobe or less
	T2b	Tumor involves more than one-half of lobe, but not both lobes
	T2c	Tumor involves both lobes
T3		Tumor extends through the prostate capsule
	T3a	Extracapsular extension
	T3b	Tumor invades seminal vesicle(s)
T4		Tumor is fixed or invades adjacent structures other than seminal vesicles, such as external sphincter, rectum, bladder, levator muscles, and/or pelvic wall
Pathologic (pT)		
T2		Organ confined
T3		Extraprostatic extension
	T3a	Extraprostatic extension or microscopic invasion of bladder neck
	T3b	Seminal vesicle invasion
pT4		Invasion of rectum, levator muscles, and/or pelvic wall
Regional lymph nodes (N)		
Clinical		
NX		Regional lymph nodes were not assessed
N0		No regional lymph node metastasis
N1		Metastasis in regional lymph node(s)
Pathologic		
pNX		Regional nodes not sampled
pN0		No positive regional nodes
pN1		Metastases in regional node(s)
Distant metastasis (M)		
M0		No distant metastasis
M1		Distant metastasis
M1a		Non-regional lymph node(s)
M1b		Bone(s)
M1c		Other site(s) with or without bone disease

Source: AJCC Cancer Staging Manual, Eighth Edition (2017), Springer, New York, Inc.

Management Options

Active Surveillance

When evaluating patients, careful attention must be given to the grade of the tumor and its apparent extent, to the serum PSA level, the Gleason score, the age of the patient, baseline urinary, bowel, and sexual function, and his comorbid health conditions and predicted life expectancy. The latter two characteristics – comorbidity and life expectancy – are key in deciding who will benefit from radical prostate cancer treatment [87]. Epidemiological data suggests that more than half of treated men who are diagnosed at age 60 years or later will die of causes other than prostate cancer within 10 years [88].

Furthermore, the likelihood that a man in the modern era with a T1–T2 tumor will die of prostate cancer at 10 years is <10% [89]. In addition, therapy itself is not benign; it may result in undesired consequences such as impotence, bowel abnormalities, urinary obstructive symptoms and/or incontinence. The most recent NCCN guidelines take this concept into account by recommending observation for carefully selected patients. Observation, or no active intervention with a plan to administer palliative therapy for the development of symptoms, is the preferred option for patients with a life expectancy less than 10 years falling into the very low-risk, low-risk, and intermediate-risk groups (see Table 27.4) [78].

Unlike observation, active surveillance (AS), as the name suggests, is an active rather than a passive strategy.

Table 27.2 AJCC prognostic stage groups.

When T is	And N is	And M is	And PSA is	And grade group is	Then the stage group is
cT1a-c, cT2a	N0	M0	<10	1	I
pT2	N0	M0	<10	1	I
cT1a-c, cT2a	N0	M0	≥10<20	1	IIA
cT2b-c	N0	M0	<20	1	IIA
T1-2	N0	M0	<20	2	IIB
T1-2	N0	M0	<20	3	IIC
T1-2	N0	M0	<20	4	IIC
T1-2	N0	M0	≥20	1-4	IIIA
T3-4	N0	M0	Any	1-4	IIIB
Any T	N0	M0	Any	5	IIIC
Any T	N1	M0	Any	Any	IVA
Any T	N0	M1	Any	Any	IVB

Note: When either PSA or Grade Group is not available, grouping should be determined by T category and/or either PSA or Grade Group as available.
Source: AJCC Cancer Staging Manual, Eighth Edition (2017), Springer, New York, Inc.

It consists of a relatively strict follow-up protocol in which the PSA is checked at least biannually, a DRE is performed at least annually, and a prostate biopsy is repeated as often as every year [78]. As a result, the patient must be carefully counseled about the importance of regular follow-up to ensure that rapid and unexpected progression is not occurring, and be amenable to likely future biopsies. There have been multiple large prospective cohort studies which have validated the safety of this approach in carefully selected patients [90, 91]. Long-term outcomes from the University of Toronto cohort showed that the 15-year risk of metastatic disease was 2.8%, and the 15-year risk of death from prostate cancer was 1.5% [91]. Increasingly, MRI is being incorporated into AS regimens to initially assess the locoregional extent of disease and/or to guide future repeat biopsies in a more targeted fashion [92].

Triggers for recommending a switch from AS to radical therapy are the subject of ongoing debate. Established triggers to prompt treatment include: progression

Table 27.3 Definition of histologic grade group.

Grade group	Gleason score	Gleason pattern
1	≤6	≤3+3
2	7	3+4
3	7	4+3
4	8	4+4
5	9 or 10	4+5, 5+4, or 5+5

Source: AJCC Cancer Staging Manual, Eighth Edition (2017), Springer, New York, Inc.

Table 27.4 Pretreatment risk stratifications.

Risk group	Clinical stage	Gleason score	PSA
Very low*	T1c	Gleason ≤6	<10 ng ml^{-1}
Low	T1–T2a	Gleason 2–6	<10 ng ml^{-1}
Intermediate**	T2b–T2c	Gleason 7	10–20 ng ml^{-1}
High**	T3a	Gleason 8–10	>20 ng ml^{-1}
Very high	T3b–T4	Any Gleason	Any PSA

*Very low-risk group must also have the following: fewer than three positive prostate biopsy cores, ≤50 % cancer in each core, and PSA density <0.15 ng ml^{-1} g^{-1}.
**Designation of intermediate and high-risk groups requires the presence of only one of the three criteria (clinical stage, Gleason, PSA).
Source: National Comprehensive Cancer Network [78]. Available at: http://www.nccn.org.

to higher Gleason score or percentage positive biopsies on repeat biopsy, development or progression of a nodule on DRE, consistently rising PSA that is suspicious for progression, and patient choice [78]. Approximately one-third of patients will undergo curative treatment for one or more of these reasons while on AS [90, 91, 93]. The risk for requiring curative treatment at some point during a patient's lifetime increases with younger age.

The ProtecT trial was a randomized controlled trial in the UK that compared AS, radical prostatectomy, and radical radiotherapy with 3-6 months hormonal therapy [93a]. The median age of patients in this study was 62, with ~90% having a PSA < 10, 77% with Gleason score of 6, and 76% with cT1 stage. The AS regimen in this study was PSA checks every 3 months for one year, then every 6 months thereafter, with a rise in PSA of ≥50% in the prior 12 months prompting a repeat PSA and referral for a discussion regarding re-biopsy or treatment.

Ten-year outcomes of the ProtecT study revealed that there was no difference in prostate cancer-specific survival or overall survival between AS and upfront definitive local therapy, although the relative risk of clinical progression (both as local progression or distant metastases) was twice as high in patients receiving AS. However, the absolute risk was still relatively low in the AS population, suggesting it is a reasonable option for many patients. Approximately 55% of patients in the AS arm ultimately underwent definitive treatment. Given that this was primarily a low-risk and favorable intermediate-risk population, the results of this study are difficult to apply to those with unfavorable intermediate-risk or high-risk disease.

While there is a great deal of data in the use of AS in low-risk prostate cancer, there are more limited data using AS in intermediate-risk patients. Although some prospective single institution AS experiences included intermediate-risk patients, and intermediate-risk patients made up a small proportion of patients in the ProtecT study, most centers do not routinely recommend it for such cases [91, 93]. Long-term results of AS from the Sunnybrook series recently presented suggest that intermediate-risk patients may have a clinically meaningful worse cause-specific survival and overall survival than low-risk patients when managed with AS, arguing that clinicians should be cautious about using AS in intermediate-risk patients [95].

As per the most recent NCCN guidelines, AS is the preferred approach for very low-risk (Table 27.4) patients with a life expectancy of 10 years or more. For low-risk patients with a life expectancy of at least 10 years, AS is considered an option along with definitive therapy [78]. Of note, only approximately 10% of men with low-risk prostate cancer choose to pursue this strategy [5]. Also, it has been shown that patients seen in a multi-disciplinary clinic are twice as likely to pursue AS as those seen by the same number of individual providers [94].

Radical Prostatectomy

Radical prostatectomy (RP) involves complete removal of the prostate and seminal vesicles with the creation of a vesicourethral anastomosis. Many technical variations and surgical approaches are practiced throughout the US. Over the past decade, the utilization of minimally invasive RP performed either laparoscopically or robotically, has risen in popularity. Such techniques possess considerable learning curves, and comparative trials are lacking [96]. Depending on the risk of lymph node involvement, surgery can be accompanied by a pelvic lymph node dissection, often involving the obturator and external iliac nodes. The risk of lymph node positivity can be predicted prior to surgery by nomograms, using clinical stage, PSA, and Gleason Score [85, 86, 97].

RP is often an effective treatment for organ-confined disease as it extirpates not only the tumor but also the prostatic epithelium within which future tumors may develop. This is an important consideration as prostate carcinoma may be multifocal not just in location, but also in time. Prostatectomy also provides prognostic information that may be useful to younger men and may guide adjuvant therapy. Extracapsular extension, positive surgical margins and seminal vesicle invasion increase the risk of local disease recurrence [98]. Based on three randomized studies, postoperative radiation therapy should be considered in patients with these risk factors [99–101]. Pathologic lymph node involvement may indicate the presence of synchronous micrometastatic disease, and thus these patients are commonly treated with long-term hormonal therapy [102]. However, multiple retrospective series suggest improved outcomes when adding salvage radiotherapy in these patients, and there is an increasing role for adding pelvic radiation therapy to long-term hormonal therapy [103–105]. Postoperatively, PSA should become undetectable, making the definition of treatment failure extremely clear. The risk of PSA failure can be predicted from the preoperative stage, Gleason score, and PSA level [106].

While RP remains the most widely used therapy for localized prostate cancer, over the past decade there has been a decline in its in low-risk cancers and a rise in its use of in intermediate-risk and high-risk prostate cancer patients [107]. Despite its utilization, there are significant potential side effects associated with RP. Approximately 50–60% of men will recover potency two years after nerve-sparing RP [108]. Potency preservation is lower when a nerve-sparing approach is not feasible. Almost 30% of patients have dripping or leaking of urine or no urinary control five years after surgery, although this risk is highly dependent on the experience of the treating surgeon and at some experienced centers it may be approximately 10% [109]. More than one in four patients with palpable disease are found to have extracapsular extension on pathologic review and thus are less likely to be cured by surgery alone [110, 111].

Two randomized studies have been conducted during the PSA era comparing prostatectomy with observation [112, 113]. The SPCG-4 trial was performed early in the PSA era and showed an improvement in prostate cancer-specific survival, overall survival and distant metastases exclusively in men aged <65 years [112]. However, 80% of patients had palpable tumors and only 12% were cT1c, suggesting a higher risk population than that seen in today's clinical practice. The PIVOT trial consisted of a PSA-screened population, and showed that there was no distant metastasis, prostate cancer-specific mortality, or overall survival benefit for the population, but there may have been subgroups with higher-risk disease who could potentially benefit [113].

Historically, recommendations were dependent on retrospective and single-arm prospective cohort studies to compare the treatment modalities. Although some series suggest better outcomes with surgery, systematic reviews of the available data and population-based cohort studies suggest that radical prostatectomy and radical radiation modalities are equally curative [114–116]. The ProtecT trial randomized radical prostatectomy, definitive EBRT with short-term hormonal therapy, and AS in primarily low-risk and favorable intermediate-risk patients. Ten year outcomes were recently reported, and revealed no difference in clinical progression (either as local progression or distant metastases), prostate-cancer specific mortality or overall survival, between prostatectomy and radiotherapy [93a]. The results of this study must cautiously be applied, as the implications on patients with unfavorable intermediate-risk and high-risk disease are less clear.

Radiation Therapy

Radiation oncologists now have a number of radiation techniques to choose from for the curative treatment of prostate cancer. The two broad categories of radical radiotherapy modalities are external beam radiation therapy (EBRT) and brachytherapy. These are both used routinely at most centers in the US, although their appropriate application depends on a number of important clinical factors. The most common form of EBRT is photon radiotherapy, and an increasing number of centers now use proton radiotherapy. Brachytherapy is delivered most commonly as LDR brachytherapy using a permanent interstitial implant of radioactive seeds, but several centers deliver HDR brachytherapy, using multiple interstitial catheters and a temporary radiation source.

There are no randomized data describing the differential disease control or toxicity outcomes of each of the radiotherapy modalities, but historically they have had relatively similar cure rates. The radiotherapeutic options for patients with prostate cancer are discussed in the flowing sections.

Historically, patients were treated with 64–70 Gy of EBRT, but several dose-escalation randomized trials have shown a benefit in PSA control of approximately 10–15% for doses ranging from 74 to 80 Gy. One study revealed a 3% benefit in distant metastases, although no benefit has been demonstrated in overall survival to dose escalation [117–121]. However, based on these level 1 data, the current standard approach to definitive EBRT is doses of 1.8–2 Gy per fraction to a total dose of 75.6 Gy or greater. More conformal methods have allowed for decreased doses to normal tissues with dose escalation to the target. There are no randomized data directly comparing IMRT with 3D conformal radiotherapy (3D-CRT) in prostate cancer; however, a planned analysis of the dose-escalation trial of RTOG 0126, in which both 3D-CRT and IMRT were allowed, revealed decreased late grade ≥ 2 gastrointestinal toxicity [122]. The use of image guidance has allowed for more accurate and reproducible set-up, and may further improve the therapeutic index [123].

There is a growing body of evidence supporting hypofractionation, or the use of a shorter radiation course with larger dose per treatment fraction. The advantages of moderate hypofractionation include patient convenience, lower treatment costs, and possible therapeutic gain due to the lower alpha/beta ratio of prostate cancer compared to other malignancies [124]. Two randomized trials evaluated this question in the non-dose-escalated era and found worse acute toxicity, with conflicting findings regarding biochemical control with hypofractionation [125, 126]. The limitations of these studies were the low biologic equivalent dose of both the conventional and hypofractionated arms (62–67 Gy in 2-Gy fractions), an absence of image guidance, and mostly 2D treatment planning. Since then, the details of several randomized trials have been published comparing standard dose-escalated conventional fractionation to hypofractionation. Most

of these trials have demonstrated similar efficacy and toxicity outcomes, but no treatment advantage for the shorter course [127–131]. These studies use higher biologically equivalent doses (74–86 Gy in 2-Gy fractions), and sophisticated treatment planning methods. RTOG 0415, which compared 73.8 Gy in 1.8 Gy per fraction with 70 Gy in 2.5 Gy per fraction in men with low-risk prostate cancer was recently presented with a median follow-up of 5.9 years, and revealed that the hypofractionated regimen was non-inferior to conventional fractionation in terms of disease-free survival and grade 3 gastrointestinal and genitourinary toxicity, but with slightly increased grade 2 genitourinary toxicity [132, 133]. The CHHiP trial (CRUK/06/016) randomized 60 Gy in 3 Gy per fraction, 57 Gy in 3 Gy per fraction, and 74 Gy in 2 Gy per fraction for low-, intermediate-, and high-risk prostate cancer patients. The five-year results revealed 60 Gy to be non-inferior to 74 Gy in terms of freedom from progression, but non-inferiority could not be met for 57 Gy compared to 74 Gy [128, 134, 135]. Acute grade ≥ 2 gastrointestinal toxicity was worse in the hypofractionated groups, but there was no difference in late grade ≥ 2 gastrointestinal or genitourinary toxicity. Similarly, the Canadian PROFIT trial randomized 78 Gy in 2 Gy per fraction with 60 Gy in 20 fractions of 3 Gy in intermediate-risk patients not receiving hormonal therapy. With median follow-up of 6 years, the hypofractionated arm was non-inferior to conventional fractionation, and actually had improved late toxicity compared to the conventionally fractionated arm [135a]. Conversely, the HYPRO study randomized 78 Gy in 2 Gy per fraction to 64.6 Gy in 19 fractions of 3.4 Gy. With 5 years median follow-up, this hypofractionated regimen was not superior to standard fractionation, and was not non-inferior in terms of grade ≥ 2 late genitourinary or gastrointestinal toxicity, and had worse grade ≥ 3 late genitourinary toxicity [135b, 135c]. Given the outcomes of these studies, it is likely that moderate hypofractionation will increasingly be used, although the optimal maximum dose per fraction may be 3 Gy, and 70 Gy in 2.5 Gy per fraction or 60 Gy in 3 Gy per fraction are preferable to 64.6 Gy in 3.4 Gy per fraction. Hypofractionation in the postoperative setting and with the treatment of the pelvic nodes is under investigation.

With the same rationale as moderate hypofractionation, extreme/ultra-hypofractionation – otherwise termed stereotactic body radiotherapy (SBRT) – is delivered over the course of one to five fractions. Most series use 4–5 fractions to deliver 33–50 Gy, with a common regimen being 36.25 Gy in five fractions. Early follow-up of prospective trials evaluating this approach are encouraging and suggest similar disease control and toxicity, though no randomized data are currently available for this approach, and the optimal dose/fractionation is unknown. Additionally, a Medicare claims-based comparative study suggested that there may be an increased risk of genitourinary toxicity in men treated with SBRT compared to IMRT, as defined by claims to Medicare associated with toxicities [136]. This same study showed considerably less overall cost to SBRT over IMRT. RTOG 0938 compared 36.25 Gy in five fractions of 7.25 Gy with 51.6 Gy in 12 fractions of 4.3 Gy to evaluate the patient-reported health-related quality of life, and showed both fractionations to have an acceptable toxicity profile [137]. Thus, these fractionations should be explored further, and potentially tested in the form of a randomized study comparing one or both of them to moderate hypofractionation.

Brachytherapy

Two forms of prostate brachytherapy are available, namely LDR brachytherapy with permanent interstitial radioactive seeds, and HDR prostate brachytherapy, using multi-catheter temporary implant with a single source iridium-192 afterloader. Patients who are candidates for brachytherapy based on American Brachytherapy Society recommendations are men with limited urinary symptoms (typically IPSS score ≤20), gland size ≤60 ml, good life expectancy, no significant TURP deficits, no prior radiotherapy, and no history of inflammatory bowel disease [138]. Patients with low-risk prostate cancer and some select patients with favorable intermediate risk can be treated with monotherapy, while patients with unfavorable intermediate-risk and high-risk disease are commonly treated with combined EBRT and brachytherapy boost if brachytherapy is desired.

LDR series suggest excellent outcomes for well-selected patients. Long-term outcomes with monotherapy reveal 15-year biochemical recurrence free-survival rates of 85.9% and 79.9% for low-risk and intermediate-risk patients, respectively [139]. When combined with EBRT, 12-year biochemical recurrence free-survival rates are 99% for intermediate-risk and 95% for high-risk patients, and 12-year metastasis-free survival rates are >90% [140, 141]. Multiple isotopes have been used, including iodine-125, palladium-103, and cesium-131. Of key importance in LDR brachytherapy is the quality of the implant, as measured by the D90, or minimum dose to 90% of the gland [142]. A multi-institutional study evaluating the D90 found that patients with a D90 <130 Gy had an eight-year PSA relapse-free survival of 76%, as compared to 93% for those with D90 ≥130 Gy [142].

Historically, HDR brachytherapy was first used in the boost setting after EBRT. RTOG 0321 evaluated 45 Gy EBRT followed by 19 Gy in two fractions of HDR brachytherapy boost. The reported early toxicity profile is promising with this approach [143]. There is also increasing experience using HDR monotherapy for the definitive management of prostate cancer. Proponents of HDR brachytherapy cite potential radiobiologic benefits, radiation safety benefits to staff, better reproducibility,

and improved dosimetry and dose certainty with this approach compared to LDR. Although newer series use one to two implants and avoid hospitalization, historically this approach has required more staff time, hospitalization, and potentially more implants than LDR.

There are no randomized data comparing the two brachytherapy approaches, although retrospective series suggest relatively similar outcomes with both approaches [144–149]. With either modality, patient selection, the quality of the implant, and practitioner expertise are likely the most important factors for patient outcome.

Follow-Up

After definitive radiation therapy, the PSA level should be measured approximately three to four months after completion of treatment, then every six months for two to five years, and then annually. A DRE is also recommended annually [78]. PSA surrogates are typically used as end points in clinical studies, given the long life expectancy of most treated patients. Historically, PSA recurrence was defined as three consecutive rises in the PSA, with the date of failure defined as halfway between the nadir and the first of the three rises. However, this was not closely associated with clinical progression or survival, and made it difficult to compare across studies with different PSA follow-up frequencies [150]. In order to create a standardized definition of biochemical failure after radiotherapy, the RTOG-ASTRO Phoenix consensus defined biochemical recurrence after radiotherapy with or without hormonal therapy as a rise in PSA by at least 2 ng ml^{-1} above the nadir PSA [150]. This is the standard definition in the modern era.

Among patients treated with brachytherapy, 33% to 40% develop a PSA bounce approximately 18–24 months after brachytherapy, making careful consideration of PSA kinetics important before determining whether a PSA rise indicates failure. The standard definition of failure is still the Phoenix definition, but the 48-month PSA has been strongly correlated with long-term prostate cancer-specific mortality [151].

Following standard radiation treatment, rebiopsy for those without biochemical failure is unnecessary. For those who fail biochemically, patients must be stratified into those who may be candidates for salvage local therapy or those who are not. Patients who are potentially candidates for salvage local therapy are those with original clinical stage T1–T2, a life expectancy >10 years, and current PSA <10 ng ml^{-1}. These patients can undergo rebiopsy, a CT or MRI of the abdomen/pelvis, bone scan, and MRI of the prostate [78]. Several novel radiotracers are being explored, such as 11-choline PET-CT, to improve the detection of occult metastases, but none of these has been incorporated into standard management. If the biopsy is positive and the imaging work-up is negative for metastases, additional local treatment options are available for well-selected patients. These options include salvage brachytherapy if EBRT was the initial treatment, as well as salvage prostatectomy or cryosurgery, although there is a significant risk of toxicity with salvage local therapy [152].

Low-Risk Disease

Patients with low-risk prostate cancer are candidates for nearly all of the treatment approaches. Active surveillance should also be considered and discussed with patients in this group, who can receive local treatment with radical prostatectomy, brachytherapy, and dose-escalated EBRT. Patients should be counseled based on their life expectancy and the potential impact of toxicities on their quality of life [153]. The disease control and toxicity results of the ProtecT study are particularly useful in counseling this cohort of patients [93a, 195b]. There is no role for hormonal therapy other than for volume reduction to improve candidacy for brachytherapy [154]. Primary hormonal therapy without local therapy has not shown any clinical benefit for this cohort of patients [155]. The dose of radiation delivered to the prostate also appears to affect outcomes significantly, and it appears a biologic equivalent dose (BED) of 200 is optimal compared to lower BEDs [156].

Intermediate-Risk Disease

The management of men with intermediate-risk prostate cancer (see Table 27.4) tends to be the most heterogeneous of the risk groups. For those with life expectancies less than 10 years, AS or observation can be considered for selected patients [78]. Definitive treatments for those with longer life expectancies include RP, brachytherapy, and EBRT. Brachytherapy as monotherapy is not typically recommended, but can be considered for patients with favorable intermediate-risk disease [139, 147]. Recently, the results of RTOG 0232, which compared LDR brachytherapy monotherapy with LDR combined with supplemental EBRT, were presented [156a]. With 6.7 years follow-up, there was no benefit in progression-free survival with the addition of supplemental EBRT, suggesting that select patients with intermediate-risk disease may not benefit from supplemental EBRT. Conversely, the ASCENDE-RT trial compared EBRT with brachytherapy boost to definitive EBRT, with both arms in the setting of 12 months androgen-deprivation therapy (ADT), and revealed a significant benefit in seven-year PSA control with the combination [157]. Whilst this was consistent with the results of several retrospective series [158, 159], it came at the cost of increased urethral toxicity and no benefit in

overall survival. Thus, a detailed discussion is needed and the risks/benefits must be weighed for each patient.

Short-course neoadjuvant and concurrent ADT using a gonadotropin-releasing hormone agonist for four to six months is commonly added to EBRT for intermediate-risk disease, particularly for those patients with unfavorable intermediate-risk disease. Three randomized trials conducted during the non-dose-escalated era revealed a 5–13% survival benefit with the addition of four to six months of ADT [154, 160, 161]. The largest trial, RTOG 9408, randomized 1979 patients (55% intermediate-risk, 35% low-risk, 10% high-risk) to 66.6 Gy EBRT alone versus EBRT and four months' ADT [154]. This resulted in an improved survival with the addition of short-term ADT, primarily in the intermediate-risk subgroup. RTOG 9910 compared ADT periods of four and nine months ADT in combination with non-dose-escalated radiotherapy, and found no benefit in extending ADT past four months [162].

The role for androgen suppression in the era of dose escalation is less clear. The recently presented Prostate Cancer Study (PCS) III trial found a benefit in PSA control and disease-free survival (DFS) with short-term ADT and dose-escalated radiotherapy, although there was no overall survival benefit (the details have yet to be published) [163]. The TROG 03.04 RADAR trial suggested a benefit to increasing hormonal therapy duration in the dose-escalated setting from six to 18 months, but the DART 01/05 randomized trial compared four and 24 months in the dose-escalated setting (≥76 Gy; median dose 78 Gy); although PSA control was better there was no survival benefit for men with intermediate-risk prostate cancer [163, 164]. The incremental benefit of short-term ADT is currently being evaluated in the RTOG 0815 trial (NCT00936390). Until these results are available, percentage positive biopsies and primary Gleason scores can be used to help risk-stratify patients for ADT use [76, 165]. Androgen suppression reliably reduces the volume of over 90% of prostate carcinomas. Tumor volume reduction prior to radiation improves the likelihood of achieving local control and reduces the radiation dose required to do so [166]. Additionally, two-year biopsy data revealed a significantly lower rate of positive biopsies with hormonal therapy compared to EBRT alone [154].

It should be noted that epidemiological studies have found an association between ADT use and myocardial infarction [167, 168]. Although some studies have suggested an increased risk of incident diabetes and cardiovascular morbidity/mortality, most have suggested no increase in the risk of cardiac mortality with the addition of ADT, including a subgroup analysis of RTOG 9408 [167–171]. RTOG 0815 has a preplanned stratification based on ACE-27 comorbidity score, and hopefully the results of the study will provide a definitive answer (NCT00936390).

High-Risk Disease

Patients with high-risk disease have worse outcomes than low-risk and intermediate-risk patients. Fortunately, only approximately 5% of patients present with clinical stage T3 or T4 disease [172]. Definitive treatment with either RP in selected patients or EBRT is recommended for men with high-risk and locally advanced disease (see Table 27.4).

There is strong evidence that the combination of EBRT with ADT is beneficial for men with high-risk disease. Two years and four months to three years of ADT have been shown to be superior to shorter courses in multiple clinical trials in the non-dose-escalated era [173, 174]. The DART 01/05 trial revealed a survival benefit for 28 months of ADT compared to four months of ADT in the setting of ≥76 Gy (median dose 78 Gy), primarily driven by high-risk patients [164, 173, 175].

Given the high risk of developing metastatic disease, the role of local therapy for patients with locally advanced disease has been questioned in some studies. Two randomized trials comparing long-term ADT with or without definitive EBRT found an 8–10% survival benefit with the addition of radiotherapy [176, 177]. Thus, for patients with high-risk locally advanced disease, randomized data support a survival advantage when combining definitive EBRT with long-term ADT (two years, four months to three years) as primary therapy.

Interestingly, the Prostate Cancer Study (PCS) IV study compared 36 months of ADT with 18 months of ADT in the setting of non-dose-escalated radiotherapy, and found no difference in biochemical control, prostate cancer-specific mortality, or overall survival at a median follow-up of 6.5 years [178]. Further follow-up of this study may alter the landscape of hormonal therapy in high-risk prostate cancer. Additionally, there may be a more favorable cohort of patients with high-risk prostate cancer, who may not require the same duration of long-term ADT as patients with T3–T4 and Gleason score 8–10 disease [80].

The addition of radiotherapy to the pelvic lymph node regions in addition to the prostate and seminal vesicles in high-risk patients is controversial. Because patients undergoing radiation typically have unknown pathologic nodal status (NX), some recommend considering pelvic nodal irradiation if the risk of lymph node involvement exceeds 15% [179]. However, three randomized trials have evaluated the incremental benefit of treating the whole pelvis and found no benefit, although there are several limitations to interpreting the results of these trials, including the older treatment techniques, the target fields used, low dose to the prostate, and statistical power [180–182]. The present authors' practice is selective treatment of the pelvic nodes in high-risk prostate cancer patients, taking into account the number of high-risk features, comorbidities, and age. Hopefully, the results of RTOG 0924 (NCT02673190), comparing long-term ADT with dose-escalated radiotherapy to the prostate and seminal vesicles with or without the pelvic nodes, will define the role of pelvic radiotherapy in prostate cancer.

The role of chemotherapy in the primary management of high-risk prostate cancer is evolving. The results of RTOG 0521, a randomized trial of standard long-term ADT and definitive EBRT to 75.6 Gy with or without six, 21-day cycles of docetaxel one month after completion of radiotherapy, was recently presented. With a median follow-up of 5.5 years, patients treated with chemotherapy had a better four-year overall survival (93% versus 89%) [183]. With longer follow-up, the results of this study may dramatically alter the treatment of high-risk prostate cancer. Additionally, there are multiple trials currently being conducted to evaluate the role of more effective hormone therapy modalities, such as enzalutamide and abiraterone.

Some patients may still elect for surgery despite high-risk features. RP with nodal dissection may be considered if there is no fixation to adjacent organs [78], although a possible disadvantage to RP in this context is that the majority of patients will not be eligible for nerve-sparing techniques, and thus near-complete erectile dysfunction may be more common [184]. Additionally, postoperative radiotherapy may be recommended in such cases, putting the patient at risk for the combined toxicity of surgery and radiotherapy.

Adjuvant and Salvage Radiation After Prostatectomy

Candidates for adjuvant radiation after RP include patients with pT3 disease (seminal vesicle involvement or extracapsular extension) or positive surgical margins. Three large randomized trials have demonstrated that adjuvant radiotherapy to 60–64 Gy improves biochemical relapse-free survival and potentially even overall survival in some patients, compared to observation. The SWOG 8794 trial enrolled patients with pT3 disease or positive surgical margins and demonstrated a clear improvement in freedom from hormone therapy and overall and metastasis-free survival, with a median follow-up of 12.5 years in the most recent update [99, 101]. The EORTC 22911 trial randomized a similar cohort of patients to 60 Gy adjuvant radiotherapy or a wait-and-see approach, and found improvements in biochemical progression-free survival and local control but not in clinical progression-free survival or overall survival. A subgroup analysis of this study found men aged <70 years and those with positive surgical margins may have a clinical progression-free survival benefit. The ARO 96-02/AUO AP 09/95 trial randomized men with pT3 disease to adjuvant radiotherapy or wait-and-see, and found a PSA progression-free survival benefit but no improvement in clinical outcomes [100]. Based on these data, the ASTRO/AUA created a guideline regarding indications for adjuvant radiotherapy use [185]. Interestingly, a recent analysis of the National Cancer Database revealed that the use of postoperative radiotherapy dropped from 9.1% to 7.3% between 2005 and 2011, despite the level 1 data and guideline recommendations [186].

However, only the ARO 96-02 study required undetectable postoperative PSA, and approximately 30–35% of patients in the SWOG and EORTC studies had a postoperative PSA level >0.2 ng ml^{-1}. Additionally, in the SWOG study, among patients who received salvage radiotherapy in the observation arm, 55% received treatment with PSA recurrence, but 41% received salvage radiotherapy after having PSA relapse and an objective recurrence; this suggested that salvage radiotherapy was delivered late in the clinical course in a large cohort [187]. The most common current clinical practice in men who do not receive adjuvant radiotherapy is to follow PSA closely and to treat when the PSA level begins to rise, while still at relatively low levels (this is otherwise known as 'early-salvage'). To date, no randomized data are available to compare adjuvant radiation with early salvage radiation, though randomized trials such as RAVES and RADICALS are currently attempting to compare these procedures (NCT00860652 and NCT00541047).

The role for salvage radiotherapy in patients with PSA or local recurrence after RP is well documented. Clinical cure is still possible, but is highly dependent on a number of factors including stage, surgical margins, and PSA level. Several nomograms are available to aid in prognostication for patients who are candidates for salvage therapy [188–190]. A systematic review of retrospective series suggested that a lower PSA of initiation and escalation of dose to >66 Gy are associated with improved outcomes, though no randomized data are available to guide physicians regarding the optimal dose or optimal PSA threshold to initiate treatment [191]. In this study, a rise in PSA of 0.1 was associated with a decline in PSA control of 2.6%, and an increase in 1 Gy from 60–70 Gy was associated with an increase in PSA control of 2% [191]. Additionally, the role of hypofractionated radiotherapy is being explored.

The roles of pelvic lymph node irradiation and ADT in the postoperative setting are unclear. Retrospective series suggest a benefit to the addition of the pelvic lymph nodes in high-risk patients, although no randomized

data are currently available addressing this issue [192]. Several retrospective series, as well as subgroup analyses of RTOG 8531, have suggested a benefit of ADT in the salvage setting for selected patients [193]. Recently reported results from RTOG 96-01, which compared salvage radiotherapy to salvage radiotherapy with two years of bicalutamide, showed that the addition of anti-androgen reduces the risk of metastatic disease and improves survival in selected patients requiring postoperative radiotherapy [194, 195]. The subgroups who benefitted most were those with PSA prior to salvage radiotherapy of 0.7 ng ml^{-1} to 4 ng ml^{-1}, positive surgical margins, or Gleason score ≥7. The current clinical practice is to substitute a gonadotropin-releasing hormone (GnRH) agonist (e.g., leuprolide, goserelin) for an anti-androgen (bicalutamide), typically for four to six months, although some institutions use a longer duration of ADT in the salvage setting. GETUG-AFU 16 was a randomized trial in men with post-operative PSA < 0.1 with a subsequent rise to 0.2-2, and compared no hormonal therapy with 6 months goserelin. Five year results revealed the addition of the GnRH agonist improved freedom from biochemical and clinical progression, with limited additional toxicity [195a]. Longer follow-up is necessary to ascertain the impact of adding short-term hormonal therapy on survival. RTOG 0534, which has completed accrual, randomized patients undergoing salvage radiotherapy to treatment to the prostate bed with or without the whole pelvis, and with or without short-term ADT, and will hopefully help to answer these questions (NCT00567580).

Node-Positive Disease

Historically, patients found to have either radiographically or pathologically positive lymph nodes had a dismal prognosis when treated with radical therapy. However, this prognosis has improved today due to decreased tumor burden in the era of PSA screening, improvements in radiation techniques allowing dose escalation, and the use of multimodality therapy [196]. Although their outcomes are worse than patients without nodal involvement, pelvic radiation with long-term ADT can be used to treat these patients with a definitive approach. There have been no randomized controlled trials exclusively evaluating EBRT with and without ADT in node-positive patients, but a trial comparing the two treatments found a significant survival benefit with EBRT plus ADT in a subanalysis of patients with N1 disease. Additional observational studies have also found that this regimen results in improved cancer-specific survival rates for node-positive patients [197, 198]. Similarly, although there is currently a trial concept in development through NRG Oncology, no randomized data are available comparing ADT with and without radiotherapy for clinically or pathologically node-positive prostate cancer. For clinically node-positive patients, population-based analyses of the Surveillance, Epidemiology, and End Results Program and National Cancer Database analyses both found a survival benefit with the addition of radiotherapy in this setting [199, 200]. As a result, EBRT with nodal irradiation and long-term ADT is a standard treatment for node-positive disease in select patients [78]. For pathologically node-positive patients, an Italian matched-pair analysis revealed a cause-specific and overall survival benefit to the addition of radiotherapy to ADT, and a subsequent study from the same institution identified patient subgroups who appear to benefit most [103, 104].

Metastatic Disease

ADT is the mainstay of treatment for metastatic disease. Symptomatic improvement is seen in 90% of patients, and PSA values usually decline to normal levels for 18–24 months on average. Patients are usually started and continued on lifelong ADT. Unfortunately, androgen independence (often referred to as castration-resistant disease) is inevitable, and the next steps in treatment, such as stronger hormonal therapy with abiraterone or enzalutamide, or chemotherapy with cabazitaxel or docetaxel, and immunotherapy, are used. A randomized trial of continuous or intermittent ADT in the metastatic setting revealed a better quality of life, but was unable to prove that intermittent therapy was non-inferior [201]. Conversely, the CHAARTED trial revealed a nearly 14-month improvement in overall survival by the addition of upfront docetaxel for newly diagnosed metastatic prostate cancer with high-volume disease, while the recently presented STAMPEDE trial revealed a similar survival benefit to upfront docetaxel [202, 203]. Thus, the role of early chemotherapy will likely continue to grow as long-term outcomes of these and similar studies are presented.

Bone pain and fatigue resulting from anemia of marrow filtration are common late clinical effects. EBRT delivered palliatively as 8 Gy in a single dose will reduce pain in two-thirds of patients with non-vertebral skeletal metastases for the remainder of the patient's life, while findings of multiple randomized trials suggest there is no benefit to going to higher doses [204]. The ASTRO Choosing Wisely campaign recommended against using palliative regimens of more than ten fractions, and encouraged using a single fraction of 8 Gy when possible [205].

When metastases are too numerous, or pain is very diffuse and poorly controlled by opiates, systemic therapy using radionucleotides, such as historically strontium-89

or samarium-153, and more recently radium-223, may be considered. Approximately one-third of men will have a subjective pain response with strontium, with a median duration of response of about four to five months, and troublesome myelosuppression, in particular thrombocytopenia, may result [206, 207]. Systemic radionuclides are therefore not suitable for patients who have diffuse marrow involvement and declining blood counts. It is important to note that strontium is not suitable for patients who are incontinent, as it is concentrated in the urine and may represent a radiation hazard.

Radium-223 dichloride, also known as Xofigo®, was compared to placebo in the Phase III randomized ALSYMPCA trial in patients with castrate-resistant prostate cancer who had received, but were not candidates for or refused, docetaxel [208, 209]. The study was stopped at interim analysis due to a superior overall survival and a prolonged time to skeletal-related events with radium-223. Importantly, EBRT has been shown to be safe to deliver for local palliation in patients receiving radium-223 [210]. Hematologic toxicities are the primary toxicity associated with radium-223.

EBRT may also be used to palliate the consequences of bulky lymphadenopathy. Patients with lower-limb edema, as a result of pelvic or para-aortic lymph node enlargement, may respond to doses of 40–44 Gy in 2-Gy fractions.

Oligometastasis

Initially coined by Hellman and Weichselbaum, the hypothesis of oligometastasis is that there exists a state during the progression of any cancer from locoregional disease to widely metastatic in which the malignancy can only involve a limited number of sites or organs due to the accumulated genetic aberrations present in the malignant clones [211]. Therefore, aggressive local therapy can result in durable long-term disease control and potential cure in selected patients. Examples of this phenomenon include the resection of lung metastases from sarcoma and liver metastases from colorectal cancer. Although most of the data have been obtained with other malignancies, several observational series have described favorable outcomes of patients treated with metastasis-directed resection or SBRT for limited skeletal, nodal or visceral metastases from prostate cancer [212, 213]. The optimal dose/fractionation has not been identified when SBRT is used, and patients are typically treated with doses of approximately 25–60 Gy in three to five fractions using sophisticated planning methods with careful attention to normal tissue dose constraints.

Based on this hypothesis and observational data from multiple malignancies, aggressive local therapy, including resection and SBRT, are increasingly being utilized in patients with metastatic cancer. However, no randomized data are currently available showing a benefit to the addition of local therapy to systemic therapy in metastatic prostate cancer. NRG Oncology BR001 (NCT02206334) is a Phase I study evaluating the safety of SBRT in the treatment of patients with two to four metastases from breast, lung, or prostate cancer, and is currently accruing. The STOMP trial (NCT01558427) is a Belgian randomized trial comparing surveillance with metastasis-directed therapy using surgery or radiation for men with up to three sites of metastatic disease after definitive treatment for prostate cancer. Hopefully, studies such as these will help to elucidate the role of local therapy in metastatic prostate cancer.

Biochemical Recurrence After Definitive Radiation

A particularly challenging cohort of patients to counsel are those who develop biochemical failure without identifiable clinical disease after definitive radiation (either EBRT or brachytherapy). The median time to prostate cancer-specific mortality after the development of biochemical failure is approximately 8–10 years, during which time a man may not even have morbidity from prostate cancer and may die of another comorbid condition [214,215]. Thus life expectancy, comorbid medical conditions, disease characteristics (particularly PSA doubling time and absolute PSA value), urinary and bowel function, and patient preference must all be considered when counseling patients on palliative or salvage treatment options.

The standard palliative treatment is ADT. The goal is to delay or potentially to avoid the morbidity/mortality associated with clinical progression, although this must be weighed against the potential impact on quality of life of ADT. Historically, patients have been treated with continuous ADT indefinitely. A randomized study compared continuous and intermittent ADT in patients with biochemical but not clinical progression after EBRT [215]. Although the study revealed that intermittent ADT was non-inferior to continuous ADT, caution must be expressed when using intermittent ADT in the subgroup of men with Gleason score 8–10, as these patients had a trend towards worse survival, though this was based on an unplanned subgroup analysis.

A select group of patients may be candidates for salvage local therapy with definitive intent – potentially those with good urinary function, long life expectancy, and favorable initial and current disease characteristics. Great caution must be taken in selecting these patients, as the chance for cure is modest and there is an increased risk of toxicity with each of the salvage options,

which include radical prostatectomy, brachytherapy, high-intensity focused ultrasound (HIFU), or cryotherapy [152]. Local disease should be pathologically identified and distant disease ruled out as best as possible prior to proceeding with one of these treatments.

Radiotherapeutic Technique

Several radiation modalities exist for the definitive treatment of localized prostate cancer, including external beam radiation with high-energy x-rays or particles, as well as LDR and HDR brachytherapy. Advances made in treatment planning and delivery allow for high doses to be delivered to the prostate while minimizing radiation to the surrounding normal tissues. In the postoperative setting, or when cancer has spread beyond the prostate, photon therapy is most often employed.

Radical External Beam Radiation

IMRT has replaced 3D-CRT in the treatment of patients with intact prostates. The use of image-guided radiation therapy (IGRT) has also increased substantially in recent years and can improve treatment accuracy by providing daily information regarding the position of the prostate and surrounding organs, and may additionally improve the therapeutic index of IMRT [123]. A variety of methods is available to obtain accurate and reliable localization and daily patient set-up, and there is no one best approach. However, some form of image-guided radiotherapy is necessary. Some centers use gold fiducials distributed throughout the prostate. During daily treatment, therapists use KV orthogonal images or cone beam CT to set up to these fiducials. Some institutions do not use fiducial markers, but rather use cone beam CT to set up to soft-tissue anatomy. Some centers use electromagnetic transponders which monitor interfraction and intrafraction motion using radiofrequency waves. Ultimately, these aspects of set-up and target verification should be based on the unique departmental resources, patient population, and set-up conditions and should be institution-dependent.

Prior to CT simulation, at institutions that use fiducial markers, these are placed using a transperineal or transrectal approach. If radiofrequency beacons are being used, these too are placed prior to CT simulation using a transperineal approach. A newer technique that is being explored at many institutions is to insert an absorbable hydrogel spacer into Denonvillier's fascia, using hydrodissection to increase the distance between the prostate and rectum, as a way to reduce the rectal dose during irradiation [216]. Based on a multicenter randomized trial, placement of this spacer may reduce late rectal toxicity [217], but not all centers use this approach given the relatively low risk of severe late rectal toxicity in patients using modern treatment approaches.

Patients are placed in the supine position during CT simulation. At this time, some centers use a rectal balloon filled with 40–60 ml of water to allow for reproducibility of the rectum and prostate position during daily treatments. Some centers ask patients to use an enema or other form of bowel preparation prior to simulation to avoid distortion of the rectum during simulation. Some institutions ask the patient to have a comfortably full bladder at the time of CT simulation and prior to each treatment. The primary rationale for a full bladder is to displace the bowel and to try to reproduce the prostate position. Some centers use a retrograde urethrogram during CT simulation to assist in identification of the prostate apex, while at other centers this is not found to be as useful and thus is not performed.

During target delineation, the prostate, seminal vesicles, bladder, rectum, and femoral heads are identified and outlined on the planning CT. If a prostate MRI has been performed, this can be used to help with prostate volume delineation, as can the ultrasound dimensions at the time of biopsy or fiducial marker placement. Careful attention is paid to the apex, anterior border, and base of the prostate gland, which can sometimes be difficult to identify on CT alone and are at risk for contouring errors [218]. Pelvic lymph node regions are also outlined if they are to be included in the treatment field.

IMRT is the standard treatment technique. There are two forms of IMRT: static field ('step and shoot') and volumetric arc therapy (VMAT). Historically, most centers used a static field approach but many institutions have transitioned to VMAT, primarily due to quicker treatment times, lower monitor units, and arguably improved dosimetry. A typical VMAT plan is shown in Figure 27.2. Adjustments to the number of beams/arc arrangement may be required depending on the patient's anatomy and the presence of hip prostheses or other metallic interfaces. Care must be taken to avoid posterior beams entering through the treatment table, which can act as a bolus to increase skin dose.

There is no one standard dose/fractionation for definitive radiotherapy, although some form of dose-escalated radiotherapy (≥ 74 Gy) should be used. When conventional fractionation is used, common dose/fractionations are 79.2 Gy in 1.8 Gy per fraction or 78 Gy in 2 Gy per fraction. When hypofractionated regimens are used, common fractionations are 70 Gy in 2.5 Gy per fraction and 60 Gy in 3 Gy per fraction. At some centers, there are two phases of treatment. The prostate and a portion of the seminal vesicles are treated to 45–50.4 Gy, after which the prostate is boosted to the definitive dose. Other institutions use a single phase of treatment and boost the prostate and target portion of the seminal vesicles to the definitive dose. Both are reasonable approaches.

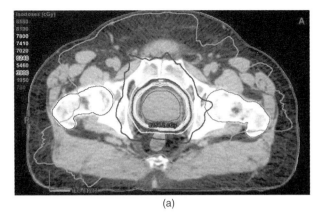

(a)

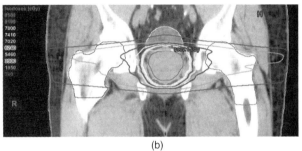

(b)

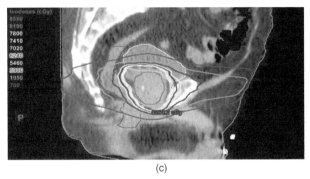

(c)

Figure 27.2 A typical definitive external beam radiotherapy isodose distribution using a VMAT plan to 78 Gy for an intermediate-risk prostate cancer patient. (a) Axial, (b) coronal, and (c) sagittal planes. The clinical target volume (CTV) is in red and the planning target volume (PTV) is in green. For a color version of this figure, see the color plate section.

Some centers treat only the prostate and omit the seminal vesicles for low-risk patients due to the low risk of seminal vesicle involvement. Pathologic data can be used to decide how much of the seminal vesicles to include in the target based on the patient's risk group, but commonly 1–2 cm of the seminal vesicles are included in intermediate-risk and high-risk patients, while some centers may treat the entire seminal vesicles in all or selected high-risk patients.

Planning target volume (PTV) expansion should be institution-specific based on the form of IGRT and intradepartmental set-up concerns. 3D expansions of 5 cm to 10 mm are commonly added to the prostate and seminal vesicle clinical target volume (CTV), as well as the pelvic node CTV if included, although some institutions use smaller or larger margins than these. Reductions in field size, fraction size, or total dose may be required for patients with comorbidities or significant underlying urinary or bowel dysfunction.

Stereotactic Body Radiotherapy

The SBRT treatment planning workflow is similar to that used for EBRT planning. The target is usually the same as for patients undergoing conventional fractionation or moderately hypofractionated EBRT. However, the pelvic nodes are usually not treated. Robust IGRT and typically smaller PTV margins are used in planning, and treatment is commonly delivered every 72 to 96 hours apart.

Particle Therapy

Charged particles such as protons and carbon-12 nuclei have been used in the treatment of localized prostate cancer since the 1970s, and have certain theoretical advantages due to their unique dose distribution. Unlike photons, which have a relatively high surface dose and deposit energy along their course through tissues, charged particles enter the body at a lower dose and deposit the majority of their energy at a specific depth. In practice, beam compensators are used to spread out the energy of the proton beam over a distance designed to correspond with the shape of the target. Two types of proton beam are used, namely passive scatter and pencil beam scanning. Most of the historic experiences utilize passive scatter beams, while scanning beams allow for intensity-modulated proton therapy (IMPT), which is increasingly being integrated into clinical practice for prostate cancer at many centers.

A dose-escalation trial using combined photon and proton treatment plans showed improved biochemical control with increased doses [119]. Patients treated with proton beam therapy are simulated in a similar fashion to IMRT patients. Daily kilovoltage (kV) imaging is used to align the treatment field based on the location of fiducial markers. Right and left lateral beam angles are used on alternating days, resulting in slightly higher doses to the hips, but lower doses to the bladder and posterior rectum compared to IMRT [219]. To ensure adequate coverage of the PTV, the entire prostatic urethra and portions of the anterior rectum and bladder neck receive the full prescription dose with either IMRT or proton beam therapy. Some centers are exploring using proton beam therapy for postoperative radiotherapy and the treatment of lymph nodes.

At present, the treatment of prostate cancer with proton beam therapy is controversial as its benefit over more conventional forms of radiation remains mainly theoretical [220, 221]. Most of the prospective series are from a single or limited number of institutions, and follow-up is relatively early (approximately 5 years or less in most series). However, the disease control and toxicity outcomes appear to be similar to those with photon EBRT [222, 223]. An analysis of patient-reported outcomes comparing 3D-CRT, IMRT, and proton therapy found that IMRT and 3D-CRT were associated with a detriment in acute bowel function in patients shortly after treatment, but proton therapy was not. With a longer follow-up, however, there was no clear difference in genitourinary or gastrointestinal function between the treatment groups [224]. A SEER-Medicare analysis comparing IMRT, 3D-CRT and proton therapy found worse gastrointestinal morbidity with proton therapy as defined by claims for gastrointestinal procedures associated with potential gastrointestinal toxicities associated with radiotherapy [220]. Another Medicare analysis comparing proton radiotherapy and IMRT revealed decreased acute genitourinary toxicity at six months with proton radiotherapy, but no difference at one year [225].

Most of these series were conducted in patients treated using passive scatter beams. Active scanning beam and IMPT may allow for further improvements in the therapeutic index in the future. The PARTIQoL Phase III randomized trial comparing high-dose IMRT versus proton beam treatment for localized prostate cancer is currently accruing patients (NCT01617161), and will hopefully identify any differences in the therapeutic index with proton radiotherapy.

Carbon ions are currently being used to treat localized and advanced prostate cancer at centers in Europe and Japan. Initial results from Phase I/II trials have been mixed and longer follow-up is needed to assess efficacy and safety [226].

Prostate Brachytherapy

Brachytherapy is an alternative to EBRT for a subset of men with localized prostate cancer as monotherapy, as well as a boost after initial EBRT. Advances in imaging and surgical techniques have led to excellent rates of disease control and minimal treatment-related morbidity in the hands of experienced providers. Both, LDR or HDR techniques can be employed, with LDR being much more common, especially in the US. Experience with HDR brachytherapy is increasing, but there are currently no randomized trials comparing HDR brachytherapy alone to other treatment modalities. Some centers are investigating the role of focal brachytherapy for well-selected patients [227].

LDR brachytherapy with iodine-125 (^{125}I) seeds is offered to carefully selected low-risk and favorable intermediate-risk patients as monotherapy. In high-risk and unfavorable intermediate-risk patients, brachytherapy monotherapy is typically not recommended due to potential occult extracapsular extension or seminal vesicle involvement, a decision to treat the pelvic nodes, and a theoretical need for a higher biologic dose. Therefore, in this latter group of patients, brachytherapy, when employed, is used as a boost after initial EBRT [228,229]. ^{125}I is a low-energy (28 keV) isotope with a half-life of 59.4 days. Paladium-103 is another commonly used isotope, with a half-life of 17 days. Cesium-131 is also seeing increasing use at some centers. The prescription dose is typically 145 Gy when ^{125}I is used and 125 Gy for ^{103}Pd. When used in the boost setting after 45–50.4 Gy, the typical dose for ^{125}I is 110 Gy, and for ^{103}Pd is 100 Gy. In the boost setting, the brachytherapy procedure is usually performed several weeks after the completion of EBRT.

There are two approaches to treatment planning in LDR brachytherapy, namely preplanning and intraoperative planning. In both cases, a volume study is performed prior to the implant with a TRUS in the lithotomy position. Serial axial images are recorded at 5-mm intervals from above the base of the prostate gland to below the apex. Each point within the prostate has a location corresponding in two transverse directions to the holes in a template grid, and in a third longitudinal direction corresponding to the 5-mm step positions of the ultrasound probe. The planning images are used to calculate optimal seed distribution required to deliver the prescribed radiation dose. Typical plans use 50–100 individual seeds contained in 20–30 needles, with each needle containing one to five seeds. Seeds contained with a single needle are often attached to other seeds or spacers in order to decrease the risk of a single seed becoming dislodged and migrating out of the prostate. A modified peripheral-loading, central-sparing technique allows adequate dose to be distributed throughout the gland while avoiding hot spots near the urethra (Figure 27.3). Some centers use intraoperative planning techniques and other forms of image guidance.

The procedure itself is performed in the operating room under general or spinal anesthesia. The patient is placed in the same position as for the planning TRUS, and the perineum is prepared under sterile conditions. The ultrasound probe is inserted into the rectum such that the images obtained correspond to those from the planning TRUS. The probe is then immobilized and needles with the preloaded ^{125}I seeds are passed through the template grid and perineum into the prostate. The seeds are deposited longitudinally from the base of the prostate to the apex under direct ultrasound guidance. A Foley catheter is placed for the procedure to allow visualization of the prostatic urethra, but is removed following completion. Patients typically return home the same day after passing a voiding trial. At approximately one month after the brachytherapy procedure, the patient returns to the department for a post-implant CT to evaluate the final dosimetry of the implant, although an acceptable variant

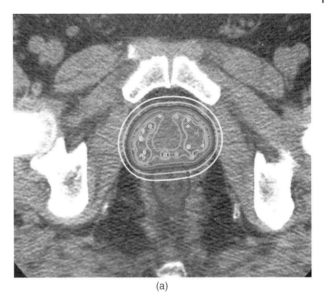

(a)

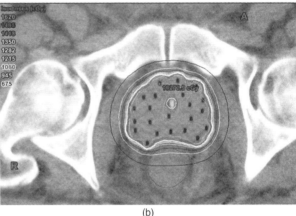

(b)

Figure 27.3 Typical isodose distributions for definitive prostate brachytherapy using (a) LDR and (b) HDR brachytherapy. The LDR plan uses iodine-125 and a modified peripheral loading, central-sparing technique. The HDR plan uses iridium-192 and dwell time/dwell position optimization after placement of the catheters. For a color version of this figure, see the color plate section.

to this is to perform the CT directly after the implant on the same day.

The key difference in the workflow in centers that use intraoperative planning is the volume study prior to the operative procedure is not necessary other than to confirm candidacy for brachytherapy. During the operative procedure, the volume study is performed first and the TRUS images are then used to generate the plan in real-time prior to and sometimes during source placement. Because the needles cannot be preloaded, they are usually loaded with sources intraoperatively.

The HDR brachytherapy procedure has several similarities to LDR brachytherapy, but several key differences. A volume study is usually not necessary other than for patient selection, as there is no pre-planning. Patients undergo implantation of ~14–22 catheters distributed throughout the prostate, extending cranially past the base to the edge of the bladder neck using either a stepper-based template or a free-hand template and TRUS guidance. Cystoscopy is sometimes used to evaluate for 'tenting' of the bladder, a sign that the catheters have been advanced appropriately without perforation into the bladder. Some centers also use fiducial markers at the apex and base and fluoroscopy to evaluate catheter placement.

After placement of the catheters, treatment planning is performed using ultrasound-based or CT-based planning. The target is defined by the physician and usually includes the prostate with or without the seminal vesicles. Some centers add several millimeters margin to the CTV to create the PTV. A treatment plan is generated to allocate the dwell times and dwell positions to be used for treatment (see Figure 27.3).

Upon completion of planning the patient is treated using a ^{192}Ir afterloader based on the plan. When treatment is complete the implant is removed and the patient is discharged. Multiple dose/fractionation regimens are used, including some that require admission and/or twice-daily treatments and some that use multiple implant procedures [230]. Commonly use boost regimens include 5.5–6.3 Gy × 3, 9–10 Gy × 2, and 15 Gy × 1, while commonly used monotherapy regimens include 6.5–7.25 Gy × 6, 9.5 Gy × 4, and 13–13.5 Gy × 2 [230,231]. When used as a boost, the HDR brachytherapy can be delivered about two weeks before or after EBRT.

Postoperative Radiation Therapy

Radiation after radical prostatectomy can be delivered in an adjuvant or salvage setting, and the optimal timing of postoperative radiation is not known. For radical prostatectomy, patients with worrisome pathologic features such as seminal vesicle involvement, extracapsular extension or positive surgical margins, adjuvant external beam radiation can be delivered in an attempt to eliminate disease that remains within the surgical bed. For other patients, postoperative radiation is delivered after objective evidence of recurrence (e.g., PSA rise, palpable nodule, or radiologic abnormality) is present.

When delivered in the adjuvant setting, radiation typically starts no earlier than four months after surgery in order to allow for the recovery of urinary function. Patients undergo CT simulation in the supine position with a similar anatomic set-up as intact patients. Some institutions use urethrograms, fiducial markers and rectal balloons, but these are optional and less common than in the intact setting. The target is contoured as a single volume and includes the vesicourethral anastomosis, seminal vesicle remnants, bladder neck and posterior

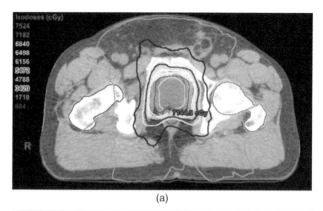

(a)

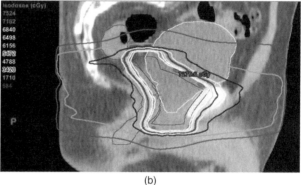

(b)

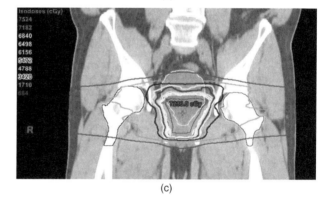

(c)

Figure 27.4 (a–c) A typical post-prostatectomy radiotherapy isodose distribution using VMAT. The clinical target volume (CTV) is shown in red, and the planning target volume (PTV) in green. (a) Axial image. (b) Sagittal image. (c) Coronal image. For a color version of this figure, see the color plate section.

wall, and peri-rectal tissue. Organs at risk, including the rectum, bladder and femoral heads, are also contoured. The target volume is typically treated in a single course to 64–66 Gy in the adjuvant setting, and 66–70 Gy in the salvage setting, using daily fractions and IMRT (Figure 27.4). Contouring atlases are available to assist with defining the areas at risk and normal anatomy [108, 109]. If felt to be at high-risk of involvement, pelvic lymph node areas are also contoured and treated to 45–50.4 Gy. The data supporting inclusion of the pelvic nodes in the salvage radiotherapy setting are primarily observational in nature, and one study suggested a benefit in biochemical relapse-free survival in high-risk patients by inclusion of the pelvic nodes [192].

Based on RTOG 9601, which demonstrated a survival benefit to adding two years of bicalutamide to salvage radiotherapy, and GETUG-AFU 16, which revealed a progression-free survival benefit to six months of ADT, many practitioners add ADT to salvage radiotherapy, usually in the form of a GnRH agonist for six months [194, 195, 195a]. The optimal patient population who benefits from salvage radiotherapy with ADT is unclear, but subgroup analysis of RTOG 9601 revealed that patients with a pre-radiotherapy PSA level of 0.7–4 ng ml^{-1}, positive surgical margins, or Gleason score 7–10 seem to benefit most, and thus it should be considered particularly in these cases.

RTOG 0534, which randomized prostate bed-only radiotherapy to prostate bed radiotherapy ± pelvic nodal radiotherapy and ± four to six months of ADT, will hopefully elucidate further the role of pelvic nodal radiotherapy and short-term ADT in the salvage radiotherapy setting.

Morbidity of Radiation Therapy

Side effects during EBRT such as fatigue, urinary frequency, slow urinary stream, dysuria, diarrhea, and occasional rectal bleeding, may occur at varying degrees in over 50% of the patients treated. These may be relieved by simple measures, such as dietary changes, anticholinergics to reduce bladder irritability and increase capacity, alpha-adrenergic blockers or 5α-reductase inhibitors to improve urinary flow, anti-inflammatory agents to relieve prostatic inflammation, and steroid suppositories.

The likelihood of early and late complications with EBRT, brachytherapy, or radical prostatectomy was documented in the PROST-QA prospective patient reported quality of life outcomes study with a median follow-up of 2.5 years [153]. At two years, weak stream was present in 10% of EBRT patients and 11% of brachytherapy patients. Hematuria was present in 1% of the EBRT and brachytherapy groups, and dysuria in 1% of EBRT patients and 5% of brachytherapy patients. Some 5% and 8% reported urinary pad use in the EBRT and brachytherapy cohorts, respectively, while 11% of EBRT patients and 8% of brachytherapy patients had overall bowel problems, with bloody stools present in <1% and 3%, respectively. Patients who received radiotherapy or brachytherapy had a higher pretreatment incidence of poor penile erection (52% and 30%), and two years after treatment poor penile erection was present in 60% of men treated with EBRT, and in 51% of those treated with brachytherapy. Large prostate size was associated with worse urinary irritative symptoms in patients

treated with brachytherapy or EBRT. The Prostate Cancer Outcomes Study (PCOS) was a longitudinal population-based study evaluating the health-related quality of life in several functional domains of patients with prostate cancer diagnosed during the 1990s and followed for 15 years [109]. Patients who underwent surgery were more likely to have urinary incontinence and erectile dysfunction at two and five years, but at 15 years there was no difference between both cohorts. Similarly, men who underwent radiotherapy were more likely to have bowel urgency than those undergoing radical prostatectomy at two and five years, but at 15 years there was no difference.

Along with disease control outcomes, the ProtecT trial performed robust patient-reported outcome assessments regarding urinary, sexual, bowel, and overall quality of life for patients receiving AS, prostatectomy, or radiotherapy at baseline and follow-up [195b]. The results of this study are particularly meaningful because the response rate remained at ~85% for the duration of the study. Six year data were published and compared the toxicity profiles of each management approach.

Urinary incontinence was worse at every time point in the surgery group compared to AS and EBRT. The was no difference in incontinence between AS and EBRT. At six months, 46% of surgery patients and 4% and 5% of patients for AS and EBRT used urinary pads; at six years these numbers were 17%, 8% and 4%. Lower urinary tract symptoms were worse with radiotherapy at six months, but then similar between all groups at one year and later.

Regarding sexual function, at baseline, 67% of men had erections firm enough for intercourse. At six months this was 52% in the AS group, 22% in the EBRT group, and 12% in the prostatectomy group. In the prostatectomy group, there was improvement up to 21% of men at 36 months, but this declined again at six years to 17%. In the EBRT group, sexual function improved up to 12 months to ~40%, and declined gradually again to 27% at six years. In the AS group, there was a gradual decline yearly with 30% having erections firm enough for intercourse at six years. Of note, the EBRT group in this study received three to six months of ADT, which is typically not used in low-risk patients in current practices, suggesting that the potential short-term decline in erectile function seen in the EBRT group may at least partially be due to ADT use as opposed to EBRT.

In terms of bowel function, there was no decline in bowel function in the prostatectomy and AS groups. In the EBRT group, bowel scores were modestly worse, particularly at 6 months. Additionally, compared to the other two groups, the proportion of men reporting bloody stools in the EBRT group was higher from 2 years on. While 3DCRT was used in this study, these rates may be improved in the contemporary era with the use of more advanced radiation delivery technologies such as IMRT.

Ultimately, there was no difference in overall health related quality of life between any of the three groups. Yet, these data are critical in helping individual patients and physicians choose the optimal management approach, and can be helpful at the societal level to evaluate the impact of these treatment modalities.

Other toxicities include pelvic insufficiency fracture, which is a relatively uncommon, but possible toxicity [232]. The risk of second malignancy induced by radiotherapy is controversial, but overall extremely rare, with an absolute increased risk likely of <1% [233–236].

Results are conflicting regarding the incremental increase in toxicity with dose escalation of EBRT. In one study, increasing the dose from 70 to 78 Gy caused the likelihood of grade 2 or greater rectal toxicity to double from 12% to 26% at six years, in spite of the use of conformal techniques [237]. No differences were found in late bladder complications. In another analysis, using patient-reported outcomes, there was no decrement in bowel, urinary, or sexual domains when using high-dose EBRT compared to conventional doses [238].

Several advances in the ability to deliver EBRT have resulted in improvements in the toxicity of EBRT. As discussed in the sections above, IMRT and IGRT have allowed for a more accurate set-up and decreased dose to the rectum and bladder, potentially contributing to decreased toxicity [122, 123]. Dosimetric parameters, such as limiting the volume of the rectum receiving 70 Gy or more (V70) to 15–20%, are commonly achievable with modern planning techniques, and have been shown to reduce the risk of toxicity [122, 239, 240]. Recently, the results of a randomized controlled trial evaluating the injection of an absorbable polyethylene glycol gel into Denonvillier's fascia to increase the distance from the prostate to the rectum were published [217]. Patients who had hydrogel spacer placement had improved dosimetry and less decline in bowel quality of life compared to those treated without the spacer.

Patient-specific factors, such as comorbid diabetes, tobacco use and anticoagulant use, have also been associated with worse toxicity [239, 241–243]. Patients with inflammatory bowel disease, particularly if active, should be treated with caution due to a potentially higher risk of gastrointestinal toxicity [224]. Phosphodiesterase inhibitors (sildenafil and tadalafil) have been evaluated for the potential prevention of EBRT-related erectile dysfunction, but there does not appear to be a consistent benefit. A randomized trial evaluating the addition of sildenafil found a benefit in erectile function at 24 years [245]. However, RTOG 0831 evaluated the addition of 24 months of tadalafil, and found no benefit in the maintenance of erectile function [246].

Radical radiation employing interstitial brachytherapy has its own unique toxicity profile. In the first week, most patients experience dysuria, urinary frequency, hematuria, and a weak urinary stream. This typically subsides, but in the second and third weeks a brisk radiation prostatitis occurs in the majority of patients, again characterized by frequency and dysuria. If there is significant prostatic swelling, urinary outflow obstruction may occur. Some patients may develop acute urinary retention after the procedure [138], and this risk increases with increasing gland size. Therefore, careful selection of patients for brachytherapy is critical. If needed, a temporary catheter may need to be placed and later removed when the patient can voluntarily void on his own. Conservative management is the most appropriate, as immediate TURP is associated with a significant risk of incontinence. In general, incontinence related to brachytherapy is low compared to prostatectomy [153]. Mild urinary symptoms may persist for three to five months, but these usually subside completely. Long-term follow-up of large brachytherapy series suggests that the risks of grade 2 genitourinary and grade 3 gastrointestinal toxicity are 27% and 10%, respectively, and the risk of grade 2 gastrointestinal toxicity and grade 3 gastrointestinal toxicity are 7.3% and 0.9% [144, 145]. A higher baseline IPSS score, a larger volume size, a greater implant D90, increasing age, and severity of acute toxicity have all been associated with late toxicity [145]. HDR brachytherapy series have a relatively shorter follow-up than LDR series, but show similar toxicity profiles [146, 147]. The combination of EBRT and brachytherapy boost, either LDR or HDR, comes at the cost of increased toxicity, particularly urinary toxicity. The ASCENDE-RT trial comparing EBRT alone or EBRT with brachytherapy boost found an increased stricture rate in the brachytherapy boost group [157]. Comparative retrospective series using HDR boost have a similar increased risk of urethral toxicity [158, 159].

Patients treated with prostate SBRT have similar toxicity profiles to those treated with brachytherapy, based on a pooled-analysis from several prospective trials [247, 248]. A Medicare claims-based analysis suggested that urinary toxicity may be higher than after conventionally fractionated IMRT, although a lack of clear dosimetric data and a lack of direct patient-reported or clinician-reported toxicity outcomes were limitations of the study [136]. Long-term outcomes with SBRT, as in RTOG 0938, are needed to identify the true toxicity profile of SBRT. As discussed in the Proton therapy section above, the long-term benefit in the toxicity profile of proton therapy is unknown. Single-institution experiences and analyses of patient-reported quality of life outcomes suggest a decreased risk of acute bowel toxicity, but no difference in late toxicity [222, 224]. However, a SEER-Medicare analysis using claims data to define late gastrointestinal toxicity found worse gastrointestinal toxicity [220]. Another Medicare analysis revealed less acute but not late genitourinary toxicity with proton therapy [225]. Long-term results of the PARTIQoL trial will be needed to identify improvements in the risk of toxicity with proton therapy (NCT01617161).

When EBRT follows RP with doses of 64–70 Gy, long-term morbidity tends to be relatively low. An analysis of health-related quality of life outcomes of patients treated on the SWOG 8794 adjuvant radiotherapy trial showed there to be an increased risk of bowel dysfunction soon after treatment compared to observation after RP, but the difference decreased over time and was minimal after two to three years. However, adjuvant radiotherapy was associated with increased urinary frequency both in the short term and long term in this study. Interestingly, there was a decline in general health-related quality of life after adjuvant radiotherapy, but after five years patients treated with adjuvant radiotherapy had better health-related quality of life scores compared to surgery-only patients, potentially due to less anxiety about recurrence and a lesser need for salvage hormonal therapy [249]. There was no impact of radiotherapy on erectile function in this study. Some would argue, however, that with modern surgical techniques the baseline risk of bowel and urinary dysfunction after surgery may be lower, potentially opening up an increased risk of deleterious urinary or bowel toxicity with adjuvant radiotherapy compared to observation. However, modern retrospective series suggest a similar low risk of toxicity with postoperative radiotherapy [250].

Conclusions

Prostate cancer is one of the most complex disease entities encountered by Radiation Oncologists, but one in which Radiation Oncologists and radiation therapy play a fundamental role. This chapter highlighted the recent updates and advances in the screening, diagnosis, radiographic imaging, and treatment of men with prostate cancer with a focus on the radiotherapeutic approaches.

There have been many advances in recent years in the treatment of prostate cancer, including the transition to dose-escalated EBRT, implementation of image-guidance, and increased sophistication of planning and refinement of planning parameters. Yet, there are many areas that require further exploration in the coming years. The optimal dose/fractionation is unknown, and the role of moderate and ultra hypofractionated regimens – both in the definitive setting and post-RP – will become more clear in the coming years. Similarly, the incremental impact on the therapeutic index with the use of particle therapy in patients with prostate cancer is currently being investigated. The role of brachytherapy, both LDR and HDR, is being elucidated both as definitive therapy as well as in the form of a boost after initial EBRT. Currently accruing and maturing trials will also further identify the optimal candidates for the addition of androgen deprivation therapy and the optimal duration based on risk-stratification. Even more unknown is the role of focal therapy in patients with localized prostate cancer and the role of radiotherapy in patients with metastatic and 'oligometastatic' prostate cancer.

Not only will new techniques and modalities in the treatment or prostate cancer evolve over time, the indications for radiotherapeutic treatment will also be further refined. All of these changes will need to adjust to changes in future screening practices and the consequent impact on stage migration. Ultimately, the most important role we will play is that of the patient's advocate and educator – using patients as vital partners in management decisions.

References

1 Siegel, R., Miller, K., Jemal, A. (2017) Cancer Statistics 2017. *CA Cancer J. Clin.*, **67**, 7–30.

2 Howlader, N., Noone, A.M., Krapcho, M., *et al.* SEER Cancer Statistics Review, 1975–2012. Available at: http://seer.cancer.gov/csr/1975_2012/, based on November 2014 SEER data submission, posted on the SEER web site, April 2015.

3 Hoffman, R.M. (2011) Screening for prostate cancer. *N. Engl. J. Med.*, **365** (21), 2013–2019.

4 Hayes, J.H., Barry, M.J. (2014) Screening for prostate cancer with the prostate-specific antigen test. *JAMA*, **311** (11), 1143.

5 Cooperberg, M.R., Broering, J.M., Carroll, P.R. (2010) Time trends and local variation in primary treatment of localized prostate cancer. *J. Clin. Oncol.*, **28** (7), 1117–1123.

6 Torre, L., Bray, F., Siegel, R.L., Ferlay, J., Lortet-tieulent, J., Jemal, A. (2015) Global Cancer Statistics. CA Cancer *J. Clin.*, **65** (2), 87–108.

7 Grönberg, H. (2003) Prostate cancer epidemiology. *Lancet*, **361** (9360), 859–864.

8 Shimizu, H., Ross, R.K., Bernstein, L., Yatani, R., Henderson, B.E., Mack, T.M. (1991) Cancers of the prostate and breast among Japanese and white immigrants in Los Angeles County. *Br. J Cancer*, **63** (6), 963–966.

9 Sundi, D., Ross, A.E., Humphreys, E.B., *et al.* (2013) African American men with very low-risk prostate cancer exhibit adverse oncologic outcomes after radical prostatectomy: should active surveillance still be an option for them? *J. Clin. Oncol.*, **31** (24), 2991–2997.

10 Sakr, W.A., Haas, G.P., Cassin, B.F., Pontes, J.E., Crissman, J.D. (1993) The frequency of carcinoma and intraepithelial neoplasia of the prostate in young male patients. *J Urol.*, **150** (2 Pt 1), 379–385.

11 Wynder, E.L., Mabuchi, K., Whitmore, W.F. (1971) Epidemiology of cancer of the prostate. *Cancer*, **28** (2), 344–360.

12 Gronberg, H., Isaacs, S.D., Smith, J.R., *et al.* (1997) Characteristics of prostate cancer in families potentially linked to the hereditary prostate cancer 1 (HPC1) locus. *JAMA*, **278** (15), 1251–1255.

13 Bruner, D.W., Moore, D., Parlanti, A., Dorgan, J., Engstrom, P. (2003) Relative risk of prostate cancer for men with affected relatives: systematic review and meta-analysis. *Int. J. Cancer*, **107** (5), 797–803.

14 Steinberg, G.D., Carter, B.S., Beaty, T.H., Childs, B., Walsh, P.C. (1990) Family history and the risk of prostate cancer. *Prostate*, **17** (4), 337–347.

15 Zheng, S.L., Sun, J., Wiklund, F., *et al.* (2008) Cumulative association of five genetic variants with prostate cancer. *N. Engl. J. Med.*, **358** (9), 910–919.

16 Leongamornlert, D., Mahmud, N., Tymrakiewicz, M., *et al.* (2012) Germline BRCA1 mutations increase prostate cancer risk. *Br. J Cancer*, **106** (10), 1697–1701.

17 Hickey, K., Do, K.A., Green, A. (2001) Smoking and prostate cancer. *Epidemiol. Rev.*, **23** (1), 115–125.

18 Rota, M., Scotti, L., Turati, F., *et al.* (2012) Alcohol consumption and prostate cancer risk: a meta-analysis of the dose–risk relation. *Eur. J. Cancer Prev.*, **21** (4), 350–359.

19 Kenfield, S.A., Meir, J., Stampfer, P.H., Chan, J.M., Giovannucci, E. (2011) Smoking and prostate cancer survival and recurrence. *JAMA*, **305** (24), 2548–2555.

20 Wilson, K.M., Kasperzyk, J.L., Rider, J.R., *et al.* (2011) Coffee consumption and prostate cancer risk and progression in the Health Professionals Follow-up Study. *J. Natl Cancer Inst.*, **103** (11), 876–884.

21 van Die, M.D., Bone, K.M., Williams, S.G., Pirotta, M.V. (2014) Soy and soy isoflavones in prostate cancer: a systematic review and meta-analysis of randomized controlled trials. *Br. J. Urol. Int.*, **113** (5b), E119–E130.

22 Ahonen, M.H., Tenkanen, L., Teppo, L., Hakama, M., Tuohimaa, P. (2000) Prostate cancer risk and prediagnostic serum 25-hydroxyvitamin D levels (Finland). *Cancer Causes Control*, **11** (9), 847–852.

23 Ahn, J., Peters, U., Albanes, D., *et al.* (2008) Serum vitamin D concentration and prostate cancer risk: a nested case-control study. *J. Natl Cancer Inst.*, **100** (11), 796–804.

24 Lippman, S.M., Klein, E.A., Goodman, P.J., *et al.* (2009) Effect of selenium and vitamin E on risk of prostate cancer and other cancers: The selenium and vitamin E cancer prevention trial (select). *JAMA*, **301** (1), 39–51.

25 Kavanaugh, C.J., Trumbo, P.R., Ellwood, K.C. (2007) The U.S. Food and Drug Administration's evidence-based review for qualified health claims: tomatoes, lycopene, and cancer. *J. Natl Cancer Inst.*, **99** (14), 1074–1085.

26 Sporn, M.B., Liby, K.T. (2013) Is lycopene an effective agent for preventing prostate cancer? *Cancer Prev. Res.*, **6** (5), 384–386.

27 MacInnis, R.J., English, D.R. (2006) Body size and composition and prostate cancer risk: systematic review and meta-regression analysis. *Cancer Causes Control*, **17** (8), 989–1003.

28 Calle, E.E., Rodriguez, C., Walker-Thurmond, K., Thun, M.J. (2003) Overweight, obesity, and mortality from cancer in a prospectively studied cohort of U.S. adults. *N. Engl. J. Med.*, **348** (17), 1625–1638.

29 Wright, M.E., Chang, S.C., Schatzkin, A., *et al.* (2007) Prospective study of adiposity and weight change in relation to prostate cancer incidence and mortality. *Cancer*, **109** (4), 675–684.

30 Stroup, S.P., Cullen, J., Auge, B.K., L'Esperance, J.O., Kang, S.K. (2007) Effect of obesity on prostate-specific antigen recurrence after radiation therapy for localized prostate cancer as measured by the 2006 Radiation Therapy Oncology Group-American Society for Therapeutic Radiation and Oncology (RTOG-ASTRO) Phoenix consensus. *Cancer*, **110** (5), 1003–1009.

31 Roddam, A.W., Allen, N.E., Appleby, P., Key, T.J. (2008) Endogenous Sex Hormones and Prostate Cancer: A Collaborative Analysis of 18 Prospective Studies. *J. Natl Cancer Inst.*, **100** (3), 170–183.

32 Fernández-Balsells, M.M., Murad, M.H., Lane, M., *et al.* (2010) Adverse effects of testosterone therapy in adult men: a systematic review and meta-analysis. *J. Clin. Endocrinol. Metab.*, **95** (6), 2560–2575.

33 Nordström, T., Clements, M., Karlsson, R., Adolfsson, J., Grönberg, H. (2015) The risk of prostate cancer for men on aspirin, statin or antidiabetic medications. *Eur. J. Cancer*, **51** (6), 725–733.

34 Farwell, W.R., D'Avolio, L.W., Scranton, R.E., Lawler, E.V., Gaziano, J.M. (2011) Statins and prostate cancer diagnosis and grade in a veterans population. *J. Natl Cancer Inst.*, **103** (11), 885–892.

35 Bansal, D., Undela, K., D'Cruz, S., Schifano, F. (2012) Statin use and risk of prostate cancer: a meta-analysis of observational studies. *PLoS One*, 7 (10), 1–11.

36 Pai, P.-Y., Hsieh, V.C.-R., Wang, C.-B., *et al.* (2015) Long term antihypertensive drug use and prostate cancer risk: A 9-year population-based cohort analysis. *Int. J. Cardiol.*, **193**, 1–7.

37 Veitonmäki, T., Tammela, T.L.J, Auvinen, A., Murtola, T.J. (2013) Use of aspirin, but not other non-steroidal anti-inflammatory drugs is associated with decreased

prostate cancer risk at the population level. *Eur. J. Cancer*, **49** (4), 938–945.

38 McNeal, J.E., Redwine, E.A., Freiha, F.S., Stamey, T.A. (1988) Zonal distribution of prostatic adenocarcinoma. Correlation with histologic pattern and direction of spread. *Am. J. Surg. Pathol.*, **12** (12), 897–906.

39 Raychaudhuri, B., Cahill, D. (2008) Pelvic fasciae in urology. *Ann. R. Coll. Surg. Engl.*, **90** (8), 633–637.

40 Montironi, R., Qian, J., Ma, J. (2008) Prostatic intraepithelial neoplasia. *Pathol. Case Rev.*, **13** (4). Available at: http://www.nature.com/modpathol/journal/v17/n3/abs/3800053a.html.

41 Epstein, J.I., Herawi, M. (2015) Prostate needle biopsies containing prostatic intraepithelial neoplasia or atypical foci suspicious for carcinoma: implications for patient care. *J. Urol.*, **175** (3), 820–834.

42 Bjartell, A. (2006) Words of wisdom. The 2005 International Society of Urological Pathology (ISUP) Consensus Conference on Gleason Grading of Prostatic Carcinoma. *Eur. Urol.*, **49** (4), 758–759.

43 Stark, J.R., Perner, S., Stampfer, M.J., *et al.* (2009) Gleason score and lethal prostate cancer: does 3 + 4 = 4 +3? *J. Clin. Oncol.*, **27** (21), 3459–3464.

44 Montironi, R., Mazzuccheli, R., Scarpelli, M., Lopez-Beltran, A., Fellegara, G., Algaba, F. (2005) Gleason grading of prostate cancer in needle biopsies or radical prostatectomy specimens: contemporary approach, current clinical significance and sources of pathology discrepancies. *Br. J. Urol. Int.*, **95** (8), 1146–1152.

45 Mosse, C.A., Magi-Galluzzi, C., Tsuzuki, T., Epstein, J.I. (2004) The prognostic significance of tertiary Gleason pattern 5 in radical prostatectomy specimens. *Am. J. Surg. Pathol.*, **28** (3), 394–398.

46 Isariyawongse, B.K., Sun, L., Banez, L.L., *et al.* (2008) Significant discrepancies between diagnostic and pathologic Gleason sums in prostate cancer: the predictive role of age and prostate-specific antigen. *Urology*, **72** (4), 882–886.

47 Epstein, J.I., Zelefsky, M.J., Sjoberg, D.D., *et al.* (2016) A contemporary prostate cancer grading system: a validated alternative to the Gleason score. *Eur. Urol.*, **69** (3), 428–435.

48 Boström, P.J., Bjartell, A.S., Catto, J.W.F., *et al.* (2015) Genomic predictors of outcome in prostate cancer. *Eur. Urol.*, **68** (6), 1033–1044.

49 Erho, N., Crisan, A., Vergara, I.A., *et al.* (2013) Discovery and validation of a prostate cancer genomic classifier that predicts early metastasis following radical prostatectomy. *PloS One*, **8** (6), e66855.

50 Den, R.B., Feng, F.Y., Showalter, T.N., *et al.* (2014) Genomic prostate cancer classifier predicts biochemical failure and metastases in patients after postoperative radiation therapy. *Radiat. Oncol. Biol.*, **89** (5), 1038–1046.

51 Den, R.B., Yousefi, K., Trabulsi, E.J., *et al.* (2015) Genomic classifier identifies men with adverse pathology after radical prostatectomy who benefit from adjuvant radiation therapy. *J. Clin. Oncol.*, **33** (8), 944–951.

52 Chao, K.K., Goldstein, N.S., Yan, D., *et al.* (2006) Clinicopathologic analysis of extracapsular extension in prostate cancer: Should the clinical target volume be expanded posterolaterally to account for microscopic extension? *Int. J. Radiat. Oncol. Biol. Phys.*, **65** (4), 999–1007.

53 Kestin, L.L., Goldstein, N.S., Vicini, F.A., Yan, D., Korman, H.J., Martinez, A. (2002) Treatment of prostate cancer with radiotherapy: Should the entire seminal vesicles be included in the clinical target volume? *Int. J. Radiat. Oncol. Biol. Phys.*, **54** (3), 686–697.

54 Howlader, N., Noone, A.M., Krapcho, M., *et al.* SEER Cancer Statistics Review, 1975–2012. Available at: http://seer.cancer.gov/csr/1975_2012/, based on November 2014 SEER data submission, posted on the SEER web site, April 2015.

55 Mistry, K., Cable, G. (2003) Meta-analysis of prostate-specific antigen and digital rectal examination as screening tests for prostate carcinoma. *J. Am. Board Fam. Pract.*, **16** (2), 95–101.

56 Chodak, G.W., Keller, P., Schoenberg, H.W. (1989) Assessment of screening for prostate cancer using the digital rectal examination. *J. Urol.*, **141** (5), 1136–1138.

57 Wolf, A.M., Wender, R.C., Etzioni, R.B., *et al.* (2010) American Cancer Society guideline for the early detection of prostate cancer: update 2010. *CA Cancer J. Clin.*, **60** (2), 70–98.

58 Catalona, W.J., Partin, A.W., Slawin, K.M., *et al.* (1998) Use of the percentage of free prostate-specific antigen to enhance differentiation of prostate cancer from benign prostatic disease: A prospective multicenter clinical trial. *JAMA*, **279** (19), 1542–1547.

59 Roobol, M.J., Kranse, R., de Koning, H.J., Schroder, F.H. (2004) Prostate-specific antigen velocity at low prostate-specific antigen levels as screening tool for prostate cancer: results of second screening round of ERSPC (ROTTERDAM). *Urology*, **63** (2), 305–309.

60 Vickers, A.J., Till, C., Tangen, C.M., Lilja, H., Thompson, I.M. (2011) An empirical evaluation of guidelines on prostate-specific antigen velocity in prostate cancer detection. *J. Natl Cancer Inst.*, **103** (6), 462–469.

61 Roobol, M.J., Schröder, F.H., van Leeuwen, P., *et al.* (2010) Performance of the Prostate Cancer Antigen 3 (PCA3) gene and prostate-specific antigen in

prescreened men: exploring the value of PCA3 for a first-line diagnostic test. *Eur. Urol.*, **58** (4), 475–481.

62 Andriole, G.L., Crawford, E.D., Grubb, R.L., *et al.* (2012) Prostate cancer screening in the randomized prostate, lung, colorectal, and ovarian cancer screening trial: Mortality results after 13 years of follow-up. *J. Natl Cancer Inst.*, **104** (2), 125–132.

63 Schröder, F.H., Hugosson, J., Roobol, M.J., *et al.* (2012) Prostate-cancer mortality at 11 years of follow-up. *N. Engl. J. Med.*, **366** (11), 981–990.

64 Hugosson, J., Carlsson, S., Aus, G., *et al.* (2010) Mortality results from the Goteborg randomised population-based prostate-cancer screening trial. *Lancet Oncol.*, **11** (8), 725–732.

65 Moyer, V.A. (2012) Screening for Prostate Cancer: U.S. Preventive Services Task Force Recommendation Statement. *Ann. Intern. Med.*, **157** (2), 120–134.

66 National Comprehensive Cancer Network (NCCN) (0000) Clinical Practice Guidelines in Oncology (NCCN Guidelines): Prostate Cancer Early Detection. Version 1.2015. Available at: www.nccn.org. Accessed on September 19 2015). NCCN Prostate Cancer Early Detection.

67 Andriole, G.L., Bostwick, D.G., Brawley, O.W., *et al.* (2010) Effect of dutasteride on the risk of prostate cancer. *N. Engl. J. Med.*, **362** (13), 1192–1202.

68 Thompson, I.M., Goodman, P.J., Tangen, C.M., *et al.* (2003) The influence of finasteride on the development of prostate cancer. *N. Engl. J. Med.*, **349** (3), 215–224.

69 Thompson, I.M., Goodman, P.J., Tangen, C.M., *et al.* (2013) Long-term survival of participants in the prostate cancer prevention trial. *N. Engl. J. Med.*, **369** (7), 603–610.

70 Cohen, Y.C., Liu, K.S., Heyden, N.L., *et al.* (2007) Detection bias due to the effect of finasteride on prostate volume: a modeling approach for analysis of the Prostate Cancer Prevention Trial. *J. Natl Cancer Inst.*, **99** (18), 1366–1374.

71 Cooperberg, M.R., Broering, J.M., Kantoff, P.W., Carroll, P.R. (2007) Contemporary trends in low risk prostate cancer: risk assessment and treatment. *J. Urol.*, **178** (3 Suppl.), S14–S19.

72 Barentsz, J., Richenberg, J., Clements, R., *et al.* (2012) ESUR prostate MR guidelines 2012. *Eur. Radiol.*, **22** (4), 746–757.

73 Pokorny, M.R., de Rooij, M., Duncan, E., *et al.* (2014) Prospective study of diagnostic accuracy comparing prostate cancer detection by transrectal ultrasound-guided biopsy versus magnetic resonance (MR) imaging with subsequent MR-guided biopsy in men without previous prostate biopsies. *Eur. Urol.*, **66** (1), 22–29.

74 Siddiqui, M., Rais-Bahrami, S., Turkbey, B., *et al.* (2015) Comparison of MR/ultrasound fusion-guided biopsy with ultrasound-guided biopsy for the diagnosis of prostate cancer. *JAMA*, **313** (4), 390–397.

75 Tonttila, P.P., Lantto, J., Pääkkö, E., *et al.* (2016) Prebiopsy multiparametric magnetic resonance imaging for prostate cancer diagnosis in biopsy-naive men with suspected prostate cancer based on elevated prostate-specific antigen values: results from a randomized prospective blinded controlled trial. *Eur. Urol.*, **69** (3), 419–425.

76 Zumsteg, Z.S., Spratt, D.E., Pei, I., *et al.* (2013) A new risk classification system for therapeutic decision making with intermediate-risk prostate cancer patients undergoing dose-escalated external-beam radiation therapy. *Eur. Urol.*, **64** (6), 895–902.

77 DeLancey, J.O., Wood, D.P, Jr, He, C., *et al.* (2013) Evidence of perineural invasion on prostate biopsy specimen and survival after radical prostatectomy. *Urology*, **81** (2), 354–357.

78 National Comprehensive Cancer Network (NCCN) Clinical Practice Guidelines in Oncology (NCCN Guidelines): Prostate Cancer. Version 1.2015., Available at: www.nccn.org (Accessed on 19 September 2015).

79 Reese, A.C., Pierorazio, P.M., Han, M., Partin, A.W. (2012) Contemporary evaluation of the national comprehensive cancer network prostate cancer risk classification system. *Urology*, **80** (5), 1075–1079.

80 Muralidhar, V., Chen, M.-H., Reznor, G., *et al.* (2015) Definition and validation of 'favorable high-risk prostate cancer': implications for personalizing treatment of radiation-managed patients. *Int. J. Radiat. Oncol. Biol. Phys.*, **93** (4), 828–835.

81 Thompson, J., Lawrentschuk, N., Frydenberg, M., Thompson, L., Stricker, P. (2013) The role of magnetic resonance imaging in the diagnosis and management of prostate cancer. *Br. J. Urol. Int.*, **112** (Suppl. 2), 6–20.

82 Boonsirikamchai, P., Choi, S., Frank, S.J., *et al.* (2013) MR imaging of prostate cancer in radiation oncology: what radiologists need to know. *RadioGraphics*, **33** (3). 741–761.

83 Oesterling, J.E., Martin, S.K., Bergstralh, E.J., Lowe, F.C. (1993) The use of prostate-specific antigen in staging patients with newly diagnosed prostate cancer. *JAMA*, **269** (1), 57–60.

84 Dall'Era, M.A., Cowan, J.E., Simko, J., *et al.* (2011) Surgical management after active surveillance for low-risk prostate cancer: pathological outcomes compared with men undergoing immediate treatment. *Br. J. Urol. Int.*, **107** (8), 1232–1237.

85 Eifler, J.B., Feng, Z., Lin, B.M., *et al.* (2013) An updated prostate cancer staging nomogram (Partin tables) based on cases from 2006 to 2011. *Br. J. Urol. Int.*, **111** (1), 22–29.

86 Briganti, A., Larcher, A., Abdollah, F., *et al.* (2012) Updated nomogram predicting lymph node invasion in patients with prostate cancer undergoing extended pelvic lymph node dissection: The essential importance of percentage of positive cores. *Eur. Urol.*, **61** (3), 480–487.

87 Williams, S.G., Zietman, A.L. (2008) Does radical treatment have a role in the management of low-risk prostate cancer? The place for brachytherapy and external beam radiotherapy. *World J. Urol.*, **26** (5), 447–456.

88 Tward, J.D., Lee, C.M., Pappas, L.M., Szabo, A., Gaffney, D.K., Shrieve, D.C. (2006) Survival of men with clinically localized prostate cancer treated with prostatectomy, brachytherapy, or no definitive treatment: impact of age at diagnosis. *Cancer*, **107** (10), 2392–2400.

89 Lu-Yao, G.L., Albertsen, P.C., Moore, D.F., *et al.* (2009) Outcomes of localized prostate cancer following conservative management. *JAMA*, **302** (11), 1202–1209.

90 Tosoian, J.J., Trock, B.J., Landis, P., *et al.* (2011) Active surveillance program for prostate cancer: an update of the Johns Hopkins experience. *J. Clin. Oncol.*, **29** (16), 2185–2190.

91 Klotz, L., Vesprini, D., Sethukavalan, P., *et al.* (2015) Long-term follow-up of a large active surveillance cohort of patients with prostate cancer. *J. Clin. Oncol.*, **33** (3), 272–277.

92 Bangma, C.H., Valdagni, R., Carroll, P.R., *et al.* (2015) Platinum Priority – Review. Prostate cancer magnetic resonance imaging in active surveillance of prostate cancer : a systematic review. *Eur. Urol.*, **67** (4), 627–636.

93 Cooperberg, M.R., Cowan, J.E., Hilton, J.F., *et al.* (2011) Outcomes of active surveillance for men with intermediate-risk prostate cancer. *J. Clin. Oncol.*, **29** (2), 228–234.

93a Hamdy, F.C., Donovan, J.L., Lane, J.A., *et al.* (2016) 10-Year outcomes after monitoring, surgery, or radiotherapy for localized prostate cancer. *N. Engl. J. Med* [Internet]. NEJMoa1606220. Available at: http://www.nejm.org/doi/10.1056/NEJMoa1606220

94 Aizer, A., Paly, J.J., Zietman, A.L., *et al.* (2012) Multidisciplinary care and pursuit of active surveillance in low-risk prostate cancer. *J. Clin. Oncol.*, **30** (25), 3071–3076.

95 Musunuru, H., Klotz, L., Vespirini, D., *et al.* (2015) Cautionary tale of active surveillance in intermediate-risk patients: Overall and cause-specific survival in the Sunnybrook experience. *J. Clin. Oncol.*, Suppl. 7, abstract 163.

96 Hu, J.C., Gu, X., Lipsitz, S.R., *et al.* (2009) Comparative effectiveness of minimally invasive vs open radical prostatectomy. *JAMA*, **302** (14), 1557–1564.

97 Katz, M.S., Efstathiou, J.A., D'Amico, A.V., *et al.* (2010) The 'CaP Calculator': an online decision support tool for clinically localized prostate cancer. *Br. J. Urol. Int.*, **105** (10), 1417–1422.

98 Karakiewicz, P.I., Eastham, J.A., Graefen, M., *et al.* (2005) Prognostic impact of positive surgical margins in surgically treated prostate cancer: Multi-institutional assessment of 5831 patients. *Urology*, **66** (6), 1245–1250.

99 Bolla, M., Van Poppel, H., Tombal, B., *et al.* (2012) Postoperative radiotherapy after radical prostatectomy for high-risk prostate cancer: Long-term results of a randomised controlled trial (EORTC trial 22911). *Lancet*, **380** (9858), 2018–2027.

100 Wiegel, T., Bartkowiak, D., Bottke, D., *et al.* (2014) Adjuvant radiotherapy versus wait-and-see after radical prostatectomy: 10-year follow-up of the ARO 96-02/AUO AP 09/95 trial. *Eur. Urol.*, **66** (2), 243–250.

101 Thompson, I.M., Tangen, C.M., Paradelo, J., *et al.* (2009) Adjuvant radiotherapy for pathological T3N0M0 prostate cancer significantly reduces risk of metastases and improves survival: long-term followup of a randomized clinical trial. *J. Urol.*, **181** (3), 956–962.

102 Messing, E.M., Manola, J., Yao, J., *et al.* (2006) Immediate versus deferred androgen deprivation treatment in patients with node-positive prostate cancer after radical prostatectomy and pelvic lymphadenectomy. *Lancet Oncol.*, **7** (6), 472–479.

103 Abdollah, F., Karnes, R.J., Suardi, N., *et al.* (2014) Impact of adjuvant radiotherapy on survival of patients with node-positive prostate cancer. *J. Clin. Oncol.*, **32** (35), 3939–3947.

104 Briganti, A., Karnes, R.J., Da Pozzo, L.F., *et al.* (2011) Combination of adjuvant hormonal and radiation therapy significantly prolongs survival of patients with pT2-4 pN+ prostate cancer: results of a matched analysis. *Eur. Urol.*, **59** (5), 832–840.

105 Da, L.F., Cozzarini, C., Briganti, A., *et al.* (2009) Long-term follow-up of patients with prostate cancer and nodal metastases treated by pelvic lymphadenectomy and radical prostatectomy: the positive impact of adjuvant radiotherapy. *Eur. Urol.*, **55** (5), 1003–1011.

106 Stephenson, A.J., Scardino, P.T., Eastham, J.A., *et al.* (2006) Preoperative nomogram predicting the 10-year probability of prostate cancer recurrence after radical prostatectomy. *J. Natl Cancer Inst.*, **98** (10), 715–717.

107 Cooperberg, M.R., Carroll, P.R. (2015) Trends in management for patients with localized prostate cancer, 1990–2013. *JAMA*, **314** (1), 80–82.

108 Saranchuk, J.W., Kattan, M.W., Elkin, E., Touijer, A.K., Scardino, P.T., Eastham, J.A. (2005) Achieving optimal

outcomes after radical prostatectomy. *J. Clin. Oncol.*, **23** (18), 4146–4151.

109 Resnick, M.J., Koyama, T., Fan, K.-H., *et al.* (2013) Long-term functional outcomes after treatment for localized prostate cancer. *N. Engl. J. Med.*, **368** (5), 436–445.

110 Ohori, M., Kattan, M.W., Koh, H., *et al.* (2004) Predicting the presence and side of extracapsular extension: a nomogram for staging prostate cancer. *J Urol.*, **171** (5), 1844–1849; discussion 1849.

111 Satake, N., Ohori, M., Yu, C., *et al.* (2010) Development and internal validation of a nomogram predicting extracapsular extension in radical prostatectomy specimens. *Int. J. Urol.*, **17** (3), 267–272.

112 Bill-Axelson, A., Holmberg, L., Ruutu, M., *et al.* (2011) Radical prostatectomy versus watchful waiting in early prostate cancer. *N. Engl. J. Med.*, **364** (18), 1708–1717.

113 Wilt, T.J., Brawer, M.K., Jones, K.M., *et al.* (2012) Radical prostatectomy versus observation for localized prostate cancer. *N. Engl. J. Med.*, **367** (3), 203–213.

114 Zelefsky, M.J., Eastham, J., Cronin, A.M., *et al.* (2010) Metastasis after radical prostatectomy or external beam radiotherapy for patients with clinically localized prostate cancer: a comparison of clinical cohorts adjusted for case mix. *J. Clin. Oncol.*, **28** (9), 1508–1513.

115 Grimm, P., Billiet, I., Bostwick, D., *et al.* (2012) Comparative analysis of prostate-specific antigen free survival outcomes for patients with low, intermediate and high risk prostate cancer treatment by radical therapy. Results from the Prostate Cancer Results Study Group. *Br. J. Urol. Int.*, **109** (Suppl.), 22–29.

116 Nepple, K.G., Stephenson, A.J., Kallogjeri, D., *et al.* (2013) Mortality after prostate cancer treatment with radical prostatectomy, external-beam radiation therapy, or brachytherapy in men without comorbidity. *Eur. Urol.*, **64** (3), 372–378.

117 Dearnaley, D.P., Jovic, G., Syndikus, I., *et al.* (2014) Escalated-dose versus control-dose conformal radiotherapy for prostate cancer: Long-term results from the MRC RT01 randomised controlled trial. *Lancet Oncol.*, **15** (4), 464–473.

118 Kuban, D., Levy, L.B., Cheung, M.R., *et al.* (2011) Long-term failure patterns and survival in a randomized dose-escalation trial for prostate cancer. Who dies of disease? *Int. J. Radiat. Oncol. Biol. Phys.*, **79** (5), 1310–1317.

119 Zietman, A.L., Bae, K., Slater, J.D., *et al.* (2010) Randomized trial comparing conventional-dose with high-dose conformal radiation therapy in early-stage adenocarcinoma of the prostate: Long-term results from Proton Radiation Oncology Group/American College Of Radiology 95-09. *J. Clin. Oncol.*, **28** (7), 1106–1111.

120 Heemsbergen, W.D., Al-Mamgani, A., Slot, A., Dielwart, M.F.H., Lebesque, J.V. (2014) Long-term results of the Dutch randomized prostate cancer trial: Impact of dose-escalation on local, biochemical, clinical failure, and survival. *Radiother. Oncol.*, **110** (1), 104–109.

121 Michalski, J.M., Moughan, J., Purdy, J., *et al.* (2015) A randomized trial of 79.2 Gy versus 70.2 Gy radiation therapy (RT) for localized prostate cancer. *J. Clin. Oncol.*, **33** (Suppl. 7), abstract 4.

122 Michalski, J.M., Yan, Y., Watkins-Bruner, D., *et al.* (2013) Preliminary toxicity analysis of 3-dimensional conformal radiation therapy versus intensity modulated radiation therapy on the high-dose arm of the Radiation Therapy Oncology Group 0126 prostate cancer trial. *Int. J. Radiat. Oncol. Biol. Phys.*, **87** (5), 932–938.

123 Zelefsky, M.J., Kollmeier, M., Cox, B., *et al.* (2012) Improved clinical outcomes with high-dose image guided radiotherapy compared with non-IGRT for the treatment of clinically localized prostate cancer. *Int. J. Radiat. Oncol. Biol. Phys.*, **84** (1), 125–129.

124 Miralbell, R., Roberts, S.A., Zubizarreta, E., Hendry, J.H. (2012) Dose-fractionation sensitivity of prostate cancer deduced from radiotherapy outcomes of 5,969 patients in seven international institutional datasets: $\alpha/\beta = 1.4$ (0.9–2.2) Gy. *Int. J. Radiat. Oncol. Biol. Phys.*, **82** (1), e17–e24.

125 Lukka, H., Hayter, C., Julian, J.A., *et al.* (2005) Randomized trial comparing two fractionation schedules for patients with localized prostate cancer. *J. Clin. Oncol.*, **23** (25), 6132–6138.

126 Yeoh, E.E., Holloway, R.H., Fraser, R.J., *et al.* (2006) Hypofractionated versus conventionally fractionated radiation therapy for prostate carcinoma: updated results of a phase III randomized trial. *Int. J. Radiat. Oncol. Biol. Phys.*, **66** (4), 1072–1083.

127 Arcangeli, S., Strigari, L., Gomellini, S., *et al.* (2012) Updated results and patterns of failure in a randomized hypofractionation trial for high-risk prostate cancer. *Int. J. Radiat. Oncol. Biol. Phys.*, **84** (5), 1172–1178.

128 Dearnaley, D., Syndikus, I., Sumo, G., *et al.* (2012) Conventional versus hypofractionated high-dose intensity-modulated radiotherapy for prostate cancer: Preliminary safety results from the CHHiP randomised controlled trial. *Lancet Oncol.*, **13** (1), 43–54.

129 Pollack, A., Walker, G., Horwitz, E.M., *et al.* (2013) Randomized trial of hypofractionated external-beam radiotherapy for prostate cancer. *J. Clin. Oncol.*, **31** (31), 3860–3868.

130 Hoffman, K.E., Voong, K.R., Pugh, T.J., *et al.* (2014) Risk of late toxicity in men receiving dose-escalated hypofractionated intensity modulated prostate

radiation therapy: Results from a randomized trial. *Int. J. Radiat. Oncol. Biol. Phys.*, **88** (5), 1074–1084.

131 Aluwini, S., Pos, F., Schimmel, E., *et al.* (2015) Hypofractionated versus conventionally fractionated radiotherapy for patients with prostate cancer (HYPRO): acute toxicity results from a randomised non-inferiority phase 3 trial. *Lancet Oncol.*, **16** (3), 274–283.

132 Lee, W.R., Dignam, J.J., Amin, M., *et al.* (2016) NRG Oncology RTOG 0415: A randomized phase III non-inferiority study comparing two fractionation schedules in patients with low-risk prostate cancer. *J. Clin. Oncol.*, **34** (Suppl.2S), abstract 1.

133 Lee, W.R., Dignam, J.J., Amin, M., *et al.* (2016) NRG Oncology RTOG 0415: A randomized phase 3 noninferiority study comparing 2 fractionation schedules in patients with low-risk prostate cancer. *Int. J. Radiat. Oncol. Biol. Phys.*, **94** (1), 3–4.

134 Dearnaley, D., Syndikus, I., Mossop, H., *et al.* (2016) Conventional versus hypofractionated high-dose intensity-modulated radiotherapy for prostate cancer: 5-year outcomes of the randomised, non-inferiority, phase 3 CHHiP trial. *Lancet Oncol*, **17** (8), 1047–1060.

135 Dearnaley, D., Syndikus, I., Mossop, H., *et al.* LATE BREAKING ABSTRACT: 5 year outcomes of a phase III randomised trial of conventional or hypofractionated high dose intensity modulated radiotherapy for prostate cancer (CRUK/06/016): report from the CHHiP Trial Investigators Group. Presentation at the European Cancer Congress 2015.

135a Catton, C.N., Lukka, H., Julian, J.A., *et al.* (2016) A randomized trial of a shorter radiation fractionation schedule for the treatment of localized prostate cancer. *J. Clin. Oncol.*, **2** (Suppl.), abstract 5003.

135b Incrocci, L., Wortel, R.C., Alemayehu, W.G., *et al.* (2016) Hypofractionated versus conventionally fractionated radiotherapy for patients with localised prostate cancer (HYPRO): final efficacy results from a randomised, multicentre, open-label, phase 3 trial. *Lancet Oncol.* [Internet], **17** (8), 1061–10699. Available at: http://www.ncbi.nlm.nih.gov/pubmed/ 27339116\nhttp://linkinghub.elsevier.com/retrieve/pii/ S1470204516300705

135c Aluwini, S., Pos, F., Schimmel, E., *et al.* (2015) Hypofractionated versus conventionally fractionated radiotherapy for patients with prostate cancer (HYPRO): acute toxicity results from a randomised non-inferiority phase 3 trial. *Lancet Oncol.* [Internet], **16** (3), 274–283. Available at: http://www.science direct.com/science/article/pii/S1470204514704826

136 Yu, J.B., Cramer, L.D., Herrin, J., Soulos, P.R., Potosky, A.L., Gross, C.P. (2014) Stereotactic body radiation therapy versus intensity-modulated radiation therapy for prostate cancer: comparison of toxicity. *J. Clin. Oncol.*, **32** (12), 1195–1201.

137 Lukka, H., Pugh, S.L., Bruner, D., *et al.* (2016) Patient reported outcomes in NRG Oncology/RTOG 0938, evaluating two ultrahypofractionated regimens (UHR) for prostate cancer (CaP). *J. Clin. Oncol.*, **34** (Suppl. S2), abstract 27.

138 Davis, B.J., Horwitz, E.M., Lee, W.R., *et al.* (2012) American Brachytherapy Society consensus guidelines for transrectal ultrasound-guided permanent prostate brachytherapy. *Brachytherapy*, **11** (1), 6–19.

139 Sylvester, J.E., Grimm, P.D., Wong, J., Galbreath, R.W., Merrick, G., Blasko, J.C. (2011) Fifteen-year biochemical relapse-free survival, cause-specific survival, and overall survival following I(125) prostate brachytherapy in clinically localized prostate cancer: Seattle experience. *Int. J. Radiat. Oncol. Biol. Phys.*, **81** (2), 376–381.

140 Taira, A.V., Merrick, G.S., Butler, W.M., *et al.* (2011) Long-term outcome for clinically localized prostate cancer treated with permanent interstitial brachytherapy. *Int. J. Radiat. Oncol. Biol. Phys.*, **79** (5), 1336–1342.

141 Taira, A.V., Merrick, G.S., Galbreath, R.W., *et al.* (2012) Distant metastases following permanent interstitial brachytherapy for patients with clinically localized prostate cancer. *Int. J. Radiat. Oncol. Biol. Phys.*, **82** (2), 225–232.

142 Zelefsky, M.J., Kuban, D., Levy, L.B., *et al.* (2007) Multi-institutional analysis of long-term outcome for stages T1-T2 prostate cancer treated with permanent seed implantation. *Int. J. Radiat. Oncol. Biol. Phys.*, **67** (2), 327–333.

143 Hsu, I.C., Bae, K., Shinohara, K., *et al.* (2010) Phase II trial of combined high-dose-rate brachytherapy and external beam radiotherapy for adenocarcinoma of the prostate: Preliminary results of RTOG 0321. *Int. J. Radiat. Oncol. Biol. Phys.*, **78** (3), 751–758.

144 Keyes, M., Spadinger, I., Liu, M., *et al.* (2012) Rectal toxicity and rectal dosimetry in low-dose-rate 125I permanent prostate implants: A long-term study in 1006 patients. *Brachytherapy*, **11** (3), 199–208.

145 Keyes, M., Miller, S., Pickles, T., *et al.* (2014) Late urinary side effects 10 years after low-dose-rate prostate brachytherapy: population-based results from a multiphysician practice treating with a standardized protocol and uniform dosimetric goals. *Int. J. Radiat. Oncol. Biol. Phys.*, **90** (3), 570–578.

146 Hauswald, H., Kamrava, M., Fallon, J.M., *et al.* (2015) High-dose-rate (HDR) monotherapy for localized prostate cancer: 10 year results. *Int. J. Radiat. Oncol. Biol. Phys.*, **94** (4), 667–674.

147 Rogers, C.L., Alder, S.C., Rogers, R.L., *et al.* (2012) High dose brachytherapy as monotherapy for intermediate risk prostate cancer. *J. Urol.*, **187** (1), 109–116.

148 Demanes, D.J., Martinez, A., Ghilezan, M., *et al.* (2011) High-dose-rate monotherapy: Safe and effective brachytherapy for patients with localized prostate cancer. *Int. J. Radiat. Oncol. Biol. Phys.*, **81** (5), 1286–1292.

149 Ghilezan, M., Martinez, A., Gustason, G., *et al.* (2012) High-dose-rate brachytherapy as monotherapy delivered in two fractions within one day for favorable/intermediate-risk prostate cancer: Preliminary toxicity data. *Int. J. Radiat. Oncol. Biol. Phys.*, **83** (3), 927–932.

150 Roach, M., 3rd, Hanks, G., Thames, H., Jr, *et al.* (2006) Defining biochemical failure following radiotherapy with or without hormonal therapy in men with clinically localized prostate cancer: recommendations of the RTOG-ASTRO Phoenix Consensus Conference. *Int. J. Radiat. Oncol. Biol. Phys.*, **65** (4), 965–974.

151 Lo, A.C., Morris, W.J., Lapointe, V., *et al.* (2014) Prostate-specific antigen at 4 to 5 years after low-dose-rate prostate brachytherapy is a strong predictor of disease-free survival. *Int. J. Radiat. Oncol. Biol. Phys.*, **88** (1), 87–93.

152 Parekh, A., Graham, P.L., Nguyen, P.L. (2013) Cancer control and complications of salvage local therapy after failure of radiotherapy for prostate cancer: A systematic review. *Semin. Radiat. Oncol.*, **23** (3), 222–234.

153 Sanda, M.G., Dunn, R.L., Michalski, J., *et al.* (2008) Quality of life and satisfaction with outcome among prostate-cancer survivors. *N. Engl. J. Med.*, **358** (12), 1250–1261.

154 Jones, C.U., Hunt, D., McGowan, D.G., *et al.* (2011) Radiotherapy and short-term androgen deprivation for localized prostate cancer. *N. Engl. J. Med.*, **365** (2), 107–118.

155 Potosky, A.L., Haque, R., Cassidy-Bushrow, A.E., *et al.* (2014) Effectiveness of primary androgen-deprivation therapy for clinically localized prostate cancer. *J. Clin. Oncol.*, **32** (13), 1324–1330.

156 Zaorsky, N.G., Palmer, J.D., Hurwitz, M.D., Keith, S.W., Dicker, A.P., Den, R.B. (2015) What is the ideal radiotherapy dose to treat prostate cancer? A meta-analysis of biologically equivalent dose escalation. *Radiother. Oncol.*, **115** (3), 295–300.

156a Prestidge, B.R., Winter, K., Sanda, M.G., *et al.* (2016) Initial Report of NRG Oncology/RTOG 0232: A Phase 3 study comparing combined external beam radiation and transperineal interstitial permanent brachytherapy with brachytherapy alone for selected patients with intermediate-risk prostatic carcinoma. *Int. J. Radiat. Oncol. Biol. Phys.* [Internet], **96** (2), Suppl. S4. Available at: http://dx.doi.org/10.1016/j.ijrobp.2016.06.026

157 Morris, W.J., Tyldesley, S., Pai, H.H., *et al.* (2015) ASCENDE-RT: A multicenter, randomized trial of dose-escalated external beam radiotherapy (EBRT-B) versus low-dose-rate brachytherapy (LDR-B) for men with unfavorable-risk localized prostate cancer. *J. Clin. Oncol.*, **33** (Suppl. 7), abstract 3.

158 Khor, R., Duchesne, G., Tai, K.H., *et al.* (2013) Direct 2-arm comparison shows benefit of high-dose-rate brachytherapy boost vs external beam radiation therapy alone for prostate cancer. *Int. J. Radiat. Oncol. Biol. Phys.*, **85** (3), 679–685.

159 Spratt, D.E., Zumsteg, Z.S., Ghadjar, P., *et al.* (2014) Comparison of high-dose (86.4Gy) IMRT vs combined brachytherapy plus IMRT for intermediate-risk prostate cancer. *Br. J. Urol. Int.*, **1140** (3), 360–367.

160 Denham, J.W., Steigler, A., Lamb, D.S., *et al.* (2011) Short-term neoadjuvant androgen deprivation and radiotherapy for locally advanced prostate cancer: 10-year data from the TROG 96.01 randomised trial. *Lancet Oncol.*, **12** (5), 451–459.

161 D'Amico, A.V., Chen, M.H., Renshaw, A.A., Loffredo, M., Kantoff, P.W. (2008) Androgen suppression and radiation vs radiation alone for prostate cancer: a randomized trial. *JAMA*, **299** (3), 289–295.

162 Pisansky, T.M., Hunt, D., Gomella, L.G., *et al.* (2014) Duration of androgen suppression before radiotherapy for localized prostate cancer: Radiation Therapy Oncology Group Randomized Clinical Trial 9910. *J. Clin. Oncol.*, **33** (4), 332–339.

163 Nabid, A., Carrier, N., Vigneault, E., *et al.* (2015) A Phase III trial of short-term androgen deprivation therapy in intermediate-risk prostate cancer treated with radiotherapy. *J. Clin. Oncol.*, **33** (Suppl.), abstract 5019.

164 Zapatero, A., Alvarez, A., Gonzalez San Segundo, C., *et al.* (2015) High-dose radiotherapy with short-term or long-term androgen deprivation in localised prostate cancer (DART01/05 GICOR): a randomised, controlled, phase 3 trial. *Lancet Oncol.*, **16** (16), 320–327.

165 Keane, F.K., Chen, M.H., Zhang, D., *et al.* (2014) The likelihood of death from prostate cancer in men with favorable or unfavorable intermediate-risk disease. *Cancer*, **120** (12), 1787–1793.

166 Zietman, A.L., Prince, E.A., Nakfoor, B.M., Park, J.J. (1997) Androgen deprivation and radiation therapy: sequencing studies using the Shionogi in vivo tumor system. *Int. J. Radiat. Oncol. Biol. Phys.*, **38** (5), 1067–1070.

167 Keating, N.L., O'Malley, A.J., Smith, M.R. (2006) Diabetes and cardiovascular disease during androgen deprivation therapy for prostate cancer. *J. Clin. Oncol.*, **24** (27), 4448–4456.

168 Saigal, C.S., Gore, J.L., Krupski, T.L., Hanley, J., Schonlau, M., Litwin, M.S. (2007) Androgen

deprivation therapy increases cardiovascular morbidity in men with prostate cancer. *Cancer*, **110** (7), 1493–1500.

169 Voog, J.C., Paulus, R., Shipley, W.U., *et al.* (2016) Cardiovascular mortality following short-term androgen deprivation in clinically localized prostate cancer: an analysis of RTOG 94-08. *Eur. Urol.*, **69** (2), 204–210.

170 Efstathiou, J.A., Bae, K., Shipley, W.U., *et al.* (2008) Cardiovascular mortality and duration of androgen deprivation for locally advanced prostate cancer: analysis of RTOG 92-02. *Eur. Urol.*, **54** (4), 816–823.

171 Efstathiou, J.A., Bae, K., Shipley, W.U., *et al.* (2009) Cardiovascular mortality after androgen deprivation therapy for locally advanced prostate cancer: RTOG 85-31. *J. Clin. Oncol.*, **27** (1), 92–99.

172 Shao, Y.H., Demissie, K., Shih, W., *et al.* (2009) Contemporary risk profile of prostate cancer in the United States. *J. Natl Cancer Inst.*, **101** (18) 1280–1283.

173 Bolla, M., de Reijke, T.M., Van Tienhoven, G., *et al.* (2009) Duration of androgen suppression in the treatment of prostate cancer. *N. Engl. J. Med.*, **360** (24), 2516–2527.

174 Horwitz, E.M., Bae, K., Hanks, G.E., *et al.* (2008) Ten-year follow-up of radiation therapy oncology group protocol 92-02: A phase III trial of the duration of elective androgen deprivation in locally advanced prostate cancer. *J. Clin. Oncol.*, **26** (15), 2497–2504.

175 Horwitz, E.M., Bae, K., Hanks, G.E., *et al.* (2008) Ten-year follow-up of radiation therapy oncology group protocol 92-02: a phase III trial of the duration of elective androgen deprivation in locally advanced prostate cancer. *J. Clin. Oncol.*, **26** (15), 2497–2504.

176 Warde, P., Mason, M., Ding, K., *et al.* (2011) Combined androgen deprivation therapy and radiation therapy for locally advanced prostate cancer: a randomised, phase 3 trial. *Lancet*, **378** (9809), 2104–2111.

177 Widmark, A., Klepp, O., Solberg, A., *et al.* (2009) Endocrine treatment, with or without radiotherapy, in locally advanced prostate cancer (SPCG-7/SFUO-3): an open randomised phase III trial. *Lancet*, **373** (9660), 301–308.

178 Nabid, A., Carrier, N., Martin, A.-G., *et al.* (2013) Duration of androgen deprivation therapy in high-risk prostate cancer: A randomized trial. *J. Clin. Oncol.*, **31** (Suppl.), abstract LBA4510.

179 Roach, M., 3rd (2008) Targeting pelvic lymph nodes in men with intermediate- and high-risk prostate cancer, and confusion about the results of the randomized trials. *J. Clin. Oncol.*, **26** (22), 3816–3818.

180 Lawton, C., DeSilvio, M., Roach, M., *et al.* (2007) An update of the Phase III trial comparing whole pelvic to prostate only radiotherapy and neoadjuvant to adjuvant total androgen suppression: updated analysis of RTOG 94-13, with emphasis on unexpected hormone/radiation interactions. *Int. J. Radiat. Oncol. Biol. Phys.*, **69** (3), 646–655.

181 Pommier, P., Chabaud, S., Lagrange, J.L., *et al.* (2007) Is there a role for pelvic irradiation in localized prostate adenocarcinoma? Preliminary results of GETUG-01. *J. Clin. Oncol.*, **25** (34), 5366–5373.

182 Asbell, S.O., Krall, J.M., Pilepich, M.V., *et al.* (1988) Elective pelvic irradiation in stage A2, B carcinoma of the prostate: analysis of RTOG 77-06. *Int. J. Radiat. Oncol. Biol. Phys.*, **15** (6), 1307–1316.

183 Sandler, H.M., Rosenthal, S.A., Sartor, O., *et al.* (2015) A phase III protocol of androgen suppression (AS) and 3DCRT/IMRT versus AS and 3DCRT/IMRT followed by chemotherapy (CT) with docetaxel and prednisone for localized, high-risk prostate cancer (RTOG 0521). *J. Clin. Oncol.*, **33** (Suppl.), abstract LBA5002.

184 Alemozaffar, M., Regan, M.M., Cooperberg, M.R., *et al.* (2011) Prediction of erectile function following treatment for prostate cancer. *N. Engl. J. Med.*, **306** (11), 1205–1214.

185 Valicenti, R.K., Thompson, I., Albertsen, P., *et al.* (2013) Adjuvant and salvage radiation therapy after prostatectomy: American Society for Radiation Oncology/American Urological Association guidelines. *Int. J. Radiat. Oncol. Biol. Phys.*, **86** (5), 822–828.

186 Sineshaw, H.M., Gray, P.J., Td, J.A., Efstathiou, I.F., Jemal, A. (2015) Platinum Priority – Prostate cancer declining use of radiotherapy for adverse features after radical prostatectomy : results from the National Cancer Data Base. *Eur. Urol.*, **68** (5), 768–774.

187 Thompson, I.M., Tangen, C.M., Paradelo, J., *et al.* (2006) Adjuvant radiotherapy for pathologically advanced prostate cancer. *JAMA*, **296** (19), 2329–2335.

188 Stephenson, A.J., Shariat, S.F., Zelefsky, M.J., *et al.* (2004) Salvage radiotherapy for recurrent prostate cancer after radical prostatectomy. *JAMA*, **291** (11), 1325–1332.

189 Stephenson, A.J., Scardino, P.T., Kattan, M.W., *et al.* (2007) Predicting the outcome of salvage radiation therapy for recurrent prostate cancer after radical prostatectomy. *J. Clin. Oncol.*, **25** (15), 2035–2041.

190 Trock, B.J., Han, M., Freedland, S.J., *et al.* (2008) Prostate cancer-specific survival following salvage radiotherapy vs observation in men with biochemical recurrence after radical prostatectomy. *JAMA*, **299** (23), 2760–2769.

191 King, C.R. (2012) The timing of salvage radiotherapy after radical prostatectomy: A systematic review. *Int. J. Radiat. Oncol. Biol. Phys.*, **84** (1), 104–111.

192 Spiotto, M.T., Hancock, S.L., King, C.R. (2007) Radiotherapy after prostatectomy: improved

biochemical relapse-free survival with whole pelvic compared with prostate bed only for high-risk patients. *Int. J. Radiat. Oncol. Biol. Phys.*, **69** (1), 54–61.

193 Corn, B.W., Winter, K., Pilepich, M.V. (1999) Does androgen suppression enhance the efficacy of postoperative irradiation? A secondary analysis of RTOG 85-31. *Urology*, **54** (3), 495–502.

194 Shipley, W.U., Seiferheld, W., Lukka, H., *et al.* (2016) Report of NRG Oncology/RTOG 9601, A Phase 3 trial in prostate cancer: Anti-androgen therapy (AAT) with bicalutamide during and after radiation therapy (RT) in patients following radical prostatectomy (RP) with pT2-3pN0 disease and an elevated PSA. *Int. J. Radiat. Oncol. Biol. Phys.*, **94** (1), 3.

195 Shipley, W.U., Seiferheld, W., Lukka, H.R., Major, P.P., Heney, N.M., Grignon, D.J., *et al.* (2017) Radiation with or without Antiandrogen Therapy in Recurrent Prostate Cancer. *N. Engl. J. Med.*, **376**, 417–428. Doi:10.1056/NEJMoa1607529.

195a Carrie, C., Hasbini, A., de Laroche, G., *et al.* (2016) Salvage radiotherapy with or without short-term hormone therapy for rising prostate-specific antigen concentration after radical prostatectomy (GETUG-AFU 16): a randomised, multicentre, open-label phase 3 trial. *Lancet Oncol.*, **17** (6), 747–756.

195b Donovan, J.L., Hamdy, F.C., Lane, J.A., *et al.* (2016) Patient-reported outcomes after monitoring, surgery, or radiotherapy for prostate cancer. Massachusetts Medical Society, *N. Engl. J. Med.* [Internet], **375** (15), 1425–1437. Available at: http://dx.doi.org/10.1056/NEJMoa1606221

196 Nguyen, O., Klein, E.A. (2012) Management of prostate cancer patients with positive regional lymph nodes, in *UpToDate* (ed. D.S. Basow), UpToDate, Waltham, MA.

197 Buskirk, S.J., Pisansky, T.M., Atkinson, E.J., *et al.* (2001) Lymph node-positive prostate cancer: evaluation of the results of the combination of androgen deprivation therapy and radiation therapy. *Mayo Clin. Proc.*, **76** (7), 702–706.

198 Granfors, T., Modig, H., Damber, J.E., Tomic, R. (1998) Combined orchiectomy and external radiotherapy versus radiotherapy alone for nonmetastatic prostate cancer with or without pelvic lymph node involvement: a prospective randomized study. *J. Urol.*, **159** (6), 2030–2034.

199 Lin, C.C., Gray, P.J., Jemal, A., Efstathiou, J. (2015) Androgen Deprivation With or Without Radiation Therapy for Clinically Node-Positive Prostate Cancer. *J. Natl Cancer Inst.*, **107** (7), pii:djv119. Doi:10.1093jnci/djv119.

200 Tward, J.D., Kokeny, K.E., Shrieve, D.C. (2013) Radiation therapy for clinically node-positive prostate adenocarcinoma is correlated with improved overall and prostate cancer-specific survival. *Pract. Radiat. Oncol.*, **3** (3), 234–240.

201 Hussain, M., Tangen, C.M., Berry, D.L., *et al.* (2013) Intermittent versus continuous androgen deprivation in prostate cancer. *N. Engl. J. Med.*, **368** (14) 1314–1325.

202 Sweeney, C.J., Chen, Y.-H., Carducci, M., *et al.* (2015) Chemohormonal therapy in metastatic hormone-sensitive prostate cancer. *N. Engl. J. Med.*, **373** (8), 737–746.

203 James, N.D., Sydes, M.R., Mason, M.D., *et al.* (2015) Docetaxel and/or zoledronic acid for hormone-naive prostate cancer: First overall survival results from STAMPEDE. *J. Clin. Oncol.*, **33** (Suppl.), abstract 5001.

204 Harstell, W.F., Scott, C.B., Bruner, D.W., *et al.* (2005) Randomized trial of short- versus long-course radiotherapy for palliation of painful bone metastases. *J. Natl Cancer Inst.*, **97** (11), 798–804.

205 Hahn, C., Kavanagh, B., Bhatnagar, A., *et al.* (2014) Choosing wisely: The American Society for Radiation Oncology's Top 5 list. *Pract. Radiat. Oncol.*, **4** (6), 349–355.

206 Oosterhof, G.O.N., Roberts, J.T., de Reijke, T.M., *et al.* (2003) Strontium-89 chloride versus palliative local field radiotherapy in patients with hormonal escaped prostate cancer: A Phase III study of the European Organisation for Research and Treatment of Cancer Genitourinary Group. *Eur. Urol.*, **44** (5), 519–526.

207 Powsner, R.A., Zietman, A.L., Foss, F.M. (1997) Bone marrow suppression after strontium-89 therapy and local radiation therapy in patients with diffuse marrow involvement. *Clin. Nucl. Med.*, **22** (3), 147–150.

208 Parker, C., Nilsson, S., Heinrich, D., *et al.* (2013) Alpha emitter radium-223 and survival in metastatic prostate cancer. *N. Engl. J. Med.*, **369** (3), 213–223.

209 Sartor, O., Coleman, R., Nilsson, S., *et al.* (2016) Effect of radium-223 dichloride on symptomatic skeletal events in patients with castration-resistant prostate cancer and bone metastases: results from a phase 3, double-blind, randomised trial. *Lancet Oncol.*, **15** (7), 738–746.

210 Finkelstein, S.E., Michalski, J.M., O'Sullivan, J., Parker, C., Garcia-Vargas, J., Sartor, O. (2016) External beam radiation therapy (EBRT) use and safety with radium-223 dichloride (Ra-223) in patients with castration-resistant prostate cancer (CRPC) and symptomatic bone metastases (mets) from the ALSYMPCA Trial. *Int. J. Radiat. Oncol. Biol. Phys.*, **93** (3), S201.

211 Hellman, S., Weichselbaum, R.R. (1995) Oligometastases. *J. Clin. Oncol.*, **13** (1), 8–10.

212 Ost, P., Jereczek-Fossa, B.A., Van As, N., *et al.* (2016) Progression-free survival following stereotactic body radiotherapy for oligometastatic prostate cancer treatment-naive recurrence: a multi-institutional analysis. *Eur. Urol.*, **69** (1), 9–12.

213 Ost, P., Bossi, A., Decaestecker, K., *et al.* (2015) Metastasis-directed therapy of regional and distant recurrences after curative treatment of prostate cancer: a systematic review of the literature. *Eur. Urol.*, **67** (5), 852–863.

214 Zumsteg, Z.S., Spratt, D.E., Romesser, P.B., *et al.* (2015) The natural history and predictors of outcome following biochemical relapse in the dose escalation era for prostate cancer patients undergoing definitive external beam radiotherapy. *Eur. Urol.*, **67** (6), 1009–1016.

215 Crook, J.M., O'Callaghan, C.J., Duncan, G., *et al.* (2012) Intermittent androgen suppression for rising PSA level after radiotherapy. *N. Engl. J. Med.*, **367** (10), 895–903.

216 Hatiboglu, G., Pinkawa, M., Vallée, J.-P., Hadaschik, B., Hohenfellner, M. (2012) Application technique: placement of a prostate–rectum spacer in men undergoing prostate radiation therapy. *Br. J. Urol. Int.*, **110** (11b), E647–E652.

217 Mariados, N., Sylvester, J., Shah, D., *et al.* (2015) Hydrogel spacer prospective multicenter randomized controlled pivotal trial: dosimetric and clinical effects of perirectal spacer application in men undergoing prostate image guided intensity modulated radiation therapy. *Int. J. Radiat. Oncol. Biol. Phys.*, **92** (5), 971–977.

218 McLaughlin, P.W., Evans, C., Feng, M., Narayana, V. (2010) Radiographic and anatomic basis for prostate contouring errors and methods to improve prostate contouring accuracy. *Int. J. Radiat. Oncol. Biol. Phys.*, **76** (2), 369–378.

219 Trofimov, A., Nguyen, P.L., Efstathiou, J.A., *et al.* (2011) Interfractional variations in the setup of pelvic bony anatomy and soft tissue, and their implications on the delivery of proton therapy for localized prostate cancer. *Int. J. Radiat. Oncol. Biol. Phys.*, **80** (3), 928–937.

220 Sheets, N.C., Goldin, G.H., Meyer, A.M., *et al.* (2012) Intensity-modulated radiation therapy, proton therapy, or conformal radiation therapy and morbidity and disease control in localized prostate cancer. *JAMA*, **307** (15), 1611–1620.

221 Lawrence, T.S., Feng, M. (2013) Protons for prostate cancer: The dream versus the reality. *J. Natl Cancer Inst.*, **105** (1), 7–8.

222 Mendenhall, N.P., Hoppe, B.S., Nichols, R.C., *et al.* (2014) Five-year outcomes from 3 prospective trials of image-guided proton therapy for prostate cancer. *Int. J. Radiat. Oncol. Biol. Phys.*, **88** (3), 596–602.

223 Slater, J.D., Rossi, C.J., Yonemoto, L.T., *et al.* (2004) Proton therapy for prostate cancer: The initial Loma Linda University experience. *Int. J. Radiat. Oncol. Biol. Phys.*, **59** (2), 348–352.

224 Gray, P.J., Paly, J.J., Yeap, B.Y., *et al.* (2013) Patient-reported outcomes after 3-dimensional conformal, intensity-modulated, or proton beam radiotherapy for localized prostate cancer. *Cancer*, **119** (9), 1729–1735.

225 Yu, J.B., Soulos, P.R., Herrin, J., *et al.* (2013) Proton versus intensity-modulated radiotherapy for prostate cancer: Patterns of care and early toxicity. *J. Natl Cancer Inst.*, **105** (1), 25–32.

226 Ishikawa, H., Tsuji, H., Kamada, T., *et al.* (2012) Carbon-ion radiation therapy for prostate cancer. *Int. J. Urol.*, **19** (4), 296–305.

227 Valerio, M., Ahmed, H.U., Emberton, M., *et al.* (2014) The role of focal therapy in the management of localised prostate cancer: a systematic review. *Eur. Urol.*, **66** (4), 732–751.

228 Spratt, D.E., Zelefsky, M.J. (2013) Point: There is a need for supplemental XRT with brachytherapy in the treatment of intermediate-risk prostate cancer patients. *Brachytherapy*, **12** (5), 389–392.

229 Stone, N.N. (2013) Counterpoint: Is there a need for supplemental XRT in intermediate-risk prostate cancer patients? *Brachytherapy*, **12** (5), 393–397.

230 Yamada, Y., Rogers, L., Demanes, D.J., *et al.* (2012) American Brachytherapy Society consensus guidelines for high-dose-rate prostate brachytherapy. *Brachytherapy*, **11** (1), 20–32.

231 Hsu, I.J., Yamada, Y., Assimos, D.G., *et al.* (2014) ACR Appropriateness Criteria high-dose-rate brachytherapy for prostate cancer. *Brachytherapy*, **13** (1), 27–31.

232 Iğdem, S., Alço, G., Ercan, T., *et al.* (2010) Insufficiency fractures after pelvic radiotherapy in patients with prostate cancer. *Int. J. Radiat. Oncol. Biol. Phys.*, **77** (3), 818–823.

233 Hamilton, S.N., Tyldesley, S., Hamm, J., *et al.* (2014) Incidence of second malignancies in prostate cancer patients treated with low-dose-rate brachytherapy and radical prostatectomy. *Int. J. Radiat. Oncol. Biol. Phys.*, **90** (4), 934–941.

234 Nam, R.K., Cheung, P., Herschorn, S., *et al.* (2014) Incidence of complications other than urinary incontinence or erectile dysfunction after radical prostatectomy or radiotherapy for prostate cancer: a population-based cohort study. *Lancet Oncol.*, **15** (2), 223–231.

235 Berrington de Gonzalez, A., Wong, J., Kleinerman, R., Kim, C., Morton, L., Bekelman, J.E. (2015) Risk of second cancers according to radiation therapy technique and modality in prostate cancer survivors. *Int. J. Radiat. Oncol. Biol. Phys.*, **91** (2), 295–302.

236 Zelefsky, M.J., Pei, X., Teslova, T., *et al.* (2012) Secondary cancers after intensity-modulated radiotherapy, brachytherapy and radical prostatectomy for the treatment of prostate cancer: incidence and cause-specific survival outcomes according to the initial treatment intervention. *Br. J. Urol. Int.*, **110** (11), 1696–1701.

237 Pollack, A., Zagars, G.K., Starkschall, G., *et al.* (2002) Prostate cancer radiation dose response: results of the M. D. Anderson phase III randomized trial. *Int. J. Radiat. Oncol. Biol. Phys.*, **53** (5), 1097–1105.

238 Talcott, J.A., Rossi, C., Shipley, W.U., *et al.* (2010) Patient-reported long-term outcomes after conventional and high-dose combined proton and photon radiation for early prostate cancer. *JAMA*, **303** (11), 1046–1053.

239 Hamstra, D., Conlon, A.S.C., Daignault, S., *et al.* (2013) Multi-institutional prospective evaluation of bowel quality of life after prostate external beam radiation therapy identifies patient and treatment factors associated with patient-reported outcomes: The PROSTQA experience. *Int. J. Radiat. Oncol. Biol. Phys.*, **86** (3), 546–553.

240 Michalski, J.M., Gay, H., Jackson, A., Tucker, S.L., Deasy, J.O. (2010) Radiation dose–volume effects in radiation-induced rectal injury. *Int. J. Radiat. Oncol. Biol. Phys.*, **76** (3 Suppl.), 123–129.

241 Solanki, A.A., Liauw, S.L. (2013) Tobacco use and external beam radiation therapy for prostate cancer: Influence on biochemical control and late toxicity. *Cancer*, **119** (15), 2807–2814.

242 Choe, K.S., Jani, A.B., Liauw, S.L. (2010) External beam radiotherapy for prostate cancer patients on anticoagulation therapy: How significant is the bleeding toxicity? *Int. J. Radiat. Oncol. Biol. Phys.*, **76** (3), 755–760.

243 Kalakota, K., Liauw, S.L. (2015) Toxicity after external beam radiotherapy for prostate cancer: an analysis of late morbidity in men with diabetes mellitus. *Urology*, **81** (6), 1196–1201.

244 Murphy, C.T., Heller, S., Ruth, K., *et al.* (2015) Evaluating toxicity from definitive radiation therapy for prostate cancer in men with inflammatory bowel disease: Patient selection and dosimetric parameters with modern treatment techniques. *Pract. Radiat. Oncol.*, **5** (3), e215–e222.

245 Zelefsky, M.J., Shasha, D., Branco, R.D., *et al.* (2014) Tadalafil for prevention of erectile dysfunction after radiotherapy for prostate cancer. *J. Urol.*, **311** (3), 1300.

246 Pisansky, T.M., Pugh, S.L., Greenberg, R.E., *et al.* (2014) Tadalafil for prevention of erectile dysfunction after radiotherapy for prostate cancer: The Radiation Therapy Oncology Group [0831] randomized clinical trial. *JAMA*, **311** (13), 1300–1307.

247 Seymour, Z., Chang, A.J., Zhang, L., *et al.* (2015) Dose–volume analysis and the temporal nature of toxicity with stereotactic body radiation therapy for prostate cancer. *Pract. Radiat. Oncol.*, **5** (5), e465–e472.

248 King, C.R., Collins, S., Fuller, D., *et al.* (2013) Health-related quality of life after stereotactic body radiation therapy for localized prostate cancer: results from a multi-institutional consortium of prospective trials. *Int. J. Radiat. Oncol. Biol. Phys.*, **87** (5), 939–945.

249 Moinpour, C.M., Hayden, K., Unger, J.M., *et al.* (2008) Health-related quality of life results in pathologic stage C prostate cancer from a Southwest Oncology Group trial comparing radical prostatectomy alone with radical prostatectomy plus radiation therapy. *J. Clin. Oncol.*, **26** (1), 112–120.

250 Corbin, K.S., Kunnavakkam, R., Eggener, S.E., Liauw, S.L. (2013) Intensity modulated radiation therapy after radical prostatectomy: Early results show no decline in urinary continence, gastrointestinal, or sexual quality of life. *Pract. Radiat. Oncol.*, **3** (2), 138–144.

28

Carcinoma of the Upper Urinary Tract

Anthony L. Zietman, Jonathan J. Paly and Jason A. Efstathiou

Renal Cell Carcinoma

Each year, 3% of new cancer cases and 3% of cancer deaths in the United States result from kidney cancer, and over 90% of adult kidney cancers are renal cell carcinomas (RCCs) [1]. The incidence of RCC in the US has been increasing by 2% per year over the past three decades. This is largely, but not totally, the result of an increased use of abdominal imaging in everyday medical practice [2, 3]. The disease is typically diagnosed later in life (median age at diagnosis 65 years), and is more common in men than women. There appear to be few racial differences in incidence but globally RCC is more frequently seen in developed nations [4].

RCC is currently classified into three major histologic subtypes: clear cell; chromophobe; and papillary. Patients with clear-cell RCC have a worse prognosis compared to patients who have papillary or chromophobe histologies, and this may be further stratified by using the nuclear Fuhrman grade. Sarcomatoid differentiation carries a particularly poor prognosis.

RCC may spread by local extension through the renal capsule into the perinephric fat or the adrenal gland [5], or by direct extension through the renal vein to the inferior vena cava (occasionally reaching the right atrium) [6] (Figure 28.1a and b). Lymphatic drainage is to the renal hilar, para-aortic, and paracaval lymph nodes [5]. RCCs may also spread by hematologic metastasis to the lung [6] or by retrograde venous drainage to the ovary or testis [5]. As for all cancers, staging is based upon the local, regional, and distant extent of the disease (Figure 28.2). The 'classic' symptoms of local tumor extension include hematuria, abdominal pain, and a flank mass, but these are now infrequently seen because of earlier detection [7].

Primary Therapy

Surgery

Radical surgical resection is the only curative treatment for localized (stage I–III) RCC, and thus is the standard of care. The kidney is removed together with its perirenal fat, the regional lymph nodes, and (for upper pole lesions) the ipsilateral adrenal gland [8]. This operation is now largely carried out laparoscopically because of the more rapid patient recovery. Partial nephrectomy, or nephron-sparing surgery (NSS), is now commonly used to treat small tumors <4 cm with a low incidence of local recurrence (<10%). Other minimally invasive ablative procedures are being developed to deal with the large numbers of small incidentally identified lesions now being found. These include radiofrequency, high-intensity focused ultrasound, and cryosurgery [9, 10].

Radiation Therapy in Primary Renal Cell Carcinoma

The data studying the use of neoadjuvant or postoperative irradiation in the management of locally advanced primary RCC are now very old, and radiation is now rarely used in this setting. Preoperative irradiation was observed to reduce the size of the tumors and increase their encapsulation [11]. In higher-stage tumors it appeared that complete resection could be more often achieved. More formal studies showed no survival advantage to preoperative therapy; indeed, in one trial patient survival was actually worse.

The role of postoperative irradiation has been evaluated both retrospectively and prospectively in multiple studies. When pooling seven major trials (five retrospective and two randomized), the retrospective

Clinical Radiation Oncology: Indications, Techniques, and Results, Third Edition. Edited by William Small Jr.
© 2017 John Wiley & Sons, Inc. Published 2017 by John Wiley & Sons, Inc.

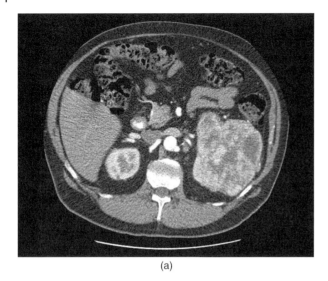

(a)

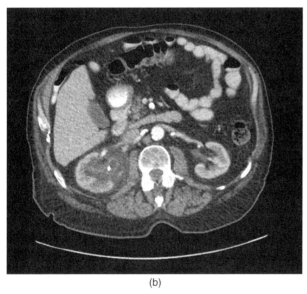

(b)

Figure 28.1 (a) Large necrotic left-sided renal cell carcinoma replacing the entire kidney. The patient presented with fever and hematuria. (b) Transitional cell carcinoma of the right renal pelvis. The renal pelvis is expanded and there is much peri-pelvis fat stranding, indicative of tumor invasion. The patient presented with flank pain and hematuria.

studies showed no or little benefit [12]. However, although one of the randomized trials showed no advantage [13] the other trial showed inferior survival [14] in the radiation arm, largely because of significant bowel or liver toxicity caused by the techniques used at that time. It is worth noting, however, that all of these studies were conducted during a period that predated the use of modern biologic targeted therapies and radiation therapy techniques such as three-dimensional conformal radiation therapy (3D-CRT) and intensity-modulated radiotherapy (IMRT). Some have called for a new look at the

role of postoperative radiation in RCC which makes use of these advances [12].

Stereotactic body radiation therapy (SBRT) is being explored for those with medically inoperable primary renal cell cancer [15]. Small series have been reported showing apparent local control. SBRT will, however, have to compete with established ablative techniques such as high-intensity focused ultrasound (HIFU) which have a more robust supportive literature.

Intraoperative radiation therapy (IORT) may have a role in the small subset of patients who experience local relapse of their disease in the renal fossa after nephrectomy. Several retrospective single-institution studies have explored the role of IORT during resection of locally recurrent RCC, and found low rates of local recurrence where higher rates might have been anticipated. Complication rates are acceptable with the addition of this therapy. In a preliminary retrospective analysis of a large multi-institutional cohort of patients treated with IORT for advanced or locally recurrent RCC ($n = 98$), the disease-specific and disease-free survival rates were found to be improved compared to a similar group managed by resection alone [16]. IORT for recurrent RCC includes 10–20 Gy delivered to a 90% isodose. Conical or elliptical collimator/applicators, generally about 10 cm at their widest axis, are positioned to cover the recurrent tumor bed and margins so as to help increase local control (Figure 28.3). Bolus and shielding are applied, and electron energies from 4 to 20 MeV are generally used.

Metastatic Renal Cell Carcinoma

Chemotherapy

RCC responds poorly to current chemotherapy, with objective response rates in clear-cell disease at less than 7%. In non-clear-cell subsets the objective responses to chemotherapy appear to be better at 10–15% when the following combinations are used: carboplatin/paclitaxel, cisplatin/gemcitabine, or doxurobicin. As a result, the mainstay of systemic treatment has historically been immunotherapy and more recently molecularly targeted therapy.

Immunotherapy

RCC is an immunologically responsive disease, with rare reports of spontaneous remission. Both, interleukin-2 (IL-2) and interferon have been studied as immune enhancers. The overall response rate to interferon-α is about 15%, with no long-term remissions [17]. Objective responses to IL-2 are slightly more frequent, with a small minority displaying long-term survival. Unfortunately IL-2 treatment carries significant morbidity and

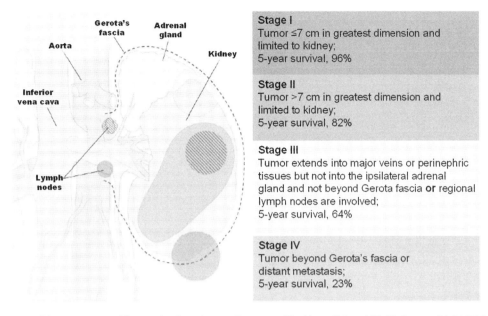

Aorta
Gerota's fascia
Adrenal gland
Kidney
Inferior vena cava
Lymph nodes

Stage I
Tumor ≤7 cm in greatest dimension and limited to kidney; 5-year survival, 96%

Stage II
Tumor >7 cm in greatest dimension and limited to kidney; 5-year survival, 82%

Stage III
Tumor extends into major veins or perinephric tissues but not into the ipsilateral adrenal gland and not beyond Gerota fascia **or** regional lymph nodes are involved; 5-year survival, 64%

Stage IV
Tumor beyond Gerota's fascia or distant metastasis; 5-year survival, 23%

Figure 28.2 Staging and five-year survival for renal cell carcinoma. Figure modified from Cohen, H.T., McGovern, F.J. (2005) Survival statistics. *N. Engl. J. Med.*, **353**, 2477–2490. Modified with permission from The NCCN Clinical Practice Guidelines in Oncology for Kidney Cancer V.2.2012. For a color version of this figure, see the color plate section.

even mortality from a capillary leak syndrome and often requires intensive care unit support for its safe administration.

Molecular-Targeted Treatment

Molecular-targeted therapies have now become central to the management of metastatic disease. Drugs such as sorafenib and sunitinib are tyrosine kinase inhibitors (TKIs), others such as everolimus are mTOR inhibitors, and the third category of VEGF-pathway inhibitors include bevacizumab. Each of these agents has shown superiority to IL-2 in randomized trials. Toxicity is less

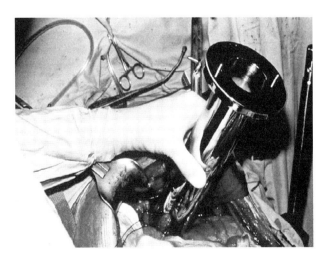

Figure 28.3 Intraoperative radiation therapy. In this image the electron cone is being aligned with the right renal bed.

than for the aggressive immunotherapies, and primarily consists of a hand–foot syndrome, nausea, and hypertension in the first-line TKIs. Trials now are geared to optimizing the dose, combination, and sequence of drugs and to exploring them in an adjuvant setting.

Radiation for metastases

Fully one-third of patients with metastatic disease present with just a solitary site of disease beyond the kidney. The three-year survival is substantially better for these patients than for those with multiple lesions.

Treatment of the solitary metastatic site has been evaluated in patients with both synchronous and metachronous solitary metastasis. Those with synchronous lesions (present at the time the primary tumor was diagnosed) fared worse than those who had a subsequent metastasis after effective management of the primary [18, 19]. Select series show that between one-third and one-half of these patients can, if their metastasis is aggressively treated, live long lives. A long disease-free interval between nephrectomy and first metastasis is prognostically very important.

Bone metastases are a common feature of metastatic RCC. They are often destructive and should be treated with complex orthopedic surgical procedures if possible and appropriate [20]. Postoperative radiation therapy should be considered in selected cases. If surgery is not possible, then higher doses of radiation should be given than in a standard palliative case. Multiple retrospective series have demonstrated that higher doses of radiation

(>50 Gy) are necessary for long-term control of bone metastases, and this is necessary in a disease that may run a protracted course. For simple palliation of pain, however, lower doses are effective. Nguyen *et al.* have shown that excellent pain relief from spinal metastases may come from stereotactic radiation therapy with either single doses of 24 Gy, 27 Gy in three fractions, or 30 Gy in five fractions. It is unclear whether this is superior to standard external beam radiation therapy [21].

The prognosis of those patients with brain metastases, particularly when multiple, is very poor despite whole-brain radiation. These patients frequently die a miserable neurologic death. Surgical resection is preferred where possible, or alternatively stereotactic radiosurgery [22]. Radiosurgery alone or in combination with whole-brain radiation therapy has been evaluated in many retrospective reports, and local tumor control rates of over 90% are routinely reported [23–26]. In a large series of over 500 treated lesions, Kano *et al.* reported that 92% of patients obtained control of the treated metastases until death (median survival 8.2 months), and 70% showed neurologic improvement or stability [27]. Multiple studies have reported that the addition of whole-brain radiation to radiosurgery improved local control and decreased distant brain failure, though there does not appear to be a survival benefit [24,28]. Recent reports have suggested that brain metastases may be irradiated at the same time as sunitinib, with no additional toxicity [29].

Few data currently exist relating to the response of soft tissues metastases to radiation, although it is well recognized to have a role in palliating symptoms of pain and bleeding in patients with massive RCC. Zelefsky *et al.* showed that SRS may have an important role in extracranial metastases generally, and demonstrated substantially better lesion control for high single doses (>24 Gy) than for lower single doses (<24 Gy) or for hypofractionated courses [30].

Surgery

Surgery for RCC cranial metastases is favored in younger patients with easily resectable tumors who have a higher performance status at presentation. The benefit of surgery in this setting includes quick neurological symptom relief, the ability to confirm pathology, and possibly longer-term control of metastatic disease.

Cancers of the Ureter and Renal Pelvis

Approximately 3000 cases of upper-urinary tract urothelial carcinoma (UC, formerly transitional cell carcinoma) are diagnosed annually in the US. Although the incidence has remained generally constant over the years, there is a more recent stage migration towards earlier tumors

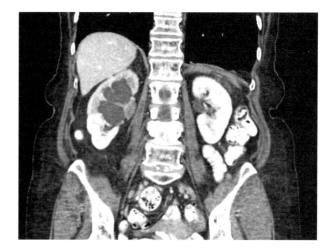

Figure 28.4 Urothelial carcinoma of the right renal pelvis. The renal calyces are expanded behind a solid tumor.

[31]. Patients who have primary UCs of the renal pelvis and/or ureter have a 20–40% incidence of either synchronous or metachronous bladder cancer. Conversely, those patients with bladder cancer have a 1–4% incidence of synchronous or metachronous upper-urinary tract UC [32,33].

Primary tumors of the upper tract occur twice as frequently in the renal pelvis as in the ureter (Figure 28.4). They occur more commonly in men, and the peak age for diagnosis is the seventh and eighth decades of life [34].

Risk factors for UC of the upper tract are the same as for all urothelial cancers: (i) chemical exposure (e.g., aniline dyes, analgesics, smoking). (ii) chronic irritation from urinary catheters or possibly stents; and (iii) geography, for example living in Taiwan or suffering from a Balkan nephropathy are associated with a higher incidence for unknown reasons.

Up to 90% of patients present with gross hematuria, and this may be accompanied by flank pain if the tumor or blood clots cause obstruction of the upper urinary tract. Hydronephrosis may also be found on work-up, or incidentally on an abdominal scan. Urinary cytology is particularly useful for high-grade tumors, with a sensitivity as high as 70%. Diagnosis is suggested by computed tomography (CT) or magnetic resonance (MR) urography, but tissue samples must obtained by cystoscopy with retrograde evaluation of the upper tracts and biopsy of visualized lesions [35, 36].

Complete staging includes further evaluation of the abdomen and pelvis and a chest CT to assess for retroperitoneal lymph node, hepatic, or pulmonary metastases. The current American Joint Committee on Cancer TNM staging for tumors of the upper urinary tract is a pathologic system that relies on the extent of invasion by the primary tumor and by microscopic evaluation of the regional lymph nodes [37].

Primary Therapy

Surgery

The standard surgical treatment for patients with transitional cell cancer of the upper urinary tract, regardless of grade or stage, is radical nephroureterectomy. The kidney is removed *in toto* along with the surrounding perirenal fat contained within Gerota's fascia and *en-bloc* removal of the ureter down to, and including, the portion of ureter within the urinary bladder [38]. A retroperitoneal lymph node dissection along the ipsilateral great vessel (the vena cava or the aorta) is performed for more complete surgical staging, especially for higher-grade and invasive cancers.

The UC is recognized to have the capacity to seed the abdomen or wound if spilled, and this has led to concern among some surgeons about the laparoscopic approach. There are, however, few reports of trocar site implantation in the literature [39].

When radical nephrectomy would result in severe renal insufficiency requiring dialysis other surgical therapies may be considered. Small tumors of the ureter, particularly low-grade tumors, may be ablated by fulguration or resection through the ureteroscope, although the success of focal resection is limited by the multicentric nature of these tumors and the common concurrent existence of carcinoma *in situ* (CIS) [40].

The success of surgery depends on the pathologic stage of the disease at the time of resection. Tumors lower in the urinary tract have a better prognosis when matched by stage with tumors higher in the ureter and pelvis [41]. Long-term results suggest five-year actuarial disease-specific survival rates close to 100% for non-invasive tumors (Ta and Tis), >90% for pT1, >70% for pT2, and approximately 40% for pT3. Long-term survival is rare for patients with T4 tumors.

Locally Advanced Cancer: Combined Modality Therapy

Despite the availability of nephroureterectomy, cure rates for patients with T3, T4, and node-positive disease are low. Whether these low survival rates can be improved by adjuvant therapy depends on the pattern of failure and the efficacy of the available treatment. Metastatic relapse appears to predominate over local relapse, and systemic cisplatin-based chemotherapy has been used, extrapolating from the experience with locally advanced bladder cancer. The true rate of locoregional failure is, however, unknown because many of the published series are old and employed pre-CT methods of intra-abdominal evaluation. The available data suggest an overall locoregional

failure of between 2% and 27%, although these figures may be an underestimate [42–44]. Cozad *et al.* reported local failure rates of 50% in stage T3 disease, rising to 60% if the tumors were high grade [45]. Brookland and Richter have reported locoregional recurrence in 45% and 62% of cases, respectively [46]. Most series report a close association between local failure and distant metastasis, although whether the association is causal or simply synchronous cannot be determined from the small numbers in the series.

Radiation has been employed as an adjuvant therapy, with mixed results having been reported in the literature. Several small Phase II studies have suggested a local control and perhaps survival advantage for adjuvant radiation [47–51]. One study reported no benefit, although the treated population was diluted with 30% early-stage patients. Another study showed no advantage for radiation, but the radiation doses given were inadequate. In others, chemotherapy was given in addition. It is therefore difficult to determine the true benefit of adjuvant radiation, if any. In a recent retrospective report from Chen *et al.* a survival advantage was seen in 67 of 133 patients receiving postoperative radiation with a median dose of 50 Gy to the tumor bed [52].

At the MGH a more aggressive approach has been taken during the past 20 years in which patients with high-risk disease were treated first with adjuvant radiation alone, and then more recently with concomitant radiation-sensitizing chemotherapy and, if tolerable, further combination chemotherapy [47]. Although the series of 31 patients is non-randomized and small, local failure was observed to be lower if chemotherapy was combined with radiation (22% versus 45%) and the survival rate at five years higher (67% versus 27%). Kwak *et al.*, in a series of 43 non-randomized patients, also suggested that cisplatin-based adjuvant chemotherapy may reduce the rate of relapse and death from disease at five years [48]. The small size of these two series, and the biases inherent in this type of retrospective review, make it difficult to draw conclusions from these data.

At present, very little published data exist to guide physicians managing patients with a local relapse following nephroureterectomy. If the relapse is bulky and metastases present elsewhere, then palliation with chemotherapy would be the most appropriate course. When the relapse appears isolated and the patient relatively vigorous, consideration can be given to an aggressive approach that holds out the chance for cure. The first step would be to downsize and perhaps improve the resectability of the recurrence using external radiation to a modest preoperative dose of 30–45 Gy, along with sensitizing chemotherapy. An attempt could then be made at resection or debulking and, if the technology were available, intraoperative radiation could then be given directly onto the tumor bed or onto an unresectable mass with the bowel and other critical organs displaced out of the field. Such an approach allows the delivery of high doses of radiation to the target without the risk of bowel injury that is present when managing such disease using external radiation treatment alone. This is a paradigm that has been used with considerable success for retroperitoneal sarcomas and locally advanced rectal cancer. Such cases are unusual and require individualized treatment that follows basic oncologic principles developed for other sites in the body. Multiple modalities are usually required, and a strong case can be made for these patients to be managed in a multidisciplinary genitourinary oncology clinic. The role of adjuvant chemotherapy in reducing relapse has not been explored in randomized fashion in this uncommon disease.

The biology of upper-tract UC is considered to be identical to that of bladder UC. Consequently, the chemotherapy regimens recommended for advanced or metastatic upper-tract UC are the same as for bladder cancer. Standard treatment is cisplatin-based combination therapy, such as gemcitabine and cisplatin or methotrexate, vinblastine, doxorubicin and cisplatin. As with bladder cancer, upper-tract UC is highly responsive to chemotherapy, but has a short median duration of response.

References

1 Eble, J.N., Sauter, G., Epstein, J.I., Sesterhenn, I.A. (2004) *World Health Organization Classification of Tumors: pathology and genetics of tumors of the urinary system and male genital organs.* IARC Press, Lyon, France.

2 Chow, W.H., Devesa, S.S., Warren, J.L., Fraumeni, J.F., Jr (1999) Rising incidence of renal cell cancer in the United States. *JAMA*, **281** (17), 1628–1631.

3 Pantuck, A.J., Zisman, A., Belldegrun, A.S. (2001) The changing natural history of renal cell carcinoma. *J. Urol.*, **166** (5), 1611–1623.

4 Parkin, D.M., Pisani, P., Ferlay, J. (1993) Estimates of the worldwide incidence of eighteen major cancers in 1985. Int. *J. Cancer*, **54** (4), 594–606.

5 Lai, P.P. (1992) Kidney, renal, pelvis and ureter, in *Principles and Practice of Radiation Oncology*, 2nd edition (eds C.A. Perez, L.W. Brady), J.B. Lippincott, Philadelphia, pp. 1025–1035.

6 Motzer, R.J., Bander, N.H., Nanus, D.M. (1996) Renal-cell carcinoma. N. Engl. *J. Med.*, **335** (12), 865–875.

7 Sokoloff, M.H., de Kernion, J.B., Figlin, R.A., Belldegrun, A. (1996) Current management of renal cell carcinoma. *CA Cancer J. Clin.*, **46** (5), 284–302.

8 Robson, C.J. (1963) Radical nephrectomy for renal cell carcinoma. *J. Urol.*, **89**, 37–42.

9 Harmon, J., Parulkar, B., Doble, A. (2004) Critical assessment of cancer recurrence following renal cryoablation: a multi-center review. *J. Urol.*, (Suppl. 4), 469; abstract 1775.

10 Shingleton, B., Sewell, P. (2004) Percutaneous renal tumor cryoablation: results in the first 90 patients. *J. Urol.*, (Suppl. 4), 463; abstract 1751.

11 Malkin, R.B. (1975) Regression of renal carcinoma following radiation therapy. *J. Urol.*, **114** (5), 782–783.

12 Tunio, M.A., Hashmi, A., Rafi, M. (2010) Need for a new trial to evaluate postoperative radiotherapy in renal cell carcinoma: a meta-analysis of randomized controlled trials. *Ann. Oncol.*, **21** (9), 1839–1845.

13 Kjaer, M., Iversen, P., Hvidt, V., *et al.* (1987) A randomized trial of postoperative radiotherapy versus observation in stage II and III renal adenocarcinoma. A study by the Copenhagen Renal Cancer Study Group. Scand. *J. Urol. Nephrol.*, **21** (4), 285–289.

14 Finney, R. (1973) The value of radiotherapy in the treatment of hypernephroma – a clinical trial. *Br. J. Urol.*, **45** (3), 258–269.

15 Siva, S., Pham, D., Gill, S., Corcoran, N.M., Foroudi, F. (2012) A systematic review of stereotactic radiotherapy ablation for primary renal cell carcinoma. *Br. J. Urol. Int.*, **110**, E737–E743

16 Paly, J.J., Hallemeier, C.L., Biggs, P.J., *et al.* (2014) Outcomes in a multi-institutional cohort of patients treated with intraoperative radiation therapy for advanced or recurrent renal cell carcinoma. *Int. J. Radiat. Oncol. Biol. Phys.*, **88** (3), 618–623

17 Motzer, R.J., Bacik, J., Murphy, B.A., Russo, P., Mazumdar, M. (2002) Interferon-alfa as a comparative treatment for clinical trials of new therapies against advanced renal cell carcinoma. *J. Clin. Oncol.*, **20** (1), 289–296.

18 O'Dea, M.J., Zincke, H., Utz, D.C., Bernatz, P.E. (1978) The treatment of renal cell carcinoma with solitary metastasis. *J. Urol.*, **120** (5), 540–542.

19 Kjaer, M. (1987) The treatment and prognosis of patients with renal adenocarcinoma with solitary metastasis. 10 year survival results. *Int. J. Radiat. Oncol. Biol. Phys.*, **13** (4), 619–621.

20 Althausen, P., Althausen, A., Jennings, L.C., Mankin, H.J. (1997) Prognostic factors and surgical treatment of osseous metastases secondary to renal cell carcinoma. *Cancer*, **80** (6), 1103–1109.

21 Nguyen, Q.N., Shiu, A.S., Rhines, L.D., *et al.* (2010) Management of spinal metastases from renal cell carcinoma using stereotactic body radiotherapy. *Int. J. Radiat. Oncol. Biol. Phys.*, **76** (4), 1185–1192.

22 Wronski, M., Arbit, E., Russo, P., Galicich, J.H. (1996) Surgical resection of brain metastases from renal cell

carcinoma in 50 patients. *Urology*, **47** (2), 187–193.

23 Sheehan, J.P., Sun, M.H., Kondziolka, D., Flickinger, J., Lunsford, L.D. (2003) Radiosurgery in patients with renal cell carcinoma metastasis to the brain: long-term outcomes and prognostic factors influencing survival and local tumor control. *J. Neurosurg.*, **98** (2), 342–349.

24 Brown, P.D., Brown, C.A., Pollock, B.E., Gorman, D.A., Foote, R.L. (2002) Stereotactic radiosurgery for patients with 'radioresistant' brain metastases. *Neurosurgery*, **51** (3), 656–665; discussion 665–657.

25 Amendola, B.E., Wolf, A.L., Coy, S.R., Amendola, M., Bloch, L. (2000) Brain metastases in renal cell carcinoma: management with gamma knife radiosurgery. *Cancer J.*, **6** (6), 372–376.

26 Shuto, T., Matsunaga, S., Suenaga, J., Inomori, S., Fujino, H. (2010) Treatment strategy for metastatic brain tumors from renal cell carcinoma: selection of gamma knife surgery or craniotomy for control of growth and peritumoral edema. *J. Neurooncol.*, **98**, 169–175.

27 Kano, H., Iyer, A., Kondziolka, D., Niranjan, A., Flickinger, J.C., Lunsford, L.D. (2011) Outcome predictors of gamma knife radiosurgery for renal cell carcinoma metastases. *Neurosurgery*, **69** (6), 1232–1239.

28 Fokas, E., Henzel, M., Hamm, K., Surber, G., Kleinert, G., Engenhart-Cabillic, R. (2010) Radiotherapy for brain metastases from renal cell cancer: should whole-brain radiotherapy be added to stereotactic radiosurgery?: analysis of 88 patients. *Strahlenther. Onkol.*, **186** (4), 210–217.

29 Staehler, M., Haseke, N., Nuhn, P., *et al.* (2011) Simultaneous anti-angiogenic therapy and single-fraction radiosurgery in clinically relevant metastases from renal cell carcinoma. *Br. J. Urol. Int.*, **108** (5), 673–678.

30 Zelefsky, M.J., Greco, C., Motzer, R., *et al.* (2012) Tumor control outcomes after hypofractionated and single-dose stereotactic image-guided intensity-modulated radiotherapy for extracranial metastases from renal cell carcinoma. *Int. J. Radiat. Oncol. Biol. Phys.*, **82** (5), 1744–1748.

31 David, K.A., Mallin, K., Milowsky, M.I., Ritchey, J., Carroll, P.R., Nanus, D.M. (2009) Surveillance of urothelial carcinoma: stage and grade migration, 1993–2005 and survival trends, 1993–2000. *Cancer*, **115** (7), 1435–1447.

32 Oldbring, J., Glifberg, I., Mikulowski, P., Hellsten, S. (1989) Carcinoma of the renal pelvis and ureter following bladder carcinoma: frequency, risk factors and clinicopathological findings. *J. Urol.*, **141** (6), 1311–1313.

33 Rabbani, F., Perrotti, M., Russo, P., Herr, H.W. (2001) Upper-tract tumors after an initial diagnosis of bladder cancer: argument for long-term surveillance. *J. Clin. Oncol.*, **19** (1), 94–100.

34 Chahal, R., Taylor, K., Eardley, I., Lloyd, S.N., Spencer, J.A. (2005) Patients at high risk for upper tract urothelial cancer: evaluation of hydronephrosis using high resolution magnetic resonance urography. *J. Urol.*, **174** (2), 478–482.

35 Walsh, I.K., Keane, P.F., Ishak, L.M., Flessland, K.A. (2001) The BTA stat test: a tumor marker for the detection of upper tract transitional cell carcinoma. *Urology*, **58** (4), 532–535.

36 Skacel, M., Fahmy, M., Brainard, J.A., *et al.* (2003) Multitarget fluorescence in situ hybridization assay detects transitional cell carcinoma in the majority of patients with bladder cancer and atypical or negative urine cytology. *J. Urol.*, **169** (6), 2101–2105.

37 Amin, M.B. (ed) American Joint Committee on Cancer (2017) *Cancer Staging Manual*, 8th edition, Springer, New York.

38 Heney, N.M., Nocks, B.N. (1982) The influence of perinephric fat involvement on survival in patients with renal cell carcinoma extending into the inferior vena cava. *J. Urol.*, **128** (1), 18–20.

39 Ong, A.M., Bhayani, S.B., Pavlovich, C.P. (2003) Trocar site recurrence after laparoscopic nephroureterectomy. *J. Urol.*, **170** (4 Pt 1), 1301.

40 Okubo, K., Ichioka, K., Terada, N., Matsuta, Y., Yoshimura, K., Arai, Y. (2001) Intrarenal bacillus Calmette–Guerin therapy for carcinoma in situ of the upper urinary tract: long-term follow-up and natural course in cases of failure. *Br. J. Urol. Int.*, **88** (4), 343–347.

41 van der Poel, H.G., Antonini, N., van Tinteren, H., Horenblas, S. (2005) Upper urinary tract cancer: location is correlated with prognosis. *Eur. Urol.*, **48** (3), 438–444.

42 Mufti, G.R., Gove, J.R., Badenoch, D.F., *et al.* (1989) Transitional cell carcinoma of the renal pelvis and ureter. *Br. J. Urol.*, **63** (2), 135–140.

43 Das, A.K., Carson, C.C., Bolick, D., Paulson, D.F. (1990) Primary carcinoma of the upper urinary tract. Effect of primary and secondary therapy on survival. *Cancer*, **66** (9), 1919–1923.

44 Vahlensieck, W., Jr, Sommerkamp, H. (1989) Therapy and prognosis of carcinoma of the renal pelvis. *Eur. Urol.*, **16** (4), 286–290.

45 Cozad, S.C., Smalley, S.R., Austenfeld, M., Noble, M., Jennings, S., Raymond, R. (1995) Transitional cell carcinoma of the renal pelvis or ureter: patterns of failure. *Urology*, **46** (6), 796–800.

46 Brookland, R.K., Richter, M.P. (1985) The postoperative irradiation of transitional cell carcinoma of the renal pelvis and ureter. *J. Urol.*, **133** (6), 952–955.

47 Czito, B., Zietman, A., Kaufman, D., Skowronski, U., Shipley, W. (2004) Adjuvant radiotherapy with and

without concurrent chemotherapy for locally advanced transitional cell carcinoma of the renal pelvis and ureter. *J. Urol.*, **172** (4 Pt 1), 1271–1275.

48 Kwak, C., Lee, S.E., Jeong, I.G., Ku, J.H. (2006) Adjuvant systemic chemotherapy in the treatment of patients with invasive transitional cell carcinoma of the upper urinary tract. *Urology*, **68** (1), 53–57.

49 Ozsahin, M., Zouhair, A., Villa, S., *et al.* (1999) Prognostic factors in urothelial renal pelvis and ureter tumours: a multicentre Rare Cancer Network study. *Eur. J. Cancer*, **35** (5), 738–743.

50 Maulard-Durdux, C., Dufour, B., Hennequin, C., *et al.* (1996) Postoperative radiation therapy in 26 patients

with invasive transitional cell carcinoma of the upper urinary tract: no impact on survival? *J. Urol.*, **155** (1), 115–117.

51 Catton, C.N., Warde, P., Gospodarowicz, M.K., *et al.* (1996) Transitional cell carcinoma of the renal pelvis and ureter: Outcome and patterns of relapse in patients treated with postoperative radiation. *Urol. Oncol.*, **2** (6), 171–176.

52 Chen, B., Zeng, Z.C., Wang, G.M., *et al.* (2011) Radiotherapy may improve overall survival of patients with T3/T4 transitional cell carcinoma of the renal pelvis or ureter and delay bladder tumour relapse. *BMC Cancer*, **11**, 297.

29

Testicular Cancer

Jonathan J. Paly and Jason A. Efstathiou

Background

Testicular cancer is the most common solid malignancy affecting men from the ages of 15 to 44 years. Approximately 8850 and >52 000 cases are diagnosed per year in the United States and globally, respectively, and the adjusted incidence is rising [1–4]. This disease, however, remains one of the most curable malignancies, with an estimated 96.8% five-year disease-specific survival (DSS) for those diagnosed between 2006 and 2012 in the US [2]. Though it constitutes 1% of all male cancers, testicular cancer produces only 0.1% of all cancer deaths in men due to treatment advances in recent years [4].

Approximately 97% of testis cancers are germ cell tumors (GCTs), while the remaining cases primarily consist of sex cord-stromal tumors and lymphomas. GCTs are broadly divided into pure seminomas and non-seminomatous GCTs (NSGCTs). Sex cord-stromal tumors originate in the supporting tissues and include Sertoli, Leydig, and granulosa cell tumors. Lymphomas overwhelmingly consist of non-Hodgkin's diffuse large B-cell lymphoma (DLBCL).

Risk factors for GCT testis cancer include cryptorchidism, Klinefelter's syndrome, HIV-positive status, maternal exposure to estrogen, advanced maternal age, polyvinyl chloride exposure, contralateral testicular tumors, family history of testis cancer, gonadal dysgenesis, and testicular microlithiasis [5]. There do not appear to be any risk factors for DLBCL aside from a family history of non-Hodgkin's lymphoma [6]. There are no known risk factors for sex cord-stromal cell tumors [7].

Patients with testis cancer generally present with a painless, firm mass in their scrotum, and are diagnosed by ultrasound. Prior to surgery, all patients with a probable diagnosis of testicular cancer should have an H&P performed, chemistry and serum tumor markers (STM) drawn, and a discussion about sperm banking. H&P,

testicular ultrasound [8]. Radical inguinal orchiectomy rather than testicular biopsy is the standard of care for testicular cancers in all cases, with the exception of diagnosis of a second metachronous testicular cancer in a patient who has already undergone orchiectomy [9]. Pathologic examination of the specimen can then identify histological classification. Following orchiectomy, patients are referred for adjuvant treatment or followed on surveillance protocols based on their histologic classification and stage. Although alpha-fetoprotein (AFP), the beta-subunit of human chorionic gonadotropin (beta-hCG), and lactate dehydrogenase (LDH) must be examined, they alone cannot diagnose disease because less than 60% of GCTs will exhibit elevated tumor markers. The American Society of Clinical Oncology (ASCO) clinical practice guidelines recommend measuring AFP and beta-hCG before orchiectomy in order to aid in diagnosis and the interpretation of post-orchiectomy results, but advises against the use of these markers to guide decisions for surgery [10]. LDH levels may be elevated in DLBCLs. In sex-cord stromal tumors, STMs such as AFP, beta-hCG and LDH will not be elevated. However, androgens or estrogens may be elevated in Leydig cell tumors, though there does not appear to be a consensus on hormone monitoring for this group [7].

Seminoma

Seminoma constitutes over 60% of GCTs, and its incidence has been increasing in Western countries during the past 40 years [3, 5, 11]. Some 85% of seminoma patients present with localized disease, and seminoma remains the most curable solid tumor with DSS rates approaching 100%. Concerns of both short- and long-term morbidity related to treatment are thus paramount to disease management decisions [12].

Clinical Radiation Oncology: Indications, Techniques, and Results, Third Edition. Edited by William Small Jr.
© 2017 John Wiley & Sons, Inc. Published 2017 by John Wiley & Sons, Inc.

Table 29.1 AJCC Clinical Staging criteria.

Stage IA/B/S	Tumor is confined to the testis*
Stage IIA	Positive nodes that are >1 cm but ≤2 cm in largest dimension
Stage IIB	Positive nodes that are >2 cm but <5 cm in largest dimension
Stage IIC	Positive nodes that are >5 cm in largest dimension
Stage III	Distant metastases, including non-regional lymph node metastases in regions such as the mediastinum and clavicular nodal chains and non-nodal metastases to regions such as the lung or bone. A positive node in combination with highly elevated STMs may indicate Stage III.

*Stage IB denotes higher pathologic tumor stage; Stage IS has elevated STMs.
Source: AJCC Cancer Staging Manual, Eighth Edition (2017), Springer, New York, Inc.

Although it remains unknown whether measuring STM concentrations improves survival or other health outcomes for seminoma patients, the ASCO recommends continuing to measure post-orchiectomy serum concentrations of beta-hCG and LDH in patients with pure seminoma and pre-orchiectomy STM elevations. However, ASCO does not recommend using post-orchiectomy STM concentrations of either beta-hCG or LDH to stage or predict prognosis of patients with positive nodes and/or metastasis [10]. Data from the Princess Margaret Hospital also suggests that STM levels do not assist in early detection of disease relapse in patients on surveillance for clinical stage I seminomas [13]. In seminomas, AFP will not be elevated, beta-hCG will be elevated in 15–20% of patients, and LDH will be elevated in 40–60% [10]. Elevated STM levels necessitate repeat testing following orchiectomy as clinical stage IS disease requires increased STMs after surgery. Additional prognostic values, such as rete testis invasion or tumor size >4 cm cannot be considered reliable clinical features for risk-adapted management [14, 15]. The most classic method for assessment and disease extent is through TNM staging using the American Joint Commission on Cancer (AJCC) TNM cancer staging system (Table 29.1). Clinical stage IA/B/S all require an absence of positive lymph nodes, defined as nodes >1 cm on their shortest axis [16]. Patients may be diagnosed as clinical stage IS if they exhibit no positive nodes but have elevated STMs before and after orchiectomy.

Management options for seminoma after orchiectomy include surveillance, adjuvant radiation, and chemotherapy. However, caution must be exercised when providing adjuvant therapy. Short-term toxicity such as gastrointestinal distress and lethargy in combination with effects on fertility and significantly increased rates of secondary malignant neoplasms (SMNs) have been reported in patients receiving adjuvant radiation therapy (ART) or adjuvant chemotherapy [12, 17]. Among 10 534 men treated with ART for seminoma, there was an overall relative risk (RR) of 2.5 for SMNs, with an average RR of 3.4 for in-field organs. This same study also found a RR for SMNs of 1.8 for testicular cancer patients treated with chemotherapy alone [18]. A publication using data from the US Surveillance, Epidemiology and End Results cancer registry found an adjusted RR of 1.43 for SMN after radiation for seminoma [19]. Others have identified a significant increase in all-cause mortality in patients treated with ART versus those managed with surveillance [20]. There are also additional concerns about the late sequela of carboplatin given the absence of long-term follow-up on these patients [12, 21].

Clinical Stage I Seminoma

Surveillance

For patients with clinical stage (CS) I disease, surveillance should be considered a preferred management option. Given the excellent salvage therapy options that exist, the late effects of adjuvant therapy may outweigh the benefits of a decreased need for salvage therapy in the 12–19% of CS I patients who will relapse [22–24]. Recent data suggest that this relapse will occur at a median of 14 months, with 92% of relapses occurring within three years [22]. The National Comprehensive Cancer Network (NCCN) suggests a surveillance computed tomography (CT) schedule with non-contrast abdominopelvic scans at 3, 6, and 12 months, every 6–12 months for year 3, and annually for years 4 and 5. STMs may be checked every 3–6 months for the first year, 6–12 months for years 2 and 3, and annually thereafter. Chest x-rays as clinically indicated may be delivered from years 1 to 5 [8]. Data from the National Cancer Data Base, which captures approximately 70% of reported new cases in the US, indicated that in 2011 the management of CS IA/B disease included post-orchiectomy surveillance for 54.0% of patients, ART for 28.8% of patients, and adjuvant chemotherapy for 16.0% [25]. At the MGH, attempts are made to risk-stratify but favor surveillance for nearly all CS I patients, with the rare exception being those who have very large tumors or extensive rete testis invasion.

Radiation

Seminoma, as opposed to non-seminoma, is an extremely radiosensitive tumor. The goal of ART in

CS I seminoma is to target the para-aortic, paracaval and retroperitoneal lymph nodes which may be harboring micrometastatic disease. The fields for CS I seminoma have evolved from large fields encompassing the supradiaphragmatic nodes and ispilateral pelvic nodes to a para-aortic strip field. Fossa *et al.* showed no inferiority when using a 'reduced' para-aortic strip field, compared to larger fields, which extends from the T10/T11 interspace to L5/S1 and is bounded laterally by the transverse processes [26]. Small renal blocks may be used [8] and it is reasonable to extend the field laterally to include the left renal hilum for left-sided tumors (Figure 29.1). Though they have not been tested in a randomized trial, modified para-aortic strip fields bounded superiorly by T11/T12 [27] or T12/L1 [28] have shown no para-aortic recurrences superior to the treatment field, suggesting that lowering the superior field borders may provide comparable disease control while sparing dose to normal tissue. A recent study that mapped nodal metastases of CS IIA/B seminoma patients has suggested that designing personalized fields based on vascular, rather than bony, landmarks may provide comparable nodal coverage while further limiting dose to normal tissue (Figure 29.2) [29]. National guidelines support this vascular-based approach to field design and have proposed a 1.2–1.9 cm expansion on the inferior vena cava (IVC) and aorta, plus set-up error and penumbra expansions, as an alternative to rectangular port fields. This field should extend from the inferior border of

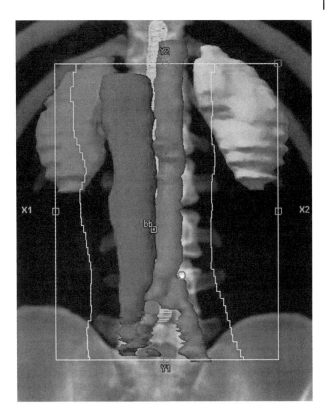

Figure 29.1 Standard para-aortic strip field. A standard para-aortic field for a CS I seminoma based on vascular anatomy. Illustration courtesy of Clair Beard, MD. For a color version of this figure, see the color plate section.

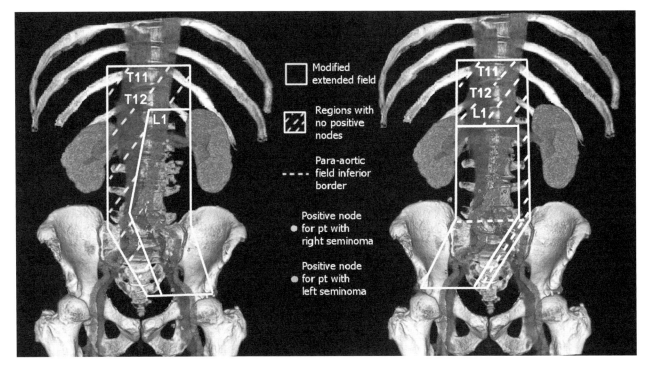

Figure 29.2 Dog-leg fields and nodal maps. The distribution of positive nodes in 90 stage IIA/B and recurrent stage I seminoma patients. Conventional and modified fields have been overlaid on the template [29]. For a color version of this figure, see the color plate section.

Table 29.2 Survival and relapse rates for Stage I seminomas.

Study/Reference	Treatment	No. of patients	Relapse-free survival	Disease-specific survival
Cummins *et al.* [36]	Surveillance	164	5-year relapse-free: 87%	98.7% at median 13.5 years follow-up
Warde *et al.* [37]	Surveillance	421	5-year relapse-free: 85.5%	99.7% at median 9.2 years follow-up
Kollmannsberger *et al.* [22]	Surveillance	1344	Total relapse-free: 87% at median 4.3 years follow-up	100% at median 4.3 years follow-up
TE10 [35]	Para-aortic field or a dog-leg field	478	5-year relapse-free rates were 96.1% in the para-aortic strip arm and 96.2% in the dogleg arm	1 death in the para-aortic arm at median 12.0 years follow-up
TE18 [35]	30 Gy in 15 fx or 20 Gy in 10 fx	1094	5-year relapse-free rates were 95.1% in the 30-Gy arm and 96.8% in the 20-Gy arm	2 deaths in 30-Gy arm and 1 death in 20-Gy arm at median 7 years follow-up
TE19 [35]	Radiation therapy or carboplatin	1477	5-year relapse-free rates were 96.0% for RT arm and 94.7% for the carboplatin arm	1 death in the radiation arm at median 6.4 years follow-up

RT, radiotherapy.

T-11 to the inferior border of L-5 [8]. In addition, it should be noted that pelvic, external iliac and inguinal nodes are considered regional when a patient received prior scrotal or inguinal surgery [16]. Thus, for patients with previous pelvic surgery, a higher rate of pelvic recurrences can be expected [30]. NCCN guidelines and the present authors' practice patterns are to recommend adjuvant therapy in the form of radiation for CS IS patients [8]. The tendency is to encourage surveillance for all CS I patients though adjuvant therapy may be considered for a CS I patient with a large primary tumor (>4 cm), given that several studies have identified a link between relapse and tumor size [15, 31, 32]. Debate persists on whether to risk-adapt treatment for CS I patients and offer radiotherapy based on tumor size and rete testis invasion, given the failure to validate the original study [14, 15].

For all CS I patients, the NCCN and European testicular cancer group recommend a dose of 20 Gy, delivered in 2-Gy fractions five times per week for two weeks and beginning once orchiectomy wound has healed [8, 23]. Some physicians choose to treat to a dose of 25.5 Gy in 17 fractions at 1.5 Gy per fraction, as this achieves a similar radiobiological effect and given that late effects may be related to fraction size. Doses less than 20 Gy are not recommended [33]. Three dimensional conformal radiation therapy rather than intensity modulated radiation therapy is utilized. All patients receiving ART should be simulated and treated with the penis and remaining testicle in clamshell shielding for protection in order to prevent effects on fertility due to dose to the contralateral testis. Care providers should discuss the issue of potential loss of fertility due to treatment or disease [34]. Semen analysis with sperm banking prior to treatment is strongly recommended. Antiemetic medications should be provided at the first sign of nausea and may be used prophylactically 1-2 hours before daily treatment.

Between 3% and 5% of patients treated with adjuvant therapy for CS I disease will relapse, usually in the pelvis for those receiving ART [35]. Survival and recurrence data for different management strategies are shown in Table 29.2 and Figure 29.3.

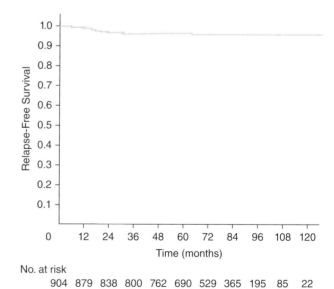

No. at risk

904 879 838 800 762 690 529 365 195 85 22

Figure 29.3 Relapse-free survival (Kaplan-Meier) in 904 patients treated with ART for stage I disease. *Source:* Oliver *et al.* 2011 [38]. Reproduced with permission of the American Society of Clinical Oncology.

Clinical Stage I Seminoma: Surveillance After Orchiectomy

	Year (at month intervals)				
	1	2	3	4	5
H&P[1,2]	Every 3–6 mo	Every 6–12 mo	Every 6–12 mo	Annually	Annually
Abdominal ± Pelvic CT[3]	At 3, 6, and 12 mo	Every 6–12 mo	Every 6–12 mo	Every 12–24 mo	
Chest x-ray	As clinically indicated, consider chest CT with contrast in symptomatic patients.				

Clinical Stage I Seminoma: Surveillance After Adjuvant Treatment (Chemotherapy or Radiation)

	Year (at month intervals)				
	1	2	3	4	5
H&P[1,2]	Every 6–12 mo	Every 6–12 mo	Annually	Annually	Annually
Abdominal ± Pelvic CT[3]	Annually	Annually	Annually	------	
Chest x-ray	As clinically indicated, consider chest CT with contrast in symptomatic patients.				

Clinical Stage IIA and Non-Bulky IIB Seminoma: Surveillance after Radiotherapy or Post-Chemotherapy[4]

	Year (at month intervals)				
	1	2	3	4	5
H&P[1,2]	Every 3 mo	Every 6 mo	Every 6 mo	Every 6 mo	Every 6 mo
Abdominal ± Pelvic CT[5]	At 3 mo, then at 6–12 mo	Annually	Annually	As clinically indicated	
Chest x-ray[6]	Every 6 mo	Every 6 mo	------		

[1]Serum tumor markers are optional.
[2]Testicular ultrasound for any equivocal exam.
[3]Without contrast.
[4]Assuming no residual mass or residual mass <3 cm and normal tumor markers.
[5]With contrast.
[6]Chest x-ray may be used for routine follow-up but chest CT with contrast is preferred in the presence of thoracic symptoms.

Figure 29.4 Follow-up guidelines for seminomas. Follow-up imaging and serum tumor marker recommendations for CS I and IIA/B patients. Adapted and reproduced with permission from The NCCN Clinical Practice Guidelines in Oncology for Testicular Cancer V.2.2017 [8].

Chemotherapy

CS I patients may also receive single-agent carboplatin for one to two cycles. This has been shown to produce non-inferior DFS when compared to ART [38], though there are concerns of late toxicity with carboplatin [12, 21]. Following adjuvant therapy, CT imaging and STM collection should be followed as per Figure 29.4 [8].

CS II seminoma

For patients who present with node-positive seminoma or relapse while on surveillance for CS I disease, ongoing surveillance is no longer an option. Those with CS IIA-B

disease (see Table 29.1) may be managed with radiation or chemotherapy.

Radiation

Radiation for CS IIA-B disease should be provided with a 'dog-leg' (or 'hockey-stick') extended field that covers the para-aortic nodes as well as ipsilateral iliac nodes. The dog-leg field mimics the para-aortic strip field above L5/S1 but extends to the cranial border of the ipsilateral acetabulum inferiorly. The lateral border of the inferior portion of the field extends from the L5 ipsilateral transverse process to the most lateral and superior aspect of the ipsilateral acetabulum. The field border then travels medially to the level of the obturator foramen, where it is drawn diagonally to the tip of the L5 contralateral transverse process (see Figure 29.2) [39].

Given the previously described acute and late sequela of treatment, a concerted effort has been made to reduce the burden of radiotherapy through the use of personalized or decreased radiation fields. Several studies have suggested that there may be a significant relationship between radiation field size and the prevalence of late effects [18, 40].

As an alternative to standard dog-leg radiation, a patient may be treated with a more personalized field based on vascular anatomy. A proposed field suggests contouring the arterial vasculature from 1.5 cm above the renal artery to the acetabulum. An expansion of 2.1 cm anterior and 2.5 cm lateral to the arterial vasculature will produce a clinical target volume (CTV) that may better approximate the region containing micrometastatic disease while limiting dose to normal tissue (see Figure 29.2). As this form of therapy is not yet validated, patients should be treated on protocol and possibly subject to increased follow-up imaging. It is notable to point out, however, the greater similarity between this modified vascular field and a retroperitoneal lymph node dissection (RPLND) used for NSGCTs (see Figure 29.5) when compared to current radiation fields [29]. National guideline recommendations now prefer a vascular-based field rather than one based on bony anatomy and recommend using an expansion of 1.2–1.9 cm around the IVC and aorta from the inferior aspect of T-11 to the superior aspect of the acetabulum [8]. Treatment planners must then add appropriate expansions to account for set-up error, patient motion, and beam penumbra to produce a planning target volume (PTV). At the present authors'

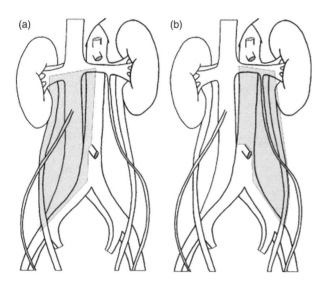

Figure 29.5 Retroperitoneal lymph node dissection (RPLND). Lymph node dissection templates for right (a) and left (b) are shown. *Source:* Jacobson and Foster 2007 [48]. Reproduced with permission of Elsevier.

institution this additional expansion is 5 mm for set-up variability and ~7 mm to account for beam penumbra.

Regardless of treatment field shape, at the MGH 20 Gy is prescribed to the dog-leg field, or PTV, with an additional 10 Gy boost to all nodal volumes in CS IIA patients (nodes are >1 cm but ≤2 cm in the largest dimension), or 16 Gy in CS IIB patients (nodes are >2 cm but <5 cm in the greatest dimension). Boost CTV includes the involved node(s) plus a 7–8 mm expansion, to which additional expansion is added for a PTV. All doses are delivered in 2.0-Gy daily fractions [41, 42]. At MGH, this is generally delivered at >6 MV on a linear accelerator, though the group has, on protocol, treated select patients with proton beam therapy in conjunction with a reduced CTV in order to reduce the prevalence of late effects in this young group of men [43]. As with CS I patients, CS IIA/B patients receiving radiation are simulated and treated with the use of scrotal clamshell shielding to reduce the risk of further fertility loss due to dose to the contralateral testis.

Relapse after dog-leg radiotherapy for CS II disease occurs in 5–11% of patients with CS IIB disease generally exhibiting a higher likelihood of recurrence [24, 39, 44]. Follow-up abdominal CT imaging and STMs should be carried out as shown in Figure 29.4.

Chemotherapy

CS IIA/B seminomas can alternatively be managed using chemotherapy. Generally, this approach is considered for CS IIB patients or used as salvage therapy for those who have relapsed after ART or who present with CS IIC or III disease. At MGH, chemotherapy is not generally offered for CS IIA patients unless the patient has recurred after prior ART. Four cycles of cisplatin and etoposide or three cycles of cisplatin, etoposide, and bleomycin (BEP) have been shown to produce good results, though these treatments may not avoid many of the late sequelae of radiotherapy [45]. Similarly, patients with CS IIC or CS III may be treated with four cycles of cisplatin and etoposide (EP) or three cycles of BEP if they contain only lymphovascular or pulmonary metastases. Those CS III patients with higher-risk disease should be managed with four cycles of BEP, rather than three. This treatment appears quite effective in preventing relapse [46]. The toxicity of EP and BEP treatments is primarily hematologic. Garcia-del-Muro *et al.* employed three cycles of BEP or four cycles of EP in the treatment of 72 patients with CS IIA/B seminoma and reported grade 3 or 4 toxicity from granulocytopenia in 13%, and febrile neutropenia in 11%. Almost half of the patients reported vomiting, though pulmonary toxicity was rare [45]. Between 60% and 80% of patients will have residual masses after chemotherapy for node-positive disease. Positron emission tomography (PET) has proved effective in determining which of these patients harbor active disease in their residual mass. For those masses exhibiting uptake on PET, surgical resection of the mass is recommended. If the resected mass is found to contain active disease, four cycles of VeIP (vinblastine, mesna, ifosamide, cisplatin) or TIP (paclitaxel, ifosfamide, mesna, cisplatin) are warranted. Irradiation of residual masses is discouraged [23, 47].

Non-Seminatomous Tumors

Non-seminatomous germ cell tumors (NSGCTs) constitute 40% of GCTs and are less radiosensitive than seminomas. They are managed by surveillance, chemotherapy, and RPLND. Survival endpoints for NSGCTs are similar to those for seminomas if salvage treatment options are exercised appropriately. Levels of AFP will be elevated in 10–60% of patients, of beta-hCG in 10–40%, and of LDH in 40–60%. The ASCO panel recommends using STMs after orchiectomy to stratify risk and help aid in treatment decisions [10].

Surveillance

For CS I non-seminomas, surveillance is an appropriate option after orchiectomy. History & Physical, STMs, and chest x-radiography should be included frequently, and abdominal CT provided at regular intervals. Approximately one-fourth of patients will relapse, though their DSS may not differ from those receiving other adjuvant therapy if they are monitored closely and are provided salvage RPLND, chemotherapy, or both [8].

RPLND

Alternatively, CS I non-seminomas can receive adjuvant RPLND in order to reduce the risk of relapse [8]. Those with positive nodes may then be managed by surveillance or adjuvant chemotherapy, which may consist of two cycles of etoposide/cisplatin or BEP. CS IS patients, who exhibit persistent elevated STMs after orchiectomy should be treated as CS II patients and managed with chemotherapy. CS II non-seminomas may be managed by either RPLND or primary chemotherapy. Second-line therapy for non-seminomas should be similar to that for seminomas. As is the case with recurrent seminoma, irradiation of residual masses is discouraged (Figure 29.5).

Sex Cord-Stromal Cell Tumors

Benign sex cord-stromal cell tumors, which represent the majority of these tumors, can be adequately controlled by orchiectomy [7, 49], though approximately 10% will be malignant [49]. Malignant sex cord-stromal cell tumors do not appear to respond to radiation, and thus this treatment must be reserved only for palliation of metastatic disease [50]. Chemotherapy regimens generally appear to be ineffective against this group of tumors, though the use of RPLND and metastasectomy may offer a benefit in some patients [49].

Lymphoma of Testis

Primary lymphoma of the testis generally occurs in men aged 60 years or more, and accounts for approximately 1–2% of all diagnoses of non-Hodgkin lymphoma. It is the most common testicular malignancy in elder men. The most common variant of this disease is DLBCL [51]. Most DLBCL patients present with early-stage disease, the median age of diagnosis being in the late 60s. LDH levels may be elevated. As with other testicular cancers, radical inguinal orchiectomy is the standard of care. Because of the high instance of bilateral disease, prophylactic scrotal radiotherapy to the contralateral testis has been shown to reduce the risk of relapse [52]. There is a high risk of central nervous system (CNS) relapse in these patients, and the administration of intrathecal methotrexate may afford protection from CNS recurrence [53]. Modern treatment techniques call for the administration of cyclophosphamide, doxorubicin, vincristine, and prednisone (CHOP) followed by radiotherapy to the contralateral testis. The addition of rituximab to CHOP (R-CHOP) has shown a benefit in survival, but a longer follow-up after this course is needed [54].

After completing induction chemo/immunotherapy and assessment of treatment response, prophylactic irradiation to the contralateral testis should be provided to all patients with a dose of 25–30 Gy. Patients with CS II disease should also receive radiotherapy with fields covering the entire involved lymph node region and, potentially, the adjacent lymph node regions. Those patients with more extensive nodal involvement should receive an inverted Y-field targeting the para-aortic lymph node region and bilateral pelvic lymph nodes. CS II patients displaying a complete response to induction therapy after R-CHOP should receive additional radiotherapy at 30–35 Gy to regional lymph nodes (and potentially to adjacent lymph node regions), while those displaying a less than complete response should receive 35–45 Gy at the conclusion of the chemoimmunotherapy program [54].

CS I/II DLBCL patients who received a course of intrathecal methotrexate, R-CHOP and radiotherapy to the contralateral testis showed a five-year progression-free survival of 74% and an overall survival of 85% [54]. Prolonged screening is absolutely necessary in this group of patients as relapses frequently occur after five years and have been identified over a decade after the initial presentation [53].

References

1 Ferlay, J., Shin, H.R., Bray, F., *et al.* GLOBOCAN 2008: Cancer incidence and mortality worldwide. IARC CancerBase No. 10 (2010) International Agency for Research on Cancer, Lyon, France.

2 Howlader, N., Noone, A.M., Krapcho, M., Miller, D., Bishop, K., Altekruse, S.F., Kosary, C.L., Yu, M., Ruhl, J., Tatalovich, Z., Mariotto, A., Lewis, D.R., Chen, H.S., Feuer, E.J., Cronin, K.A. (eds). *SEER Cancer Statistics Review, 1975–2013*, National Cancer Institute. Bethesda, MD, Available at http://seer.cancer.gov/csr/1975_2013/.

3 Purdue, M.P., Devesa, S.S., Sigurdson, A.J., McGlynn, K.A. (2005) International patterns and trends in testis cancer incidence. *Int. J. Cancer,* **115** (5), 822–827.

4 Siegel, R.L., Miller, K.D. and Jemal, A. (2017) Cancer statistics, 2017. *CA Cancer J. Clin.,* **67** (1), 730.

5 Manecksha, R.P., Fitzpatrick, J.M. (2009) Epidemiology of testicular cancer. *Br. J. Urol. Int.,* **104** (9 Pt B), 1329–1333.

6 Goldin, L.R., Landgren, O., McMaster, M.L., *et al.* (2005) Familial aggregation and heterogeneity of non-Hodgkin lymphoma in population-based samples. *Cancer Epidemiol. Biomarkers Prev.,* **14** (10), 2402–2406.

7 Al-Agha, O.M., Axiotis, C.A. (2007) An in-depth look at Leydig cell tumor of the testis. *Arch. Pathol. Lab. Med.,* **131** (2), 311–317.

8 National Comprehensive Cancer Network. Testicular Cancer (V.2.2017). Available at: http://www.nccn.org/professionals/physician_gls/pdf/testicular.pdf. Accessed February 24, 2017.

9 Whitmore, W.F., Jr (1979) Surgical treatment of adult germinal testis tumors. *Semin. Oncol.,* **6** (1), 55–68.

10 Gilligan, T.D., Seidenfeld, J., Basch, E.M., *et al.* (2010) American Society of Clinical Oncology Clinical Practice Guideline on uses of serum tumor markers in adult males with germ cell tumors. *J. Clin. Oncol.,* **28** (20), 3388–3404.

11 Ruf, C.G., Isbarn, H., Wagner, W., Fisch, M., Matthies, C., Dieckmann, K.P. (2013) Changes in epidemiologic features of testicular germ cell cancer: age at diagnosis and relative frequency of seminoma are constantly and significantly increasing. *Urol. Oncol.,* **32** (1), e31–e36.

12 Travis, L.B., Beard, C., Allan, J.M., *et al.* (2010) Testicular cancer survivorship: research strategies and recommendations. *J. Natl Cancer Inst.,* **102** (15), 1114–1130.

13 Vesprini, D., Chung, P., Tolan, S., *et al.* (2012) Utility of serum tumor markers during surveillance for stage I seminoma. *Cancer,* **118** (21), 5245–5250.

14 Chung, P., Warde, P. (2011) Stage I seminoma: adjuvant treatment is effective but is it necessary? *J. Natl Cancer Inst.,* **103** (3). 194–196.

15 Chung, P.W., Daugaard, G., Tyldesle, S., *et al.* (2010) Prognostic factors for relapse in stage I seminoma managed with surveillance: A validation study. *J. Clin. Oncol.,* **18** (15 Suppl.), abstract 4535.

16 Amin, M.B. and American Joint Committee on Cancer (2017) *AJCC Cancer Staging Manual,* 8th edition. Springer, New York.

17 Oliver, R.T., Mason, M.D., Mead, G.M., *et al.* (2005) Radiotherapy versus single-dose carboplatin in adjuvant treatment of stage I seminoma: a randomised trial. *Lancet,* **366** (9482), 293–300.

18 Travis, L.B., Fossa, S.D., Schonfeld, S.J., *et al.* (2005) Second cancers among 40,576 testicular cancer patients: focus on long-term survivors. *J. Natl Cancer Inst.,* **97** (18), 1354–1365.

19 de Gonzalez, A.B., Curtis, R.E., Kry, S.F., *et al.* (2011) Proportion of second cancers attributable to radiotherapy treatment in adults: a cohort study in the US SEER cancer registries. *Lancet Oncol.,* **12** (4), 353–360.

20 Beard, C.J., Travis, L.B., Chen, M.H., *et al.* (2013) Outcomes in stage I testicular seminoma: a population-based study of 9193 patients. *Cancer,* **119** (15), 2771–2777.

21 Bosl, G.J., Patil, S. (2011) Carboplatin in clinical stage I seminoma: too much and too little at the same time. *J. Clin. Oncol.,* **29** (8), 949–952.

22 Kollmannsberger, C., Tandstad, T., Bedard, P.L., *et al.* (2014) Patterns of relapse in patients with clinical stage I testicular cancer managed with active surveillance. *J Clin. Oncol.,* **33** (1), 51–57.

23 Krege, S., Beyer, J., Souchon, R., *et al.* (2008) European consensus conference on diagnosis and treatment of germ cell cancer: a report of the second meeting of the European Germ Cell Cancer Consensus group (EGCCCG): part I. *Eur. Urol.,* **53** (3), 478–496.

24 Kollmannsberger, C., Tyldesley, S., Moore, C., *et al.* (2011) Evolution in management of testicular seminoma: population-based outcomes with selective utilization of active therapies. *Ann. Oncol.,* **22** (4), 808–814.

25 Gray, P.J., Lin, C.C., Sineshaw, H., Paly, J.J., Jemal, A., Efstathiou, J.A. (2014) Management trends in stage I testicular seminoma: Impact of race, insurance status, and treatment facility. *Cancer,* **121** (5), 681–687.

26 Fossa, S.D., Horwich, A., Russell, J.M., *et al.* (1999) Optimal planning target volume for stage I testicular seminoma: A Medical Research Council randomized trial. Medical Research Council Testicular Tumor Working Group. *J. Clin. Oncol.,* **17** (4), 1146.

27 Bruns, F., Bremer, M., Meyer, A., Karstens, J.H. (2005) Adjuvant radiotherapy in stage I seminoma: is there a role for further reduction of treatment volume? *Acta Oncol.*, **44** (2), 142–148.

28 Kiricuta, I.C., Sauer, J., Bohndorf, W. (1996) Omission of the pelvic irradiation in stage I testicular seminoma: a study of postorchiectomy paraaortic radiotherapy. *Int. J. Radiat. Oncol. Biol. Phys.*, **35** (2), 293–298.

29 Paly, J.J., Efstathiou, J.A., Hedgire, S.S., *et al.* (2013) Mapping patterns of nodal metastases in seminoma: rethinking radiotherapy fields. *Radiother. Oncol.*, **106** (1), 64–68.

30 Klein, F.A., Whitmore, W.F., Jr, Sogani, P.C., Batata, M., Fisher, H., Herr, H.W. (1984) Inguinal lymph node metastases from germ cell testicular tumors. *J. Urol.*, **131** (3), 497–500.

31 von der Maase, H., Specht, L., Jacobsen, G.K., *et al.* (1993) Surveillance following orchidectomy for stage I seminoma of the testis. *Eur. J. Cancer.*, **29A** (14), 1931–1934.

32 Warde, P., Specht, L., Horwich, A., *et al.* (2002) Prognostic factors for relapse in stage I seminoma managed by surveillance: a pooled analysis. *J. Clin. Oncol.*, **20** (22), 4448–4452.

33 Classen, J., Dieckmann, K., Bamberg, M., *et al.* (2003) Radiotherapy with 16 Gy may fail to eradicate testicular intraepithelial neoplasia: preliminary communication of a dose-reduction trial of the German Testicular Cancer Study Group. *Br. J. Cancer*, **88** (6), 828–831.

34 Huyghe, E., Matsuda, T., Daudin, M., *et al.* (2004) Fertility after testicular cancer treatments: results of a large multicenter study. *Cancer*, **100** (4), 732–737.

35 Mead, G.M., Fossa, S.D., Oliver, R.T., *et al.* (2011) Randomized trials in 2466 patients with stage I seminoma: patterns of relapse and follow-up. *J. Natl Cancer Inst.*, **103** (3), 241–249.

36 Cummins, S., Yau, T., Huddart, R., Dearnaley, D., Horwich, A. (2009) Surveillance in Stage I seminoma patients: a long-term assessment. *Eur. Urol.*, **57** (4), 673–678.

37 Warde, P.R., Chung, P., Sturgeon, J., Panzarella, T., Giuliani, M. (2005) Should surveillance be considered the standard of care in stage I seminoma? *J. Clin. Oncol. (Meeting Abstracts)*, **23** (16 Suppl.), 4520.

38 Oliver, R.T., Mead, G.M., Rustin, G.J., *et al.* (2011) Randomized trial of carboplatin versus radiotherapy for Stage I seminoma: mature results on relapse and contralateral testis cancer rates in MRC TE19/EORTC 30982 study (ISRCTN27163214). *J. Clin. Oncol.*, **29** (8), 957–962.

39 Classen, J., Schmidberger, H., Meisner, C., *et al.* (2003) Radiotherapy for stages IIA/B testicular seminoma: final report of a prospective multicenter clinical trial. *J. Clin. Oncol.*, **21** (6), 1101–1106.

40 van den Belt-Dusebout, A.W., Aleman, B.M., Besseling, G., *et al.* (2009) Roles of radiation dose and chemotherapy in the etiology of stomach cancer as a second malignancy. *Int. J. Radiat. Oncol. Biol. Phys.*, **75** (5), 1420–1429.

41 Wilder, R.B., Buyyounouski, M.K., Efstathiou, J.A., Beard, C.J. (2012) Radiotherapy treatment planning for testicular seminoma. *Int. J. Radiat. Oncol. Biol. Phys.*, **83** (4), e445–e452.

42 Schmoll, H.J., Jordan, K., Huddart, R., *et al.* (2010) Testicular seminoma: ESMO Clinical Practice Guidelines for diagnosis, treatment and follow-up. *Ann. Oncol.*, **21** (Suppl. 5), 140–146.

43 Efstathiou, J.A., Paly, J.J., Lu, H.M., *et al.* (2012) Adjuvant radiation therapy for early stage seminoma: Proton versus photon planning comparison and modeling of second cancer risk. *Radiother. Oncol.*, **103** (1), 12–17.

44 Chung, P.W., Gospodarowicz, M.K., Panzarella, T., *et al.* (2004) Stage II testicular seminoma: patterns of recurrence and outcome of treatment. *Eur. Urol.*, **45** (6), 754–759; discussion 759–760.

45 Garcia-del-Muro, X., Maroto, P., Guma, J., *et al.* (2008) Chemotherapy as an alternative to radiotherapy in the treatment of stage IIA and IIB testicular seminoma: a Spanish Germ Cell Cancer Group Study. *J. Clin. Oncol.*, **26** (33), 5416–5421.

46 de Wit, R., Louwerens, M., de Mulder, P.H., Verweij, J., Rodenhuis, S., Schornagel, J. (1999) Management of intermediate-prognosis germ-cell cancer: results of a phase I/II study of Taxol-BEP. *Int. J. Cancer*, **83** (6), 831–833.

47 Lavery, H.J., Bahnson, R.R., Sharp, D.S., Pohar, K.S. (2009) Management of the residual post-chemotherapy retroperitoneal mass in germ cell tumors. *Ther. Adv. Urol.*, **1** (4), 199–207.

48 Jacobsen, N.E., Foster, R.S. (2007) The role of surgery in the management of recurrent or persistent non-seminomatous germ cell tumors. *EAU-EBU Update Series*, **5** (4), 163–176.

49 Acar, C., Gurocak, S., Sozen, S. (2009) Current treatment of testicular sex cord-stromal tumors: critical review. *Urology*, **73** (6), 1165–1171.

50 Young, R.H., Koelliker, D.D., Scully, R.E. (1998) Sertoli cell tumors of the testis, not otherwise specified: a clinicopathologic analysis of 60 cases. *Am. J. Surg. Pathol.*, **22** (6), 709–721.

51 Ahmad, S.S., Idris, S.F., Follows, G.A., Williams, M.V. (2012) Primary Testicular Lymphoma. *Clin. Oncol. (R. Coll. Radiol.)*, **24** (5), 358–365.

52 Park, B.B., Kim, J.G., Sohn, S.K., *et al.* (2007) Consideration of aggressive therapeutic strategies for

primary testicular lymphoma. *Am. J. Hematol.*, **82** (9), 840–845.

53 Zucca, E., Conconi, A., Mughal, T.I., *et al.* (2003) Patterns of outcome and prognostic factors in primary large-cell lymphoma of the testis in a survey by the International Extranodal Lymphoma Study Group. *J. Clin. Oncol.*, **21** (1), 20–27.

54 Vitolo, U., Chiappella, A., Ferreri, A.J., *et al.* (2011) First-line treatment for primary testicular diffuse large B-cell lymphoma with rituximab-CHOP, CNS prophylaxis, and contralateral testis irradiation: final results of an international phase II trial. *J. Clin. Oncol.*, **29** (20), 2766–2772.

30

Penile Cancer

Kent W. Mouw, Anthony L. Zietman and Jason A. Efstathiou

Introduction

Penile cancer is rare in the United States and Europe, with an incidence of 0.58–1.3 cases per 100 000 population [1–4]. The incidence is several-fold higher in some Asian and South American countries, and penile cancer has been reported to represent up to 17% of new male cancer diagnoses in some populations [5,6]. Risk increases with age, and most patients are aged between 50 and 70 years at diagnosis.

Multiple factors have been associated with the risk of developing penile cancer. Circumcision is protective, with penile cancer rates significantly lower among cultures that routinely circumcise male infants [7–9]. Phimosis, smoking, and photochemotherapy (PUVA) therapy have been shown to increase risk [8, 10, 11]. Premaligant lesions, including condyloma acuminata, leukoplakia, balanitis xerotica obliterans, erythroplasia of Queyrat (carcinoma *in-situ* of the glans or prepuce), and Bowen's disease (carcinoma *in-situ* of the shaft epithelium) are associated with an increased risk of developing invasive cancer [12]. Men with human papilloma virus (HPV) infection are at increased risk. The prevalence of HPV infection in penile cancer patients in one series was 47%, significantly higher than in healthy men [13–15]. HPV subtypes 16 and 18 are the most common.

Over 95% of penile cancers are squamous cell carcinomas; other tumors including basal cell, lymphoma, sarcoma, melanoma, and metastases are far less common [16]. Several squamous cell histologic variants have been characterized, with some correlation of histologic type and biologic behavior noted [17, 18]. Basaloid and warty appear to be the most frequent HPV-associated types [15].

Patients often present with a visible or palpable penile lesion, sometimes accompanied by itching or burning (Figures 30.1A and 30.2A). Pain is less common at presentation. The glans is the most common site of involvement, followed by the prepuce, and least commonly the shaft [19]. Involvement is limited to the penis at presentation in approximately two-thirds of cases.

The primary lymphatic drainage of the penis is to the inguinal nodes. Several studies have shown a poor correlation between clinical and pathologic assessment of inguinal lymph nodes. The percentage of men with clinically positive inguinal nodes varies widely across series; however, only one-half of men with positive inguinal nodes by clinical criteria have nodal disease on pathologic assessment [20–22]. Conversely, the risk of pathologic involvement of clinically negative inguinal nodes is approximately 20% [23, 24]. The risk of nodal involvement increases with increasing tumor stage and grade [23]. Distant spread typically occurs late, and less than 10% of patients present with non-regional metastases. Sites of spread include the lung, liver, skeleton, and brain.

Patients presenting with a penile lesion suspicious for penile squamous cell carcinoma (SCC) should undergo work-up including examination, biopsy of the lesion, urethroscopy, and imaging with pelvis computed tomography (CT) and/or magnetic resonance imaging (MRI) [25]. Suspicious lymph nodes can be sampled and, if positive, should prompt a metastatic survey including chest x-radiography and abdominal CT. The utility of positron emission tomography (PET) in identifying involved inguinal lymph nodes in men without clinical evidence of inguinal metastases varies across series [26–28]. A study by Graafland *et al.* found that in men with known inguinal metastases, PET was useful in identifying involved pelvic nodes [29].

Clinical Radiation Oncology: Indications, Techniques, and Results, Third Edition. Edited by William Small Jr.
© 2017 John Wiley & Sons, Inc. Published 2017 by John Wiley & Sons, Inc.

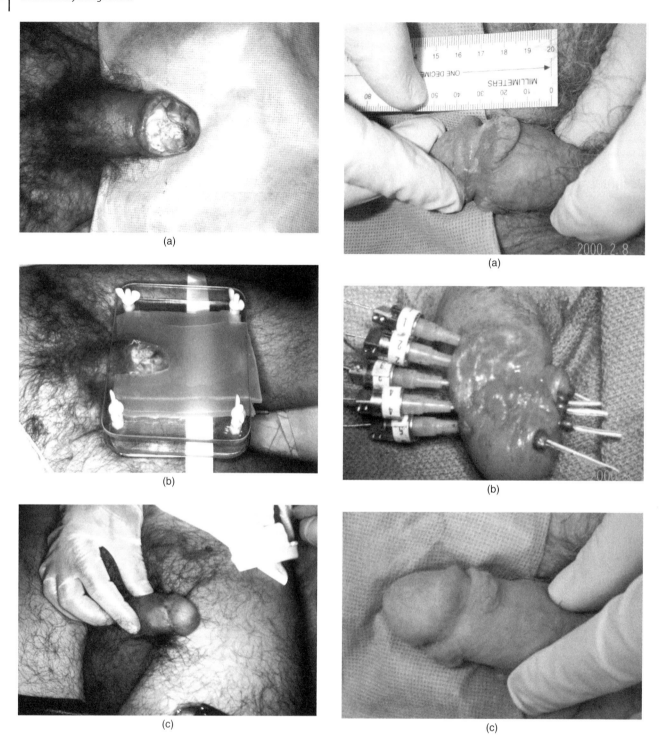

Figure 30.1 (a) Primary lesion of glans. (b) EBRT patient set-up with penis within a lucite 'sandwich'. The lucite acts as a bolus and additional bolus material is packed around the sides of the glans. A lead shield lies below to block the transmission to the testes. (c) One year post-EBRT. There is a well-healed, pale scar at the primary site. For a color version of this figure, see the color plate section.

Figure 30.2 (a) Primary lesion of the corona radiata. (b) Interstitial, single-plane brachytherapy with catheters placed perpendicular to the penile shaft. The patient is catheterized and care is taken to avoid the urethra. (c) One year post-brachytherapy. For a color version of this figure, see the color plate section.

Table 30.1 Rates of penile preservation. Adapted from *Clinical Radiation Oncology*, 3rd edition (eds L.L. Gunderson, J.E. Tepper), Elsevier, Philadelphia, PA (2012), and Crook, J.M., *et al.* (2013) American Brachytherapy Society - Groupe Européen de Curietherapie - European Society of Therapeutic Radiation Oncology (ABS-GEC-ESTRO) Consensus Statement for penile brachytherapy. *Brachytherapy*, **12**, 191–198.

EBRT

Author	Year	No. of patients	Dose	Follow-Up, Mo. (Range)	5 Yr Local Control	5 Yr Cause-Specific Survival	Penile Preservation	Complications
Gotsadze *et al.*	2000	155	40-60 Gy (2 Gy/fx)	78	65%	86%	65%	1% necrosis, 7% stenosis
McLean *et al.*	1993	26	35 Gy/10 fx - 60 Gy/25 fx	116 (84-168)	61.5%	69%	66% (crude)	28% (unspecified)
Neave *et al.*	1993	20	50-55 Gy (20-22 fx)	≥36	69.7%	58%	60%	10% stenosis
Sarin *et al.*	1997	59	60 Gy/30 fx	62 (2-264)	55%	66%	50% (crude)	3% necrosis, 14% stenosis
Zouhair *et al.*	2001	23	45-74 Gy/25-37 fx	12 (5-139)	41%	nr	36%	10% stenosis

Brachytherapy

Author	Year	No. of patients	Dose (Gy)	Follow-Up, Mo. (Range)	Local Control	5 yr Cause-Specific Survival	Penile Preservation	Necrosis/Stenosis
Chaudhary *et al.*	1999	23	50	21 (4-117)	70% (8 yr)	nr	70% (8 yr)	0%/9%
Crook *et al.*	2009	67	60	48 (6-194)	87% (5 yr), 72% (10 yr)	83.6%	88% (5 yr), 67% (10 yr)	12%/9%
de Crevoisier *et al.*	2009	144	65	68 (6-348)	80% (10 yr)	92% (10 yr)	72% (10 yr)	26%/29%
Delannes *et al.*	1992	51	50-65	65 (12-144)	86% (crude)	85%	75%	23%/45%
Kiltie *et al.*	2000	31	64	61.5	81% (5 yr)	85.4%	75%	8%/44%
Mazeron *et al.*	1984	50	60-70	36-96	78% (crude)	nr	74%	6%/19%
Rozan *et al.*	1995	184	59	139	86% (5 yr)	88%	78%	21%/45%
Sarin *et al.*	1997	102	61-70	111	77% (5 yr)	72%	72% (6 yr)	nr/nr
Delaunay *et al.*	2013	47	42-70	80 (13-190)	60% crude	87.6%	66%	nr/42%

*7 patients treated with brachytherapy boost.
fx, fractions.
nr, not reported.

Historically, penile cancer has been managed surgically with penile-sparing surgery or penectomy (partial or complete), and the extent of surgery is dependent on tumor size, location, and grade [21, 22, 30]. Local control rates following penectomy typically exceed 90% when adequate margins can be obtained; however, functional and psychological sequelae can be significant [31]. Penile-sparing surgery is associated with improved postsurgical function and quality of life, and rates of penile-sparing surgery have increased over time. Although local recurrence rates are higher following penile-sparing surgery, most recurrences can be salvaged with penectomy, and no impact on survival has been observed [32].

Radiation therapy with external beam radiotherapy (EBRT) or brachytherapy can also be used in the primary treatment of penile cancer, and can allow for the complete preservation of an intact penis [33]. There are no randomized clinical trials comparing surgical treatment with radiation. A large series of patients treated by EBRT over a 30-year period showed a 65% rate of penile preservation and a five-year cancer-specific survival of 86%. Local control for Stage 1 and 2 disease ranges from 65% to 90% in other series [34–40] (Table 30.1).

Circumcision should always be performed prior to penile irradiation. Typical EBRT doses are 65–70 Gy using conventional fractionation, and include 40–50 Gy to the entire shaft plus a boost of 10–20 Gy to the gross tumor volume (GTV) plus a margin. The use of a bolus is usually required to achieve an adequate skin dose unless kilovoltage therapy is employed (Figure 30.1B). Acute side effects can include pain, swelling, and skin erythema or desquamation. Late reactions include telangiectasia, urethral stricture, meatal stenosis, and necrosis (Figures 30.1C and 30.3).

Brachytherapy is used more commonly in Europe and can be delivered via a fitted penile mold or an interstitial implant. Low-dose rate (LDR), pulse-dose rate (PDR), and high-dose rate (HDR) techniques have been described [41]. Penile molds with embedded seeds or catheters are crafted to closely fit the patient's surface anatomy, and surface doses of 50–60 Gy are typically prescribed. Interstitial implants are more common and are often used to treat invasive tumors (Figure 30.2A). Catheters are inserted perpendicular to the long axis of the penis and an iridium-192 source delivers prescription doses of 50–65 Gy (Figure 30.2B) [42]. Local control rates using these techniques are reported as 60–90% in published series, with similar rates of penile preservation [33, 38, 43–48] (Table 30.1). Acute urinary symptoms are common, and up to 40% of men require urethral dilation after treatment. Desquamated skin may take months to fully heal, especially for larger ulcerated lesions (Figure 30.2C). However, many men maintain sexual potency following brachytherapy [34, 39].

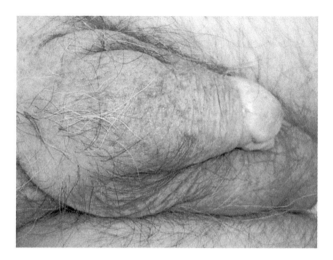

Figure 30.3 Post-treatment effects can include telangiectasia and penile swelling. The latter can result from the direct effect of radiation on the penile lymphatics or from irradiation of the inguinal lymph nodes. For a color version of this figure, see the color plate section.

Patients with pathologically confirmed inguinal involvement should undergo bilateral inguinal lymph node dissection [49, 50]. Adjuvant radiation has been shown to decrease recurrence rates following lymphadenectomy, especially in cases where multiple nodes are involved or extranodal extension is present [51–53]. There is no consensus regarding target volumes, and published reports range from treating only the pathologically involved region to treating bilateral inguinal and pelvic nodal regions.

Management of the clinically uninvolved groin is controversial. The likelihood of inguinal nodal involvement increases with increasing T stage and grade, and nomograms have been developed to predict the risk of occult involvement [20, 24, 54, 55]. Patients with greater than or equal pT2 disease or a grade 2–3 pT1 tumor are often considered for upfront inguinal lymph node dissection, and the use of inguinal lymph node dissection has been increasing according to a recent SEER analysis [49]. Sentinel node biopsy is emerging as a less-invasive alternative, and has been shown in several studies to be both sensitive and specific [56–58].

EBRT alone is unlikely to control disease in patients with unresectable primary or nodal disease. Neoadjuvant cisplatin-based chemotherapy can induce significant response rates in patients with bulky nodal disease, and may be followed with definitive local therapy with surgery and/or radiation [59, 60]. Although direct evidence is lacking, extrapolation from randomized trials involving other squamous cell cancers has led to the use of concurrent chemotherapy and radiation in some settings. Finally, the majority of penile squamous cell tumors express epidermal growth factor receptor (EGFR) at high levels, and several reports have suggested that anti-EGFR compounds may be active in a subset of tumors [61, 62].

Stage at presentation is the strongest predictor of outcome in patients with penile cancer. Long-term survival rates greater than 80% have been achieved in patients with disease confined to the penis [3, 63, 64]. Nodal metastases confer a significantly worse prognosis, with five-year survival rates of approximately 50% [65–68]. Data from a large European study shows that lymphovascular invasion (LVI) and grade are independent predictors for occult metastases [24]. Tumor grade has also been shown to be associated with recurrence risk and outcomes [69], and both tumor grade and LVI are included in the 2017 AJCC staging system for penile cancer [70]. Molecular determinants of prognosis are also being identified. The overexpression of p16(INK4A) is highly correlated with infection by high-risk HPV genotypes, and is associated with improved cancer-specific survival [71, 72].

References

1 Baldur-Felskov, B., *et al.* (2012) Increased incidence of penile cancer and high-grade penile intraepithelial neoplasia in Denmark 1978–2008: a nationwide population-based study. *Cancer Causes Control*, **23** (2), 273–280.

2 Barnholtz-Sloan, J.S., *et al.* (2007) Incidence trends in primary malignant penile cancer. *Urol. Oncol.*, **25** (5). 361–367.

3 Visser, O., *et al.* (2011) Incidence and survival of rare urogenital cancers in Europe. *Eur. J. Cancer*, **48**, 456–464.

4 Graafland, N.M., *et al.* (2011) Incidence trends and survival of penile squamous cell carcinoma in the Netherlands. *Int. J. Cancer*, **128** (2). 426–432.

5 Ornellas, A.A. (2008) Management of penile cancer. *J. Surg. Oncol.*, **97** (3), 199–200.

6 Riveros, M., Lebron, R.F. (1963) Geographical pathology of cancer of the penis. *Cancer*, **16**, 798–811.

7 Chaux, A., *et al.* (2011) Epidemiologic profile, sexual history, pathologic features, and human papillomavirus status of 103 patients with penile carcinoma. *World J. Urol.*, **31**, 861–867.

8 Dillner, J., *et al.* (2000) Etiology of squamous cell carcinoma of the penis. *Scand. J. Urol. Nephrol. Suppl.*, **205**, 189–193.

9 Kochen, M., McCurdy, S. (1980) Circumcision and the risk of cancer of the penis. A life-table analysis. *Am. J. Dis. Child.*, **134** (5), 484–486.

10 Calmon, M.F., *et al.* (2011) Penile carcinoma: risk factors and molecular alterations. *Sci. World J.*, **11**, 269–282.

11 Minhas, S., *et al.* (2010) Penile cancer – prevention and premalignant conditions. *Urology*, **76** (2 Suppl. 1), S24–S35.

12 Schellhammer, P.F., *et al.* (1992) Premalignant lesions and nonsquamous malignancy of the penis and carcinoma of the scrotum. *Urol. Clin. North. Am.*, **19** (1). 131–142.

13 Grussendorf-Conen, E.I., *et al.* (1987) Occurrence of HPV genomes in penile smears of healthy men. *Arch. Dermatol. Res.*, **279** (Suppl.), S73–S75.

14 Hartwig, S., *et al.* (2012) Estimation of the epidemiological burden of human papillomavirus-related cancers and non-malignant diseases in men in Europe: a review. *BMC Cancer*, **12** (1), 30.

15 Miralles-Guri, C., *et al.* (2009) Human papillomavirus prevalence and type distribution in penile carcinoma. *J. Clin. Pathol.*, **62** (10). 870–878.

16 Moses, K.A., *et al.* (2013) Non-squamous cell carcinoma of the penis: single-center, 15-year experience. *World J. Urol.*, **32**, 1347–1353.

17 Chaux, A., *et al.* (2011) Distribution and characterization of subtypes of penile intraepithelial neoplasia and their association with invasive carcinomas: a pathological study of 139 lesions in 121 patients. *Hum. Pathol.*, **43**, 1020–1027.

18 Cubilla, A.L., *et al.* (2001) Histologic classification of penile carcinoma and its relation to outcome in 61 patients with primary resection. *Int. J. Surg. Pathol.*, **9** (2), 111–120.

19 Hernandez, B.Y., *et al.* (2008) Burden of invasive squamous cell carcinoma of the penis in the United States, 1998–2003. *Cancer*, **113** (10 Suppl.), 2883–2891.

20 Hughes, B.E., *et al.* (2010) Lymph node metastasis in intermediate-risk penile squamous cell cancer: a two-centre experience. *Eur. Urol.*, **57** (4), 688–692.

21 Guimaraes, G.C., *et al.* (2009) Penile squamous cell carcinoma clinicopathological features, nodal metastasis and outcome in 333 cases. *J. Urol.*, **182** (2), 528–534; discussion 534.

22 Ornellas, A.A., *et al.* (1994) Surgical treatment of invasive squamous cell carcinoma of the penis: retrospective analysis of 350 cases. *J. Urol.*, **151** (5), 1244–1249.

23 Solsona, E., *et al.* (2001) Prospective validation of the association of local tumor stage and grade as a predictive factor for occult lymph node micrometastasis in patients with penile carcinoma and clinically negative inguinal lymph nodes. *J. Urol.*, **165** (5), 1506–1509.

24 Graafland, N.M., *et al.* (2010) Prognostic factors for occult inguinal lymph node involvement in penile carcinoma and assessment of the high-risk EAU subgroup: a two-institution analysis of 342 clinically node-negative patients. *Eur. Urol.*, **58** (5), 742–747.

25 McDougal, W.S., *et al.* (2014) Case records of the Massachusetts General Hospital. Case 2-2014. A 44-year-old man with a lesion on the penis. *N. Engl. J. Med.*, **370** (3), 263–271.

26 Schlenker, B., *et al.* (2012) Detection of inguinal lymph node involvement in penile squamous cell carcinoma by 18F-fluorodeoxyglucose PET/CT: A prospective single-center study. *Urol. Oncol.*, **30** (1), 55–59.

27 Souillac, I., *et al.* (2012) Prospective evaluation of (18)f-fluorodeoxyglucose positron emission tomography-computerized tomography to assess inguinal lymph node status in invasive squamous cell carcinoma of the penis. *J. Urol.*, **187** (2), 493–497.

28 Leijte, J.A., *et al.* (2009) Prospective evaluation of hybrid 18F-fluorodeoxyglucose positron emission tomography/computed tomography in staging clinically node-negative patients with penile carcinoma. *Br. J. Urol. Int.*, **104** (5), 640–644.

29 Graafland, N.M., *et al.* (2009) Scanning with 18F-FDG-PET/CT for detection of pelvic nodal involvement in inguinal node-positive penile carcinoma. *Eur. Urol.*, **56** (2), 339–345.

30 Feldman, A.S., McDougal, W.S. (2011) Long-term outcome of excisional organ sparing surgery for carcinoma of the penis. *J. Urol.*, **186** (4), 1303–1307.

31 Opjordsmoen, S., Fossa, S.D. (1994) Quality of life in patients treated for penile cancer. A follow-up study. *Br. J. Urol.*, **74** (5), 652–657.

32 Hegarty, P.K., *et al.* (2013) Penile Cancer: Organ-sparing techniques. *Br. J. Urol. Int.*, **114**, 799–805.

33 Crook, J., Ma, C., Grimard, L. (2009) Radiation therapy in the management of the primary penile tumor: an update. *World J. Urol.*, **27** (2), 189–196.

34 Gotsadze, D., *et al.* (2000) Is conservative organ-sparing treatment of penile carcinoma justified? *Eur. Urol.*, **38** (3), 306–312.

35 McLean, M., *et al.* (1993) The results of primary radiation therapy in the management of squamous cell carcinoma of the penis. *Int. J. Radiat. Oncol. Biol. Phys.*, **25** (4), 623–628.

36 Neave, F., *et al.* (1993) Carcinoma of the penis: a retrospective review of treatment with iridium mould and external beam irradiation. *Clin. Oncol. (R. Coll. Radiol.)*, **5** (4), 207–210.

37 Ozsahin, M., *et al.* (2006) Treatment of penile carcinoma: to cut or not to cut? *Int. J. Radiat. Oncol. Biol. Phys.*, **66** (3), 674–679.

38 Sarin, R., *et al.* (1997) Treatment results and prognostic factors in 101 men treated for squamous carcinoma of the penis. *Int. J. Radiat. Oncol. Biol. Phys.*, **38** (4), 713–722.

39 Zouhair, A., *et al.* (2001) Radiation therapy alone or combined surgery and radiation therapy in squamous-cell carcinoma of the penis? *Eur. J. Cancer*, **37** (2), 198–203.

40 Delaunay, B., *et al.* (2013) Brachytherapy for penile cancer: Efficacy and impact on sexual function. *Brachytherapy*, **13**, 380–387.

41 Van Poppel, H., *et al.* (2013) Penile cancer: ESMO Clinical Practice Guidelines for diagnosis, treatment and follow-up. *Ann. Oncol.*, **24** (Suppl. 6), 115–124.

42 Crook, J., Jezioranski, J., Cygler, J.E. (2010) Penile brachytherapy: technical aspects and postimplant issues. *Brachytherapy*, **9** (2), 151–158.

43 Chaudhary, A.J., *et al.* (1999) Interstitial brachytherapy in carcinoma of the penis. *Strahlenther. Onkol.*, **175** (1), 17–20.

44 de Crevoisier, R., *et al.* (2009) Long-term results of brachytherapy for carcinoma of the penis confined to the glans (N- or NX). *Int. J. Radiat. Oncol. Biol. Phys.*, **74** (4), 1150–1156.

45 Delannes, M., *et al.* (1992) Iridium-192 interstitial therapy for squamous cell carcinoma of the penis. *Int. J. Radiat. Oncol. Biol. Phys.*, **24** (3), 479–483.

46 Kiltie, A.E., *et al.* (2000) Iridium-192 implantation for node-negative carcinoma of the penis: the Cookridge Hospital experience. Clin. *Oncol. (R. Coll. Radiol.)*, **12** (1), 25–31.

47 Mazeron, J.J., *et al.* (1984) Interstitial radiation therapy for carcinoma of the penis using iridium 192 wires: the Henri Mondor experience (1970–1979). *Int. J. Radiat. Oncol. Biol. Phys.*, **10** (10), 1891–1895.

48 Rozan, R., *et al.* (1995) Interstitial brachytherapy for penile carcinoma: a multicentric survey (259 patients). *Radiother. Oncol.*, **36** (2), 83–93.

49 Thuret, R., *et al.* (2011) A contemporary population-based assessment of the rate of lymph node dissection for penile carcinoma. *Ann. Surg. Oncol.*, **18** (2), 439–446.

50 Graafland, N.M., *et al.* (2011) Inguinal recurrence following therapeutic lymphadenectomy for node positive penile carcinoma: outcome and implications for management. *J. Urol.*, **185** (3), 888–893.

51 Chen, M.F., *et al.* (2004) Contemporary management of penile cancer including surgery and adjuvant radiotherapy: an experience in Taiwan. *World J. Urol.*, **22** (1), 60–66.

52 Franks, K.N., *et al.* (2011) Radiotherapy for node positive penile cancer: experience of the Leeds teaching hospitals. *J. Urol.*, **186** (2), 524–529.

53 Graafland, N.M., *et al.* (2010) Prognostic significance of extranodal extension in patients with pathological node positive penile carcinoma. *J. Urol.*, **184** (4), 1347–1353.

54 Ficarra, V., *et al.* (2006) Nomogram predictive of pathological inguinal lymph node involvement in patients with squamous cell carcinoma of the penis. *J. Urol.*, **175** (5), 1700–1704; discussion 1704–1705.

55 Alkatout, I., *et al.* (2011) Squamous cell carcinoma of the penis: predicting nodal metastases by histologic grade, pattern of invasion and clinical examination. *Urol. Oncol.*, **29** (6), 774–781.

56 Leijte, J.A., *et al.* (2009) Two-center evaluation of dynamic sentinel node biopsy for squamous cell carcinoma of the penis. *J. Clin. Oncol.*, **27** (20), 3325–3329.

57 Neto, A.S., *et al.* (2011) Dynamic sentinel node biopsy for inguinal lymph node staging in patients with penile cancer: a systematic review and cumulative analysis of the literature. *Ann. Surg. Oncol.*, **18** (7), 2026–2034.

58 Sadeghi, R., *et al.* (2012) Accuracy of sentinel lymph node biopsy for inguinal lymph node staging of penile squamous cell carcinoma: systematic review and meta-analysis of the literature. *J. Urol.*, **187** (1), 25–31.

59 Haas, G.P., *et al.* (1999) Cisplatin, methotrexate and bleomycin for the treatment of carcinoma of the penis: a Southwest Oncology Group study. *J. Urol.*, **161** (6), 1823–1825.

60 Pagliaro, L.C., *et al.* (2010) Neoadjuvant paclitaxel, ifosfamide, and cisplatin chemotherapy for metastatic penile cancer: a phase II study. *J. Clin. Oncol.*, **28** (24), 3851–3857.

61 Gou, H.F., *et al.* (2013) Epidermal growth factor receptor (EGFR)-RAS signaling pathway in penile squamous cell carcinoma. *PLoS One*, **8** (4), e62175.

62 Brown, A., *et al.* (2014) Epidermal growth factor receptor-targeted therapy in squamous cell carcinoma of the penis: a report of 3 cases. *Urology*, **83** (1), 159–165.

63 Ornellas, A.A., *et al.* (2008) Surgical treatment of invasive squamous cell carcinoma of the penis: Brazilian National Cancer Institute long-term experience. *J. Surg. Oncol.*, **97** (6), 487–495.

64 Rippentrop, J.M., Joslyn, S.A., Konety, B.R. (2004) Squamous cell carcinoma of the penis: evaluation of data from the surveillance, epidemiology, and end results program. *Cancer*, **101** (6), 1357–1363.

65 Srinivas, V., *et al.* (1987) Penile cancer: relation of extent of nodal metastasis to survival. *J. Urol.*, **137** (5), 880–882.

66 Pandey, D., Mahajan, V., Kannan, R.R. (2006) Prognostic factors in node-positive carcinoma of the penis. *J. Surg. Oncol.*, **93** (2), 133–138.

67 Ficarra, V., *et al.* (2011) Prognostic factors in penile cancer. *Urology*, **76** (2 Suppl. 1), S66–S73.

68 Marconnet, L., Rigaud, J., Bouchot, O. (2010) Long-term followup of penile carcinoma with high risk for lymph node invasion treated with inguinal lymphadenectomy. *J. Urol.*, **183** (6), 2227–2232.

69 Escudero, R.M., *et al.* (2011) Predictive factors for recurrence in clinically localized squamous cell carcinoma of the penis. Analysis of our case series. *Arch. Esp. Urol.*, **64** (6), 525–532.

70 Amin, M.B. (ed) (2017) *AJCC Cancer Staging Manual*, 8th edition, Springer, New York.

71 Cubilla, A.L., *et al.* (2011) Value of p16(INK)(a) in the pathology of invasive penile squamous cell carcinomas: A report of 202 cases. *Am. J. Surg. Pathol.*, **35** (2), 253–261.

72 Gunia, S., *et al.* (2012) p16(INK4a) is a marker of good prognosis for primary invasive penile squamous cell carcinoma: a multi-institutional study. *J. Urol.*, **187**, 899–907.

Section 6

Gynecological Malignancies

Section Editor: William Small Jr.

31

Endometrium

Ann Klopp and Patricia Eifel

Epidemiology

Cancers of the uterine corpus are the most common female genital tract cancers in the United States, impacting 757,190 women in 2016 [1]. Uterine cancers represent approximately 50% of new cases of gynecologic cancer and 20% of deaths due to female genital tract cancers [1].

Endometrial cancer is classically divided into two separate biological entities: type I endometrial cancer, which is most common and has a better prognosis; and type II endometrial cancer, which includes uterine serous carcinoma, carcinosarcoma (malignant mixed Mullerian tumor; MMMT), and clear cell carcinoma (Table 31.1). Type I cancers typically arise in the setting of a hyperplastic endometrium, while type II cancers typically arise in the atrophic endometria of older women. The two types of endometrial cancer also differ with respect to mutations in signaling pathways: type I cancers frequently have mutations in the PTEN pathway, while type II cancers are more likely than type I cancers to have mutation of p53 [2].

Type I endometrial cancers most commonly have endometrioid histology and are associated with excess exogenous or endogenous [3] estrogen exposure. The most common cause of increased endogenous estrogen exposure is obesity. Biochemical changes in peripheral adipose tissue result in high serum estrogen and androgen levels and relatively lower progesterone levels. Excess intra-abdominal obesity is also associated with increased endometrial cancer risk [4]. Obesity and a sedentary lifestyle are strongly correlated with an increased incidence of endometrioid endometrial cancer [5, 6]. Other causes of increased endogenous estrogen exposure include estrogen-secreting tumors, low parity, early menarche, and late menopause [7, 8].

Exogenous estrogen without concurrent progesterone (unopposed estrogen) is clearly associated with an increased incidence of endometrial hyperplasia and abnormal bleeding. Unopposed estrogen replacement therapy may also be associated with an increased risk of endometrial cancer, but has not been clearly demonstrated to cause an increased risk of endometrial cancer mortality [9, 10]. Tamoxifen, a selective estrogen receptor modulator, used in the treatment and prevention of breast cancer, increases the risk of endometrial cancer [11]. Combination treatment with estrogen and progesterone has not been demonstrated to increase the risk of endometrial cancer and may in fact be protective [8].

Type II endometrial cancers include uterine serous carcinoma, clear cell carcinoma, and carcinosarcoma. They are generally not associated with estrogen exposure and have a worse prognosis than type I endometrial cancers. P53 mutations are seen more frequently in type II than type I endometrial cancers.

The Cancer Genome Atlas (TCGA) project recently identified new molecular subsets of endometrial cancer using an integrated genomic analysis of 373 endometrial cancers [12]. A favorable prognosis group with mutations in the catalytic subunit of DNA polymerase epsilon was identified. These very favorable prognosis tumors are often high-grade or serous, contain more tumor-infiltrating T-cells and a high rate of mutations throughout the genome [13]. The TCGA analysis also identified a poor prognosis group with a high rate of changes in the number of copies of genes ('copy number high'). This group had frequent mutations in p53 and included serous tumors as well as 25% of grade 3 endometrioid cancers, and also had the lower rates of survival. In the future, these molecular subtypes may find clinical utility in the management of endometrial cancer.

Clinical Radiation Oncology: Indications, Techniques, and Results, Third Edition. Edited by William Small Jr.
© 2017 John Wiley & Sons, Inc. Published 2017 by John Wiley & Sons, Inc.

Table 31.1 Clinical and molecular characteristics of type I and II endometrial cancers.

Characteristic	Type I	Type II
Percent of cases	80–90	10–20
Histology	Endometrioid	Serous, clear-cell, carcinosarcoma
Risk factors	Obesity, excessive estrogen exposure	More common in African-American women
Menopausal status	Perimenopausal women	Post-menopausal women
Endometrial environment	Arise from endometrial hyperplasia	Arise from atrophic endometrium
Pathways effects	More frequent mutations in PTEN, PIK3CA, KRAS, and β-catenin.	Mutant p53, HER-2/neu, p16, and E-cadherin

The incidence of endometrial cancer is lower in black women than in non-Hispanic whites. Although the incidence in white women has been stable since 1992, that in black women has increased at a rate of approximately 1.7% per year [1]. Black women also have a significantly higher uterine cancer death rate than other groups. This disparity appears to be associated with many factors; black women are more likely to be diagnosed with unfavorable histologic types of uterine cancer and tend to have more advanced stage disease at diagnosis. Social disparities and a greater incidence of serious comorbid diseases may also contribute to the relatively high death rate in black women with uterine cancer [14].

Other clinical factors that have been associated with an increased risk of uterine cancer are diabetes, hypertension, late menopause (age >52 years), and a prior history of radiation therapy. Long-term tamoxifen exposure is associated with a significantly increased risk of endometrial cancer, particularly uterine serous carcinoma and carcinosarcoma [15]. Aromatase inhibitors are associated with a significantly lower risk of second uterine cancers than is tamoxifen [16].

About 5% of uterine cancers appear to be related to a genetic cause. The most common genetic predisposition is Lynch syndrome, or hereditary non-polyposis colorectal cancer, which is characterized by a germline mutation in DNA mismatch repair genes. Lynch syndrome results in an increased risk of developing cancer, particularly colon cancer and, in women, endometrial cancer. It is estimated that female mutation carriers have a lifetime risk of developing endometrial cancer of 40–60% [17, 18]. Women with Lynch-associated uterine cancer tend to be younger than the average endometrial cancer patient, and are more likely to have tumors involving the lower uterine segment. In a review of women with lower uterine segment tumors, Westin et al. [19] found that 29% had Lynch syndrome. Hysterectomy is an effective means of reducing the risk of endometrial cancer for women with Lynch syndrome [20].

It has been reported that uterine cancers which develop in women with a history of breast cancer are more likely to be serous carcinomas than are those which develop in women without a history of breast cancer [21]. Although tamoxifen exposure has been associated with an increased risk of uterine cancer, the increased rate of uterine serous carcinoma seen in women treated with tamoxifen may also reflect an association with *BRCA* mutations. Several studies have now suggested that *BRCA* mutation carriers, who are known to be at high risk for developing breast and ovarian cancer, also may have an increased risk of developing uterine serous carcinoma [22].

Interestingly, both smoking and drinking coffee have been correlated with a lower risk of endometrial cancer. Smoking at least 20 cigarettes per day has been associated with a 28% reduction in the risk of endometrial cancer among women in general, and with a greater reduction among obese women [23]. Needless to say, the toxic and carcinogenic effects of tobacco outweigh any association with a lower risk of endometrial cancer. Additionally, drinking more than three or four cups of coffee per day has been associated with a lower risk of endometrial cancer, perhaps through decreasing circulating estrogen or insulin levels [24, 25].

Prognostic Factors

Histologic Subtype and Grade

Approximately 80% of uterine cancers are classified as endometrioid, which means that the tumor has a histologic appearance that recapitulates, in its differentiated features, normal or hyperplastic endometrial glandular tissue [26]. Typical endometrioid carcinomas consist of tubular glands lined by stratified or pseudostratified columnar cells with rounded nuclei and varying degrees of pleomorphism. Although most endometrioid cancers fit into this 'typical' category, there are a number of variants, which can sometimes be the source of important problems with differential diagnosis. In particular, villoglandular endometrioid carcinomas have a papillary pattern that has sometimes been confused with papillary serous carcinoma, although villoglandular cancers generally lack the fibrous stromal cores, high-grade nuclei, and highly aggressive behavior typical of serous neoplasms. Occasionally, endometrioid variants have prominent glycogen vacuoles within the neoplastic cells or nests of prominent glycogenated squamous cells; the clear appearance of these cells should not cause them to be confused with clear cell carcinomas of the endometrium.

Prognosis is strongly correlated with tumor grade. The 1988 International Federation of Gynecology and Obstetrics (FIGO)/International Society of Gynecological Pathologists grading system for endometrioid tumors classified tumors by pattern and nuclear features (International Federation of Gynecology and Obstetrics, 1989). Tumors that have less than 5% solid growth pattern are grade 1, tumors that are 5–50% solid are grade 2, and tumors more than 50% solid are grade 3. This grading is based only on the glandular component; it excludes areas of squamous differentiation. Tumors that are architecturally grade 1 or 2 may have their grade increased by 1 if they have high-grade nuclear features (e.g., marked nuclear pleomorphism, coarse chromatin, or prominent nucleoli); this criterion may encourage more realistic grading of special variants such as papillary serous carcinoma but probably contributes to subjective variations in grading practice.

The 20% of uterine cancers that are not classified as endometrioid represent a diverse group of special variants with a range of histologic appearances and behaviors [27]. The most important of these variants is serous carcinoma of the uterus, which was first established as a distinct clinicopathologic entity during the early 1980s [27–29]. Serous carcinomas account for 5–10% of uterine cancers but are responsible for a much higher percentage of deaths from uterine cancer. Serous carcinomas tend to occur in older women, and the median age at diagnosis of serous carcinoma is about 10 years older than the median age at diagnosis of endometrioid cancer. Histologically, uterine serous tumors are similar to high-grade ovarian serous neoplasms. Typically, the cells have highly pleomorphic nuclei, scant cytoplasm, and macronucleoli; the cells are usually, but not always, arranged in striking papillae on fibrovascular stalks. Some tumors arise in polyps. The behavior of uterine serous cancers is aggressive, and metastasis – particularly intraperitoneal metastasis – is common. Relapse rates for stage I disease have been reported to be as high as 50%, although in reports of patients who have been meticulously staged and aggressively treated, outcomes have been better [30, 31]. Although serous tumors are frequently admixed with other types, the prognosis of tumors with a mix of types tends to be similar to that of pure serous carcinoma if more than 10–25% of the tumor is serous [27].

Other special variants are rare. Clear cell carcinomas usually occur in older women and often have a papillary structure. However, the cells generally have abundant cytoplasm and the nuclear features tend to be somewhat lower-grade than those of serous tumors [27, 32]. The prognosis is less well-defined but appears to be better than that of serous cancers [32]. Although primary mucinous carcinomas have been reported to account for up to 10% of endometrial cancers, most are admixed with endometrioid cancer [27]. Pure mucinous endometrial cancers tend to be small and have a good prognosis. Other, very rare variants include squamous carcinoma, adenosarcoma, lapatransitional cell carcinoma, and large- or small-cell undifferentiated carcinoma.

Carcinosarcoma, or MMMT, is characterized by the combination of adenocarcinoma (which can be endometrioid, serous, or clear cell) and a mesenchymal sarcomatoid component. Carcinosarcomas are thought to be high-grade carcinomas that undergo differentiation into a sarcomatous/stromal cell tumor [33]. This suggestion is supported by molecular evidence showing that most, but not all, carcinosarcomas are monoclonal in origin [33]. Carcinosarcomas typically have a worse prognosis than endometrioid tumors and a higher rate of intraperitoneal dissemination [34, 35].

Myometrial and Cervical Invasion

The depth of myometrial infiltration is one of the most important predictors of lymph node involvement and prognosis. In the Gynecologic Oncology Group (GOG) 33 study, patients with clinical stage I endometrial cancer underwent total abdominal hysterectomy with bilateral salpingo-oophorectomy with pelvic and para-aortic lymph node dissection. The depth of myometrial invasion was an independent predictor of having involved lymph nodes [36]. Furthermore, the depth of invasion is independently predictive of overall survival [37]. However, in women with type II endometrial cancer, minimal invasion does not portend a good prognosis. Uterine serous carcinoma may behave aggressively in the absence of demonstrable myometrial invasion [29].

Tumors that involve the endocervical stroma are classified by FIGO as stage II. In the updated 2009 FIGO staging system, involvement of only the endocervical glands does not qualify disease as stage II. This 2009 modification to the staging system was made because patients with only endocervical gland involvement have a relatively good prognosis, probably similar to that of patients with tumors of similar grade and depth that are confined to the fundus [3]. The decision to deliver pelvic radiation for patients with endocervical gland involvement without stromal invasion involvement is generally made on the basis of other risk factors, such as depth of invasion, grade, and presence of lymphovascular space invasion (LVSI).

Tumors which involve the endocervical stroma have a higher likelihood of extrauterine involvement and disease recurrence than tumors which involve only the endocervical glands. Presumably, involvement of the endocervical stroma gives the tumor access to regional routes of spread, placing pelvic nodes at relatively greater risk of tumor involvement. As a result, patients with endocervical stromal invasion that is detected on pathologic examination but not initial pelvic examination, are generally treated with pelvic radiation therapy. The optimal treatment of patients with gross cervical involvement is discussed below.

Lymphovascular Space Invasion

Lymphovascular space invasion is a strong independent predictor of lymph node involvement [36] and, ultimately, of survival [38]. In a study from the Mayo Clinic that included patients with ≤50% invasion and grade 1 or 2 tumors, those without LVSI had a five-year cancer-related survival rate of 98% compared to 77% for patients with LVSI (P <0.0001) [38]. The presence of LVSI was found to predict for the presence of isolated para-aortic lymph node metastasis [39]. In addition, GOG 99 identified LVSI as one of the critical criteria to identify patients at 'high intermediate risk' who would benefit from pelvic radiation therapy [40]. The extent of LVSI has also been reported to have prognostic value: extensive LVSI is more highly correlated with lymph node involvement than is focal LVSI [41].

Tumor Size

Tumor size has been reported to be an independent predictor of lymph node metastasis. Patients with tumors smaller than 2 cm with minimal invasion, endometrioid histology, and low or moderate grade have been reported to have very low rates of nodal involvement [38]. In a series of 187 patients with clinical stage I endometrial cancer who underwent lymphadenectomy, no nodal metastasis was detected among patients with these pathologic characteristics [38]. It has been proposed that this group of patients can avoid a lymph node dissection.

Lymph Node Involvement

The survival rate at five years is significantly lower for patients with positive lymph nodes (ca. 50–80% for patients with endometrioid cancer) than for those with uterine-confined disease (80–95%). The 2009 FIGO staging system separates patients with positive pelvic lymph nodes only (stage IIIC1) from patients with positive para-aortic nodes with or without positive pelvic nodes (stage IIIC2). Reports are mixed as to the prognostic implications of positive para-aortic nodes [42], but in the present authors' experience of patients treated with appropriately tailored radiation fields, para-aortic node involvement did not portend a worse prognosis than pelvic node involvement [43].

Adnexal Invasion and Synchronous Primary Tumors

About 5% of women with endometrial cancer are found to have concurrent involvement of one or both ovaries with cancer [44, 45]. Synchronous involvement of the uterus and fallopian tubes also occurs but is very rare [46]. Ovarian involvement with adenocarcinoma in a patient with endometrial cancer can represent either metastasis from the endometrium or a simultaneous separate primary tumor. Features that suggest simultaneous primary tumors are minimal myometrial invasion, an absence of LVSI, and the presence of atypical hyperplasia in the uterus and, in the ovarian tumor, parenchymal as opposed to surface or predominantly hilar location and presence of background endometriosis [45]. The presence of locally advanced uterine involvement and ovarian hilar or multinodular surface involvement suggests that the adnexal lesions may represent metastasis. In the future, molecular studies may be able to determine if two lesions arose independently or represent metastasis. Molecular studies will need to account for intratumoral heterogeneity which may otherwise limit the interpretation of these findings.

Women who present with synchronous endometrial and ovarian endometrioid cancers tend to be young and nulliparous. For women diagnosed with endometrial cancer before the age of 45 years, the incidence of a synchronous ovarian tumor may be as high as 25%. This risk must be considered when patients are being counseled about possible ovarian preservation.

The treatment for patients with synchronous endometrial and ovarian endometrioid tumors is based on the features of the tumors at each site. A woman who has a grade 1 endometrioid cancer that minimally invades the myometrium and a small low-grade ovarian cancer may have an excellent outcome without any adjuvant treatment. Women who have high-grade endometrioid or type 2 endometrial cancers or ovarian tumor features that suggest metastasis usually require adjuvant treatment with chemotherapy, radiation, or both.

Pretreatment Investigation

Initial Presentation

Vaginal bleeding is by far the most common presenting symptom of endometrial cancer. Other less common symptoms include anemia and pelvic cramping.

The presence of pain or urinary or bowel complaints suggests the presence of a more advanced cancer.

Diagnostic Techniques and Initial Evaluations after Diagnosis

The evaluation of any woman with postmenopausal vaginal bleeding requires a biopsy. An endometrial biopsy involves inserting a pipelle endometrial suction currette into the endometrial cavity to obtain a sample of endometrial tissue. This procedure can be performed safely in the clinic setting. If findings on endometrial biopsy are negative for malignancy but bleeding persists, a dilation and curettage should be performed to ensure that a malignancy was not missed because of a sampling error. Endometrial biopsy is generally accompanied by a Pap smear and an endocervical curettage to evaluate for a cervical abnormality. If cervical involvement is suspected on the basis of cytology or physical examination, a cervical biopsy should be performed.

Evaluation of patients diagnosed with endometrial cancer should include a careful history and physical examination, complete blood cell count and serum chemistry studies, liver function tests, and chest radiography. CA-125 level is sometimes checked, especially for patients with serous cancer, since CA-125 level can predict advanced disease [47]. Further studies are generally indicated only in patients with abnormal findings on pelvic examination or high-risk histologies. Stage is determined after hysterectomy and abdominal exploration using surgical staging schema.

Presurgical Imaging

For a woman with endometrial biopsy findings positive for endometrioid endometrial cancer, and with normal findings on physical examination and a typical clinical presentation, no presurgical imaging is required. Transvaginal sonography is often used to evaluate the thickness of the endometrial lining and has high sensitivity in the detection of endometrial cancer in postmenopausal women because of abnormal thickening of the endometrial stripe [48]. However, transvaginal sonography is generally unnecessary in the evaluation of women with postmenopausal bleeding since a biopsy is needed for evaluation in this setting.

Currently, the standard approach for women with biopsy findings positive for endometrial cancer is to proceed with total abdominal hysterectomy with bilateral salpingo-oophorectomy with or without lymph node dissection. Computed tomography (CT) can detect gross nodal metastasis or distant metastasis in patients with concerning clinical findings or high-risk histology, such as uterine serous carcinoma. Magnetic resonance imaging (MRI) provides more information than CT about local tumor extension, including cervical involvement,

and bladder or rectal involvement. As a result, MRI can be particularly useful for patients with abnormal findings on physical examination [49]. MRI may be useful for patients with a cervical mass in whom there is a question about whether the lesion arose in the cervix or endometrium [50]. MRI can also be used to evaluate the extent of myometrial invasion [49, 51]. This information has the potential to help the surgeon decide whether to proceed with a node dissection, which is often not performed in patients with low-grade tumors with minimal invasion. However, MRI has not been incorporated into routine practice at most institutions since myometrial invasion can be accurately assessed with intraoperative frozen section examination.

Surgical Treatment and Staging

Hysterectomy

A type I extrafascial hysterectomy with bilateral salpingo-oophorectomy is the standard surgical approach for women with endometrial cancer. The ovaries are usually removed because most women are postmenopausal or perimenopausal at diagnosis, and because women with endometrial carcinoma are at significant risk for ovarian metastasis or independent primary ovarian cancer. A radical hysterectomy is rarely justified unless a primary surgical approach is being used for a patient with gross cervical involvement.

Techniques have been developed for laparoscopic hysterectomy and lymph node dissection. The Gynecologic Oncology Group conducted a randomized study to compare laparoscopy to laparotomy for surgical staging of uterine cancer [52]. Approximately 25% of cases that were planned for laparoscopy were converted to laparotomy because a greater access was required for excision of the cancer, because of poor visibility, or due to bleeding. The rate of grade 2 or more severe postoperative complications was lower in the laparoscopy arm (14% versus 21%; P <0.001). These results suggested that laparoscopic surgical staging for uterine cancer is feasible and safe in terms of short-term outcomes and results in fewer complications and a shorter hospital stay. The impact of laparoscopic surgery on complications following pelvic radiation therapy remains unknown.

Surgical Lymph Node Assessment

The current FIGO staging system for endometrial cancer requires surgical evaluation of the abdomen and regional lymph nodes, but there is no consensus about the superior extent of node dissection or the number of nodes to be removed.

Most clinicians identify a subset of patients, based on biopsy grade and intraoperative assessment of the hysterectomy specimen, who have a negligible risk of regional metastasis and thus do not require full node dissection. Mariani *et al.* [38] have identified the intrauterine pathologic findings that predict for nodal involvement. On the basis of their findings, these authors concluded that nodal dissection can be omitted for patients with FIGO grade 1 or 2 uterine-confined endometrioid corpus cancer with greatest surface dimension ≤2 cm, myometrial invasion ≤50%, and no intraoperative evidence of macroscopic disease.

The therapeutic benefit of performing a lymphadenectomy for any patient with stage I endometrial cancer has been called into question by two recently reported randomized studies. Both of these studies randomized women with clinical stage I endometrial cancer to lymph node sampling or lymph node dissection [53,54]. No benefit of lymphadenectomy was detected in either study with respect to local control, overall survival, or disease-free survival (DFS). The findings of these randomized trials conflict with the findings of retrospective studies reporting that removal of a higher number of lymph nodes was associated with improved survival [55, 56]. This discrepancy between the results of prospective and retrospective studies could be explained by either selection bias to remove more nodes in patients with less adverse medical or disease findings in retrospective studies, or by better nodal dissections in the retrospective studies. The former explanation is supported by an analysis of Surveillance, Epidemiology and End Results (SEER) data demonstrating that patients who underwent a more extensive lymphadenectomy were less likely to die of any cause, suggesting that more nodes were removed in healthier patients [56]. In the randomized trials, lymphadenectomy increased the rates of postoperative complications, including lymphedema and ileus [53,54].

Despite this question about the therapeutic benefit of lymphadenectomy, node dissection continues to be essential in identifying those patients who have positive nodes because these patients require intensified treatment. Sentinel lymph node biopsy has the potential to provide diagnostic information without the toxicity of full node dissection and is being actively investigated [57].

When lymphadenectomy is performed for diagnostic benefit, it is essential to evaluate the para-aortic nodes so that radiation fields can be tailored appropriately. An alternative approach is to consider prophylactic treatment of para-aortic nodes in patients with involved pelvic nodes who have not undergone a para-aortic node dissection.

Evaluation of sentinel lymph nodes has the potential to identify patients with positive nodes while sparing patients with negative lymph nodes the toxicity of lymphadenectomy. In recent years, sentinel lymph node evaluation has been tested in endometrial cancer [58]. This approach involves injecting a tracer dye into the cervix or uterine corpus and then identifying the node or nodes which drains the uterus by identifying the node that contains the tracer. The sentinel lymph node approach is based on the concept that lymphatic dissemination is predictable, so that the sentinel node will be involved before malignant cells spread to other adjacent lymph nodes. Early experiences with endometrial cancer suggest that sentinel nodes can be identified in up to 90% of cases and false negatives are rare with experienced surgeons [59].

Adjuvant Treatment

The majority of women diagnosed with uterine cancer have early-stage, low-grade type I endometrial cancers. These women are usually cured with hysterectomy alone; most require no adjuvant treatment. A small percentage of patients present with very advanced disease metastatic to peritoneal surfaces or distant sites; these are usually treated with multiagent chemotherapy, although they are rarely curable.

Between 5% and 10% of women who are surgically staged are found to have evidence of lymph node metastases. These patients have a high risk of recurrence, and although the optimal use of chemotherapy and radiation therapy is still controversial, most clinicians agree that women with lymph node metastases require fairly intensive adjuvant treatment. The remaining 20–25% of women have tumors confined to the uterus that exhibit one or more high-risk features, including high nuclear grade, type 2 histology, LVSI, or deep muscle or cervical stromal invasion. These women form a heterogeneous group whose risk of recurrence and patterns of failure vary widely. Variations in the extent of surgical staging add to this heterogeneity. Although several randomized trials have focused on this group of patients, their optimal treatment continues to be a subject of considerable controversy.

Low- and Intermediate-Risk Disease

Most clinicians categorize type I tumors that are grade 1 or grade 2, that are minimally invasive, and that lack other high-risk features such as LVSI or cervical stromal involvement as 'low risk.' For patients with these early tumors, the risk of recurrence after hysterectomy is less than 5–10% [34,60]. Also, for patients with these low-risk tumors, local recurrence can be treated successfully in about 70% of cases if it does occur [61, 62]. In patients with low-risk tumors, the risks of adjuvant treatment, particularly pelvic irradiation, generally outweigh the potential benefits. A randomized study investigating brachytherapy versus no adjuvant treatment in this population, found that rates of vaginal recurrence are predictably low without brachytherapy, and as a result no significant benefit to cuff irradiation was detected[63]. This study supports the recommendation to treat these patients without any adjuvant therapy.

More controversial is the treatment of patients who have disease that is apparently confined to the uterus but who have one or more risk factors for recurrence. In recent years, several randomized trials, including GOG 99 [34], the PORTEC (Post Operative Radiation Therapy for Endometrial Cancer) trials 1 and 2 [64–66], and the ASTEC trial [67], have attempted to define the role of adjuvant pelvic radiation in this 'intermediate-risk' group. These trials have refined the present understanding of the role of adjuvant radiation therapy in women with intermediate-risk disease, and have led to a significant shift towards less use of pelvic external beam irradiation. However, they have left many questions unanswered, particularly for patients whose tumors are high-grade or demonstrate multiple risk factors for pelvic recurrence.

To draw practical conclusions from the results of these trials, it is important to understand their limitations. Probably the greatest limitations arise from the heterogeneity of the eligibility criteria and the inclusion of many patients whose tumors were low-risk or fell in the relatively low-risk range of the intermediate-risk spectrum.

The GOG 99 study [40], which compared adjuvant pelvic radiation therapy with no adjuvant treatment in 392 women who had total abdominal hysterectomy with bilateral salpingo-oophorectomy and lymph node staging, demonstrated decreased pelvic recurrence but failed to demonstrate a significant overall benefit from adjuvant pelvic radiation therapy. However, more than 40% of the patients in this trial had invasion of less than one-third of the myometrial thickness, and more than 40% had grade 1 disease; for these patients, the margin for improvement with pelvic radiation therapy would be expected to be very small. Although there was no up-front stratification into subgroups by risk, the authors did identify a 'high intermediate risk' subset of 132 patients (one-third of the study group) who accounted for two-thirds of the cancer-related deaths in the trial (Table 31.1; Figure 31.1). For patients in this group who had no adjuvant treatment, the four-year survival rate was 72%; in contrast, for patients in this group who had pelvic radiation therapy, the four-year survival rate was 88%, similar to that of patients in the low intermediate risk group (Figure 31.1). Patients in the low intermediate risk group had excellent local control and survival rates with or without adjuvant radiation therapy.

In 2000, the PORTEC investigators [64] published results of PORTEC-1 (updated in 2005 [66]) in which 704 patients with endometrial cancer were randomized after

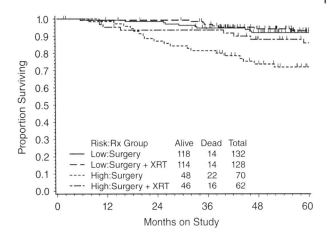

Figure 31.1 Survival by randomized treatment group and risk group in Gynecologic Oncology Group trial GOG 99. *Source*: Keys *et al.*, 2004 [40]. Reproduced with permission of Elsevier.

hysterectomy to receive pelvic radiation therapy (46 Gy) or no further treatment. This trial also failed to demonstrate any survival benefit of radiation therapy, although there was a significant reduction in the rate of local recurrence for patients who received radiation therapy. The eligibility criteria for this trial were even more favorable than those of GOG 99: patients were eligible if they had FIGO (1988) stage IC grade 1 or 2 disease or stage IB grade 2 or 3 disease. Unlike GOG 99, patients with deeply invasive grade 3 disease and patients with stage II disease were excluded, while patients with relatively favorable stage IB grade 2 disease were included; surgical staging was not systematically performed. Even more important, a pathology review performed after the initial analysis demonstrated that the initial grade assignments (frequently made in small community facilities) were often incorrect (Figure 31.2). For the 569 patients whose specimens were available, following pathology review, the percentage deemed to have grade 1 disease increased from 21% to 69%; 24% of the cases reviewed did not meet the trial's eligibility criteria because they had minimally invasive grade 1 disease. The assigned depth of invasion was not reviewed, so the accuracy of this measure is unknown. Unfortunately, the number of patients in this trial who had intermediate-risk grade 2–3 disease was small, and therefore any possible impact of adjuvant treatment in this subgroup would have been difficult to detect.

A third study, published in 2009 [67], was reported as a meta-analysis of 905 patients gathered from a small National Cancer Institute of Canada trial and an ASTEC trial that accrued some patients through the ASTEC lymphadenectomy trial and other patients from outside the lymphadenectomy trial. Patients were randomized after hysterectomy to receive adjuvant pelvic radiation therapy or 'observation.' However, more than half of the patients

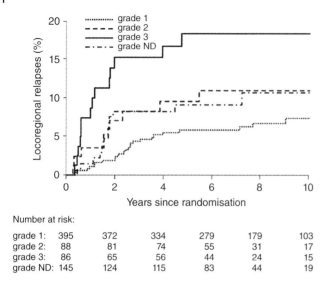

Number at risk:

grade 1:	395	372	334	279	179	103
grade 2:	88	81	74	55	31	17
grade 3:	86	65	56	44	24	15
grade ND:	145	124	115	83	44	19

Figure 31.2 Impact of grade on local-regional relapse. Reproduced from Ref. [58] with permission from Elsevier.

in the 'observation' arm had vaginal cuff brachytherapy. In general, patients were eligible if they had FIGO (1988) stage IC or IIA (any grade) or stage IA-B grade 3 disease; however, patients found at surgical staging to have positive nodes or peritoneal washings were not excluded, so some patients with stage III disease were included in the trial. Most patients did not have surgical staging, and as with the PORTEC trials, there was no central pathology review. The results of the trial were similar to those of GOG 99 and PORTEC-1; patients who had pelvic radiation therapy had a decreased local recurrence rate, but there was no significant difference in overall survival between the two treatment arms.

All three of these trials, then, demonstrated an improvement in local control without a significant improvement in overall survival when adjuvant pelvic radiation therapy was added to hysterectomy. In all three trials, there was a significantly higher rate of treatment-related side effects, particularly bowel side effects, in patients who had adjuvant radiation therapy [40, 64, 67]. It is safe to conclude that, at least for patients with low intermediate risk disease, the benefit of pelvic radiation therapy is at most very slight and does not justify the side effects of pelvic radiation therapy. A subset analysis of GOG 99 did suggest that patients who had high intermediate risk disease may benefit from radiation therapy [40]. Unfortunately, the broad eligibility criteria for all three trials and the lack of central pathology review in the PORTEC and ASTEC trials limited the ability of these trials to ascertain the value of pelvic radiation therapy in patients with high intermediate risk disease – specifically those with combinations of deep myometrial invasion, LVSI, high grade, or advanced age.

In these trials, the most frequent site of local recurrence was the vagina. It was therefore logical to ask

whether vaginal cuff irradiation could achieve a similar local control benefit with fewer side effects than pelvic radiation therapy. This question had been addressed in a very early trial from the Norwegian Radium Hospital, published in 1980 [68]. The trial appeared to demonstrate an improvement in pelvic disease control, but no difference in survival when adjuvant irradiation of the vaginal cuff and pelvis was compared with adjuvant irradiation of the vaginal cuff only; subset analysis suggested a possible advantage for patients with deeply invasive grade 3 disease. However, most of the patients in this trial had very favorable disease, and the number of patients was small; these and other factors limited the generalizability of the results to modern practice.

The question of whether vaginal cuff irradiation was equivalent to pelvic irradiation in terms of local control was asked again in PORTEC-2, a trial that randomly assigned patients with 'high intermediate risk' endometrial cancer to receive either pelvic external beam or vaginal cuff irradiation after hysterectomy [65]. When the trial was analyzed in 2010, the primary endpoint of vaginal recurrence rate was not significantly different between the two arms. The overall rate of pelvic recurrence was only 4% in the vaginal cuff radiation therapy arm, but was less than 1% with pelvic radiation therapy (P = 0.02); however, the projected overall survival rates were not significantly different at five years. An important question is whether the patients in this trial really should have been termed high intermediate risk. The outcome of those treated with pelvic radiation therapy was nearly identical to the outcome of patients in the similar arm of PORTEC-1. From the start, the PORTEC definition of 'high intermediate risk' differed from that used by the GOG (Table 31.2), most notably in the exclusion of patients who had deeply invasive grade 3 disease. Central pathology review was not performed before patient entry, and as in PORTEC-1 the subsequent pathology review revealed very poor agreement between the reviewing pathologists' and the community practitioners' diagnoses. In particular, after pathology review, the percentage of patients with grade 1 disease shifted from 48.5% to 78.6%; after review, only 9% of patients had grade 2 disease and 12% had grade 3 disease. The accuracy of the outside assessments of depth of myometrial invasion was not assessed. PORTEC-2 did indicate that vaginal cuff brachytherapy is as effective as pelvic radiation therapy in many cases. However, because of the small number of patients with grade 2 or 3 disease, the trial failed to provide clear guidance about the role of radiation therapy in such patients.

Although robust level-1 data to guide treatment of some subgroups are still lacking, trials completed during the past decade have helped clinicians reduce the number of patients exposed unnecessarily to the side effects of radiation therapy. Patients with ≤50% myometrial invasion, grade 1 disease rarely, if ever, require any

Table 31.2 High intermediate risk criteria according used in the Gynecologic Oncology Group (GOG) and PORTEC studies.

Gynecologic Oncology Group:
- Any patient with grade 2–3, LVSI, and outer-third myometrial invasion.
- Aged ≥50 years with two of these features.
- Aged ≥70 years with one of these features.

PORTEC-2:
- Aged >60 years with grade 3 or outer-half myometrial invasion.*
- Any patient with stage IIA disease†

*Patients with deeply invasive grade 3 disease were not eligible for the trial.
†Patients with FIGO IIA disease at the time of this trial would now be classified as having FIGO (2009) stage I disease. Patients who had FIGO (1988) stage IIB disease (now classified as FIGO (2009) stage II disease) were not eligible for the PORTEC-2 trial.

form of radiation therapy. Those with grade 2 disease with ≤50% myometrial invasion can be observed or treatment with vagina cuff brachytherapy. Without cuff irradiation, the risk of vaginal recurrence may be as high as 25–30% for patients with grade 3 disease, even with minimal myometrial invasion [64]. Vaginal cuff radiation therapy is probably also sufficient for patient with grade 1 disease with >50% myometrial invasion, particularly in the absence of LVSI or other high-risk features. The optimal treatment for patients with deeply invasive grade 2 or 3 disease is still uncertain. Most of these patients should receive at least vaginal cuff irradiation; the decision whether to treat the whole pelvis is generally influenced by the number and nature of adverse features present in the hysterectomy specimen, and the extent of the surgical staging. Patients with deeply invasive grade 2 or 3 tumors who have not had a node dissection are generally treated with pelvic radiation, since the potential for microscopically involved nodes is significant [69]. These patients should receive a pelvic and abdomen CT prior to radiation, to ensure that no grossly involved lymph nodes are identified.

The role of chemotherapy for patients with high intermediate risk disease is as yet untested. In 2008, the Japanese Gynecologic Oncology Group published results of a randomized trial [70] comparing adjuvant pelvic radiation therapy versus chemotherapy (cisplatin, doxorubicin, and cyclophosphamide) for patients with intermediate-risk or high-risk endometrial cancer. The number of patients was relatively small (385 of the 475 enrolled patients were deemed eligible and evaluable for analysis), the eligibility criteria were broad (stage IC–IIIC), and there was no central pathology review. There was no significant difference in progression-free or overall survival between patients in the two arms, although a subset analysis of 101 patients in the higher-risk categories suggested a possible benefit from chemotherapy. GOG 0249 compared pelvic radiation therapy versus a combination of vaginal cuff irradiation and chemotherapy with carboplatin and paclitaxel in patients with high intermediate risk disease. Early reports on this study

reported no significant difference in outcome between the two arms with a higher rate of acute toxicity in patients treated with chemotherapy (SGO 2014).

High-Risk Disease

Various definitions of high-risk endometrial cancer have been applied in clinical trials. Stage III cancers are generally included, in addition to some lower-stage cancers with high-risk histology such as serous and clear-cell cancers. As a result, patients with high-risk disease are a highly diverse group with a wide range of risks for pelvic recurrence. This heterogeneity can make it difficult to interpret results of trials of 'high-risk' disease. Stage IIIA is a particularly diverse group, which includes patients with ovarian involvement and involvement of the uterine serosa. In the FIGO staging system, patients with tumor cells in peritoneal washings were classified as having stage III disease until 2009, when peritoneal washings were removed from the staging system; as a result, many published studies of stage III endometrial cancer include patients who would not be considered stage III in the current staging system. Partially on account of this heterogeneity, the optimal treatment for high-risk endometrial cancer remains poorly defined [36].

Pelvic or para-aortic metastasis is the most common reason for classification of endometrial cancer as stage III. Some 8% of all patients with endometrial cancer present with positive nodes. The FIGO 2009 staging system split stage IIIC into stage IIIC1, which includes patients with pelvic but not para-aortic metastasis, and stage IIIC2, which includes patients with para-aortic metastasis with or without pelvic metastasis. Pelvic metastasis without para-aortic metastasis is the most common presentation of IIIC disease. Approximately 25% of patients present with both pelvic and para-aortic disease, and less than one-fourth of patients present with para-aortic disease only. This distribution of disease suggests that it is important to surgically evaluate both the pelvic and para-aortic nodes at the time of lymphadenectomy. Interestingly, compared to patients with lymphatic metastasis and other pathologic findings indicating stage III disease, such as ovarian or uterine serosal invasion, patients with lymphatic metastasis without such other pathologic findings have a better prognosis. Five-year survival rates >80% have been reported for these patients with best therapy, highlighting the importance of aggressive treatment of patients with stage IIIC cancer.

Adjuvant Therapy for Stage III Disease

Although the optimal adjuvant therapy for patients with stage III disease remains a subject of much debate, the best evidence suggests that combined-modality adjuvant therapy with site-directed radiation therapy and chemotherapy provides the best outcomes.

Radiation therapy and chemotherapy were compared in GOG 122. This study randomized 388 patients with stage III or IV endometrial cancer to adjuvant chemotherapy (doxorubicin and cisplatin) or whole-abdomen radiation therapy. Whole-abdomen radiation therapy was delivered to 30 Gy in 20 fractions, with an additional boost of 15 Gy delivered to the pelvis or extended fields including para-aortic nodes. Rates of progression-free survival were significantly higher in the chemotherapy arm than in the whole-abdomen radiation therapy arm (five-year progression-free survival rate, 50% versus 38%). The proportion of patients with stage IV disease was higher in the chemotherapy arm, so the reported results were 'stage-adjusted,' which is the type of post hoc analysis that is generally avoided in randomized Phase III studies. A major limitation of the study was the inclusion of patients with intraperitoneal disease, including unresected lesions up to 2 cm. These patients are unlikely to benefit from radiation therapy because the whole abdomen is limited to 30 Gy which is not an adequate dose to treat microscopic disease, and gross disease within the peritoneum is difficult if not impossible to treat to tumoricidal doses without excessive toxic effects. As a result, the radiation therapy doses were inadequate for many patients. Despite the limitations of this study, it established a role for chemotherapy in the treatment of endometrial cancer.

This study and others have reported that 30–50% of patients with node-positive endometrial cancer who are treated with chemotherapy without external beam will develop a pelvic relapse [43, 71, 72]. This result suggests that adjuvant radiation therapy should be combined with adjuvant chemotherapy in patients with stage III disease.

Two other prospective randomized studies have been reported that compared chemotherapy to radiation therapy for high-risk endometrial cancer. Maggi *et al.* [73] conducted a randomized trial comparing adjuvant chemotherapy to adjuvant radiation therapy. The study enrolled 345 patients with deeply invasive grade 3 tumors and stage III endometrial cancer limited to the pelvis.

Chemotherapy consisted of five cycles of cisplatin, doxorubicin, and cyclophosphamide. Patients on the radiation therapy arm received 45–50 Gy to the pelvis. There was no significant difference in overall or progression-free survival between the pelvic radiation therapy and chemotherapy arms, but there was a non-significant trend towards delayed metastasis in the chemotherapy arm and delayed pelvic relapse in the radiation therapy arm. This study enrolled a more homogeneous group of patients than GOG 122: patients with uterine serous carcinoma or peritoneal disease were not included. Additionally, the radiation therapy was more similar to the current standard pelvic or extended-field radiation therapy. The pattern-of-relapse data suggested that combined-modality treatment may be the optimal approach, which is the focus of ongoing investigations. The second randomized study comparing chemotherapy to pelvic radiation therapy for high-risk endometrial cancer was conducted in Japan. In this trial, patients were randomized to cyclophosphamide, doxorubicin, and cisplatin or pelvic radiation therapy [74]. This study enrolled patients with stage 1C endometrial cancer with >50% invasion through stage IIIC endometrial cancer. The majority (77.4%) of the registered patients had stage IC or II lesions, and only 11.9% had stage IIIC lesions. There was no significant difference between the chemotherapy and radiation therapy groups in overall or progression-free survival, or pattern of relapse. A high-risk subset was identified that had improved progression-free survival with chemotherapy. However, the study was not stratified for analysis of this subset, nor was this a planned subset analysis, which limits the utility of this observation.

Hogberg *et al.* [75] reported on the role of combined radiation therapy and chemotherapy delivered using a sequential approach for patients with high-risk endometrial cancer. These investigators conducted two independent randomized studies: one was conducted in Milan at the Instituted Mario Negri, and the other was conducted by the European Organization for Research and Treatment of Cancer. There were differences in the eligibility criteria and the chemotherapy regimen used, but both studies included patients with high-risk stage I–III endometrial cancer with no residual tumor following hysterectomy. Patients were randomized to radiation therapy alone or radiation therapy followed by chemotherapy. The patients who received combined-modality treatment had a 36% reduction in recurrence and improved cancer-specific survival.

The optimal sequencing of combined-modality treatment remains unknown. A retrospective study at Duke University compared the outcome of women treated with different sequences of chemotherapy and radiation therapy. After controlling for stage, age, grade, race, histology, and cytoreduction status, overall survival was best in patients treated with chemotherapy followed by radiation therapy followed by additional chemotherapy (referred to as the 'sandwich approach') [76]. This strategy has the advantage of ensuring that radiation therapy does not compromise the ability to deliver adjuvant chemotherapy. A disadvantage is that radiation therapy is that radiotherapy is delayed beyond the immediate postoperative period, which may negatively impact local control.

Concurrent chemotherapy and radiotherapy followed by adjuvant chemotherapy was studied in a Phase II trial conducted by the Radiation Therapy Oncology Group [77] and was found to be feasible with acceptable toxicity. This regimen is also being used in GOG 0258, which is comparing combined-modality treatment to chemotherapy alone for patients with high-risk endometrial cancer. While awaiting maturation of these data, the optimal adjuvant treatment for high-risk endometrial cancer is tailored radiation therapy with or without concurrent cisplatin chemotherapy and adjuvant chemotherapy, which may be delivered following radiation therapy or both before and after radiation therapy (the 'sandwich' arrangement).

Technique

External Beam Radiation Therapy

Pelvic radiation therapy for adjuvant treatment of endometrial cancer targets the vaginal apex and pelvic lymphatics, and is typically delivered with either IMRT or a four-field approach using at least 10-MV photons. The superior border for a patient with negative nodes or involvement of only pelvic nodes is typically set at L4/5 or the aortic bifurcation. In a patient with positive para-aortic nodes, the superior border is extended to the top of T12. The lateral borders are generally set 2 cm lateral to the internal pelvic brim. The inferior border is at the inferior aspect of the obturator foramen, which results in treatment of 4-6 cm of the vagina. The anterior border of the lateral field is at the tip of the pubic symphysis, and the posterior border is set at the posterior aspect of S2. If the cervix is grossly involved, the posterior border can be moved back at least one vertebral body to the back of S3.

Toxicity of Pelvic Radiation Therapy

Acute gastrointestinal symptoms during pelvic radiation therapy typically involve varying degrees of diarrhea, cramping, and abdominal pain, which can negatively affect quality of life during treatment. Between 50% and 90% of patients treated with standard pelvic radiation therapy develop diarrhea that necessitates medication [78]. Chronic gastrointestinal symptoms are also not uncommon: approximately one-half of patients treated with standard pelvic radiation therapy have at least mild chronic bowel symptoms [79]. The impact on quality of life was studied in PORTEC-2, which randomized patients to vaginal brachytherapy versus pelvic radiation therapy. Patients treated with pelvic irradiation had higher rates of diarrhea limiting daily activities, which affected social functioning during radiation therapy [80].

Intensity-modulated radiotherapy (IMRT) may be useful in reducing the toxicity of pelvic radiation therapy. IMRT can be used to limit the dose to the bladder, bowel, and bone marrow while treating the vagina and pelvic lymphatics. The volume of bowel irradiated to 30–45 Gy can be reduced by 50–67% compared to the volume irradiated with standard four-field treatment [81–83]. A comparison of the dose distribution in a standard plan as compared to IMRT is shown in Figure 31.3. The target volumes, the nodal CTV and vaginal PTV, lie within the border of standard fields used for pelvic radiation (Figure 31.4). Clinical studies suggest that the reduction in dose to the small bowel with IMRT is associated with lower

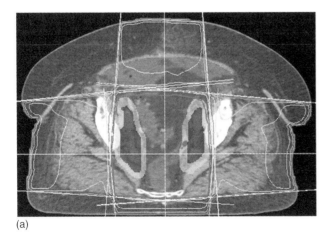
(a)

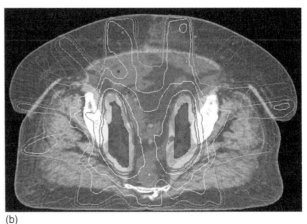
(b)

Figure 31.3 Standard three-dimensional conformal irradiation (a) requires treatment of small bowel (contoured in brown) which can be spared with IMRT (b). For a color version of this figure, see the color plate section.

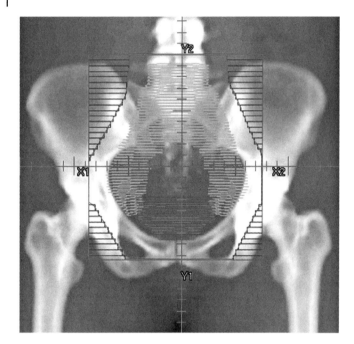
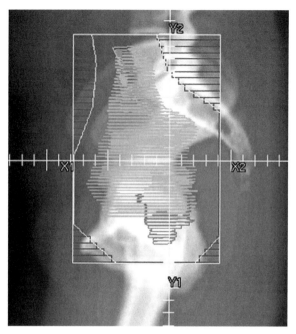

Figure 31.4 Examples of standard AP and lateral fields for pelvic radiation. Contours used for IMRT planning are shown as wireframe on the DRRs. The green contours represent the pelvic nodal CTV and the red volume is the vaginal CTV. For a color version of this figure, see the color plate section.

rates of both acute and chronic gastrointestinal symptoms. Mundt *et al.* reported a lower rate of acute grade 2 gastrointestinal side effects in 40 patients treated with IMRT than in patients treated at the same institution with conventional whole-pelvis radiation therapy (60% versus 91%, P = 0.002) [78] In addition, IMRT appears to reduce chronic gastrointestinal symptoms [79,84]. IMRT can also be used to spare the bone marrow, which can reduce rates of hematologic toxic effects [85]. The feasibility of delivering pelvic IMRT was investigated on the RTOG 0418 study [86]. NRG 1203 (TIME-C) randomized patients with endometrial and cervical cancer with indications for postoperative pelvic radiation to IMRT or standard four-field radiation. Patients receiving IMRT had less gastrointestinal and urinary toxicity as compared to patients treated with standard four-field radiation [87].

Vaginal Brachytherapy

Intracavitary vaginal brachytherapy can be used to treat the vaginal mucosa to prevent recurrence. Vaginal brachytherapy can be used as the only component of radiation therapy for patients in whom the vaginal cuff, and not the pelvis, is the primary site of recurrence risk. Vaginal cuff brachytherapy can also be used in addition to pelvic radiation therapy to deliver additional radiation to the vaginal apex.

The primary technical concern is ensuring that the vaginal dome abuts the vaginal apex and is in contact with the mucosal surface [88,89]. Several types of vaginal applicators have been developed to accomplish this. The vagina after surgery is typically cylindrical and is often treated with a vaginal cylinder containing a single central line of sources. Vaginal cylinders generally range in size from 2 to 4 cm. The size of the dome should be optimized. A dome too large will not pass to the apex, while a dome which is too small may allow the vaginal mucosa to collapse and form pockets of vaginal mucosa, which will not receive an adequate dose. When the incision creates a pocket at the right and left aspects of the vaginal apex, ovoids may provide better coverage of apical vaginal mucosa. Imaging should be performed to verify that the dome is up against the apex. One approach to accomplish this is to place a radio-opaque marker at the apex of the vagina and verify that the cylinder abuts the marker using an anteroposterior film. Alternatively, CT can be performed to verify placement. Imaging can also be used to evaluate doses to normal tissues and to optimize dwell positions. CT planning allows optimization of doses delivered to the bladder and rectum [88].

Vaginal brachytherapy when planned with standard regimens delivers a minimal dose to the bladder, rectum and bowel, and the risk of complications is consequently low. In a randomized study in patients with low-risk endometrial cancer treated with no therapy or vaginal brachytherapy, vaginal brachytherapy had minimal side effects [90]. A small increase in mild vaginal and urinary side effects, but not gastrointestinal side effects, was seen in the brachytherapy arm compared to the untreated control arm. Given these low rates of side effects, there is little opportunity for dosimetric optimization to produce a measurable reduction in toxicity [89, 90].

A wide range of regimens have been recommended for prophylactic vaginal apex brachytherapy [89]. The American Brachytherapy Society recommends that the dose delivered be reported to the surface as well as to 0.5 mm. Commonly prescribed regimens include 7 Gy in three fractions prescribed to 5 mm depth, or 6 Gy in five fractions prescribed to the vaginal surface, as is used at M.D. Anderson. When a regimen of 7 Gy in three fractions is prescribed, it is most commonly delivered weekly, whereas the M.D. Anderson regimen (6 Gy in five fractions) is delivered every other day over one-and-a-half weeks. Sorbe *et al.* [90] demonstrated that the delivery of a higher dose increased the toxicity of treatment but did not have a detectable effect on disease control. A total of 290 patients was randomized to either 5 Gy in five fractions prescribed to 5 mm, or 2.5 Gy in five fractions prescribed to 5 mm [91]. No difference in vaginal recurrence rates was detected. Vaginal length, as measured with colpometry, was significantly reduced in patients who received the higher dose per fraction, and rates of mucosal atrophy and bleeding were also higher in the group that received the higher dose per fraction.

At least the upper third of the vagina is treated to cover the scar and a margin around it. For patients at high risk, such as patients with grade 3 tumor or serous cancers, a longer length of vagina may be treated.

Radiation Therapy for Patients with Inoperable Disease

Although hysterectomy with or without adjuvant radiation therapy is the standard treatment for clinical stage I endometrial carcinoma, patients who are at very high risk for major complications from surgery can be effectively treated with radiation therapy alone. With this approach, disease-specific survival rates of 80% and uterine control rates of 70–80% have been reported [92–95]. Prognosis tends to be correlated with clinical stage and grade, but intercurrent disease is the most common cause of death in these patients [93].

Before the decision can be made whether to proceed with definitive radiation therapy for endometrial cancer, surgical risks as well as risks due to radiation treatment must be considered. In general, if the risks of major morbidity and mortality from surgery are greater than 5–10%, radiation therapy alone should be strongly considered as a treatment option. If there is a post-radiation therapy uterine recurrence, the risk-benefit ratio for surgery should be reconsidered.

For definitive radiation therapy, a combination of pelvic radiation therapy and brachytherapy is most commonly used. Some patients with a small uterus and low-grade tumors have been treated with brachytherapy without external beam radiation therapy (EBRT) [93]. However, since the risk of nodal involvement is very difficult to assess with clinical staging, the most common approach is to treat the pelvis to approximately 45 Gy and then deliver brachytherapy. Brachytherapy for endometrial cancer is different in several ways from brachytherapy for cervical cancer. A broader radiation dose distribution in the region of the fundus is typically required. In a woman with a small uterus, this can be accomplished with differential loading of the tip of an intrauterine tandem. In a woman with a larger uterus, two tandems curving away from one another into the cornua of the uterus can be used. A series of Y-shaped applicators have been designed with two diverging curved intrauterine tandems that lock together in the vagina [94]. Alternatively, the uterus can be filled with Heyman's capsules, which are placed throughout the uterine cavity to provide a broader dose distribution, especially for women with a larger uterine cavity. However, limited availability of these sources has reduced the use of this approach [94, 95]. Generally, the vagina and parametrium are not at significant risk and require lower doses than are delivered with brachytherapy for cervical cancer.

A variety of different methods have been described for prescribing dose in patients treated with definitive radiation therapy[12]. When available, CT and MRI may allow optimization of dose to improve target coverage and reduce the dose to normal tissues [96]. With this approach using fractionated HDR, the mean D_{90} to the CTV encompassing the uterus and upper 1–2 cm of the vagina was 72 Gy (EQD2) when EBRT was combined with brachytherapy. The D_{90} EQD2 dose to the GTV for these patients was 172.3 ± 59.6 Gy, reflecting the small GTV volumes for many patients with small tumors in the endometrial cavity lying along the length of the tandem. The two-year local control and survival in this cohort was 90.6% and 94.4%, respectively. With low-dose-rate irradiation, uterine applicators are commonly loaded with 45- to 50-mg radium equivalents for two 48-h treatments after 40–45 Gy is delivered to the whole pelvis. With this approach, reported control rates have been high and complication rates low. Alternatively, some investigators prescribe a dose at 1 cm from the sources or, when a 'Y' applicator is used, to a uterine point midway between the tip of the two intrauterine tandems [97]. The vagina does not require as high a dose as in patients with cervical cancer unless there is cervical stromal involvement. For a clinical stage I tumor, source loadings that yield a vaginal surface dose of 60–90 Gy should be sufficient to prevent vaginal recurrence in most patients.

References

1 Miller, K.D., *et al.* (2016) Cancer treatment and survivorship statistics, 2016. *CA Cancer J. Clin.*, **66** (4), 271–289.

2 Di Cristofano, A., Ellenson, L.H. (2007) Endometrial carcinoma. *Annu. Rev. Pathol.*, **2**, 57–85.

3 Creasman, W. (2009) Revised FIGO staging for carcinoma of the endometrium. *Int. J. Gynaecol. Obstet.*, **105**, 109.

4 Friedenreich, C., Cust, A., Lahmann, P.H., *et al.* (2007) Anthropometric factors and risk of endometrial cancer: the European prospective investigation into cancer and nutrition. *Cancer Causes Control*, **18**, 399–413.

5 Fader, A.N., Arriba, L.N., Frasure, H.E., von Gruenigen, V.E. (2009) Endometrial cancer and obesity: epidemiology, biomarkers, prevention and survivorship. *Gynecol. Oncol.*, **114**, 121–127.

6 Schouten, L.J., Goldbohm, R.A., van den Brandt, P.A. (2004) Anthropometry, physical activity, and endometrial cancer risk: results from the Netherlands Cohort Study. *J. Natl Cancer Inst.*, **96**, 1635–1638.

7 Brinton, L.A., Berman, M.L., Mortel, R., *et al.* (1992) Reproductive, menstrual, and medical risk factors for endometrial cancer: results from a case-control study. *Am. J. Obstet. Gynecol.*, **167**, 1317–1325.

8 Dossus, L., Allen, N., Kaaks, R., *et al.* (2010) Reproductive risk factors and endometrial cancer: the European Prospective Investigation into Cancer and Nutrition. *Int. J. Cancer*, **127**, 442–451.

9 Beral, V., Banks, E., Reeves, G. (2002) Evidence from randomised trials on the long-term effects of hormone replacement therapy. *Lancet*, **360**, 942–944.

10 Nelson, H.D., Humphrey, L.L., Nygren, P., Teutsch, S.M., Allan, J.D. (2002) Postmenopausal hormone replacement therapy: scientific review. *JAMA*, **288**, 872–881.

11 Davies, C., *et al.* (2013) Long-term effects of continuing adjuvant tamoxifen to 10 years versus stopping at 5 years after diagnosis of oestrogen receptor-positive breast cancer: ATLAS, a randomised trial. *Lancet*, **381** (9869), 805–816.

12 Cancer Genome Atlas Research (2013) Integrated genomic characterization of endometrial carcinoma. *Nature*, **497** (7447), 67–73.

13 Hussein, Y.R., *et al.* (2015) Clinicopathological analysis of endometrial carcinomas harboring somatic POLE exonuclease domain mutations. *Mod. Pathol.*, **28** (4), 505–514.

14 Yap, O.W., Matthews, R.P. (2006) Racial and ethnic disparities in cancers of the uterine corpus. *J. Natl Med. Assoc.*, **98**, 1930–1933.

15 Hoogendoorn, W.E., Hollema, H., van Boven, H.H., *et al.* (2008) Prognosis of uterine corpus cancer after tamoxifen treatment for breast cancer. *Breast Cancer Res. Treat.*, **112**, 99–108.

16 Amir, E., Seruga, B., Niraula, S., Carlsson, L., Ocana, A. (2011) Toxicity of adjuvant endocrine therapy in postmenopausal breast cancer patients: a systematic review and meta-analysis. *J. Natl Cancer Inst.*, **103**, 1299–1309.

17 Lu, K.H. (2008) Hereditary gynecologic cancers: differential diagnosis, surveillance, management and surgical prophylaxis. *Fam. Cancer*, **7**, 53–58.

18 Lynch, H.T., Lynch, P.M., Lanspa, S.J., *et al.* (2009) Review of the Lynch syndrome: history, molecular genetics, screening, differential diagnosis, and medicolegal ramifications. *Clin. Genet.*, **76**, 1–18.

19 Westin, S.N., Lacour, R.A., Urbauer, D.L., *et al.* (2008) Carcinoma of the lower uterine segment: a newly described association with Lynch syndrome. *J. Clin. Oncol.*, **26**, 5965–5971.

20 Schmeler, K.M., Lynch, H.T., Chen, L.M., *et al.* (2006) Prophylactic surgery to reduce the risk of gynecologic cancers in the Lynch syndrome. *N. Engl. J. Med.*, **354**, 261–269.

21 Gehrig, P.A., Bae-Jump, V.L., Boggess, J.F., *et al.* (2004) Association between uterine serous carcinoma and breast cancer. *Gynecol. Oncol.*, **94**, 208–211.

22 Lavie, O., Ben-Arie, A., Segev, Y., *et al.* (2010) BRCA germline mutations in women with uterine serous carcinoma – still a debate. *Int. J. Gynecol. Cancer*, **20**, 1531–1534.

23 Polesel, J., Serraino, D., Zucchetto, A., *et al.* (2009) Cigarette smoking and endometrial cancer risk: the modifying effect of obesity. *Eur. J. Cancer Prev.*, **18**, 476–481.

24 Gunter, M.J., Schaub, J.A., Xue, X., *et al.* (2011) A prospective investigation of coffee drinking and endometrial cancer incidence. *Int. J. Cancer*, **15**, 530–536.

25 Je, Y., Hankinson, S.E., Tworoger, S.S., Devivo, I., Giovannucci, E. (2011) A prospective cohort study of coffee consumption and risk of endometrial cancer over a 26-year follow-up. *Cancer Epidemiol. Biomarkers Prev.*, **20**, 2487–2495.

26 Clement, P.B., Young, R.H. (2002) Endometrioid carcinoma of the uterine corpus: a review of its pathology with emphasis on recent advances and problematic aspects. *Adv. Anat. Pathol.*, **9**, 145–184.

27 Clement, P.B., Young, R.H. (2004) Non-endometrioid carcinomas of the uterine corpus: a review of their pathology with emphasis on recent advances and problematic aspects. *Adv. Anat. Pathol.*, **11**, 117–142.

28 Goldberg, H., Miller, R.C., Abdah-Bortnyak, R., *et al.* (2008) Outcome after combined modality treatment for uterine papillary serous carcinoma: a study by the Rare Cancer Network (RCN). *Gynecol. Oncol.*, **108**, 298–305.

29 Hendrickson, M., Ross, M., Eifel, P., Martinez, A., Kempson, R. (1982) Uterine papillary serous carcinoma. A highly malignant form of endometrial adenocarcinoma. *Am. J. Surg. Pathol.*, **6**, 93–108.

30 Bristow, R.E., Asrari, F., Trimble, E.L., Montz, F.J. (2001) Extended surgical staging for uterine papillary serous carcinoma: survival outcome of locoregional (Stage I–III) disease. *Gynecol. Oncol.*, **81**, 279–286.

31 Nguyen, N.P., Sallah, S., Karlsson, U., *et al.* (2001) Prognosis for papillary serous carcinoma of the endometrium after surgical staging. *Int. J. Gynecol. Cancer*, **11**, 305–311.

32 Carcangiu, M.L., Chambers, J.T. (1995) Early pathologic stage clear cell carcinoma and uterine papillary serous carcinoma of the endometrium: comparison of clinicopathologic features and survival. *Int. J. Gynecol. Pathol.*, **14**, 30–38.

33 Wada, H., Enomoto, T., Fujita, M., *et al.* (1997) Molecular evidence that most but not all carcinosarcomas of the uterus are combination tumors. *Cancer Res.*, **57**, 5379–5385.

34 Bansal, N., Herzog, T.J., Seshan, V.E., *et al.* (2008) Uterine carcinosarcomas and grade 3 endometrioid cancers: evidence for distinct tumor behavior. *Obstet. Gynecol.*, **112**, 64–70.

35 Callister, M., Ramondetta, L.M., Jhingran, A., Burke, T.W., Eifel, P.J. (2004) Malignant mixed Mullerian tumors of the uterus: analysis of patterns of failure, prognostic factors, and treatment outcome. *Int. J. Radiat. Oncol. Biol. Phys.*, **58**, 786–796.

36 Creasman, W.T., Morrow, C.P., Bundy, B.N., *et al.* (1987) Surgical pathologic spread patterns of endometrial cancer. A Gynecologic Oncology Group Study. *Cancer*, **60**, 2035–2041.

37 Zaino, R.J., Kurman, R.J., Diana, K.L., Morrow, C.P. (1996) Pathologic models to predict outcome for women with endometrial adenocarcinoma: the importance of the distinction between surgical stage and clinical stage – a Gynecologic Oncology Group study. *Cancer*, **77**, 1115–1121.

38 Mariani, A., Webb, M.J., Keeney, G.L., Haddock, M.G., Calori, G., Podratz, K.C. (2000) Low-risk corpus cancer: is lymphadenectomy or radiotherapy necessary? *Am. J. Obstet. Gynecol.*, **182**, 1506–1519.

39 Chang, S.J., Kong, T.W., Kim, W.Y., *et al.* (2011) Lymph-vascular space invasion as a significant risk factor for isolated para-aortic lymph node metastasis in endometrial cancer: a study of 203 consecutive patients. *Ann. Surg. Oncol.*, **18**, 58–64.

40 Keys, H.M., Roberts, J.A., Brunetto, V.L., *et al.* (2004) A phase III trial of surgery with or without adjunctive external pelvic radiation therapy in intermediate risk endometrial adenocarcinoma: a Gynecologic Oncology Group study. *Gynecol. Oncol.*, **92**, 744–751.

41 Hachisuga, T., Kaku, T., Fukuda, K., *et al.* (1999) The grading of lymphovascular space invasion in endometrial carcinoma. *Cancer*, **86**, 2090–2097.

42 Garg, G., Morris, R.T., Solomon, L., *et al.* (2011) Evaluating the significance of location of lymph node metastasis and extranodal disease in women with stage IIIC endometrial cancer. *Gynecol. Oncol.*, **123**, 208–213.

43 Klopp, A.H., Jhingran, A., Ramondetta, L., Lu, K., Gershenson, D.M., Eifel, P.J. (2009) Node-positive adenocarcinoma of the endometrium: outcome and patterns of recurrence with and without external beam irradiation. *Gynecol. Oncol.*, **115**, 6–11.

44 Eifel, P., Hendrickson, M., Ross, J., Ballon, S., Martinez, A., Kempson, R. (1982) Simultaneous presentation of carcinoma involving the ovary and the uterine corpus. *Cancer*, **50**, 163–170.

45 Singh, N. (2010) Synchronous tumours of the female genital tract. *Histopathology*, **56**, 277–285.

46 Culton, L.K., Deavers, M.T., Silva, E.G., Liu, J., Malpica, A. (2006) Endometrioid carcinoma simultaneously involving the uterus and the fallopian tube: a clinicopathologic study of 13 cases. *Am. J. Surg. Pathol.*, **30**, 844–849.

47 Dotters, D.J. (2000) Preoperative CA 125 in endometrial cancer: is it useful? *Am. J. Obstet. Gynecol.*, **182**, 1328–1334.

48 Jacobs, I., Gentry-Maharaj, A., Burnell, M., *et al.* (2011) Sensitivity of transvaginal ultrasound screening for endometrial cancer in postmenopausal women: a case-control study within the UKCTOCS cohort. *Lancet Oncol.*, **12**, 38–48.

49 Shin, K.E., Park, B.K., Kim, C.K., Bae, D.S., Song, S.Y., Kim, B. (2011) MR staging accuracy for endometrial cancer based on the new FIGO stage. *Acta Radiol.*, **52**, 818–824.

50 Ramirez, P.T., Frumovitz, M., Milam, M.R., *et al.* (2010) Limited utility of magnetic resonance imaging in determining the primary site of disease in patients with inconclusive endometrial biopsy. *Int. J. Gynecol. Cancer*, **20**, 1344–1349.

51 Spencer, J.A., Messiou, C., Swift, S.E. (2008) MR staging of endometrial cancer: needed or wanted? *Cancer Imaging*, **8**, 1–5.

52 Walker, J.L., Piedmonte, M.R., Spirtos, N.M., *et al.* (2009) Laparoscopy compared with laparotomy for comprehensive surgical staging of uterine cancer: Gynecologic Oncology Group Study LAP2. *J. Clin. Oncol.*, **27**, 5331–5336.

53 Benedetti Panici, P., Basile, S., Maneschi, F., *et al.* (2008) Systematic pelvic lymphadenectomy vs. no lymphadenectomy in early-stage endometrial carcinoma: randomized clinical trial. *J. Natl Cancer Inst.*, **100**, 1707–1716.

54 Kitchener, H., Swart, A.M., Qian, Q., Amos, C., Parmar, M.K. (2009) Efficacy of systematic pelvic lymphadenectomy in endometrial cancer (MRC ASTEC trial): a randomised study. *Lancet*, **373**, 125–136.

55 Chan, J.K., Urban, R., Cheung, M.K., *et al.* (2007) Lymphadenectomy in endometrioid uterine cancer staging: how many lymph nodes are enough? A study of 11,443 patients. *Cancer*, **109**, 2454–2460.

56 Smith, D.C., Macdonald, O.K., Lee, C.M., Gaffney, D.K. (2008) Survival impact of lymph node dissection in endometrial adenocarcinoma: a surveillance, epidemiology, and end results analysis. *Int. J. Gynecol. Cancer*, **18**, 255–261.

57 Kang, S., Yoo, H.J., Hwang, J.H., Lim, M.C., Seo, S.S., Park, S.Y. (2011) Sentinel lymph node biopsy in endometrial cancer: meta-analysis of 26 studies. *Gynecol. Oncol.*, **123**, 522–527.

58 Abu-Rustum, N.R. (2014) Update on sentinel node mapping in uterine cancer: 10-year experience at Memorial Sloan-Kettering Cancer Center. *J. Obstet. Gynaecol. Res.*, **40** (2), 327–334.

59 Khoury-Collado, F., *et al.* (2009) Improving sentinel lymph node detection rates in endometrial cancer: how many cases are needed? *Gynecol. Oncol.*, **115** (3), 453–455.

60 Morrow, C.P., Bundy, B.N., Kurman, R.J., *et al.* (1991) Relationship between surgical-pathological risk factors and outcome in clinical stage I and II carcinoma of the endometrium: a Gynecologic Oncology Group study. *Gynecol. Oncol.*, **40**, 55–65.

61 Creutzberg, C.L., van Putten, W.L., Koper, P.C., *et al.* (2003) Survival after relapse in patients with endometrial cancer: results from a randomized trial. *Gynecol. Oncol.*, **89**, 201–209.

62 Jhingran, A., Burke, T.W., Eifel, P.J. (2003) Definitive radiotherapy for patients with isolated vaginal recurrence of endometrial carcinoma after hysterectomy. *Int. J. Radiat. Oncol. Biol. Phys.*, **56**, 1366–1372.

63 Sorbe, B., *et al.* (2009) Intravaginal brachytherapy in FIGO stage I low-risk endometrial cancer: a controlled randomized study. *Int. J. Gynecol. Cancer*, **19** (5), 873–878.

64 Creutzberg, C.L., van Putten, W.L., Koper, P.C., *et al.* (2000) Surgery and postoperative radiotherapy versus surgery alone for patients with stage-1 endometrial carcinoma: multicentre randomised trial. PORTEC Study Group. Post Operative Radiation Therapy in Endometrial Carcinoma. *Lancet*, **355**, 1404–1411.

65 Nout, R.A., Smit, V.T., Putter, H., *et al.* (2010) Vaginal brachytherapy versus pelvic external beam radiotherapy for patients with endometrial cancer of high-intermediate risk (PORTEC-2): an open-label, non-inferiority, randomised trial. *Lancet*, **375**, 816–823.

66 Scholten, A.N., van Putten, W.L., Beerman, H., *et al.* (2005) Postoperative radiotherapy for Stage 1 endometrial carcinoma: Long-term outcome of the randomized PORTEC trial with central pathology review. *Int. J. Radiat. Oncol. Biol. Phys.*, **63**, 834–838.

67 Blake, P., Swart, A.M., Orton, J., *et al.* (2009) Adjuvant external beam radiotherapy in the treatment of endometrial cancer (MRC ASTEC and NCIC CTG EN.5 randomised trials): pooled trial results, systematic review, and meta-analysis. *Lancet*, **373**, 137–146.

68 Aalders, J., Abeler, V., Kolstad, P., Onsrud, M. (1980) Postoperative external irradiation and prognostic parameters in stage I endometrial carcinoma: clinical and histopathologic study of 540 patients. *Obstet. Gynecol.*, **56**, 419–427.

69 Klopp, A., *et al.* (2014) The role of postoperative radiation therapy for endometrial cancer: Executive summary of an American Society for Radiation Oncology evidence-based guideline. *Pract. Radiat. Oncol.*, **4** (3), 137–144.

70 Susumu, N., *et al.* (2008) Randomized phase III trial of pelvic radiotherapy versus cisplatin-based combined chemotherapy in patients with intermediate- and high-risk endometrial cancer: a Japanese Gynecologic Oncology Group study. *Gynecol. Oncol.*, **108** (1), 226–233.

71 Mundt, A.J., McBride, R., Rotmensch, J., Waggoner, S.E., Yamada, S.D., Connell, P.P. (2001) Significant pelvic recurrence in high-risk pathologic stage I–IV endometrial carcinoma patients after adjuvant chemotherapy alone: implications for adjuvant radiation therapy. *Int. J. Radiat. Oncol. Biol. Phys.*, **50**, 1145–1153.

72 Randall, M.E., Spirtos, N.M., Dvoretsky, P. (1995) Whole abdominal radiotherapy versus combination chemotherapy with doxorubicin and cisplatin in advanced endometrial carcinoma (phase III): Gynecologic Oncology Group Study No. 122. *J. Natl Cancer Inst. Monogr.*, 13–15.

73 Maggi, R., Lissoni, A., Spina, F., *et al.* (2006) Adjuvant chemotherapy vs radiotherapy in high-risk endometrial carcinoma: results of a randomised trial. *Br. J. Cancer*, **95**, 266–271.

74 Susumu, N., Sagae, S., Udagawa, Y., Niwa, K., Kuramoto, H., Satoh, S., Kudo, R. (2008) Randomized phase III trial of pelvic radiotherapy versus cisplatin-based combined chemotherapy in patients with intermediate- and high-risk endometrial cancer: a Japanese Gynecologic Oncology Group study. *Gynecol. Oncol.*, **108**, 226–233.

75 Hogberg, T., Signorelli, M., de Oliveira, C.F., *et al.* (2010) Sequential adjuvant chemotherapy and radiotherapy in endometrial cancer – results from two randomised studies. *Eur. J. Cancer*, **46**, 2422–2431.

76 Secord, A.A., Havrilesky, L.J., O'Malley, D.M., *et al.* (2009) A multicenter evaluation of sequential multimodality therapy and clinical outcome for the treatment of advanced endometrial cancer. *Gynecol. Oncol.*, **114**, 442–447.

77 Greven, K., Winter, K., Underhill, K., Fontenesci, J., Cooper, J., Burke, T. (2004) Preliminary analysis of RTOG 9708: Adjuvant postoperative radiotherapy combined with cisplatin/paclitaxel chemotherapy after surgery for patients with high-risk endometrial cancer. *Int. J. Radiat. Oncol. Biol. Phys.*, **59**, 168–173.

78 Mundt, A.J., Lujan, A.E., Rotmensch, J., *et al.* (2002) Intensity-modulated whole pelvic radiotherapy in women with gynecologic malignancies. *Int. J. Radiat. Oncol. Biol. Phys.*, **52**, 1330–1337.

79 Mundt, A.J., Mell, L.K., Roeske, J.C. (2003) Preliminary analysis of chronic gastrointestinal toxicity in gynecology patients treated with intensity-modulated whole pelvic radiation therapy. *Int. J. Radiat. Oncol. Biol. Phys.*, **56**, 1354–1360.

80 Nout, R.A., Putter, H., Jurgenliemk-Schulz, I.M., *et al.* (2009) Quality of life after pelvic radiotherapy or vaginal brachytherapy for endometrial cancer: first results of the randomized PORTEC-2 trial. *J. Clin. Oncol.*, **27**, 3547–3556.

81 Heron, D.E., Gerszten, K., Selvaraj, R.N., *et al.* (2003) Conventional 3D conformal versus intensity-modulated radiotherapy for the adjuvant treatment of gynecologic malignancies: a comparative dosimetric study of dose-volume histograms small star, filled. *Gynecol. Oncol.*, **91**, 39–45.

82 Portelance, L., Chao, K.S., Grigsby, P.W., Bennet, H., Low, D. (2001) Intensity-modulated radiation therapy (IMRT) reduces small bowel, rectum, and bladder doses in patients with cervical cancer receiving pelvic and para-aortic irradiation. *Int. J. Radiat. Oncol. Biol. Phys.*, **51**, 261–266.

83 Roeske, J.C., Lujan, A., Rotmensch, J., Waggoner, S.E., Yamada, D., Mundt, A.J. (2000) Intensity-modulated whole pelvic radiation therapy in patients with gynecologic malignancies. *Int. J. Radiat. Oncol. Biol. Phys.*, **48**, 1613–1621.

84 Hasselle, M.D., *et al.* (2011) Clinical outcomes of intensity-modulated pelvic radiation therapy for carcinoma of the cervix. *Int. J. Radiat. Oncol. Biol. Phys.*, **80** (5), 1436–1445.

85 Mell, L.K., Schomas, D.A., Salama, J.K., *et al.* (2008) Association between bone marrow dosimetric parameters and acute hematologic toxicity in anal cancer patients treated with concurrent chemotherapy and intensity-modulated radiotherapy. *Int. J. Radiat. Oncol. Biol. Phys.*, **70**, 1431–1437.

86 Klopp, A.H., *et al.* (2013) Hematologic toxicity in RTOG 0418: a phase 2 study of postoperative IMRT for gynecologic cancer. *Int. J. Radiat. Oncol. Biol. Phys.*, **86** (1), 83–90.

87 Klopp, A.H., Yeung, A.R., Deshmukh, S., *et al.* (2016) A Phase III randomized trial comparing patient-reported toxicity and quality of life (QOL) during pelvic intensity modulated radiation therapy as compared to conventional radiation therapy. *Int. J. Radiat. Oncol. Biol. Phys.*, **96** (2S), S3.

88 Kim, H., Houser, C., Beriwal, S. (2012) Is there any advantage to three-dimensional planning for vaginal cuff brachytherapy? *Brachytherapy*, **11** (5), 398–401.

89 Small, W., Jr, Beriwal, S., Demanes, D.J., *et al.* (2012) American Brachytherapy Society consensus guidelines for adjuvant vaginal cuff brachytherapy after hysterectomy. *Brachytherapy*, **11**, 58–67.

90 Sorbe, B., Nordstrom, B., Maenpaa, J., *et al.* (2009) Intravaginal brachytherapy in FIGO stage I low-risk endometrial cancer: a controlled randomized study. *Int. J. Gynecol. Cancer*, **19**, 873–878.

91 Sorbe, B., Straumits, A., Karlsson, L. (2005) Intravaginal high-dose-rate brachytherapy for stage I endometrial cancer: a randomized study of two dose-per-fraction levels. *Int. J. Radiat. Oncol. Biol. Phys.*, **62**, 1385–1389.

92 Inciura, A., Atkocius, V., Juozaityte, E., Vaitkiene, D. (2010) Long-term results of high-dose-rate brachytherapy and external-beam radiotherapy in the primary treatment of endometrial cancer. *J. Radiat. Res. (Tokyo)*, **51**, 675–681.

93 Podzielinski, I., Randall, M.E., Breheny, P.J., *et al.* (2012) Primary radiation therapy for medically inoperable patients with clinical stage I and II endometrial carcinoma. *Gynecol. Oncol.*, **124**, 36–41.

94 Shenfield, C.B., Pearcey, R.G., Ghosh, S., Dundas, G.S. (2009) The management of inoperable Stage I endometrial cancer using intracavitary brachytherapy alone: a 20-year institutional review. *Brachytherapy*, **8**, 278–283.

95 Schwarz, J.K., *et al.* (2015) Consensus statement for brachytherapy for the treatment of medically inoperable endometrial cancer. *Brachytherapy*, **14** (5), 587–599.

96 Coon, D., Beriwal, S., Heron, D.E., *et al.* (2008) High-dose-rate Rotte 'Y' applicator brachytherapy for definitive treatment of medically inoperable endometrial cancer: 10-year results. *Int. J. Radiat. Oncol. Biol. Phys.*, **71**, 779–783.

97 Beriwal, S., Kim, H., Heron, D.E., Selvaraj, R. (2006) Comparison of 2D vs. 3D dosimetry for Rotte 'Y' applicator high dose rate brachytherapy for medically inoperable endometrial cancer. *Technol. Cancer Res. Treat.*, **5**, 521–527.

32

Vulva

Kanokpis Townamchai, Caitlin Newhouse and Akila N. Viswanathan

Etiology and Epidemiology

Vulvar carcinoma occurs in only 2% of women with gynecologic cancer, making it one of the least common types, following uterine and cervical cancer. Most affected women are post-menopausal women with a median age of 65–70 years [1, 2]. Although no single etiologic factor exists, research has identified several potential risk factors for vulvar carcinoma. One such risk factor is a history of malignant or premalignant lesions of the genital tract [3, 4]. Between 2% and 5% of vulvar intraepithelial neoplasms can progress to invasive carcinoma [5]. Several infectious agents have been proposed as possible etiologic agents in vulvar carcinoma, including granulomatous infections, syphilis, herpes simplex virus, and human papillomavirus (HPV) [6]. Immunocompromised patients, such as those with organ transplantation or human immunodeficiency virus (HIV) infection, also have an increased risk of vulvar cancer [7–14].

Recently, investigators have focused on the types of HPV which are associated with neoplasia; one study found that HPV-16 and -18 are most commonly associated with vulvar cancer [15–18]. HPV DNA can be identified in approximately 70% of intraepithelial lesions, but in less than 50% of invasive lesions [19]. Several studies found the p53 mutation to be associated with vulvar cancer, in particular, HPV-negative vulvar carcinomas [18, 20]. However there was no relationship between p53 mutation status and tumor stage [21]. Smoking has been found to increase the risk of vulvar cancer, especially when the patient also has a history of HPV, genital warts, or HIV infection [19, 22].

Both chronic vulvar inflammatory lesions, such as vulvar dystrophy or lichen sclerosis, and squamous intraepithelial lesions have been suggested as precursors of invasive squamous cancers [23]. However, less than 5% of patients with these epithelial alterations will eventually progress to invasive vulvar malignancy [24].

Pathology

Squamous cell carcinoma is the predominant type of vulvar carcinoma, with 90% of cases having squamous features [25]. There are three ways to describe tumor growth patterns for squamous cell carcinoma [25]:

- *Confluent growth* is characteristic of deeply invasive tumors and is associated with stromal desmoplasia.
- *Compact growth* indicates a well-defined tumor and usually minimal stromal desmoplasia.
- *Spray, diffuse or poorly differentiated growth* is characterized by a trabecular appearance, with small islands of poorly differentiated tumor cells found within the dermis or submucosa; it is typically associated with a desmoplastic stromal response and a lymphocytic inflammatory cell infiltration [26].

There are several histopathologic subtypes of squamous cell carcinoma, of which non-keratinizing is the most common. Other common subtypes are keratinizing and basaloid carcinoma. Warty (condylomatous) carcinoma is a subtype associated with HPV, primarily HPV-16. A less-common subtype is acantholytic squamous cell carcinoma (carcinoma with pseudoglandular features), which may have a more aggressive clinical behavior [27]. *Verrucous carcinoma* is an uncommon variant of squamous cell carcinoma with a pushing growth pattern (tumor–dermal interface with minimal stroma between the epithelial elements). Verrucous tumors may be associated with HPV-6 [28]. These tumors typically have an excellent prognosis, and metastasis is uncommon.

Clinical Radiation Oncology: Indications, Techniques, and Results, Third Edition. Edited by William Small Jr.
© 2017 John Wiley & Sons, Inc. Published 2017 by John Wiley & Sons, Inc.

Vulvar malignant melanomas account for approximately 10% of all primary malignant neoplasms on the vulva. Most cases arise in women aged 60–70 years, while only 30% arise in women aged under 50 years [29]. Vulvar malignant melanomas may be subclassified into three specific categories: superficial spreading; nodular; and mucosal lentiginous melanoma. Prognosis is correlated with depth of invasion and regional nodal spread [30–33].

Pathway of Spread

Invasive vulvar cancer can spread in three ways: by infiltration to adjacent organs; through lymphatic channels; or via hematogenous spread. The vulvar area has rich lymphatic and blood supplies. The first echelon of lymph nodes from the vulva includes superficial inguinal and femoral lymph nodes. The primary lymphatic drainage from the clitoris goes to the superficial femoral nodes as well as the deep femoral and pelvic (obturator and external iliac) nodes [34,35]. In patients with small, well-lateralized lesions, contralateral node metastasis without the presence of ipsilateral groin node metastasis is very infrequently seen. However, in patients with advanced lesions the frequency may be as high as 15% [36–40]. Hematogenous spread is most commonly found in patients with a prior positive inguinal lymph node, especially with more than three positive nodes. The most common sites of metastasis from hematogenous spread are lung and bone [41,42].

Prognostic Factors

The strongest factor in predicting the outcome of treatment of vulvar cancer is inguinal lymph node involvement [43–46]. The five-year overall survival rate for patients with negative lymph nodes ranges from 80% to 100%, compared to 30–70% for those with positive nodes [42, 47–49]. Other prognostic features related to nodal involvement include the volume of tumor in the involved nodes, the presence of extracapsular extension, and the number of positive nodes [50,51]. Depth of invasion and size of tumor are also associated with regional metastasis and locoregional recurrence (Table 32.1). The size of the tumor margin after surgery has been found to be predictive of local recurrence; several reports [27,51,52] have described a clear association between the risk of vulvar recurrence and the width of surgical resection margins [53]. Local recurrence has been observed in patients when microscopic margins are close, described as less than 8 mm by Heaps *et al.* (Table 32.2) [27,51–53]. This 8-mm pathologic formalin-fixed tissue margin correlates with a 1-cm margin in normal tissue.

Table 32.1 Incidence of groin-node metastasis correlated with size and depth.

Size (cm)	%	Depth (mm)	%
0–1	7	<1	0
1.1–2	22	1.1–2.0	7
2.1–3	27	2.1–3.0	8
3.1–5	34	3.1–5.0	23
Any size beyond vulva	54	>5	37

Pooled data from Refs [36,37,91,156,202].

Clinical Manifestations

Most women with vulvar cancer present with a mass or ulcer in the vulvar area and may have a history of pruritus or pain. Symptoms, including bleeding, discharge, dysuria and constipation, can occur because of the location and extension of the tumor. Unfortunately, some patients present with advanced disease without any symptoms. Others may present with inguinal-node involvement that causes groin tenderness, ulceration or lower-extremity edema.

Patient Evaluation and Staging System

The International Federation of Gynecology and Obstetrics (FIGO) published a modified surgical staging system for vulvar cancer in 2009 (Table 32.3) which was a revision of the previous system introduced in 1988. As per the FIGO system, all patients with invasive disease must be carefully evaluated with a physical examination, including a complete pelvic examination, measurement of the primary tumor and assessment of extension to adjacent organs. Special attention should also be paid to the clinical examination to assess for enlargement of lymph nodes.

Histopathologic confirmation is required for the diagnosis of vulvar cancer. Some lesions are difficult to biopsy, such as when chronic vulvar dystrophy or multifocal dysplasia is present. In this case, multiple biopsies should be taken, including both the cutaneous lesion and underlying stroma, to assess the depth of invasion. Colposcopy can be used to identify abnormal areas with difficult-to-visualize lesions and may increase accuracy for directed biopsies. Excisional biopsies should be avoided in patients with small lesions prior to a sentinel node biopsy because this can compromise the accuracy of the sentinel node procedure.

Diagnostic imaging may assist in evaluating lymph node status in the inguinofemoral region, with a sensitivity of 80–85% with magnetic resonance imaging (MRI) or ultrasound [55–61]. Although positron emission

Table 32.2 FIGO staging 2009: Carcinoma of the vulva.

Stage		
I		Tumor confined to the vulva
	IA	Lesions ≤2 cm, confined to the vulva or perineum and with stromal invasion ≤1.0 mm*; no nodal metastasis
	IB	Tumor of any size with extension to adjacent perineal structures (one-third lower urethra, one-third lower vagina, anus) with negative nodes
II		Tumor of any size with or without extension to adjacent perineal structures (one-third lower urethra, one-third lower vagina, anus) with positive inguinofemoral lymph nodes.
III		Tumor of any size with or without extension to adjacent perineal structures (one-third lower urethra, one-third lower vagina, anus) with positive inguinofemoral lymph nodes.
	IIIA	(i) With one lymph node metastasis (≥5 mm), or (ii) One to two lymph node metastasis(es) (<5 mm)
	IIIB	(i) With two or more lymph node metastases (≥5 mm), or (ii) Three or more lymph nodes metastases (<5 mm)
	IIIC	With positive nodes with extracapsular spread
IV		Tumor invades other regional (two-thirds upper urethra, one-third upper vagina), or distant structures
	IVA	Tumor invades any of the following: (i) Upper urethral and/or vaginal mucosa, bladder mucosa, rectal mucosa or fixed to pelvic bone, or (ii) Fixed or ulcerated inguinofemoral nodes
	IVB	Any distant metastasis including pelvic lymph nodes

*The depth of invasion is defined as the measurement of the tumor from the epithelial stromal junction of the adjacent most superficial dermal papilla to the deepest point of invasion.
Source: Pecorelli, S. (2009) Revised FIGO staging for carcinoma of the vulva, cervix, and endometrium. *Int. J. Gynaecol. Obstet.*, **105**, 103–104. Reproduced with permission of Elsevier.

tomography (PET) is not a standard procedure, it is useful in detecting nodal or distant metastases [62]. Computed tomography (CT), when used alone, may be less sensitive for evaluating inguinal nodes because large nodes, regardless of their cancer status, are usually detected [63]. 3D imaging may assist with needle-guided biopsy of suspicious nodes. For primary vulvar lesions, although CT and PET/CT can provide only limited data, MRI can detect extension to adjacent structures. However, MRI has limited value with small lesions [64]. FIGO staging does not change on the basis of diagnostic imaging.

Surgical dissection usually confirms the status of lymph nodes. Recently, sentinel lymph node biopsy has increased in use; the procedure requires the injection of blue dye and a radiocolloid in the vulvar tumor, followed by selective excisional biopsy of the highlighted node [65–69]. Cystoscopy and proctoscopy should be performed in patients with a tumor near the bladder or rectum.

Treatment

For many years, radical vulvectomy (*en bloc* resection) with inguinofemoral lymphadenectomy was the standard treatment for invasive vulvar cancer. In this procedure, tissue around the vulvar and groin areas is resected, including all of the skin bridging the vulva and groin. Successful radical resection is associated with five-year survival rates of approximately 80–90% for patients who receive the treatment [47, 70]. However, several postoperative morbidities are associated with this extensive surgery, such as leg edema, wound breakdown, pelvic relaxation, organ prolapse, vaginal incontinence, and psychosexual impairment. During the past few decades, the management of invasive vulvar cancer has shifted to limiting the extent of surgery in order to decrease morbidities without compromising the efficacy of the treatment [71, 72]. Currently, more limited resections such as wide local excision or partial vulvectomy are acceptable in early, less-extensive disease [34, 40, 73–75]. Radical

Table 32.3 Local recurrence related to surgical margin.

Study/Reference	Margin <8 mm		Margin ≥8 mm	
	No	(%)	No	(%)
Heaps *et al.* [27]	21/44	48	0/91	0
De Hullu *et al.* [52]	9/40	23	0/39	0
Chan *et al.* [78]	13/61	21	0/29	0
Viswanathan *et al.* [53]	39/101	39	5/15	30%

surgery is frequently ineffective in curing patients with bulky tumors or positive groin nodes. Multimodality treatment, which includes preoperative or definitive radiation with or without concurrent chemotherapy, potentially followed by limited surgery, has been used to treat more advanced disease, with the goal of improving outcome without increasing morbidity [76].

Surgical Management

In early-stage vulvar cancer, surgery can be effective when adequate negative margins of the tumor are obtained, or by completely removing the entire vulva. Radical local excision, or removal of the tumor with an adequate margin, has become a much more common form of vulvar surgery, in particular for small lesions [77–79]. This is combined with lymph node dissection as the treatment of choice for early-stage lesions. One surgical approach used to reduce morbidity while preserving adequate local control is the *triple incision* technique, which utilizes separate groin and vulvar incisions. No prospective randomized controlled trials have compared radical vulvectomy (*en-bloc* resection) with inguinofemoral lymphadenectomy to the triple incision technique. However, several groups have proposed in retrospective studies that the triple incision technique provides similar outcomes to *en-bloc* resection with a butterfly incision, with less morbidity and a low risk of skin-bridge recurrence [77,80,81].

Wide local excision is widely accepted as an alternative approach in the treatment of small lesions. The first successful conservative resection was described in tumors measuring 1 cm or less with invasion of less than 5 mm [34]. There are additional reports which tend to use wide local excision for larger lesions with deep invasion [40,74,75,82,83].

Surgery for primary invasive tumors should extend to obtain a margin of at least 1–2 cm. Although the optimal extent of the surgical margin is uncertain, several studies have shown that for cases in which the surgical margin is >8 mm in the fixed state, local control rates are high and are equivalent to those of cases with a 1-cm margin on fresh tissue postoperatively [78,84]. Another study indicates that a critical threshold of 5 mm correlated with higher local control rates [53].

Radical lymphadenectomy – surgical removal of the inguinal lymph nodes – has typically been considered standard treatment. This procedure includes superficial and deep inguinofemoral node dissections. Complications of radical lymphadenectomy are common and include wound breakdown, lymphangitis or lymphocyst formation, and chronic lower-extremity lymphedema [48, 85, 86]. These complications occur even with the triple-incision approach [87,88].

Superficial inguinal nodes are the sentinel lymph nodes for vulvar cancer and, as such, are evaluated first for lymphatic metastases. Rarely are patients found with deep inguinal node metastasis without also having spread to the superficial nodes. Because it involves only removing the sentinel nodes, ipsilateral superficial groin-node dissection is the most conservative surgical approach [87, 89]. In patients with tumors larger than 2 cm and with invasion of more than 5 mm, the incidence of node metastasis may be up to 30%. An ipsilateral inguinal node dissection should be performed in these cases [90, 91]. Contralateral inguinal node dissection may be unnecessary for early lateralized lesions less than 2 cm without ipsilateral node metastasis; the risk of contralateral node metastases is less than 1% [92, 93]. However for midline lesions, bilateral superficial dissections should be performed [75].

Sentinel lymphadenectomy is another surgical concept used to define the true sentinel groin nodes. The routine study of sentinel nodes might reduce the risk of groin recurrence by identifying patients with direct lymphatic pathways to deep nodes so that they can receive early treatment [65, 67, 69, 80, 94–96]. The detection rate of sentinel node biopsy in vulvar cancer is very high, ranging up to 100% in some studies [96–98]. Inguinofemoral lymphadenectomy after sentinel node biopsy in several studies showed a low rate of false-negative identification of the sentinel node when using technetium-labeled nanocolloid or combined technetium nanocolloid with blue dye, and when the tumor size was <4 cm [97, 99–102]. However, large tumors or multifocal lesions were usually excluded from these studies.

The first large observational multicenter study, GROningen INternational Study on Sentinel nodes in Vulvar cancer (GROINSS-V), involved patients with early-stage vulvar cancer whose tumors measured <4 cm [103]. The study split patients by result of the sentinel node biopsy: patients with a negative sentinel node biopsy did not undergo lymphadenectomy, whereas those with a positive sentinel node biopsy did. With a median follow-up time of 35 months, inguinal recurrences occurred in 2.3% of patients; this is comparable to groin recurrence rates in patients treated with inguinal node dissection in previous studies [104–106]. Based on the convincing results of the GROINSS-V trial, vulvar cancer patients with tumors smaller than 4 cm, unifocal disease, and clinically negative groins may undergo sentinel node dissection. In a recent update, with a median follow up of 105 months, the overall local recurrence rate was 27.2% at 5 years and 39.5% at 10 years. Most importantly, patients that had a vulvar relapse had an approximately 50% risk of death from vulvar cancer [107].

The Gynecologic Oncology Group (GOG) conducted a multi-institutional study (GOG 173) of the diagnostic accuracy of sentinel node biopsies in tumors with a diameter of 2–6 cm. The false-negative rate for primary tumors 4–6 cm in size (14%) was almost twice that for tumors <2 cm (6.9%) [66]. Because tumors larger than 4 cm have a higher likelihood of false-negative results with sentinel node detection, the conclusions of this study suggested that sentinel node lymphoscintigraphy should not be performed on tumors larger than 4 cm [101]. There is an unknown risk of micrometastases and isolated tumor cells when a sentinel node is detected, and so bilateral inguinofemoral lymphadenectomy should be performed in these cases.

An ongoing study, GROINSS-V II, includes patients with unifocal squamous lesions smaller than 4 cm and negative groin nodes, both of which are identified by clinical examination and imaging [108]. No further treatment is given in patients with negative sentinel nodes; however, chemoradiation or radiation is given in patients with positive sentinel nodes.

Surgery alone, even radical vulvectomy (*en-bloc*), is ineffective in controlling locally advanced disease. In the latter situation, surgery is integrated into a multimodality treatment; less-extensive surgery can be used after radiation or chemoradiation to reduce the tumor volume. Radical wide excision with adequate margins can be as effective as radical vulvectomy, but without compromising the function of the vulva. The risk of complications associated with extensive groin dissection may be reduced by initial surgery to debulk an enlarged node, combined with later radiation with or without chemotherapy. One retrospective analysis reported that debulking lymph nodes prior to irradiation provided equivalent outcomes to complete lymphadenectomy followed by radiation [109].

Radiation Therapy

Radiation therapy is accepted as an important part of the multimodality management of locally advanced vulvar cancer and the postoperative treatment of early-stage lesions with high-risk features. Advances in technology and the recognition of dose fractionation and organ tolerance have decreased morbidity and improved local control rates and survival. Radiation has also been used for palliation in patients who have extensive disease, or who are medically inoperable [110–113].

Adjuvant Postoperative Radiation Therapy
Postoperative radiation therapy aims to improve local control in patients with a high risk of recurrence and nodal metastasis. It is important to distinguish between radiation for the primary vulvar region and radiation to the inguinal and pelvic nodal regions. Various surgico-pathologic nodal features have been associated with a higher risk of nodal recurrence. Three such predictors of poor prognosis include the involvement of any lymph nodes, evidence of extracapsular nodal spread, and large

nodal metastases [44, 51]. In one study it was reported that patients with no positive nodes had a better prognosis than node-positive patients, even if involvement consisted of microscopic lymph nodes without extracapsular extension. Worse outcomes can be expected in patients with multiple node metastasis [114]. With regards to the primary vulvar lesion, an increased risk of recurrence has been seen in patients with close or positive margins, lymphovascular space invasion, large tumor size, and deep tumor penetration [115]. The risk of recurrence is lower for patients with close vulvar margins treated with ≥56 Gy [53].

A GOG randomized trial (GOG 37) showed the benefits of adjuvant nodal irradiation in a postoperative setting. Patients with positive groin nodes, detected through inguinal node dissection, were split into two groups: one arm received pelvic and groin irradiation, and the other arm received ipsilateral pelvic node resection. The patients who received radiation therapy experienced a significantly reduced groin recurrence rate (24% versus 5%). The radiation therapy arm had fewer cancer-related deaths at the six-year follow-up mark (29% versus 51%). In that trial, postoperative radiation therapy had overall better outcomes than pelvic node dissection. The largest advantage was seen in patients with two or more involved nodes, extracapsular extension or grossly involved nodes [116, 117]. Additional data confirms that patients with one grossly positive node with extracapsular extension or multiple involved nodes should benefit from postoperative radiation [118, 119]. For patients with positive or close margins (<8 mm), postoperative radiation therapy has been shown to improve local control [87].

Postoperative radiation therapy is suggested for patients with positive inguinal nodes or nodal extracapsular extension. Other high-risk features for recurrence at the primary site and groin-node metastasis include positive or close margins (<8 mm), depth of invasion >5 mm, and lymphovascular invasion. Patients with these risk factors require postoperative radiation therapy. In patients with a single nodal metastasis, postoperative radiation therapy improves disease-specific survival but not overall survival. When fewer than 12 nodes have been removed, adjuvant radiation treatment may improve survival in this group [120]. The utility of postoperative radiation therapy in patients with one positive lymph node must be assessed individually, though many centers do typically irradiate for one positive lymph node given the high risk of mortality seen in patients suffering from a subsequent nodal failure.

The recommended prescribed dose for adjuvant radiation depends on the indication. In one series of 205 postoperative vulvar cancer patients, 116 had close margins (defined as ≤1 cm); the greatest risk for recurrence was found in those who had margins ≤5 mm, though recurrences were noted with margins up to 9 mm [53].

For patients with a close surgical margin, ≥56 Gy is recommended [53]. For patients with positive postoperative margins, a dose of 63–70 Gy is attempted, with concurrent weekly cisplatin as tolerated.

For patients with positive groin nodes and high-risk features in the vulva other than close margins, such as lymphovascular invasion or large tumor size alone, treating the vulva to 45–50.4 Gy is recommended, given the high risk of tumor cells in the region of the remaining vulvar tissue. For patients receiving preoperative radiation for locally advanced disease, a dose of 45–50.4 Gy is attempted. If the tumor remains unresectable, a definitive dose of approximately 70 Gy, attempted with concurrent weekly cisplatin 40 mg m^{-2}, is administered. For patients with involved lymph nodes that have been completely excised without extracapsular extension present, the involved groin and pelvic region should receive approximately 45–54 Gy. If extracapsular extension is present, a dose of 63–65 Gy is recommended. For those patients with gross residual nodal disease, a dose of 65–70 Gy should be attempted. Treatment of the undissected contralateral groin is reasonable, particularly if the lesion approaches midline or is large, or if lymphovascular invasion is present, given the high risk of contralateral nodal disease.

Preoperative Radiation and Chemoradiation

Preoperative radiation was first recognized as an effective method of treatment during the 1970s, when several studies reported that no residual disease was found in vulvectomy specimens after the patient had received 30–55 Gy of preoperative radiation therapy [121, 122]. However, despite the success of these early trials radiation still was not used as primary treatment. Several studies during the chemoradiation era reported encouraging results when employing preoperative chemoradiation before conservative resection in patients with locally advanced or locally recurrent vulvar cancer [123, 124]. One study in particular marks the beginning of the chemoradiation era: GOG protocol 101, a prospective Phase II study for locally advanced vulvar cancer that demonstrated compelling data in support of preoperative concurrent chemoradiation. Under GOG 101, preoperative radiation of 47.6 Gy in once- or twice-daily fractions of 1.7 Gy given with two courses of infusional 5-fluorouracil (5-FU) and cisplatin, was followed by excision of the residual primary tumor and bilateral inguinofemoral lymph node dissection in stage III–IV patients [125]. At the time of surgery, 46% of patients had no visible disease, and 36% had experienced a pathologic complete response. These results suggest that preoperative chemoradiation is feasible and can allow the use of less extensive surgery for locally advanced vulvar cancer.

A GOG protocol also studied the effectiveness of preoperative chemoradiation in patients with positive inguinofemoral nodes (N2, N3). For this, 46 patients were treated with preoperative chemoradiation with the same chemotherapy and radiation dose schema as GOG 101, but the radiation also included pelvic and groin nodes. Some 95% of patients had resectable disease after completing preoperative chemoradiation. Among patients who underwent surgery, 40% (15/37) had pathologically negative nodes. Of those 37 patients, 19 experienced recurrent or metastatic disease, and only one patient had a lymph node recurrence. The study concluded that, in patients with extensive nodal involvement, preoperative chemoradiation may increase the local control rate and result in a higher rate of resectable tumors [126].

Another study (GOG protocol 205), a prospective Phase II trial, treated patients with locally advanced vulvar cancer. The patients received preoperative weekly cisplatin 40 mg m−2 concurrent with radiation (45 Gy to vulvar, inguinofemoral node, lower pelvic node with the superior border at the inferior sacroiliac joint and 57.6 Gy to gross disease, without a planned treatment break). At the conclusion of chemoradiation, 37 of 58 patients (64%) had a complete clinical response and 29 (50%) had a pathologic complete response. The locoregional recurrence rate was 17% (5/29) in the complete-response patients. The study concluded that concurrent chemoradiation with a relatively high radiation dose and short treatment time is feasible, and results in a high complete-response rate [127]. The main criticism of the trial is that most centers routinely use concurrent chemotherapy and radiation to a higher dose (i.e., ca. 65–70 Gy to involved sites of gross disease), which may increase the complete-response rate.

After preoperative chemoradiation, surgical resectability should be evaluated and a more conservative, less-extensive procedure considered. If a patient's disease is not resectable with conservative surgery, even after initial preoperative chemoradiation, an additional limited field of radiation to the residual disease with or without chemotherapy can be used. For patients with clinically positive nodes, the grossly involved node may be debulked prior to preoperative chemoradiation. If the node is not debulked and there is residual disease after chemoradiation, a limited resection may be performed.

The preoperative dose to the area of the primary tumor and lymph nodes should be 45–54 Gy. Dose escalation to 65–70 Gy is required for patients not able to undergo surgery. One study reported a recurrence rate of 65% for patients treated with <54 Gy as compared to 15% for those receiving >54 Gy [128].

Primary Radiation Therapy or Chemoradiation

Given the success of primary chemoradiation in other sites such as the cervix [129], several studies have analyzed the use of chemoradiation in vulvar cancer [130]. Some report no significant difference in progression-free

Table 32.4 Pelvic-node metastasis in patients with inguinal-node metastasis.

Study/Reference	Positive inguinal nodes	Positive pelvic nodes	
		No	(%)
Collins *et al.* [202]	31	9	29
Curry *et al.* [203]	40	9	23
Hacker *et al.* [106]	31	1	19
Podratz *et al.* [70]	47	7	15
Homesley *et al.* [115]	53	15	28

survival between patients treated with primary chemoradiation and those treated with primary surgery [131,132]. Another study suggests that patients may be cured with definitive chemoradiation [133,134]. This definitive treatment is increasingly being used in patients with small midline lesions to preserve the critical structure from surgery; however, this does not mean that chemoradiation can replace surgery in a multimodal treatment approach. The benefit of concurrent chemoradiation used either preoperatively or as primary definitive treatment in locally advanced disease is shown in Table 32.4 [26, 76, 84, 123–125, 134–143].

Studies have used a variety of chemotherapy drugs in conjunction with radiation therapy; most used a combination of 5-FU and cisplatin or mitomycin. GOG 205 used weekly cisplatin in combination with definitive radiation, and reported a 64% complete clinical response rate and a 50% pathologic complete response rate. The locoregional recurrence rate was 17% in the complete-response patients [127]. In one retrospective study, radiation with weekly cisplatin was compared to radiation plus three or four weeks of 5-FU-based chemotherapy. No significant differences were found in response, recurrence, or survival rates between the two regimens [130]. Weekly cisplatin caused fewer significant gastrointestinal side effects. Single-agent bleomycin has also been used with evidence of good response, but is not commonly used in vulvar cancer.

Prophylactic Inguinal Radiation Treatment

The role of prophylactic inguinal radiation is not well established [87, 144–150]. One GOG study evaluated the potential role of prophylactic inguinal radiation in patients with clinically negative nodes in order to avoid inguinal lymphadenectomy. Patients with clinically negative nodes were randomly assigned to one of two treatment arms: radical lymphadenectomy or inguinal node radiation. If a positive node was found during radical lymphadenectomy, additional postoperative radiation was given. Unfortunately, the radiation treatment prescription to a depth of 3 cm was inadequate to cover the

inguinal region. Not surprisingly therefore, the interim results demonstrated significantly higher inguinal node recurrence and death rates in patients assigned to the radiation therapy arm and the trial was closed early [87]. However, the GOG later criticized its own study for failing to eliminate confounding factors that may have caused high rates of failure after prophylactic inguinal radiation. First, patients who received radiation alone may have received an inadequate dose to the groin area (the prescribed dose to the groin nodes was at a depth 3 cm below the skin). Second, the determination of groin node involvement relied on physical examination only. Lastly, distal pelvic nodes were not included in the radiation field. A review of inguinal node depth from another study demonstrated that approximately 30% of patients had a superficial inguinal node depth of more than 3 cm, and all deep inguinal nodes were more than 3 cm below the surface of the skin [151]. Koh *et al.* reported a mean potential groin node depth of 6.1 cm. The same group also recalculated the dose of five patients from the GOG study who had recurrent disease; the received doses for all five were lower than the prescribed doses, and in three of five cases it was 30% less than prescribed [152]. Lymphadenectomy patients may have achieved better results because patients in this study were clinically evaluated for positive groin nodes, but macroscopic groin metastasis in a deep region may not be detectable by clinical examination alone.

Radiographic imaging can be used to help detect macroscopic lymph nodes and to direct measurement of the depth of the inguinal area for radiation prescription dose. Petereit *et al.*, in 48 women with squamous cell carcinoma of vulva with clinically negative groin nodes, found no difference in the three-year nodal control and cause-specific survival rates between 23 patients who underwent groin irradiation and 25 patients who underwent groin dissection after radical vulvectomy. In addition, the patients in the radiation group had a lower incidence of lymphadenectomy-related morbidity, such as lymphedema, seroma, infection and wound separation [150]. Katz *et al.* retrospectively studied the effects of different modalities of groin node treatment. In that study, the inguinal node recurrence rate was 16% in patients treated with dissection, and 11% in those treated with radiation [144]. Currently, CT-based imaging is used in treatment planning. This technique can improve the detection of groin node involvement, which can be missed by physical examination, and can increase the likelihood of adequate dose coverage of the groin node region. In summary, groin node radiation may be an alternative for patients who are not suitable candidates for surgery.

Another GOG study, GOG 37, suggested that radiation therapy can be used to control microscopic regional disease. That observational study reported that radiation therapy was effective in controlling microscopic disease in those with clinically negative nodes. There were no groin relapses in patients who elected to receive inguinal node radiation. Additional chemotherapy with radiation may increase effectiveness [136,153,154]. A retrospective study reviewed 23 patients with clinically negative lymph nodes who received radiation combined with 5-FU with or without cisplatin. The results showed no recurrences in the inguinal lymph nodes [153].

Treatment Algorithms and Approaches

Treatment decisions for patients with primary vulvar cancer are typically based on all clinical characteristics of the disease, including primary tumor extension and regional node metastasis. Patient age, comorbidities and quality of life are also considered in treatment decision-making.

Early Invasive Disease

Wide local excision can be used to treat small, favorable, non-midline primary tumors without sacrificing the function of the urethra, clitoris, vagina, and rectum. The results of wide local excision for these small lesions are similar to those achieved with radical vulvectomy: local recurrence rates of 6–7% and DFS rates of 98–99% [34, 40,74,83]. To be eligible for conservative surgery, patients do not need to match precise criteria, but rather should have a small lesion (<2 cm) and a depth of invasion not more than 5 mm [34, 40, 74, 83, 155]. Ipsilateral groin node dissections are recommended except for patients with a tumor smaller than 2 cm and with a depth of invasion <1 mm, due to the very small risk of lymph node involvement. Ipsilateral groin node dissections can also be foregone when a successful sentinel node study has confirmed at least one negative sentinel node [36,37,156]. Contralateral groin node dissection may not be necessary when ipsilateral groin node dissection is negative. Small lateralized tumors with negative ipsilateral groin nodes have a less than 1% risk of contralateral groin metastasis [39,155,157].

It is recommended that patients with high-risk features, including close or positive margins, receive postoperative radiation treatment. The benefits of postoperative radiation treatment are shown in retrospective studies in which these high-risk groups experienced improvements in local control and survival [79]. The other risk factors for local recurrence include deep invasion (>5 mm) and lymphovascular invasion, though radiation is not typically recommended for these risk features unless in combination with positive lymph nodes. For patients with two or more lymph node metastases or one

macroscopic node with extracapsular extension, postoperative bilateral radiation to the groin is recommended according to GOG 37. Whether to irradiate the contralateral groin in patients receiving radiation for one positive unilateral node is unknown.

Another controversial issue involves routine radiation to the tumor bed in addition to radiation treatment to the groin and pelvic nodes. One report suggested including the primary tumor with groin radiation due to an increase in the local recurrence rate when radiation to the groin is performed with a shielded primary region [158]. Given the relatively low rate of late of life-threatening toxicity from 45 Gy to the vulva, and the difficulty with matching treatments in the event of a vulvar recurrence, it is recommended to treat the primary vulvar region when treatment is given to the groin. Algorithms for management of patients with early, lateralized disease are shown in Figure 32.1.

Adjuvant Postoperative Irradiation

The volume of the radiation field in adjuvant postoperative radiation is dependent on the patient's indication for adjuvant treatment. To lower the risk of local recurrence in cases with positive surgical margins or similar indicators, the radiation field may be limited to the vulvar scar and the limited residual vulvar area. In this way, uninvolved vulvar tissues may be conserved and potential future complications from radiation prevented. Such patients should receive appositional radiation, via electron beam or a low-energy photon beam radiation, in the lithotomy position, and the radiation should be directed at the resected region of the tumor. The energy of the beam should be chosen to ensure that the lesion is completely covered from the surface to the deepest point. Bolus can be used to ensure the delivery of the prescribed tumor dose to the surface.

Postoperative radiation to pelvic and groin nodes, as established in GOG 37, can be used in patients with metastases to the inguinofemoral nodes. External-beam radiation therapy (EBRT) should be directed bilaterally to the inguinofemoral area and pelvic nodes. Patients with inguinal node metastasis are more at risk for pelvic node involvement (Table 32.5). The benefits of using radiation to higher nodes or contralateral nodes to improve survival are uncertain. Radiation doses of 45–50 Gy in 1.8–2.0 Gy fractions are prescribed for microscopic disease.

The 'frogleg' position may be used for treatment to minimize skin reaction in the upper medial thigh and skin folds. The superior border of the pelvic field should extend from L5–S1 to cover the external iliac nodes. The inferior border should cover the entire vulva, 6–8 cm inferior to the inguinal skin crease or ligament. There are no data available regarding lymphadenectomy scar recurrence, but the common practice also includes the

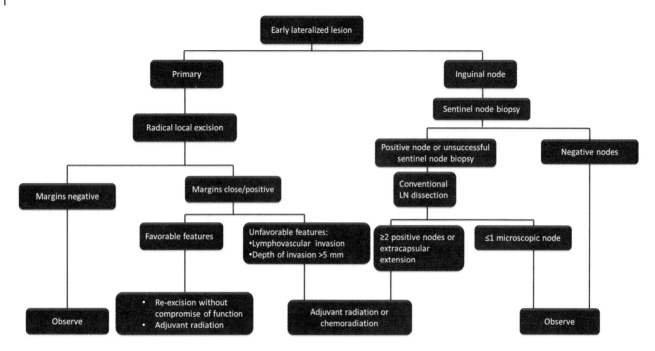

Figure 32.1 Algorithm for the management of an early-stage lateralized lesion.

lymphadenectomy scar in the field. Bolus may be used to ensure an adequate dose into the groin.

One study of patients with node-positive vulvar cancer reported a high local recurrence rate when the midline structure was blocked [158]. Therefore, radiation to the midline structure should be omitted only if risk factors for local recurrence are minimal. The prescription depth for the inguinofemoral nodes is defined as the depth beneath the inguinal ligament, where the femoral artery passes. One study evaluated the depth of inguinal

Table 32.5 Concurrent chemoradiation therapy for patients with locally advanced vulvar cancer.

Study/ Reference	No. of patients	Chemotherapy regimen	RT dose (Gy)	Complete response rate (%)	Follow-up time (months)	Recurrent and persistent (%)
Levin *et al.* [122]	6	5-FU+Mito-C	18–60	100	1–25	0
Thomas *et al.* [123]	9	5-FU+Mito-C	40–60	67	5–45	30
Sebag-Montefiore *et al.* [134]	37	5-FU+Mito-C	45–50	47	6–36	
Whalen *et al.* [135]	19	5-FU+Mito-C	45–50	53	34	5
Lupi *et al.* [136]	24	5-FU+Mito-C	36		22–73	23
Landoni *et al.* [137]	41	5-FU+Mito-C	54	31	4–48	22
Evans *et al.* [138]	4	5-FU+Mito-C	25–70	50	5–43	50
Koh *et al.* [139	20	5-FU+/−Mito-C or CDDP	30–54	57	1–75	30
Han *et al.* [133]	10	5-FU+/−Mito-C or CDDP	40–62	71	3.5–273	50
Russell *et al.* [26]	18	5-FU+/−Mito-C or CDDP	47–56	89	4–52	24
Berek *et al.* [84]	12	5-FU+ CDDP	45–54	67	7–60	25
Eifel *et al.* [140]	12	5-FU+ CDDP	40–50	42	17–30	50
Cunningham *et al.* [76]	14	5-FU+ CDDP	50–65	64	7–81	29
Moore *et al.* [124]	73	5-FU+ CDDP	47.6	46	22–72	21
Gerszten *et al.* [141]	18	5-FU+ CDDP	44.6	67	1–55	16
Beriwal *et al.* [142]	18	5-FU+ CDDP	42.8–46.4	72	4–31	33
Mak *et al.* [129]	16	CDDP	22–75	58.8	31	43
	28	5-FU+/−Mito-C or CDDP		53.8		46
Moore *et al.* [126]	58	CDDP	57.6	64	24	44

5FU, 5-fluorouracil; CDDP, cisplatin; Mito-C, mitomycin C; RT, radiation therapy.

nodes in gynecologic malignancy: superficial inguinal nodes were deeper than 3 cm in 29% of cases, and all deep inguinal nodes were at least 3 cm below the surface [151]. Imaging, such as MRI, CT or ultrasonography, should be used to confirm the nodal volume.

Radiation dose to the femoral area should be reduced to decrease femoral complications [159]; various techniques are available to do this. One approach, termed *partial transmission block*, uses both a wide anterior field with low-energy photons, which includes the inguinal and pelvic area, and a narrow posterior field with high-energy photons to cover the pelvic area [144]. The inguinal area is treated separately by adding an electron field, with careful attention paid to the junction of fields that lies on the femoral neck. A partial transmission block is placed on the anterior field over the pelvic and vulvar areas. Beam attenuation is calculated to the deep pelvic node, which receives a homogeneous dose from the anterior and posterior fields.

The *modified segmental boost technique* uses a combination of the wide anterior field with a narrow posterior field. A separate boost is then given to the bilateral inguinal fields. The bilateral inguinal fields are angled to align with the divergence of the posterior field. This technique provides a more homogeneous dose distribution [160, 161].

Intensity-modulated radiation therapy (IMRT) has been used to treat vulvar cancer. The rationale behind the use of IMRT for adjuvant postoperative radiation is that it decreases the doses to normal tissues, including to the rectum, bladder, small bowel, and femoral head. The doses to the normal structures are related to late toxicity. Beriwal *et al.* reported 18 cases using IMRT [143], where the clinical target volume (CTV) included the entire vulva with a 1-cm margin, any nodes with a

1- to 2-cm margin, and the gross tumor volume with a 1-cm margin. The CTV was then expanded 5–10 mm to obtain the planning target volume (PTV). The superior border was at L5–S1. This technique appears to be very precise and to have the benefit of high reproducibility, although it requires extreme precision, especially in daily set-up. The technique also requires further evaluation and individualized decision-making on whether to treat potentially at-risk regions such as the skin bridge. A consensus atlas was published describing recommendations for vulvar cancer contouring for IMRT [162]. Key points included that the CTV for nodal contours should not extend behind the femoral vessels; a 0.7–1 cm margin should be given for the PTV expansion.

For lesions with bulky vaginal invasion, an interstitial brachytherapy implant can be used as a boost after EBRT. Randomized data to evaluate benefit and toxicity are unavailable, but retrospective data show good local control (25%) with acceptable toxicity (27%) [163]. The radiation plan of a patient who received a 3D conformal first course followed by IMRT and a subsequent interstitial boost is shown in Figure 32.2.

Small Midline Primary Tumors

Midline tumors can be treated with primary radiation or chemoradiation. Although surgical excision is the standard treatment for early-stage lesions, surgery can impair the function of the vulva and have negative cosmetic and psychological results. Because of these potential consequences of radical surgery of midline primary tumors, evaluation after preoperative chemoradiation to determine the feasibility of more conservative surgery, that would not impair function and cosmesis, should be considered.

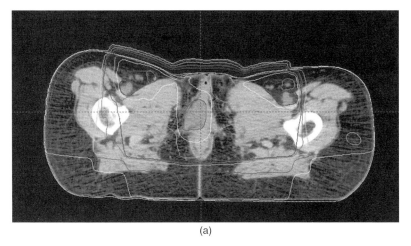
(a)
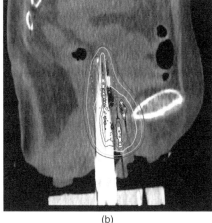
(b)

Figure 32.2 Dose distribution in a patient with vulvar cancer. Vaginal involvement was treated with IMRT (a) and interstitial brachytherapy (b). The external beam target volume included elective treatment of groin nodes with bolus covering the vulvar and groin areas. The interstitial brachytherapy boost dose is to the primary tumor, which involves the vagina. For a color version of this figure, see the color plate section.

Preoperative or Definitive Vulvar Irradiation

For locally advanced primary or groin tumors, the target volume should include the vulva and the pelvic and bilateral groin areas. A technique similar to that described for adjuvant therapy may be used. A break-in treatment can be offered to patients with severe skin desquamation to allow epithelial regeneration before completion of the definite treatment plan. However, plans that include split-course radiation increase the total treatment time, and can allow the tumor time to proliferate during the break. One way to reduce total treatment time after treatment is interrupted is to use twice-daily fractionation during the boost course.

Locally Advanced Disease

Patients with locally advanced disease, including those with extensive primary tumors, should be evaluated for radical resection, unless there is involvement of the anal sphincter or extensive urethral involvement. Resection of the anal sphincter or more than 1 cm of the urethra may result in highly morbid incontinence and should be avoided. Surgery alone has poor results when pelvic exenteration plus radical vulvectomy are performed. Associated morbidities include psychological impairment [164–167]. Combined modality treatment, involving radiation with or without chemotherapy and surgery, has benefits and is often used to manage tumors with adjacent organ invasion.

Patients with locally advanced nodal disease (bulky, fixed or ulcerated nodes) commonly present with locally advanced primary tumors. Initial radiation or chemoradiation is often the treatment of choice. One retrospective study compared outcomes in two arms of patients: one arm underwent complete groin dissection followed by radiation, while the other arm underwent debulking surgery followed by radiation. The inguinal recurrence rate was not significantly different between the two arms. Debulking the node before radiation might be optimal for treating patients with at least one positive groin node [109]. The algorithm for management of patients with locally advanced vulvar cancer, with or without locally extensive groin metastases, is shown in Figure 32.3.

Recurrence and Metastatic Cancer

Outcomes for patients with recurrent vulvar cancer depend heavily on the site of recurrence, regardless of primary treatment received by the patient. Isolated vulvar recurrence results in a better outcome than other recurrences, particularly when the recurrent tumor can be resected with a negative margin. Recurrence-free survival is obtained in 70% of patients after recurrence followed by surgery [168, 169]. Radiation therapy or chemoradiation for local recurrence is also an option, particularly when surgery cannot obtain an adequate margin without compromising function [26, 124]. In one study from 1997, the two-year survival rate after recurrence was only 25% after salvage radiation [79]. However,

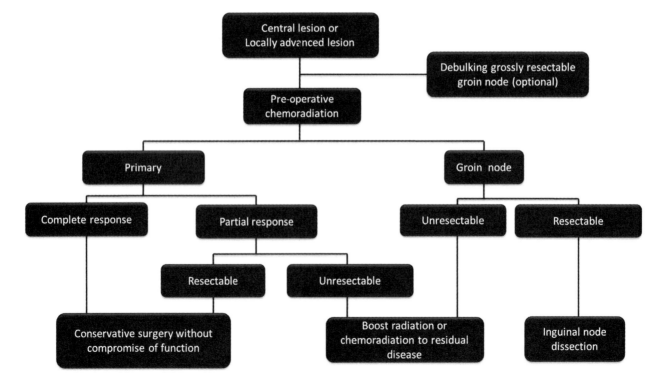

Figure 32.3 Algorithm for the management of a locally advanced or midline lesion.

modern radiation therapy has shown a five-year survival rate of 62.6% [145].

Regional nodal recurrence for patients with vulvar cancer is often fatal. Resection of bulky disease and radiation or chemoradiation may be used for local control, but few such patients experience long-term survival [169–173]. For patients with distant metastases, active systemic chemotherapy agents, which are often offered against squamous cell cancers, are associated with poor response rates and response durations [170, 174].

Sequelae of Treatment

Surgical Complications

Treatment may result in acute and/or chronic complications. These side effects depend on the treatment sites and modalities used.

Acute surgical wound adverse effects include seroma, hematoma, infection, wound necrosis and wound breakdown. Side effects can be greater when more extensive surgery is performed. In a separate-incision operation, the overall incidence of wound breakdown, necrosis and infection was 15%. Other potential side effects include deep-vein thrombosis, pulmonary embolism and numbness of the thigh from femoral nerve injury.

Lymphedema of the lower extremities is a common chronic complication, the degree of edema being related to the extent of groin dissection. Other side effects are chronic cellulitis, inguinal stenosis, and inguinal hernia.

Radiation Complications

The most common acute effects of radiation, either alone or combined with chemotherapy, are skin and mucosal reactions, even when a preoperative dose of 45–50 Gy is used. Almost all patients have moist desquamation in the irradiated area, including the perineal and groin regions. The severity of desquamation can vary from patchy to moist, and may be associated with radiation dose fractionation and the details of chemotherapy administration. Other acute effects include urethritis and cystitis, which present with symptoms of urgency, frequency, and dysuria. Vaginal effects include pruritus and vaginal discharge. Effects on the anorectal area, which include proctitis and diarrhea, may occur. Patients who develop loose stools should be counseled very early in the course to start anti-diarrheal medications daily as a preventive measure and to continue them until the conclusion of radiation.

Prophylaxis and management of acute radiation side effects should be undertaken. A Sitz bath twice daily will keep the affected area of skin clean and provide a healing effect. Topical steroid cream/ointment and pain medication can be used for the relief of pain symptoms in the desquamated area. A topical medication for hemorrhoid treatment may have benefit in some patients. For treatment and prophylaxis of fungal infections in the vaginal area, an antifungal drug such as fluconazole (Diflucan®) should be administered during the second week of radiation. Some patients who have symptoms of urinary irritation and discomfort may respond to a urinary analgesic drug such as phenazopyridine (Pyridium®). Foley catheter placement during treatment may be required in patients who have moist desquamation with difficulties when urinating. Radiation should be discontinued for a short period in patients who suffer from severe toxicity.

Late Sequelae of Treatment

There are many possible late effects of treatment, such as hyperpigmentation, telangiectasia, fibrosis, atrophy of the skin, sexual dysfunction including vaginal stenosis, and prolonged wound complications. Cellulitis and lower-extremity edema can be found after radical node dissection and radiation [70, 175]. Sentinel node biopsy may lead to significantly fewer surgical complications than node dissection [26]. Avascular necrosis of the femoral head has been reported as an effect of radiation or chemoradiation [125]. Fracture in the pelvic area has been found in patients who received pelvic and groin radiation, with an incidence of 9%; hip fracture is the most common site (90% of reported pelvic fractures) [176]. Femoral-head fractures have also occasionally been reported in some studies, with an 11% five-year fracture rate [124, 154, 175]. The risk of fracture may not be correlated only with the dose delivered to the femur, but also with other factors such as osteoporosis [159]. However, limiting the dose to the head of the femur should reduce the overall risk of femur fracture.

Rare Histologies

Malignant Melanoma

Malignant vulvar melanoma is the second most common vulvar neoplasm [177, 178], accounting for approximately 10% of all vulvar tumors [179]. Patients usually present with asymptomatic pigmented lesions or masses. Biopsies provide a definitive diagnosis. The three biologic subtypes of vulvar malignant melanomas include: superficial spreading, lentigo maligna, and nodular. Of these, superficial spreading melanomas are the most common while nodular melanomas are the most aggressive.

The prognoses of vulvar melanomas are parallel to those of cutaneous malignant melanomas. Prognosis is correlated with depth of invasion by Clark's methodology, and is also correlated with tumor thickness or depth of invasion by Breslow's classification [31, 180, 181]. The staging system for vulvar melanomas uses the TNM classifications for cutaneous malignant melanoma.

Surgery is the primary treatment for vulvar melanoma. Radical vulvectomy with bilateral groin node dissection is still considered the standard of care, but there has been a trend towards more conservative surgical options [182, 183]. In order to reduce complications without decreasing survival, limited surgery is recommended; however, only observational studies of this approach have been reported [183, 184]. For lesions with a depth of invasion <1 mm, the risk of nodal metastasis is small, and wide local excision may be adequate [30, 185]. Sentinel node biopsy has been used frequently for squamous cell carcinomas of the vulva, but the data for its use in malignant melanoma are insufficient.

The overall five-year survival rate in women with vulvar melanoma is approximately 50% [183, 186]. Radiation therapy has played a limited role in vulvar melanoma because the tumor is radioresistant, the perineal skin of the vulva has poor tolerance, and the rate of death due to distant metastatic disease is high despite local radiation. Radiation therapy may be used for palliation of unresectable, symptomatic recurrent or metastatic disease.

Verrucous Carcinoma

Verrucous carcinomas are slow-growing, locally invasive and rarely metastatic tumors [187]. Patients may present with a 'cauliflower' mass. Radical local excision is often curative and is considered the standard of care [188–190]. Inguinal node metastases are uncommon and inguinal node dissection is indicated if such metastases are documented. However, suspicious groin nodes are usually caused by inflammatory processes; in the case of suspicious nodes, fine-needle aspiration or excisional biopsy should be performed. Radiation therapy generally has been ineffective, and in some cases has been reported to cause anaplastic transformations [191]. While surgery remains the treatment of choice, radiation does have limited use for patients in whom curative surgery is not possible.

Vulvar Sarcomas

Primary sarcomas of the vulva account for approximately 1–2% of vulvar cancers. There are many histopathologic types, including leiomyosarcoma, fibrosarcoma, epithelioid sarcoma, synovial sarcoma, and rhabdomyosarcoma [192]. Nielsen *et al.* reported that having three or more of the following features indicates a possible sarcoma diagnosis: tumor size at least 5 cm; an infiltrative margin; five or more mitotic figures per 10 high-power fields; and moderate to severe cytologic atypia [193].

Wide local excision is the treatment of choice. Ulutin *et al.* reported no recurrences of tumor in their vulvar sarcoma series with a median follow-up time of 127 months [192]. Adjuvant radiation may be used for high-grade tumors or for locally recurrent high-grade lesions.

Leiomyosarcoma is the most common type. An enlarged painless mass in the labia majora or minora is usually present [194]. Negative prognostic factors for recurrence are tumor size >5 cm, an infiltrating margin, more than 10 mitotic figures per high-power field, and the presence of tumoral necrosis [195]. Nodal metastases are uncommon for this type of tumor. Radiation treatment should be considered when there is a high risk for recurrence [196].

Epithelioid sarcoma is an extremely rare tumor in the vulvar area, occurring more often in young women. This tumor behaves more aggressively in the vulvar region than it does in an extragenital area [197]. Wide local excision or radical vulvectomy with ipsilateral inguinal node dissection is usually performed [196]. Approximately 70–77% of patients have local recurrence, but this may be prevented by adjuvant radiation. Systemic therapy is ineffective [198]. Synovial sarcoma of the vulva treated with a multimodal approach has also been reported [199].

Lymphoma

Primary lymphoma of the vulva is uncommon, with only a few reported cases. It is staged according to the Ann Arbor staging system. The majority of cases are non-Hodgkin lymphoma (NHL), and the most common subtype is diffuse large B-cell lymphoma. Patients usually present with systemic involvement. In an M.D. Anderson Cancer Center report, two of six patients with localized NHL of the vulva treated with chemotherapy and radiation therapy had complete remission, but both relapsed within one year and died within two years, similar to a previous report [200, 201]. Systemic disease is usually treated with chemotherapy.

References

1 Beller, U., Quinn, M.A., Benedet, J.L., *et al.* (2006) Carcinoma of the vulva. FIGO 26th Annual Report on the Results of Treatment in Gynecological Cancer. *Int. J. Gynaecol. Obstet.*, **95** (Suppl. 1), S7–27.

2 Ries, L.G., Pollack, E.S., Young, J.L., Jr (1983) Cancer patient survival: Surveillance, Epidemiology, and End Results Program, 1973–79. *J. Natl Cancer Inst.*, **70** (4), 693–707.

3 Marill, J.A.R.N. (1961) Cancer of the vulva. *Cancer,* **1961**, 13–20.

4 Mabuchi, K., Bross, D.S., Kessler, I.I. (1985) Epidemiology of cancer of the vulva. A case-control study. *Cancer,* **55** (8), 1843–1848.

5 Buscema, J., Woodruff, J.D., Parmley, T.H., Genadry, R. (1980) Carcinoma in situ of the vulva. *Obstet. Gynecol.,* **55** (2), 225–230.

6 Franklin, E.W. 3rd, Rutledge, F.D. (1972) Epidemiology of epidermoid carcinoma of the vulva. *Obstet. Gynecol.,* **39** (2), 165–172.

7 Abercrombie, P.D., Korn, A.P. (1998) Vulvar intraepithelial neoplasia in women with HIV. *AIDS Patient Care STDS,* **12** (4), 251–254.

8 Caterson, R.J., Furber, J., Murray, J., McCarthy, W., Mahony, J.F., Sheil, A.G. (1984) Carcinoma of the vulva in two young renal allograft recipients. *Transplant Proc.,* **16** (2), 559–561.

9 Halpert, R., Fruchter, R.G., Sedlis, A., Butt, K., Boyce, J.G., Sillman, F.H. (1986) Human papillomavirus and lower genital neoplasia in renal transplant patients. *Obstet. Gynecol.,* **68** (2), 251–258.

10 Korn, A.P., Abercrombie, P.D., Foster, A. (1996) Vulvar intraepithelial neoplasia in women infected with human immunodeficiency virus-1. *Gynecol. Oncol.,* **61** (3), 384–386.

11 Wright, T.C., Koulos, J.P., Liu, P., Sun, X.W. (1996) Invasive vulvar carcinoma in two women infected with human immunodeficiency virus. *Gynecol. Oncol.,* **60** (3), 500–503.

12 Porreco, R., Penn, I., Droegemueller, W., Greer, B., Makowski, E. (1975) Gynecologic malignancies in immunosuppressed organ homograft recipients. *Obstet. Gynecol.,* **45** (4), 359–364.

13 Giaquinto, C., Del Mistro, A., De Rossi, A., *et al.* (2000) Vulvar carcinoma in a 12-year-old girl with vertically acquired human immunodeficiency virus infection. *Pediatrics,* **106** (4), E57.

14 Adami, J., Gabel, H., Lindelof, B., *et al.* (2003) Cancer risk following organ transplantation: a nationwide cohort study in Sweden. *Br. J. Cancer,* **89** (7), 1221–1227.

15 Sutton, B.C., Allen, R.A., Moore, W.E., Dunn, S.T. (2008) Distribution of human papillomavirus genotypes in invasive squamous carcinoma of the vulva. *Mod. Pathol.,* **21** (3), 345–354.

16 Gissmann, L., Schwarz, E. (1986) Persistence and expression of human papillomavirus DNA in genital cancer. *Ciba Found. Symp.,* **120**, 190–207.

17 Buscema, J., Naghashfar, Z., Sawada, E., Daniel, R., Woodruff, J.D., Shah, K. (1988) The predominance of human papillomavirus type 16 in vulvar neoplasia. *Obstet. Gynecol.,* **71** (4), 601–606.

18 Hording, U., Junge, J., Daugaard, S., Lundvall, F., Poulsen, H., Bock, J.E. (1994) Vulvar squamous cell carcinoma and papillomaviruses: indications for two different etiologies. *Gynecol. Oncol.,* **52** (2), 241–246.

19 Brinton, L.A., Nasca, P.C., Mallin, K., Baptiste, M.S., Wilbanks, G.D., Richart, R.M. (1990) Case-control study of cancer of the vulva. *Obstet. Gynecol.,* **75** (5), 859–866.

20 Lee, Y.Y., Wilczynski, S.P., Chumakov, A., Chih, D., Koeffler, H.P. (1994) Carcinoma of the vulva: HPV and p53 mutations. *Oncogene,* **9** (6), 1655–1659.

21 Woelber, L., Choschzick, M., Eulenburg, C., *et al.* (2011) Prognostic value of pathological resection margin distance in squamous cell cancer of the vulva. *Ann. Surg. Oncol.,* **18** (13), 3811–3818.

22 Madeleine, M.M., Daling, J.R., Carter, J.J., *et al.* (1997) Cofactors with human papillomavirus in a population-based study of vulvar cancer. *J. Natl Cancer Inst.,* **89** (20), 1516–1523.

23 Carli, P., De Magnis, A., Mannone, F., Botti, E., Taddei, G., Cattaneo, A. (2003) Vulvar carcinoma associated with lichen sclerosus. Experience at the Florence, Italy, Vulvar Clinic. *J. Reprod. Med.,* **48** (5), 313–318.

24 Jones, R.W., Sadler, L., Grant, S., Whineray, J., Exeter, M., Rowan, D. (2004) Clinically identifying women with vulvar lichen sclerosus at increased risk of squamous cell carcinoma: a case-control study. *J. Reprod. Med.,* **49** (10), 808–811.

25 Hunter, D.J. (1975) Carcinoma of the vulva: a review of 361 patients. *Gynecol. Oncol.,* **3** (2), 117–123.

26 Russell, A.H., Mesic, J.B., Scudder, S.A., *et al.* (1992) Synchronous radiation and cytotoxic chemotherapy for locally advanced or recurrent squamous cancer of the vulva. *Gynecol. Oncol.,* **47** (1), 14–20.

27 Heaps, J.M., Fu, Y.S., Montz, F.J., Hacker, N.F., Berek, J.S. (1990) Surgical-pathologic variables predictive of local recurrence in squamous cell carcinoma of the vulva. *Gynecol. Oncol.,* **38** (3), 309–314.

28 Rando, R.F., Sedlacek, T.V., Hunt, J., Jenson, A.B., Kurman, R.J., Lancaster, W.D. (1986) Verrucous carcinoma of the vulva associated with an unusual type 6 human papillomavirus. *Obstet. Gynecol.,* **67** (3 Suppl.), 70S–75S.

29 Panizzon, R.G. (1996) Vulvar melanoma. *Semin. Dermatol.,* **15** (1), 67–70.

30 Breslow, A. (1978) Tumor thickness in evaluating prognosis of cutaneous melanoma. *Ann. Surg.,* **187** (4), 440.

31 Breslow, A. (1980) Prognosis in cutaneous melanoma: tumor thickness as a guide to treatment. *Pathol. Ann.,* **15** (Pt 1), 1–22.

32 McGovern, V.J., Mihm, M.C. Jr, Bailly, C., *et al.* (1973) The classification of malignant melanoma and its histologic reporting. *Cancer,* **32** (6), 1446–1457.

33 Mihm, M.C. Jr, Lopansri, S. (1979) A review of the classification of malignant melanoma. *J. Dermatol.,* **6** (3), 131–142.

34 DiSaia, P.J., Creasman, W.T., Rich, W.M. (1979) An alternate approach to early cancer of the vulva. *Am. J. Obstet. Gynecol.*, **133** (7), 825–832.

35 Plentl, A.A., Friedman, E.A. (1971) Lymphatic system of the female genitalia. The morphologic basis of oncologic diagnosis and therapy. *Major Probl. Obstet. Gynecol.*, **2**, 1–223.

36 Parker, R.T., Duncan, I., Rampone, J., Creasman, W. (1975) Operative management of early invasive epidermoid carcinoma of the vulva. *Am. J. Obstet. Gynecol.*, **123** (4), 349–355.

37 Hacker, N.F., Berek, J.S., Lagasse, L.D., Nieberg, R.K., Leuchter, R.S. (1984) Individualization of treatment for stage I squamous cell vulvar carcinoma. *Obstet. Gynecol.*, **63** (2), 155–162.

38 Krupp, P.J., Bohm, J.W. (1978) Lymph gland metastases in invasive squamous cell cancer of the vulva. *Am. J. Obstet. Gynecol.*, **130** (8), 943–952.

39 Iversen, T., Abeler, V., Aalders, J. (1981) Individualized treatment of stage I carcinoma of the vulva. *Obstet. Gynecol.*, **57** (1), 85–89.

40 Burke, T.W., Stringer, C.A., Gershenson, D.M., Edwards, C.L., Morris, M., Wharton, J.T. (1990) Radical wide excision and selective inguinal node dissection for squamous cell carcinoma of the vulva. *Gynecol. Oncol.*, **38** (3), 328–332.

41 Hacker, N.F. (1990) Current treatment of small vulvar cancers. *Oncology (Williston Park)*, **4** (8), 21–25; discussions 26, 28, 33.

42 Homesley, H.D., Bundy, B.N., Sedlis, A., *et al.* (1991) Assessment of current International Federation of Gynecology and Obstetrics staging of vulvar carcinoma relative to prognostic factors for survival (a Gynecologic Oncology Group study). *Am. J. Obstet. Gynecol.*, **164** (4), 997–1003, discussion 1003–1004.

43 Boyce, J., Fruchter, R.G., Kasambilides, E., Nicastri, A.D., Sedlis, A., Remy, J.C. (1985) Prognostic factors in carcinoma of the vulva. *Gynecol. Oncol.*, **20** (3), 364–377.

44 Raspagliesi, F., Hanozet, F., Ditto, A., *et al.* (2006) Clinical and pathological prognostic factors in squamous cell carcinoma of the vulva. *Gynecol. Oncol.*, **102** (2), 333–337.

45 Kurzl, R., Messerer, D. (1989) Prognostic factors in squamous cell carcinoma of the vulva: a multivariate analysis. *Gynecol. Oncol.*, **32** (2), 143–150.

46 Homesley, H.D., Bundy, B.N., Sedlis, A., *et al.* (1993) Prognostic factors for groin node metastasis in squamous cell carcinoma of the vulva (a Gynecologic Oncology Group study). *Gynecol. Oncol.*, **49** (3), 279–283.

47 Morley, G.W. (1976) Infiltrative carcinoma of the vulva: results of surgical treatment. *Am. J. Obstet. Gynecol.*, **124** (8), 874–888.

48 Green, T.H. Jr (1978) Carcinoma of the vulva. A reassessment. *Obstet. Gynecol.*, **52** (4), 462–469.

49 Benedet, J.L., Turko, M., Fairey, R.N., Boyes, D.A. (1979) Squamous carcinoma of the vulva: results of treatment, 1938 to 1976. *Am. J. Obstet. Gynecol.*, **134** (2), 201–207.

50 Raspagliesi, F., Ditto, A., Paladini, D., *et al.* (2000) Prognostic indicators in melanoma of the vulva. *Ann. Surg. Oncol.*, **7** (10), 738–742.

51 van der Velden, J., van Lindert, A.C., Lammes, F.B., *et al.* (1995) Extracapsular growth of lymph node metastases in squamous cell carcinoma of the vulva. The impact on recurrence and survival. *Cancer*, **75** (12), 2885–2890.

52 De Hullu, J.A., Hollema, H., Lolkema, S., *et al.* (2002) Vulvar carcinoma. The price of less radical surgery. *Cancer*, **95** (11), 2331–2338.

53 Viswanathan, A.N., Pinto, A.P., Schultz, D., Berkowitz, R., Crum, C.P. (2013) Relationship of margin status and radiation dose to recurrence in post-operative vulvar carcinoma. *Gynecol. Oncol.*, **130** (3), 545–549.

54 Wo, J.Y., Tanaka, C., Schultz, D., Viswanathan, A.N. (2008) Predictors of vulvar recurrence: The effect of margin status. *Int. J. Radiat. Oncol. Biol. Phys.*, **72** (1), S20.

55 Singh, K., Orakwue, C.O., Honest, H., Balogun, M., Lopez, C., Luesley, D.M. (2006) Accuracy of magnetic resonance imaging of inguinofemoral lymph nodes in vulval cancer. *Int. J. Gynecol. Cancer*, **16** (3), 1179–1183.

56 Bipat, S., Fransen, G.A., Spijkerboer, A.M., *et al.* (2006) Is there a role for magnetic resonance imaging in the evaluation of inguinal lymph node metastases in patients with vulva carcinoma? *Gynecol. Oncol.*, **103** (3), 1001–1006.

57 Montana, G.S. (2004) Carcinoma of the vulva: combined modality treatment. *Curr. Treat. Options Oncol.*, **5** (2), 85–95.

58 Cohn, D.E., Dehdashti, F., Gibb, R.K., *et al.* (2002) Prospective evaluation of positron emission tomography for the detection of groin node metastases from vulvar cancer. *Gynecol. Oncol.*, **85** (1), 179–184.

59 Hall, T.B., Barton, D.P., Trott, P.A., *et al.* (2003) The role of ultrasound-guided cytology of groin lymph nodes in the management of squamous cell carcinoma of the vulva: 5-year experience in 44 patients. *Clin. Radiol.*, **58** (5), 367–371.

60 Sohaib, S.A., Moskovic, E.C. (2003) Imaging in vulval cancer. *Best Pract. Res. Clin. Obstet. Gynaecol.*, **17** (4), 543–556.

61 Barton, D.P., Moskovic, E., Sohaib, A. (2007) Accuracy of magnetic imaging of inguinofemoral lymph nodes in vulval cancer. *Int. J. Gynecol. Cancer*, **17** (5), 1179; author reply 1180.

62 Viswanathan, A.N., Tanaka, C.K. (2008) The impact of positron emission tomography on the diagnosis and management of vulvar cancer. *Int. J. Radiat. Oncol. Biol. Phys.*, **72** (1), S360.

63 Land, R., Herod, J., Moskovic, E., *et al.* (2006) Routine computerized tomography scanning, groin ultrasound with or without fine needle aspiration cytology in the surgical management of primary squamous cell carcinoma of the vulva. *Int. J. Gynecol. Cancer*, **16** (1), 312–317.

64 Sohaib, S.A., Richards, P.S., Ind, T., *et al.* (2002) MR imaging of carcinoma of the vulva. *Am. J. Roentgenol.*, **178** (2), 373–377.

65 Rob, L., Robova, H., Pluta, M., *et al.* (2007) Further data on sentinel lymph node mapping in vulvar cancer by blue dye and radiocolloid Tc99. *Int. J. Gynecol. Cancer*, **17** (1), 147–153.

66 Levenback, C.F. (2008) How safe is sentinel lymph node biopsy in patients with vulvar cancer? *J. Clin. Oncol.*, **26** (6), 828–829.

67 Decesare, S.L., Fiorica, J.V., Roberts, W.S., *et al.* (1997) A pilot study utilizing intraoperative lymphoscintigraphy for identification of the sentinel lymph nodes in vulvar cancer. *Gynecol. Oncol.*, **66** (3), 425–428.

68 Ansink, A.C., de Hullu, J.A., van der Zee, A.G. (2003) Re: Further data on the usefulness of sentinel lymph node identification and ultrastaging in vulvar squamous cell carcinoma. *Gynecol. Oncol.*, **88** (1), 29–34; *Gynecol. Oncol.*, **90** (3), 688–689; author reply 689–690.

69 Terada, K.Y., Shimizu, D.M., Wong, J.H. (2000) Sentinel node dissection and ultrastaging in squamous cell cancer of the vulva. *Gynecol. Oncol.*, **76** (1), 40–44.

70 Podratz, K.C., Symmonds, R.E., Taylor, W.F., Williams, T.J. (1983) Carcinoma of the vulva: analysis of treatment and survival. *Obstet. Gynecol.*, **61** (1), 63–74.

71 Magrina, J.F., Gonzalez-Bosquet, J., Weaver, A.L., *et al.* (1998) Primary squamous cell cancer of the vulva: radical versus modified radical vulvar surgery. *Gynecol. Oncol.*, **71** (1), 116–121.

72 Lin, J.Y., DuBeshter, B., Angel, C., Dvoretsky, P.M. (1992) Morbidity and recurrence with modifications of radical vulvectomy and groin dissection. *Gynecol. Oncol.*, **47** (1), 80–86.

73 Thomas, G.M., Dembo, A.J., Bryson, S.C., Osborne, R., DePetrillo, A.D. (1991) Changing concepts in the management of vulvar cancer. *Gynecol. Oncol.*, **42** (1), 9–21.

74 Berman, M.L., Soper, J.T., Creasman, W.T., Olt, G.T., DiSaia, P.J. (1989) Conservative surgical management of superficially invasive stage I vulvar carcinoma. *Gynecol. Oncol.*, **35** (3), 352–357.

75 Burke, T.W., Levenback, C., Coleman, R.L., Morris, M., Silva, E.G., Gershenson, D.M. (1995) Surgical therapy of T1 and T2 vulvar carcinoma: further experience with radical wide excision and selective inguinal lymphadenectomy. *Gynecol. Oncol.*, **57** (2), 215–220.

76 Cunningham, M.J., Goyer, R.P., Gibbons, S.K., Kredentser, D.C., Malfetano, J.H., Keys, H. (1997) Primary radiation, cisplatin, and 5-fluorouracil for advanced squamous carcinoma of the vulva. *Gynecol. Oncol.*, **66** (2), 258–261.

77 Hacker, N.F., Leuchter, R.S., Berek, J.S., Castaldo, T.W., Lagasse, L.D. (1981) Radical vulvectomy and bilateral inguinal lymphadenectomy through separate groin incisions. *Obstet. Gynecol.*, **58** (5), 574–579.

78 Chan, J.K., Sugiyama, V., Pham, H., *et al.* (2007) Margin distance and other clinico-pathologic prognostic factors in vulvar carcinoma: a multivariate analysis. *Gynecol. Oncol.*, **104** (3), 636–641.

79 Faul, C.M., Mirmow, D., Huang, Q., Gerszten, K., Day, R., Jones, M.W. (1997) Adjuvant radiation for vulvar carcinoma: improved local control. *Int. J. Radiat. Oncol. Biol. Phys.*, **38** (2), 381–389.

80 Ansink, A., van der Velden, J. (2000) Surgical interventions for early squamous cell carcinoma of the vulva. *Cochrane Database Syst. Rev.* 2000 (2), CD002036.

81 Siller, B.S., Alvarez, R.D., Conner, W.D., *et al.* (1995) T2/3 vulva cancer: a case-control study of triple incision versus en bloc radical vulvectomy and inguinal lymphadenectomy. *Gynecol. Oncol.*, **57** (3), 335–339.

82 Wharton, J.T., Gallager, S., Rutledge, F.N. (1974) Microinvasive carcinoma of the vulva. *Am. J. Obstet. Gynecol.*, **118** (2), 159–162.

83 Stehman, F.B., Bundy, B.N., Dvoretsky, P.M., Creasman, W.T. (1992) Early stage I carcinoma of the vulva treated with ipsilateral superficial inguinal lymphadenectomy and modified radical hemivulvectomy: a prospective study of the Gynecologic Oncology Group. *Obstet. Gynecol.*, **79** (4), 490–497.

84 Berek, J.S., Heaps, J.M., Fu, Y.S., Juillard, G.J., Hacker, N.F. (1991) Concurrent cisplatin and 5-fluorouracil chemotherapy and radiation therapy for advanced-stage squamous carcinoma of the vulva. *Gynecol. Oncol.*, **42** (3), 197–201.

85 McKelvey, J.L. (1970) Carcinoma of the vulva: classification, treatment and results. *Proc. Natl Cancer Conf.*, **6**, 361–364.

86 Figge, D.C., Gaudenz, R. (1974) Invasive carcinoma of the vulva. *Am. J. Obstet. Gynecol.*, **119** (3), 382–395.

87 Stehman, F.B., Bundy, B.N., Thomas, G., *et al.* (1992) Groin dissection versus groin radiation in carcinoma of the vulva: a Gynecologic Oncology Group study. *Int. J. Radiat. Oncol. Biol. Phys.*, **24** (2), 389–396.

88 Petereit, D.G., Mehta, M.P., Buchler, D.A., Kinsella, T.J. (1993) A retrospective review of nodal treatment for vulvar cancer. *Am. J. Clin. Oncol.*, **16** (1), 38–42.

89 Morris, J.M. (1977) A formula for selective lymphadenectomy. Its application to cancer of the vulva. *Obstet. Gynecol.*, **50** (2), 152–158.

90 Sedlis, A., Homesley, H., Bundy, B.N., *et al.* (1987) Positive groin lymph nodes in superficial squamous cell vulvar cancer. A Gynecologic Oncology Group Study. *Am. J. Obstet. Gynecol.*, **156** (5), 1159–1164.

91 Gonzalez Bosquet, J., Kinney, W.K., Russell, A.H., Gaffey, T.A., Magrina, J.F., Podratz, K.C. (2003) Risk of occult inguinofemoral lymph node metastasis from squamous carcinoma of the vulva. *Int. J. Radiat. Oncol. Biol. Phys.*, **57** (2), 419–424.

92 DeSimone, C.P., Van Ness, J.S., Cooper, A.L., *et al.* (2007) The treatment of lateral T1 and T2 squamous cell carcinomas of the vulva confined to the labium majus or minus. *Gynecol. Oncol.*, **104** (2), 390–395.

93 Gonzalez Bosquet, J., Magrina, J.F., Magtibay, P.M., *et al.* (2007) Patterns of inguinal groin metastases in squamous cell carcinoma of the vulva. *Gynecol. Oncol.*, **105** (3), 742–746.

94 Levenback, C., Burke, T.W., Morris, M., Malpica, A., Lucas, K.R., Gershenson, D.M. (1995) Potential applications of intraoperative lymphatic mapping in vulvar cancer. *Gynecol. Oncol.*, **59** (2), 216–220.

95 Rodier, J.F., Janser, J.C., Routiot, T., *et al.* (1999) Sentinel node biopsy in vulvar malignancies: a preliminary feasibility study. *Oncol. Rep.*, **6** (6), 1249–1252.

96 Levenback, C.F., Ali, S., Coleman, R.L., *et al.* (2012) Lymphatic mapping and sentinel lymph node biopsy in women with squamous cell carcinoma of the vulva: a gynecologic oncology group study. *J. Clin. Oncol.*, **30** (31), 3786–3791.

97 Sliutz, G., Reinthaller, A., Lantzsch, T., *et al.* (2002) Lymphatic mapping of sentinel nodes in early vulvar cancer. *Gynecol. Oncol.*, **84** (3), 449–452.

98 De Cicco, C., Sideri, M., Bartolomei, M., *et al.* (2000) Sentinel node biopsy in early vulvar cancer. *Br. J. Cancer*, **82** (2), 295–299.

99 Akrivos, N., Rodolakis, A., Vlachos, G., *et al.* (2011) Detection and credibility of sentinel node in vulvar cancer: a single institutional study and short review of literature. *Arch. Gynecol. Obstet.*, **284** (6), 1551–1556.

100 Devaja, O., Mehra, G., Coutts, M., *et al.* (2011) A prospective study of sentinel lymph node detection in vulval carcinoma: is it time for a change in clinical practice? *Int. J. Gynecol. Cancer*, **21** (3), 559–564.

101 Lindell, G., Jonsson, C., Ehrsson, R.J., *et al.* (2010) Evaluation of preoperative lymphoscintigraphy and sentinel node procedure in vulvar cancer. *Eur. J. Obstet. Gynecol. Reprod. Biol.*, **152** (1), 91–95.

102 Hampl, M., Hantschmann, P., Michels, W., Hillemanns, P. (2008) Validation of the accuracy of the sentinel lymph node procedure in patients with vulvar cancer: results of a multicenter study in Germany. *Gynecol. Oncol.*, **111** (2), 282–288.

103 Van der Zee, A.G., Oonk, M.H., De Hullu, J.A., *et al.* (2008) Sentinel node dissection is safe in the treatment of early-stage vulvar cancer. *J. Clin. Oncol.*, **26** (6), 884–889.

104 Rodolakis, A., Diakomanolis, E., Voulgaris, Z., Akrivos, T., Vlachos, G., Michalas, S. (2000) Squamous vulvar cancer: a clinically based individualization of treatment. *Gynecol. Oncol.*, **78** (3 Pt 1), 346–351.

105 Bell, J.G., Lea, J.S., Reid, G.C. (2000) Complete groin lymphadenectomy with preservation of the fascia lata in the treatment of vulvar carcinoma. *Gynecol. Oncol.*, **77** (2), 314–318.

106 Hacker, N.F., Berek, J.S., Lagasse, L.D., Leuchter, R.S., Moore, J.G. (1983) Management of regional lymph nodes and their prognostic influence in vulvar cancer. *Obstet. Gynecol.*, **61** (4), 408–412.

107 Oonk, M.H., van der Zeee, A.G. (2013) GROINSS-V: GROningen International Study on Sentinel Nodes in Vulvar Cancer. *Ned. Tijdschr. Oncol.*, **10**, 77–79.

108 Hyde, S.E., Valmadre, S., Hacker, N.F., Schilthuis, M.S., Grant, P.T., van der Velden, J. (2007) Squamous cell carcinoma of the vulva with bulky positive groin nodes-nodal debulking versus full groin dissection prior to radiation therapy. *Int. J. Gynecol. Cancer*, **17** (1), 154–158.

109 Tod, M.C. (1949) Radium implantation treatment of carcinoma vulva. *Br. J. Radiol.*, **22** (261), 508–512.

110 Frischbier, H.J., Thomsen, K., Schmermund, H.J., Oberheuser, F., Hohne, G., Lohbeck, H.U. (1985) [Radiotherapy of vulvar cancer. Treatment results of electron therapy in 446 patients 1956 to 1978]. *Geburtshilfe Frauenheilkd.*, **45** (1), 1–5.

111 Backstrom, A., Edsmyr, F., Wicklund, H. (1972) Radiotherapy of carcinoma of the vulva. *Acta Obstet. Gynecol. Scand.*, **51** (2), 109–115.

112 Helgason, N.M., Hass, A.C., Latourette, H.B. (1972) Radiation therapy in carcinoma of the vulva. A review of 53 patients. *Cancer*, **30** (4), 997–1000.

113 Oonk, M.H., de Hullu, J.A., van der Zee, A.G. (2010) Current controversies in the management of patients with early-stage vulvar cancer. *Curr. Opin. Oncol.*, **22** (5), 481–486.

114 Husseinzadeh, N., Wesseler, T., Schneider, D., Schellhas, H., Nahhas, W. (1990) Prognostic factors and the significance of cytologic grading in invasive squamous cell carcinoma of the vulva: a clinicopathologic study. *Gynecol. Oncol.*, **36** (2), 192–199.

115 Homesley, H.D., Bundy, B.N., Sedlis, A., Adcock, L. (1986) Radiation therapy versus pelvic node resection

for carcinoma of the vulva with positive groin nodes. *Obstet. Gynecol.*, **68** (6), 733–740.

116 Kunos, C., Simpkins, F., Gibbons, H., Tian, C., Homesley, H. (2009) Radiation therapy compared with pelvic node resection for node-positive vulvar cancer: a randomized controlled trial. *Obstet. Gynecol.*, **114** (3), 537–546.

117 Origoni, M., Sideri, M., Garsia, S., Carinelli, S.G., Ferrari, A.G. (1992) Prognostic value of pathological patterns of lymph node positivity in squamous cell carcinoma of the vulva stage III and IVA FIGO. *Gynecol. Oncol.*, **45** (3), 313–316.

118 Ansink, A.C., van Tinteren, H., Aartsen, E.J., Heintz, A.P. (1991) Outcome, complications and follow-up in surgically treated squamous cell carcinoma of the vulva 1956–1982. *Eur. J. Obstet. Gynecol. Reprod. Biol.*, **42** (2), 137–143.

119 Parthasarathy, A., Cheung, M.K., Osann, K., *et al.* (2006) The benefit of adjuvant radiation therapy in single-node-positive squamous cell vulvar carcinoma. *Gynecol. Oncol.*, **103** (3), 1095–1099.

120 Jafari, K., Magalotti, F., Magalotti, M. (1981) Radiation therapy in carcinoma of the vulva. *Cancer*, **47** (4), 686–691.

121 Acosta, A.A., Given, F.T., Frazier, A.B., Cordoba, R.B., Luminari, A. (1978) Preoperative radiation therapy in the management of squamous cell carcinoma of the vulva: preliminary report. *Am. J. Obstet. Gynecol.*, **132** (2), 198–206.

122 Levin, W., Goldberg, G., Altaras, M., Bloch, B., Shelton, M.G. (1986) The use of concomitant chemotherapy and radiotherapy prior to surgery in advanced stage carcinoma of the vulva. *Gynecol. Oncol.*, **25** (1), 20–25.

123 Thomas, G., Dembo, A., DePetrillo, A., *et al.* (1989) Concurrent radiation and chemotherapy in vulvar carcinoma. *Gynecol. Oncol.*, **34** (3), 263–267.

124 Moore, D.H., Thomas, G.M., Montana, G.S., Saxer, A., Gallup, D.G., Olt, G. (1998) Preoperative chemoradiation for advanced vulvar cancer: a phase II study of the Gynecologic Oncology Group. *Int. J. Radiat. Oncol. Biol. Phys.*, **42** (1), 79–85.

125 Montana, G.S., Thomas, G.M., Moore, D.H., *et al.* (2000) Preoperative chemo-radiation for carcinoma of the vulva with N2/N3 nodes: a gynecologic oncology group study. *Int. J. Radiat. Oncol. Biol. Phys.*, **48** (4), 1007–1013.

126 Moore, D.H., Ali, S., Koh, W.J., *et al.* (2011) A phase II trial of radiation therapy and weekly cisplatin chemotherapy for the treatment of locally-advanced squamous cell carcinoma of the vulva: A gynecologic oncology group study. *Gynecol. Oncol.*, **124** (3), 529–533.

127 Jhingran, A., Levenback, C., Katz, A., Eifel, P. (2003) Radiation therapy for vulvar carcinoma: predictors of vulvar recurrence. *Int. J. Radiat. Oncol. Biol. Phys.*, **57** (2), S193.

128 Morris, M., Eifel, P.J., Lu, J., *et al.* (1999) Pelvic radiation with concurrent chemotherapy compared with pelvic and para-aortic radiation for high-risk cervical cancer. *N. Engl. J. Med.*, **340** (15), 1137–1143.

129 Mak, R.H., Halasz, L.M., Tanaka, C.K., *et al.* (2011) Outcomes after radiation therapy with concurrent weekly platinum-based chemotherapy or every-3-4-week 5-fluorouracil-containing regimens for squamous cell carcinoma of the vulva. *Gynecol. Oncol.*, **120** (1), 101–107.

130 Landrum, L.M., Skaggs, V., Gould, N., Walker, J.L., McMeekin, D.S. (2008) Comparison of outcome measures in patients with advanced squamous cell carcinoma of the vulva treated with surgery or primary chemoradiation. *Gynecol. Oncol.*, **108** (3), 584–590.

131 Maneo, A., Landoni, F., Colombo, A. (2003) Randomised study between neoadjuvant chemoradiotherapy and primary surgery for the treatment of advanced vulval cancer. *Int. J. Gynecol. Cancer*, **13** (Suppl. 1), 6.

132 Perez, C.A., Grigsby, P.W., Chao, C., *et al.* (1998) Irradiation in carcinoma of the vulva: factors affecting outcome. *Int. J. Radiat. Oncol. Biol. Phys.*, **42** (2), 335–344.

133 Han, S.C., Kim, D.H., Higgins, S.A., Carcangiu, M.L., Kacinski, B.M. (2000) Chemoradiation as primary or adjuvant treatment for locally advanced carcinoma of the vulva. *Int. J. Radiat. Oncol. Biol. Phys.*, **47** (5), 1235–1244.

134 Sebag-Montefiore, D.J., McLean, C., Arnott, S.J., *et al.* (1994) Treatment of advanced carcinoma of the vulva with chemoradiotherapy – can exenterative surgery be avoided? *Int. J. Gynecol. Cancer*, **4** (3), 150–155.

135 Wahlen, S.A., Slater, J.D., Wagner, R.J., *et al.* (1995) Concurrent radiation therapy and chemotherapy in the treatment of primary squamous cell carcinoma of the vulva. *Cancer*, **75** (9), 2289–2294.

136 Lupi, G., Raspagliesi, F., Zucali, R., *et al.* (1996) Combined preoperative chemoradiotherapy followed by radical surgery in locally advanced vulvar carcinoma. A pilot study. *Cancer*, **77** (8), 1472–1478.

137 Landoni, F., Maneo, A., Zanetta, G., *et al.* (1996) Concurrent preoperative chemotherapy with 5-fluorouracil and mitomycin C and radiotherapy (FUMIR) followed by limited surgery in locally advanced and recurrent vulvar carcinoma. *Gynecol. Oncol.*, **61** (3), 321–327.

138 Evans, L.S., Kersh, C.R., Constable, W.C., Taylor, P.T. (1988) Concomitant 5-fluorouracil, mitomycin-C, and radiotherapy for advanced gynecologic malignancies. *Int. J. Radiat. Oncol. Biol. Phys.*, **15** (4), 901–906.

139 Koh, W.J., Wallace, H.J. 3rd, Greer, B.E., *et al.* (1993) Combined radiotherapy and chemotherapy in the management of local-regionally advanced vulvar cancer. *Int. J. Radiat. Oncol. Biol. Phys.*, **26** (5), 809–816.

140 Eifel, P.J., Morris, M., Burke, T.W., Levenback, C., Gershenson, D.M. (1995) Prolonged continuous infusion cisplatin and 5-fluorouracil with radiation for locally advanced carcinoma of the vulva. *Gynecol. Oncol.*, **59** (1), 51–56.

141 Gerszten, K., Selvaraj, R.N., Kelley, J., Faul, C. (2005) Preoperative chemoradiation for locally advanced carcinoma of the vulva. *Gynecol. Oncol.*, **99** (3), 640–644.

142 Beriwal, S., Coon, D., Heron, D.E., *et al.* (2008) Preoperative intensity-modulated radiotherapy and chemotherapy for locally advanced vulvar carcinoma. *Gynecol. Oncol.*, **109** (2), 291–295.

143 Katz, A., Eifel, P.J., Jhingran, A., Levenback, C.F. (2003) The role of radiation therapy in preventing regional recurrences of invasive squamous cell carcinoma of the vulva. *Int. J. Radiat. Oncol. Biol. Phys.*, **57** (2), 409–418.

144 Boronow, R.C., Hickman, B.T., Reagan, M.T., Smith, R.A., Steadham, R.E. (1987) Combined therapy as an alternative to exenteration for locally advanced vulvovaginal cancer. II. Results, complications, and dosimetric and surgical considerations. *Am. J. Clin. Oncol.*, **10** (2), 171–181.

145 Frankendal, B., Larsson, L.G., Westling, P. (1973) Carcinoma of the vulva. Results of an individualized treatment schedule. *Acta Radiol. Ther. Phys. Biol.*, **12** (2), 165–174.

146 Lee, W.R., McCollough, W.M., Mendenhall, W.M., Marcus, R.B. Jr, Parsons, J.T., Million, R.R. (1993) Elective inguinal lymph node irradiation for pelvic carcinomas. The University of Florida experience. *Cancer*, **72** (6), 2058–2065.

147 Manavi, M., Berger, A., Kucera, E., Vavra, N., Kucera, H. (1997) Does T1, N0-1 vulvar cancer treated by vulvectomy but not lymphadenectomy need inguinofemoral radiation? *Int. J. Radiat. Oncol. Biol. Phys.*, **38** (4), 749–753.

148 Perez, C.A., Grigsby, P.W., Galakatos, A., *et al.* (1993) Radiation therapy in management of carcinoma of the vulva with emphasis on conservation therapy. *Cancer*, **71** (11), 3707–3716.

149 Petereit, D.G., Mehta, M.P., Buchler, D.A., Kinsella, T.J. (1993) Inguinofemoral radiation of N0,N1 vulvar cancer may be equivalent to lymphadenectomy if proper radiation technique is used. *Int. J. Radiat. Oncol. Biol. Phys.*, **27** (4), 963–967.

150 Kalidas, H. (1995) Influence of inguinal node anatomy on radiation therapy techniques. *Med. Dosim.*, **20** (4), 295–300.

151 Koh, W.J., Chiu, M., Stelzer, K.J., *et al.* (1993) Femoral vessel depth and the implications for groin node radiation. *Int. J. Radiat. Oncol. Biol. Phys.*, **27** (4), 969–974.

152 Leiserowitz, G.S., Russell, A.H., Kinney, W.K., Smith, L.H., Taylor, M.H., Scudder, S.A. (1997) Prophylactic chemoradiation of inguinofemoral lymph nodes in patients with locally extensive vulvar cancer. *Gynecol. Oncol.*, **66** (3), 509–514.

153 Henderson, R.H., Parsons, J.T., Morgan, L., Million, R.R. (1984) Elective ilioinguinal lymph node irradiation. *Int. J. Radiat. Oncol. Biol. Phys.*, **10** (6), 811–819.

154 Hacker, N.F., Van der Velden, J. (1993) Conservative management of early vulvar cancer. *Cancer*, **71** (4 Suppl.), 1673–1677.

155 Magrina, J.F., Webb, M.J., Gaffey, T.A., Symmonds, R.E. (1979) Stage I squamous cell cancer of the vulva. *Am. J. Obstet. Gynecol.*, **134** (4), 453–459.

156 Buscema, J., Stern, J.L., Woodruff, J.D. (1981) Early invasive carcinoma of the vulva. *Am. J. Obstet. Gynecol.*, **140** (5), 563–569.

157 Dusenbery, K.E., Carlson, J.W., LaPorte, R.M., *et al.* (1994) Radical vulvectomy with postoperative irradiation for vulvar cancer: therapeutic implications of a central block. *Int. J. Radiat. Oncol. Biol. Phys.*, **29** (5), 989–998.

158 Grigsby, P.W., Roberts, H.L., Perez, C.A. (1995) Femoral neck fracture following groin irradiation. *Int. J. Radiat. Oncol. Biol. Phys.*, **32** (1), 63–67.

159 Moran, M., Lund, M.W., Ahmad, M., Trumpore, H.S., Haffty, B., Nath, R. (2004) Improved treatment of pelvis and inguinal nodes using modified segmental boost technique: dosimetric evaluation. *Int. J. Radiat. Oncol. Biol. Phys.*, **59** (5), 1523–1530.

160 Moran, M.S., Castrucci, W.A., Ahmad, M., *et al.* (2010) Clinical utility of the modified segmental boost technique for treatment of the pelvis and inguinal nodes. *Int. J. Radiat. Oncol. Biol. Phys.*, **76** (4), 1026–1036.

161 De Ieso, P.B., Mullassery, V., Shrimali, R., Lowe, G., Bryant, L., Hoskin, P.J. (2011) Image-guided vulvovaginal interstitial brachytherapy in the treatment of primary and recurrent gynecological malignancies. *Brachytherapy*, **11** (4), 306–310.

162 Gaffney, D., King, B., Viswanathan, A.N., *et al.* (2016) Consensus recommendations for radiation therapy contouring and treatment of vulvar carcinoma. *Int. J. Radiat. Oncol. Biol. Phys.*, **95** (4), 1191–1200.

163 Cavanagh, D., Shepherd, J.H. (1982) The place of pelvic exenteration in the primary management of advanced carcinoma of the vulva. *Gynecol. Oncol.*, **13** (3), 318–322.

164 Gleeson, N., Baile, W., Roberts, W.S., *et al.* (1994) Surgical and psychosexual outcome following vaginal reconstruction with pelvic exenteration. *Eur. J. Gynaecol. Oncol.*, **15** (2), 89–95.

165 Roberts, W.S., Cavanagh, D., Bryson, S.C., Lyman, G.H., Hewitt, S. (1987) Major morbidity after pelvic exenteration: a seven-year experience. *Obstet. Gynecol.*, **69** (4), 617–621.

166 Benn, T., Brooks, R.A., Zhang, Q., *et al.* (2011) Pelvic exenteration in gynecologic oncology: a single institution study over 20 years. *Gynecol. Oncol.*, **122** (1), 14–18.

167 Hopkins, M.P., Reid, G.C., Morley, G.W. (1990) The surgical management of recurrent squamous cell carcinoma of the vulva. *Obstet. Gynecol.*, **75** (6), 1001–1005.

168 Piura, B., Masotina, A., Murdoch, J., Lopes, A., Morgan, P., Monaghan, J. (1993) Recurrent squamous cell carcinoma of the vulva: a study of 73 cases. *Gynecol. Oncol.*, **48** (2), 189–195.

169 Podratz, K.C., Symmonds, R.E., Taylor, W.F. (1982) Carcinoma of the vulva: analysis of treatment failures. *Am. J. Obstet. Gynecol.*, **143** (3), 340–351.

170 Tilmans, A.S., Sutton, G.P., Look, K.Y., Stehman, F.B., Ehrlich, C.E., Hornback, N.B. (1992) Recurrent squamous carcinoma of the vulva. *Am. J. Obstet. Gynecol.*, **167** (5), 1383–1389.

171 Krupp, P.J., Lee, F.Y., Bohm, J.W., Batson, H.W., Diem, J.E., Lemire, J.E. (1975) Prognostic parameters and clinical staging criteria in the epidermoid carcinoma of the vulva. *Obstet. Gynecol.*, **46** (1), 84–88.

172 Prempree, T., Amornmarn, R. (1984) Radiation treatment of recurrent carcinoma of the vulva. *Cancer*, **54** (9), 1943–1949.

173 Srivannaboon, S., Boonyanit, S., Vatananusara, C., Sophak, P. (1973) A clinical trial of bleomycin on carcinoma of the vulva: a preliminary report. *J. Med. Assoc. Thai.*, **56** (2), 101–108.

174 Hacker, N.F., Berek, J.S., Juillard, G.J., Lagasse, L.D. (1984) Preoperative radiation therapy for locally advanced vulvar cancer. *Cancer*, **54** (10), 2056–2061.

175 Baxter, N.N., Habermann, E.B., Tepper, J.E., Durham, S.B., Virnig, B.A. (2005) Risk of pelvic fractures in older women following pelvic irradiation. *JAMA*, **294** (20), 2587–2593.

176 Morrow, C.P., Rutledge, F.N. (1972) Melanoma of the vulva. *Obstet. Gynecol.*, **39** (5), 745–752.

177 Jaramillo, B.A., Ganjei, P., Averette, H.E., Sevin, B.U., Lovecchio, J.L. (1985) Malignant melanoma of the vulva. *Obstet. Gynecol.*, **66** (3), 398–401.

178 Verschraegen, C.F., Benjapibal, M., Supakarapongkul, W., *et al.* (2001) Vulvar melanoma at the M. D. Anderson Cancer Center: 25 years later. *Int. J. Gynecol. Cancer*, **11** (5), 359–364.

179 Clark, W.H., Jr, From, L., Bernardino, E.A., Mihm, M.C. (1969) The histogenesis and biologic behavior of primary human malignant melanomas of the skin. *Cancer Res.*, **29** (3), 705–727.

180 Breslow, A. (1970) Thickness, cross-sectional areas and depth of invasion in the prognosis of cutaneous melanoma. *Ann. Surg.*, **172** (5), 902–908.

181 Phillips, G.L., Bundy, B.N., Okagaki, T., Kucera, P.R., Stehman, F.B. (1994) Malignant melanoma of the vulva treated by radical hemivulvectomy. A prospective study of the Gynecologic Oncology Group. *Cancer*, **73** (10), 2626–2632.

182 Trimble, E.L., Lewis, J.L. Jr, Williams, L.L., *et al.* (1992) Management of vulvar melanoma. *Gynecol. Oncol.*, **45** (3), 254–258.

183 Davidson, T., Kissin, M., Westbury, G. (1987) Vulvo-vaginal melanoma—should radical surgery be abandoned? *Br. J. Obstet. Gynaecol.*, **94** (5), 473–476.

184 Look, K.Y., Roth, L.M., Sutton, G.P. (1993) Vulvar melanoma reconsidered. *Cancer*, **72** (1), 143–146.

185 Podratz, K.C., Gaffey, T.A., Symmonds, R.E., Johansen, K.L., O'Brien, P.C. (1983) Melanoma of the vulva: an update. *Gynecol. Oncol.*, **16** (2), 153–168.

186 Gallousis, S. (1972) Verrucous carcinoma. Report of three vulvar cases and review of the literature. *Obstet. Gynecol.*, **40** (4), 502–507.

187 Japaze, H., Van Dinh, T., Woodruff, J.D. (1982) Verrucous carcinoma of the vulva: study of 24 cases. *Obstet. Gynecol.*, **60** (4), 462–466.

188 Foye, G., Marsh, M.R., Minkowitz, S. (1969) Verrucous carcinoma of the vulva. *Obstet. Gynecol.*, **34** (4), 484–488.

189 Lucas, E.W., Jr, Branton, P., Mecklenburg, F.E., Moawad, G.N. (2009) Ectopic breast fibroadenoma of the vulva. *Obstet. Gynecol.*, **114** (2 Pt 2), 460–462.

190 Proffitt, S.D., Spooner, T.R., Kosek, J.C. (1970) Origin of undifferentiated neoplasm from verrucous epidermal carcinoma of oral cavity following irradiation. *Cancer*, **26** (2), 389–393.

191 Ulutin, H.C., Zellars, R.C., Frassica, D. (2003) Soft tissue sarcoma of the vulva: A clinical study. *Int. J. Gynecol. Cancer*, **13** (4), 528–531.

192 Nielsen, G.P., Rosenberg, A.E., Koerner, F.C., Young, R.H., Scully, R.E. (1996) Smooth-muscle tumors of the vulva. A clinicopathological study of 25 cases and review of the literature. *Am. J. Surg. Pathol.*, **20** (7), 779–793.

193 Gonzalez-Bugatto, F., Anon-Requena, M.J., Lopez-Guerrero, M.A., Baez-Perea, J.M., Bartha, J.L., Hervias-Vivancos, B. (2009) Vulvar leiomyosarcoma in Bartholin's gland area: a case report and literature review. *Arch. Gynecol. Obstet.*, **279** (2), 171–174.

194 Tavassoli, F.A., Norris, H.J. (1979) Smooth muscle tumors of the vulva. *Obstet. Gynecol.*, **53** (2), 213–217.

195 Tjalma, W.A., Hauben, E.I., Deprez, S.M., Van Marck, E.A., van Dam, P.A. (1999) Epithelioid sarcoma of the vulva. *Gynecol. Oncol.*, **73** (1), 160–164.

196 Ulbright, T.M., Brokaw, S.A., Stehman, F.B., Roth, L.M. (1983) Epithelioid sarcoma of the vulva. Evidence suggesting a more aggressive behavior than extra-genital epithelioid sarcoma. *Cancer*, **52** (8), 1462–1469.

197 Chiyoda, T., Ishikawa, M., Nakamura, M., Ogawa, M., Takamatsu, K. (2011) Successfully treated case of epithelioid sarcoma of the vulva. *J. Obstet. Gynaecol. Res.*, **37** (12), 1856–1859.

198 Holloway, C.L., Russell, A.H., Muto, M., Albert, M., Viswanathan, A.N. (2007) Synovial cell sarcoma of the vulva: multimodality treatment incorporating preoperative external-beam radiation, hemivulvectomy, flap reconstruction, interstitial brachytherapy, and chemotherapy. *Gynecol. Oncol.*, **104** (1), 253–256.

199 Vang, R., Medeiros, L.J., Malpica, A., Levenback, C., Deavers, M. (2000) Non-Hodgkin's lymphoma involving the vulva. *Int. J. Gynecol. Pathol.*, **19** (3), 236–242.

200 Swanson, S., Innes, D.J., Jr, Frierson, H.F., Jr, Hess, C.E. (1987) T-immunoblastic lymphoma mimicking B-immunoblastic lymphoma. *Arch. Pathol. Lab. Med.*, **111** (11), 1077–1080.

201 Wilkinson, E.J., Rico, M.J., Pierson, K.K. (1982) Microinvasive carcinoma of the vulva. *Int. J. Gynecol. Pathol.*, **1** (1), 29–39.

202 Collins, C.G., Lee, F.Y., Roman-Lopez, J.J. (1971) Invasive carcinoma of the vulva with lymph node metastasis. *Am. J. Obstet. Gynecol.*, **109** (3), 446–452.

203 Curry, S.L., Wharton, J.T., Rutledge, F. (1980) Positive lymph nodes in vulvar squamous carcinoma. *Gynecol. Oncol.*, **9** (1), 63–67.

33

Ovary

Charles A. Kunos

Introduction

Epithelial ovarian cancer ranks first among the most frequently lethal forms of gynecologic cancer. The American Cancer Society estimates that 22 440 American women will be newly diagnosed in 2017, with 14 080 fatalities attributed to ovarian cancer disease progression [1]. Age-specific incidence of the disease rises with age such that the peak incidence occurs between age 65 and 69 years, but 52% of women are aged <65 years when diagnosed [2, 3].

Here, the rationale, logistics, and technical aspects of radiotherapy are discussed as pertaining to ovarian cancer management. Clinical outcomes are reviewed, with comments on future plans for novel radiation therapy delivery systems and radiotherapy coadministered with novel anticancer agents.

Epidemiology

A unifying hypothesis for the pathogenesis of epithelial ovarian cancer remains elusive. Environmental, dietary, reproductive, embryological, endocrine, and genetic factors are all implicated in the epidemiology of epithelial ovarian cancer.

Factors that reduce the number of ovulatory cycles may be protective against developing ovarian cancer, while factors that increase the lifetime number of ovulations may increase risk. This has led to the contentious hypothesis that epithelial ovarian cancer may be the result of reparative error of the ovary surface epithelium after ovulatory cycle rupture and subsequent healing. For instance, parity inversely associates with risk related to ovarian cancer, with relative risk declining with increasing number of pregnancies [4, 5]. Breast feeding

[5] and oral contraceptive use [6,7] both lower the risk of ovarian cancer due to suppression of ovulatory cycling. Ovulatory infertility and its associated futile cycling of the epithelium may be associated with an elevated ovarian cancer risk [8]. The use of ovulation-inducing fertility drugs raises the relative risk of ovarian cancer [8, 9]. Molecular studies of human ovarian carcinomas are increasingly finding perturbed molecular pathways associated with neoplasia and eventual carcinogenesis [10, 11].

Hereditary (familial) ovarian cancer occurs in Lynch type II cancer family syndromes (also known as hereditary non-polyposis colorectal cancer). Hereditary ovarian cancers account for 5–10% of the total number of cancers found among families with this syndrome [12]. In addition, hereditary ovarian–breast cancer syndromes are associated with mutations in DNA repair genes *BRCA1* and *BRCA2* [13, 14]. The *BRCA1* breast cancer susceptibility gene suppresses tumors by actively participating in DNA double-strand break repair through homologous recombination [15], nucleotide excision repair [16], and base-excision repair of oxidative DNA damage [17]. The *BRCA2* (*FANCD1*) tumor suppressor gene product binds, in a critical step, the homologous recombination repair protein *RAD51* to single-strand DNA. The disruption of *BRCA2* function antagonizes DNA repair and promotes carcinogenesis. Inheritance of mutant alleles for *BRCA1* or *BRCA2* predisposes cancer development when the remaining wild-type allele is damaged or inactivated. It is thought that a second mutation or irreparable change in the remaining wild-type allele would be needed for 'phenotypic' expression. Women with familial ovarian cancer are frequently diagnosed in their forties, in contrast to women with sporadic ovarian cancer who are typically in their sixties. Once thought to be rare, familial ovarian cancer may be more common than originally appreciated [18]. Increased awareness has

Clinical Radiation Oncology: Indications, Techniques, and Results, Third Edition. Edited by William Small Jr.
© 2017 John Wiley & Sons, Inc. Published 2017 by John Wiley & Sons, Inc.

Table 33.1 Carcinoma of the ovary: FIGO staging and TNM classification.

FIGO	TNM category			Description
Stage I				Growth limited to ovaries
IA	T1a			Growth limited to one ovary; no ascites containing malignant cells; no tumor on external surface; capsule intact
IB	T1b			Growth limited to both ovaries; no ascites containing malignant cells; no tumor on external surface, capsule intact
IC	T1c			Tumor limited to one or both ovaries, but with tumor on surface of one or both ovaries, or capsule ruptured, or malignant ascites or malignant peritoneal washings
Stage II				Growth involving one or both ovaries with pelvic extension
IIA	T2a			Extension and/or metastases to the uterus and/or fallopian tubes
IIB	T2b			Extension to other pelvic tissues
IIC	T2c			Tumor extension to uterus, fallopian tubes, or other pelvic tissues, but with tumor on surface of one or both ovaries, or capsule ruptured, or malignant ascites or malignant peritoneal washings
Stage III				Tumor involving one or both ovaries with histologically confirmed peritoneal implants outside the pelvis and/or regional lymph nodes. Superficial liver metastases equals stage III. Tumor is limited to the true pelvis, but with histologically proven malignant extension to small bowel or omentum.
IIIA	T3a			Tumor grossly limited to the true pelvis with negative lymph nodes, but with histologically confirmed microscopic seeding of abdominal peritoneal surfaces, or histologically proven extension to small bowel or mesentery
IIIB	T3b			Tumor of one or both ovaries with histologically confirmed implant, peritoneal metastasis of abdominal peritoneal surfaces, none exceeding 2 cm in diameter; lymph nodes are negative
IIIC	T3c	N1		Peritoneal metastasis beyond the pelvis >2 cm in diameter and/or positive regional lymph nodes
Stage IV			M1	Growth involving one or both ovaries with distant metastases. If pleural effusion is present, there must be positive cytology to allot stage IV classification. Parenchymal liver metastases equals stage IV.

Adapted from [47] and [158].

led to better risk estimation among hereditary ovarian cancer syndrome cohorts.

Ovarian cancer is usually diagnosed at an advanced stage at initial surgery (Table 33.1), often attributed to asymptomatic 'silent' dissemination of disease throughout the abdominal cavity. Efforts to prevent ovarian cancer have included oral contraceptive use and prophylactic oophorectomy. Five years of oral contraceptive use lowers risk in nulliparous women to risk levels comparable to those in parous women who have not used oral contraceptives [19]. Ten years of oral contraceptive use in women having hereditary ovarian cancer syndromes reduces risk levels to lower than women without family history and no oral contraceptive use [19]. Prophylactic oophorectomy has been advocated for women with a validated family history of ovarian cancer (i.e., two or more first-degree relatives affected) [20–22]. This is not straightforward since the removal of histologically normal ovaries does not eliminate the risk of primary peritoneal carcinomatosis, which may be cytopathologically identical and clinically interchangeable with ovarian cancers [23].

Non-invasive imaging modalities and tumor markers have been investigated for the early detection of ovarian cancer. Diagnostic transvaginal ultrasound (used due to its independence from ionizing radiation for image contrast) has been met with dubious sensitivity for detecting abnormal cell clusters in the ovary [24]. Ultrasound contrast agents, such as microbubbles (1–8 μm diameter) and nanobubbles (170–250 nm diameter) of inert gas cores surrounded by lipid, protein, or polymer shells, are improving the sensitivity and the specificity of detecting early ovarian abnormalities. Yet, ultrasound utilizing bubble contrast agents has not yet found widespread clinical relevance for the early detection of cancer [25, 26]. The manner in which bubbles detect intrinsic abnormalities of the ovary depends upon bubble vibration or 'bounce' under ultrasound acoustic pressure (i.e., bubbles shrink at high pressure and expand under low pressure). Acoustic impedance mismatch between host tissue and bubbles produces ultrasound image contrast. Nanobubble ultrasound imaging agents are capable of detecting cancer target receptors, and this revelation has accelerated clinical development of bubble contrast agents.

Serum biomarkers for early detection of ovarian cancer also have been considered. The blood serum carbohydrate antigen 125 (CA-125) serves as a biomarker for epithelial ovarian cancer, although a rise in CA-125 occurs in benign disease such as endometriosis, uterine fibroids, pelvic inflammatory disease, or other medical conditions irritating peritoneal surfaces. An elevation in CA-125 greater than 65 U/ml (normal detectable range 0–35 U/ml) has a sensitivity of 97% and specificity of 78% for ovarian cancer, but this measure is less reliable in premenopausal women [27]. A clinical trial randomized 78 216 women undergoing screening for ovarian cancer to have routine health examination or to routine health examination plus annual CA-125 testing and pelvic transvaginal ultrasound [24]. In the CA-125 plus ultrasound group, 212 ovarian cancers were found. This compared non-significantly with the 176 ovarian cancers found by routine examination. Survival attributed to the CA-125 plus ultrasound intervention group was not improved significantly. No national consensus has been reached on CA-125 testing or ultrasound, alone or together, for comprehensive screening of early-stage ovarian cancer. CA-125 may be useful to monitor disease state and potential relapse; however, when elevated post-therapy as a signal for early relapse after anticancer treatment, a threshold for initiating treatment in an otherwise asymptomatic woman remains the subject of debate [28]. A recent clinical trial has shown routine surveillance of CA-125 postoperatively does not affect long-term survival [29].

Human epididymal secretory protein E4 (HE4) is a new serological biomarker for the diagnosis of ovarian cancer. As compared to CA-125 and other biomarkers, HE4 is sensitive for the detection of early ovarian cancer [30,31], while the HE4-encoding protein whey-acidic polypeptide (WAP) four-disulfide core domain protein 2 (WFDC2) may be selectively expressed in serous and endometrioid ovarian cancers [32, 33]. Measuring both HE4 and CA-125 together provides a more accurate tool for differentiating ovarian cancer from normal ovaries (93% sensitivity) and from ovarian endometriotic cysts (79% sensitivity) in healthy women [34].

Histology and Molecular Biology

The histological classification of ovarian tumors is complex. The most widely accepted classifications are listed in Table 33.2, as recommended by the World Health Organization. Tumors are categorized further as serous, mucinous, endometrioid, clear cell, and transitional (Brenner) cell tumor (Table 33.3) [35]. Other categories included mixed tumors and undifferentiated carcinomas. Within each category except for the undifferentiated carcinomas, tumors may be either benign or malignant.

Table 33.2 Frequency of ovarian neoplasms.*

Class	Frequency (%)
Epithelial stromal tumors	65
Germ cell tumors	20–25
Sex cord-stromal tumors	6
Lipid (lipoid) cell tumors	<0.1
Gonadoblastoma	<0.1
Unclassified	<0.1
Secondary (metastatic) tumors	5

*World Health Organization Classification.

Histological grade in malignant tumors ranges from 1 to 3, corresponding to the progressive loss of differentiation. Mixed epithelial and sarcomatous tumors exist. There are variants that include homologous and heterologous mesodermal (Müllerian) mixed tumors, stromal sarcomas, and tumors of germ and sex-cord-stromal origin [35]. Attention in this chapter is focused predominantly on the epithelial tumors.

It is essential for the treating physician to appreciate that a label of 'borderline' or low-malignant potential tumor occurs within the categories of serous, mucinous, clear-cell and endometrioid variants of ovarian cancer. Labeling tumors borderline may be a subtle distinction, requiring evaluation by experienced gynecologic pathologists able to integrate operative and histopathologic findings. Because borderline tumors behave in an indolent manner, there is a lack of persuasive evidence that therapy, other than surgery, alters prognosis. Death attributable to borderline tumor progression is unusual in stage I or II patients regardless of whether adjuvant therapy was utilized [36]. Among those patients with stage III or IV borderline tumors, physicians are often reluctant to refrain from therapy. Survival at five years post-therapy is not indicative of freedom-from-disease, as relapses may occur after more than five years and disease-related mortality approaches 25–35% [37, 38]. Data suggest that DNA content may simply segregate indolent from aggressive borderline tumors. For

Table 33.3 Epithelial ovarian tumor cell types.

	Approximate Frequency	
Type	All Neoplasms	Cancers
Serous	20–50	35–40
Mucinous	15–25	6–10
Endometrioid	5	15–25
Clear-cell (mesonephroid)	<5	5
Transitional cell (Brenner)	2–3	<1

Source: Rustin 2010 [29]. Reproduced with permission of Elsevier.

example, women aged ≥60 years with diploid borderline tumors had a 15-year survival of 75% compared to similarly aged women with aneuploid tumors whose 15-year survival was 20% [39]. Molecular studies of borderline ovarian cancers have not yet uncovered reliable biomarkers that predict biologic behavior [40]. Emerging evidence suggests that chemotherapy administration may coax aneuploid tumors out of dormant or proliferation-arrested conditions due to the selective pressure of recruiting cellular machinery to repair damaged DNA [41]. Further investigations are required in this area.

Endometrioid carcinomas of the ovary introduce other management challenges. Up to 25% of women with endometrioid ovarian cancers will have a synchronous cancer of the uterus, which itself may represent an independent primary neoplasm and multifocal malignant transformation of the Müllerian tract, or may represent metastasis from the uterus (classifying stage IIIA disease) [42, 43]. Endometrioid carcinoma of the ovary may also arise from a site of benign endometriosis, as a consequence of unopposed estrogen used for replacement therapy in postmenopausal women, and is less often associated with abdominal dissemination of disease [44, 45]. Indeed, women with localized endometrioid cancers of the ovary were once considered 'radiocurable,' through the use of opposed radiation anteroposterior and posteroanterior portals limited to just the ovary or volume-directed parametria [46].

Surgery

Staged assignment of ovarian cancer relies on operative findings, except for those women with extra-abdominal disease such as cytology-confirmed malignant pleural effusion (see Table 33.1) [47]. Exploration of the abdomen should be performed through an incision permitting access to the entire peritoneal cavity such that all sites of disease are removed. Ascites should be sampled. Peritoneal washes of the pelvis, pericolonic gutters, and undersurfaces of the liver and diaphragm also should be obtained. Encapsulated ovarian masses should be removed without rupture, if technically feasible. Vigorous surgical efforts should be made to remove all accessible sites of disease. In the absence of clinically apparent disease, a rigorous abdominal exploration should be carried out to evaluate all surfaces of the peritoneum. Random biopsies of 'normal' areas and areas of 'benign' adhesions should be obtained to evaluate for carcinoma. Omentectomy, para-aortic and pelvic node sampling, and biopsies of the cul-de-sac, pericolonic gutters, and undersurface of the diaphragm should be routinely performed. With rare exception, total hysterectomy and bilateral salpingo-oophorectomy should be carried

out. Following this, 31% of patients who are clinically stage I or II will be upstaged to stage III [48]. Moreover, women with small-volume disease of the ovary (<1 cm) have a better recurrence-free interval and survival than those with large-volume disease of the ovary (>1 cm) [49]. Cytoreduction to less than 1.5 cm of disease at surgery was first found to impact post-therapy survival [50], but today the extirpation of disease to <1 cm is considered optimal cytoreductive surgery and continues to have prognostic significance for post-therapy survival outcome [51].

Second-Look Surgery

Second-look surgery was popularized as a means to identify patients without identifiable residual tumor for whom discontinuation of chemotherapy might be feasible. In addition to acute toxicities, a late induction of leukemia has been linked to the prolonged use of alkylating chemotherapeutic drugs [52,53]. Despite refinements in body imaging, the most reliable method for assessing whether morphologically persistent cancer is present after chemotherapy remains second surgery. Even when a CA-125 level in a marker-positive patient has fallen to within normal limits, persistent cancer can be identified in up to 62% of women [54, 55]. Second-look surgery has not been adopted as a means of improving ultimate patient survival. Despite negative findings at second surgery, 50% of women with negative second-look procedures after platinum-containing chemotherapy will relapse [56, 57]. The likelihood of relapse correlates with a higher initial ovarian cancer stage, a higher histological grade, and the extent of residual disease after initial surgery [56, 57]. While second-look surgery may be used to select patients after response to first-line chemotherapy and before consolidative therapies such as intraperitoneal chemotherapy, radiophosphorus, or radiochemotherapy, the benefit of second-look surgery has been marginal since no generally accepted consolidative therapy has provided convincing evidence that such therapy alters survival or relapse rates.

Women who relapse after negative second surgery, particularly if the interval to relapse is more than 12 months, will have a significant chance of response to second-line chemotherapy. Similarly, women may remain sensitive to the agents that induced the initial complete clinical response seen at second-look surgery. However, curative management remains elusive. Women with persistent disease detected at second laparotomy or by radiographic imaging may be candidates for additional systemic cytotoxic therapies, possibly including new biologic agents, dose-intense chemotherapy, or radiochemotherapy. There is no national standard of care for these patients at present.

Robotic-Assisted Surgery

Whether robotic-assisted surgery improves upon the ability to surgically cytoreduce ovarian cancer is an open question. While the improved ergonomics may aid in these types of radical surgery, other limitations inherent in the robotic platform – namely the inability to simultaneously operate in the pelvis and abdomen – remain a significant disadvantage.

Robotic surgery for ovarian cancer management remains relatively untested. In the limited experience to date, blood loss and postoperative complications of bowel injury and wound dehiscence are infrequent. Port site relapses have not been reported routinely among the early investigational studies. A single manuscript has compared robotic surgery to traditional means of ovarian cancer staging surgery [58]. In this case-control study, 25 patients undergoing primary staging for epithelial ovarian cancers were matched to patients treated by laparoscopy and by laparotomy. In the authors' view, laparoscopic surgery or robotic surgery provided adequate surgical access to sites of potential disease and allowed reasonable maximal safe tumor excision in women not requiring extensive bowel or upper abdominal debulking during their ovarian cancer staging procedures. It must be emphasized that these patients were highly selected and their results are not likely to apply to all women with ovarian cancer. While robotic surgery reduces postoperative surgery-related complications and shortens patient recovery time, (thereby dropping interval wait times for start of chemotherapy),

robotic surgery may limit a surgeon's ability to detect and excise tumor. Additionally, robotic surgical instruments may seed tumor elsewhere. These limitations have not been meticulously investigated. To this end, the use of robotic surgery in the setting of ovarian cancer management is not recommended until further study suggests otherwise.

Chemotherapy

Women undergoing laparotomy for ovarian cancer often receive post-surgical cytotoxic chemotherapy. Women with grade 1 or 2, stage IA or IB ovarian cancer based on vigorous surgical staging can be observed closely as survival exceeds 90% in this group of patients [59]. Women with grade 3 ovarian cancer or higher operative stage are recommended to have combination systemic chemotherapy selected from a variety of agents targeting molecular pathways (Table 33.4).

The standard therapy regimen for women with ovarian cancer includes surgery followed by a platinum–taxane combination chemotherapy infusion every three weeks for six cycles [60]. For two decades, intravenous combination chemotherapy regimens with platinum (cisplatin, carboplatin) and paclitaxel have been the standard post-surgical treatment for women with ovarian cancer [61]. Platinum and paclitaxel therapies are associated with normal tissue sequelae, and these sequelae may be substantial [60]. For example, they may be severe enough to disrupt the completion of scheduled infusions,

Table 33.4 Efficacy of anticancer agents in platinum-sensitive and -resistant ovarian cancer.

Agent	Platinum-sensitive response rate	Platinum-resistant response rate	Progression-free survival (weeks)	Molecular target	Main toxicity
Paclitaxel	20–41	14–26	28	Mitotic spindle	Myelosuppression
Docetaxel	28–38	22–25	20	Mitotic spindle	Myelosuppression
Vinorelbine	15–29	15–21	16	Mitotic spindle	Myelosuppression
Pegylated liposomal doxorubicin	19–28	14–26	22	DNA	Mucositis, palmar-plantar erythrodysthesia
Hexamethylmelamine	10–27	10–18	16	DNA	Nausea and emesis
Ifosfamide	12–15	12–15	17	DNA	Hemorrhagic cystitis, neurotoxicity
Gemcitabine	16–22	13–22	19	Ribonucleotide reductase	Myelosuppression
Topotecan	24–33	14–18	23	Topoisomerase	Myelosuppression
Etoposide	27–35	16–27	17	Topoisomerase	Myelosuppression
Tamoxifen	10–15	10–15	16	Estrogen receptor blockade	Hot flashes and thromboembolic events
Anastrozole	10–15	10–15	16	Estrogen receptor blockade	Osteopenia and muscle aches

resulting in poorer long-term outcomes. The introduction of topotecan, gemcitabine, and bevacizumab have advanced ovarian cancer management; yet, long-term rates of disease control attributed to cytoreductive surgery paired with systemic chemotherapy remain in the region of 20% [62]. A regimen of the antiangiogenic agent bevacizumab plus chemotherapy may extend survival in women with recurrent epithelial ovarian cancer [63]. Preliminary Phase III results of six cycles of carboplatin and paclitaxel with bevacizumab followed by single-agent bevacizumab every three weeks for 12 additional cycles showed a two-month improvement in median duration of progression-free survival [64]. A second Phase III clinical trial (OCEANS) has shown a four-month improvement in median progression-free survival after six to 10 cycles of carboplatin and gemcitabine plus bevacizumab followed by additional bevacizumab in women with platinum-sensitive recurrent epithelial ovarian, peritoneal, or fallopian tube cancers [65]. Chemotherapy plus bevacizumab may hold promise in the setting of persistent or recurrent epithelial ovarian cancer.

In an attempt to lengthen survival, lower risk of relapse, and preserve quality of life through the reduction of treatment-related sequelae, members of the National Cancer Institute proposed the direct instillation of chemotherapy into the peritoneal cavity [66]. Today, the insertion of an intraperitoneal drug delivery catheter (fenestrated or Port-A-Cath) has become a routine surgical procedure among gynecologic oncologists and usually only adds 15–30 min to the operative time [67]. The pharmacologic advantage of ovarian tumor cells bathing in the instilled chemotherapy has proven to be substantial in Phase I [68, 69] and Phase 2 [70–72] testing. Three Phase III randomized clinical trials have been conducted, using intraperitoneal cisplatin plus intravenous cyclophosphamide (Southwest Oncology Group [SWOG 8501]/Gynecologic Oncology Group [GOG 0104]) [73], intraperitoneal cisplatin plus intravenous paclitaxel (GOG 0114) [74], and intraperitoneal cisplatin plus both intravenous and intraperitoneal paclitaxel (GOG 0172) [75]. From these three studies, intraperitoneal instillation of chemotherapy provided median overall survival gains of eight months (SWOG 8501/GOG 0104), 11 months (GOG 0114), and 16 months (GOG 0172). Intraperitoneal therapies instilled directly into the abdomen have been associated with mixed toxicity results [67]. As such, the National Cancer Institute issued a Clinical Announcement in January 2006 recommending that women with optimally resected stage III ovarian cancer be counseled about the survival benefits associated with the combination of intravenous and intraperitoneal chemotherapy [76].

New anticancer agents effective against ovarian cancer are emerging. Trabectedin plus pegylated liposomal doxorubicin has been tested effectively in women with partially platinum-sensitive ovarian cancer [77]. Trabectedin chemically fits within the DNA minor groove and alkylates the N2 amino group of guanine, with predilection for RC-rich sequences, and bends DNA toward the major groove [78]. A randomized study of 672 women with recurrent ovarian cancer after failure of first-line, platinum-based chemotherapy found a median improvement in progression-free survival of 1.5 months after trabectedin and pegylated doxorubicin (hazard ratio 0.79 [95% CI 0.65–0.96], $P = 0.019$) versus pegylated doxorubicin alone [77]. For women with platinum-sensitive ovarian cancer, the response rate was higher with the trabectedin and pegylated doxorubicin combination (35%) as compared to pegylated doxorubicin alone (23%, $P = 0.004$) [77]. Toxicities were transient and non-cumulative, suggesting tolerance of the regimen [77]. This non-platinum-based regimen may be considered a new treatment option for women with advanced ovarian cancer after failure of platinum-based chemotherapy, particularly for women with an interval to relapse of 12 months or less [79].

Also, it has been established that ribonucleotide reductase (RNR) is crucial to intracellular DNA damage response occurring after cytotoxic chemotherapies [80, 81]. Pharmacological blockade of the RNR subunit M1 by gemcitabine [82], or the RNR subunits M2 or M2b (p53R2) by hydroxyurea or 3-aminopyridine-2-carboxaldehyde thiosemicarbazone (3-AP) [81] renders RNR inactive. The long-lived M1 subunit has a catalytic site that the suicide-inhibitor gemcitabine can bind covalently and inactivate RNR. Both, the M2 and p53M2b subunits house a tyrosine free radical stabilized by diferric iron moieties. Hydroxyurea or 3-AP quenches the M2/p53M2b free radical, impeding regeneration of the M1 catalytic site during ribonucleotide reduction reaction. Ovarian [83] cancers have relatively high levels of RNR. Indeed, when ovarian cancer RNR is blocked by 3-AP, RNR inhibition restored platinum-chemosensitivity in an otherwise platinum-resistant ovarian cancer cell model [84]. A better understanding of the interrelated cellular mechanisms regulating RNR activity will guide the selection of RNR inhibitors to best combat ribonucleotide reduction for repair of DNA damage after cytotoxic chemotherapy.

Chromosome assembly and packing occurring the G2-M-phase transition makes cells not only vulnerable to deadly DNA damage from cytotoxic chemotherapy, but also sensitive to 'poisons' of the mitotic spindle. Plant alkaloids, such as vinorelbine and vincristine, block the assembly of tubulin causing toxic destruction of the mitotic spindle. Paclitaxel (and its synthetic analog docetaxel) is derived from the bark of the Western yew tree (*Taxus baccata*), and inhibits the depolymerization of tubulin at the conclusion of mitosis. The taxane

Figure 33.1 Disease-free survival was estimated for two platinum-containing hypothetical treatments in women with ovarian cancer, measuring time intervals from date of enrollment to date of first relapse, death, or censored follow-up. Three conceptual categories for women and their disease response emerge: (i) those that are platinum-insensitive (0–6-month post-therapy disease-related relapse or death); (ii) those that are partially platinum-sensitive (6–18-month post-therapy disease-related relapse or death); and (iii) those that are platinum-sensitive (≥18-month post-therapy disease-related relapse or death. Opportunities for targeted biologic chemotherapy, cytotoxic chemotherapy, and radiotherapeutic intervention are noted.

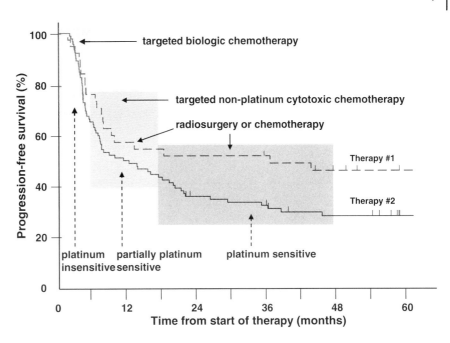

cabazitaxel promotes tubulin assembly and stabilizes microtubules against depolymerization in cells, acting similarly in mechanism to paclitaxel. Cabazitaxel has been shown to sensitize ovarian cancer cells to the effects of radiation due to cell cycle redistribution, and best when cabazitaxel was given 24 h before radiation [85]. The epipodophyllotoxin etoposide (derived from the root of the May apple) stabilizes DNA strand breaks made by topoisomerase 2 during supercoiling of DNA. Camptothecin (and its semisynthetic derivatives topotecan and irinotecan) is obtained from a Tibetan deciduous tree (*Camptotheca accuminata*) and blocks topoisomerase I, an enzyme that relaxes DNA structural tension by propagating single-strand breaks. Lastly, the process of connecting mitotic spindle poles to kinetichores at the centromeres of each chromosome is regulated by Aurora A-C serine/threonine kinases. Pharmacological agents targeting Aurora kinases are being studied for their anticancer properties [86]. Further study is warranted in the role of these agents in the treatment of ovarian cancer.

Patients too infirm for initial operative intervention or with stage IV disease or non-resectable disease may gain clinical benefit from neoadjuvant chemotherapy approaches. Opportunities to decrease morbidity through less substantial surgery, to allow improvement in performance of daily living activities, and to achieve optimal surgical results all have been mentioned as benefits of such an approach. In a matched one neoadjuvant-to-one cytoreductive surgery case series of 60 patients, optimal cytoreduction was achieved equally (76% versus 60%) as well in both, despite the neoadjuvant cohort being older and more infirm [87]. In this particular study, progression-free and overall survival outcomes were found to be similar in both cohorts. Long-term

results have not established a clear role for neoadjuvant chemotherapy in the management of advanced ovarian cancer [88], but it is a good therapeutic option in the appropriately selected patient.

Importantly, long-term freedom from disease is the most unambiguous outcome for women with ovarian cancer. The goal of improving long-term outcome has translated into the use of overall survival as the primary end point in therapy trials (Figure 33.1). A five-year survival end point has the advantage of being simple to measure, easy to interpret, straightforward to explain, and clinically meaningful. A disadvantage of a five-year end point is extended follow-up. Metrics for judging the success of particular treatment for ovarian cancer may be considered in context of cancer sensitivity to platinum: women having persistence or relapse within six months of platinum therapy are considered having platinum-insensitive disease, women having disease recur between six and 18 months as having partially platinum-sensitive disease, and women having disease relapse 18 months or greater from initial platinum therapy as having platinum-sensitive disease (Figure 33.1). Ovarian cancers are radiosensitive, with treatment effectively controlling therapy-naïve and early or late chemorefractory disease [89–92]. Attention is now focused on radiotherapeutic interventions for women with ovarian cancer.

Radiotherapy

The use of radiation to treat patients with ovarian cancer has a long and storied history. The ovary and its associated malignancies are exquisitely sensitive to the effects of radiation [89–92]. In the past, radiation has been used as: (i) primary therapy following surgical diagnosis with or without cytoreduction; (ii) consolidation after complete response to surgery and chemotherapy; (iii) a chemosensitizer for persistent or recurrent disease; and (iv) second-line therapy for persistent disease after surgery and chemotherapy. Radiation by external beam radiotherapy (EBRT) has targeted the entire abdominopelvic cavity, the pelvis, or other tumor-directed volumes of the peritoneal cavity. Intraperitoneal isotopes have been administered to treat entire peritoneal surfaces. Clearly radiation is an active agent in ovarian cancer, but the goal of identifying clinical circumstances when radiation can be used with predictable clinical benefit remains obscure.

Radiophosphorus

The intraperitoneal instillation of colloidal suspensions of radioactive isotopes of gold (^{198}Au) and phosphorus (^{32}P) has been a theoretically attractive means of treatment for ovarian cancer patients. Ovarian cancer can be expected to manifest diffuse dissemination to multiple foci scattered throughout the peritoneal surfaces, without demonstrating extra-abdominal spread until late in the clinical course of the disease. Intraperitoneal isotope administration 'coats' all peritoneal surfaces with sufficient radiation dose to sterilize the tumor cells without undue gastrointestinal toxicity, hematopoietic suppression and marrow ablation, and time commitments to fractionated whole-abdominopelvic radiation.

Due to partial γ-emission of ^{198}Au and concerns about radiation exposure to individuals other than the patient, ^{198}Au is no longer routinely used for intraperitoneal therapy. As a pure β-emitter, ^{32}P has become the radioisotope of choice ($t_{1/2}$ = 14.3 days). Radiophosphorus has been used as post-surgical therapy for ovarian cancer whose tumor: (i) ruptures during surgery; (ii) is found on the surface of the ovary; (iii) is associated with malignant ascites; or (iv) is confined to the ovary and has high-grade histology. However, a randomized Gynecologic Oncology Group clinical trial comparing ^{32}P and melphalan in stage I or II patients with such characteristics found no survival benefit for one therapy compared to the other at five years [59]. While associated with favorable survival, treatment with adjuvant ^{32}P carries a higher risk of bowel sequelae than treatment with systemic chemotherapy [93].

A prospective randomized trial in Norway compared radiophosphorus to six courses of cisplatin as a single agent in women with thoroughly staged, completely resected stage I, II, and III epithelial ovarian cancers [94]. There was no statistically significant difference in relapse-free survival, but there was a 5% rate of bowel

obstruction requiring surgical intervention among the group treated with ^{32}P. The rate of bowel obstruction requiring surgery was 1% in the cisplatin-treated group. The Gynecologic Oncology Group conducted a prospective randomized trial comparing ^{32}P to three cycles of cisplatin and cyclophosphamide (GOG-0095) for patients with selected unfavorable stage IA and IB ovarian cancers or for patients with stage IC, stage IIA-C disease [95]. On study, there was a 3% risk for small bowel perforation after ^{32}P intraperitoneal administration. A non-significant cumulative incidence of recurrence at 10 years of 35% after ^{32}P versus 28% (P = 0.15) after chemotherapy led the investigators to conclude that platinum-based combinations were the preferred less-toxic adjuvant therapy for early ovarian cancer. Such data was repeated in an Italian study that randomized women with stage IC disease to six courses of cisplatin or intraperitoneal ^{32}P [96]. In stage III ovarian cancer patients who had received chemotherapy and then had a negative second-look laparotomy, the intraperitoneal instillation of ^{32}P did not lower the risk of relapse and did not lengthen survival as compared to no further therapy [97].

The methodological administration of ^{32}P (chromic phosphate suspension is not for intravascular use) has hampered its anticancer clinical development. Because of these technical concerns, ^{32}P has largely been abandoned in the setting of early stage or completely resected ovarian cancer. This radioisotope emits β-particles with a mean energy of 0.695 MeV, which will potentially treat 3 mm deep into peritoneal surface tissues. Predictably, deposits of ovarian cancer greater than 5 mm in depth or metastasis to retroperitoneal lymph nodes will not be affected by ^{32}P radiation dose. Because inflammatory adhesions form within days after surgery, radioisotope suspensions of ^{32}P are not distributed by the free flow of ascites fluid. Multi-perforated peritoneal catheters used for administration should be placed within hours of surgery, with first instillations of therapeutic doses of the isotope accomplished shortly thereafter. The sequence of administration is usually as follows: (i) 250 ml of normal saline is infused by catheter into the abdomen to ensure catheter function; (ii) ^{99}m-technetium injection followed by anterior and lateral abdominopelvic scans to ensure that loculation has not occurred; (iii) infusion of 15 mCi of chromic phosphate suspension in 500 ml of normal saline; (iv) flush of 250 ml normal saline (bringing the total infusion to 1000 ml); (v) removal of the catheter to prevent leakage of the chromic phosphate suspension. A carefully choreographed sequence of patient positional changes (e.g., every 10 min the patient rolls to her left side, onto her back, into Trendelenburg, into reverse Trendelenburg, and to her right side for 2 h) is needed to ensure uniform distribution of the radioisotope (Figure 33.2). Failure to observe all of these precautions

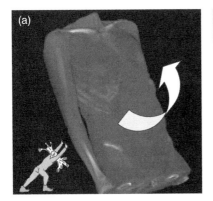 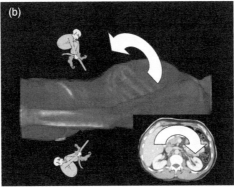 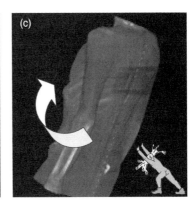

Figure 33.2 ^{32}P choreography. ^{32}P administration (15 mCi) necessitates patient movement every 10 min to ensure homogeneous delivery of the radioisotope. Movements generally include 10-min rolls to the left side (a), onto the back and into Trendelenburg or reverse Trendelenburg (b), and to her right side (c). These movements may occur for up to 2 h.

usually results in the under-dosage of peritoneal surfaces, loculation of radioisotope with focal soft-tissue injury usually manifesting as bowel obstruction, and ineffective treatment [98, 99]. The combination of ^{32}P and pelvic radiation has been met with unacceptably high toxicity and should be avoided [100].

In summary, the radioisotope ^{32}P has been used in ovarian cancer management to consolidate chemotherapy at the time of second-look laparotomy [97] or to treat small-volume persistent disease [101]. Overall, trial results have been conflicting, with sequelae outweighing perceived therapeutic benefits. No standard role for ^{32}P has been established. The methodological administration of ^{32}P and its minimal depth of treatment ($\sim$3 mm) appear to offer the greatest challenge for future anti-cancer clinical development.

External Radiation

Historically, external radiation administered to the whole abdomen or a portion of the abdomen has been used as first-line therapy following maximal surgical resection for women with stage I, II, or III ovarian cancer [102]. Currently, however, most patients are treated with chemotherapy, as this will often prolong survival for these patients without recognized late sequelae of bowel injury or obstruction. Chemotherapy doublets or other combinations are difficult, if not practically impossible, to administer following wide-field radiation due to profound effects on hematopoietic stem cell renewal. Thus, chemotherapy has assumed primacy in the post-surgical management of epithelial ovarian cancer, and the use of radiotherapy limited to isolated relapses or palliative measures.

Early efforts to lower the risk of relapse from ovarian cancer employed pelvic radiation. While successful in limiting disease relapse in pelvic tissue, the high frequency of extrapelvic and upper abdominal disease

recurrences limited its widespread application. Rigorous analysis of treatment and subsequent relapse patterns made it apparent that the appropriate target volume for first-line radiotherapeutic management of ovarian cancer is the whole abdominopelvic cavity [103, 104].

Because of limited radiation dose tolerance by sensitive organs such as the kidney, liver, and small bowel (100–150 cGy), bulky ovarian cancer disease may sustain only sublethal radiation-related DNA damage and be inadequately sterilized. In an effort to overcome this treatment barrier, abdominopelvic radiation by means of a 'moving-strip' technique or by open field encompassing the domes of the diaphragm to the pelvic floor sequentially blocked has been used. The strip technique originated when therapy machines could not generate fields large enough to encompass the whole abdomen in continuity. Treatment strips in 225 cGy doses theoretically decreased treatment time and improved local effectiveness, assuming that the cancer targets did not move between fractions. Cancer control outcomes associated with the moving-strip or with the open technique are equivalent, but consequential late effects of normal tissue have consistently been more pronounced with the moving strip technique [105, 106]. Examples of radiation portals, dose and fractionation guidelines are shown in Figure 33.3.

The best available lines of evidence for abdominopelvic irradiation as first-line therapy originate from Canada [103] and Australia [107, 108]. Consistently, risk of relapse and survival are better for women with no residual disease following surgery than for women with residual disease more than 2 cm in summed diameter. As such, the general consensus regarding whole-abdominopelvic radiation is that women with residual pelvic disease 2 cm or larger, or residual macroscopic disease in the upper abdomen, should not be managed in this fashion. Similarly, women with stage III disease should be managed only when chemotherapeutics cannot be given and if the ovarian cancer is grade 1. Following

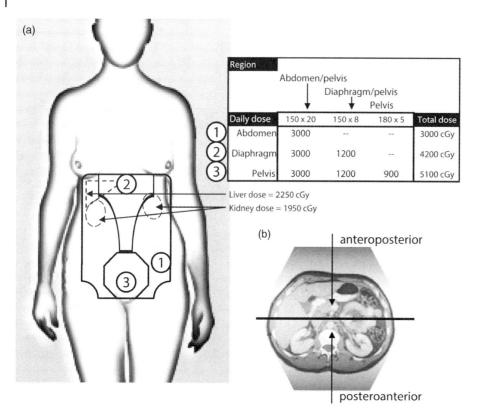

Region	Abdomen/pelvis	Diaphragm/pelvis	Pelvis	
Daily dose	150 × 20	150 × 8	180 × 5	**Total dose**
Abdomen	3000	--	--	3000 cGy
Diaphragm	3000	1200	--	4200 cGy
Pelvis	3000	1200	900	5100 cGy

Liver dose = 2250 cGy
Kidney dose = 1950 cGy

(b)

anteroposterior

posteroanterior

Figure 33.3 Abdominopelvic radiation for ovarian cancer. (a) Large-volume ① treatment fields are intended to cover the entire peritoneal cavity, including the vagina and pelvic floor. Expiratory and inspiratory gating, designed with the assistance of fluoroscopy or computed tomography, is done to ensure both leaves of the diaphragm are covered with respiratory motion. Lateral flash of the abdomen is preferred to provide adequate coverage of the peritoneal cavity, but is not always achieved. Prescriptions for volume ① are typically 3000 cGy. A T-shaped ② plus pelvic ③ volume encompasses the right and left diaphragmatic crus where the peritoneal lymphatics coalesce, the para-aortic nodes and pelvic lymph nodes for an additional 1200 cGy. The true pelvis ③ may receive a cone-down boost of 900 cGy. A daily radiation dose of 150 cGy is recommended. The right lateral edge of the liver should be shielded such that it receives a tolerable maximum of 2250 cGy. The right and left kidneys should be shielded (commonly with posterior beam five half-value layer lead or equivalent) for a tolerable maximum of 1950 cGy. (b) Radiation beam arrangements are typically opposed anteroposterior and posteroanterior.

these guidelines, outcomes from abdominopelvic radiation may not be inferior to polyagent chemotherapy [109–113]. Attempts to conduct prospective clinical trials have been unsuccessful, probably because treatments are so different that patient and investigator bias preclude adequate numbers of patients to complete a trial. Also, retrospective comparisons are hampered by the bulk of the radiation data antedating the era of vigorous surgical staging now performed in ovarian cancer patients. Women with comparable volumes of residual disease after laparotomy without debulking, as opposed to laparotomy with maximal effort at surgical cytoreduction, may fall into different prognostic groups. Moreover, there is a misconception that late radiation sequelae attributed to abdominopelvic radiation in modest doses are more frequent than in fact they are. Bowel obstruction is a complication of abdominopelvic radiation, but it also is a common event in the natural history of recurrent ovarian cancer. Bowel obstruction after abdominopelvic radiation, in the absence of tumor recurrence, is actually

an uncommon event. Among more than 600 women treated by abdominopelvic radiation as first-line therapy, between 2% and 6% required operative intervention for bowel complications [106, 107]. The relative merits of radiation for first-line post-surgical therapy are likely to continue to be debated.

Whole-Abdomen Radiation Technique

Irradiation of the entire abdominal contents is best planned with either a fluoroscopic or four-dimensional computed tomography (4-D CT) simulator to assure adequate coverage of the diaphragm throughout the respiratory cycle. 4-D CT scanners are state-of-the-art for integration of respiratory motion into the planning of abdominopelvic radiation fields [114, 115]. Care must also be taken to include the entirety of the peritoneum, meaning that superior borders are set 1.5 cm superior to the diaphragm and 1.5 cm inferior to the ischial tuberosities of the pelvis (Figure 33.3). Normally, the use of secondary collimation in an effort to shield non-critical normal tissue can risk marginal miss, particularly when patients are treated at an extended distance in the supine and prone positions. Because there are no critical tissues lateral to the peritoneum and the fraction size and total doses are modest, there is no major contraindication to treating the abdomen without collimation (so-called 'flashing' the skin) so that lateral radiation dose fall-off assures full coverage of the peritoneum. Posterior kidney shields (five half-value layers) have been used to limit the bilateral kidneys to dose ranges of 1800–2200 cGy, if the dose to the abdomen will be higher. Depending on the total abdominopelvic radiation dose prescribed, a portion of the liver may be shielded to restrict the dose to 2400–2700 cGy if 150 cGy per day doses are employed. Liver shielding is not needed if the abdominopelvic dose is 2250–2500 cGy if fractions of 100–125 cGy are used. Limited volumes may be escalated in dose, including: (i) medial leaves of the diaphragm where lymphatics coalesce; (ii) para-aortic lymph nodes in women with confirmed nodal metastases; and (iii) pelvis. Cumulative radiation doses to limited boost volumes may be as high as 5100 cGy, with boost fractions administered in 180–200 cGy fraction sizes.

Abdominopelvic radiation fields result in substantial hematopoietic suppression and gastrointestinal sequelae. Lowered blood counts will delay treatment in 27% of chemotherapy-naïve patients [116], but will interrupt treatment more frequently in patients treated by chemotherapy [117]. Treating physicians should consider holding therapy if absolute neutrophil counts are lower than 500 mm^{-3} or if platelet counts are lower than 35 000 mm^{-3} [118]. Gastroenteritis (20%), bowel obstruction (9–14%), or hepatitis (hepatic veno-occlusive disease, 3%) can manifest [119]. Scarring of the lung bases with rare pneumonitis (1%) can occur. Renal injury is uncommon if shielding is correctly used [120].

Intensity-Modulated and Helical Tomotherapy Radiation Techniques

Efforts to reduce abdominopelvic radiation treatment-related sequelae have incorporated the use of new, sophisticated radiation delivery systems. Historical limitations of crude radiation shielding in early years of abdominopelvic irradiation and the use of shrinking radiation treatment portal techniques have been replaced by more sophisticated radiation dose sculpting by beam collimation [111–113] and by more suitable large-field radiation techniques such as helical tomotherapy [121,122].

A first approach utilizes intensity-modulated radiation therapy (IMRT). This technique applies a non-uniform photon fluency among multiple angled radiation treatment beams to produce relative high-dose radiation in targeted tissues at the cost of exposing more intervening tissues to low radiation doses [111–113]. Current techniques deliver modest radiation dose to intervening abdominal organs and bowel, substantially lowering gastrointestinal, genitourinary, and marrow toxicities [123]. Consensus guidelines for delineation of target and organ at-risk volumes for pelvic IMRT are emerging [124]. Extended radiation beam field lengths often >40 cm, multiple dose isocenters in the abdomen and pelvis, and treatment complexity all limit the widespread practicality of IMRT for abdominopelvic radiation [111–113].

A second approach incorporates computer-guided planning and advanced treatment beam collimation such that 'shaped' beams conform to targeted tissue [121,122]. One such delivery system incorporates a linear accelerator coupled to a helical CT scanner for image-guided radiation therapy, a system termed 'helical tomotherapy' (Figure 33.4) [125]. The clinical use of helical tomotherapy has focused on radiation 'dose-painting,' where volumes of tumor tissue are targeted by a full 360° treatment arc. Helical tomotherapy treatment obviates extended beam field lengths and multiple dose isocenters due its continuous helical delivery of radiation. *Abdominopelvic tomotherapy* offers another advantage of improved radiation dose homogeneity while simultaneously providing high-priority radiation dose avoidance to critical organs at risk. As such, radiation dose hot spots common within bowel following conventional abdominopelvic radiation are avoided, lessening the risk of long-term bowel adverse events.

There are no clinical trials evaluating conventional abdominopelvic radiation with IMRT or helical tomotherapy techniques. While many dosimetry comparisons have been made [126–128], data validating such approaches remain sparse. Clearly, further investigative studies of these new abdominopelvic radiation techniques are warranted to fully scrutinize their capabilities of lowering radiation-related sequelae and their clinical benefit of control of ovarian cancer disease.

Radiochemotherapy

Radiation as adjuvant therapy: The integration of radiochemotherapy into mainstream treatment of ovarian cancer remains controversial. In a Phase II trial, women with stage II or III ovarian cancer underwent optimal surgical cytoreduction and six cycles of cisplatin-based chemotherapy, followed by abdominopelvic radiation [129]. As opposed to matched control patients with radiation alone, the median survival was 2.4 years versus 5.7 years, and relapse-free survival was 22% versus 43% at five years, favoring radiochemotherapy. No benefit [130] or minor benefit [131–133] of consolidative conventional abdominopelvic radiation has been observed in other clinical trials with few patients. Hyperfractionated abdominopelvic radiation after surgery and chemotherapy in women with stage III ovarian cancer has been attempted in a Phase II clinical trial conducted by the

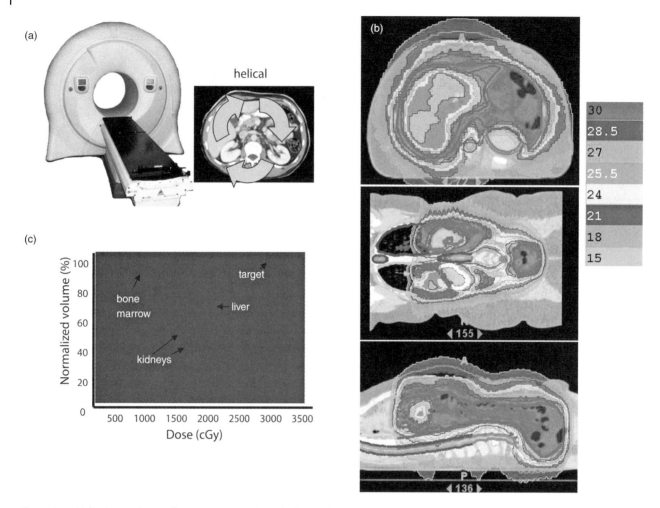

Figure 33.4 Helical tomotherapy for ovarian cancer. (a) Helical tomotherapy involves gradual passage through a circular bore with radiation delivered in helical arcs. (b) Avoidance structures (e.g., central liver parenchyma excluding 1 cm peripheral rim, central kidney excluding 1 cm peripheral rim) can be identified and prioritized for radiation dose exclusion. In this way, peritoneal surfaces are dosed by radiation, while underlying organ at-risk parenchyma are relatively spared from excessive radiation dose. For a color version of this figure, see the color plate section.

Gynecologic Oncology Group [134]. Of 37 patients with known disease status after post-surgical chemotherapy and second-look laparotomy, 21 (57%) had macroscopic persistent disease, four (11%) had microscopic disease, and 12 (32%) had no evidence of disease. Objective responses after abdominopelvic radiation were seen in eight (23%) of 35 treated women. Consistently across multiple studies, post-surgical chemotherapy and abdominopelvic radiation have been difficult to administer due to hematological toxicities. Up to one-third of patients are unable to complete planned therapies [132, 134, 135]. Partial abdominal radiation directed to limited volumes of persistent disease after surgery and chemotherapy makes sense if only one or two discrete targets are treated by radiation, and thus, consequential radiation-related acute and late toxicities are minimized.

Radiation as a chemosensitizer: Around the world, ovarian cancer remains a leading cause of cancer-related mortality among women, in part due to a greater than 65% incidence of persistent disease or less than six-month disease relapse after platinum chemotherapy [75,136]. Chemotherapeutic strategies to overcome platinum resistance have included coadministered paclitaxel or docetaxel [60,74,137], but whether other therapeutics such as radiation may restore platinum cytotoxicity in platinum-resistant ovarian cancer is uncertain. Patients with macroscopic disease at second-look laparotomy, even if cytoreduced to microscopic disease, fared substantially less well than patients with only microscopically persistent disease [138]. Radiochemotherapy may be of clinical benefit when women have macroscopic disease after primary surgery and chemotherapy.

It has been observed that low-dose radiation (50 cGy × four fractions) increased cell death in p53-mutated colon cancer when compared to single-fraction (200 cGy) radiation [139]. It was speculated that a first-dose radiation fraction arrested cells in a radiosensitive G2/M phase of the cell cycle and subsequent low-dose fractions resulted in cell cytotoxicity [140]. This led to the testable hypothesis that hyperfractionated low-dose abdominopelvic radiation may enhance the sensitivity of ovarian cancers to the antitumor effect of the cytotoxic G2/M anticancer agent docetaxel. In a Gynecologic Oncology Group Phase I study,140 women with persistent or recurrent advanced ovarian, peritoneal, or fallopian tube cancer underwent weekly docetaxel chemotherapy (20 mg m^{-2}) coadministered with twice-daily low-dose (60 cGy) whole-abdominopelvic radiation given twice weekly for six weeks. All 13 women on trial experienced hematological toxicities (majority grade 1 or 2), with thrombocytopenia (77%) the most frequent adverse event. Of 10 women with measureable disease prior to the start of trial therapy, three (30%) had no evidence of disease-progression at six months. It was concluded that radiochemotherapy was well tolerated, and indicated a possible chemosensitization effect. While this approach is intuitively reasonable, the validation of single-agent chemotherapeutics plus low-dose radiation data are needed to substantiate a chemosensitization radiation-drug effect.

Stereotactic Radiosurgery

In settings where surgery and first-line chemotherapy results in persistent small-volume chemorefractory ovarian cancer disease, stereotactic radiosurgery has emerged as an effective radiotherapeutic treatment modality [141]. One stereotactic radiosurgery system uses a linear accelerator mounted on an industrial robotic arm (Cyberknife®; Accuray Inc., Sunnyvale, CA), offering radiotherapeutic advantages in increased freedom in the number and in the angle of non-coplanar treatment beam trajectories to focus high-dose radiation on localized area(s) of disease while simultaneously distributing low-dose radiation to critical organs (Figure 33.5). Sub-millimeter accuracy (~0.4 mm) of radiosurgery delivery has been verified by end-to-end radiation dose phantoms [142–144]. A Phase II clinical trial enrolling 16 women with chemorefractory ovarian cancer (of 35 enrollees at the time of preliminary reporting) used an ablative stereotactic radiosurgery dose of 2400 cGy (800 cGy × three fractions) to sterilize abdominopelvic ovarian cancer targets [145]. Through a median follow-up of 12 months (range: 6–21 months), only one patient (6%) developed manageable hyperbilirubinemia when radiosurgery targeted an ovarian cancer metastasis to the liver. Otherwise, treatment has been safe and well-tolerated. Preliminary data show a 94% rate of radiosurgical ovarian cancer target response. Immature follow-up data have indicated a greater than 50% non-radiosurgical target rate of disease progression. The rise of occult chemorefractory metastatic ovarian cancer disease has stimulated interest in the coadministration of carboplatin and gemcitabine plus stereotactic radiosurgery in a pilot Phase I clinical trial. Further definition of the role of stereotactic radiosurgery in the overall management of ovarian cancer is needed.

Radiation for Rare Ovarian Neoplasms

Dysgerminoma is a germ cell line neoplasm that is exquisitely sensitive to radiation and can be considered analogous in radiation response to testicular seminoma in males. Dysgerminomas occur in women in their twenties and may involve both ovaries in 20% of cases. In women with bulky stage I disease, radiotherapy has been used with success [146, 147]. The most common application of radiation has been in the setting of primary disease of the ovary with disease metastases to para-aortic nodes (with consideration of prophylactic radiation to the mediastinum and supraclavicular fossae). Over the years, the chemotherapy regimen bleomycin, etoposide, and cisplatin (BEP) has replaced radiotherapy due to concerns of infertility [148, 149].

Dermoid cysts are mature cystic teratomas composed of epidermis and skin appendages. While mature tissue elements derived from all three embryonic germ cell layers may be present, primitive neural and squamous cells may undergo malignant transformation. These rare cancers are locally aggressive and spread early to regional node-bearing tissues. Radiotherapy may be useful in stage II or III patients (local extension of disease and/or regional nodal disease without diffuse peritoneal dissemination), although the heterogeneity of these uncommon patients precludes generalization concerning radiotherapeutic target volumes, doses, or fractionations. Other tumor arising in dermoids include malignant neural tumors, malignant thyroid tumors, melanoma, sarcoma, carcinoids, and basal cell carcinomas.

Granulosa cell tumors are malignant stromal tumors of the ovary affecting female infants, children, adolescents, and adult alike. The adult form of the disease is histologically distinct from that of the rare childhood form, is found in women in their fifties, and represents 5% of ovarian cancer incidence. Adult granulosa cell tumors are hormonally active and produce circulating estrogens such that there are associated menstrual cycle irregularities. Progesterone production can be detected. Hirsuitism, virilization, and oligomenorrhea may occur from androgen production within tumors. Granulosa cell tumor may be associated with uterine pathology in more than half of patients, with endometrial hyperplasia or endometrial cancer arising in response to prolonged unopposed estrogen exposure [150, 151]. Granulosa tumors are indolent, with relapses or metastases occurring many years after initial surgery [150–152]. Hormonal symptoms may antedate clinical tumor relapse or

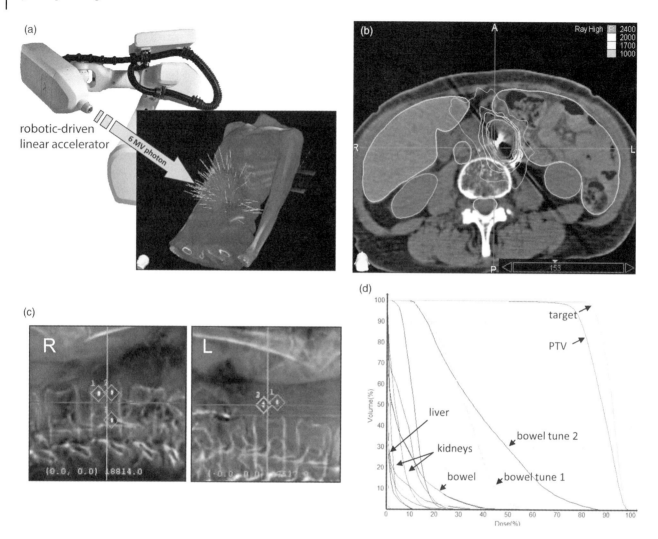

Figure 33.5 Stereotactic radiosurgery for ovarian cancer. (a) Depicted is a robotic stereotactic body radiosurgery system (Cyberknife®; Accuray, Sunnyvale, CA). The system allows for increased freedom in the number and in the angle of non-coplanar treatment beam trajectories (blue vectors) to focus high-dose radiation on localized area(s) of disease. (b) Robotic systems have submillimeter accuracy such that highly conformal radiation dose plans sparing normal tissues from excessive radiation dose per fraction can be achieved. Pictured is a radiosurgery plan for a para-aortic relapse of ovarian cancer with a gold fiducial placed within the target. (c) Orthogonal right (R) and left (L) fluoroscopic images taken by treatment room cameras allow on-board real-time tracking of implanted gold fiducials (green diamonds). (d) Dose–volume histograms indicate high percentage target coverage (red) while simultaneously distributing low radiation dose to critical organs (such as bowel, liver, and kidneys). For a color version of this figure, see the color plate section.

metastasis. Extirpated stage I disease is associated with a 90% disease-free survival, obviating indications for adjuvant therapy. Up-front adjuvant radiotherapy has been used with equivocal results [150,153,154]. As such, the role of radiotherapy has been limited to palliation with no real sense of curative salvage potential.

Ovarian clear cell carcinomas are uncommon cases of ovarian cancer (incidence 4–14%), with an apparently higher prevalence in Japanese women [155]. This disease occurs in young women, remains contained almost exclusively in the pelvis, associates with endometriosis, and portends a poor cancer-related outcome [155]. A five-year disease-free survival benefit of 20% was found in those women with stage IC or II disease receiving

three cycles of carboplatin (AUC 5–6) and paclitaxel (175 mg m^{-2}) every three to four weeks, then pelvic radiation (22.5 Gy to pelvis in 10 fractions over two weeks followed by 22.5 Gy in 22 fractions over four-and-one-half weeks delivered to the whole abdomen and pelvis), as compared to historical control (41–66%) [155]. Whether this opens the door for therapeutic radiation in women with ovarian clear cell carcinomas remains to be seen.

Because of histopathological features favoring a positive radiation therapy effect, it remains attractive to consider women having hypercalcemic-type small-cell ovary cancer [156] or with squamous cell ovary cancer [157] as candidates for radiation treatment. However, the role of radiation therapy in these ovarian cancer variants remains to be established.

Future Directions for Radiochemotherapy

Exciting early clinical trials show clinical promise of maximal safe resection of ovarian cancer disease followed by first-line combinatorial cytotoxic agent and antiangiogenic agent chemotherapy. Continued clinical development of impressive new radiotherapy devices presage improved radiation delivery to small-volume chemorefractory ovarian cancer targets in the next five years. Results from prospective studies and clinical trials of abdominopelvic radiation delivered by IMRT, helical tomotherapy, and robotic stereotactic radiosurgery will at least in part differentiate post-surgical patients with chemorefractory disease into: (i) patient cohorts expected to have long-term disease-free clinical benefit from targeted radiotherapy alone; and (ii) patient cohorts that may need target-directed radiochemotherapy. Interest in radiotherapy techniques that can be safely administered with novel small-molecule inhibitors of ribonucleotide reductase, poly(ADP-ribose) polymerase, and signaling pathway kinases likely will direct radiochemotherapy research over the next decade. Clinical trials incorporating such approaches are eagerly awaited over the next five to ten years.

References

1 Siegel, R., Miller, K., Jemal, A. (2017) Cancer Statistics 2017. *CA Cancer J. Clin.*, **67**, 7–30.

2 Yancik, R., Ries, L., Yates, J. (1986) Ovarian cancer in the elderly: An analysis of Surveillance, Epidemiology, and End Results program data. *Am. J. Obstet. Gynecol.*, **154** (3), 639–647.

3 Yancik, R. (2005) Population aging and cancer: a cross-national concern. *Cancer J.*, **11** (6), 427–441.

4 Greene, M., Clark, J., Blayney, D. (1984) The epidemiology of ovarian cancer. *Semin. Oncol.*, **11** (3), 209–226.

5 Braem, M., Onland-Moret, N., van den Brandt, P., *et al.* (2010) Reproductive and hormonal factors in association with ovarian cancer in the Netherlands cohort study. *Am. J. Epidemiol.*, **172** (10), 1181–1189.

6 The Cancer and Steroid Hormone Study of the Centers for Disease Control and the National Institute for Child Health and Human Development (1987) The reduction in risk of ovarian cancer associated with oral-contraceptive use. *N. Engl. J. Med.*, **316**, 650–655.

7 Rosenblatt, K., Thomas, D., Noonan, E. (1992) High-dose and low-dose combined oral contraceptives: Protection against epithelial ovarian cancer and the length of the protective effect. The WHO Collaborative Study of Neoplasia and Steroid Contraceptives. *Eur. J. Cancer.*, **28A**, 1872–1976.

8 Devesa, M., Barri, P., Coroleu, B. (2010) Assisted reproductive technology and ovarian cancer. *Minerva Endocrinol.*, **35** (4), 247–257.

9 Rossing, M., Daling, J., Weiss, N., Moore, D., Self, S. 91994) Ovarian tumors in a cohort of infertile women. *N. Engl. J. Med.*, **331** (12), 771–776.

10 Wiegand, K., Shah, S., Al-Agha, O., *et al.* (2010) ARID1A mutations in endometriosis-associated ovarian carcinomas. *N. Engl. J. Med.*, **363** (16), 1532–1543.

11 Sato, N., Tsunoda, H., Nishida, M., *et al.* (2000) Loss of heterozygosity on 10q23.3 and mutation of the tumor suppressor gene PTEN in benign endometrial cyst of the ovary: possible sequence progression from benign endometrial cyst to endometrioid carcinoma and clear cell carcinoma of the ovary. *Cancer Res.*, **60** (24), 7052–7056.

12 Watson, P., Lynch, H. (1993) Extracolonic cancer in hereditary nonpolyposis colorectal cancer. *Cancer*, **71** (3), 677–685.

13 Ford, D., Easton, D., Bishop, D., Narod, S., Goldgar, D., Breast Cancer Linkage Consortium (1994) Risks of cancer in *BRCA1*-mutation carriers. *Lancet*, **343** (8899), 692–695.

14 Wooster, R., Neuhausen, S., Mangion, J., *et al.* (1994) Localization of a breast cancer susceptibility gene, *BRCA2*, to chromosome 13q12-13. *Science*, **265** (5181), 2088–2090.

15 Zhang, J., Powell, S. (2005) The role of the *BRCA1* tumor suppressor in DNA double-strand break repair. *Mol. Cancer Res.*, **3** (10), 531–539.

16 Hartman, A., Ford, J. (2002) *BRCA1* induces DNA damage recognition factors and enhances nucleotide excision repair. *Nat. Genet.*, **32** (1), 180–184.

17 Alli, E., Sharma, V., Sunderesakumar, P., Ford, J. (2009) Defective repair of oxidative DNA damage in triple-negative breast cancer confers sensitivity to inhibition of poly(ADP-ribose) polymerase. *Cancer Res.*, **69** (8), 3589–3596.

18 Hemminki, K., Sundquist, J., Brandt, A. (2011) Incidence and mortality in epithelial ovarian cancer by family history of any cancer. *Cancer*, **117** (17), 3972–3980.

19 Gross, T., Schlesselman, J. (1994) The estimated effect of oral contraceptive use on the cumulative risk of epithelial ovarian cancer. *Obstet. Gynecol.*, **83** (3), 419–424.

20 Struewing, J., Watson, P., Easton, D., Ponder, B., Lynch, H., Tucker, M. (1995) Prophylactic oophorectomy in inherited breast/ovarian cancer families. *J. Natl Cancer Inst. Monogr.*, **17**, 33–35.

21 Finch, A., Beiner, M., Lubinski, J., *et al.* (2006) Salpingo-oophorectomy and the risk of ovarian, fallopian tube, and peritoneal cancers in women with a *BRCA1* or *BRCA2* mutation. *J. Am. Med. Assoc.*, **296** (2), 185–192.

22 Salhab, M., Bismohun, S., Mokbel, K. (2010) Risk-reducing strategies for women carrying *BRCA1/2* mutations with a focus on prophylactic surgery. *BMC Womens Health*, **10**, 28.

23 Piver, M., Jishi, M., Tsukada, Y., Nava, G. (1993) Primary peritoneal carcinoma after prophylactic oophorectomy in women with a family history of ovarian cancer. *Cancer*, **71** (9), 2751–2755.

24 Buys, S., Partridge, E., Black, A., *et al.* (2011) Effect of screening on ovarian cancer mortality: the Prostate, Lung, Colorectal, and Ovarian (PLCO) cancer screening randomized control trial. *J. Am. Med. Assoc.*, **305** (22), 2295–2303.

25 Fleischer, A., Lyshchik, A., Jones, H.J., *et al.* (2008) Contrast-enhanced transvaginal sonography of benign versus malignant ovarian masses: preliminary findings. *J. Ultrasound Med.*, **27** (7), 1019–1021.

26 Gao, Z., Kennedy, A., Christensen, D., Rapoport, N. (2008) Drug-loaded nano/microbubbles for combining ultrasonography and targeted chemotherapy. *Ultrasonics*, **48** (4), 260–270.

27 Malkasian, G.J., Knapp, R., Lavin, P., *et al.* (1988) Preoperative evaluation of serum CA-125 levels in premenopausal and postmenopausal patients with pelvic masses: Description of benign from malignant disease. *Am. J. Obstet. Gynecol.*, **159** (2), 341–346.

28 Prat, A., Parera, M., Adamo, B., *et al.* (2009) Risk of recurrence during follow-up for optimally treated advanced epithelial ovarian cancer (EOC) with a low-level increase of serum CA-125 levels. *Ann. Oncol.*, **20** (2), 294–297.

29 Rustin, G., van der Burg, M., Griffin, C., *et al.* (2010) Early versus delayed treatment of relapse ovarian cancer (MRC OV05/EORTC 55955): a randomised trial. *Lancet*, **376** (9747), 1155–1163.

30 Havrilesky, L., Whitehead, C., Rubatt, J., *et al.* (2008) Evaluation of biomarker panels for early stage ovarian cancer detection and monitoring for disease recurrence. *Gynecol. Oncol.*, **10**, 374–382.

31 Moore, R., Brown, A., Miller, M., *et al.* (2008) The use of multiple novel tumor biomarkers for the detection of ovarian carcinoma with a pelvic mass. *Gynecol. Oncol.*, **108**, 402–408.

32 Drapkin, R., von Horstein, H., Lin, Y., *et al.* (2005) Human epididymis protein 4 (HE4) is a secreted glycoprotein that is overexpressed by serous and endometrioid ovarian carcinomas. *Cancer Res.*, **65**, 2162–2169.

33 Galgano, M., Hampton, G., Frierson, H. (2006) Comprehensive analysis of HE4 expression in normal and malignant human tissues. *Mod. Pathol.*, **19**, 847–853.

34 Huhtinen, K., Suvitie, P., Hiissa, J., *et al.* (2009) Serum HE4 concentration differentiates malignant ovarian tumours from ovarian endometriotic cysts. *Br. J. Cancer*, **100** (8), 1315–1319.

35 Scully, R., Young, R., Clemens, P. (1998) Tumors of the ovary, maldeveloped gonads, fallopian tube, and broad ligament, in *Atlas of Tumor Pathology*. Vol. 23, series 3. Armed Forces Institute of Pathology, Washington, DC.

36 Creasman, W., Park, R., Norris, H., Disaia, P., Morrow, C., Hreshchyshyn, M. (1982) Stage 1 borderline ovarian tumors. *Obstet. Gynecol.*, **59** (1), 93–96.

37 Chambers, J., Merino, M., Kohom, E., Schwartz, P. (1988) Borderline ovarian tumors. *Am. J. Obstet. Gynecol.*, **159** (5), 1088–1094.

38 Silva, E., Gershenson, D., Malpica, A., Deavers, M. (2006) The recurrence and the overall survival rates of ovarian serous borderline neoplasms with noninvasive implants is time dependent. *Am. J. Surg. Pathol.*, **30** (11), 1367–1371.

39 Kaern, J., Trope, C., Kjorstad, K., Abeler, V., Petersen, E. (1990) Cellular DNA content as a new prognosis tool in patients with borderline tumors of the ovary. *Gynecol. Oncol.*, **38** (3), 452–457.

40 Trope, C., Davidson, B., Paulsen, T., Abeler, V., Kaern, J. (2009) Diagnosis and treatment of borderline ovarian neoplasms – 'the state of the art'. *Eur. J. Gynaecol. Oncol.*, **30** (5), 471–482.

41 Kusumbe, A., Bapat, S. (2009) Cancer stem cells and aneuploid populations within developing tumors are the major determinants of tumor dormancy. *Cancer Res.*, **69** (24), 9245–9253.

42 Pearl, M., Johnston, C., Frank, T., Roberts, J. (1993) Synchronous dual primary ovarian and endometrial carcinomas. *Int. J. Gynaecol. Oncol.*, **43** (3), 305–312.

43 Soliman, P., Slomovitz, B., Broaddus, R., *et al.* (2004) Synchronous primary cancers of the endometrium and ovary: a single institution review of 84 cases. *Gynecol. Oncol.*, **94** (2), 456–462.

44 Heaps, J., Neiberg, R., Berek, J. (1990) Malignant neoplasms arising in endometriosis. *Obstet. Gynecol.*, **75** (6), 1023–1028.

45 Leiserowitz, G., Gumbs, J., Oi, R., *et al.* (2003) Endometriosis-related malignancies. *Int. J. Gynecol. Oncol.*, **13** (4), 466–471.

46 Martinez, A., Schray, M., Howes, A., Bagshaw, M. (1985) Postoperative radiation therapy for epithelial ovarian cancer: the curative role based on a 24-year experience. *J. Clin. Oncol.*, **3** (7), 901–911.

47 FIGO Committee on Gynecologic Oncology. (2009) Current FIGO staging for cancer of the vagina, fallopian tube, ovary, and gestational trophoblastic neoplasia. *Int. J. Gynaecol. Obstet.*, **105** (1), 3–4.

48 Young, R., Decker, D., Wharton, J., *et al.* (1983) Staging laparotomy in early ovarian cancer. *J. Am. Med. Assoc.*, **250** (22), 3072–3076.

49 Hoskins, W., Bundy, B., Thigpen, J., Omura, G. (1992) The influence of cytoreductive surgery on recurrence-free interval and survival in small-volume stage III epithelial ovarian cancer: a Gynecologic Oncology Group study. *Gynecol. Oncol.*, **47** (2), 159–166.

50 Griffiths, C. (1975) Surgical resection of tumor bulk in the primary treatment of ovarian carcinoma. *J. Natl Cancer Inst. Monogr.*, **42**, 101–104.

51 Bristow, R., Tomacruz, R., Armstrong, D., Trimble, E., Montz, F. (2002) Survival effect of maximal cytoreductive surgery for advanced ovarian carcinoma during the platinum era: a meta-analysis. *J. Clin. Oncol.*, **20** (5), 1248–1259.

52 Reimer, R., Hoover, R., Faumeni, J.J., Young, R. (1977) Acute leukemia after alkylating agent therapy for ovarian cancer. *N. Engl. J. Med.*, **297** (4), 177–181.

53 Kaldor, J., Day, N., Pettersson, F., *et al.* (1990) Leukemia following chemotherapy for ovarian cancer. *N. Engl. J. Med.*, **322** (1), 1–6.

54 Rubin, S., Hoskins, W., Hakes, T., *et al.* (1989) Serum CA-125 levels and surgical findings in patients undergoing second operations for epithelial ovarian cancer. *Am. J. Obstet. Gynecol.*, **160** (3), 667–671.

55 Berek, J., Knapp, R., Malkasian, G.J., *et al.* (1986) CA-125 serum levels correlated with second-look operations among ovarian cancer patients. *Obstet. Gynecol.*, **67** (5), 685–689.

56 Rubin, S., Hoskins, W., Hakes, T., Markman, M., Cain, J., Lewis, J.J. (1988) Recurrence after negative second-look laparotomy for ovarian cancer: Analysis of risk factors. *Am. J. Obstet. Gynecol.*, **159** (5), 1094–1098.

57 Rubin, S., Randall, T., Armstrong, K., Chi, D., Hoskins, W. (1999) Ten-year follow-up of ovarian cancer patients after second-look laparotomy with negative findings. *Obstet. Gynecol.*, **93** (1), 21–24.

58 Magrina, J., Zanagnolo, V., Noble, B., Kho, R., Magitbay, P. (2011) Robotic approach for ovarian cancer: perioperative and survival results and comparison with laparoscopy and laparotomy. *Gynecol. Oncol.*, **121** (1), 100–105.

59 Young, R., Walton, L., Ellenberg, S., *et al.* (1990) Adjuvant therapy in stage 1 or 2 epithelial ovarian cancer. Results of two prospective randomized trials. *N. Engl. J. Med.*, **322** (15), 1021–1027.

60 Ozols, R., Bundy, B., Greer, B., *et al.* (2003) Phase 3 trial of carboplatin and paclitaxel compared with cisplatin and paclitaxel in patients with optimally resected stage 3 ovarian cancer: a Gynecologic Oncology Group study. *J. Clin. Oncol.*, **21** (17), 3194–3200.

61 McGuire, W., Hoskins, W., Brady, M., *et al.* (1996) Cyclophosphamide and cisplatin compared with paclitaxel and cisplatin in patients with stage 3 and stage 4 ovarian cancer. *N. Engl. J. Med.*, **334** (1), 1–6.

62 Alberts, D. (2006) Intraperitoneal chemotherapy: Changing the paradigm for the management of ovarian cancer. Introduction. *Semin. Oncol.*, **33** (6, Suppl. 12), S1–S2.

63 Burger, R., Sill, M., Monk, B., Greer, B., Sorosky, J. (2007) Phase II trial of bevacizumab in persistent or recurrent epithelial ovarian cancer or primary peritoneal cancer: a Gynecologic Oncology Group study. *J. Clin. Oncol.*, **25** (33), 5165–5171.

64 London, S. (2011) Bevacizumab shows promise for high-risk and recurrent ovarian cancer. *Commun. Oncol.*, **8** (7), 332–333.

65 Aghajanian, C., Blank, S., Goff, B., *et al.* (2012) OCEANS: a randomized, double-blind, placebo-controlled phase III trial of chemotherapy with or without bevacizumab in patients with platinum-sensitive recurrent epithelial ovarian, peritoneal, or fallopian-tube cancer. *J. Clin. Oncol.*, **30** (17), 2039–2045.

66 Dedrick, R., Myers, C., Bungay, P., DeVita, V. (1978) Pharmacokinetic rationale for peritoneal drug administration in the treatment of ovarian cancer. *Cancer Treat. Rep.*, **62** (1), 1–11.

67 Alberts, D., Delforge, A. (2006) Maximizing the delivery of intraperitoneal therapy while minimizing drug toxicity and maintaining quality of life. *Semin. Oncol.*, **33** (6, Suppl. 12), S8–S17.

68 Francis, P., Rowinsky, E., Schneider, J., Hakes, T., Hoskins, W., Markman, M. (1995) Phase 1 feasibility and pharmacologic study of weekly intraperitoneal paclitaxel: a Gynecologic Oncology Group pilot study. *J. Clin. Oncol.*, **13** (12), 2961–2967.

69 Markman, M., Rowinsky, E., Hakes, T., *et al.* (1992) Phase 1 trial of intraperitoneal taxol: a Gynecologic Oncology Group study. *J. Clin. Oncol.*, **10** (9), 1485–1491.

70 Barakat, R., Almadrones, L., Venkatraman, E., *et al.* (1998) A phase 2 trial of intraperitoneal cisplatin and etoposide as consolidation therapy in patients with stage 2-4 epithelial ovarian cancer following surgical assessment. *Gynecol. Oncol.*, **69** (1), 17–22.

71 Markman, M., George, M., Hakes, T., *et al.* (1990) Phase 2 trial of intraperitoneal mitoxantrone in the management of refractory ovarian cancer. *J. Clin. Oncol.*, **8** (1), 146–150.

72 Markman, M., Brady, M., Spirtos, N., Hanjani, P., Rubin, S. (1998) Phase 2 trial of intraperitoneal paclitaxel in carcinoma of the ovary, tube, and peritoneum: a Gynecologic Oncology Group study. *J. Clin. Oncol.*, **16** (8), 2620–2624.

73 Alberts, D., Liu, P., Hannigan, E., *et al.* (1996) Intraperitoneal cisplatin plus intravenous cyclophosphamide versus intravenous cisplatin plus intravenous cyclophosphamide for stage 3 ovarian cancer. *N. Engl. J. Med.*, **335** (26), 1950–1955.

74 Markman, M., Bundy, B., Alberts, D., *et al.* (2001) Phase 3 trial of standard-dose intravenous cisplatin plus paclitaxel versus moderately high-dose carboplatin followed by intravenous paclitaxel and intraperitoneal cisplatin in small-volume stage 3 ovarian carcinoma: an intergroup study of the Gynecologic Oncology Group, Southwestern Oncology Group, and Eastern Cooperative Oncology Group. *J. Clin. Oncol.*, **19** (4), 1001–1007.

75 Armstrong, D., Bundy, B., Wenzel, L., *et al.* (2006) Intraperitoneal cisplatin and paclitaxel in ovarian cancer. *N. Engl. J. Med.*, **354** (1), 34–43.

76 Trimble, E. (2006) Concluding remarks: Optimal treatment for women with ovarian cancer. *Semin. Oncol.*, **33** (6, Suppl. 12), S25–S26.

77 Monk, B., Herzog, T., Kaye, S., *et al.* (2010) Trabectedin plus pegylated liposomal Doxorubicin in recurrent ovarian cancer. *J. Clin. Oncol.*, **28** (19), 3107–3114.

78 D'Incalci, M., Galmarini, C. (2010) A review of trabectedin (ET-743): a unique mechanism of interaction. *Mol. Cancer Ther.*, **9**, 2157–2163.

79 Poveda, A., Vergote, I., Tjulandin, S., *et al.* (2011) Trabectedin plus pegylated liposomal doxorubicin in relapsed ovarian cancer: outcomes in the partially platinum-sensitive (platinum-free interval 6–12 months) subpopulation of OVA-301 phase III randomized trial. *Ann. Oncol.*, **22** (1), 39–48.

80 Kolberg, M., Strand, K.R., Graff, P., Andersson, K.K. (2004) Structure, function, and mechanism of ribonucleotide reductases. *Biochim. Biophys. Acta*, **1699** (1–2), 1–34.

81 Kunos, C., Radivoyevitch, T., Pink, J., *et al.* (2010) Ribonucleotide reductase inhibition enhances chemoradiosensitivity of human cervical cancers. *Radiation Res.*, **174** (5), 574–581.

82 Wang, J., Lohman, G., Stubbe, J. (2009) Mechanism of inactivation of human ribonucleotide reductase with p53R2 by gemcitabine 5'-diphosphate. *Biochemistry*, **48** (49), 11612–11621.

83 Ferrandina, G., Mey, V., Nannizzi, S., *et al.* (2010) Expression of nucleoside transporters, deoxycytidine kinase, ribonucleotide reductase regulatory subunits, and gemcitabine enzymes in primary ovarian cancer. *Cancer Chemother. Pharmacol.*, **65** (4), 679–686.

84 Kunos, C., Radivoyevitch, T., Abdul-Karim, F., *et al.* (2012) Ribonucleotide reductase inhibition restores platinum-sensitivity in platinum-resistant ovarian cancer: a Gynecologic Oncology Group study. *J. Transl. Med.*, **10** (1), 79.

85 Kunos, C., Stefan, T., Jacobberger, J. (2013) Cabazitaxel-induced stabilization of microtubules enhances radiosensitivity in ovarian cancer cells. *Front. Oncol.*, **3**, 226.

86 Kamei, H., Jackson, R., Zheleva, D., Davidson, F. (2010) An integrated pharmacokinetic-pharmacodynamic model for an Aurora kinase inhibitor. *J. Pharmacokinet. Pharmacodyn.*, **37**, 407–434.

87 Loizzi, V., Cormio, G., Resta, L., *et al.* (2005) Neoadjuvant chemotherapy in advanced ovarian cancer: a case-control study. *Int. J. Gynecol. Cancer*, **15** (2), 217–223.

88 Schwartz, P., Rutherford, T., Chambers, J., Kohorn, E., Thiel, R. (1999) Neoadjuvant chemotherapy for advanced ovarian cancer: long-term survival. *Gynecol. Oncol.*, **72** (1), 93–99.

89 Fuller, L., Painter, R. (1988) A Chinese hamster ovary cell line hypersensitive to ionizing radiation and deficient in repair replication. *Mutat. Res.*, **193** (2), 109–121.

90 Baker, T. (1971) Radiosensitivity of mammalian oocytes with particular reference to the human female. *Am. J. Obstet. Gynecol.*, **110** (5), 746–761.

91 Wallace, W., Thomson, A., Kelsey, T. (2003) The radiosensitivity of the human oocyte. *Hum. Reprod.*, **18** (1), 117–121.

92 Adriaens, I., Smitz, J., Jacquet, P. (2009) The current knowledge on radiosensitivity of ovarian follicle development stages. *Hum. Reprod. Update.*, **15** (3), 359–377.

93 Condra, K., Mendenhall, W., Morgan, L., Marcus, R.J. (1997) Adjuvant 32P in the treatment of ovarian carcinoma. *Radiat. Oncol. Invest.*, **5** (6), 300–304.

94 Vergote, I., Vergote-DeVos, L., Abeler, V., *et al.* (1992) Randomized trial comparing cisplatin with radioactive phosphorus or whole abdominal irradiation as adjuvant treatment of ovarian cancer. *Cancer*, **69** (3), 741–749.

95 Young, R., Brady, M., Nieberg, R., *et al.* (2003) Adjuvant treatment for early ovarian cancer: a randomized phase III trial of intraperitoneal 32P or intravenous cyclophosphamide and cisplatin – a Gynecologic Oncology Group study. *J. Clin. Oncol.*, **21** (23), 4350–4355.

96 Bolis, G., Colombo, N., Pecorelli, S., *et al.* (1995) Adjuvant treatment for early epithelial ovarian cancer: results of two randomised clinical trials comparing cisplatin to no further treatment or chromic phosphate (32P). Gruppo Interregionale Collaborativo in Ginecologia Oncologica. *Ann. Oncol.*, **6** (9), 887–893.

97 Varia, M., Stehman, F., Bundy, B., *et al.* (2003) Intraperitoneal radioactive phosphorus (32P) versus observation after negative second-look laparotomy for stage III ovarian carcinoma: a randomized trial of the Gynecologic Oncology Group. *J. Clin. Oncol.*, **21** (15), 2849–2855.

98 Spanos, W.J., Day, T., Abner, A., Jose, B., Paris, K., Pursell, S. (1992) Complications in the use of intra-abdominal 32P for ovarian carcinoma. *Gynecol. Oncol.*, **45** (3), 243–247.

99 Walton, L., Yadusky, A., Rubinstein, L. (1991) Intraperitoneal radioactive phosphate in early ovarian carcinoma: An analysis of complications. *Int. J. Radiat. Oncol. Biol. Phys.*, **20** (5), 939–944.

100 Klaassen, D., Starreveld, A., Shelly, W., *et al.* (1985) External beam pelvic radiotherapy plus intraperitoneal radioactive chromic phosphate in early stage ovarian cancer: a toxic combination. A National Cancer Institute of Canada Clinical Trials Group report. *Int. J. Radiat. Oncol. Biol. Phys.*, **11** (10), 1804–1804.

101 Soper, J., Wilkinson, R.J., Bandy, L., Clarke-Pearson, D., Creasman, W. (1987) Intraperitoneal chromic phosphate P-32 as salvage therapy for persistent carcinoma of the ovary after surgical restaging. *Am. J. Obstet. Gynecol.*, **156** (5), 1153–1158.

102 Thomas, G. 91994) Radiotherapy for early ovarian cancer. *Gynecol. Oncol.*, **55** (3 Pt 2), S73–S79.

103 Dembo, A., Bush, R., Beale, F., *et al.* (1979) Ovarian carcinoma: Improved survival following abdominopelvic irradiation in patients with a completed pelvic operation. *Am. J. Obstet. Gynecol.*, **134**, 793–800.

104 Dembo, A. (1992) Epithelial ovarian cancer: The role of radiotherapy. *Int. J. Radiat. Oncol. Biol. Phys.*, **22** (5), 835–845.

105 Fyles, A., Dembo, A., Bush, R., *et al.* Analysis of complications in patients treated with abdominopelvic radiation therapy for ovarian carcinoma. *Int. J. Radiat. Oncol. Biol. Phys.*, **22** (5), 867–874.

106 Fazekas, J., Maier, J. (1974) Irradiation of ovarian carcinomas. A prospective comparison of the open-field and moving-strip techniques. *Am. J. Roentgenol. Radium Ther. Nucl. Med.*, **120** (1), 118–123.

107 Hruby, G., Bull, C., Langlands, A., Gebski, V. (1997) WART revisited: The treatment of epithelial ovarian cancer by whole abdominal radiotherapy. *Australas. Radiol.*, **41** (3), 276–280.

108 MacGibbon, A., Bucci, J., MacLeod, C., *et al.* (1999) Whole abdominal radiotherapy following second-look laparotomy for ovarian carcinoma. *Gynecol. Oncol.*, **75**, 62–67.

109 Thomas, G. (1994) Radiotherapy in early ovarian cancer. *Gynecol. Oncol.*, **55** (3 Pt 2), S73–S79.

110 Rochet, N., Kieser, M., Sterzing, F., *et al.* (2011) Phase II study evaluating consolidation whole abdomen intensity-modulated radiotherapy (IMRT) in patients with advanced ovarian cancer stage FIGO III – the OVAR-IMRT-02 study. *BMC Cancer*, **11**, 41.

111 Rochet, N., Sterzing, F., Jensen, A., *et al.* (2010) Intensity-modulated whole abdominal radiotherapy after surgery and carboplatin/taxane chemotherapy for advanced ovarian cancer: Phase 1 study. *Int. J. Radiat. Oncol. Biol. Phys.*, **76** (5), 1382–1389.

112 Garsa, A., Andrade, R., Heron, D., *et al.* (2007) Four-dimensional computed tomography-based respiratory-gated whole-abdominal intensity-modulated radiation therapy for ovarian cancer: a feasibility study. *Int. J. Gynecol. Cancer.*, **17**, 55–60.

113 Hong, L., Alektiar, K., Chui, C., *et al.* (2002) IMRT of large fields: Whole-abdomen irradiation. *Int. J. Radiat. Oncol. Biol. Phys.*, **54** (1), 278–289.

114 Yang, D., Lu, W., Low, D., Deasy, J., Hope, A., El Naga, I. (2008) 4D-CT motion estimation using deformable image registration and 5D respiratory motion modeling. *Med. Phys.*, **35** (10), 4577–4590.

115 Li, G., Citrin, D., Camphausen, K., *et al.* (2008) Advances in 4D medical imaging and 4D radiation therapy. *Technol. Cancer Res. Treat.*, **7** (1), 67–81.

116 Schray, M., Martinez, A., Howes, A. (1989) Toxicity of open-field whole abdominal irradiation as primary postoperative treatment in gynecologic malignancy. *Int. J. Radiat. Oncol. Biol. Phys.*, **16** (2), 397–403.

117 Firat, S., Murray, K., Erickson, B. (2003) High-dose whole abdominal and pelvic irradiation for treatment of ovarian carcinoma: long-term toxicity and outcomes. *Int. J. Radiat. Oncol. Biol. Phys.*, **57** (1), 201–207.

118 Schray, M., Martinez, A., Howes, A., *et al.* (1986) Advanced epithelial ovarian cancer: toxicity of whole abdominal irradiation after operation, combination chemotherapy, and reoperation. *Gynecol. Oncol.*, **24** (1), 68–80.

119 Whelan, T., Dembo, A., Bush, R., *et al.* (1992) Complications of whole abdominal and pelvic radiotherapy following chemotherapy for advanced ovarian cancer. *Int. J. Radiat. Oncol. Biol. Phys.*, **22** (5), 853–858.

120 Irwin, C., Fyles, A., Wong, C., Cheung, C., Zhu, Y. (1996) Late renal function following whole abdominal irradiation. *Radiother. Oncol.*, **38** (3), 257–261.

121 Rochet, N., Sterzing, F., Jensen, A., *et al.* (2008) Helical tomotherapy as a new treatment technique for whole abdominal irradiation. *Strahlenther. Onkol.*, **184** (3), 145–149.

122 Swamidas, V., Mahantshetty, U., Goel, V., *et al.* (2009) Treatment planning of epithelial ovarian cancers using

helical tomotherapy. *J. Appl. Clin. Med. Phys.*, **10** (4), 96–105.

123 Mell, L., Roeske, J., Mehta, N., Mundt, A. (2005) Gynecologic Cancer: Overview, in *Intensity-Modulated Radiation Therapy: A Clinical Perspective*, Vol. 1 (eds A. Mundt, J. Roeske), BC Decker Inc., London, pp. 492–505.

124 Small, W.J., Mell, L., Anderson, P., *et al.* (2008) Consensus guidelines for delineation of clinical target volume for intensity-modulated pelvic radiotherapy in postoperative treatment of endometrial and cervical cancer. *Int. J. Radiat. Oncol. Biol. Phys.*, **71** (2), 428–434.

125 Mackie, T., Holmes, T., Swerdloff, S., *et al.* (1993) Tomotherapy: a new concept for the delivery of dynamic conformal radiotherapy. *Med. Phys.*, **20** (6), 1709–1719.

126 Sterzing, F., Schubert, K., Sroka-Perez, G., Kalz, J., Debus, J., Herfarth, K. (2008) Helical tomotherapy: experiences of the first 150 patients in Heidelberg. *Strahlenther. Onkol.*, **184** (1), 8–14.

127 Kim, Y., Kim, J., Jeong, K., Seong, J., Suh, C., Kim, G. (2009) Dosimetric comparisons of three-dimensional conformal radiotherapy, intensity-modulated radiotherapy, and helical tomotherapy in whole abdominopelvic radiotherapy for gynecologic malignancy. *Technol. Cancer Res. Treat.*, **8** (5), 369–377.

128 Soisson, E., Hoban, P., Kammeyer, T., *et al.* (2011) A technique for stereotactic radiosurgery treatment planning with helical tomotherapy. *Med. Dosim.*, **36** (1), 46–56.

129 Ledermann, J., Dembo, A., Sturgeon, J., *et al.* (1991) Outcome of patients with unfavorable optimally cytoreduced ovarian cancer treated with chemotherapy and whole abdomen radiation. *Gynecol. Oncol.*, **41** (1), 30–35.

130 Fuks, Z., Rizel, S., Biran, S. (1988) Chemotherapeutic and surgical induction of pathologic complete remission and whole abdominal irradiation for consolidation does not enhance the cure of stage III ovarian cancer. *J. Clin. Oncol.*, **6** (3), 509–516.

131 Goldhirsch, A., Greiner, R., Deher, E., *et al.* (1988) Treatment of advanced ovarian cancer with surgery, chemotherapy, and consolidation of response by whole-abdomen radiotherapy. *Cancer*, **62** (1), 40–47.

132 Petit, T., Velten, M., d'Hombres, A., *et al.* (2007) Long-term survival of 106 stage III ovarian cancer patients with minimal residual disease after second-look laparotomy and consolidation radiotherapy. *Gynecol. Oncol.*, **104** (1), 104–108.

133 Sorbe, B., Swedish-Norwegian Ovarian Cancer Study Group (2003) Consolidation treatment of advanced (FIGO sage III) ovarian carcinoma in complete surgical remission after induction chemotherapy: A randomized, controlled clinical trial comparing whole abdominal radiotherapy, chemotherapy, and no further treatment. *Int. J. Gynecol. Cancer*, **13**, 278–286.

134 Randall, M., Barrett, R., Spirtos, N., *et al.* (1996) Chemotherapy, early surgical reassessment, and hyperfractionated abdominal radiotherapy in stage III ovarian cancer: results of a Gynecologic Oncology Group study. *Int. J. Radiat. Oncol. Biol. Phys.*, **34** (1), 139–147.

135 Buser, K., Bacchi, M., Goldhirsch, A., *et al.* (1996) Treatment of ovarian cancer with surgery, short-course chemotherapy and whole abdominal radiation. *Ann. Oncol.*, **7** (1), 65–70.

136 Thigpen, J., Vance, R., McGuire, W., Hoskins, W., Brady, M. (1995) The role of paclitaxel in the management of coelomic epithelial carcinoma of the ovary: a review with emphasis on the Gynecologic Oncology Group experience. *Semin. Oncol.*, **22** (6 Suppl. 14), 23–31.

137 du Bois, A., Luck, H., Meier, W., *et al.* (2003) A randomized clinical trial of cisplatin/paclitaxel versus carboplatin/paclitaxel as first-line treatment of ovarian cancer. *J. Natl Cancer Inst.*, **95** (17), 1329–1329.

138 Schray, M., Martinez, A., Howes, A., *et al.* (1988) Advanced epithelial ovarian cancer: Salvage whole abdominal irradiation for patients with recurrent or persistent disease after combination chemotherapy. *J. Clin. Oncol.*, **6** (9), 1433–1439.

139 Chendil, D., Oakes, R., Alcock, R., *et al.* (2000) Low dose fractionated radiation enhances the radiosensitization effect of paclitaxel in colorectal tumor cells with mutant p53. *Cancer*, **89** (9), 1893–1900.

140 Kunos, C., Sill, M., Buekers, T., *et al.* (2011) Low-dose abdominal radiation as a docetaxel chemosensitizer for recurrent epithelial ovarian cancer: a phase 1 study of the Gynecologic Oncology Group. *Gynecol. Oncol.*, **120** (2), 224–228.

141 Mayr, N., Huang, Z., Sohn, J., *et al.* (2011) Emerging application of stereotactic body radiation therapy for gynecologic malignancies. *Expert Rev. Anticancer Ther.*, **11** (7), 1071–1077.

142 Hoogeman, M., Prévost, J.-B., Nuyttens, J., Pöll, J., Levandag, P., Heijmen, B. (2009) Clinical accuracy of the respiratory tumor tracking system of the Cyberknife: Assessment by analysis of log files. *Int. J. Radiat. Oncol. Biol. Phys.*, **74** (1), 297–303.

143 Antypas, C., Pantelis, E. (2008) Performance evaluation of a CyberKnife® G4 image-guided robotic stereotactic radiosurgery system. *Phys. Med. Biol.*, **53**, 4697–4718.

144 Wilcox, E., Daskalov, G. (2007) Evaluation of GAFCHROMIC EBT film for Cyberknife® dosimetry. *Med. Phys.*, **34** (6), 1967–1974.

145 Kunos, C., Brindle, J., Waggoner, S., *et al.* (2012) Phase II clinical trial of robotic stereotactic body radiosurgery for metastatic gynecologic malignancies. *Front. Oncol.*, **2012** (2), 181.

146 Lawson, A., Adler, G. (1988) Radiotherapy in the treatment of ovarian dysgerminoma. *Int. J. Radiat. Oncol. Biol. Phys.*, **14** (3), 431–434.

147 Krepart, G., Smith, J., Rutledge, F., Delclos, L. (1978) The treatment of dysgerminoma of the ovary. *Cancer*, **41** (3), 986–990.

148 Williams, S., Blessing, J., Hatch, K., Homesley, H. (1991) Chemotherapy of advanced germinoma: Trials of the Gynecologic Oncology Group. *J. Clin. Oncol.*, **9** (11), 1950–1955.

149 Gershenson, D., Morris, M., Cangir, A., *et al.* (1990) Treatment of malignant germ cell tumors of the ovary with bleomycin, etoposide, and cisplatin. *J. Clin. Oncol.*, **8** (4), 715–720.

150 Evans, A., Gaffey, T., Malkasian, G.J., Anegers, J. (1980) Clinicopathologic review of 118 granulosa and 82 theca cell tumors. *Obstet. Gynecol.*, **55** (2), 231–238.

151 Gusberg, S., Kardon, P. (1971) Proliferative endometrial response to theca-granulosa-cell tumors. *Am. J. Obstet. Gynecol.*, **111** (5), 633–643.

152 Bjorkholm, E., Silfversward, C. (1981) Prognostic factors in granulosa-cell tumors. *Gynecol. Oncol.*, **11** (3), 261–274.

153 Ohel, G., Kaneti, H., Schenker, J. (1983) Granulosa-cell tumors in Israel: a study of 172 cases. *Gynecol. Oncol.*, **15** (2), 278–286.

154 Wolf, J., Mullen, J., Eifel, P., Burke, T., Levenback, C., Gershenson, D. (1999) Radiation treatment of advanced or recurrent granulosa cell tumor of the ovary. *Gynecol. Oncol.*, **73** (1), 35–41.

155 Hoskins, P., Le, N., Gilks, B., *et al.* (2012) Low-stage ovarian clear cell carcinoma: Population-based outcomes in British Columbia, with evidence for a survival benefit as a result of irradiation. *J. Clin. Oncol.*, **30** (14), 1656–1662.

156 Stephens, B., Anthony, S., Han, H., *et al.* (2012) Molecular characterization of a patient's small cell carcinoma of the ovary of hypercalcemic type. *J. Cancer*, **3**, 58–66.

157 Hackethal, A., Brueggmann, D., Bohlmann, M., Franke, F., Tinneberg, H., Münstedt, K. (2008) Squamous-cell carcinoma in mature cystic teratoma of the ovary: systematic review and analysis of published data. *Lancet Oncol.*, **9** (12), 1173–1180.

158 Edge, S.B., Byrd, D.R., Compton, C.C. (eds) (2010) *AJCC Cancer Staging Manual*, 7th edition. Springer, New York.

34

Vagina

Charles A. Kunos

Introduction

Malignancies of the vagina are uncommon. The American Cancer Society (ACS) projects that 4810 women in the United States (0.5% of 852 630 new cancers) will be identified as having vaginal cancer in 2017 [1]. Moreover, the ACS estimates that 1240 (26%) deaths will occur due to disease progression of vaginal cancer [1]. Staging systems for vaginal cancer (Table 34.1) classify those neoplasms extending from the vagina to reach the cervix as cervical cancer [2]. Vaginal cancer staging also labels those neoplasms reaching any portion of the vulva as vulvar cancers [2]. These dictums unavoidably catalog some cancers whose bulk occupies the proximal vagina as stage II or higher cervical cancer. Vice versa, some cancers whose bulk originates in the distal vagina are identified as stage III or higher vulvovaginal cancers. In this way, 80–90% of vaginal neoplasms are considered secondary neoplasms, but only if the adjacent cervix and vulva can be excluded as the tissue of origin, preferably by tissue sampling, can an invasive vaginal cancer be listed as a primary cancer site [3]. Because of this particular nomenclature, the uncommon stage IIIA cervical cancer may indeed reflect peculiarities of vaginal cancer staging rather than a tellingly separate disease entity. Moreover, it may not be possible to clinically distinguish between synchronous but separate squamous cell cancers of the vagina and cervix, which by convention would be scored a cervical cancer of higher stage. Similarly, metachronous appearance of vaginal cancer after treatment for cervical cancer would be conventionally counted as recurrence or metastasis unless two years have elapsed from the time of preinvasive disease, or five or more years have elapsed between the two invasive cancer diagnoses.

In this chapter, guidelines for radiotherapy are commented on as pertaining to vaginal cancer management. Standardized radiotherapeutic approaches are infrequently found. As such, common clinical procedures and cancer control outcomes are reviewed for women with vaginal cancer. Comment on new radiotherapeutic delivery systems is offered.

Epidemiology

Malignancies of the vagina are typically (90%) squamous cell in origin (Table 34.2) [4, 5]. While not much is known, low income, low educational status and a history of genital condyloma infection appear to be risk factors for vaginal cancer [6–11]. Women with vaginal intraepithelial neoplasia (VAIN) may often have simultaneous cervical intraepithelial neoplasia (CIN) or invasive cervical cancer [12]. Immunosuppression predisposes to lower-vaginal tract neoplasia [13, 14], although a higher incidence of vaginal cancer attributed to VAIN resulting from immunosuppression has not been demonstrated.

Accord has not been reached regarding the usefulness of vaginal Papanicolaou smears of the vaginal vault after hysterectomy for the early detection of vaginal cancer. Based on the low incidence of the disease and the limited effectiveness of vaginal cytology alone to confirm or to refute cancer, there is a lack of evidence for routine vaginal smear screening for cancer among women having had hysterectomy for benign disease [15,16]. National screening has not been found to be cost-effective [17]. To this day, treating physicians still are supported in the notion of repeated vaginal Papanicolaou smears in women at-risk for vaginal cancer as they age. However,

Clinical Radiation Oncology: Indications, Techniques, and Results, Third Edition. Edited by William Small Jr.
© 2017 John Wiley & Sons, Inc. Published 2017 by John Wiley & Sons, Inc.

Table 34.1 Carcinoma of the vagina: FIGO staging and TNM classification.*

FIGO	TNM Category			Description
Stage I	T1			Carcinoma is confined to the vagina
Stage II	T2			Carcinoma invades paravaginal tissues but not the pelvic side wall
Stage III	T3			Carcinoma involves the pelvic side wall
		N1		Carcinoma has spread to lymph nodes
Stage IV				
IVA	T4			Carcinoma involves the mucosa of the bladder or rectum (bullous edema does not qualify)
IVB			M1	Carcinoma has spread outside of the pelvis

*Carcinoma involving the cervix are cervical cancers; carcinomas involving the vulva are vulvar cancers.

treating physicians also must be reminded that speculums may obscure beginning or sessile vaginal lesions, and careful visual same-time manual inspections of the entire length of the vagina are a must. Women whose vaginal cancer is detected by vaginal smear cytology are more likely to have early stage disease and favorable clinical outcome.

Histology and Molecular Biology

Cytological criteria for the diagnosis of VAIN and invasive cancer follow those for cervical cancer. Delineating dysplasia and inflammatory change from neoplasia can be tedious [18]. Features of vaginal mucosal atrophy and afterward irradiation cellular change can mirror characteristics of neoplasia [19]. The role of VAIN as a predisposing factor for vaginal malignancies has not been entirely clarified, but an association between VAIN and progression to vaginal cancer has been suggested [20, 21]. The continuum describing the pathogenesis of VAIN appears to implicate human papillomavirus (HPV), perhaps inducing a viral 'field' multifocal transformation effect upon sizeable areas of anogenital epithelial cells. A randomized study reporting 42 months of follow-up in 17 622 HPV-naïve women (aged 16–26 years) has shown that prophylactic quadrivalent HPV vaccine administered on day 1, month 2, and month 6

Table 34.2 Frequency of vaginal neoplasms and age.

Class	Frequency (%)	Age (years)
Endodermal sinus tumor (adenocarcinoma)	<1	<2
Sarcoma botryoides	<1	<8
Clear-cell adenocarcinoma	2	>14
Melanoma	6	>50
Squamous cell carcinoma	90	>50

sustains immunoprotection against HPV16- and HPV18-associated VAIN in those receiving vaccine (0 cases) versus those receiving placebo (18 cases) [22].

Physicians should be aware of the HPV life cycle as it pertains to VAIN and invasive cancers of the vagina. HPVs are small, non-enveloped DNA viruses capable of inducing host cell proliferation, especially in the cutaneous and mucosal epithelium of the anogenital tract [23]. HPV proliferates by making ineffective a host cell's signal for cell cycle termination. As HPV replication depends on host cell enzymes for DNA synthesis, processes modified by HPV-E6 and HPV-E7 proteins do not allow host cells to exit the cell cycle when they normally would during passage from the basal to superficial epithelial strata. Repetitive, possibly error-prone, DNA turnover and replication may lead to oncogenic phenotypes [23]. To explain this phenomenon, it is important to examine the way in which HPV molecularly manipulates the cell cycle. The HPV-E6 protein consists of 150 amino acids forming two zinc-finger motifs [24, 25]. HPV-E6 disrupts the role of p53 in regulating the cell cycle, essentially removing the G1/S cell-cycle checkpoint by binding p53 to its annihilation ubiquitin ligase E6AP [26–28]. Elimination of the G1/S restriction checkpoint, and activation of telomerase [29], allows continuous DNA synthesis, viral DNA replication, and increase in HPV-infected cell number. The HPV-E7 protein consists of 98 amino acids facilitating union with retinoblastoma (RB) tumor suppressor proteins and two zinc-finger motifs. HPV-E7 binds and degrades hypophosphorylated RB proteins through a proteosome-dependent pathway [30], and thus promotes unchecked E2F transcription factor activation [31]. E2F transcription factors turn on critical S-phase proteins for DNA replication. Consequences of HPV viral proteins overriding cellular checkpoint mechanisms include genomic instability, which predisposes to neoplasia and cancer alike. The higher incidence of CIN predisposing to invasive cervical cancer as opposed to VAIN predisposing to vaginal cancer appears to relate to the vulnerability of the cervical transformation zone to viral-mediated carcinogenesis [32, 33].

Surgery, Chemotherapy, and Radiotherapy Treatment

Overviews regarding therapeutic interventions for women with vaginal cancer commonly are restricted to discussions of treatment of VAIN and invasive squamous cell carcinoma. There have been no prospective randomized trials evaluating the clinical benefits of surgery, chemotherapy, or radiation for women with vaginal cancer. Surgical therapy is often selected for women with vaginal neoplasia in an effort to avoid perceived late consequential effects of endocrine and reproductive ablation and vaginal stenosis associated with radiotherapy. In general, physician treatment recommendations for invasive vaginal cancer have been extrapolated from results of randomized radiochemotherapy trials in cervical cancer [34].

Vaginal Intraepithelial Neoplasia

Prior to deciding on a treatment course for VAIN, it is critical to carefully examine vaginal tissues and consider saturation biopsies (e.g., sampling tissue along the canal at hourly positions of a clock face) to exclude invasive disease and to map areas of neoplasia. In the interests of preserving vaginal function, surgical extirpation of the entire vagina is avoided.

Topical 5-fluorouracil (5-FU) cream [35, 36] disrupts cell turnover and conservatively limits VAIN disease progression, especially in previously irradiated tissue [37]. Self-administration of 5-FU cream (ca. 5 g) is done with the aid of a vaginal applicator inserted into the vagina, preferably with the patient in a lying position at bedtime. Because the cream may be irritating to the skin, zinc oxide ointment applied to the vulva protects the skin. Treatment lasts for a seven-day cycle and should be discontinued if excessive irritation occurs. 5-FU cream treatment may be repeated for a second cycle, three to four weeks later if VAIN persists. Lesions with hyperkeratosis (thick white crust) are less sensitive to topical 5-FU cream therapy. In one study, 24 of 27 women were free of disease at 12 months (see Ref. [44]). Typical response rates are 80–90%. High patient motivation is needed to complete therapy, and may be the single most commonly cited drawback of therapy.

Focal laser vaporization (15–20 W) focused on a controlled depth of the lamina propria (2–3 mm) eliminates the vaginal mucosa with a nominal harmful effect on vaginal elasticity and functional caliber [38, 39]. Treating physicians must take care not to vaporize vaginal epithelial layers too deeply because of the closeness of the bowel and bladder, especially in elderly or infirm women whose atrophied vaginal epithelium may be quite thin. Post-therapy, a vaginal discharge may persist for up to two to four weeks and an eschar (scar) may form. Laser vaporization has a 60–85% response rate. Repeated laser treatments are tolerated and often done because of the indolent nature of the disease. Laser vaporization is indicated when the full margins of disease are readily demarcated, and probably will not be effectual when VAIN lies buried in the proximal vaginal cuff after hysterectomy [39]. Nowadays, the use of a high-energy, precise argon plasma jet stream emanating from a surgical wand has emerged as a novel alternative to laser vaporization [40, 41]. When the plasma stream is applied to tissue (5 s, 1 cm away from the surface), tissue shrinkage and coagulation are observed. Histological sectioning usually identifies a carbonized layer (5–15 μm), a spongy necrotic layer (300 μm) and a deep necrotic layer (up to 1600 μm) [41]. The advantages of a plasma jet system include plasma that is electrically neutral, no flow of electrical current through the patient, electrical ground pads are unnecessary, and controlled coagulation can be achieved without the typical eschar seen with other laser vaporization systems. Mature experience for plasma vaporization is materializing [40], and studies using this new surgical technology for management of VAIN are eagerly awaited.

Total vaginectomy with split-thickness skin grafting has been done as a surgical intervention for women with multifocal and recurrent disease [42]. Such a surgical approach is reserved usually for relapses after less morbid interventions, and for circumstances in which minimal VAIN disease is anticipated at the time of surgery.

Endocavitary radiation delivering mucosal doses of 6500–8000 cGy using low-dose-rate techniques, and of 1500–4500 cGy using high-dose-rate techniques, will control VAIN in a substantial proportion of women with disease (Figure 34.1) [43–49]. The treating physician must be aware that treatments may result in: (i) ovarian ablation in premenopausal women; (ii) vaginal inelasticity; and (iii) vaginal stenosis and dyspareunia [43–49]. Vaginal brachytherapy should not be used unless conventional methods have been tried and disease persists. If endocavitary brachytherapy is done for VAIN disease, the most often-used applicator is either a high-dose-rate vaginal cylinder inserted gently into the vaginal canal after hysterectomy, or a tandem and ovoid applicator after a supracervical hysterectomy, or a high-dose-rate tandem and ovoid applicator when the cervix and vaginal fornices are intact. The techniques for endocavitary brachytherapy are discussed later in this chapter.

Invasive Cancer of the Vagina

Administration of therapy for invasive disease of the vagina relies on tumor stage, tumor size, and physical morphology. Physicians also consider age, parity, vaginal caliber, desires for sexual health and future fertility, and medical co-morbid conditions when selecting

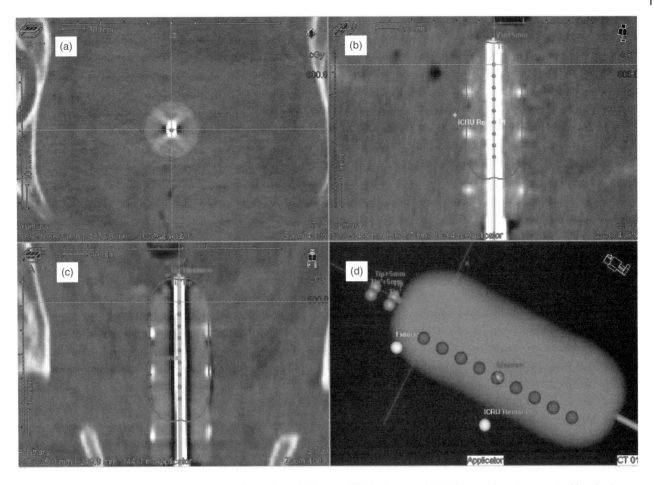

Figure 34.1 Endocavitary vaginal brachytherapy. (a–c) Three-field view of high-dose-rate 192-iridium endocavitary vaginal brachytherapy to deliver 3000 cGy in five divided fractions of 600 cGy radiation prescribed to the vaginal surface for a woman with vaginal intraepithelial neoplasia. (d) Optimization points along the vaginal surface (blue circles) and the vaginal apex (green circles) are depicted. The rectal International Commission on Radiation Units (ICRU) point is indicated (yellow circle). A fiducial (yellow circle) was placed in the right proximal vaginal apex pretherapy to ensure proper radiotherapy device placement during dosimetry planning. For a color version of this figure, see the color plate section.

and recommending therapies. Surgery and radiation have involved a myriad of techniques [34, 43–49].

Invasive vaginal cancers may be managed either by surgery or by radiation. Invasive vaginal disease less than 2 cm in diameter may be cut out by transmural local excision with good results. Excision of posterior lesions overlying the rectovaginal septum may not achieve adequate (>2 mm) deep surgical margins. Excision of anterior lesions lying beneath the bladder and urethra are similarly constrained. Lesions residing at the vaginal fornices are generally approached with an upper vaginectomy. Wide local excision usually removes lesions of the lateral walls and distal lesions nearing the vaginal introitus. Skin grafting may be required rather than primary surgical closure, so that vaginal caliber is not narrowed intentionally. Young women diagnosed with diethylstilbestrol (DES)-associated clear-cell cancer of the vagina are often concerned with preserving endocrine and reproductive function and sexual health,

such that limited surgery is desired for early-stage disease. Conversely, postmenopausal women with invasive disease less than 2 cm may opt for radiation rather than a surgical intervention. In some circumstances, extensive surgical procedures may adversely affect vaginal function more than carefully sculpted radiotherapy, which provides cancer control in 75–80% of women [43–49].

For invasive vaginal cancers with limited thickness, radiation may be applied using brachytherapy alone, or transvaginal cone external beam radiation. Endocavitary brachytherapy devices such as colpostats, cylinders, and molds effectively irradiate 5 mm-thick tumors and present a high-quality technical therapy for flat, sessile tumors of limited diameter. When performing endocavitary brachytherapy for invasive vaginal cancer, use should be made of the largest comfortable device to lower radiation dose inhomogeneity within the targeted tumor. The greater the distance between brachytherapy sources and vaginal mucosa, the lower the mucosal dose required delivering radiation dose at a depth where the targeted tumor is thickest. Endocavitary brachytherapy has also been selected as the desired treatment modality if the radiation dose achieved at depth is 75% or greater of the calculated mucosal (surface) radiation dose [50]. This guideline applies to brachytherapy alone, or to brachytherapy when employed as a supplement to fractionated radiation. If this ratio cannot be attained, transperineal interstitial and vaginal endocavitary radiation is performed [50] (see discussion of interstitial brachytherapy below).

When invasive vaginal cancer extends to paravaginal tissues, radiotherapy should start with external beam teletherapy prior to brachytherapy [51–53]. Prior surgical series indicate that lymph node metastases are detected in 6% (1/17) of women with stage I disease and 26% (8/31) women with stage II disease [51]. External beam radiation field design depends on the location of vaginal disease and whether nodal metastases have been detected by surgery, by magnetic resonance imaging (MRI), or by ^{18}F-fluorodeoxyglucose (FDG) positron emission tomography and computed tomography (FDG PET/CT) [54]. The lymphatic drainage of the upper third of the vagina is through parametrial tissues to pelvic lymph nodes, while lymphatic drainage of the distal third of the vagina occurs via pathways to inguinofemoral lymph nodes and cephalad to pelvic nodes. Imaging by MRI, CT or ultrasound may be needed to determine the depth of inguinofemoral nodes, as the depth of such nodes notoriously has been underestimated by palpation [55, 56]. Groin or pelvic nodes >1 cm in size should be assessed using CT-guided fine-needle aspiration or surgical excision to assess their appropriateness for inclusion in radiation fields. For tumors confined entirely to the upper third of the vagina, external beam radiation ports need to cover only pelvic nodes caudal to the bifurcation of the common iliac arteries (approximately the L5–S1 vertebral interspace). If pelvic node metastases are confirmed, external beam borders may be extended to cover para-aortic nodal tissues. For tumors confined to the middle and lower thirds of the vagina, women are positioned frog-legged and external beam radiation ports are widened for inguinofemoral node coverage. Typical radiation fields are shown in Figure 34.2.

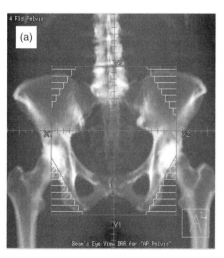
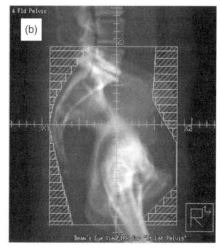
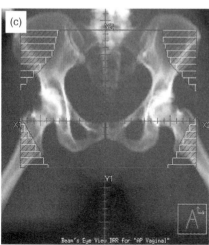
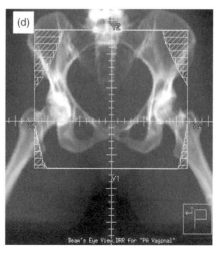

Figure 34.2 Pelvic radiotherapy for vaginal cancer. (a,b) Anteroposterior and right lateral portal images for conventional four-field radiation are shown for treatment of the vagina and pelvic lymph nodes. (c,d) Anteroposterior and posteroanterior portal images are depicted for two-field radiation treatment of the vagina, pelvic lymph nodes, and inguinal lymph nodes. Care must be taken to ensure that inguinal nodes (occasionally lying 3 cm or deeper in groin tissue) are adequately covered by radiation dose. Supplemental electron or photon fields to boost radiation dose to the groins may be needed. For a color version of this figure, see the color plate section.

Typical external beam radiation doses are 4500–5040 cGy in divided 180-cGy fractions, and are delivered to the primary disease and nodal groups confirmed as or suspected of harboring tumor. Using shrinking volumes, radiation doses up to 7020 cGy in divided 180-cGy fractions are given to bulky nodal basins. The radiation dose is escalated by interstitial and intracavitary radiation. Total doses of 6500–7500 cGy are given. The upper limit of radiation dose is not necessarily that which is delivered to the primary disease, but is constrained by radiation dose delivered unavoidably to abutting normal tissue.

For stage II to stage IV disease, where the intent of therapy is to provide pelvic control of disease, interstitial and endocavitary brachytherapy is a mainstay of therapy. Before any therapy, the treating physicians should conduct examinations under anesthesia with cystoscopy and proctosigmoidoscopy as clinically indicated to fully map-out the disease. During the third or fourth week of external beam radiation, women undergo pelvic CT and MRI imaging with a vaginal obturator and geometric template positioned for preplanning tumor delineation prior to brachytherapy. The CT and MRI images are overlaid, and the treating physician draws contours for tumor targets and organs at-risk. Radiation physicists, certified medical dosimetrists, and physicians together determine a individualized configuration of needles capable of holding strands of equidistant radioactive sources into concentric rings parallel along the vaginal wall and parallel to a vaginal obturator (cylinder) housing a central linear radioactive source in a tandem (Figure 34.3).

Therapeutic gain from implantable interstitial and intracavitary brachytherapy arises from its highly conformal radiation dose permeation. For this procedure, afterloading metallic needles or Teflon catheters with metallic guides are positioned into deep pelvic tissues by a transperineal approach aided by grid templates (Figure 34.3). For implants of the vagina itself, single- or double-circle arrangements are used. If a single-circle implant is implanted, full intensity sources are required, but if a double-circle is implanted the inner ring should have half-intensity sources and the peripheral ring should have full-intensity sources. For implants of the vagina and surrounding paravaginal tissue, individualized configurations of needles are needed. Typically, a central tandem eventually holding equidistant radioactive sources (2 cm) is positioned in the vaginal canal and a template for positioning of concentric rings of hollow needles (1.0 cm cylindrical center-to-center apart) is applied. Fluoroscopy [57, 58] or laparoscopy [59] may be used when needles are introduced percutaneously through the perineal skin, then tumor and cephalad into the pelvic floor. Realizing that positioning of needles is tailored to each examination and cancer presentation at the time of the procedure, conventional needle placement starts a

1 o'clock on the patient's left side and at 11 o'clock on the right side. A planned implantation of at least one-half the vaginal circumference inclusive of the cancer target is recommended [52, 60, 61]. At the time of operative procedure, transrectal ultrasound [58, 62, 63], fluoroscopy [57, 58], endorectal coil MRI [59] or laparoscopy [59] may be used when needles are introduced percutaneously through the perineal skin, then tumor and cephalad into the pelvic floor. Laparoscopy may be a preferred technical adjunct to assure a minimal risk of bowel perforation when needles penetrate the pelvic floor. The risk of bowel injury is highest when antecedent hysterectomy has been performed. As clinically indicated, cystoscopy and a careful rectal examination are performed on completion of the procedure to ensure that no catheters are residing in the bladder mucosa or rectal mucosa. Thereby, excessive radiation dose may be avoided such that fistula rates are uncommon.

Following the procedure and operative recovery, CT image acquisition verifies the position of the needles relative to vaginal cancer targets, and allows final dosimetry calculations. Once brachytherapy plans are approved, sources may be loaded into individual needles and the cylinder tandem. Interstitial and endocavitary brachytherapy will permit dose escalation to 7000–8000 cGy without exceeding the tolerance of normal tissues. To ensure tumor cell cytoreduction without harm to normal cells, interstitial and endocavitary brachytherapy is typically prescribed to a 50 cGy to 80 cGy per hour radiation dose rate contour [52, 60, 61]. Pelvic control without disease progression occurs in one-half to one-third of stage II or stage III patients [52]. Less than 20% of stage IV patients will be disease-free at five years [52].

Vaginal Adenocarcinoma

Epithelial squamous strata of the vagina lack substantial glandular tissue, lowering the incidence of true adenocarcinomas. Estimates for non-DES-associated adenocarcinoma of the vagina range from 10% to 20% of all vaginal cancer patient presentations [64, 65]. Women presenting with an adenocarcinoma of the vagina have a poorer prognosis than women with squamous cell cancers [66], a finding at first attributed to failure to recognize some lesions as metastases from other organs and subsequently attributed to inadequate treatment response. Smaller tumors, superficial death of invasion, and pelvic lymph nodes free of tumor associate with favorable prognosis. Long-term disease-free survival after treatment for stage II to IVa adenocarcinoma of the vagina ranges from 65% to 80%, which is considerably lower than the more than 90% survival rate seen among women having stage I disease [67–70].

The clustered appearance of clear-cell adenocarcinomas in adolescent and young adult women led to the

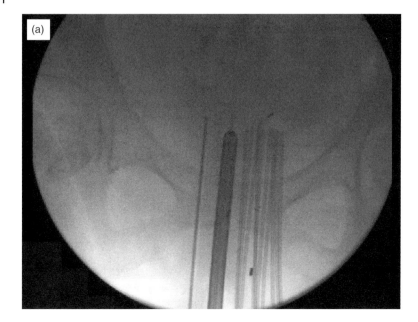

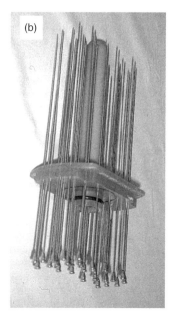

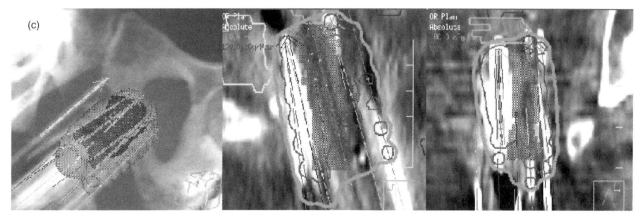

Figure 34.3 Vaginal interstitial brachytherapy. (a) Intraoperative anteroposterior radiograph of 192-iridium needle and 137-cesium tandem interstitial implant in a woman with stage II squamous cell carcinoma of the left lateral wall of the upper to mid-vagina having undergone pelvic radiation (4500 cGy). Four gold seed markers are implanted around the periphery of the disease to guide needle positioning. A central obturator with tandem for 137-cesium sources has been positioned in the vagina. Ten hollow interstitial needles for 192-iridium sources have been introduced percutaneously using a Syed–Neblett grid template (b, example of fully deployed template) according to preoperative CT/MRI planning. (c) Depicted is interstitial implant dosimetry of six 192-iridium sources 1 cm apart in 10 needles supplemented with five 137-cesium tandem sources to deliver 4000 cGy over 50 h (80 cGy h–1 isodose line, green outline). For a color version of this figure, see the color plate section.

link of *in-utero* exposure to DES [67,71]. DES-associated clear-cell carcinomas are found in women aged 40 years younger than the usual patients with other histologies of vaginal cancer. Older females have a more favorable prognosis in comparison to younger adolescents (aged <15 years), an outcome linked to the more common tubulocystic variety of clear-cell carcinoma seen in older females. Waggoner and colleagues [38] found that females with clear-cell adenocarcinomas, and whose mothers had been exposed to DES, fared better with therapies than those females with clear-cell adenocarcinomas without a maternal DES history. DES-associated clear-cell carcinomas are commonly seen accompanied by vaginal adenosis, which may be composed of elements from endocervical, endometrial, or tubal Müllerian epithelia. Malignant transformation of extraovarian endometriosis is rare and occurs typically along the rectovaginal septum. For DES-associated clear-cell carcinomas, radiation alone, vaginectomy alone, or wide local excision alone plus radiation all provide pelvic control in early-stage disease [69,70].

Vaginal Melanoma

Management of melanoma of the vagina is personalized, based primarily on the treating physician and patient bias rather than widely accepted clinical evidence. Melanoma of the vagina has a high mortality rate (90%) regardless of therapeutic intervention, with equal likelihood of locoregional and distant relapses. Vigorous attempts at surgical extirpation have been justified by the presumed radioresistance of melanoma to conventional radiation dose. The poor prognosis of vaginal melanoma may relate to delay in diagnosis as compared to more early detection of cutaneous melanoma. Prognosis associates with melanoma depth of invasion into the wall of the vagina. The elevated mortality risk from vaginal melanoma, despite aggressive surgical intervention including partial and total vaginectomy with anterior, posterior, or total pelvic exenteration, should prompt a diligent search for tumor dissemination before embarking on disfiguring surgery. FDG PET/CT may aid in this endeavor as this imaging modality has been well correlated with clinical course and histopathology [72,73]. The documentation of metastatic melanoma should lessen enthusiasm for surgical procedures that may diminish the patient's quality of life without any realistic prospect for a lengthy disease-free survival interval. Conversely, overall poor results should not be a foundation for therapeutic nihilism justifying the undertreatment of women for whom surgery and radiotherapy could provide clinical benefit. Demonstrable benefit with novel chemotherapies and new radiation delivery systems may extend disease-free intervals.

Vaginal Tumors of Infants and Children

Endodermal sinus tumors (yolk-sac tumors) are rare germ-cell tumors that secrete α-fetoprotein, and arise in the vagina of infants (<2 years of age). These tumors have an aggressive untreated natural history and are usually treated with surgery, radiation, and chemotherapy (vincristine, actinomycin D, and cyclophosphamide; VAC) with modest clinical efficacy [74–76].

Sarcoma botryoides (embryonal rhabdomyosarcoma) is a rare vaginal sarcoma occurring in female children (aged <8 years). Vaginal bleeding with a mass (resembling a cluster of grapes) at the introitus is commonplace. Strap cells of eosinophilic rhabdomyoblasts with cross-striations are intermingled with loose myomatous stroma and malignant pleomorphic cells in this disease. Because tumors often are multicentric and expand to fill the vagina, surgeries may be radical and disfiguring. Exenterations have been performed in children with this disease to provide local control [77]. Today, multimodality approaches including wide local excision coupled with radiochemotherapy (VAC) have been found effective [78]. In one such study [78], 17 children with sarcoma botryoides underwent multimodality therapy; 15 of the children were free from disease at the time of reporting. With long-term follow-up, 11 of 12 treated pubescent females retained menses and two of 12 had a record of conceiving and of delivering healthy infants.

High-Dose-Rate Brachytherapy

Remote afterloading technology for high-dose-rate brachytherapy offers advantages of: (i) shortened brachytherapy times for outpatient service; (ii) precise control of radiation depth-dose; and (iii) perhaps ultimately better preservation of vaginal function [43–49]. High-dose-rate endocavitary radiation may be carried out in women who receive all or a portion of their radiation by brachytherapy. Long-term, vaginal elasticity will depend intimately on the vaginal volume irradiated. Usually, endocavitary brachytherapy is directed towards the entire vaginal length to address propensity for disease multifocality and possible occult dissemination of disease in the vaginal mucosa or lymphatics. However, endocavitary brachytherapy does not necessarily need to fully dose the vagina in its entirety, with high-dose-rate techniques capable of tapering dose in vaginal tissue where disease is less likely. Tapering of radiation dose is achieved by carefully selecting reduced dwell times of miniaturized radiation source (i.e., on the order of a grain of rice). Flexibility in designing isodose distributions that narrowly conform to disease allows less vaginal tissue to be irradiated. Equivalent dose distributions are difficult to achieve with more cumbersome low-dose-rate sources that are often larger size and variable source activity.

Afterloaded high-dose-rate techniques provide short treatment times on the order of minutes. Patients are reproducibly immobilized for high-dose-rate therapy. Women may tolerate a more tightly fit endocavitary applicator if it is applied for minutes rather than hours to days. A larger-diameter cylinder or colpostats decreases the mucosal dose relative to cancer target dose at depth. Despite best efforts, low-dose-rate interstitial and endocavitary brachytherapy plans must account for some patient motion when treatments last for hours to days; accounting for patient motion is minimal when high-dose-rate techniques are employed. Inserting cylinders into the vagina under modest tension and securing the device to a locking base plate allows portions of the long axis of the vagina to be irradiated under computer-assisted control. Well-circumscribed lesions may be amenable to commercial, partially shielded applicators. Such applicators may spare up to 75% of the vaginal circumference from treatment, preserving vaginal elasticity and function through a reduction in vaginal fibrosis, stenosis, and mucosal atrophy. Preservation of anatomic form and function represent primary aims for radiation. Often, these aims form a rationale for management by radiotherapy rather than more radical surgery. Careful practice must be exercised to limit areas of high radiation dose (>100 Gy) to an anatomy that has need of it.

Radiochemotherapy

For many decades, bulky stage II, stage III, or stage IV vaginal cancers have been treated with radiochemotherapy [79–81]. Early on, radiochemotherapy involved 5-FU, cisplatin, and mitomycin-C chemotherapy, as well as external beam radiation [79–83]. A variety of techniques, radiation and chemotherapy doses, and also schedules of administration, have been explored to the advantage of women with genitoanal cancers [34]. Naturally, squamous cell cancer of the vagina responds favorably to these combinations. Radiochemotherapy usage for the treatment of vaginal cancer, extracted from the Surveillance, Epidemiology, and End Results (SEER) and Medicare database, has risen since 1999 but has not translated to a substantial gain in clinical survival benefit when analyzed at a population-based interrogative level.

It is important to note that external radiation plus chemotherapy manifests rapid tumor regression [84]. Bulky lesions flatten quickly, and this in turn allows a substantial reduction in cancer targets for 'boost' radiation doses. Brachytherapy applications become less cumbersome and can often be achieved with endocavitary techniques treating sessile lesions after radiochemotherapy, reserving interstitial brachytherapy for persistently bulky lesions [80, 84]. Indeed, cancers have been controlled using cumulative radiation doses that, if given in isolation, would be thought of as subtherapeutic. It is estimated that radiation doses are 10–15% lower when given with chemotherapy, as opposed to when radiation is administered alone [79]. While consequential acute (<30 days) normal tissue reactions are more brisk, anticipated late consequential reactions are less severe when radiochemotherapy is given [85]. Vaginal effects have been mild, with some women having dyspareunia from initial bulky tumors, maintaining regular sexual intercourse without discomfort after radiochemotherapy [80, 84]. It seems plausible that radiochemotherapy will gain wider acceptance as more women are treated [34]. The unsatisfactory outcomes for women with stage III and IV vaginal cancers warrant innovative radiochemotherapy approaches. Radiation dose escalation likely provides a modest gain in local control at an increased hazard in treatment-related complications [79].

Stereotactic Radiosurgery

Whether stereotactic radiosurgery can serve as a brachytherapy alternative in selected patients remains to be studied. For women with vaginal cancer, the considerable therapeutic advantage of interstitial and endocavitary brachytherapy relies on its narrowly confined radiation dose permeation and its brisk radiation dose fall-off. These characteristics successfully limit nearby tissues from excessive radiation dose that may cause tissue injury. Implanted radioactive sources are also not subject to organ motion because of their 'fixed' proximity to vaginal cancer targets.

However, there are women with vaginal cancer who have undergone radiation or radiochemotherapy whose tumor may not easily be covered by interstitial brachytherapy, or whose comorbidities preclude the invasive placement of interstitial applicators or protracted therapy. Stereotactic radiosurgery may provide a non-invasive alternative to brachytherapy [86–89]. Forms of brachytherapy alternatives involving intensity-modulated radiation therapy (IMRT) or helical arc therapy (tomotherapy) for vaginal cancer management have not been developed substantially [90]. Clinical experience has emerged in the use of stereotactic radiosurgery to deliver additional radiation dose to the vagina in clinical situations where interstitial brachytherapy may not be feasible [91]. While in its clinical infancy, robotic stereotactic radiosurgery has been used to target metastatic gynecologic lesions appearing in the vagina after prior pelvic irradiation [86]. Ablative radiosurgery doses of 2400 cGy in three divided daily doses of 800 cGy (biologically effective dose nearly 6170 cGy, assuming an α/β ratio of 10) have been used safely and successfully when directed to the vagina [86]. And yet, front-line stereotactic radiosurgery of treatment-naïve vaginal cancer has not been studied. Stereotactic radiosurgery for vaginal cancer treatment would best be investigated in multi-institutional collaborative clinical trials.

Future Directions for Vaginal Cancer Management

Radiochemotherapy has emerged as an important treatment consideration for women with vaginal cancer as it potentially addresses: (i) an improved locoregional pelvic control of disease; and (ii) a lower risk of occult disease progression. Optimal radiochemotherapy agent combinations, schedules, and intensity are anticipated over the next decade of vaginal cancer clinical research. However, clinical trials restricted to vaginal cancer disease may not be feasible due to the rarity of the disease and to a lack of molecular pathways that are clearly amenable to targeted anticancer therapy. Clinical benefits from surgery, chemotherapy and radiation are likely to be extrapolated from cervical cancer clinical trials also enrolling women with vaginal cancers. Further technical improvements of radiation dose delivery by brachytherapy and by stereotactic radiosurgery hold promise.

References

1 Siegel, R., Miller, K., Jemal, A. (2017) Cancer Statistics 2017. *CA Cancer J. Clin.*, **67**, 7–30.

2 FIGO Committee on Gynecologic Oncology (2009) Current FIGO staging for cancer of the vagina, fallopian tube, ovary, and gestational trophoblastic neoplasia. *Int. J. Gynaecol. Obstet.*, **105** (1), 3–4.

3 Henson, D., Tarone, R. (1977) A epidemiologic study of cancer of the cervix, vagina, and vulva based on the Third National Cancer Survey in the United States. *Am. J. Obstet. Gynecol.*, **29** (5), 525–532.

4 Rubin, S., Young, J., Mikuta, J. (1985) Squamous carcinoma of the vagina: Treatment, complications, and long-term follow-up. *Gynecol. Oncol.*, **20** (3), 1346–1353.

5 Benedet, J., Murphy, K., Fairey, R., Boyes, D. (1983) Primary invasive carcinoma of the vagina. *Obstet. Gynecol.*, **62** (6), 715–719.

6 Reyes-Ortiz, C., Camacho, M., Amador, L., Velez, L., Ottenbacher, K., Markides, K. (2007) The impact of education and literacy on cancer screening among older Latin American and Caribbean adults. *Cancer Control*, **14** (4), 388–395.

7 Barzon, L., Militello, V., Pagni, S., *et al.* (2010) Distribution of human papillomavirus types in the anogenital tract of females and males. *J. Med. Virol.*, **82** (8), 1424–1430.

8 McAlearney, A., Song, P., Rhoda, D., *et al.* (2010) Ohio Appalachian women's perceptions of the cost of cervical cancer screening. *Cancer*, **116** (20), 4727–4734.

9 McKinnon, B., Harper, S., Moore, S. (2011) Decomposing income-related inequality in cervical screening in 67 countries. *Int. J. Public Health.*, **56** (2), 139–152.

10 Brunner, A., Grimm, C., Polterauer, S., *et al.* (2011) The prognostic role of human papillomavirus in patients with vaginal cancer. *Int. J. Gynaecol. Cancer.*, **21** (5), 923–929.

11 Mahdi, H., Kumar, S., Hanna, R., *et al.* (2011) Disparities in treatment and survival between African-American and white women with vaginal cancer. *Gynecol. Oncol.*, **122** (1), 38–41.

12 Brinton, L., Nasca, P., Mallin, K., *et al.* (1990) Case-control study of in situ and invasive carcinoma of the vagina. *Gynecol. Oncol.*, **38** (1), 49–54.

13 Jamieson, D., Paramsothy, P., Cu-Uvin, S., Duerr, A. (2006) HIV epidemiology research study group. Vulvar, vaginal, and perianal intraepithelial neoplasia in women with or at risk for human immunodeficiency virus. *Obstet. Gynecol.*, **107** (5), 1023–1028.

14 Patemoster, D., Cester, M., Resente, C., *et al.* (2008) Human papillomavirus infection and cervical intraepithelial neoplasia in transplanted patients. *Transplant. Proc.*, **40** (6), 1877–1880.

15 Fetters, M., Fischer, G., Reed, B. (1996) Effectiveness of vaginal Papanicolaou smear screening after total hysterectomy for benign disease. *JAMA*, **275** (12), 940–947.

16 Pearce, K., Haefner, H., Sarwar, S., Nolan, T. (1996) Cytopathological findings on vaginal Papanicolaou smears after hysterectomy for benign gynecologic disease. *N. Engl. J. Med.*, **335** (21), 1559–1562.

17 Fetters, M., Lieberman, R., Abrahamse, P., Sanghvi, R., Sonnad, S. (2003) Cost-effectiveness of pap smear screening for vaginal cancer after total hysterectomy for benign disease. *J. Low. Genit. Tract Dis.*, **7** (3), 194–202.

18 Robboy, S., Szyfelbein, W., Goeliner, J., *et al.* (1981) Dysplasia and cytologic findings in 4,589 young women enrolled in diethylstibestrol-adenosis (DESAD) project. *Am. J. Obstet. Gynecol.*, **140** (5), 579–586.

19 Liao, J., Jean, S., Wilkinson-Ryan, I., *et al.* (2011) Vaginal intraepithelial neoplasia (VAIN) after radiation therapy for gynecologic malignancies: a clinically recalcitrant entity. *Gynecol. Oncol.*, **120** (1), 108–112.

20 Aho, M., Vesterinen, E., Meyer, B., Purola, E., Paavonen, J. (1991) Natural history of vaginal intraepithelial neoplasia. *Cancer*, **68** (1), 195–197.

21 Smith, J., Backes, D., Hoots, B., Kurman, R., Pimenta, J. (2009) Human papillomavirus type-distribution in vulvar and vaginal cancers and their associated precursors. *Obstet. Gynecol.*, **113** (4), 917–924.

22 Dillner, J., Kjaer, S., *et al.* the FUTURE I/II Study Group. (2010) Four-year efficacy of prophylactic human papillomavirus quadrivalent vaccine against low grade cervical, vulvar, and vaginal intraepithelial neoplasia and anogenital warts: randomised controlled trial. *Br. Med. J.*, **341**, c3493.

23 Hebner, C., Laimins, L. (2006) Human papillomaviruses: basic mechanisms and pathogenesis and oncogenicity. *Rev. Med. Virol.*, **16** (2), 83–97.

24 Cole, S., Danos, O. (1987) Nucleotide sequence and comparative analysis of the human papillomavirus type 18 genome: phylogeny of papillomaviruses and repeated structure of the E6 and E7 gene products. *J. Mol. Biol.*, **193** (4), 599–608.

25 Barbosa, M., Lowy, D., Schiller, J. (1989) Papillomavirus polypeptides E6 and E7 are zinc-binding proteins. *J. Virol.*, **63** (3), 1404–1407.

26 Werness, B., Levine, A., Howley, P. (1990) Association of human papillomavirus type 16 and 18 E6 proteins with p53. *Science*, **248** (4951), 76–79.

27 Scheffner, M., Werness, B., Huibregtse, J., Levine, A., Howley, P. (1990) The E6 oncoprotein encoded by human papillomavirus types 16 and 18 promotes the degradation of p53. *Cell*, **63** (6), 1129–1136.

28 Huibregtse, J., Scheffner, M., Howley, P. (1991) A cellular protein mediates association of p53 with the E6 oncoprotein of human papillomavirus types 16 or 18. *EMBO J.*, **10** (13), 4129–4135.

29 Klingelhutz, A., Foster, S., McDougall, J. (1996) Telomerase activation by the E6 gene product of human papillomavirus type 16. *Nature*, **380** (6569), 79–82.

30 Gonzalez, S., Stremlau, M., He, X., Baile, J., Münger, K. (2001) Degradation of the retinoblastoma tumor suppressor by the human papillomavirus type 16 E7 oncoprotein is important for functional inactivation and is separable from proteosomal degradation of E7. *J. Virol.*, **75** (16), 7583–7591.

31 Huang, P., Patrick, D., Edwards, G., *et al.* (1993) Protein domains governing interactions between E2F, the retinoblastoma gene product, and human papillomavirus type 16 E7 protein. *Mol. Cell. Biol.*, **13** (2), 953–960.

32 Auborn, K., Woodworth, C., DiPaolo, J., Bradlow, H. (1990) The interaction between HPV infection and estrogen metabolism in cervical carcinogenesis. *Int. J. Cancer*, **49** (6), 867–869.

33 Elson, D., Riley, R., Lacey, A., Thordarson, G., Talamantes, F., Arbreit, J. (2000) Sensitivity of the cervical transformation zone to estrogen-induced squamous carcinogenesis. *Cancer Res.*, **60** (5), 1267–1275.

34 Ghia, A., Gonzalez, V., Tward, J., Stroup, A., Pappas, L., Gaffney, D. (2011) Primary vaginal cancer and chemoradiotherapy: a patterns-of-care analysis. *Int. J. Gynecol. Cancer*, **21** (2), 378–384.

35 Woodruff, J., Parmley, T., Julian, C. (1975) Topical 5-fluorouracil in the treatment of vaginal carcinoma *in situ*. *Gynecol. Oncol.*, **3** (2), 124–132.

36 Calgar, H., Hertzog, R., Hreshchyshyn, M. (1981) Topical 5-fluorouracil treatment of vaginal intraepithelial neoplasia. *Obstet. Gynecol.*, **58** (5), 580–583.

37 Piver, M., Barlow, J., Tsukada, Y., Gamarra, M., Saudecki, A. (1979) Postirradiation squamous cell carcinoma of the vagina: treatment by topical 20 percent 5-fluorouracil cream. *Am. J. Obstet. Gynecol.*, **135** (3), 377–380.

38 Kim, H., Park, N., Park, I., *et al.* (2009) Risk factors for recurrence of vaginal intraepithelial neoplasia in the vaginal vault after laser vaporization. *Lasers Surg. Med.*, **41** (3), 196–202.

39 Jobson, W., Campion, M. (1991) Vaginal laser surgery. *Obstet. Gynecol. Clin. North Am.*, **18** (3), 511–524.

40 Madhuri, T., Paptheodorou, D., Tailor, A., Sutton, C., Butler-Manuel, S. (2010) First clinical experience of argon neutral plasma energy in gynaecological surgery in the UK. *Gynecol. Surg.*, **7** (4), 423–425.

41 Sonoda, Y., Olvera, N., Chi, D., Brown, C., Abu-Rustum, N., Levine, D. (2010) Pathological analysis of ex vivo plasma energy tumor destruction in patients with ovarian or peritoneal cancer. *Int. J. Gynecol. Cancer*, **20** (8), 1326–1330.

42 Indemaur, M., Martino, M., Fiorica, J., Roberts, W., Hoffman, M. (2005) Upper vaginectomy for the treatment of vaginal intraepithelial neoplasia. *Am. J. Obstet. Gynecol.*, **193** (2), 577–580.

43 Perez, C., Camel, H. (1982) Long-term follow-up in radiation therapy of carcinoma of the vagina. *Cancer*, **49** (6), 1308–1315.

44 MacLeod, C., Fowler, A., Dalrymple, C., Atkinson, K., Elliott, P., Carter, J. (1997) High dose-rate brachytherapy in the management of high-grade intraepithelial neoplasia of the vagina. *Gynecol. Oncol.*, **65** (1), 74–77.

45 Ogino, I., Kitamura, T., Okajima, H., Matsubara, S. (1998) High-dose-rate intracavitary brachytherapy in the management of cervical and vaginal intraepithelial neoplasia. *Int. J. Radiat. Oncol. Biol. Phys.*, **40** (4), 881–887.

46 Perez, C., Grigsby, P., Garipagaoglu, M., Mutch, D., Lockett, M. (1999) Factors affecting long-term outcome of irradiation in carcinoma of the vagina. *Int. J. Radiat. Oncol. Biol. Phys.*, **44** (1), 37–45.

47 Graham, K., Wright, K., Cadwallader, B., Reed, N., Symonds, R. (2007) 20-year retrospective review of medium dose rate intracavitary brachytherapy in VAIN3. *Gynecol. Oncol.*, **106** (1), 105–111.

48 Blanchard, P., Monnier, L., Dumas, I., *et al.* (2011) Low-dose-rate definitive brachytherapy for high-grade vaginal epithelial neoplasia. *Oncologist*, **16** (2), 182–188.

49 Beriwal, S., Heron, D., Mogus, R., Edwards, R., Kelley, J., Sukumvanich, P. (2008) High-dose rate brachytherapy (HDRB) for primary or recurrent cancer in the vagina. *Radiat. Oncol.*, **13** (3), e1–e7.

50 Demanes, D., Rege, S., Rodriguez, R., Schutz, K., Altieri, G., Wong, T. (1999) The use and advantages of a multichannel vaginal cylinder in high-dose-rate brachytherapy. *Int. J. Radiat. Oncol. Biol. Phys.*, **44** (1), 211–219.

51 Davis, K., Stanhope, C., Garton, G., Arkinson, E., O'Brien, P. (1991) Invasive vaginal carcinoma: analysis of early-stage disease. *Gynecol. Oncol.*, **42** (2), 131–136.

52 Tewari, K., Cappuccini, F., Puthawala, A., *et al.* (2001) Primary invasive carcinoma of the vagina: treatment with interstitial brachytherapy. *Cancer*, **91** (4), 758–770.

53 Sinha, B., Stehman, F., Schilder, J., Clark, L., Cardenes, H. (2009) Indiana University experience in the management of vaginal cancer. *Int. J. Gynecol. Cancer*, **19** (4), 686–693.

54 Basu, S., Li, G., Alavi, A. (2009) PET and PET-CT imaging of gynecological malignancies: present role and future promise. *Expert Rev. Anticancer Ther.*, **9** (1), 75–96.

55 Petereit, D., Mehta, M., Buchler, D., Kinsella, T. (1993) Inguinofemoral radiation of N0,N1 vulvar cancer may

be equivalent to lymphadenectomy if proper radiation technique is used. *Int. J. Radiat. Oncol. Biol. Phys.*, **27** (4), 963–967.

56 Frumovitz, M., Gayed, I., Jhingran, A., *et al.* (2008) Lymphatic mapping and sentinel lymph node detection in women with vaginal cancer. *Gynecol. Oncol.*, **108** (3), 478–481.

57 Demanes, D., Rodriguez, R., Altieri, G. (2000) High dose rate prostate brachytherapy: The California Endocurietherapy (CET) method. *Radiother. Oncol.*, **57** (3), 289–296.

58 Demanes, D., Rodriguez, R., Bendre, D., Ewing, T. (1999) High dose rate transperineal interstitial brachytherapy for cervical cancer: high pelvic control and low complication rates. *Int. J. Radiat. Oncol. Biol. Phys.*, **45** (1), 105–112.

59 Corn, B., Lanciano, R., Rosenblum, N., Schnall, M., King, S., Epperson, R. (1995) Improved treatment planning for the Syed–Neblett template using endorectal-coil magnetic resonance and intraoperative (laparotomy/laparoscopy) guidance: A new integrated technique for hysterectomized women with vaginal tumors. *Gynecol. Oncol.*, **56** (2), 255–261.

60 Fleming, P., Nisar Syed, A., Neblett, D., Puthawala, A., George, Fr., Townsend, D. (1980) Description of an afterloading 192 Ir interstitial-intracavitary technique in the treatment of carcinoma of the vagina. *Obstet. Gynecol.*, **55** (4), 525–530.

61 Kumar, P., Good, R., Scott, J., Jones, E. (1988) Choice of afterloading endocurietherapy techniques for vaginal carcinoma. *Radiat. Med.*, **6** (2), 71–78.

62 Prestidge, B., Butler, E., Shaw, D., McComas, V. (1994) Ultrasound guided placement of transperineal prostatic afterloading catheters. *Int. J. Radiat. Oncol. Biol. Phys.*, **28** (1), 263–266.

63 Stock, R., Chan, K., Terk, M., Dewyngaert, J., Stone, N., Dottino, P. (1997) A new technique for performing Syed–Neblett template interstitial implants for gynecologic malignancies using transrectal-ultrasound. *Int. J. Radiat. Oncol. Biol. Phys.*, **37** (4), 819–825.

64 Frank, S., Deavers, M., Jhingran, A., Bodurka, D., Eifel, P. (2007) Primary adenocarcinoma of the vagina not associated with diethylstilbestrol (DES) exposure. *Gynecol. Oncol.*, **105** (2), 470–474.

65 Creasman, W., Phillips, J., Menck, H. (1998) The national cancer data base report on cancer of the vagina. *Cancer*, **83** (5), 1033–1040.

66 Chyle, V., Zagars, G., Wheeler, J., Wharton, J., Delclos, L. (1996) Definitive radiotherapy for carcinoma of the vagina: outcome and prognostic factors. *Int. J. Radiat. Oncol. Biol. Phys.*, **35** (5), 891–905.

67 Waggoner, S., Mittendorf, R., Biney, N., Anderson, D., Herbst, A. (1994) Influence of in utero diethylstilbestrol exposure on the prognosis and biologic behavior of vaginal clear-cell adenocarcinoma. *Gynecol. Oncol.*, **55** (2), 238–244.

68 Senekjian, E., Frey, K., Stone, C., Herbst, A. (1988) An evaluation of stage II vaginal clear cell adenocarcinoma according to substage. *Gynecol. Oncol.*, **31** (1), 56–64.

69 Senekjian, E., Frey, K., Anderson, D., Herbst, A. (1987) Local therapy in stage I clear cell adenocarcinoma of the vagina. *Cancer*, **60** (6), 1319–1324.

70 Renaud, M., Plante, M., Gregoire, J., Roy, M. (2009) Primitive clear cell carcinoma of the vagina treated conservatively. *J. Obstet. Gynaecol. Cancer*, **31** (1), 54–56.

71 Goodman, A., Schorge, J., Greene, M. (2011) The long-term effects of *in utero* exposures – the DES story. *N. Engl. J. Med.*, **364** (22), 2083–2084.

72 Oudoux, A., Rousseau, T., Bindji, B., Resche, I., Rousseau, C. (2004) Interest of F-18 fluorodeoxyglucose positron emission tomography in the evaluation of vaginal malignant melanoma. *Gynecol. Oncol.*, **95** (3), 765–768.

73 Husain, A., Akhurst, T., Larson, S., Alektiar, K., Barakat, R., Chi, D. (2007) A prospective study of the accuracy of 18Fluorodeoxyglucose positron emission tomography (18FDG PET) in identifying sites of metastasis prior to pelvic exenteration. *Gynecol. Oncol.*, **106** (1), 177–180.

74 Kohorn, E., McIntosh, S., Lytton, B., Knowlton, A., Merino, M. (1985) Endodermal sinus tumor of the infant vagina. *Gynecol. Oncol.*, **20** (2), 196–203.

75 Young, R., Scully, R. (1984) Endodermal sinus tumor of the vagina: a report of nine cases and review of the literature. *Gynecol. Oncol.*, **18** (3), 380–392.

76 Collins, H., Burke, T., Heller, P., Olson, T., Woodward, J., Park, R. (1989) Endodermal sinus tumor the infant vagina treated exclusively by chemotherapy. *Obstet. Gynecol.*, **73** (3 Pt 2), 507–509.

77 Mahesh Kumar, A., Wrenn, E.J., Fleming, I., Omar Hustu, H., Pratt, C. (1976) Combined therapy to prevent complete pelvic exenteration for rhabdomyosarcoma of the vagina or uterus. *Cancer*, **37** (1), 118–122.

78 Flamant, F., Gerbaulet, A., Nihoul-Fekete, C., Valteau-Couanet, D., Chassagne, D., Lemerle, J. (1990) Long-term sequelae of conservative treatment by surgery, brachytherapy, and chemotherapy for vulvar and vaginal rhabdomyosarcoma in children. *J. Clin. Oncol.*, **8** (11), 1847–1853.

79 Dalrymple, C., Russell, A., Lee, S., *et al.* (2004) Chemoradiation for primary invasive squamous cell carcinoma of the vagina. *Int. J. Gynecol. Cancer*, **14** (1), 110–117.

80 Samant, R., Lau, B., EC, Le, T., Tam, T. (2007) Primary vaginal cancer treated with concurrent chemoradiation using cis-platinum. *Int. J. Radiat. Oncol. Biol. Phys.*, **69** (3), 746–750.

81 Kirkbride, P., Fyles, A., Rawlings, G., *et al.* (1995) Carcinoma of the vagina – experience at the Princess Margaret Hospital (1974–1989). *Gynecol. Oncol.*, **56** (3), 435–443.

82 Mundt, A., Rotmensch, J., Waggoner, S., Quiet, C., Fleming, G. (1999) Phase 1 trial of concomitant chemoradiotherapy for cervical cancer and other advanced pelvic malignancies. *Gynecol. Oncol.*, **72** (1), 45–50.

83 Roberts, W., Hoffman, M., Kavanagh, J., *et al.* (1991) Further experience with radiation therapy and concomitant intravenous chemotherapy in advanced carcinoma of the lower female genital tract. *Gynecol. Oncol.*, **43** (3), 233–236.

84 Kunos, C., Waggoner, S., Zanotti, K., *et al.* (2011) Phase 2 trial of pelvic radiation, weekly cisplatin, and 3-aminopyridine-2-carboxaldehyde thiosemicarbazone (3-AP, NSC #663249) for locally advanced cervical and vaginal cancer. *J. Clin. Oncol.*, **29** (Suppl.), abstract #5034.

85 Grigsby, P., Russell, A., Bruner, D., *et al.* (1995) Late injury of cancer therapy on the female reproductive tract. *Int. J. Radiat. Oncol. Biol. Phys.*, **31** (5), 1281–1299.

86 Kunos, C., Chen, W., DeBernardo, R., *et al.* (2009) Stereotactic body radiosurgery for pelvic relapse of gynecologic malignancies. *Technol. Cancer Res. Treat.*, **8** (5), 393–400.

87 Mollà, M., Escude, L., Nouet, P., *et al.* (2005) Fractionated stereotactic radiotherapy boost for gynecologic tumors: an alternative to brachytherapy? *Int. J. Radiat. Oncol. Biol. Phys.*, **62** (1), 118–124.

88 Jorcano, S., Molla, M., Escude, L., *et al.* (2010) Hypofractionated extracranial stereotactic radiotherapy boost for gynecologic tumors: a promising alternative to high-dose rate brachytherapy. *Technol. Cancer Res. Treat.*, **9** (5), 509–514.

89 Guckenberger, M., Bachmann, J., Wulf, J., *et al.* (2010) Stereotactic body radiotherapy for local boost irradiation in unfavourable locally recurrent gynaecological cancer. *Radiother. Oncol.*, **94** (1), 53–59.

90 Chan, P., Milosevic, M., Paterson, J., Yeo, I., Fyles, A. (2005) Cervical cancer not suitable for brachytherapy, in *Intensity-Modulated Radiation Therapy*, Vol. 1 (eds A. Mundt, J. Roeske), BC Decker, Inc., London, pp. 518–522.

91 Mayr, N., Huang, Z., Sohn, J., *et al.* (2011) Emerging application of stereotactic body radiation therapy for gynecologic malignancies. *Expert Rev. Anticancer Ther.*, **11** (7), 1071–1077.

35

Cervix

Charles A. Kunos

Incidence and Mortality

Worldwide, 1.1 million women were diagnosed with a gynecologic cancer and an estimated 494 000 (45%) died of their disease in 2014 [1]. Of those 1.1 million women diagnosed, nearly 528 000 had new cancers of the uterine cervix, and 266 000 women (50% of newly diagnosed women) died of uterine cervix cancer [1]. The American Cancer Society (ACS) estimates that 12 820 American women will develop cervical cancer in 2017, and 4210 (32%) would die of it [2, 3]. The probability of developing invasive cervical cancers over selected age intervals in American women between 2011 and 2013 was 0.6 (1 in 161) from birth to death [2]. As of 2011, there was a precipitous rise in probability for invasive cancer of the uterine cervix, from 0.15 (1 in 656) in the birth to 39 years old age range, to 0.27 (1 in 377) from 40 to 59 years old age range [3]. Since 2003, and after the widespread implementation of cisplatin radiochemotherapy for advanced-stage cervical cancer, overall mortality rates have remained flat at 30% of diagnosed [3].

While organized screening programs based on the Papinicolaou (Pap) exfoliative cytology smear [4, 5] have lowered incidence figures for invasive disease and mortality attributed to cervical cancer, this malignant disease remains a leading cause of death in developing nations. Factors contributing to these observations are likely manyfold, but are commonly linked to differences in regional demographics and access to medical resources. A most effective strategy to reduce mortality due to cervical cancer remains an early diagnosis of precursor lesions, lesions that may be detectable during five to 20 years before the onset of invasive disease [6]. Carcinoma *in situ* is acknowledged as the harbinger of invasive disease, and is readily detected by exfoliative cytology [7]. Current reporting of exfoliative cytology

follows a National Cancer Institute consensus statement with refinement [8, 9]. Worldwide, the likelihood that a woman undergoes regular health examination that includes a Pap smear remains small (30%), despite coordinated World Health Organization, international, and humanitarian foundation effort to reverse this trend [10–12]. Even in the US, regional demographic differences reveal that age, race, socioeconomic factors and the practical logistics of medical practice such as adequate patient insurance coverage, service reimbursement and the experience of medical staff, contribute to the complexity of cervical cancer screening and the implementation of anticancer therapies [13–17].

Epidemiology of Uterine Cervix Cancers

The epidemiology of cervical cancer has long been linked to sexual activity, although the precise molecular events involved in its pathogenesis remain uncharacterized. Factors such as early age of first intercourse [18], multiple sexual partners or male partners with multiple partners [19], and a history of sexually transmitted disease [20] correlate with the risk of developing cervical cancer. Uterine cervix cancer is rare among females not sexually active [21]. Surrogates reflecting vulnerability to a sexually transmitted agent, such as low income, low educational status, and a history of genital condyloma infection, appear to be risk factors for cervical cancer [22–26]. Smoking may be a cofactor for and/or promoter of malignant transformation of cervix cells [14,27,28].

Several lines of evidence have implicated human papillomavirus (HPV) infection as a causative agent for the onset of cervical cancer neoplasia (Table 35.1). HPV subtypes 16, 18, and 45 are the most common viral forms associated with grade 3 cervical intraepithelial neoplasia and cancer [25]. Up to 90% of the worldwide incidence of

Clinical Radiation Oncology: Indications, Techniques, and Results, Third Edition. Edited by William Small Jr.
© 2017 John Wiley & Sons, Inc. Published 2017 by John Wiley & Sons, Inc.

Table 35.1 Oncogenic human papillomavirus (HPV) genotypes.

Low-risk HPV genotypes	High-risk HPV genotypes
6, 11, 42, 43, 44	16, 18, 31, 33, 35, 45, 51, 52, 56, 58, 59

cervical cancer is related to HPV [25]. While HPV infection may be cleared in some individuals or remain latent in others, the immunologic competence of the infected female plays a role in the process of carcinogenesis [29–31]. When both human immunodeficiency virus and cervical cancer are detected, a cervical cancer diagnosis becomes an acquired immunodeficiency syndrome (AIDS)-defining event [32, 33]. HPV screening has emerged as a sufficiently discriminatory biomarker for the risk of developing cervical cancer, with a sensitivity of 96% and a specificity of 92% [34]. The strong negative predictive power of HPV screening has been argued for justifying long five-year intervals between screens. For comparison, exfoliative cytology has a modest sensitivity of 53% and specificity of 97%, which suggests that sampling detects cancer not because of diagnostic accuracy but rather because smears are performed often [34]. The proportion of women developing carcinoma *in situ* grade 2 or worse is 0.48% at three years after negative exfoliative cytology, and 0.23% at six years after HPV testing [35]. According to the 2009 consensus guidelines of the American Society for Colposcopy and Cervical Pathology, women over the age of 30 years who undergo exfoliative cytology and HPV testing and are found to have negative cytology, and a patient with a positive high-risk HPV (HPV16 or HPV18) test may either have both tests repeated in 12 months or undergo HPV genotyping [36]. If the genotyping assay is positive, women should submit to timely colposcopy.

HPV may produce a viral 'field' multifocal transformation effect upon many regions of anogenital epithelial cells. Because of this phenomenon, an opportunity for reduced mortality from cervical cancer may include prophylactic vaccination. A randomized study reporting 42 months of follow-up in 17 622 HPV-naïve women (aged 16–26 years) has shown that prophylactic quadrivalent HPV (types 6, 11, 16, 18) vaccine administered at day 1, month 2, and month 6 within the vaccination program sustains immunoprotection against HPV16- and HPV18-associated intraepithelial neoplasia in those receiving vaccine versus those receiving placebo [37]. High efficacy, immunogenicity, and acceptable safety in women aged 24–45 years have been confirmed [38]. In 2007, Australia was the first nation to introduce an extensive, funded national HPV vaccination program with the quadrivalent vaccine as a continuing component of a 12–13-year-old schoolgirl health program, plus two catch-up

programs targeting 13–17-year-old school adolescents and 18–26-year-old women in general practice and community settings [39]. After introduction of the vaccination program, a decrease in population-wide incidence of cervical intraepithelial neoplasia grade 2 or worse or carcinoma *in situ* by 0.38% (95% CI 0.61–0.16, $p = 0.05$) was observed in the vaccinated cohort between 2007 and 2009, compared to incidence found in the Victorian Cervical Cytology registry (Australia, 2003–2009). The efficacy of HPV vaccination against high-grade cervical neoplasia remains high [37–40].

Symptoms Leading to Diagnosis

A thorough history should be obtained from each patient before diagnostic assessments are initiated, since focused questions will often assist in determining the direction of histopathological and imaging work-up. Medical attention is often sought for vaginal spotting or bleeding associated with intercourse. Sexual health and partnering should be obtained; screening for HIV should be considered in women with relevant risk factors. Such lines of questioning also establish a baseline sexual history and expectations that may be important to counseling regarding planned interventions and post-therapy sexual rehabilitation. Solicited accounts of irregular or excessive bleeding may be telling of tumor vascularity rather than perceptions of cyclical bleeding attributed by patients to fluctuating hormone levels. A malodorous cloudy yellow or gray discharge accompanies necrotic and saprophytic infected cervical tumors. Pain is unusual when disease is confined to the cervix, and so when noted it may be indicative of disease extension along the pelvic floor or to lymph nodes compressing the sacral nerve plexus. Cramping pains reminiscent of uterine contractions may signal either occlusion of the endocervical canal and accumulation of blood (hematometra) within the uterine cavity, or invasion of the lower uterine segment by disease. Fever, chills, and intense pelvic pain may identify infection of the uterine cavity (pyometria), which should be drained transvaginally (perhaps, under ultrasound guidance) followed by antibiotic therapy. Lateralized pain in the groin may accompany parametrial extension with obstruction of the ureter. Pain in the buttock or along the length of the leg usually indicates pelvic sidewall disease-by-disease spreading along the cardinal suspensory ligaments or extensive metastases to pelvic and obturator lymph nodes. Compression of pelvic veins due to bulky pelvic lymph nodes elicits lower-extremity edema and deep venous thromboses. Thrombophlebitis may ensue. Changes in micturition such as urinary frequency, urgency, or dysuria most commonly are due to a mass blocking urinary outflow and less frequently to direct bladder invasion. Frank hematuria is uncommon and normally necessitates cystoscopy, while spurious hematuria from admixture of urine and vaginal blood is common. Painful defecation and alteration in defecation pattern may be experienced with bulky cervical cancers and consequent pressure on the midrectum. Passage of frank blood (hematochezia) mandates proctoscopy. Constitutional symptoms including anorexia, dysgeusia, and weight loss reflect advanced disease.

Cancers of the uterine cervix may be preceded by pre-cancerous cervical intraepithelial neoplasia (CIN). Conventional smear or liquid-based cytology methods are acceptable for sampling [41]. For diagnosis, the cells of the uterine cervix are taken by spatula and/or endocervical brush, and then rinsed in a container with fixative and processed either by filtration and vacuum-packed on a membrane/glass slide (ThinPrep® or Cytyc®) or by centrifugation and sedimentation through a gradient density (Surepath® or Tripath Imaging®). Up to 5000 cells may be evaluated for liquid smears, as compared to 8000–12 000 cells that must be present for the evaluation of conventional smears [42]. If inflammation, blood, and cellular debris cloud more than 75% of a smear, it should be considered unsatisfactory [42].

Histopathology of the Uterine Cervix

Squamous cell cancers are the predominant variant of cervical cancer, accounting for 70% of disease. Squamous cell cancers usually arise in the transformation zone and manifest an exophytic component recognized on speculum examination of the vagina. Squamous cell cancers are triaged into keratinizing, non-keratinizing, verrucous, basaloid, papillary (transitional), squamo-transitional, and lymphoepithelioma-like variants by the World Health Organization (WHO) [43]. Efforts to correlate stage of cancer and prognosis with histological category has not yet been reproducible or accepted. Discrimination of growth patterns and natural history does not provide a suitable foundation for selection of anti-cancer intervention. The verrucous variant of squamous cell cancer is strikingly exophytic and well-differentiated with exuberant keratinization. Verrucous squamous cell cancers seldom spread to lymph nodes, and tend to relapse locally after surgery and persist after radiation [44, 45]. Lymphoepithelioma-like carcinoma presents marked infiltration of inflammatory cells in the stroma (not Epstein–Barr virus-driven, which is unlike other lymphoepithelial cancers except for those occurring in Asian populations). Lymphoepithelioma-like carcinomas carry more favorable prognoses than other cervical cancer varieties when stratified by cancer stage [46].

Adenocarcinoma of the uterine cervix has increased its proportional representation to 25% of cervical cancers over the past 50 years. This may in part be due to screening programs detecting precursor squamous cell lesions leading to an apparent drop in the squamous cell cancer incidence rate. The WHO classifies adenocarcinomas of the cervix into mucinous (endocervical, intestinal, signet ring, minimal deviation, and villoglandular subtypes), endometrioid, clear-cell, serous, and mesonephric variants [43]. Over 70% of adenocarcinomas are of the endocervical type, with a complex glandular architecture often intermingled with adenocarcinoma *in situ.* Adenocarcinomas carry a more ominous prognosis, but this adverse effect associates with bulky stage I tumors 4 cm or larger or stage II tumors [47, 48]. The finding of spread to regional nodes in patients with adenocarcinoma treated by surgery carries a higher risk of relapse than is found in comparable patients with squamous cell cancer [49, 50]. Women matched stage-for-stage and treated by radiation alone for adenocarcinoma of the cervix fare marginally worse in recurrence and cancer-related death than women with squamous cervical cancers [51]. The decrement in prognosis for women with larger adenocarcinomas of the cervix appears due to a higher rate of nodal metastases than extrapelvic visceral metastases, rather than an ability to control pelvic disease with radiation.

Clear-cell adenocarcinoma of the cervix isolated to the ectocervix are found in girls and adolescents having had exposure to *in-utero* diethylstilbestrol (DES) [52]. These same females are susceptible to vaginal clear-cell carcinomas [53, 54]. Treatment for clear-cell adenocarcinoma of the cervix follows that of other cervical cancer subtypes, except that very young age typically directs surgical intervention rather than radiation treatment.

The minimal deviation (adenoma malignum) variant of cervical adenocarcinoma is rare. Its paradoxical appellation has been "…justified by a deceptively bland histologic appearance (adenoma) accompanied by a bad prognosis (malignum)" [55]. This lesion is often misdiagnosed as benign and is often an incidental finding in hysterectomy specimens carried out for other reasons. Delay in diagnosis or placid treatment occasioned by low histological grade likely impact the apparent post-therapy high risk of relapse and cancer-related mortality attributed to this disease [56].

A diagnosis of adenosquamous cancer hinges on the identification of admixtures of malignant glandular and malignant squamous tumor components. Adenosquamous cancers are associated with a poorer prognosis since the glandular component may be of worse grade and spread early. Glassy cell cancers are an aggressive subtype of adenosquamous cancer, with explosive growth and bulky, exophytic growth pattern [57]. Adenosquamous cancers are usually treated by surgery and radiochemotherapy as most are diagnosed at stage I with high local relapse risk [58, 59]. Basaloid adenocarcinomas consist of well-differentiated nests of basaloid cells with focal squamous or glandular differentiation. It is often an incidental finding in the absence of a mass lesion, and may be a precursor for adenoid cystic carcinoma (<1% of adenocarcinomas of the cervix). Basaloid cancers tend to grow in a polypoid fashion and are treated similar to other cervical cancers.

Accounting for 5% of cervical epithelial cancers, small-cell neuroendocrine cancers have a high nuclear-to-cytoplasm ratio with secretory granules and immunohistochemistry positive for chromogranin and synaptophysin. Malignant small-cell cancers of the cervix are aggressive and may manifest endocrine paraneoplastic syndromes. These cancers are not to be confused with the rare carcinoid tumor of the cervix, which tends to be less aggressive and more easily controlled with anticancer interventions. Neuroendocrine cancers classically form barrel-shaped circumferential expansion of the cervix. Clinical management of small-cell cervical cancer follows cisplatin plus etoposide radiochemotherapy recommendations for other neuroendocrine tumors (e.g., small-cell cancer of the lung).

Lastly, hematological malignancies such as leukemia and lymphoma arise more often in the cervix than elsewhere in the Müllerian tract, and if they do, cause barrel-shaped circumferential expansion of the cervix [60]. Metastatic cancer arising in the parenchyma of the cervix is very rare (with the exception of primary uterine malignancies). A clue to a metastatic origin is often extensive lymphovascular space invasion in the absence of a defined mass within the cervix [60].

Anatomy of the Uterine Cervix

The cervix may be considered the neck of the uterus. The cervix consists of the *portio vaginalis*, that part consisting of the ectocervix and the transformation zone that protrudes into the vaginal vault, and the *portio supravaginalis*, which contains the endocervical canal. The latter is lined by columnar glandular epithelium that extends through a transformation zone (squamocolumnar junction) to squamous epithelium that covers the ectocervix. The cervix is separated from the uterine body by a narrow isthmus that broadens to form the muscular uterine body. The uterus and cervix are retained in the pelvis by a lattice of connective tissue through which course smooth muscle, nerves, and blood and lymph vessels. The paired uterosacral ligaments extend posterolaterally from the caudal portion of the uterus to pass along the rectouterine peritoneal folds to insert on the deep lateral aspect of the sacrum. The transverse cardinal ligaments originate at the upper, lateral portions of the cervix and insert into the fascia that covers the pelvic diaphragm laterally. Regional spread of cervical cancer through these structures can result in the presence of cancer significantly

posterior to the cervix. This fact must be taken into consideration when a four-field radiation technique is used [61]. The uterine corpus is attached to the lateral pelvic wall by the broad ligament and secured anterolaterally by the round ligaments. The broad ligament consists of a two-layered fold of peritoneum, sandwiching a layer of connective tissue termed the *parametria*, which extends from the lateral uterus to the pelvic sidewalls, with the fallopian tubes lying along the superior border of this structure. The round ligaments originate anterolaterally on the uterine fundus and course laterally and anteriorly over the pelvic brim to the internal inguinal ring, then pass through the canal to merge with the fascia of the labia majora. The rare cervical cancer metastasis to inguinal nodes in the absence of vaginal extension is believed to represent spread through lymphatic channels in the round ligaments.

The primary lymphatics of the cervix course through the parametria, which contain small lymphoid aggregates that may harbor secondary cancer deposits as an early manifestation of metastatic spread. Lymphatic drainage proceeds initially to the obturator nodes lying at the superior pole of the obturator foramen, and then to the internal iliac and external iliac nodes, which lie along the course of their associated named vessels. Subsequent lymphatic drainage is to the common iliac nodes and the para-aortic or aortocaval nodes, which lie in parallel with their associated blood vessels. Lymphatics of the uterine body may drain through the parametria to pelvic nodes, but portions of the uterine fundus, including the corneal areas, have draining lymphatics that course through the broad ligament to merge with the ovarian lymphatics running through the infundibulopelvic ligament and parallel to the ovarian vessels. Thus, metastases in right-sided para-aortic nodes, and metastases in left-sided para-aortic nodes or the left renal hilum, may be first-echelon nodes in women with cervical cancer extending to the uterine fundus. Yet, upper retroperitoneal nodes harbor metastases in the absence of concurrent or prior malignant pelvic lymph nodes. Para-aortic lymphatics coalesce at the cysterna chyli lying as high as the level of the 12th thoracic vertebra. Lymph flow progresses through the thoracic duct to empty most commonly in the left subclavian vein, accounting for metastases to the supraclavicular nodal chain. Appreciation of nodal chains by the treating physician meaningfully impacts design of radiation treatment portals and facilitates communication with surgeons and diagnostic radiologists.

In most females, the aorta bifurcates into the common iliac arteries at the 3rd to 4th vertebrae. Common iliac arteries bifurcate above the lumbosacral promontory in 87% of patients [61]. The internal iliac vessels run posteriorly in the pelvis, and the use of a four-field box technique for pelvic radiotherapy will hazard underdosing the associated nodes if the posterior border on the lateral fields is not positioned sufficiently behind the sacrum.

The lymphatics of the upper vagina drain through the cervical lymphatics. The rare, apparently discontinuous, spread of cervical cancer to the vagina is believed to represent retrograde lymphatic dissemination. In general, the radiotherapy target volume should include the full length of the vagina when cervical cancer extends caudally below the vaginal fornix to involve the vaginal wall. To ensure this, a vaginal fiducial could be implanted at the distal tip of the cervical cancer. As the distal half of the vagina has direct lymphatic drainage to the inguinofemoral nodes, radiotherapy portals must be adjusted to encompass inguinofemoral nodes when cervical cancer extends to the distal vagina.

The arterial supply of the uterus is from the uterine arteries, which are branches of the internal iliac arteries. The uterine arteries run through the broad ligament to cross the ureters at points just above and slightly lateral to the vaginal fornix within the medial parametria. These arteries shortly thereafter branch into small arteries supplying the vagina, uterine fundus, fallopian tubes, and small branches of the medial ovary.

On each side of the cervix, the point at which the uterine artery and ureter cross is designated 'point A' and is arbitrarily assigned to lie 2 cm lateral to a point 2 cm cephalad to the cervical os, measured along the axis of the endocervical canal (i.e., parallel to the uterine tandem). The right point A and left point A have been the prescription points for intracavitary brachytherapy. Dose to these points are labeled medial parametrial dose or 'para-central dose.'

The point at the pelvic sidewall (or, internal iliac lymph nodes) is designated 'point B' and is arbitrarily positioned to lie 5 cm lateral to a point 2 cm cephalad to the cervical os, measured from the mid-sacrum meridian.

Molecular Biology of Uterine Cervix Cancers

To sharpen thinking about cervical cancer, a discussion of the molecular biology of HPV is needed. HPVs are non-enveloped, double-stranded closed circular DNA viruses proliferating in the cutaneous and mucosal epithelium of the female and the male anogenital tract [62]. The circular HPV genome is organized into eight open-reading frames that encode six early proteins (E1, E2, E4–E7) and two late protein (L1, L2) [62]. When perturbed to increase viral copy number, HPV disrupt the host cell signals for cell cycle termination and hijacks host cell enzymes for DNA synthesis. First, HPV-E6 (a 150-amino acid protein) [63,64] binds p53 and shuttles it to its annihilation ubiquitin ligase E6AP, essentially lifting restrictions at the G1/S cell cycle checkpoint [65–67].

Also, HPV-E7 degrades hypophosphorylated RB proteins through a proteosome-dependent pathway [68], and thus, promotes unchecked E2F transcription factor activation [69]. E2F transcription factors turn on critical S-phase proteins for DNA replication. In effect, and after the activation of telomerase [70], HPV proteins allow unhindered DNA synthesis, viral DNA replication, and an increase in HPV-infected cell number. The consequences of HPV viral proteins overriding cell checkpoints include genomic instability and predisposition to neoplasia and oncogenic phenotypes [62].

Emerging evidence has identified that the consumption and renewal of $2'$-deoxyribonucleoside triphosphates (dNTPs) is a critical molecular pathway in cervical cancer (Figure 35.1) [71–76]. Two molecular pathways form dNTPs used for DNA synthesis and repair. The main pathway involves *de-novo* ribonucleotide reductase (RNR) enzyme reduction of intracellular ribonucleoside diphosphates to their corresponding deoxyribonucleosides [77, 78]. A complementary pathway recycles deoxynucleosides through deoxynucleoside kinases [79]. Cells synchronize the *de-novo* and salvage pathways such that dNTP supply matches dNTP demand, with disproportions in dNTP pools avoided because of resultant disruptive genotoxic stress [80].

RNR acts in cells as a rate-limiting heterotetrameric enzyme harboring two active site large subunits (M1) and two small catalytic subunits (M2 or p53R2 [M2b]) [77]. Protein M1 is a long-lived protein and can be found in all cell cycle phases [77]. A M1–M2 complex is tasked to reduce ribonucleotides during S-phase only, as it is abruptly dismantled in late mitosis due to a KEN-box sequence favoring proteosome-dependent elimination of M2 [81,82]. A M1–M2b complex has been detected in all cell cycle phases, and has been suggested to act as a DNA damage response protein, with both its transcription and activity regulated by p53 [81–83]. Sources of dNTPs after DNA-damaging insults such as ionizing radiation include ribonucleotide reduction through a M1–M2b-mediated process first, and subsequently through a M1–M2 mechanism [72,84]. HPV-E6, by degrading p53, allows RNR to generate dNTPs unchecked (Figure 35.1).

In the salvage dNTP pathway, deoxynucleoside kinases act as rate-limiting dNTP supply enzymes. These enzymes [TK1 and/or dCK in the cytosol, and thymidine kinase 2 (TK2) and deoxyguanosine kinase (dGK) in mitochondria; Figure 35.1] phosphorylate deoxyribonucleosides to produce deoxyribonucleoside monophosphates (dNMPs) [85]. TK1 is S-phase-specific through a mechanism similar to that of M2; the other three deoxynucleoside kinases are constitutively active across the cell cycle. Deoxynucleoside kinases are variably expressed in human normal and cancer tissues, with TK1 being elevated in cervical cancers [86]. The substrates of these salvage enzymes, deoxynucleosides, enter cells and

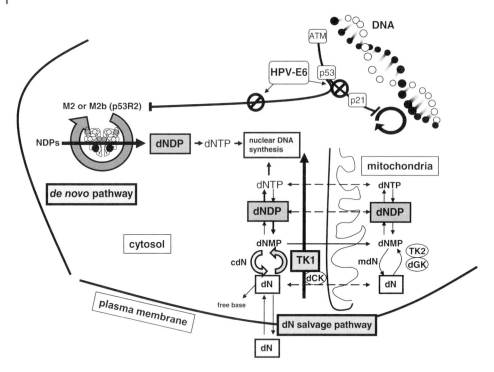

Figure 35.1 Cervical cancer molecular biology. Two biomolecular pathways generate 2′-deoxyribonucleoside diphosphates (dNDPs) used for DNA synthesis and DNA repair. The *de-novo* path utilizes ribonucleotide reductase (RNR) as the rate-limiting step. A M1–M2 complex reduces ribonucleotides during S-phase only, as it is abruptly dismantled in late mitosis due to a KEN-box sequence favoring proteosome-dependent elimination. A M1–M2b complex has been detected in all cell cycle phases and acts as a DNA damage response protein, with both its transcription and activity regulated by p53. A salvage deoxynucleoside (dN) path complements the *de-novo* generator, with deoxynucleoside kinases (e.g., thymidine kinase [TK1]) act as rate-limiting dNTP suppliers. TK1 happens to be S-phase-specific through a mechanism similar to that of M2. Levels of M2, M2b and TK1 become elevated after radiation and may be implicated in the facile repair of radiation-mediated DNA damage. Lastly, human papillomavirus (HPV) protein E6 disrupts p53, releasing the G1-S phase restriction point and allowing RNR M2b to freely associate with M1 to produce dNTPs. NDP, nucleoside diphosphate; dNTM, deoxynucleoside monophosphate; dNTP, deoxynucleoside triphosphate; ATM, ataxia-telangiectasia mutation protein

mitochondria passively by plasma membrane equilibrative nucleoside transporters [87]. TK1 levels become elevated after radiation and may be implicated in the facile repair of radiation-mediated DNA damage [88].

A better appreciation of the molecular signatures of cervical cancer provides sharper insight into the clinical behavior and anticipated response to therapy. An understanding of the interaction of radiochemotherapeutic interventions and the underlying biology of cervical cancer will become the rationale for targeted prevention, screening, and treatment.

Staging of Uterine Cervix Cancers

The extent of disease at diagnosis is a meaningful indicator of the efficacy of public health efforts in education and screening. Correction for clinical stage is important in the assessment of prognostic factors such as tumor histology, histopathologic indices such as semi-quantified protein immunohistochemistry or DNA gene microarray data, and immune competence. Clinical stage assignment prior to anticancer intervention permits the comparison of cancer control and treatment morbidity achieved by means of alternative therapeutic strategies, and aids in the international assessment of innovative surgical, chemotherapy, and radiation therapies.

The most widely accepted international staging system is that of the International Federation of Gynecology and Obstetrics, with the latest revision in 2009 [89]. The FIGO staging system (Table 35.2) permits the grouping of women with uterine cervix cancer worldwide based on local tumor extent prior to major therapeutic intervention. It must be recognized that cervical cancer is most prevalent among women in geographic regions associated with poverty, limited access to modern medical imaging, and communities that are economically constrained for providing medical resources. A staging system must describe its constituency, and must be useful in practical clinical settings; hence, high-technology modalities for the detection of disease are not well positioned to contribute elaborate staging systems and

Table 35.2 Carcinoma of the Uterine Cervix: FIGO staging* and TNM classification.

FIGO	TNM category			Description
Stage IA				Invasive cancers diagnosed by microscopy only
IA1	T1a1			Measured stromal invasion ≤3.0 mm in depth and extension of ≤7.0 mm
IA2	T1a2			Measured stromal invasion >3.0 mm in depth and extension of not >7.0 mm
Stage IB				Clinical visible lesions limited to the cervix
IB1	T1b1			Clinical visible lesion ≤4.0 cm in greatest dimension
IB2	T1b2			Clinical visible lesion >4.0 cm in greatest dimension
Stage II				Invasive cancers extending beyond the uterus, but not to the pelvic wall or the lower one-third of the vagina
IIA1	T2a1			Clinical visible lesion ≤4.0 cm in greatest dimension without parametrial invasion
IIA2	T2a2			Clinical visible lesion >4.0 cm in greatest dimension without parametrial invasion
IIB	T2b			Clinical visible lesion with obvious parametrial invasion
Stage III				Invasive cancer extends to the pelvic sidewall and/or lower one-third of the vagina and/or causes hydronephrosis
IIIA	T3A			Cancer involves the lower one-third of the vagina without extension to the pelvic sidewall
IIIB	T3B	N1		Cancer extends to pelvic sidewall and/or causes hydronephrosis and/or non-functioning kidney
Stage IV				Invasive cancer involves organs of pelvis or has spread outside the true pelvis
IVA	T4a			Cancer involves the mucosa of the bladder or rectum (bullous edema does not categorized lesion as IVA)
IVB			M1	Cancer spreads to distant organs

*International Federation of Gynecology and Obstetrics, 2009 [89].

treatment algorithms. It cannot be overemphasized that FIGO stage assignment does not provide sufficient information to predicate a course of treatment based all or in part on radiation therapy.

Imaging goals for women with cervical cancer include a better definition of local tumor invasiveness, its dissemination to lymph nodes, detection of hydronephrosis, and distant metastatic disease. Computed tomography (CT) uses low-dose ionizing radiation to detect differences in tissue density to generate anatomic images with a resolution of 5 mm. Hydronephrosis detected on CT can be used to classify stage IIIb cervical cancer disease. In contrast, magnetic resonance imaging (MRI) applies strong magnetic fields (no ionizing radiation) across cellular water in tissues such that uniform spin and then differential relaxation allows images with high soft-tissue contrast to be made. The ability of examination under anesthesia (EUA), CT and MRI to detect parametrial extension is low; findings indicated that the FIGO staging EUA had the highest specificity for parametrial tissue invasion by cervix cancer [90]. The sensitivity of CT or MRI to detect early-stage cervical cancer disease is 30–40% [91], but these techniques may not be useful for detecting lymphatic spread due to limits of nodal size criteria for CT and impractical back-to-back 1- to 2-h scanning times for MRI to evaluate pelvic and then para-aortic nodes.

Positron emission tomography (PET) relies on the coincident detection of gamma ray photons occurring from positron-emitting radioisotope decay. The most commonly used radioisotope is 2-deoxy-2-[^{18}F]fluoro-D-glucose ([^{18}F]-FDG), a molecule which is trapped in cells when hexokinase adds a phosphate to the glucose. [^{18}F]-FDG PET has been shown to be more effective in describing cervical cancer dissemination than CT through its portrayal of accurate whole-body images and its high specificity in advanced-stage disease [92, 93]. [^{18}F]-FDG PET has also become useful in the assessment of cervical cancer treatment [94–96] and the detection of asymptomatic relapses [97]. However, one wonders whether the [^{18}F]-FDG trap is sufficient to detect malignancy? Radiolabeled glucose may be metabolized through the glycolysis pathway, but also may be funneled to nucleoside biosynthesis or to fatty acid biosynthesis. This is the Warburg effect of glucose metabolism in cancer cells; sugar may not be just accumulated for 'energy' but rather used to make the building blocks for the next generation of cells. A new radioisotope for PET imaging is 3-deoxy-3-[^{18}F]fluorothymidine ([^{18}F]-FLT) [98]. This molecule may be a more important discriminator of proliferating malignant cells because cells that salvage deoxynucleosides to make DNA incorporate [^{18}F]-FLT readily. Here, TK1 adds three phosphates to the radiolabeled pyrimidine nucleoside, fluorothymidine. TK1 is restricted to the S-phase fraction of cancers, and is commonly interpreted loosely as a marker of proliferation. Note that TK1 rises after radiation treatment [88] and that the deoxynucleoside salvage pathway can be used in DNA repair after radiation or DNA-damaging chemotherapy [76]. Clinical investigations of [^{18}F]-FLT are currently under way.

Radiation Therapy for Uterine Cervix Cancers

Selection of Target Volume

The FIGO staging system (see Table 35.2) for cervical cancers recognizes the potential contributions of diagnostic imaging by allowing the results of chest radiography, skeletal radiography, excretory urography (intravenous pyelogram; IVP), and barium enema to be considered at the time of assignment to clinical stage. With the exception of the IVP, these assessments are most useful in defining disease extent for patients with very advanced cancer. While tumor size and presence and the level of lymph node metastases are acknowledged to be of prognostic importance, the FIGO staging system largely ignores these factors [99–101].

Except for the use of linear dimensions for stratification within stage IA and IB to serve as surrogates for primary tumor size, tumor volume is not considered in the FIGO system. The assessment of regional lymph node status is also largely irrelevant in the FIGO staging classification. However, these parameters may be of pivotal importance in making decisions for patients whose treatment will be radiation-based. Sophisticated contemporary imaging modalities demonstrate that verifiable regional and remote cancer spread substantially exceeds that of imaging modalities permitted in the FIGO staging formalism. Information gleaned from such studies should be integrated into clinical decision-making, but it should not alter clinical stage assignment. Nowadays, [^{18}F]-FDG PET results are not considered in the FIGO staging formalism, but [^{18}F]-FDG PET findings are being used to guide radiation therapy field design and implementation [102]. In addition, an American College of Surgeons Commission on Cancer studied the pretherapy diagnostic tools used to assess the spread of disease among 9338 women of known clinical stage determined between 1984 and 1990 [103]. The study identified a substantially greater than before utilization of CT and MRI technologies because of their high likelihood of informative findings due to cancer that balanced the key rejection of historically important FIGO staging procedures, including cystoscopy, proctoscopy, barium enema, excretory urography (IVP), bone scintography, and lymphangiography. An update from the American College of Radiology Imaging Network has concluded that there is a large gap between FIGO-recommended diagnostic tests and the actual tests used by physicians for cervical cancer staging. This signifies a call for the reassessment of FIGO guidelines for a more contemporary and relevant clinical practice in the US [104].

The FIGO clinical stage does not alone inform the treating physician regarding target volume, fractionation, total radiation dose, and brachytherapy dose distribution. Failure to include the entirety of disease is usually lethal. This mandates that sites of possible gross cancer involvement by direct extension (bladder, rectum, parametria, uterus, and suspensory ligaments) and by spread to regional pelvic nodes must be encompassed by radiation treatment fields. The risk of extrapelvic nodal spread must be carefully weighed against the relative toxicity hazard of extending the treatment volume to cover extrapelvic nodal sites. Defining target volumes becomes critical in an era of radiochemotherapy, especially when intensity-modulated radiation therapy (IMRT) is considered for postoperative [105, 106] and definitive [107, 108] treatment. Certainly, IMRT reduces acute and long-term gastrointestinal [109, 110] and hematological [111, 112] toxicity. It seems at first reckless to extend conventional pelvic fields to provide coverage of para-aortic nodes when the majority of stage IB2 to IIIB have uninvolved nodes; however, with the possibility of field-matching a four-field pelvic box and an IMRT para-aortic nodal field [113], women with confirmed para-aortic nodes or deemed to show sufficient clinical suspicion for para-aortic nodes may have next-echelon para-aortic nodes treated for curative intent. The long-term surveillance of relapse patterns after cisplatin radiochemotherapy has shown a steady rise in para-aortic nodal relapses when radiation is restricted to the pelvis, and cisplatin alone must be used to tackle occult para-aortic nodal disease [114]. Even in the new era of biologic plus cytotoxic radiochemotherapy, it may be unwise to confine radiation to a pelvic target volume when there is evidence of pelvic nodal metastases, and treatment of the next-echelon para-aortic nodes in an extended volume would be entirely consistent with radiotherapeutic custom and convention for primary cancers of other anatomic sites.

Surgical Assessment of Lymph Nodes Prior to Radiation

In many instances, relapses detected early after primary radiochemotherapy are related to undiagnosed, and thus undertreated, lymph node metastases [114–118]. Some would argue that the definition of nodal targets for radiotherapy (pelvic versus para-aortic extended-field radiation) may be most accurately accomplished by an extraperitoneal surgical assessment of retroperitoneal nodes [119]. While it appears that projectional imaging is being replaced by cross-sectional imaging such as CT and MRI [90], the contemporary use of routine extraperitoneal surgical staging prior to radiation therapy in patients with bulky or locally advanced disease remains controversial. Surgical cytoreduction may increase the probability of cancer control otherwise compromised by limited radiotherapy dose that can be prudently directed at grossly contaminated nodes [115–118, 120]. Supporters of surgical staging cite an ability to detect and then treat metastatic disease beyond typical radiation fields [115, 116]. It has been found that surgical lymphadenectomy provides superior informative data to guide subsequent radiotherapy than CT scans, with up to 40% of radiation portal treatment modifications occurring as a result [121,122]. Such concepts may in theory extend to a potential benefit of the removal of large nodal metastases beyond the ability of standard radiation doses to sterilize disease. Surgical assessment of retroperitoneal lymph nodes will upstage nearly 40% of those with stage IB to stage IIB disease [123]. Detractors of surgical staging claim that such staging may delay radiochemotherapy, and that only a small proportion of patients will benefit from extended-field radiation, basing these beliefs on the pretence that patients with advanced-stage disease die from local relapse, making distant control irrelevant [124, 125]. Yet, evidence identifies a survival advantage both in women with para-aortic lymph node metastases who receive radiation [126] and in women who receive prophylactic para-aortic radiation despite having negative or unevaluated para-aortic lymph nodes [127]. Balancing the advantages of nodal surgery and the disadvantages of delaying treatment initiation, as well as costs and the potential for surgical morbidity must be carefully weighed. It is hoped that the GOG-0233/ACRIN 6671 study will resolve some of these issues through the evaluation of preoperative [18F]-FDG PET/CT imaging in identifying metastases to retroperitoneal lymph nodes.

When feasible, the surgical assessment of retroperitoneal lymph nodes should be conducted through an extraperitoneal approach to reduce the subsequent hazard of bowel obstruction occasioned by adhesions and aggressive radiotherapy. Late bowel sequelae of radiochemotherapy can be lessened with an extraperitoneal approach. It is held that, with the exception of removal of clinically enlarged grossly contaminated nodes, the operative intervention should be understood as a primarily diagnostic procedure. Complete nodal stripping involving the extirpation of adventitia overlying major blood vessels only increases the risk of acute complications (e.g., bleeding, infection, lymphocele, deep-vein thrombosis) and late consequential leg lymphedema. The removal of a single para-aortic node (verified by intraoperative frozen section) will suffice to define the need for extended field radiation. A further dissection of clinically normal nodes typically included in radiotherapy fields is probably superfluous, and likely to increase the risk of adverse sequelae without a compensatory increase in treatment success.

Teletherapy

The design of radiation treatment portals is most effectively accomplished by integrating an understanding of normal anatomy with information concerning cancer extent in a particular patient. Morbid anatomy, distorted by the mass effects of tumor, reactive inflammation and scaring, intrauterine hemorrhage or infection, and adnexal pathology, may differ substantially from the normal anatomy (as illustrated in Refs [128, 129]). The radiation technique must be predicated on knowing where anatomic structures are as opposed to where they ought to be. Guidelines in reference texts should be understood to be only guidelines, not rigid formulations, and not a substitute for an intimate knowledge of disease distribution in an individual patient. It is impossible to overstate the concept that there exist no such entities as 'standard' radiation treatment volumes, 'standard' portal design, or 'standard' field sizes. To assert otherwise is the intellectual equivalent of arguing that one size and style of shoe will fit all feet [130].

The most common arrangement of external beam radiation portals is anterior, posterior and opposed lateral ports to deliver 4500 cGy in 25 divided daily fractions of 180 cGy (commonly, five weeks of Monday through Friday therapy). The careful design of rectangular fields with secondary collimation will reduce the radiation dose and the risk of collateral injury to normal tissues. Sparing of the bowel anteriorly may be achieved in this way, but this comes at the price of more radiation dose delivered to the iliac wings (and bone marrow), skin, and subcutaneous tissue than would be accomplished with anteroposterior and posteroanterior opposed fields using high-energy beams. A four-field arrangement offers no superior treatment advantage in slim women, but will permit a reduction of maximal bowel dose for women with protuberant abdomens and for women needing an extended external beam treatment field.

Tailored four-field radiation portals allow the delivery of higher doses that can be achieved under the limitations imposed by anteroposterior and posteroanterior opposed fields. Nevertheless, a four-field technique increases the hazard of inadequately covering disease at the lateral margins of the fields [128–131]. Cervical cancer disease coverage may be accomplished with greater security by CT-based dosimetry planning paired with advanced imaging overlays (e.g., [18F]-FDG PET or MRI) [132, 133]. Portals designed to shield the posterior rectal wall and portions of the sacrum and coccyx will hazard marginal relapses in internal iliac lymph nodes, presacral nodes, and uterosacral ligaments [128, 129]. Anterior shielding may cause the under-dosage of external iliac nodes [131]. Treating slightly expanded pelvic volumes to assure adequate geographic coverage does not appear to augment late normal tissue sequelae compared to

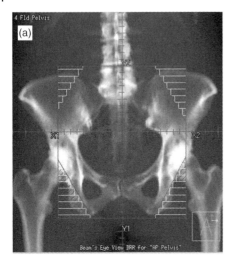
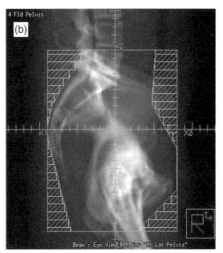
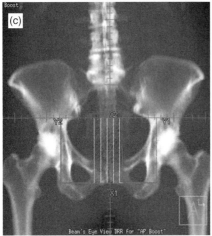
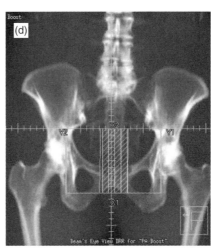

Figure 35.2 Pelvic radiotherapy for cervical cancer. (a,b) Anteroposterior and right lateral portal images for conventional four-field radiation are shown for treatment of the uterine cervix and pelvic lymph nodes. (c,d) Anteroposterior and posteroanterior portal images are depicted for two-field parametrial boost sparing the central portion of the bladder and rectum. Dose to tumor not covered by these fields is made up with intracavitary brachytherapy. For a color version of this figure, see the color plate section.

the treatment of traditional fields. Sample four-field external beam portals are illustrated in Figure 35.2.

The superior border of the four-field treatment will be set by the extent of nodal involvement as determined by surgery or non-invasive imaging. In the absence of radiopaque markers, the superior border of the fields may be set at the L4–L5 vertebral bodies if only nodes below the bifurcation of the common iliac arteries are to be included. The superior border may be positioned at the L2–L3 vertebral bodies if coverage of the common iliac nodes is to be assured.

The inferior border of the four-field treatment will be determined by the extent of vaginal wall invasion, occasionally marked by implanted fiducials. The bottom of the obturator space may serve as one landmark. With extension of disease limited to the proximal one-third of the vagina, a 3-cm margin of normal vagina distal to the tumor will suffice. When cancer extends to the mid-vagina, it is wise to cover the entire vaginal length, with the length marked by a fiducial at the time of simulation. Usually, the inguinofemoral lymph nodes are electively treated when the distal one-third of the vagina is involved

with disease. The infrequent patient will have one or more foci of discontinuous vaginal disease representing retrograde lymphatic spread of disease through the vaginal walls. Under these situations, the entire vagina must be treated. Some women will have an exuberant exophytic primary tumor, which extends to the distal vagina, but does not invade the vaginal wall. Here, the insertion of a radiopaque marker will aid in assuring adequate inferior margin. This technique is also useful when women have pelvic floor muscle relaxation and uterine prolapse.

The anterior and posterior fields will have lateral borders most accurately defined by body imaging, location of hemostatic clips placed at operation, or vascular/late filling images of a lymphangiogram. Along vertebral bodies, fields should be drawn to the tips of the transverse processes. In the pelvis, fields should be drawn such that field edges are 2 cm lateral to the inner edge of the bony pelvis at its maximal aperture. Low in the pelvis, field margins should shield the femoral heads and necks while including obturator lymph nodes that lie superior and lateral to the corners of the obturator foraminae. It is typically not feasible to shield the entire femoral head, since to do so would limit the margins of these nodes. When invasion of the lower one-third vagina is encountered, anterior fields are expanded to include the inguinofemoral nodes but employing a posterior field that does not. Compensatory dose to the inguinofemoral nodes may be delivered with small anterior photon or high-energy electron fields to lower dose delivered to the femoral necks.

For lateral fields, the anterior border will most accurately be determined by a combination of sagittal CT or MRI images. Fields must encompass external and internal iliac nodes as well as the uterus in the lateral projection. In women with direct invasion of tumor into the posterior bladder wall the bladder dome should be included. To ensure the coverage of external iliac nodes, it has been commonly held that a line drawn from the caudal border of the L4 vertebra extended to the apex of the pubic arch will mark the course of these nodes. Fields shielding bowel with at least a 2 cm margin displaced anteriorly will provide sufficient coverage. If the uterine fundus is not adequately encompassed by such an anterior border, then the field should be widened to do so at the expense of less bowel shielding. The posterior border of lateral fields should course behind the L4 vertebral body and should pass behind the sacrum and coccyx silhouette to assure inclusion of the internal iliac and presacral nodes as well as the posterior uterosacral ligaments where disease may creep. At the caudal extent of the posterior lateral portal, the field may be tapered (maintaining a minimum 2 cm margin on primary tumor) so that the buttock, a portion of the posterior rectum, anal canal, and intergluteal fold are shielded. Radiopaque markers may aid in this endeavor.

The reduced volumes of an anteroposterior and posteroanterior parametrial boost supplements dose delivered by brachytherapy while limiting midline dose to the rectum and bladder (see Figure 35.2). This is accomplished by reducing the superior border to 1 cm above the inferior aspect of the sacroiliac joint. The inferior and lateral borders remain the same as in the initial four-field field. A midline 4 cm block, customized relative to and accommodating dose from the brachytherapy implant, is carried through the entire center portion of the fields shielding the rectum and bladder. Note that such a beam arrangement does not dose the primary cervical tumor, but the primary cervical tumor will receive its full radiation dose at the time of brachytherapy.

In the clinical scenario, when an extended field is desired, a modification of the four-field technique may be utilized. The superior border is typically positioned at the top of the T12 vertebrae. The inferior border remains the same. The lateral margins of the anterior and posterior margin are drawn at the tips of the transverse processes of T12 through L5 vertebrae, with the caudal portion of the field the same. On lateral fields, the anterior border passes 3 cm anterior to the anterior edge of the T12 to L5 vertebrae and the posterior border passes through the mid-portion of the T12 to L5 vertebrae. Again, the caudal pelvic portion of the field remains the same. An updated technique for extended field radiation involves matching an intensity-modulated radiation therapy (IMRT) field to a four-field pelvic field arrangement. This is accomplished by setting up a four-field pelvis as described above, but rather than the isocenter being positioned in the pelvis it is raised to the L4/L5 vertebral interspace with the superior field edge closed (Figure 35.3). By creating a flat beam edge, an IMRT field can be matched at the L4/L5 interspace and extended to the top of T12. This is done in an effort to reduce late consequential gastrointestinal sequelae [110]. Such a pelvic plus IMRT field arrangement may become more commonplace in an era of testing doublet cytotoxic or doublet biologic–cytotoxic radiochemotherapy in advanced-stage cervical cancer.

Intensity-Modulated Radiation Therapy (IMRT)

To which patients IMRT should be offered remains debatable [105–108]. In practice, IMRT may replace all external beam teletherapy approaches performed for gynecologic cancer targets; however, the outcome data remain limited almost exclusively to postoperative pelvic radiation [134, 135]. IMRT is increasingly being used to treat cervical cancer and has the potential for an improved therapeutic ratio because of its ability to escalate the radiation dose while sparing any abutting healthy normal tissue [136]. Early reported series of women treated by cervical cancer have shown dosimetry and clinical benefits, with reduction in gastrointestinal and hematopoietic toxicity. Consensus indications for postoperative IMRT are emerging [106].

Although effective, IMRT has a number of practical limitations that must be recognized. Uncertainties in target volume definition when using IMRT techniques have been identified [137, 138]. Commonly, relatively large radiation portals are required to cover gynecologic cancer targets, and thereby may exceed the travel limits of IMRT multileaf collimators. In this situation, radiation portals are often split into two or more collimator carriage movements that dose subpopulations of tumor cells while simultaneously contributing additive scatter and leakage radiation dose to normal tissues [139]. Likewise, respiratory motion and differential filling of the bladder and rectum cause intrafraction and interfraction motion of pelvic cancer targets, obscuring fine delineation of radiation target volumes [140, 141]. Postoperative organ motion has a median range of 6 mm and a 95% confidence interval of 16 mm, perhaps attributed to shifting bladder and rectal volumes [142, 143]. Although priority is given to cancer targets, small volumes of the target should be allowed to receive below the prescription

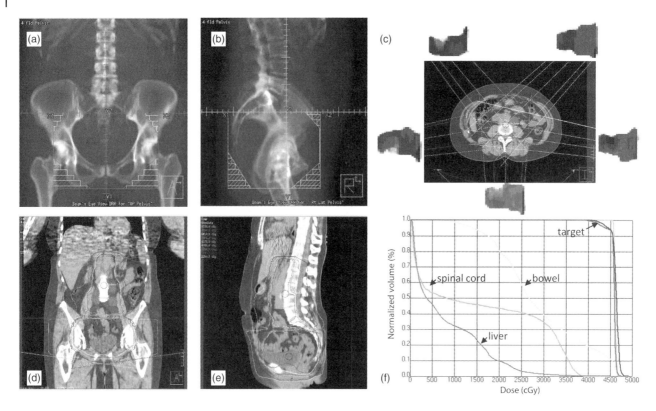

Figure 35.3 Extended field para-aortic intensity-modulated radiation therapy (IMRT) matched to four-field pelvic radiotherapy for cervical cancer. (a,b) Half-beam anteroposterior and right lateral portal images for four-field radiation are shown for treatment of the uterine cervix and pelvic lymph nodes. (c) A matched IMRT field is applied in five fields. Opening density matrices modeling the intensity of each control point are depicted for each beam. Coronal (d) and sagittal (e) dosimetry images for the composite pelvic plus IMRT para-aortic treatment fields. The heavy red contour identifies the 4500 cGy isodose line for which the daily prescription of 180 cGy was given for 25 divided fractions. (f) Dose–volume histogram plots for cancer targets and critical structures for this technique. For a color version of this figure, see the color plate section.

dose to account for motion, with a suggestion that ≥98% of the planning target volume (PTV) receives the prescription radiation dose [105]. Indeed, variation in organ position during IMRT can result in a marked transposition of cancer target volumes, ultimately exposing organs at-risk (e.g., small and large bowel) to higher than anticipated radiation doses. It is speculated that a daily repositioning of women prior to radiation delivery, using such devices as on-board cone beam CT, will adjust for organ motion [140]. Although IMRT treatment delivery is desired when the bladder is full and the rectal vault empty, women may be inconsistent in their pre-therapy water consumption for bladder filling, and in their pre-therapy defecation for evacuation of stool and bowel gas.

It is for these reasons that postoperative IMRT use for women with cervical cancer remains under scrutiny. Clinical trials for women with cervical cancer are slowly incorporating IMRT techniques because of their favorable gastrointestinal [109] and hematological [111] toxicity profiles. Indeed, considering the favorable normal tissue toxicity profile of IMRT, its use paired with additive cisplatin plus novel radiosensitizing biologic anticancer

chemotherapy is tantalizing. If the efficacy of IMRT is judged ultimately not to inferior with conventional four-field therapy [144], IMRT may become more commonplace in at least the postoperative setting, if not also in the definitive radiation setting. At present, IMRT remains an active area of research in cervical cancer management.

Brachytherapy

Low-Dose-Rate

As the cervix, uterine body, and upper vagina are tolerant of high radiation dose, this makes brachytherapy an ideal method for the management of cervical cancer, as sterilizing and permissible radiation doses can be delivered to cancer targets without undue injury to normal tissues. Endocavitary brachytherapy has a long and rich history [145] thanks in part to the pioneering studies of the Curies, who discovered the radioactivity of radium in 1898, and to Becquerel, who shortly afterwards noted skin erythema due to carrying radium in his waistcoat pocket. Brachytherapy for cervical cancer treatment was first performed in 1902. Impressively, Alexander

Graham Bell suggested the interstitial implantation of radioisotopes to treat cancers in 1903, and radium needle parametrial implantation was popularized during the 1940s. Since these early efforts, technology has become increasingly refined, now permitting elegant dose distributions to cancer targets based on cross-sectional CT or MRI imaging. Computer calculations rooted in sophisticated dosimetry algorithms now guide absorbed radiation dose delivery. Commercial CT and MRI brachytherapy devices are in routine clinical use, allowing the three-dimensional reconstruction of cancer and normal tissue volumes with the brachytherapy device *in situ* and limited device artifact.

Nowadays, a working knowledge of techniques and outcomes of low-dose-rate (LDR) brachytherapy utilizing 137-cesium (^{137}Cs) provides the context for modern brachytherapy [146]. Stereotypical LDR doses are expressed in milligram–hours, or the mathematical product of total number of milligrams radium or radium-equivalent ^{137}Cs and the duration of the implant in hours. The LDR dose is prescribed to point A, providing a reference standard against which new techniques should be compared for cancer control and late normal tissue sequelae. However, empiric prescriptions evolving in an era without sophisticated computational algorithms and cross-sectional imaging should not be viewed as immutable dogma. Brachytherapy allows the practitioner to selectively exploit radioisotope administration of a radiation dose higher to cancer targets than to adjacent normal tissue. The object is to create isodose lines that parallel and encompass cancer targets with high conformity.

Teletherapy is coordinated with one or two LDR tandem and ovoid insertions such that the total treatment time is 56 days. It has been estimated that for every day over 56 days, the chances for survival decrease by 0.6% per day, and for pelvic control fall by 0.7% per day [147]. Dose from brachytherapy is recorded at points A and B. However, it must be stressed that the single most important determinant of radiation dose is the gross tumor felt by the treating physician at time tandem and ovoid insertion, and not the projectional or cross-sectional imaging anatomy used in dosimetry algorithm computations of the radiation dose. Whilst brachytherapy cannot overdose the tumor, any vulnerable abutting normal tissue can be overdosed.

For this discussion, a Henschke tandem and ovoid applicator serves as one illustrative example of the procedure (Figure 35.4). Insertions are made at the time of an examination under anesthesia. With control of the cervix by single-tooth tenaculum, and after a Foley catheter has been positioned in the bladder (7 ml of saline or radiopaque solution), the cervix is dilated. The uterine cavity is sounded and measured. The keel of the tandem is locked 0.5–1.0 cm less than the measured length of the uterine cavity. The tandem is inserted into the uterine cavity through the cervical os. Two ovoid colpostats with intrinsic anterior and posterior shields (providing ~10% dose reduction to bladder and rectum) are locked to the tandem, such that the tandem bisects the colpostats. Using the largest of colpostats comfortably fitting in the vaginal canal causes the bladder and rectum to be physically displaced away from the radiation sources, and improves the homogeneity of brachytherapy dose delivery. Once placed, vaginal packing secures the brachytherapy device, but the practitioner is cautioned to not position packing above or below the colpostats. Typically, a composite teletherapy plus brachytherapy radiation dose limit of 7500 cGy may be delivered safely to the posterior bladder. Dose to the bladder may be tailored by the choice of intrauterine tandem curvature, with the more curved tandems delivering higher doses to the posterior bladder wall and bladder dome. Likewise, more-curved tandems will direct radiation away from the anterior rectal wall, which usually has a composite radiation dose limit of 7000 cGy. In this way, one or two tandem and ovoid insertions raise the dose to point A of 4000 cGy or more. When added to the typical 4500 cGy delivered by four-field teletherapy, cumulative doses to point A should be 8500 cGy.

Brachytherapy doses are recorded to several standardized points: Point A (2 cm superior and 2 cm lateral to the cervical os in the plane of the tandem); Point B (2 cm superior to the cervical os and 5 cm lateral to the mid-sacrum meridian); a bladder maximum (the most posterior point of the Foley balloon to the intrauterine tandem); a bladder average (the center of the Foley balloon); and a rectal point (the closest point between a rectal marker and the intrauterine tandem). How long an implant doses cancer targets is determined conventionally by the average of point A dose rate. A ratio for the assessment of favorable geometry may be calculated, and is one-half the arithmetic sum of right and left Point A dose rates divided by the higher of dose rate to the average bladder or rectum points. A favorable geometry has a ratio of 1.6 or higher. When cancer extends to the uterine cavity, the full length of the tandem will be dosed with the source that has the most activity. If a cervical cancer is exophytic and minimally involves parametria, the highest positions of the uterine tandem need not be loaded – a measure that will spare the small bowel and sigmoid colon from unnecessary radiation exposure. Orthodox weightings of brachytherapy sources are not employed, as strict conformality of isodose lines to identified cancer targets guides source deployment, which is often personalized for each woman. It is not uncommon to load a single 2-cm spacer followed by four 2-cm ^{137}Cs sources along the intrauterine tandem, paired with a single 2-cm ^{137}Cs source in the right and left colpostats to achieve adequate lateral dose distribution (Figure 35.4).

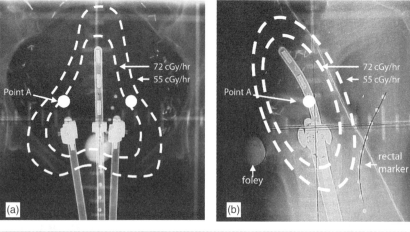

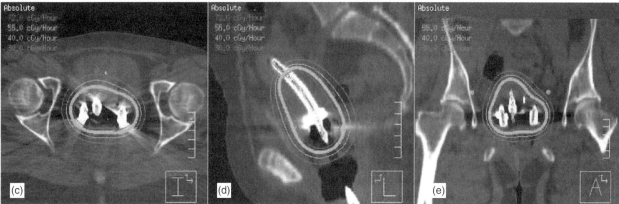

Figure 35.4 Intracavitary low-dose-rate brachytherapy for cervical cancer. (a,b) Anteroposterior and left lateral portal images are shown for a Henschke device low-dose-rate 137-cesium implant. Typical isodose contours are depicted with labeled dashed lines when five sources are loaded in the uterine tandem and one source is positioned in each ovoid colpostat. The point A prescription point is identified. (c–e) 3-D computed tomography dosimetry is shown for a low-dose-rate implant to deliver 4000 cGy, with a source not loaded in the first tandem position to spare bowel. Prescription point A (red circle) and point B (green circle) are shown for this implant dosing at a rate of 55 cGy h^{-1} (thick green line). For a color version of this figure, see the color plate section.

High-Dose-Rate

Robotic remote-afterloading technology using high-activity 192-iridium (^{192}Ir) has provided an opportunity to conduct outpatient high-dose-rate (HDR) brachytherapy for women with cervical cancer (Figure 35.5). For discussion here, a Henschke tandem and ovoid HDR applicator and its placement procedure are described, although various devices (e.g., tandem and ring) and techniques are acceptable. Women undergo five tandem and ovoid insertions, usually within the outpatient clinic. To facilitate outpatient service, a closed-sleeve, sutured button-sized temporary guide is placed pre-brachytherapy by the gynecologic oncologist within the cervical os and uterine canal. Sometimes the procedure is carried out in the operating room to allow for ultra-sound guidance for tandem placement when the cervical os is obstructed by tumor or when anatomic landmarks are obscured from treatment effect.

Five fractions of intrauterine HDR brachytherapy are integrated into the radiation course. The first brachytherapy insertion typically is done the third week of teletherapy and the final insertion is to coincide with the end of teletherapy treatment. Teletherapy treatments are not delivered on days when brachytherapy is given. As such, brachytherapy insertions are made usually on the fifth day of a weekly cycle (i.e., Friday of a Monday through Friday five-day schedule). When done in this way, teletherapy and brachytherapy are complete by day 56 (8 weeks), as is conventional practice. An alternate fractionation schedule is to complete all teletherapy treatments, and then perform twice-weekly HDR brachytherapy treatments (with 72 h between HDR insertions). This accomplishes brachytherapy delivery in $2^{1}/_{2}$ weeks so that all radiation dose is given by day 56. Usually, no interruptions in treatment are planned. The treating radiation oncologist must be aware that HDR

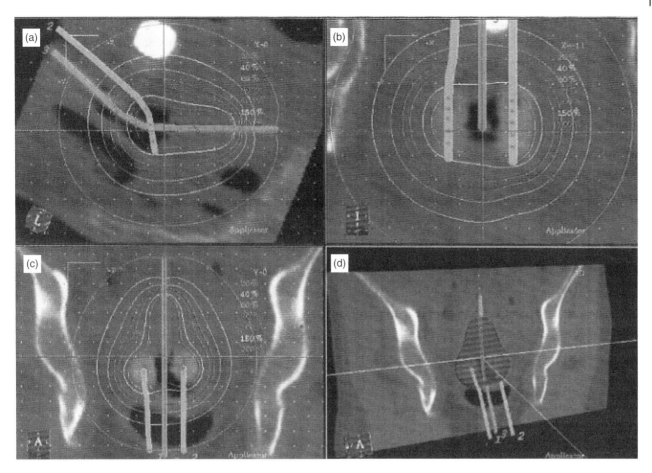

Figure 35.5 Intracavitary high-dose-rate brachytherapy for cervical cancer. (a–c) Cross-plane digital reconstructed radiographs obtained by computed tomography (CT)-based dosimetry planning are shown for a Henschke device high-dose-rate 192-iridium implant. Isodose contours are depicted after tailored dwell point dose calculations. (d) 3-D CT isodose contour (blue) for delivery of 600 cGy delivered for one of five fractions of brachytherapy. For a color version of this figure, see the color plate section.

may be associated with a more brisk cell-killing effect both in cancer targets and normal tissues, such that the therapeutic window of HDR brachytherapy is narrow. Relative to brachytherapy administered by ^{137}Cs LDR, ^{192}Ir HDR uses a 25% reduction in total brachytherapy dose to spare the bladder and rectum late consequential sequelae due to the higher dose rate effects. In analogous fashion to LDR brachytherapy, doses are recorded to points A and points B, but dose distribution is personalized based on physical examination and cross-plane imaging (preferably MRI, or CT). A recognized dose of 600 cGy for five fractions is prescribed, although up to 800 cGy for three fractions per fraction has been given [148]. Doses to the bladder and rectal points should not exceed 400 cGy per insertion, and generally no more than two fractions of 400 cGy are given to either organ at-risk during a series of five insertions. Customarily, total brachytherapy dose to the bladder and rectum do not exceed 1875 cGy if 4500 cGy is planned for teletherapy to the whole pelvis. The average dose to points A has been between 2600 cGy and 3500 cGy, but usually

this falls in a narrower range of 3000–3300 cGy. With this formalism, late radiation sequelae (14% at two years) have been higher than after conventional therapy [149] but not excessively so [150]. Because of the flexibility to tailor dose distribution made possible by the use of high-intensity, miniaturized sources with multiple dwell positions 5 mm apart, more favorable ratios of dose prescribed to points A to dose-limiting normal structures may be attained. A ratio of 1.75, as calculated for LDR brachytherapy above, is considered favorable.

Controversy continues to surround the issue of whether HDR brachytherapy is isoeffective with conventional LDR brachytherapy [149, 150]. When appropriate radiobiological corrections are applied and care is taken to exploit the ability to optimize HDR dose distribution, late consequential sequelae attributable to HDR are not encountered frequently [149] and do not appear appreciably different from those seen with LDR [151, 152]. Improved dose distributions appear to compensate for the inherent hazards to normal tissues posed by the increased dose rate. Adaptive brachytherapy utilizing shrinking volumes based on [^{18}F]-FDG imaging, assuming that hypermetabolic signal associates with active disease, limits normal tissue toxicity while maintaining ablative therapy to cancer targets [153, 154]. Clinical trials, such as the Australian and New Zealand Gynecologic Oncology Group (ANZGOG-0902) Phase III trial of radiochemotherapy and randomized adjuvant carboplatin/paclitaxel chemotherapy in node-negative cervical cancer, and RTOG 0724 studying radiochemotherapy plus adjuvant carboplatin/paclitaxel in node-positive cervical cancer, recognize both LDR (4000 cGy) and HDR (3000 cGy) as isoeffective brachytherapy techniques.

Pulse-Dose-Rate

A relatively new clinical brachytherapy technique involves pulse-dose-rate brachytherapy (PDR) utilizing a ^{192}Ir source. A basic tenet of brachytherapy is that, for a given dose, decreasing the dose rate (or increasing the number of fractions) will lower consequential late effects in normal tissue much more than reducing cancer target control [155]. When changing from continuous LDR to pulsed brachytherapy, it is the tissue with reduced repair times that will be relatively more damaged by the pulsed-radiation dose [156]. PDR brachytherapy is typically carried out with a miniaturized stepping source of 1 Ci of ^{192}Ir (37 GBq, 0.428 cGy h^{-1} at 1 m) or less, in contrast to HDR brachytherapy which utilizes a miniaturized source of 10 Ci (370 GBq) [157]. For PDR treatment, overall mean dose rates are 300 cGy h^{-1} if a 10-min pulse is given at one pulse every hour [157]. Larger cell-kill proportions in cancer and normal tissue are noted to occur for larger doses per pulse, so that keeping to small doses per pulse is a safer policy when concerned for normal tissue late consequential sequelae [157]. It is speculated that small pulses of brachytherapy synchronize cells at radiosensitive G1/S and G2/M phases of the cell cycle, and thus render cells more susceptible to the DNA-damaging effects of radiation

[155, 158]. This mechanism of radiosensitization is still under investigation.

Clinically, PDR has been used to treat cervical cancer [159–161]. PDR has been given in continuous hourly pulses of 55 cGy h^{-1} (range 40–70 cGy per hour) in one or two tandem and ovoid device insertions for a prescription of ~2475 cGy to Point A (45 h total around the clock treatment time) when given ~5040 cGy by teletherapy prior to brachytherapy [159, 160]. A median bladder point dose rate of 39 cGy h^{-1} and a median rectal point dose rate of 29 cGy h^{-1} were accepted [159, 160]. Compared to conventional progression-free rates (65%), PDR resulted in a 69% progression-free rate in women with stage IIIb-IVa cervical cancer [160]. Noted less than 30-day post-therapy complication rates were low, with five (7%) of 72 procedures [159] and three (6%) of 52 procedures [160] producing grade 3 or 4 sequelae. Long-term sequelae are not chronicled as of yet. Given that LDR ^{137}Cs sources expose attendant medical staff to radiation dose while at the bedside, and are more difficult to renew for higher-activity material, techniques using ^{192}Ir, which not only biologically mimic the efficacy of LDR ^{137}Cs without unnecessary exposure to attendant medical staff but are also more easily replaced, may become more commonplace with further study and experience.

Teletherapy Replacing Brachytherapy

On occasion, brachytherapy may be unfeasible due to an obliterated cervical os or uterus unable to accept a uterine brachytherapy device. In this situation, a reduced multiple teletherapy arrangement of beams may be used to dose-escalate cancer targets identified on cross-sectional imaging (preferably CT and MRI overlays). Daily fractionated doses of 180 cGy may be given for an additional 13 fractions for a total 2340 cGy. When added to the pelvic radiation dose (4500 cGy), a dose of 6840 cGy is recommended based on cumulative data (Table 35.3) [162–165]. Data for radiation alone in

Table 35.3 Central/pelvic relapses associated with radiotherapy method.

Study Stages	Reference		Incidence of central/pelvic relapse (%)	Significance
1st PoC Study stage III	[162]	External beam only	86	<0.001
		External beam plus Intracavitary brachytherapy	50	
University of North Carolina stage III	[163]	External beam only	40	0.6725
		External beam plus Intracavitary brachytherapy	32	
M.D. Anderson Cancer Center stage IIIB	[164]	External beam only	45	<0.001
		External beam plus Intracavitary brachytherapy	24	
Tokyo stage II–IV	[165]	External beam only	80	
		External beam plus Intracavitary brachytherapy	NR	
2nd PoC Study stage I–III	[166]	External beam only	53	<0.010
		External beam plus Intracavitary brachytherapy	22	

cervical cancer management shows that survival (67% at four years) and pelvic tumor control (78%) are better when teletherapy and brachytherapy are given together than survival (36% at four years) and pelvic tumor control (53%) when teletherapy alone is performed [166]. Two intracavitary LDR brachytherapy insertions were associated with higher survival (73% at four years) and pelvic tumor control (83%) compared to survival (60% at four years) and to pelvic tumor control (71%) after a single intracavitary application [166]. Dose escalation remains critical for pelvic control, but treatment results remain less optimal (Table 35.3) [162–166].

Treatment of Uterine Cervix Cancer by Stage

In the US, women with early-stage cervical cancer (*in situ*, stage IA and IB) may be managed by surgery, with controversy confined to the extent of the surgical procedure required to reliably affect cure while minimizing functional surgical sequelae. Women having advanced-stage cervical cancers (IIA to IVA) – those cancers invading pelvic tissues and organs rendering them not amenable to radical hysterectomy – are aggressive malignancies marked by higher rates of metastases and poorer disease-specific survival [167] than organ-confined cervical cancers [168]. Patients with bulky (>6 cm) cervical cancers treated weekly with cisplatin coadministered with daily radiation have lower rates of response (60%) [167] than patients with organ-confined (<6 cm) cervical cancer (90%) [169]. Cervical cancer disease that is unresponsive to standard-of-care cisplatin radiochemotherapy foreshadows a very poor prognosis, with median patient survival less than two years [169].

Evidence-based behavior for the treatment of women with uterine cervix cancer follows critical appraisal of quality surgery and radiochemotherapy clinical trial results, and applying it to a specific patient. For the purposes of this chapter, clinical efficacy is discussed relative to progression-free survival (PFS), a metric that directly measures the efficacy of initial therapy unaffected by life-prolonging treatment at disease progression. This metric often is defined as central/pelvic, regional nodal, para-aortic nodal, or extrapelvic distant relapse, as well as all-cause death measured from the date of enrollment/randomization to the date of first relapse or last censored follow-up. A drawback of this metric is that PFS often relies on clinical or imaging detection of disease relapse, both of which have subjectivity (i.e., erroneous declaration of disease progression) and influence of previous therapy (e.g., surgery, radiation, chemotherapy), influence of imaging technique, and influence of observe bias. Nevertheless, conceptual categories emerge regarding the efficacy of therapeutic intervention (Figure 35.6): (i) women whose disease is refractory to initial therapy; (ii) early progressors whose disease relapses

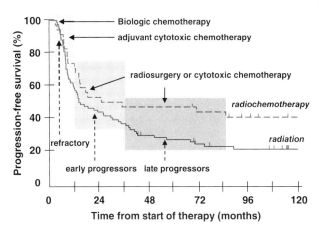

Figure 35.6 Simulated progression-free survival (PFS) in uterine cervix cancer. PPFS may be defined as central/pelvic, regional nodal, para-aortic nodal, or extrapelvic distant relapse, as well as all-cause death measured from date of enrollment/randomization to date of first relapse or last censored follow-up. Conceptual groupings emerge regarding therapeutic efficacy: (a) women whose disease is refractory to primary therapy; (b) early progressors whose disease relapses 12–36 months after initial therapy; and (c) late progressors whose disease relapses more than 36 months after initial therapy. Opportunities for biologic and cytotoxic chemotherapy as well as stereotactic body radiosurgery are indicated.

12–36 months after initial therapy; and (iii) late progressors whose disease relapses more than 36 months after initial therapy. Opportunities for targeted biologic chemotherapy, cytotoxic chemotherapy and radiotherapeutic intervention are noted and mentioned throughout this chapter (Figure 35.6).

In-situ Carcinoma and Stage IA-IB1 Uterine Cervix Cancer
In situ, stage IA, and stage IB1 diseases are managed by surgery, with PFS rates in population-based databases of 98% [170]. Patients with small-volume cervical cancer disease are unlikely to harbor occult nodal metastases (12/1127; 1%) [171], and so extrafascial hysterectomy is highly likely to affect cure with minimal probability of complications. Selected patients desiring the conservation of reproductive integrity may be managed by cervical conization or radical trachelectomy, with central/pelvic relapses of about 3% when the initial tumors measured ≤2 cm [172,173].

Women having *in-situ*, stage IA and stage IB1 disease can also be treated with radiation alone [174,175]. Treatment may be successfully carried out with brachytherapy alone (8640–13 680 radium mg·h) for patients with *in-situ* or stage IA1 disease, with no relapses (0/41), and four relapses among women with stage IB (<1 cm) disease (4/93; 4%) [174]. Bulkier stage IB (>1 cm) disease treated by intracavitary brachytherapy alone was met with more central/pelvic relapse (3/17; 18%), perhaps due to a non-negligible risk of parametrial spread [174].

Complications arising from brachytherapy alone have been infrequent (grade 3: 3/151; 2%) [174].

Stage IB2 Uterine Cervix Cancer

Vigorous controversy surrounds surgical or radiotherapeutic treatment selection and interpretation of outcomes for women with stage IB2 cervical cancer. Alleged superior survival results for surgery will sometimes reflect case selection, in that women with small cancers may opt for surgery while women with larger cancers may be relegated to radiation due to perceptions of surgical complication risk. Practice finds that women surgically explored and found to have gross metastatic adenopathy may have radical surgery aborted and subsequently dropped from analyses of surgical outcome. The inclusion of such women in radiation outcome analyses will obscure the interpretation of therapeutic radiation intervention.

A prospective clinical trial of women with either stage IB or stage IIA ($n = 343$) was conducted in Milan (1986–1991), randomizing women to surgery ($n = 172$, class 3 radical abdominal hysterectomy) or pelvic radiation plus LDR brachytherapy ($n = 171$, median point A dose 7600 cGy) [176]. PFS estimates at five years were 80% for surgery and 82% for radiation among women with tumors 4 cm or less, and were 63% for surgery and 57% for radiation for women whose tumors measured more than 4 cm ($P > 0.05$). To interpret the results of this trial, it must be appreciated that postoperative radiation was offered to women with surgical stage IIA (TIIa), with less than 3 mm of uninvolved cervical stroma, with cut-through surgery, or with documented lymph node metastases. These criteria led to adjuvant radiation treatment in 62 (54%) of 114 women with tumors ≤4 cm, and 46 (84%) of 55 women with tumors ≥4 cm. Consequential late sequelae were encountered in 24% of women (15/62) after surgery, in 15% (25/171) after radiation, and in 29% (31/108) after surgery plus radiation.

Non-randomized studies also have guided the selection of women recommended to undergo surgery or to have radiation [177–179]. Consideration for radiation following inadvertent hysterectomy in the setting of invasive cancer may occur as a surprise finding in a woman operated on for benign pathology, such as uterine myomata, or have the true pathologic extent of the disease underestimated by cervical conization performed by cold-knife excision or a loop electrocautery excision procedure (LEEP). The misinterpretation of pathology results and failure to recognize positive surgical margins do occur. When careful study of the operative specimen reveals cancer invasion of ≤3 mm, and ≤7 mm horizontal spread without lymphovascular space invasion, the vast majority of patients can be followed without further intervention. Yet, depth of invasion in the outer fractional third of the cervix consistently has been associated with

nodal metastasis more than absolute millimeters [177]. Outer-third cervical cancer led to nodal positivity in 26% of women (60/227) in a large surgicopathological study conducted by the Gynecologic Oncology Group (GOG) [177]. Among women with stage IB and occult stage IIA disease, it appears that nodal positivity found at the time of surgery (even when combined with radiation) lowers by one-half the likelihood PFS at three years, as compared to women without nodal metastases [177–179].

A single randomized study has shown improved PFS with radiation after radical hysterectomy. Building on their previous experience [177], the GOG randomized 277 women to observation after radical hysterectomy ($n = 140$) or to pelvic radiation ($n = 137$; 4600–5040 cGy) [180, 181]. A reduced hazard of relapse or death was observed after radiation (ratio: 0.58, 90% CI 0.4–0.85; $P = 0.009$) [181]. The three-year PFS was higher among women undergoing radiation after surgery (88%) as compared to those only having surgery (72%). Adverse toxicities (grade 3 or higher) came to pass in nine women (7%) after radiation, and in three (2%) after surgery. Regardless of the merits of the radiation argument, the use of surgery alone has increased for women with lower-stage cervical cancer coincident with the increasing involvement of gynecologic oncologists in the management of these patients [130, 182].

For women with stage IB2 cervical cancer, surgery has been found to be the most common form of treatment, although survival rates after radiation and after surgery are equivalent [130]. Because pelvic relapse is uncommonly salvaged, particularly when lymph nodes were originally involved [183–185], adjuvant radiation has been used in an effort to lower the hazards of central/pelvic relapses of cervical cancer. The potential survival benefit attributed to radiation has not necessarily been apparent in case-controlled or matched-pair retrospective series [186]. Studies have identified high-risk factors for relapse (nodal metastasis, parametrial extension, and positive surgical margins) [187], and intermediate-risk factors for relapse (large tumor volume, outer-third stromal invasion, and lymphovascular space invasion) [180] are found frequently among women with stage IB2 cervical cancer. A retrospective study of 58 women with stage IB2 lesions treated with surgery found that, based on current risk factor criteria, 52% of women would require postoperative radiation and an additional 36% would require radiochemotherapy, leaving only 12% adequately treated with surgery alone [188].

In an effort to enhance central/pelvic control of cervical cancer disease and reduce distant extrapelvic metastases among women with stage IB2 cervical cancer expected to have substantial survivorship, investigators have sought to intensify therapy. Four strategies have emerged. Building on data from a retrospective series in 49 women [189], the Radiation Therapy Oncology

Group (RTOG) embarked on a randomized study of pelvic radiation alone (4000–5000 cGy) or extended para-aortic plus pelvic radiation (4400–4500 cGy), followed by brachytherapy (3000–4000 cGy) for 367 women with bulky stage IB or IIA and stage IIB cervical cancers (1979–1986) [127]. A lower cumulative incidence for first distant failure was observed in the para-aortic arm than the pelvic-only arm ($P = 0.053$), translating to a reduction in cumulative incidence of death due to cervical cancer at 10 years of 29% after para-aortic plus pelvic radiation, and 41% after pelvic-only radiation ($P = 0.01$) [127]. It has been argued that in bulky stage IB2 disease, and when radiation alone is planned, prophylactic para-aortic plus pelvic radiation should be used to lower the incidence of distant extrapelvic relapses and cancer-related death.

In 1999, the GOG released the results of a randomized clinical trial of cisplatin (40 mg m^{-2}, once weekly) radiochemotherapy (median point A dose of 7500 cGy pelvic radiation plus brachytherapy) and adjuvant hysterectomy compared with radiation and adjuvant hysterectomy for bulky stage IB cervical carcinoma (GOG #0123) [190]. The study is now updated [168, 169]. The six-year PFS among women with stage IB2 disease was 71% after radiochemotherapy plus hysterectomy, versus 60% after radiation plus hysterectomy (hazard ratio: 0.61, 95% CI 0.43–0.85, $P < 0.015$). Based on the mature results of a prior randomized trial (GOG #0071), investigators have suggested that the clinical benefit of post-radiation hysterectomy was doubtful, and radiochemotherapy should be adequate for women with bulky stage IB2 cervical cancers [191]. Combined data from GOG #0071 and #0123 suggest a cumulative 10-year risk of pelvis, cervix, or vagina relapse of 9% (16/175) after radiochemotherapy, versus 17% (50/289) after radiation alone [169]. The management of women with stage IB2 or 'barrel-shaped' cancer has become a source of conflict between radiation oncologists and gynecologic oncologists, possibly owing to rigid orthodoxy where none need exist. It is probably not helpful to surgically remove a cervix and uterus when radiochemotherapy has sterilized the disease. Neither is it sensible to leave *in situ* a cervix suspected of holding persistent cancer because adjunctive hysterectomy has not had a measurable impact on survival statistics.

Extrapolating from stage IIA to IVA cervical cancer clinical trials, radiochemotherapy has materialized as an initial therapeutic strategy for women with bulky barrel-shaped cervical cancers [192, 193]. Undeniably, community comprehensive cancer center networks are increasingly utilizing a radiochemotherapeutic approach for women with stage IB2 cervical cancer due to the more routine cooperation of radiation, gynecologic, and medical oncologists [15, 16]. If there has been substantial, objective shrinkage of tumor in response to radiochemotherapy, it is reasonable to complete treatment by brachytherapy. Cumulative doses are 7500–8500 cGy. Conversely, if minimal tumor shrinkage is achieved by radiation plus brachytherapy, it would seem prudent to proceed with an extrafascial hysterectomy.

In the postoperative setting, women undergoing radical hysterectomy for bulky stage IB2 disease may be counseled on radiochemotherapy if high-risk factors for relapse (nodal metastasis, parametrial extension, and positive surgical margins) are found [187]. The Southwest Oncology Group (SWOG), GOG, and RTOG all recruited women, whose operative findings included parametrial extension (pT2b), positive metastatic pelvic lymph nodes, and positive surgical margins, to a randomized study of adjuvant pelvic radiation versus adjuvant radiochemotherapy (two cycles of concurrent cisplatin plus 5-fluorouracil [5-FU]), followed by two additional cycles of cisplatin and 5-FU [187]. The four-year PFS was 80% after radiochemotherapy plus cisplatin/5-FU versus 63% after radiation alone (hazard ratio: 2.0, $P = 0.003$) [187]. Sites of first relapse for all women on the study were within the pelvis 9% (11/127) after radiochemotherapy, and 22% (25/116) after radiation alone [187]. This strategy should limit the hazards of surgical and radiochemotherapy to selected higher-risk patients who are most likely to benefit, and for whom potentially more complex therapy can be justified. Data fully characterizing cancer outcomes for women with stage IB2 disease are lacking.

Stage IIA–IVA Uterine Cervix Cancer

The management of women diagnosed with stage IIA to IVA cervical cancer is radiation-based. The role of surgery is limited. Extraperitoneal surgical assessment of regional nodes may assist in the planning of radiation portals [119, 194]. The rare patient with stage IVA disease presenting with vesicovaginal or rectovaginal fistula may be appropriately treated by exenterative surgery, often coordinated with radiation. Current interventions for women diagnosed with stage IIA to IVA cervical cancer focus upon radiochemotherapy, especially after the publication in 1999 of randomized trials showing the clinical benefit of adding cisplatin chemotherapy to daily radiation [195–197]. But why was the DNA-damaging cisplatin anticancer drug selected among various agents with activity in cervical cancer disease? In 1981, the GOG (#0026C) revealed results of a Phase II trial of cisplatin 50 mg m^{-2} administered once every three weeks, that showed a response rate of 50% in women with advanced or recurrent cancer who were naïve to chemotherapy, and a response rate of 17% in women who had cisplatin in their initial therapy ($P = 0.059$) [198]. In a similar patient population, the GOG (#0043) explored the use of dose-dense cisplatin 20 mg m^{-2} for five consecutive days repeated every 21 days, 50 mg m^{-2} once every 21 days, and 100 mg m^{-2} once every 21 days, and found response rates of 25%, 21%, and 31%, respectively [199]. A comparison of PFS among the regimens gave non-significant results, with median survivals of 3.9 months, 3.7 months, and 4.6 months, respectively [199]. In a Phase III clinical trial conducted by the GOG (#0077) in treatment-naïve, advanced-stage cervical cancer patients, response rates for analogs of cisplatin, carboplatin (15%) and iproplatin (11%), were inferior to those of the parent compound [200]. As such, most treating physicians have accepted cisplatin as the dominant compound in this setting. There is controversial interest of re-comparing the weekly dose (40 mg m^{-2}) [197] versus every 21-day (100 mg m^{-2}) [198] in modern radiochemotherapy settings. A Phase II trial has shown safety and efficacy of tri-weekly cisplatin (75 mg m^{-2}) doses delivered during radiation [286]. A Phase III clinical trial of tri-weekly administration of cisplatin in locally advanced cervical cancer (TACO) currently randomizes women with stage IB2, IIB, IIIB, or IVA cervical cancer to cisplatin during radiation given as six weekly doses (40 mg m^{-2}) versus three tri-weekly doses (75 mg m^{-2}).

The broadest effort to improve outcomes for women with stage IIA to IVA cervical cancer has been directed at the use of chemotherapy administered in a coordinated fashion with radiation. A radiochemotherapy approach avoids any delay in the initiation of radiation and avoids concerns of treatment-selected clonogen cross-resistant chemotherapy on the one hand or radiation on the other hand. Initially, oral hydroxyurea was known to impair ribonucleotide reductase [201–203], rendering G1-S-phase transition arrest and allowing cytotoxic synergism. Three-year disease-free survivals ranged from 25% to 60% after hydroxyurea radiochemotherapy, versus 10% to 55% after placebo plus radiation [204, 205]. Profound hematopoietic toxicity became dose-limiting. Between 1986 and 1990, the GOG and SWOG conducted a Phase III trial randomizing 368 eligible women to radiation with oral hydroxyurea versus radiation potentiated with cisplatin and 5-FU (GOG #0085) [196]. This study found a three-year PFS benefit conferred by cisplatin and 5-FU (60%) compared to hydroxyurea (50%) for stage IIB to IVA patients (hazard ratio: 0.79, 90% CI 0.62–0.99, $P = 0.033$). The next clinical trial (GOG #0120) randomized 526 eligible women to one of three radiochemotherapy regimens: daily pelvic radiation plus either weekly cisplatin (40 mg m^{-2}); or day 1 or day 29 cisplatin (50 mg m^{-2}) plus 96-h infusion of 5-FU (4 g) plus twice weekly oral hydroxyurea (2 g m^{-2}); or twice weekly oral hydroxyurea (3 g m^{-2}) [197]. At 30 months, radiochemotherapy by cisplatin (63%), by cisplatin + 5-FU, and hydroxyurea (62%), and by hydroxyurea (42%) resulted in differential PFSs. The relative risk of disease progression or death was 0.57 (95% CI 0.42–0.78, $P < 0.001$) for weekly cisplatin radiochemotherapy, and 0.55 (95% CI 0.40–0.75, $P < 0.001$) for cisplatin + 5-FU and hydroxyurea radiochemotherapy, as compared

to hydroxyurea radiochemotherapy. Thus, a weekly cisplatin radiochemotherapy strategy has been adopted widely because of its long-term durable outcome data [167].

Between 1990 and 1997, the RTOG carried out a Phase III trial randomizing 388 women with stage IIB to IVA cervical cancers (or IB to IIA cancers with a diameter of at least 5 cm or involvement of pelvic lymph nodes) to receive either 4500 cGy of pelvic plus para-aortic radiation ($n = 193$) or 4500 cGy of pelvic radiation ($n = 195$) plus two cycles of day 1 and day 22 cisplatin (75 mg m^{-2}) plus 5-FU (4 g over 96-h infusion) [195]. Women were then to receive one or two applications of LDR intracavitary brachytherapy (mean point A dose 8900 cGy), with a third cycle of chemotherapy planned for the second intracavitary procedure in the radiochemotherapy cohort. Long-term outcome data from RTOG #90-01 have been updated [114]. The eight-year PFS values were 61% for radiochemotherapy and 36% for pelvic plus para-aortic radiation, reducing the hazard for disease progression by 51% (HR 0.49, 95% CI 0.36–0.66, $P < 0.0001$). A remarkable statistic from the long-term analysis shows that para-aortic node relapse rose from 7% (95% CI 3–11%) at five years to 9% (95% CI 4–13%) at eight years after radiochemotherapy, compared to a flat 4% (95% CI 1–7%) rate at five and eight years after pelvic plus para-aortic radiation ($P = 0.15$). The investigators duly noted that radiochemotherapy did not eliminate the risk for late para-aortic nodal relapse. Consequential late effects of radiation were infrequent, with grade 3 or 4 toxicities, especially in the bowels, seen in 13% (24/191) after radiochemotherapy and in 10% (20/194) after pelvic plus para-aortic radiation at eight years [114]. In another study of pelvis plus para-aortic radiation, four-year PFS was not substantially different after pelvic radiation (50%) versus after pelvis plus para-aortic radiation (53%) [206]. On this trial, more para-aortic relapses occurred in the pelvis-only treatment arm.

Trends for reductions in first distant failures in women whose para-aortic lymph nodes have been irradiated enticed radiation oncologists to consider extending radiation portals to encompass para-aortic nodal basins. Patients most likely to benefit from extended volume radiation would seem to be the subset of women with evidence of pelvic or para-aortic metastasis, without evidence of hematogenous dissemination. Identification of this subset of patients may not be straightforward, but may be aided by radiotracer PET/CT imaging [92, 93, 194]. Cisplatin (50 mg m^{-2}) and 5-FU (1 g m^{-2} per day over 96-h infusion) coadministered with daily pelvis plus para-aortic radiation has been attempted, and deemed feasible in women with cervical cancer metastatic to para-aortic lymph nodes [207]. The three-year progression-free rate on GOG protocol #0125 was 34% for all enrollees, with grade 3 or grade 4 gastrointestinal (19%) and hematologic (15%) toxicities noted.

Table 35.4 Randomized cisplatin radiochemotherapy trials in cervical cancer.

Study Stages	Reference		3-year PFS (%)	Relative hazard of disease relapse or death	Significance
RTOG-9001	[195]	Extended-field radiation	40	0.48	<0.001
IIB-IVA		Pelvic radiation/5-fluorouracil infusion/cisplatin bolus	67		
GOG-0085	[196]	Pelvic radiation/oral hydroxyurea	57	0.79	0.033
IIB-IVA		Pelvic radiation/5-fluorouracil infusion/cisplatin bolus	67		
GOG-0120	[197]	Pelvic radiation/weekly cisplatin infusion	67	0.51	<0.001
IIB-IVA		Pelvic radiation/oral hydroxyurea	47		
		Pelvic radiation/5-fluorouracil/cisplatin bolus/oral hydroxyurea	64	0.57	
GOG-0123	[190]	Pelvic radiation/hysterectomy	74	0.54	<0.001
IB2		Pelvic radiation/weekly cisplatin infusion/hysterectomy	83		
GOG-0109	[187]	Radical hysterectomy/radiation/cisplatin/5-fluorouracil	63	0.50	0.003
IA2-IIA		Radical hysterectomy/radiation/cisplatin/5-fluorouracil + adjuvant 5-fluorouracil/cisplatin ×2 courses	80		
National Cancer Institute of Canada	[208]	Pelvic radiation	58	NR	0.42
IB-IVA		Pelvic radiation/cisplatin	62		
B9E-MC-JHQS	[210]	Pelvic radiation/weekly gemcitabine/weekly cisplatin	65	0.68	0.029
IIB-IVA		Pelvic radiation/weekly gemcitabine/weekly cisplatin + adjuvant gemcitabine/cisplatin q3week ×2 courses	74		

PFS, progression-free survival; NR, not reported.

A single clinical trial failed to show any advantage of adding cisplatin to radiation for women with stage IB to IVA cervical cancer (1991–1996) [208]. To be eligible for this Canadian study, women ($n = 253$) must have had tumors measuring ≥5 cm, parametrial or pelvic sidewall or pelvic visceral disease (TIIb–TIVa), or confirmed malignant pelvic lymph nodes. Women were randomized to pelvic radiation (4500 cGy, followed by a compacted schedule of LDR [3500 cGy], or medium-dose-rate [2700 cGy], or HDR [2400 cGy] brachytherapy), or to the same radiation plus once-weekly cisplatin (40 mg m^{-2}). Through a median follow-up of 82 months, non-significant differences in six-year PFS were 62% after radiochemotherapy and 58% after radiation [208]. The investigators reckoned that cisplatin added little to the radiotherapeutic effect because the median total treatment time on this study was 51 days [208], as compared to 58 days [195], 62 days [197], and 64 days [196] for other studies. Indeed, the clinical benefits of coadministered therapies can be exaggerated when primary radiation is suboptimal, and perhaps, the cisplatin administered during radiation therapy makes up for the subtle differences in technique and treatment delays. Criticisms of the Canadian study include the compact brachytherapy schedule (one to three treatments, all radiation recommended to be done in under 56 days), higher hemoglobin eligibility criterion (11 g dl^{-1} versus typical 10 g dl^{-1} [209]), relatively small analyzable sample size given larger statistical variance and confidence intervals, abdominal staging by CT only (versus lymphangiography or surgical staging in GOG and RTOG trials). All in all, the most compelling evidence for cervical cancer radiochemotherapy rests with cisplatin coadministered with daily radiation (Table 35.4).

Are we making progress? Since 2003 and after the widespread implementation of cisplatin radiochemotherapy for advanced-stage cervical cancer, worldwide mortality rates have remained flat (30%) [3]. Results from prospective evaluations of coadministered radiosensitizing chemotherapies during cisplatin radiochemotherapy are now coming to fruition. A randomized comparison of gemcitabine added to cisplatin radiochemotherapy plus adjuvant cisplatin and gemcitabine versus cisplatin radiochemotherapy has been reported [210]. Eligible treatment-naïve women (stage IIB to IVA) were assigned to once-weekly cisplatin (40 mg m^{-2}) plus gemcitabine (125 mg m^{-2}) for six weeks during pelvic radiation (5040 cGy), then brachytherapy (3000–3500 cGy to point A) followed by two adjuvant 21-day cycles of cisplatin (50 mg m^{-2}, day 1) plus gemcitabine (1 g m^{-2}, days 1 and 8). Alternatively, eligible women were assigned to once-weekly cisplatin (40 mg m^{-2}) and the same radiation. Three-year PFS values were 74% (95% CI 68–80%) after gemcitabine plus cisplatin radiochemotherapy, and 65% (95% CI 59–71%) after cisplatin radiochemotherapy. A significant reduced hazard for cervical cancer relapse or death of 32% (HR 0.68; 95% CI 0.49–0.95, $P = 0.023$) was observed. Controversy exists regarding a gemcitabine plus cisplatin radiochemotherapy clinical benefit, as treatment-related grade 3 or 4 gastrointestinal (diarrhea 18% versus 5%; emesis 8% versus 3%) and hematological (72% versus 24%) toxicities have been high [210]. In a GOG effort (GOG-9912), this regimen was deemed toxic [211]. Because two scientific questions were posed in the gemcitabine plus cisplatin radiochemotherapy trial – namely that of (i) adding a radiosensitizing chemotherapy with intrinsic and additive anticancer effect, and (ii) adjuvant gemcitabine plus cisplatin chemotherapy – it remains unclear whether the treatment in the study arm simply delayed relapse or cured more patients [212]. Also, no missing data describing how many women were lost to follow-up during the planned 48-month observation period. Phase I and phase II studies involving more-potent and less-toxic inhibitors of ribonucleotide reductase such as triapine hold promise [74, 288, 289].

A rationale for sequential neoadjuvant chemotherapy followed by radiation includes the potential to cytoreduce pelvic cancer, thus improving anatomy for brachytherapy and decreasing the number of clonogens requiring sterilization by radiation. Neoadjuvant chemotherapy is less likely to complicate or delay radiation completion once it has started, and neoadjuvant chemotherapy will address the problem of occult micrometastases without delay and without dilution of chemotherapy anticancer effect. Phase II studies of neoadjuvant chemotherapy for cervical cancer have been conducted [213–215], but Phase III testing of chemotherapy before surgery or radiation remains uniformly disappointing [216, 217]. In one Italian study the five-year PFS was improved with neoadjuvant chemotherapy then surgery (55%) as compared to radiation only (41%, median point A dose 7000 cGy) [216], although by modern standards the radiation dose employed was low. There has been no compensatory improvement in pelvic control with neoadjuvant chemotherapy [217], and this line of investigation has been largely abandoned. A single Phase III clinical trial (INTERLACE) currently randomizes 770 women with locally advanced cervical cancer to either weekly carboplatin and paclitaxel neoadjuvant chemotherapy for six weeks, followed by standard cisplatin radiochemotherapy or to standard cisplatin radiochemotherapy alone.

Stage IVB Uterine Cervix Cancer

For women with metastatic stage IVB cervical cancer, monotherapy has not achieved much clinical benefit (Table 35.5). Durable responses after monotherapy last

Table 35.5 Efficacy of anticancer agents in cervical cancer.

Study	Agent	Molecular target	Response rate (%)	Progression-free survival (months)	Significance	Reference
	Cyclophosphamide	DNA	15			
	Ifosfamide	DNA	22			
	Carboplatin	DNA	15			
	Cisplatin	DNA	23			
	Doxorubicin	DNA	17			
	Pemetrexed	Ribonucleotide reductase	15			
	Topotecan	Topoisomerase	19			
	Paclitaxel	Mitotic poison	17			
GOG-0110						[196]
	Cisplatin	DNA	18	3.2		
	Cisplatin/mitolactol	DNA/DNA	21	3.3	0.835	
	Cisplatin/ifosphamide	DNA/DNA	31	4.6	0.003	
GOG-0169						[197]
	Cisplatin	DNA	19	2.8		
	Cisplatin/paclitaxel	DNA/mitotic poison	36	4.8	<0.001	
GOG-0179						[198]
	Cisplatin	DNA	13	2.9		
	Cisplatin/topotecan	DNA/topoisomerase	27	4.6	0.014	
GOG-0204						[199]
	Cisplatin/paclitaxel	DNA/mitotic poison	29	5.8		
	Cisplatin/vinorelbine	DNA/mitotic poison	26	4.0	0.060	
	Cisplatin/gemcitabine	DNA/ribonucleotide reductase	22	4.7	0.040	
	Cisplatin/topotecan	DNA/topoisomerase	23	4.6	0.190	

only for a few weeks to a few months. Conversely, doublet therapies have been met with more clinical benefit, with survival measured in months [218–221]. Combinations of cisplatin plus paclitaxel (36%) [219] and cisplatin plus topotecan (26%) [220] have reasonable anticancer response rates (sum of partial plus complete responses). In Phase III testing, a trend in response, PFS and overall survival favors a paclitaxel and cisplatin doublet, with pre-existing morbidity and toxicity important in regimen selection [221]. Recently, a Gynecologic Oncology Group clinical trial #240 reported a Phase III two-by-two factorial designed clinical trial of cisplatin–paclitaxel versus paclitaxel–topotecan with or without anti-VEGF bevacizumab (15 mg kg^{-1} body weight) in women with metastatic, persistent, or recurrent uterine cervix cancer [287]. After a median follow-up of 21 months in 452 enrollees, either chemotherapy plus bevacizumab significantly lengthened overall survival (17 months versus 13.3 months, HR 0.71, 98% CI: 0.54–0.82, p = 0.004). Both, PFS (8.2 months versus 5.9 months; p = 0.002) and response rate (48% versus 36%; p = 0.008) favored chemotherapy plus bevacizumab. Adverse events attribute to bevacizumab effects included grade 2 or higher hypertension (25%), grade 3 or higher gastrointestinal or genitourinary fistula (6%), and grade 3 or higher thromboembolism (8%). Genitourinary or gastrointestinal bleeding was infrequent.

Special Circumstances for Radiotherapy in Uterine Cervix Cancer Management

Bleeding, Anemia, and the Need for Urgent Radiation

In an effort to secure hemostasis, a woman with massive hemorrhage may urge the radiation oncologist to initiate radiation precipitously to an arbitrarily selected tumor volume. Hasty selection of a high-dose-per-fraction volume may compromise the eventual completion of a carefully fractionated treatment course. Once absorbed, radiation dose cannot be forgiven. When bleeding slows, it is natural to credit this change to the radiation dose delivered; however, most cervical cancers bleed spontaneously and unpredictably, with reliable stimulants being manipulation with manual pelvic examination or instrument-guided cervical biopsy. It is the exceptional patient in whom bleeding cannot be slowed to non-life-threatening pace through intervention by superficial cauterization, vaginal packing with Monsel's solution (active ingredients: ferrous sulfate, sulfuring acid, nitric acid), and bed rest. The topical application of acetone causes a prompt cessation of bleeding from the ecto-cervix. In rare instances, when conservative measures cannot arrest bleeding, urgent radiation can be applied

using parallel-opposed anteroposterior and posteroanterior pelvic fields. Field margins, and thus beam edges, are unlikely to transect gross tumor. The risk of late normal tissue injury by use of high dose per fraction radiation is avoided when women are transitioned expediently over two or three days to normal radiation dose fractionation. In this way, up to 1080 Gy can be given within 36 h of starting radiation at 180 cGy for three daily fractions over two days, with each fraction separated by 6 h or more. Two daily doses of 400 cGy separated by 24 h achieves similar results.

Cancer of Cervical Stump

Cancer of the cervical stump following remote supracervical hysterectomy has become less frequent as that operation has declined in popularity. In the hands of the surgeon, cancer of the cervical stump can be treated by radical trachelectomy and lymphadenectomy when disease is confined to the upper vagina. Commonly, a woman presenting with cancer of the cervical stump will be elderly, and the potential advantage of surgery in the younger woman largely irrelevant. With more extensive disease, radiation is frequently curative but will require modifications in technique because of a lesser ability to achieve satisfactory lateral dose distribution to the parametria and suspensory ligaments due to the short tandem length. A decrease in brachytherapy dose and increase in teletherapy dose solves this technical problem. Radiochemotherapy by 'shrinking-field' techniques (i.e., targeting progressively smaller volumes of disease) provides effective therapy when brachytherapy cannot be achieved. Radiochemotherapy followed by trachelectomy may be a solution for women with bulky central disease and poor brachytherapy anatomy. It is important to realize that, following supracervical hysterectomy, the bowel may become situated much lower in the pelvis in the space usually occupied by the uterus. Not surprisingly, bowel complications are more common in patients in whom unfavorable brachytherapy geometry is found [222]. Stage-by-stage matching, women with cancer of the cervical stump have similar prognoses as those with an intact uterine anatomy [223, 224].

Metastatic Adenopathy at the Time of Hysterectomy

The controversial notion to perform completion hysterectomy in women who are found intraoperatively to have clinically apparent pelvic or para-aortic adenopathy is not settled. One option involves the completion of a modified radical hysterectomy, followed by adjuvant radiochemotherapy [28, 187]. Another option after open dialogue between the operating gynecologic oncologist and gynecologic radiation oncologist is to abort the planned surgical procedure and complete radiochemotherapy with the cervix and uterus intact. Matched-pair analyses [225] could discern no advantage to completion hysterectomy, noting a trend for improved local control with radiotherapy in this study. Women with early-stage cervical cancer and undergoing extirpation of grossly involved lymph nodes fare well, with only modest benefit of adjuvant radiation seen when given for ominous histopathological findings [226]. No consensus resolution exists for this debate; practice follows the biases of treating physicians.

Cervical Cancer During Pregnancy

Invasive cervical cancers may be detected in 1–1.5% of women who are pregnant. Management is contingent upon the clinical stage of disease at diagnosis, gestational age, and whether continuation of the pregnancy is desired. An initial evaluation of the disease may be tempered by a need to reduce the intensity of investigation to avoid injurious radiation exposure to the fetus engendered during medical testing. A former practice of transvaginal radiation to diminish bleeding from cervical cancer has been abandoned due to fetal exposure that may be leukemogenic. Treatment may be delayed until fetal maturity [227] (assessed biochemically and by ultrasound), with only rare instances of progression during observation [228]. A cervix obliterated by cancer will not dilate at term, and delivery will normally occur by cesarean section rather than vaginal delivery to avoid obstructed labor and tumor transplantation to site of episotomy [229]. Delivery by hysterectomy avoids these concerns. Stage-by-stage, pregnant women with cervical cancer fare equally well as non-gravid women [229,230]. Most American women are diagnosed at stage IA or stage IB, and will be amenable to surgical intervention alone, with a cure rate exceeding 90% [182,231]. For pregnant women with more advanced disease at diagnosis, irradiation in the first trimester of pregnancy inevitably results in fetal death and spontaneous abortion with expulsion of the products of conception. This may prove emotionally challenging for the patient and the treating radiation oncologist. Pretherapy surgical evacuation is preferred by some. New innovations in surgical application of the trachelectomy and chemotherapy prove more useful.

Cervical cancer detected in the second trimester has been managed by conization between the 12th and 20th weeks of pregnancy [232]. Pregnant women between the 13th and 24th weeks of pregnancy and having tumors ≤2 cm may undergo two-step surgical procedures including first lymphadenectomy, and if lymph node-negative, then trachelectomy by a vaginal approach with placement of cerclage [233,234]. Pregnant women with tumors ≥2 cm may undergo lymphadenectomy, followed by three to six cycles of chemotherapy

(e.g., carboplatin [area under the curve 6] and paclitaxel [175 mg m^{-2}]) up to the 34th–36th week of pregnancy may be given with caution [235]. The interval between chemotherapy and delivery (with delivery by cesarean section followed by radical hysterectomy being the preferred procedure) should not be shorter than three weeks, as the highest risk for fetal hematotoxicity when born within two weeks of the last chemotherapy administration [236].

Cervical cancer detected in the third trimester may indicate a desired pregnancy, and treatment may be delayed with observation and monitoring of tumor progression by means of ultrasound or MRI.

The accurate quantification of hazards in the delay of treatment is challenging. Delay of treatment may not incur major incremental risk of cancer-related death. Options for treatment must be weighed in the context of patient's desire for pregnancy, and of the patient's ethical and religious principles regarding the termination of pregnancy. Individualization of care is the appropriate rule for the management of pregnant women with cervical cancer.

Radiotherapy Late Effects

Following radiation therapy, the radiation oncologist should play a role in the recognition and management of normal tissue sequelae and cancer surveillance [237]. Recommended schedules for follow-up are arbitrary, but often meet the needs of management and surveillance when performed every three months for years 1 and 2, and every six months for years 3 to 5. Interval medical and sexual health histories are taken and complemented by physical examination, including pelvic examination. Post-therapy three-month PET/CT scans are obtained to assess treatment response [94,95]. Scans are not obtained typically in asymptomatic patients. Exfoliative cytology (Pap smears) may be obtained at the three-month and six-month evaluations, but often include statements regarding radiation-induced atypia, which creates confusion rather than the early detection of recurrent disease.

Sequelae of teletherapy and brachytherapy are designated early or late in reference to the time after all of the radiation dose has been delivered. For the purpose of this chapter, early adverse events occur 30 days or less from radiation dose administration, while late adverse events occur greater than 30 days from radiation dose delivery. Important to the treating physician is to identify critical tissues and organ systems at risk of radiation damage, approximate tolerance of tissues to radiation dose, and the radiation dose fraction size.

Early effects most commonly result from cell death in a large population of normally functioning cells. The skin overlying teletherapy targets can be visibly marked by reddening (erythema) and loss of hair (epilation) where the teletherapy beams enter the body. Erythema may progress to dry or moist skin breakdown or desquamation due to a loss of the actively proliferating basal layer of the epidermis which renews the overlying epithelium. Medical management for treatment-related skin desquamation includes non-metal-containing creams and emollients during treatment, and 1% silvadene cream after treatment. Discomfort resolves and healing occurs usually within two weeks after completion of radiation. Late skin fibrosis may produce a rough, leathery texture to the skin in the irradiated field, but occurs rarely. Pentoxifylline (Trental®; 400 mg by mouth three times daily) may be used to decrease blood viscosity by altering the erythrocyte membrane properties so that oxygen is delivered to injured tissues [238]. Hyperbaric oxygen as daily medical treatment of radiation-induced skin or mucosal injury accelerates cell renewal and healing, but is logistically complex (up to 12 weeks of daily fractionated therapy) and should be reserved for the failure of simpler management strategies [239].

In a similar respect to the skin, radiation injury to the epithelial strata of the vagina manifests as desquamation, ulceration, and fistula formation. Radiation-related vaginitis includes the spectrum of pale, atrophic vaginal mucosa to severe inflammation and necrosis. Pressure injury from vaginal packing at the time of brachytherapy will predispose women to vaginal adhesions and obliteration of the upper vagina. Functional sequelae of radiation vaginitis are better prevented than treated. As such, daily or every-other-day use of a vaginal dilator (10 min) immediately after treatment minimizes the risk of agglutination and obliteration of the vaginal canal. Bacteria-containing plain yogurt, applied topically to the vaginal mucosa by hand or by a vaginal dilator, soothes vaginal canal irritation, promotes healing, and replenishes pH-balancing lactobacilli [240]. Women who are not sexually active should use the dilator regularly to minimize vaginal narrowing and foreshortening, both contributing to perceived and actual dyspareunia. Indeed, adherers to vaginal dilation report more worry about their sex lives, or lack thereof, than non-adherers ($P = 0.047$) [241]. Moreover, after irradiation of the vaginal mucosa, the basal layers of cells may take months to regenerate the normal layered strata of the vagina. Estrogen given systemically does not reliably renew epithelial cells, nor does it mature stratified squamous epithelium; topical estrogen administration has proven to be the most effective delivery route for the prevention of mucosal atrophy [242, 243]. It has been recommended that estrogen therapy begin at 1 g applied topically and daily for three to six weeks, and then reduced in frequency to two or three times weekly as maintenance. Systemic absorption of estrogen may be sufficient to elicit breast tenderness in postmenopausal women.

Because of the cell renewal pattern of the bladder, rectum, and large and small bowel, these tissues are at risk of radiation-induced normal tissue damage when treating cervical cancer. Depletion of the basal layer diploid cells of the bladder epithelium slows a replenishment of overlying transitional cells. Since the latter are periodically sloughed off during urination, radiation cystitis ensues. Smoking during therapy may exacerbate cystitis [27]. Pyridium (which contains an orange dye) may lessen symptoms of painful micturition (dysuria). Hematuria after radiation is very uncommon, and so evaluations of other malignancies such as bladder cancer should be conducted. Sclerosing solutions or fulguration through a cystoscope, which often needs to be used with bladder injury, have not been reported [244]. Chronic radiation cystitis, bladder fibrosis, or reduced bladder capacity leading to frequent urination occur in 3% of radiation-treated patients at four years [244]. Chronic radiation cystitis mimics the symptoms of recurrent urinary tract infections, and if not recognized as such may lead to the ineffective prescription of antibiotic therapy [244]. The urothelium has as one of its constituent macromolecules, glyosaminoglycan, which protects the bladder wall from toxic substances excreted in the urine leaking past the transitional epithelium. When radiation-induced mucosal injury permits leakage, inflammation and hemorrhage result. Pentosan polysulfate sodium (Elmiron®), a macromolecular carbohydrate that chemically resembles natural glyosaminoglycans, is used to replenish depleted epithelial polysaccharides and render a therapeutic effect. The prescription is an oral dose of 100 mg three times daily for six weeks, and if effective it may be continued for another 12 weeks [245].

Renewable stem cells of the intestine are located in the crypts of Lieberkuhn. Within two to four days after the start of radiation, these cells may become depleted, and atrophy of the intestinal mucosa follows. The resulting inflammation (sigmoiditis or gastroenteritis) may lead to increased bowel motility or diarrhea in up to 30% of patients. It also may be rarely associated with severe bleeding and cramping pain. Symptoms of urgency and pain with defecation may require low-roughage diets and antispasmodic medications when less severe. In conventionally treated patients, those women with radiation-induced bowel complications not requiring operation may have vitamin B_{12} and bile acid malabsorption. Most late bowel complications manifest within two years after treatment [244]. Intermittent rectal bleeding due to small-vessel vascular damage in the epithelium can be treated with topical steroid enemas; diagnostic evaluations for other sources of bleeding should be conducted. Biopsy or fulguration should be avoided as fistulas could arise. Bowel stenosis or obstructions related to late tissue fibrosis will be highest in women undergoing pretherapy laparotomy (actuarial risk 14.5% at 10 years), as opposed to women who have undergone non-operative assessment (actuarial risk 3.7% at 10 years) [244]. The risk of bowel injury rises when women undergo extended field radiation, as compared to those women who undergo pelvic radiation alone [127]. When women acquire radiation-related enteric or rectovaginal fistulas, bypass surgeries of the intestine are needed to allow healing. As a general rule, extensive dissection of irradiated tissue should be avoided. Experienced surgeons, comfortable working in heavily irradiated tissue, should take an active role.

A lowering of circulating lymphocytes, granulocytes, platelets, and red blood cells can be seen with pelvic or with pelvic plus para-aortic radiation therapy. The stem cells of the bone marrow in an adult (estimated 25%) reside in the axial skeleton (vertebrae, ribs, and pelvis) [246, 247]. Hematopoietic growth factor-stimulating medicines may be given prior to radiation if chemotherapy precedes radiation treatment. However, caution is warranted for the coadministration of red cell growth factors due to a possible risk of cancer cell stimulation [248] and thromboembolism [249]. Granulocyte colony-stimulating factors have been administered with cisplatin radiochemotherapy, without undue injury [250].

Microfractures in the pelvic girdle are complications of pelvic radiation that are difficult to diagnose and manage. Symptoms of pain and findings on isotope bone scans mimic cancer relapse. Many fractures are asymptomatic, may appear in pelvic MRI in up to 89% of treated women without late consequential effect, and heal either without knowledge of their presence or without intervention [251]. The best imaging modalities are bone window CT or MRI. Such microfractures are often multiple and symmetrical. Findings on isotope bone scans may suggest insufficiency fracture rather than cancer when abnormal signals are confined to the radiation portal utilized for treatment. The irradiation of extended fields has been associated with insufficiency fractures in the lumbar vertebrae which sometimes are severe enough to lead to vertebral collapse [252]. Dietary and medical interventions aiding bone health are recommended.

Systemic hormone replacement therapy should be considered in all premenopausal women who have not had surgical displacement of at least one ovary away from the irradiated volume. Oophoropexy will not always result in viable endocrine function, and is associated with an accelerated rate of premature ovarian failure when ovaries are transposed out of the pelvis [253, 254]. Scatter dose to ovaries transposed outside the direct radiation beam may be sufficient to accelerate ovarian failure in 29% to 83% of women, depending on the volume irradiated [253, 254]. Oophoropexy is underused [255]. In women treated for cervical cancer where the uterus remains intact, hormonally responsive endometrial linings may persist despite brachytherapy [256, 257]. Unopposed estrogen may cause intrauterine bleeding, but if brachytherapy results in obliteration of the cervical os, a hematometra with cramping pain results and a hysterectomy may be needed for symptom relief. These symptoms may be adverted by treatment with progesterone three weeks prior to the commencement of estrogen/progesterone replacement therapy. Estrogen alone may be used in patients who have undergone hysterectomy, but combined hormone replacement therapy should be used in individuals with a history of endometriosis.

Sexual dysfunction following radiotherapy is common, and a result of complex psychosocial and physical factors [241, 258–260]. The diagnosis of cancer and anxieties concerning prognosis may precipitate depression and loss of libido. Loss of procreative capacity may have unpredictable consequences on sexual health and function. In some cultures, the perceived worth of a woman is inextricably linked to her procreative prowess, and general cultural background and religious convictions will be important in this regard. Loss of sexual confidence may precipitate physical change. Endocrine ablation and menopausal symptoms may convince some women that they have lost their sexual attractiveness. As some women may be aware that sexual contact may predispose to HPV transmission, concerns about the transmission of disease to their partner may diminish enthusiasm for intercourse. Psychological factors that may curtail opportunities for sexual enjoyment may compound consequential physical change. Decrease in vaginal length and caliber, as well as a loss of spontaneous lubrication, will lead to dyspareunia, and subsequent anticipatory pain may involuntarily contract the muscles of the pelvic floor. Alterations in coital positioning may alleviate some of these stressors, with the female-astride position serving to limit penetration and control vigor of the sexual encounter. Intercourse with the thighs adducted following penetration will serve to stimulate greater vaginal depth, allowing the male partner to perceive full penetration without female discomfort in the context of a foreshortened vaginal length. Open conversations between the patient, her sexual partner, and treating physicians both before and after therapy provide the best opportunity for counseling women with cervical cancer regarding sexual health in the survivorship period.

Future Directions for Radiochemotherapy

Radiosurgery

For women with cervical cancer, therapeutic gain from implantable interstitial and intracavitary brachytherapy arises from its highly conformal radiation dose

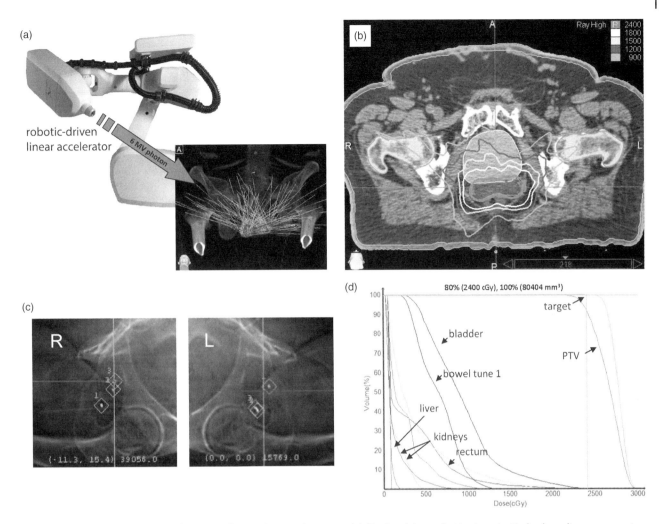

Figure 35.7 Stereotactic body radiosurgery for uterine cervix cancer. (a) Depicted is a robotic stereotactic body radiosurgery system (CyberKnife®; Accuray, Sunnyvale, CA). The robotic system increases freedom in the number and in the angle of non-coplanar treatment beam trajectories (blue vectors) to focus high-dose radiation on localized area(s) of disease. (b) Robotic systems have submillimeter accuracy such that highly conformal radiation dose plans sparing normal tissues from excessive radiation dose per fraction can be achieved. Pictured is a radiosurgery plan for a vaginal relapse of cervical cancer. (c) Orthogonal right (R) and left (L) fluoroscopic images taken by treatment room cameras allow on-board real-time tracking of implanted gold fiducials (green diamonds). (d) Dose–volume histograms indicate a high percentage of target coverage (light blue) while simultaneously distributing low radiation dose to critical organs (e.g., rectum, bladder, small bowel, liver, and kidneys). For a color version of this figure, see the color plate section.

permeation. Robotic stereotactic radiosurgery has been explored to deliver ablative radiosurgery doses of 2400 cGy in three divided daily doses of 800 cGy (biological effective dose nearly 6170 cGy [assuming an α/β ratio of 10]) to relapsed cervical cancer in a previously irradiated treatment field (Figure 35.7). The radiation emitted from a robotic stereotactic radiosurgery linear accelerator is collimated either by using one of 12 fixed tungsten circular collimators (5–60 mm) or by using a tungsten–copper alloy segmented hexagon IRIS collimator [261]. End-to-end phantom studies provide evidence that robotic radiosurgery systems can deliver radiation dose with sub-millimeter (0.4 mm) accuracy [262–264]. Preliminary cervical cancer-specific stereotactic

radiosurgery disease control rates are 95% (10/11) [265]. Only one (2%, 1/50) probable late stereotactic radiosurgery-related fistula has been identified through a median follow-up of 12 months.

Patients with metastatic gynecologic cancer have median survival times of 6–10 months [14]. Systemic interventions, usually implemented by chemotherapy, benefit only 10–15% of patients with metastatic disease, and even fewer patients experience durable benefits that affect survival. It is hoped that by radiosurgical targeting of metastatic disease not responding to chemotherapy, or occurring in previously irradiated tissues, it might be possible to render durable disease control. Whether stereotactic radiosurgery can be combined with chemotherapies to effect local and distant disease control simultaneously is an active area of research in clinical trials.

Biologic and Cytotoxic Chemotherapy

In 1999, a National Cancer Institute clinical alert advocated the use of cisplatin-based radiochemotherapy for the treatment of women with advanced-stage cervical cancer [266]. In women whose cancer persists after radiochemotherapy or whose cancer relapses, the use of chemotherapy remains challenging due to an often occurrence of obstructive uropathy and renal impairment which alters the excretion of chemotherapeutic agents. Chemotherapies that have some single- and double-agent activity are listed in Table 35.5. Cisplatin may be administered in patients with renal impairment at a 25% (for creatinine clearance [CC] = 46–60 ml min^{-1}) to 50% (for CC = 31–45 ml min^{-1}) dose reduction. Ifosfamide may also be given at a reduced dose (25–50% reduction for creatinine 2.1–3.0 mg dl^{-1} and held for creatinine >3.0 mg dl^{-1}). The kidney clears topotecan, and so a 50% dose reduction is administered for a CC of 30–40 ml min^{-1}. Dose-reduction guidelines for gemcitabine have not been developed.

Doublet cytotoxic or cytotoxic–biologic therapies have been met with more clinical benefit, often with survival measured in months rather than weeks [218–221]. GOG-0204 evaluated four randomized cisplatin doublet combinations (Table 35.5). Interim analyses after recruiting 513 patients suggest that novel therapeutics paired with cisplatin were no better than the reference arm of cisplatin plus paclitaxel [221]. PFS hazard ratios relative to the cisplatin plus paclitaxel control arm were 1.35 (CI: 0.97–1.90) for cisplatin plus vinorelbine, 1.43 (CI: 1.02–2.01) for cisplatin plus gemcitabine, and 1.28 (CI: 0.91–1.80) for cisplatin plus topotecan. Based on these findings, a Phase III trial testing the efficacy of cisplatin plus paclitaxel versus carboplatin plus paclitaxel is underway in Japan [267]. Non-cisplatin doublets have been studied in the recurrent disease setting due to anticipated cisplatin resistance occurring during primary radiochemotherapy. Topotecan plus paclitaxel, when given together, has a response rate of 54% and survival of 8.6 months [268]. Docetaxel plus gemcitabine achieved clinical benefit (complete + partial + stable disease patients) in 61% of patients (11/18) despite substantial treatment-related neutropenia eliminating day 8 gemcitabine in 41% of treated women [269].

The search for even more effective therapies now focuses on targeted biologic agents. Agents with anticancer activity against cervical cancer have ranged from ribonucleotide reductase inhibitors (RNRi), poly(adenosine diphosphate[ADP]-ribose) polymerase inhibitors (PARPi), Ras-Raf-MEK-ERK cascade inhibitors (MEKi),

aurora kinase inhibitors (AKi), and inhibitors of vascular endothelial growth factor (VEGFi). A brief discussion of each follows.

Ribonucleotide reductase (RNR) is pivotal to the cellular response to DNA damage [77]. Pharmacological blockade of either the M1 or M2 or M2b (p53R2) renders RNR inactive, with timing of the inhibitor and DNA damage important to prolonged DNA damage repair [72, 73]. Gemcitabine disrupts the catalytic subunit of M1 to impair DNA damage repair, and is useful against cervical cancer when paired with cisplatin [270, 271]. Hydroxyurea and 3-aminopyridine-2-carboxaldehyde thiosemicarbazone (3-AP) both quench the M2/M2b free radical, barring renewal of the M1 catalytic site during the ribonucleotide reduction reaction [72, 73]. Clofarabine as a purine nucleoside antimetabolite inhibits the RNR dATP active site. 5-FU obstructs thymidylate synthase, in due course upsetting the deoxyribonucleotide feedback ladder modulating the selectivity site of RNR. As cervical cancers express relatively high levels of RNR [73], a better knowledge of the interconnected cellular pathways regulating RNR activity will guide the selection of RNR is to contest purposeful ribonucleotide reduction for repair of chemotherapy-related DNA damage.

Of the 17 nuclear proteins in the PARP superfamily, PARP-1 and PARP-2 are generally recognized as tankyrase enzymes that are primarily involved in base-excision repair (BER) [272, 273]. The enzymatic activity of PARP-1 is enhanced 500-fold by its binding to DNA strand breaks; in the absence of such binding synthesis of poly(ADP-ribose) polymers (PAR) is negligible [274]. In knockout mouse models, 80–90% of PARP-dependent repair activity is significantly blocked with the deletion of PARP-1 [275]. Residual PARP-dependent repair is due to PARP-2 [272, 273]. Data suggest that only PARP-1/2 needs to be inhibited to impair BER [276]. The expression of PARP is twofold higher in cervical cancer cells, and its elevated level in cells is linked to cytotoxic drug resistance [277]. Further study is warranted.

The extracellular signal-regulated kinase (ERK) mitogen-activated protein (MAP) kinase cascade is integral to cancer cell proliferation and metastasis. Ionizing radiation rapidly activates a Ras-Raf-MAP/ERK kinase (MEK)-ERK pathway to promote cell survival [278]. The Ras-Raf-MEK-ERK cascade provides feed-forward protein–protein binding-partner regulation of RNR [279]. A new investigational agent AZD6244 (selumetinib) is a highly selective inhibitor of MEK1/2 in the Ras-Raf-MEK-ERK cascade by a drug–protein interaction not competitive with ATP [280]. Not only is there potential for enhanced cytotoxicity after a SBRT–AZD6244 combination, but there may be single-agent systemic activity of AZD6244 against cervical cancers which over-express MEK1/2 [281]. Further study of molecular crosstalk of Ras-Raf-MEK-ERK intermediates, and DNA damage responses in turn, will disclose possible clinical significances of an approach of MEK1/2 inhibition.

Chromosome assembly and packing occurring at the G2/M-phase transition renders cells susceptible not only to mitotic spindle poisons (e.g., paclitaxel) but also to processes involved in connecting mitotic spindle poles to kinetichores at the centromeres of each chromosome. These processes are regulated by Aurora A-C serine/threonine kinases (AKis), which are being studied for their anticancer properties [282].

The overexpression of VEGF has been associated with tumor progression and poor prognosis in cervical cancer patients. Bevacizumab is a human monoclonal antibody directed against the VEGF-A factor that stimulates endothelial cell mitogenesis and cell migration. It is thought that antibodies directed against VEGF bind the molecule so that the endothelial receptor remains unoccupied, endothelial growth is halted, and blood vessel permeability is stabilized [283]. GOG-0227 evaluated bevacizumab as monotherapy in 46 women with persistent or metastatic cervical cancer, and found a 10.9% partial response rate translating to a PFS benefit in 11 women (24%) [284]. A recent report of Radiation Therapy Oncology Group clinical trial 0417 provided Phase II clinical trial data on 49 women with stage IB-IIIB cervical cancer [285]. This trial evaluated three-cycle anti-VEGF bevacizumab (10 mg kg^{-1} body weight) added to cisplatin radiochemotherapy. The trial found no serious adverse events for the combination over a median follow-up of 12 months. Fourteen women (29%) had blood or bone marrow toxicity, but there were no grade 4 gastrointestinal adverse events. Three-year overall and disease-free survival estimates were 81% (95% CI: 67–90%) and 69% (95% CI: 54–80%), respectively. However, a 23% locoregional control failure rate was noted because six women had persistent cervix cancer at the 12-month post-therapy evaluation.

Summary

Recent data of teletherapy and brachytherapy in cervical cancers have provided a rationale for therapy targeting altered molecular pathways in disease, in an effort to induce significant tumor regression and sometimes to affect a durable anticancer response. Whether innovative radiation delivery systems complemented by novel biologic therapeutics can improve treatment response through enhanced radiochemosensitivity remains to be determined. Radiochemotherapy treatment selections perhaps are to be guided by tailored interrogations of cervical cancer tissue in the near future. Clinical trials of radiation coadministered with novel anticancer therapies should provide answers to the questions of whether or not this approach improves overall survival in comparison to other therapeutic regimens. The greatest challenge may be considered to lie in a better understanding of the molecular biology underlying cervical cancer cell resistance to therapy, and of the next steps that best combat this resistance.

References

1 Ferlay, J., Soerjomataram, I., Ervik, M., et al. GLOBOCAN 2012 v1.0, Cancer Incidence and Mortality Worldwide: IARC CancerBase No. 11 [Internet]. Lyon, France: International Agency for Research on Cancer; 2013. Available at: http://globocan.iarc.fr, Accessed November 10, 2014.

2 Siegel, R., Miller, K., Jemal, A. (2017) Cancer Statistics 2017. CA Cancer J. Clin., 67, 7–30.

3 American Cancer Society (2015) Cancer Facts & Figures 2015. American Cancer Society, Atlanta.

4 Papanicolaou, G. (1954) Atlas of Exfoliative Cytology. Commonwealth Fund, University Press, Boston, Massachusetts.

5 Guzick, D. (1978) Efficacy of screening for cervical cancer: A review. Am. J. Public Health, 68, 125–134.

6 Kashigarian, M., Dunn, J. (1970) The duration of intraepithelial and preclinical squamous cell carcinoma of the cervix. Am. J. Epidemiol., 92, 211–222.

7 Kolstad, P., Klem, V. (1976) Long-term follow-up of 1121 cases of carcinoma in situ. Obstet. Gynecol., 48, 125–129.

8 Kurman, R., Solomon, D. (1994) The Bethesda System for reporting cervical/vaginal cytologic diagnoses: Definitions, criteria, and explanatory notes for terminology and specimen adequacy. Springer-Verlag, New York.

9 Solomon, D., Davey, D., Kurman, R., et al. (2002) The 2001 Bethesda System. Terminology for reporting results of cervical cytology. JAMA, 287, 2114–2119.

10 Lazcano-Ponce, E., Palacio-Mejia, L., Allen-Leigh, B., et al. (2008) Decreasing cervical cancer mortality in Mexico: effect of Papanicolaou coverage, birthrate, and the importance of diagnostic validity of cytology. Cancer Epidemiol. Biomarkers Prev., 17 (10), 2808–2817.

11 Hoque, M., Hoque, E., Kader, S. (2008) Evaluation of cervical cancer screening program at a rural

community of South Africa. *East Afr. J. Public Health*, **5** (2), 111–116.

12 von Zuben, M., Derchain, S., Sarian, L., Westin, M., Thuler, L., Zeferino, L. (2007) The impact of a community intervention to improve cervical cancer screening uptake in the Amazon region of Brazil. *Sao Paulo Med. J.*, **125** (1), 42–45.

13 McLaughlin, C., Wyszewianski, L. (2002) Access to care: remembering old lessons. *Health Serv. Res.*, **37** (6), 1441–1443.

14 Waggoner, S.E. (2003) Cervical cancer. *Lancet*, **361** (9376), 2217–2225.

15 Kunos, C., Gibbons, H., Simpkins, F., Waggoner, S. (2008) Chemotherapy administration during pelvic radiation for cervical cancer patients aged ≥ 55 years in the SEER-Medicare population. *J. Oncol.*, **2008** (Article 931532), 1–7.

16 Kunos, C., Ferris, G., Waggoner, S. (2010) Implementing chemoradiation treatment for patients with cervical cancer in a comprehensive cancer center community oncology practice. *Commun. Oncol.*, 7, 446–450.

17 McAlearney, A., Song, P., Rhoda, D., *et al.* (2010) Ohio Appalachian women's perceptions of the cost of cervical cancer screening. *Cancer*, **116** (20), 4727–4734.

18 Plummer, M., Peto, J., Franceschi, S.; International Collaboration of Epidemiological Studies of Cervical Cancer (2011) Time since first sexual intercourse and the risk of cervical cancer. *Int. J. Cancer*, **130** (11), 2638–2644.

19 Lu, B., Viscidi, R., Lee, J., *et al.* (2011) Human papillomavirus (HPV) 6, 11, 16, and 18 seroprevalence is associated with sexual practice and age: results from the multinational HPV Infection in Men Study (HIM Study). *Cancer Epidemiol. Biomarkers Prev.*, **20** (5), 990–1002.

20 Svare, E., Kjaer, S., Worm, A, *et al.* (1998) Risk factors for HPV infection in women from sexually transmitted disease clinics: comparison between two areas with different cervical cancer incidence. *Int. J. Cancer*, **75** (1), 1–8.

21 Taylor, R., Carroll, B., Lloyd, J. (1959) Mortality among women in three Catholic religious orders with special references to cancer. *Cancer*, **12**, 1207–1225.

22 Reyes-Ortiz, C., Camacho, M., Amador, L., Velez, L., Ottenbacher, K., Markides, K. (2007) The impact of education and literacy on cancer screening among older Latin American and Caribbean adults. *Cancer Control*, **14** (4), 388–395.

23 McKinnon, B., Harper, S., Moore, S. (2011) Decomposing income-related inequality in cervical screening in 67 countries. *Int. J. Public Health*, **56** (2), 139–152.

24 Barzon, L., Militello, V., Pagni, S., *et al.* (2010) Distribution of human papillomavirus types in the anogenital tract of females and males. *J. Med. Virol.*, **82** (8), 1424–1430.

25 Munoz, N., Bosch, F.X., de Sanjose, S., *et al.* (2003) Epidemiologic classification of human papillomavirus types associated with cervical cancer. *N. Engl. J. Med.*, **348** (6), 518–527.

26 Lai, C., Chang, C., Huang, H. (2007) Role of human papillomavirus genotype in prognosis of early-stage cervical cancer undergoing primary surgery. *J. Clin. Oncol.*, **25** (24), 3628–3634.

27 Eifel, P., Jhingran, A., Bodurka, D., Levenback, C., Thames, H. (2002) Correlation of smoking history and other patient characteristics with major complications of pelvic radiation therapy for cervical cancer. *J. Clin. Oncol.*, **20**, 3651–3657.

28 Waggoner, S., Darcy, K., Fuhrman, B., *et al.* (2006) Association between cigarette smoking and prognosis in locally advanced cervical carcinoma treated with chemoradiation: a Gynecologic Oncology Group study. *Gynecol. Oncol.*, **103** (3), 853–858.

29 Patemoster, D., Cester, M., Resente, C., *et al.* (2008) Human papillomavirus infection and cervical intraepithelial neoplasia in transplanted patients. *Transplant Proc.*, **40** (6), 1877–1880.

30 Auborn, K., Woodworth, C., DiPaolo, J., Bradlow, H. (1990) The interaction between HPV infection and estrogen metabolism in cervical carcinogenesis. *Int. J. Cancer*, **49** (6), 867–869.

31 Elson, D., Riley, R., Lacey, A., Thordarson, G., Talamantes, F., Arbreit, J. (2000) Sensitivity of the cervical transformation zone to estrogen-induced squamous carcinogenesis. *Cancer Res.*, **60** (5), 1267–1275.

32 Fruchter, R., Maiman, M., Sedlis, A., Bartley, L., Camilien, L., Arrastia, C. (1996) Multiple recurrences of cervical intraepithelial neoplasia in women with the human immunodeficiency virus. *Obstet. Gynecol.*, **87**, 338–344.

33 Maiman, M., Fruchter, R., Clark, M., Arrastia, C., Mathews, R., Gates, E. (1997) Cervical cancer as an AIDS-defining illness. *Obstet. Gynecol.*, **89**, 76–80.

34 Cuzick, J., Clavel, C., Petry, K.-U., *et al.* (2006) Overview of the European and North American studies on HPV testing in primary cervical cancer screening. *Int. J. Cancer*, **119** (5), 1095–1101.

35 Mesher, D., Szarewski, A., Cadman, L., *et al.* (2010) Long-term follow-up of cervical disease in women screened by cytology and HPV testing: results from the HART study. *Br. J. Cancer*, **102** (9), 1405–1420.

36 American Society for Colposcopy and Cervical Pathology (2009) HPV genotyping clinical update. Available at: http://www.asccp.org/Consensus

Guidelines/HPVGenotypingClinicalUpdate/tabid/
5963/Default.aspx. Accessed September 11, 2011.

37 Dillner, J., Kjaer, S., *et al.*, the FUTURE I/II Study Group (2010) Four year efficacy of prophylactic human papillomavirus quadrivalent vaccine against low grade cervical, vulvar, and vaginal intraepithelial neoplasia and anogenital warts: randomised controlled trial. *Br. Med. J.*, **341**, c3493.

38 Castellsague, X., Munoz, N., Pitisuttithum, P., *et al.* (2011) End-of-study safety, immunogenicity, and efficacy of quadrivalent HPV (types 6, 11, 16, 18) recombinant vaccine in adult women 24–45 years of age. *Br. J. Cancer*, **105** (1), 28–37.

39 Brotherton, J., Fridman, M., May, C., Chappell, G., Saville, A., Gertig, D. (2011) Early effects of the HPV vaccination programme on cervical abnormalities in Victoria, Australia: an ecological study. *Lancet*, **377**, 2085–2092.

40 Kjaer, S., Sigurdsson, K., Iverson, O., *et al.* (2009) A pooled analysis of continued prophylactic efficacy of quadrivalent human papillomavirus (types 6/11/16/18) vaccine against high-grade cervical and external genital lesions. *Cancer Prev. Res.*, **2** (10), 868–878.

41 Ronco, G., Cuzick, J., Pierotti, P., *et al.* (2007) Accuracy of liquid based versus conventional cytology: overall results of new technologies for cervical cancer screening: a randomised controlled trial. *Br. Med. J.*, **335** (7609), 28

42 Arbyn, M., Bergeron, C., Klinkhamer, P., Martin-Hirsch, P., Siebers, A., Bulten, J. (2008) Liquid compared to cervical cytology: a systematic review and meta-analysis. *Obstet. Gynecol.*, **111**, 167–177.

43 Wells, M., Oster, A., Crum, C., *et al.* (2003) Epithelial tumors, in *World Health Organization Classification of Tumors: Pathology and Genetics of Tumors of the Breast and Female Genital Organs* (eds F. Tavassoli, P. Devilee), IARC Press, Lyon, France.

44 Kraus, F., Perez-Mesa, C. (1966) Verrucous carcinoma: Clinical and pathological study of 105 cases involving oral cavity, larynx, and genitalia. *Cancer*, **19**, 26–38.

45 Lucas, W., Benirschke, K., Lebherz, T. (1974) Verrucous carcinoma of the female genital tract. *J. Obstet. Gynecol.*, **119**, 435–440.

46 Hasumi, K., Sugano, H., Sakamoto, G., Masubuchi, K., Kubo, H. (1977) Circumscribed carcinoma of the uterine cervix with marked lymphocytic infiltration. *Cancer*, **39**, 2503–2507.

47 Eifel, P., Burke, T., Morris, M., Smith, T. (1995) Adenocarcinoma as an independent risk factor for disease recurrence in patients with stage IB cervical carcinoma. *Gynecol. Oncol.*, **59**, 38–44.

48 Eifel, P., Morris, M., Oswald, M., Wharton, J., Delclos, L. (1990) Adenocarcinoma of the uterine cervix:

Prognosis and patterns of failure in 367 cases. *Cancer*, **65**, 2507–2514.

49 Shingleton, H., Bell, M., Fremgen, A., *et al.* (1995) Is there really a difference in survival of women with squamous cell carcinoma, adenocarcinoma, and adenosquamous cell carcinoma of the cervix? *Cancer*, **76** (Suppl. 10), 1948–1955.

50 Samlal, R., van der Velden, J., Schilthuis, M., *et al.* (1997) Identification of high risk groups among node-positive patients with stage IB and IIA cervical carcinoma. *Gynecol. Oncol.*, **64**, 463–467.

51 Grigsby, P., Perez, C., Kuske, R., *et al.* (1988) Adenocarcinoma of the uterine cervix: Lack of evidence for a poor prognosis. *Radiother. Oncol.*, **12**, 289–296.

52 Herbst, A., Robboy, S., Scully, R., Poskanzer, D. (1974) Clear-cell adenocarcinoma of the vagina and cervix in girls: Analysis of 170 Registry cases. *Am. J. Obstet. Gynecol.*, **119**, 713–724.

53 Robboy, S., Szyfelbein, W., Goeliner, J., *et al.* (1981) Dysplasia and cytologic findings in 4,589 young women enrolled in diethylstibestrol-adenosis (DESAD) project. *Am. J. Obstet. Gynecol.*, **140** (5), 579–586.

54 Waggoner, S., Mittendorf, R., Biney, N., Anderson, D., Herbst, A. (1994) Influence of in utero diethylstilbestrol exposure on the prognosis and biologic behavior of vaginal clear-cell adenocarcinoma. *Gynecol. Oncol.*, **55** (2), 238–244.

55 Mulvaney, N., Monostori, S. (1997) Adenoma malignum of the cervix: a reappraisal. *Pathology*, **29**, 17–20.

56 Gilks, C., Young, R., Aguirre, P., DeLellis, R., Scully, R. (1989) Adenoma malignum (minimal deviation adenocarcinoma) of the uterine cervix. A clinicopathological and immunohistochemical analysis of 26 cases. *Am. J. Surg. Pathol.*, **13**, 717–729.

57 Glucksman, A., Cherry, C. (1956) Incidence, histology, and response to radiation of mixed carcinoma (adenocanthoma) of the uterine cervix. *Cancer*, **9**, 971–979.

58 Tamimi, H., Ek, M., Hesla, J., Cain, J., Figge, D., Greer, B. (1988) Glassy cell carcinoma of the cervix redefined. *Obstet. Gynecol.*, **71**, 837–841.

59 Lotocki, R., Krepart, G., Paraskevas, M., Vadas, G., Heywood, M., Fung Kee Fung, M. (1992) Glassy cell carcinoma of the cervix: A bimodal treatment strategy. *Gynecol. Oncol.*, **44**, 254–259.

60 Scott, M. (2011) The pathology of the cervix, in *Textbook of Gynaecology Oncology* (eds A. Ayhan, N. Reed, M. Gultekin, J. Dunn), Günes Publishing, Ankara, pp. 328–332.

61 Greer, B., Koh, W.-J., Figge, D., Russell, A., Cain, J., Tamimi, H. (1990) Gynecological radiotherapy fields

defined by intraoperative measurements. *Gynecol. Oncol.*, **38**, 421–424.

62 Hebner, C., Laimins, L. (2006) Human papillomaviruses: basic mechanisms and pathogenesis and oncogenicity. *Rev. Med. Virol.*, **16** (2), 83–97.

63 Cole, S., Danos, O. (1987) Nucleotide sequence and comparative analysis of the human papillomavirus type 18 genome: phylogeny of papillomaviruses and repeated structure of the E6 and E7 gene products. *J. Mol. Biol.*, **193** (4), 599–608.

64 Barbosa, M., Lowy, D., Schiller, J. (1989) Papillomavirus polypeptides E6 and E7 are zinc-binding proteins. *J. Virol.*, **63** (3), 1404–1407.

65 Werness, B., Levine, A., Howley, P. (1990) Association of human papillomavirus type 16 and 18 E6 proteins with p53. *Science*, **248** (4951), 76–79.

66 Scheffner, M., Werness, B., Huibregtse, J., Levine, A., Howley, P. (1990) The E6 oncoprotein encoded by human papillomavirus types 16 and 18 promotes the degradation of p53. *Cell*, **63** (6), 1129–1136.

67 Huibregtse, J., Scheffner, M., Howley, P. (1991) A cellular protein mediates association of p53 with the E6 oncoprotein of human papillomavirus types 16 or 18. *EMBO J.*, **10** (13), 4129–4135.

68 Gonzalez, S., Stremlau, M., He, X., Baile, J., Münger, K. (2001) Degradation of the retinoblastoma tumor suppressor by the human papillomavirus type 16 E7 oncoprotein is important for functional inactivation and is separable from proteosomal degradation of E7. *J. Virol.*, **75** (16), 7583–7591.

69 Huang, P., Patrick, D., Edwards, G., *et al.* (1993) Protein domains governing interactions between E2F, the retinoblastoma gene product, and human papillomavirus type 16 E7 protein. *Mol. Cell. Biol.*, **13** (2), 953–960.

70 Klingelhutz, A., Foster, S., McDougall, J. (1996) Telomerase activation by the E6 gene product of human papillomavirus type 16. *Nature*, **380** (6569), 79–82.

71 Kuo, M.-.L, Kinsella, T. (1998) Expression of ribonucleotide reductase after ionizing radiation in human cervical carcinoma cells. *Cancer Res.*, **58**, 2245–2252.

72 Kunos, C., Chiu, S., Pink, J., Kinsella, T. (2009) Modulating radiation resistance by inhibiting ribonucleotide reductase in cancers with virally or mutationally silenced p53 protein. *Radiation Res.*, **172** (6), 666–676.

73 Kunos, C., Radivoyevitch, T., Pink, J., *et al.* (2010) Ribonucleotide reductase inhibition enhances chemoradiosensitivity of human cervical cancers. *Radiation Res.*, **174** (5), 574–581.

74 Kunos, C., Waggoner, S., Von Gruenigen, V., *et al.* (2010) Phase I trial of intravenous 3-aminopyridine-2-carboxaldehyde thiosemicarbazone (3-AP, NSC #663249) in combination with pelvic radiation therapy and weekly cisplatin chemotherapy for locally advanced cervical cancer. *Clin. Cancer Res.*, **16** (4), 1298–1306.

75 Kunos, C., Colussi, V., Pink, J., Radivoyevitch, T., Oleinick, N. (2011) Radiosensitization of human cervical cancer cells by inhibiting ribonucleotide reductase: enhanced radiation response at low dose rates. *Int. J. Radiat. Oncol. Biol. Phys.*, **80** (4), 1198–1204.

76 Kunos, C., Ferris, G., Pyatka, N., Pink, J., Radivoyevitch, T. (2011) Deoxynucleoside salvage facilitates DNA repair during ribonucleotide reductase blockade in human cervical cancers. *Radiat. Res.*, **176**, 425–433.

77 Kolberg, M., Strand, K.R., Graff, P., Andersson, K.K. (2004) Structure, function, and mechanism of ribonucleotide reductases. *Biochim. Biophys. Acta*, **1699** (1-2), 1–34.

78 Hakansson, P., Hofer, A., Thelander, L. (2006) Regulation of mammalian ribonucleotide reduction and dNTP pools after DNA damage and in resting cells. *J. Biol. Chem.*, **281** (12), 7834–7841.

79 Sandrini, M., Piskur, J. (2005) Deoxyribonucleoside kinases: two enzyme families catalyze the same reaction. *Trends Biochem. Sci.*, **30** (5), 225–228.

80 Weinberg, G., Ullman, D., Martin, D., Jr (1981) Mutator phenotypes in mammalian cell mutants with distinct biochemical defects and abnormal deoxyribonucleoside triphosphate pools. *Proc. Natl Acad. Sci. USA*, **78** (4), 2447–2451.

81 Eriksson, S., Graslund, A., Skog, S., Thelander, L. (1984) Cell cycle-dependent regulation of mammalian ribonucleotide reductase. The S phase-correlated increase in subunit M2 is regulated by de novo protein synthesis. *J. Biol. Chem.*, **259**, 11695–11700.

82 Chabes, A., Thelander, L. (2000) Controlled protein degradation regulates ribonucleotide reductase activity in proliferating mammalian cells during the normal cell cycle and in response to DNA damage and replication blocks. *J. Biol. Chem.*, **275** (23), 17747–17753.

83 Tanaka, H., Arakawa, H., Yamaguchi, T., *et al.* (2000) A ribonucleotide reductase gene involved in a p53-dependent cell-cycle checkpoint for DNA damage. *Nature*, **404** (6773), 42–49.

84 Zhou, B., Liu, X., Mo, X., *et al.* (2003) The human ribonucleotide reductase subunit hRRM2 complements p53R2 in response to UV-induced DNA repair in cells with mutant p53. *Cancer Res.*, **63** (20), 6583–6594.

85 Eriksson, S., Munch-Petersen, B., Johansson, K., Eklund, H. (2002) Structure and function of cellular deoxyribonucleoside kinases. *Cell. Mol. Life Sci.*, **59** (8), 1327–1346.

86 Fujiwaki, R., Hata, K., Moriyama, M., *et al.* (2001) Clinical value of thymidine kinase in patients with cervical carcinoma. *Oncology*, **61** (1), 47–54.

87 Belt, J., Marina, N., Phelps, C., Crawford, C. (1993) Nucleoside transport in normal and neoplastic cells. *Adv. Enzyme Regul.*, **33**, 235–252.

88 Boothman, D., Davis, T., Sahijdak, W. (1994) Enhanced expression of thymidine kinase in human cells following ionizing radiation. *Int. J. Radiat. Oncol. Biol. Phys.*, **30**, 391–398.

89 FIGO Committee On Gynecologic Oncology (2009) Revised FIGO staging for carcinoma of the vulva, cervix, and endometrium. *Int. J. Gynecol. Obstet.*, **105**, 103–104.

90 Hricak, H., Gatsonis, C., Chi, D., *et al.* (2005) Role of imaging in pretreatment evaluation of early invasive cervical cancer: Results of the intergroup study American College of Radiology Imaging Network 6651-Gynecologic Oncology Group 183. *J. Clin. Oncol.*, **23**, 9329–9337.

91 Grigsby, P. (2011) Imaging in gynecologic oncology, in *Textbook of Gynaecological Oncology* (eds A. Ayhan, N. Reed, M. Gultekin, P. Dursun), Günes Publishing, Ankara, pp. 261–263.

92 Rose, P.G., Adler, L.P., Rodriguez, M., Faulhaber, P.F., Abdul-Karim, F.W., Miraldi, F. (1999) Positron emission tomography for evaluating para-aortic nodal metastasis in locally advanced cervical cancer before surgical staging: a surgicopathologic study. *J. Clin. Oncol.*, **17** (1), 41–45.

93 Grigsby, P., Siegel, B., Dehdashti, F. (2001) Lymph node staging by positron emission tomography in patients with carcinoma of the cervix. *J. Clin. Oncol.*, **19** (17), 3745–3749.

94 Schwartz, J., Grigsby, P., Dehdashti, F., Delbeke, D. (2009) The role of 18F-FDG PET in assessing therapy response in cancer of the cervix and ovaries. *J. Nucl. Med.*, **50** (5 Suppl.), 64S–73S.

95 Schwartz, J., Siegel, B., Dehdashti, F., Grigsby, P. (2007) Association of post-therapy positron emission tomography with tumor response and survival in cervical carcinoma. *JAMA*, **298** (19), 2289–2295.

96 Kunos, C., Radivoyevitch, T., Abdul-Karim, F., Faulhaber, P. (2011) 18F-fluoro-2-deoxy-d-glucose positron emission tomography standard uptake value as an indicator of cervical cancer chemoradiation therapeutic response. *Int. J. Gynecol. Oncol.*, **21** (6), 1117–1123.

97 Brooks, R., Rader, J., Dehdashti, F., *et al.* (2009) Surveillance FDG-PET detection of asymptomatic recurrences in patients with cervical cancer. *Gynecol. Oncol.*, **112**, 104–109.

98 Shields, A., Briston, D., Chandupatla, S., *et al.* (2005) A simplified analysis of [18F]3′-deoxy-3′-

fluorothymidine metabolism and retention. *Eur. J. Nucl. Med. Mol. Imaging*, **32** (11), 1269–1275.

99 Piver, M., Chung, W. (1975) Prognostic significance of cervical lesion size and pelvic node metastases in cervical cancer. *Obstet. Gynecol.*, **46** (5), 507–510.

100 Homesley, H., Raben, M., Blake, D., *et al.* (1980) Relationship of lesion size to survival in patients with stage 1b squamous cell carcinoma of the cervix uteri treated by radiation therapy. *Surg. Gynecol. Obstet.*, **150** (4), 529–531.

101 Perez, C., Grigsby, P., Nene, S., *et al.* (1992) Effect of tumor size on the prognosis of carcinoma of the uterine cervix treated with irradiation alone. *Cancer*, **69** (11), 2796–2806.

102 Kidd, E., Siegel, B., Dehdashti, F., *et al.* (2010) Clinical outcomes of definitive intensity-modulated radiation therapy with fluorodeoxyglucose-positron emission tomography simulation in patients with locally advanced cervical cancer. *Int. J. Radiat. Oncol. Biol. Phys.*, **77** (4), 1085–1091.

103 Russell, A., Shingleton, H., Jones, W., *et al.* (1996) Diagnostic assessments in patients with invasive cancer of the cervix: a national patterns of care study of the American College of Surgeons. *Gynecol. Oncol.*, **63** (2), 159–165.

104 Amendola, M., Hricak, H., Mitchell, D., *et al.* (2005) Utilization of diagnostic studies in the pretreatment evaluation of invasive cervical cancer in the United States: results of intergroup protocol ACRIN 6651/GOG 183. *J. Clin. Oncol.*, **23** (30), 7454–7459.

105 Mell, L., Roeske, J., Mehta, N., Mundt, A. (2005) Gynecologic Cancer: Overview, in *Intensity-Modulated Radiation Therapy: A Clinical Perspective* (eds A. Mundt, J. Roeske), B.C. Decker, Inc., London, pp. 492–505.

106 Small, W.J., Mell, L., Anderson, P., *et al.* (2008) Consensus guidelines for delineation of clinical target volume for intensity-modulated pelvic radiotherapy in postoperative treatment of endometrial and cervical cancer. *Int. J. Radiat. Oncol. Biol. Phys.*, **71** (2), 428–434.

107 Lim, K., Small, W.J., Portelance, L., *et al.* (2011) Consensus guidelines for delineation of clinical target volume for intensity-modulated pelvic radiotherapy for the definitive treatment of cervix cancer. *Int. J. Radiat. Oncol. Biol. Phys.*, **79** (2), 348–355.

108 Toita, T., Ohno, T., Kaneyasu, Y., *et al.* (2011) A consensus-based guideline defining clinical target volume for primary disease in external beam radiotherapy for intact uterine cervical cancer. *Jpn. J. Clin. Oncol.*, **41** (9), 1119–1126.

109 Portelance, L., Winter, K., Jhingran, A., *et al.* (2009) Post-operative pelvic intensity modulated radiation therapy (IMRT) with chemotherapy for patients with cervical carcinoma/RTOG 0418 phase II study. *Int. J.*

Radiat. Oncol. Biol. Phys., **75** (3), S640–S641 (abstract 3022).

110 Mundt, A., Mell, L., Roeske, J. (2003) Preliminary analysis of chronic gastrointestinal toxicity in gynecology patients treated with intensity-modulated whole pelvic radiation therapy. *Int. J. Radiat. Oncol. Biol. Phys.*, **56**, 1354–1360.

111 Klopp, A., Moughan, J., Portelance, L., *et al.* (2013) Hematologic toxicity in RTOG 0418: a phase 2 study of postoperative IMRT for gynecologic cancer. *Int. J. Radiat. Oncol. Biol. Phys.*, **86** (1), 83–90.

112 Brixey, C., Roeske, J., Lujan, A., Yamada, S., Rotmensch, J., Mundt, A. (2002) Impact of intensity-modulated radiotherapy on acute hematologic toxicity in women with gynecological malignancies. *Int. J. Radiat. Oncol. Biol. Phys.*, **54** (5), 1388–1396.

113 Salama, J., Mundt, A., Roeske, J., Mehta, N. (2006) Preliminary outcome and toxicity report of extended-field, intensity modulated radiation therapy for gynecologic malignancies. *Int. J. Radiat. Oncol. Biol. Phys.*, **65** (4), 1170–1176.

114 Eifel, P., Winter, K., Morris, M., *et al.* (2004) Pelvic irradiation with concurrent chemotherapy versus pelvic and para-aortic irradiation for high-risk cervical cancer: an update of radiation therapy oncology group trial (RTOG) 90-01. *J. Clin. Oncol.*, **22** (5), 872–880.

115 Potish, R., Downey, G., Adcock, L., Prem, K., Twiggs, L. (1989) The role of surgical debulking in cancer of the uterine cervix. *Int. J. Radiat. Oncol. Biol. Phys.*, **17** (5), 979–984.

116 Downey, G., Potish, R., Adcock, L., Prem, K., Twiggs, L. (1989) Pretreatment surgical staging in cervical carcinoma: therapeutic efficacy of pelvic lymph node resection. *Am. J. Obstet. Gynecol.*, **160** (5 Pt 1), 1055–1061.

117 Hacker, N., Wain, G., Nicklin, J. (1995) Resection of bulky positive lymph nodes in patients with cervical carcinoma. *Int. J. Gynecol. Cancer*, **5** (4), 250–256.

118 Odunsi, K., Lele, S., Gharmande, S., Seago, P., Driscoll, D. (2001) The impact of pre-therapy extraperitoneal surgical staging on the evaluation and treatment of patients with locally advanced cervical cancer. *Eur. J. Gynaecol. Oncol.*, **22** (5), 325–330.

119 Weiser, E., Bundy, B., Hoskins, W., *et al.* (1989) Extraperitoneal versus transperitoneal selective paraaortic lymphadenectomy in the pretreatment surgical staging of advanced cervical carcinoma (A Gynecologic Oncology Group Study). *Gynecol. Oncol.*, **33** (3), 283–289.

120 Inoue, T., Chihara, T., Morita, K. (1984) The prognostic significance of the size of the largest nodes in metastatic carcinoma of the uterine cervix. *Int. J. Radiat. Oncol. Biol. Phys.*, **19** (2), 187–193.

121 Goff, B., Muntz, H., Paley, P., Tamimi, H., Koh, W.-J., Greer, B. (1999) Impact of surgical staging in women with locally advanced cervical cancer. *Gynecol. Oncol.*, **74** (3), 436–442.

122 Berman, M., Lagasse, L., Ballon, S., Watring, W., Tesler, A. (1978) Modification of radiation therapy following operative evaluation of patients with cervical carcinoma. *Gynecol. Oncol.*, **6** (4), 328–332.

123 Marnitz, S., Köhler, C., Roth, C., Füller, J., Hinkelbein, W., Schneider, A. (2005) Is there a benefit of pretreatment laparoscopic transperitoneal surgical staging in patients with advanced cervical cancer? *Gynecol. Oncol.*, **99** (3), 536–544.

124 Kademian, M., Bosch, A. (1977) Is staging laparotomy in cervical cancer justifiable? *Int. J. Radiat. Oncol. Biol. Phys.*, **2** (11-12), 1235–1238.

125 Holcomb, K., Abulafia, O., Mathews, R., Gabbur, N., Lee, Y., Buhl, A. (1999) The impact of pretreatment staging laparotomy on survival in locally advanced cervical carcinoma. *Eur. J. Gynaecol. Oncol.*, **20** (2), 90–93.

126 Grigsby, P., Heydon, K., Mutch, D., Kim, R., Eifel, P. (2001) Long-term follow-up of RTOG 92-10: cervical cancer with positive para-aortic lymph nodes. *Int. J. Radiat. Oncol. Biol. Phys.*, **51** (4), 982–987.

127 Rotman, M., Pajak, T., Choi, K., *et al.* (1995) Prophylactic extended-field irradiation of para-aortic nodes in stages IIB and bulky IB and IIA cervical carcinomas. Ten year results of RTOG 79-20. *JAMA*, **274** (5), 387–393.

128 Russell, A., Walter, J., Anderson, M., Zukowski, C. (1992) Sagittal magnetic resonance imaging in the design of lateral radiation treatment portals for patients with locally advanced squamous cancer of the cervix. *Int. J. Radiat. Oncol. Biol. Phys.*, **23**, 449–455.

129 Kim, R., McGinnis, L., Spencer, S., Meredith, R., Jenelle, R., Salter, M. (1995) Conventional four-field pelvic radiotherapy technique without computed tomography – Treatment planning in cancer of the cervix: potential for geographic miss and its impact on pelvic control. *Int. J. Radiat. Oncol. Biol. Phys.*, **31**, 109–112.

130 Russell, A. (2000) Cervix, in *Clinical Radiation Oncology: Indications, Techniques, and Results* (ed. C. Wang), Wiley-Liss, New York, pp. 519–564.

131 Chun, M., Timmerman, R., Mayer, R., Ling, M., Sheldon, J., Fishman, E. (1994) Radiation therapy of external iliac lymph nodes with lateral pelvic portals: Identification of patients at risk for inadequate regional coverage. *Radiology*, **194**, 147–150.

132 Kruser, T., Bradley, K., Bentzen, S., *et al.* (2009) The impact of hybrid PET-CT scan on overall oncologic management, with a focus on radiotherapy planning: a prospective, blinded study. *Technol. Cancer Res. Treat.*, **8** (2), 149–158.

133 Thomas, L., Chacon, B., Kind, M., *et al.* (1997) Magnetic resonance imaging in the treatment planning of radiation therapy in carcinoma of the cervix treated with the four-field pelvic technique. *Int. J. Radiat. Oncol. Biol. Phys.*, **37** (4), 827–832.

134 Mundt, A., Lujan, A., Rotmensch, J., *et al.* (2002) Intensity-modulated whole pelvic radiotherapy in women with gynecologic malignancies. *Int. J. Radiat. Oncol. Biol. Phys.*, **52**, 1330–1337.

135 Mundt, A., Roeske, J., Lujan, A., *et al.* (2001) Initial clinical experience with intensity-modulated whole-pelvis radiation therapy in women with gynecologic malignancies. *Gynecol. Oncol.*, **82** (3), 456–463.

136 Loiselle, C., Koh, W. (2010) The emerging use of IMRT for treatment of cervical cancer. *J. Natl Compr. Cancer Network*, **8** (12), 1425–1434.

137 Weiss, E., Ruichter, S., Krauss, T., *et al.* (2003) Conformal radiotherapy planning of cervic carcinoma: differences in the delineation of the clinical target volume. A comparison between gynaecologic and radiation oncologists. *Radiother. Oncol.*, **67** (1), 87–95.

138 Han, Y., Shin, E., Huh, S., Lee, J., Park, W. (2006) Interfractional dose variation during intensity-modulated radiation therapy for cervical cancer assessed by weekly CT evaluation. *Int. J. Radiat. Oncol. Biol. Phys.*, **65** (2), 617–623.

139 Hong, L., Alektiar, K., Chui, C., *et al.* (2002) IMRT of large fields: Whole-abdomen irradiation. *Int. J. Radiat. Oncol. Biol. Phys.*, **54** (1), 278–289.

140 Tyagi, N., Lewis, J., Yashar, C., *et al.* (2011) Daily online cone beam computed tomography to assess interfraction motion in patients with intact cervical cancer. *Int. J. Radiat. Oncol. Biol. Phys.*, **80** (1), 272–280.

141 Hasselle, M., Rose, B., Kochanski, J., *et al.* (2011) Clinical outcome of intensity-modulated pelvic radiation therapy for carcinoma of the cervix. *Int. J. Radiat. Oncol. Biol. Phys.*, **80** (5), 436–446.

142 Jhingran, A., Salehpour, M., Sam, M., Levy, L., Eifel, P. (2012) Vaginal motion and bladder and rectal volumes during pelvic intensity-modulated radiation therapy after hysterectomy. *Int. J. Radiat. Oncol. Biol. Phys.*, **82** (1), 256–262.

143 Harris, E., Latifi, K., Rusthoven, C., Javedan, K., Forster, K. (2011) Assessment of organ motion in postoperative endometrial and cervical cancer patients treated with intensity-modulated radiation therapy. *Int. J. Radiat. Oncol. Biol. Phys.*, **81** (4), e645–e650.

144 Portelance, L., Radiation Therapy Oncology Group (2011) A phase II multi-institutional study of postoperative pelvic intensity-modulated radiation therapy (IMRT) with weekly cisplatin in patients with cervical carcinoma: Two year efficacy results of the RTOG 0418. *Int. J. Radiat. Oncol. Biol. Phys.*, **81** (2, Suppl.1), abstract #5.

145 Corscaden, J. (1956) *Gynecologic Cancer*. Williams & Wilkins, Baltimore.

146 Nag, S., Chao, C., Erickson, B., *et al.* (2002) The American Brachytherapy Society recommendations for low-dose-rate brachytherapy for carcinoma of the cervix. *Int. J. Radiat. Oncol. Biol. Phys.*, **52** (1), 33–48.

147 Petereit, D., Sakaria, J., Chappell, R., *et al.* (1995) The adverse effect of treatment prolongation in cervical carcinoma. *Int. J. Radiat. Oncol. Biol. Phys.*, **32** (5), 1301–1307.

148 Nag, S., Erickson, B., Thomadsen, B., Orton, C., Demanes, J., Petereit, D. (2000) The American Brachytherapy Society recommendation for high-dose-rate brachytherapy for carcinoma of the cervix. *Int. J. Radiat. Oncol. Biol. Phys.*, **48** (1), 201–2011.

149 Forrest, J., Ackerman, I., Barbera, L., *et al.* (2010) Patient outcome study of concurrent chemoradiation, external beam radiotherapy, and high-dose-rate brachytherapy in locally advanced carcinoma of the cervix. *Int. J. Gynecol. Cancer*, **20** (6), 1074–1078.

150 Falkenberg, E., Kim, R., Meleth, S., de Los Santos, J., Spencer, S. (2006) Low-dose-rate vs. high-dose-rate intracavitary brachytherapy for carcinoma of the cervix: The University of Alabama at Birmingham (UAB) experience. *Brachytherapy*, **5** (1), 49–55.

151 Kapp, K., Stuecklschweiger, G., Kapp, D., Poschauko, J., Pickel, H., Hackl, A. (1997) Carcinoma of the cervix: analysis of complications after primary external beam radiation and IR-192 HDR brachytherapy. *Gynecol. Oncol.*, **42** (2), 143–153.

152 Han, I., Malviya, V., Chuba, P., *et al.* (1996) Multifractionated high-dose-rate brachytherapy with concomitant daily teletherapy for cervical cancer. *Gynecol. Oncol.*, **63** (1), 71–77.

153 Mutic, S., Grigsby, P.W., Low, D.A., *et al.* (2002) PET-guided three-dimensional treatment planning of intracavitary gynecologic implants. *Int. J. Radiat. Oncol. Biol. Phys.*, **52** (4), 1104–1110.

154 Malyapa, R.S., Mutic, S., Low, D.A., *et al.* (2002) Physiologic FDG-PET three-dimensional brachytherapy treatment planning for cervical cancer. *Int. J. Radiat. Oncol. Biol. Phys.*, **54** (4), 1140–1146.

155 Brenner, D., Hall, E., Huang, Y., Sachs, R. (1994) Optimizing the time course of brachytherapy and other accelerated radiotherapeutic protocols. *Int. J. Radiat. Oncol. Biol. Phys.*, **29** (4), 893–901.

156 Fowler, J. (1993) Why shorter half-times of repair lead to greater damage in pulsed brachytherapy. *Int. J. Radiat. Oncol. Biol. Phys.*, **26** (2), 353–356.

157 Fowler, J., van Limbergen, E. (1997) Biological effect of pulsed dose rate brachytherapy with stepping sources

if short half-times of repair are present in tissue. *Int. J. Radiat. Oncol. Biol. Phys.*, **37** (4), 877–883.

158 Chen, C.-Z., Huang, Y., Hall, E., Brenner, D. (1997) Pulsed brachytherapy as a substitute for continuous low dose rate: an *in vitro* study with human carcinoma cells. *Int. J. Radiat. Oncol. Biol. Phys.*, **37** (1), 137–143.

159 Swift, P., Purser, P., Roberts, L., Pickett, B., Powell, C., Phillips, T. (1997) Pulsed low-dose-rate brachytherapy for pelvic malignancies. *Int. J. Radiat. Oncol. Biol. Phys.*, **37** (4), 811–817.

160 Rogers, C., Freel, J., Speiser, B. (1999) Pulsed low-dose-rate brachytherapy for uterine cervix carcinoma. *Int. J. Radiat. Oncol. Biol. Phys.*, **43** (1), 95–100.

161 Charra-Brunaud, C., Peiffert, D. (2008) Preliminary results of a French prospective-multicentric study of 3D pulsed dose-rate brachytherapy for cervix carcinoma. *Cancer Radiother.*, **12** (6-7), 527–531.

162 Hanks, G., Herring, D., Kramer, S. (1983) Patterns of care outcome studies. Results of the national practice in cancer of the cervix. *Cancer*, **51** (5), 959–967.

163 Montana, G., Fowler, W., Varia, M., Walton, L., Mack, Y., Shemanski, L. (1986) Carcinoma of the cervix, stage III. Results of radiation therapy. *Cancer*, **57** (1), 148–154.

164 Logsdon, M., Eifel, P. (1999) FIGO IIIB squamous cell of the cervix: an analysis of prognostic factors emphasizing the balance between external beam and intracavitary radiation therapy. *Int. J. Radiat. Oncol. Biol. Phys.*, **43** (4), 763–765.

165 Akine, Y., Hashida, I., Kajiura, Y., *et al.* (1986) Carcinoma of the uterine cervix treated with external irradiation alone. *Int. J. Radiat. Oncol. Biol. Phys.*, **12** (9), 1611–1616.

166 Coia, L., Won, M., Lanciano, R., Marcial, V., Martz, K., Hanks, G. (1990) The Patterns of Care Outcome Study for cancer of the uterine cervix. Results of the second national practice survey. *Cancer*, **66** (12), 2451–2456.

167 Rose, P., Ali, S., Watkins, E., *et al.* (2007) Long-term follow-up of a randomized trial comparing concurrent single agent cisplatin, cisplatin-based combination chemotherapy, or hydroxyurea during pelvic irradiation for locally advanced cervical cancer: A Gynecologic Oncology Group Study. *J. Clin. Oncol.*, **25** (19), 2804–2810.

168 Stehman, F., Ali, S., Keys, H., *et al.* (2007) Radiation therapy with or without weekly cisplatin for bulky stage 1B cervical carcinoma: follow-up of a Gynecologic Oncology Group trial. *Am. J. Obstet. Gynecol.*, **197**, **503**, e501–e503, e506.

169 Kunos, C., Ali, S., Abdul-Karim, F., Stehman, F., Waggoner, S. (2010) Posttherapy residual disease associates with long-term survival after chemoradiation for bulky stage 1B cervical carcinoma:

a Gynecologic Oncology Group study. *Am. J. Obstet. Gynecol.*, **203** (4), 351, e351–e358.

170 Webb, J., Key, R., Qualls, C., Smith, H. (2001) Population-based study of microinvasive adenocarcinoma of the uterine cervix. *Obstet. Gynecol.*, **97** (5, Pt 1), 701–706.

171 Whitney, C., Stehman, F. (2000) The abandoned radical hysterectomy: a Gynecologic Oncology Group Study. *Gynecol. Oncol.*, **79** (3), 350–356.

172 Diaz, J., Sonoda, Y., Leitao, M., *et al.* (2008) Oncologic outcome of fertility-sparing radical trachelectomy versus radical hysterectomy for stage 1B1 cervical carcinoma. *Gynecol. Oncol.*, **111** (2), 255–260.

173 Einstein, M., Park, K., Sonoda, Y., *et al.* (2009) Radical vaginal versus abdominal trachelectomy for stage IB1 cervical cancer: a comparison of surgical and pathologic outcomes. *Gynecol. Oncol.*, **112** (1), 73–77.

174 Hamberger, A., Fletcher, G., Wharton, J. (1978) Results of treatment of early stage 1 carcinoma of the uterine cervix with intracavitary radium alone. *Cancer*, **41** (3), 980–985.

175 Grigsby, P., Perez, C. (1991) Radiotherapy alone for medically inoperable carcinoma of the cervix: stage 1A and carcinoma in situ. *Int. J. Radiat. Oncol. Biol. Phys.*, **21** (2), 375–378.

176 Landoni, F., Maneo, A., Colombo, A., *et al.* (1997) Randomized study of radical surgery versus radiotherapy for stage Ib-IIa cervical cancer. *Lancet*, **350** (9077), 535–540.

177 Delgado, G., Bundy, B., Fowler, W., *et al.* (1989) A prospective surgical pathological study of stage 1 squamous carcinoma of the cervix: A Gynecologic Oncology Group Study. *Gynecol. Oncol.*, **35** (3), 314–320.

178 Piver, M., Marchetti, D., Patton, T., Halpern, J., Blumenson, L., Driscoll, D. (1988) Radical hysterectomy and pelvic lymphadenectomy versus radiation therapy for small (less than or equal to 3 cm) stage IB cervical carcinoma. *Am J. Clin. Oncol.*, **11** (1), 21–24.

179 Perez, C., Camel, H., Kao, M., Hederman, M. (1987) Randomized study of preoperative radiation and surgery or irradiation alone in the treatment of stage IB and IIA carcinoma of the cervix: final report. *Gynecol. Oncol.*, **27** (2), 129–140.

180 Sedlis, A., Bundy, B., Rotman, M., Lentz, S., Muderspach, L., Zaino, R. (1999) A randomized trial of pelvic radiation therapy versus no further therapy in selected patients with stage IB carcinoma of the cervix after radical hysterectomy and pelvic lymphadenectomy: A Gynecologic Oncology Group Study. *Gynecol. Oncol.*, **73** (2), 177–183.

181 Rotman, M., Sedlis, A., Piedmonte, M., *et al.* (2006) A phase III randomized trial of postoperative pelvic irradiation in stage IB cervical carcinoma with poor

prognostic features: follow-up of a Gynecologic Oncology Group study. *Int. J. Radiat. Oncol. Biol. Phys.*, **65** (1), 169–176.

182 Jones, W., Shingleton, H., Russell, A., *et al.* (1996) Cervical carcinoma and pregnancy. A national patterns of care study of the American College of Surgeons. *Cancer*, **77**, 1479–1488.

183 Russell, A., Tong, D., Figge, D., Tamimi, H., Greer, B., Elder, S. (1984) Adjuvant postoperative pelvic radiation for carcinoma of the uterine cervix: Pattern of cancer recurrence in patients undergoing elective radiation following radical hysterectomy and pelvic lymphadenectomy. *Int. J. Radiat. Oncol. Biol. Phys.*, **10**, 211–214.

184 Fuller, A., Elliott, N., Kosloff, C., Hoskins, W., Lewis, J.J. (1989) Determinations of increased risk for recurrence in patients undergoing radical hysterectomy for stage IB and IIA carcinoma of the cervix. *Gynecol. Oncol.*, **33**, 34–39.

185 Larson, D., Copeland, L., Stringer, C., Gershenson, D., Malone, J., Edwards, C. (1988) Recurrent cervical carcinoma after radical hysterectomy. *Gynecol. Oncol.*, **30**, 381–387.

186 Kinney, W., Alvarez, R., Reid, G., *et al.* (1989) Value of adjuvant whole-pelvis irradiation after Wertheim hysterectomy for early-stage squamous carcinoma of the cervix with pelvic nodal metastasis: A matched-control study. *Gynecol. Oncol.*, **34**, 258–262.

187 Peters, W.I., Liu, P., Barrett, R., *et al.* (2000) Cisplatin and 5-fluorouracil plus radiation therapy are superior to radiation therapy as adjunctive in high-risk early stage carcinoma of the cervix after radical hysterectomy and pelvic lymphadenectomy: Report of a phase III intergroup study. *J. Clin. Oncol.*, **18** (8), 1606–1613.

188 Yessaian, A., Magistris, A., Burger, R., Monk, B. (2004) Radical hysterectomy followed by tailored postoperative therapy in the treatment of stage 1B2 cervical cancer: feasibility and indications for adjuvant therapy. *Gynecol. Oncol.*, **94** (1), 61–66.

189 Rotman, M., Moon, S., John, M., Choi, K., Sall, S. (1978) Extended field para-aortic radiation in cervical carcinoma: the case for prophylactic treatment. *Int. J. Radiat. Oncol. Biol. Phys.*, **4** (9-10), 795–799.

190 Keys, H.M., Bundy, B.N., Stehman, F.B., *et al.* (1999) Cisplatin, radiation, and adjuvant hysterectomy compared with radiation and adjuvant hysterectomy for bulky stage IB cervical carcinoma. *N. Engl. J. Med.*, **340** (15), 1154–1161.

191 Keys, H.M., Bundy, B.N., Stehman, F.B., *et al.* (2003) Radiation therapy with and without extrafascial hysterectomy for bulky stage IB cervical carcinoma: a randomized trial of the Gynecologic Oncology Group. *Gynecol. Oncol.*, **89** (3), 343–353.

192 Goksedef, B., Kunos, C., Belinson, J., Rose, P. (2009) Concurrent cisplatin-based chemoradiation for International Federation of Gynecology and Obstetrics stage IB2 cervical carcinoma. *Am. J. Obstet. Gynecol.*, **200**, 175, e171–e175.

193 Choi, I., Cha, M., Park, E., (2008) *et al.* The efficacy of concurrent cisplatin and 5-flurouracil chemotherapy and radiation therapy for locally advanced cancer of the uterine cervix. *J. Gynecol. Oncol.*, **19** (2), 129–134.

194 Gold, M., Tian, C., Whitney, C., Rose, P., Lanciano, R. (2008) Surgical versus radiographic determination of para-aortic lymph node metastases before chemoradiation for locally-advanced cervical carcinoma. A Gynecologic Oncology Group Study. *Cancer*, **112**, 1954–1963.

195 Morris, M., Eifel, P., Lu, J., *et al.* (1999) Pelvic radiation with concurrent chemotherapy compared with pelvic and para-aortic radiation for high-risk cervical cancer. *N. Engl. J. Med.*, **340** (15), 1137–1143.

196 Whitney, C.W., Sause, W., Bundy, B.N., *et al.* (1999) Randomized comparison of fluorouracil plus cisplatin versus hydroxyurea as an adjunct to radiation therapy in stage IIB-IVA carcinoma of the cervix with negative para-aortic lymph nodes: a Gynecologic Oncology Group and Southwest Oncology Group study. *J. Clin. Oncol.*, **17** (5), 1339–1348.

197 Rose, P.G., Bundy, B.N., Watkins, E.B., *et al.* (1999) Concurrent cisplatin-based radiotherapy and chemotherapy for locally advanced cervical cancer. *N. Engl. J. Med.*, **340** (15), 1144–1153.

198 Thigpen, J., Shingleton, H., Homesley, H., Lagasse, L., Blessing, J. (1981) Cis-platinum in treatment of advanced or recurrent squamous cell carcinoma of the cervix: a phase II study of the Gynecologic Oncology Group. *Cancer*, **48** (4), 899–903.

199 Bonomi, P., Blessing, J.A., Stehman, F.B., DiSaia, P.J., Walton, L., Major, F.J. (1985) Randomized trial of three cisplatin dose schedules in squamous-cell carcinoma of the cervix: a Gynecologic Oncology Group study. *J. Clin. Oncol.*, **3** (8), 1079–1085.

200 McGuire, W.I., Arseneau, J., Blessing, J.A., *et al.* (1989) A randomized comparative trial of carboplatin and iproplatin in advanced squamous cell carcinoma of the uterine cervix: a Gynecologic Oncology Group Study. *J. Clin. Oncol.*, **7** (10), 1462–1468.

201 Nyholm, S., Thelander, L., Graslund, A. (1993) Reduction and loss of the iron center in the reaction of the small subunit of mouse ribonucleotide reductase with hydroxyurea. *Biochemistry*, **32** (43), 11569–11574.

202 Sinclair, W. (1968) The combined effect of hydroxyurea and x-rays on Chinese hamster cell *in vitro*. *Cancer Res.*, **28**, 198–201.

203 Piver, M., Howes, A., Suit, H., Marshall, N. (1972) Effect of hydroxyurea on the radiation response of

C3H mouse mammary tumors. *Cancer*, **55**, 2123–2130.

204 Hreshchyshyn, M.M., Aron, B.S., Boronow, R.C., Franklin, E.W., 3rd, Shingleton, H.M., Blessing, J.A. (1979) Hydroxyurea or placebo combined with radiation to treat stages IIIB and IV cervical cancer confined to the pelvis. *Int. J. Radiat. Oncol. Biol. Phys.*, **5** (3), 317–322.

205 Piver, M., Vongtama, V., Emrich, L. (1987) Hydroxyurea plus pelvic radiation versus placebo plus pelvic radiation in surgically staged IIIB cervical cancer. *J. Surg. Oncol.*, **35**, 129–134.

206 Haie, C., Pejovic, M., Gerbaulet, A., *et al.* (1988) Is prophylactic para-aortic radiation worthwhile in the treatment of advanced cervical carcinoma? Results of a controlled clinical trial of the EORTC radiotherapy group. *Radiother. Oncol.*, **11** (2), 101–112.

207 Varia, M.A., Bundy, B.N., Deppe, G., *et al.* (1998) Cervical carcinoma metastatic to para-aortic nodes: extended field radiation therapy with concomitant 5-fluorouracil and cisplatin chemotherapy: a Gynecologic Oncology Group study. *Int. J. Radiat. Oncol. Biol. Phys.*, **42** (5), 1015–1023.

208 Pearcy, R., Brundage, M., Drouin, P., *et al.* (2002) Phase III trial comparing radical radiotherapy with and without cisplatin chemotherapy in patients with advanced squamous cell cancer of the cervix. *J. Clin. Oncol.*, **20** (4), 966–972.

209 Winter, W.R., Maxwell, G., Tian, C., *et al.* (2004) Association of hemoglobin level with survival in cervical carcinoma patients treated with concurrent cisplatin and radiotherapy: a Gynecologic Oncology Group Study. *Gynecol. Oncol.*, **94** (2), 495–501.

210 Duenas-Gonzalez, A., Zarba, J., Patel, F., *et al.* (2011) A phase III, open-label, randomized study comparing concurrent gemcitabine plus cisplatin and radiation followed by adjuvant gemcitabine and cisplatin versus concurrent cisplatin and radiation in patients with stage IIB to IVA carcinoma of the cervix. *J. Clin. Oncol.*, **29** (13), 1678–1685.

211 Rose, P., DeGeest, K., McMeekin, S., Fusco, N. (2007) A phase I study of gemcitabine followed by cisplatin concurrent with whole pelvic radiation therapy in locally advanced cervical cancer: A Gynecologic Oncology Group study. *Gynecol. Oncol.*, **107**, 274–279.

212 Thomas, G. (2011) Are we making progress in curing advanced cervical cancer? *J. Clin. Oncol.*, **29** (13), 1654–1656.

213 Sardi, J., Sananes, C., Giaroli, A., *et al.* (1993) Results of a prospective randomized trial with neoadjuvant chemotherapy in stage IB, bulky squamous cell carcinoma of the cervix. *Gynecol. Oncol.*, **49**, 156–165.

214 Hwang, Y., Moon, H., Cho, S., *et al.* (2001) Ten-year survival of patients with locally-advanced, stage IB-IIB cervical cancer after neoadjuvant chemotherapy and radical hysterectomy. *Gynecol. Oncol.*, **82**, 88–93.

215 Cho, Y., Kim, D., Kim, J., Kim, Y., Kim, Y., Nam, J. (2009) Comparative study of neoadjuvant chemotherapy before radical hysterectomy and radical surgery alone in stage IB2-IIA bulky cervical cancer. *J. Gynecol. Oncol.*, **20** (1), 22–27.

216 Benedetti-Panici, P., Greggi, S., Colombo, A., *et al.* (2002) Neoadjuvant chemotherapy and radical surgery versus exclusive radiotherapy in locally advanced squamous cell cervical cancer: Results from the Italian multicenter randomized study. *J. Clin. Oncol.*, **20** (1), 179–188.

217 Eddy, G., Bundy, B.N., Creasman, W., *et al.* (2007) Treatment of ('bulky') stage IB cervical cancer with or without neoadjuvant vincristine and cisplatin prior to radical hysterectomy and pelvic/para-aortic lymphadenectomy: a phase III trial of the Gynecologic Oncology Group. *Gynecol. Oncol.*, **106** (2), 362–369.

218 Omura, G., Blessing, J., Vaccarella, S., *et al.* (1997) Randomized trial of cisplatin versus cisplatin plus mitolactol versus cisplatin plus ifosphamide in advanced squamous carcinoma of the cervix: a Gynecologic Oncology Group study. *J. Clin. Oncol.*, **15** (1), 165–171.

219 Moore, D., Blessing, J., McQuellon, R., *et al.* (2004) Phase III study of cisplatin with and without paclitaxel in stage IVB, recurrent, or persistent squamous cell carcinoma of the cervix: a Gynecologic Oncology Group study. *J. Clin. Oncol.*, **22** (15), 3113–3119.

220 Long, H.R., Bundy, B., Grendys, E.J., *et al.* (2005) Randomized phase III trial of cisplatin with or without topotecan in carcinoma of the uterine cervix: a Gynecologic Oncology Group study. *J. Clin. Oncol.*, **23** (21), 4626–4633.

221 Monk, B., Sill, M., McMeekin, D., *et al.* (2009) Phase III trial of four cisplatin-containing doublet combinations in stage IVB, recurrent, or persistent cervical carcinoma: a Gynecologic Oncology Group study. *J. Clin. Oncol.*, **27** (28), 4649–4655.

222 Wimbush, P., Fletcher, G. (1969) Radiation therapy of carcinoma of the cervical stump. *Radiology*, **93**, 655–658.

223 Kovalic, J., Grigsby, P., Perez, C., Lockett, M. (1991) Cervical stump carcinoma. *Int. J. Radiat. Oncol. Biol. Phys.*, **20**, 933–938.

224 Wolff, J., Lacour, J., Chassagne, D., Berend, M. (1972) Cancer of the cervical stump: a study of 173 patients. *Obstet. Gynecol.*, **39**, 10–16.

225 Potter, M., Alvarez, R., Shingleton, H., Soong, S., Hatch, K. (1990) Early invasive cervical cancer with pelvic lymph node involvement: To complete or not to

complete radical hysterectomy? *Gynecol. Oncol.*, **37**, 78–81.

226 Kinney, W., Hodge, D., Egorshin, E., Ballard, D., Podratz, K. (1995) Surgical treatment of patients with stage IB and IIA carcinoma of the cervix and palpably positive lymph nodes. *Gynecol. Oncol.*, **57**, 145–149.

227 Greer, B., Easterling, T., McLennan, D., *et al.* (1989) Fetal and maternal consideration in the management of stage 1-B cervical cancer during pregnancy. *Gynecol. Oncol.*, **34**, 61–65.

228 Dudan, R., Yon, J.J., Ford, J.J., Averette, H. (1973) Carcinoma of the cervix and pregnancy. *Gynecol. Oncol.*, **1**, 283–289.

229 Hopkins, M., Morley, G. (1992) The prognosis and management of cervical cancer associated with pregnancy. *Gynecol. Oncol.*, **80**, 9–13.

230 Creasman, W., Rutledge, F., Fletcher, G. (1970) Carcinoma of the cervix associated with pregnancy. *Obstet. Gynecol.*, **36**, 495–501.

231 Magrina, J. (1996) Primary surgery for stage IB-IIA cervical cancer, including short-term and long-term morbidity and treatment in pregnancy. *J. Natl Cancer Inst. Monogr.*, **21**, 53–59.

232 Robova, H., Rob, L., Pluta, M., *et al.* (2005) Squamous intraepithelial lesions-microinvasive carcinoma of the cervix during pregnancy. *Eur. J. Gynaecol. Oncol.*, **26**, 611–614.

233 Plante, M., Gregoire, J., Renaud, M., Roy, M. (2011) The vaginal radical trachelectomy: an update of a series of 125 cases and 106 pregnancies. *Gynecol. Oncol.*, **121** (2), 290–297.

234 Knight, L., Acheson, N., Kay, T., Rennison, J., Shepherd, J., Taylor, M. (2010) Obstetric management following fertility-sparing radical vaginal trachelectomy for cervical cancer. *J. Obstet. Gynecol.*, **30** (8), 784–789.

235 Amant, F., van Calsteren, K., Halaska, M.J., *et al.* (2009) Gynecologic cancers in pregnancy: guidelines of an international consensus meeting *Int. J. Gynecol. Cancer*, **19** (Suppl. 1), S1–S12.

236 Rob, L., Pluta, M., Skapa, P., Robova, H. (2010) Advances in fertility-sparing surgery for cervical cancer. *Expert Rev. Anticancer Ther.*, **10** (7), 1101–1114.

237 Grigsby, P., Russell, A., Bruner, D., *et al.* (1995) Late injury of cancer therapy on the female reproductive tract. *Int. J. Radiat. Oncol. Biol. Phys.*, **31** (5), 1281–1299.

238 Chiao, T.B., Lee, A.J. (2005) Role of pentoxifylline and vitamin E in attenuation of radiation-induced fibrosis. *Ann. Pharmacother.*, **39** (3), 516–522.

239 Feldmeier, J. (2008) Hyperbaric oxygen therapy for delayed radiation injuries, in *Physiology and Medicine of Hyperbaric Oxygen Therapy* (eds T. Neuman,

S. Thom), Saunders-Elsevier, Philadelphia, PA, pp. 231–256.

240 Hughes, V., Hillier, S. (1990) Microbiological characteristics of Lactobacillus products used for colonization of the vagina. *Obstet. Gynecol.*, **75** (2), 244–248.

241 Friedman, L., Abdallah, R., Schluchter, M., Panneerselvam, A., Kunos, C. (2011) Adherence to vaginal dilation following high dose rate brachytherapy for endometrial cancer. *Int. J. Radiat. Oncol. Biol. Phys.*, **80** (3), 751–757.

242 Pitkin, R., Bradbury, J. (1965) The effect of topical estrogen on irradiated vaginal epithelium. *Am. J. Obstet. Gynecol.*, **92**, 175–182.

243 Pitkin, R., van Voorhis, L. (1971) Postirradiation vaginitis. An evaluation of prophylaxis with topical estrogen. *Radiology*, **99** (2), 417–421.

244 Eifel, P., Levenback, C., Wharton, J., Oswald, M. (1995) Time course and incidence of late complications in patients treated with radiation therapy for FIGO stage IB carcinoma of the uterine cervix. *Int. J. Radiat. Oncol. Biol. Phys.*, **32** (5), 1289–1300.

245 Davis, E., El Khoudary, S., Talbott, E., Davis, J., Regan, L. (2008) Safety and efficacy of the use of intravesical and oral pentosan polysulfate sodium for interstitial cystitis: a randomized double-blind clinical trial. *J. Urol.*, **179** (1), 177–185.

246 Liang, Y., Messer, K., Rose, B., *et al.* (2010) Impact of bone marrow radiation dose on acute hematologic toxicity in cervical cancer: principal component analysis on high dimensional data. *Int. J. Radiat. Oncol. Biol. Phys.*, **78** (3), 912–919.

247 Rose, B., Aydogan, B., Liang, Y., *et al.* (2011) Normal tissue complication probability modeling of acute hematologic toxicity in cervical cancer patients treated with chemoradiotherapy. *Int. J. Radiat. Oncol. Biol. Phys.*, **79** (3), 800–807.

248 Shenouda, G., Mehio, A., Souhami, L., *et al.* (2006) Erythropoietin receptor expression in biopsy specimens from patients with uterine cervix squamous cell carcinoma. *Int. J. Gynecol. Cancer*, **16** (2), 752–756.

249 Thomas, G., Ali, S., Hoebers, F., *et al.* (2008) Phase III trial to evaluate the efficacy of maintaining hemoglobin levels above 12.0g/dL with erythropoietin vs above 10.0 g/dL without erythropoietin in anemic patients receiving concurrent radiation and cisplatin for cervical cancer. *Gynecol. Oncol.*, **108** (2), 317–325.

250 Vokes, E., Haraf, D., Drinkard, L., *et al.* (1995) A phase I trial of concomitant chemoradiotherapy with cisplatin dose intensification and granulocyte-colony stimulating factor support for advanced malignancies of the chest. *Cancer Chemother. Pharmacol.*, **35** (4), 304–312.

251 Blomlie, V., Rofstad, E., Talle, K., Sundfør, K., Winderen, M., Lien, H. (1996) Incidence of radiation-induced insufficiency fractures of the female pelvis: evaluation with MR imaging. *Am. J. Roentgenol.*, **167** (5), 1205–1210.

252 Chatani, M., Matayoshi, Y., Masaki, N., Narumi, Y., Teshima, T., Inoue, T. (1995) Prophylactic irradiation of para-aortic lymph nodes in carcinoma of the uterine cervix. A randomized study. *Strahlenther. Onkol.*, **171** (11), 655–660.

253 Owens, S., Roberts, W., Fiorica, J., Hoffman, M., LaPolla, J., Cavanaugh, D. (1989) Ovarian management at the time of radical hysterectomy for cancer of the cervix. *Gynecol. Oncol.*, **35**, 349–351.

254 Feeney, D., Moore, D., Look, K., Stehman, F., Sutton, G. (1995) The fate of the ovaries after radical hysterectomy and ovarian transposition. *Gynecol. Oncol.*, **56** (1), 3–7.

255 Han, S., Kim, Y., Lee, S., *et al.* (2011) Underuse of ovarian transposition in reproductive-aged cancer patients treated by primary or adjuvant pelvic irradiation. *J. Obstet. Gynaecol. Res.*, **37** (7), 825–829.

256 Barnhill, D., Heller, P., Dames, J., Hoskins, W., Gallup, D., Park, R. (1985) Persistence of endometrial activity after radiation therapy for cervical carcinoma. *Obstet. Gynecol.*, **66**, 805–808.

257 McKay, M., Bull, C., Houghton, C., Langlands, A. (1990) Persisting cyclical uterine bleeding in patients treated with radical radiation therapy and hormonal replacement for carcinoma of the cervix. *Int. J. Radiat. Oncol. Biol. Phys.*, **18**, 921–925.

258 Andersen, B. (1996) Stress and quality of life following cervical cancer. *J. Natl Cancer Inst. Monogr.*, **21**, 65–70.

259 Levin, A., Carpenter, K., Fowler, J., Brothers, B., Andersen, B., Maxwell, G. (2010) Sexual morbidity associated with poorer psychological adjustment among gynecological cancer survivors. *Int. J. Gynecol. Cancer*, **20** (3), 461–470.

260 Carpenter, K., Fowler, J., Maxwell, G., Andersen, B. (2010) Direct and buffering effects of social support among gynecologic cancer survivors. *Ann. Behav. Med.*, **39** (1), 79–90.

261 Echner, G., Kilby, W., Lee, M., *et al.* (2009) The design, physical properties and clinical utility of an iris collimator for robotic radiosurgery. *Phys. Med. Biol.*, **54**, 5359–5380.

262 Hoogeman, M., Prévost, J.-B., Nuyttens, J., Pöll, J., Levandag, P., Heijmen, B. (2009) Clinical accuracy of the respiratory tumor tracking system of the CyberKnife: Assessment by analysis of log files. *Int. J. Radiat. Oncol. Biol. Phys.*, **74** (1), 297–303.

263 Antypas, C., Pantelis, E. (2008) Performance evaluation of a CyberKnife® G4 image-guided robotic stereotactic radiosurgery system. *Phys. Med. Biol.*, **53**, 4697–4718.

264 Wilcox, E., Daskalov, G. (2007) Evaluation of GAFCHROMIC EBT film for CyberKnife® dosimetry. *Med. Phys.*, **34** (6), 1967–1974.

265 Kunos, C., Brindle, J., Zhang, Y., DeBernardo, R. (2011) A prospective phase 2 evaluation of stereotactic body radiosurgery for gynecologic malignancies. *CyberKnife Robotic Radiosurgery Summit*, 12 February 2011, San Francisco, CA.

266 McNeil, C. (1999) New standard of care for cervical cancer sets stage for next questions. *J. Natl Cancer Inst.*, **91** (6), 500–501.

267 Saito, I., Kitagawa, R., Fukuda, H., *et al.* (2010) A phase III trial of paclitaxel plus carboplatin versus paclitaxel plus cisplatin in stage IVB, persistent of recurrent cervical cancer: Gynecologic Cancer Study Group/Japan Clinical Oncology Group Study (JCOG0505). *Jpn. J. Clin. Oncol.*, **40** (1), 90–93.

268 Tiersten, A., Selleck, M., Hershman, D., *et al.* (2004) Phase II study of topotecan and paclitaxel for recurrent, persistent, or metastatic cervical carcinoma. *Gynecol. Oncol.*, **92** (2), 635–638.

269 Symonds, R., Davidson, S., Chan, S., *et al.* (2011) SCOTCERV: A phase II trial of decetaxel and gemcitabine as second line chemotherapy in cervical cancer. *Gynecol. Oncol.*, **123** (1), 105–109.

270 Wang, J., Lohman, G., Stubbe, J. (2009) Mechanism of inactivation of human ribonucleotide reductase with p53R2 by gemcitabine 5′-diphosphate. *Biochemistry*, **48** (49), 11612–11621.

271 Duenas-Gonzalez, A., Lopez-Graniel, C., Gonzalez-Enciso, A., *et al.* (2002) Concomitant chemoradiation versus neoadjuvant chemotherapy in locally advanced cervical carcinoma: results from two consecutive phase II studies. *Ann. Oncol.*, **13** (8), 1212–1219.

272 Ame, J., Rolli, V., Schreiber, V., *et al.* (2004) PARP-2, a novel mammalian DNA damage-dependent poly(ADP-ribose) polymerase. *J. Biol. Chem.*, **274**, 17860–17868.

273 Ame, J., Spenlehauer, C., de Murcia, G. (2004) The PARP superfamily. *BioEssays*, **26** (8), 882–893.

274 Benjamin, R., Gill, D. (1980) ADP-ribosylation in mammalian cell ghosts. Dependence on poly(ADP-ribose) synthesis on strand breakage in DNA. *J. Biol. Chem.*, **255**, 10493–10501.

275 Fernet, M., Ponette, V., Deniaud-Alexandre, E., *et al.* (2000) Poly(ADP-ribose) polymerase, a major determinant of early cell response to ionizing radiation. *Int. J. Radiat. Oncol. Biol. Phys.*, **76** (12), 1621.

276 Schreiber, V., Ame, J., Dollie, P., *et al.* (2002) Poly(ADP-ribose) polymerase-2 (PARP-2) is required for efficient base excision repair in association with

PARP-1 and XRCC1. *J. Biol. Chem.*, **277** (25), 23028–23036.

277 Fukushima, M., Kuzuya, K., Ota, K., Ikai, K. (1981) Poly(ADP-ribose) synthesis in human cervical cancer cell-diagnostic cytological usefulness. *Cancer Lett.*, **14** (3), 227–236.

278 Bernhard, E., Stanbridge, E., Gupta, S., *et al.* (2000) Direct evidence for the contribution of activated *N-ras* and *K-ras* oncogenes to increased intrinsic radiation resistance in human tumor cell lines. *Cancer Res.*, **60**, 6597–6600.

279 Piao, C., Jin, M., Lee, S., *et al.* (2009) Ribonucleotide reductase small subunit p53R2 suppresses MEK-ERK activity by binding to ERK kinase 2. *Oncogene*, **28**, 2173–2184.

280 Chung, E., Brown, A., Asano, H., *et al.* (2009) *In vitro* and *in vivo* radiosensitization with AZD6244 (ARRY-142886), an inhibitor of mitogen-activated protein kinase / extracellular signal-related kinase 1/2 kinase. *Clin. Cancer Res.*, **15** (9), 3050–3057.

281 Branca, M., Ciotti, M., Santini, D., *et al.* (2004) Activation of the ERK/MAP kinase pathway in cervical intraepithelial neoplasia is related to grade of the lesion but not to high-risk human papillomavirus, virus clearance, or prognosis in cervical cancer. *Am. J. Clin. Pathol.*, **122**, 902–911.

282 Kamei, H., Jackson, R., Zheleva, D., Davidson, F. (2010) An integrated pharmacokinetic-pharmacodynamic model for an Aurora kinase inhibitor. *J. Pharmacokinet. Pharmacodyn.*, **37**, 407–434.

283 Eichholz, A., Merchant, S., Gaya, A. (2010) Anti-angiogenesis therapies: their potential in cancer management. *Oncol. Targets Ther.*, **3**, 69–82.

284 Monk, B., Sill, M., Burger, R., Gray, H., Buekers, T., Roman, L. (2009) Phase II trial of bevacizumab in the treatment of persistent or recurrent squamous cell carcinoma of the cervix: a Gynecologic Oncology Group study. *J. Clin. Oncol.*, **27** (7), 1069–1074.

285 Schefter, T., Winter, K., Kwon, J.S., *et al.* (2014) RTOG 0417: efficacy of bevacizumab in combination with definitive radiation therapy and cisplatin chemotherapy in untreated patients with locally advanced cervical carcinoma. *Int. J. Radiat. Oncol. Biol. Phys.*, **88** (1), 101–105.

286 Ryu, S.Y., Lee, W.M., Kim, K., *et al.* (2011) Randomized clinical trial of weekly vs. tri-weekly cisplatin-based chemotherapy concurrent with radiotherapy in the treatment of locally advanced cervical cancer. *Int. J. Radiat. Oncol. Biol. Phys.*, **81** (4), 577–581.

287 Tewari, K., Sill, M., Long, H.R., *et al.* (2014) Improved survival with bevacizumab in advanced cervical cancer. *N. Engl. J. Med.*, **370** (8), 734–743.

288 Kunos, C., Radivoyevitch, T., Waggoner, S., *et al.* (2013) Radiochemotherapy plus 3-aminopyridine-2-carboxaldehyde thiosemicarbazone (3-AP, NSC #663249) in advanced-stage cervical and vaginal cancers. *Gynecol. Oncol.*, **130** (1), 75–80.

289 Kunos, C.A., Sherertz, T.M. (2014) Long-term disease control with triapine-based radiochemotherapy for patients with stage IB2-IIIB cervical cancer. *Front. Oncol.*, **4**, 184.

Section 7

Miscellaneous Sites

Section Editor: William Small, Jr

36

Cancer of the Skin

Justin Lee, Elizabeth Barnes, May Tsao and Phillip Devlin

Introduction

Cancers of the skin are the most commonly diagnosed form of human malignancy and occur more than all other types of cancer combined; if detected at an early stage, the majority of skin tumours are highly curable [1]. Radiotherapy is an effective treatment option for many patients which can be utilized as the primary curative modality, or in the form of postoperative adjuvant treatment or for palliation of symptoms. In this chapter, attention is focused on the role of radiotherapy in the treatment of skin cancer, with a review of relevant radiation physics, planning and dosimetric issues, brachytherapy techniques as well as a discussion of approaches to commonly treated anatomic regions.

Basal cell carcinoma (BCC) and squamous cell carcinoma (SCC) comprise the majority of skin tumors treated by radiation oncologists, and therefore the discussion is focused on those tumor types, although the principles of radiation physics and planning are relevant to all non-melanoma skin cancer (NMSC). A brief review of radiotherapy for malignant melanoma and Merkel cell carcinoma (MCC) complete the chapter.

The skin is a complex and rapidly proliferating organ. The basic structure consists of the epidermis where BCCs and SCCs originate, and the underlying subdermis, which contains melanocytes, microvasculature, lymphatics and adnexal structures which may also give rise to abnormal growth or malignancy. Ideally, patients with a complex skin malignancy should be seen by a multidisciplinary team consisting of a dermatologist, pathologist, plastic/reconstructive surgeon, and radiation oncologist. At the present authors' practice, the multidisciplinary team evaluates in excess of 500 new patients each year; it has been found that this model can help patients to understand and compare various treatment options during a single consultation, and to

better navigate multimodality treatment pathways, such as surgical excision followed by adjuvant radiotherapy. For the radiation oncologist, a multidisciplinary assessment provides the opportunity to evaluate the tumor preoperatively which can guide adjuvant radiotherapy (XRT). Clinical photographs are a useful resource for documenting treatment, outcomes and toxicity.

A complete history and physical examination should be performed with special focus on previous malignancies, chronic immune suppression (often related to transplant, hematologic disorder, or HIV) and the use of anti-platelet or anti-coagulant medications. Overall performance status and medical comorbidities are also important for evaluating fitness for major surgery or prolonged courses of radiotherapy. Absolute and relative contraindications to radiotherapy, such as Gorlin's syndrome, ataxia telangiectasia, xeroderma pigmentosum, pregnancy, connective tissue diseases and prior irradiation, must also be assessed prior to treatment.

Diagnosis and Staging

Biopsy is essential in order to direct treatment and investigations. For BCC, the rate of lymph node and distant metastases is exceedingly rare; Computed tomography (CT) scanning or magnetic resonance imaging (MRI) are only performed to assess locally advanced tumors where there is clinical suspicion of bone or cartilage invasion, or perineural invasion. SCC staging is based on tumor size and invasion of deep structures, with increasing recognition that other prognostic factors including tumor thickness (>4 mm), perineural or lymphovascular invasion, desmoplastic growth, primary location (ear, lip) and immunosuppression must be considered [2, 3]. Clinically node-negative patients with multiple high-risk features should be considered for staging investigations

Clinical Radiation Oncology: Indications, Techniques, and Results, Third Edition. Edited by William Small Jr.
© 2017 John Wiley & Sons, Inc. Published 2017 by John Wiley & Sons, Inc.

of regional lymphatics. The optimal staging modality for SCC is not well defined; CT or ultrasound are routinely utilized, while sentinel lymph node biopsy is not standard of care but may be considered for carefully selected, high-risk patients [4].

Treatment Options

For relatively small NMSCs, stage T1–T2N0, a number of treatment options with a high chance of cure exist. Surgery continues to be the mainstay of treatment for small, skin tumors where the tumor can be resected with adequate margins and cosmetic outcome is expected to be acceptable. Surgery has advantages of relatively low resource requirements, short treatment times, patient preferences, and the ability to assess surgical resection margins.

Surgical Treatment Options

Moh's Micrographic Surgery (MMS)
This technique involves excision with immediate mapping of the tumor extent and the examination of frozen sections by the treating surgeon/dertmato-pathologist to determine which margin(s) require further excision. This sequence is repeated until negative margins are achieved, which helps to minimize the volume of tissue removed in cosmetically sensitive locations. Reported cure rates with MMS are as high as 97.5% at five years in some studies [5].

Surgical Excision
This approach is a mainstay of treatment for many NMSCs where a wide normal tissue margin of 3–5 mm will not result in unacceptable cosmetic outcomes. A randomized study comparing 612 primary or recurrent BCCs located on the face, treated with MMS or surgical excision for BCC of the face, failed to demonstrate any significant difference in recurrence rates at five years: 2.5% versus 4.0% for MMS and surgical excision, respectively [5].

Electrodessication and Curettage (EDC)
EDC is a simple in-office technique which should be considered only for very small, low-risk, BCC lesions [6, 7]. Reported cure rates vary widely and likely depend on patient selection as well as EDC technique. Silverman *et al.* observed five-year recurrence rates of 17.5% for BCC of the face [8].

Non-Surgical Treatment Options

Cryotherapy
Cryotherapy utilizes the direct application of liquid nitrogen spray to the lesion to cause the tissue temperature to decrease rapidly to between −50 and −60°C in order to cause cell damage through the process of freezing and thawing. Hall *et al.* prospectively studied cryotherapy compared with radiotherapy for the treatment of BCC, and found an unacceptably high recurrence rate; 39% of patients in the cryotherapy group developed recurrence after two years' follow-up, compared to 4% recurrence rate in the radiotherapy arm [9].

Photodynamic Therapy (PDT)
PDT requires the application of a topical photosensitizer (porphyrin) followed by exposure to light of a specific wavelength to activate the drug and cause localized damage to dysplastic and malignant cells. Current indications for PDT include Bowen's disease (SCC *in-situ*) and selected superficial or nodular BCC tumors, with reported response rates between 70% and 90% [10]. The depth of penetration is limited by the wavelength of the photoactivating light, and is typically <2 mm, which may limit the clinical utility of PDT for the treatment of thicker or deeply invasive lesions. One randomized controlled, three-arm trial compared PDT versus topical imiquimod versus topical 5-fluorouracil (5-FU) for the treatment of 601 patients with superficial BCC [11]. Tumor control rates were inferior with PDT when compared to imiquimod (72.8% versus 83.4%, p = 0.021), while 5-FU was deemed to be non-inferior (80.1% control rate).

Topical Treatment/Medical Management
The topical treatment and medical management of NMSC can be considered for superficial BCC lesions, but is not well studied for SCC. Topical anti-neoplastic treatments include 5-FU, imiquimod, intra-lesional interferon, and other agents. A Cochrane Collaboration found short-term response rates of 87% for superficial BCC to imiquimod applied daily for six weeks, and 76% for nodular BCC [12]. The authors, after systematic review of interventions for BCC, suggested that surgery and radiotherapy appeared overall to be the most effective treatments [12]. Bath-Hextall *et al.* also led a multicenter, randomized, non-inferiority study of imiquimod 5% cream versus surgery for nodular and superficial BCC. The treatment success rates were 98% and 84% for surgery and imiquimod, respectively (RR = 0.84, p < 0.0001). At three years, 401 patients were evaluated based on an intention-to-treat analysis; based on pre-defined criteria, imiquimod was found to be inferior to surgery [13]. A non-randomized, multicenter, two-cohort study using hedgehog pathway inhibitors has demonstrated benefit in some patients with metastatic, locally advanced and recurrent BCC, and is approved for use [14]. The response rates for patients with metastatic, and locally advanced BCC were 30% and 43%, respectively, with a median duration of response of 7.6 months. Although

hedgehog inhibitors represents an important systemic treatment option for patients with locally advanced and metastatic BCC, the majority of cases can be treated effectively with surgery and/or radiotherapy.

Radiotherapy for Skin Cancer: Indications

Radiotherapy represents a non-invasive, versatile and effective treatment in the management of non-melanoma carcinoma of the skin. Tumor cure rates with radiotherapy are similar to those achieved with surgery, although direct comparison may be limited by patient selection bias and retrospective design. One prospective randomized study comparing surgical excision with radiotherapy was initiated in 1982 and reported by Avril *et al.* [15]. A significant difference in four-year failure rate was detected favoring surgery over radiotherapy (0.7% versus 7.5%). The majority of patients receiving radiotherapy in the study underwent either interstitial brachytherapy (55%) or 50 kV 'contact therapy' (33%), which delivers high doses to a relatively shallow depth of approximately 2 mm compared with higher-energy orthovoltage units. In general, for small, simple lesions, surgery is preferred due to a shorter treatment time, lower cost, and the ability to assess microscopic margins. Clinical indications for radiotherapy include:

- Critical anatomic regions where surgery would result in a worse cosmetic outcome unacceptable to the patient, or require significant reconstruction with associated risks of anesthesia (often in the head and neck region – tumors of the ear, nose, eyelid, scalp).
- Patients who are unfit for surgery or refuse surgery.
- Palliative treatment with incurable locally advanced or metastatic skin cancer where the primary tumor is causing symptoms such as pain, bleeding or ulceration.
- Postoperative, adjuvant radiotherapy for tumors at high risk of local recurrence due to positive/close margins, perineural invasion, lymphovascular invasion, multiple recurrences [3].

The clinical aspects of radiotherapy for the treatment of NMSC are discussed below. Technical set-up, radiation physics and tumor biology are all important factors for the radiation oncologist to consider when determining the treatment of this diverse and challenging disease site.

External Beam Radiation Treatment Techniques

Curative external beam radiotherapy (EBRT) treatment of non-melanomatous skin cancer can be delivered through the use of orthovoltage, electrons, and megavoltage photon therapy. The beam characteristics of common external beam radiation modalities used in the treatment of NMSC are summarized in Table 36.1. Patient selection, planning and treatment techniques used for skin brachytherapy are described in the following sections of this chapter.

Kilovoltage Radiation Treatment (Orthovoltage/Superficial XRT)

Kilovoltage radiotherapy techniques can be separated into three general categories:

- Contact therapy utilizes 40–50 kV with a very short focus to surface distance (FSD), typically <5 cm; it is effective for treatment to approximately 2 mm depth.
- Superficial therapy between 50 and 150 kV energy, 5–10 mm depth.
- Orthovoltage or 'Deep' kilovoltage therapy range between 150 and 300 kV, with maximum FSD to 50 cm; this has a clinically effective depth of up to 15 mm.

Kilovoltage therapy offers the most simple and direct radiation treatment approach for NMSC. Planning and target delineation can be done with a marking pen, and is entirely dependent on clinical examination and knowledge of clinicopathological features. This technique offers a simple clinical set-up and allows for frail or non-ambulatory patients to be treated in a seated or semi-reclined supine position, without a customized treatment table or immobilization devices. The skin surface dose is 100%, obviating the need for tissue-equivalent bolus or compensators. The set-up is checked visually every day rather than by portal imaging, and the penumbra is relatively small, allowing for maximal sparing of adjacent, uninvolved tissues.

Special Considerations for Kilovoltage Treatment

Maximum Depth of Penetration
The 90% depth dose is limited to approximately 10–12 mm, with maximum energy of 250–300 kV and standard FSD. With an extended FSD, specific filters and large field sizes, the depth may approach 15 mm. This is adequate for most superficial lesions of the nose, eyelids, lips and ear, but may be insufficient when treating bulky, raised, or deeply invading tumors. At higher orthovoltage energy, the thickness of lead shielding required, which is typically placed directly on the skin surface, may be uncomfortable for the patient or it may be difficult to shape to the patient's anatomy.

Convex, Irregular Surfaces
The dose delivered to convex, protuberant structures or oblique surfaces may be inhomogeneous due to differences in the distance from the treatment source to

Table 36.1 Comparison of beam characteristics for kV, electron, and MV treatments.

Beam energy/Quality	Surface dose (%)	D_{max} (cm)	d_{90} (cm)	d_{50} (cm)	Dose at 10 cm (%)	Penumbra 90–50% (mm)	Pb shielding for <5% transmission
75 kVp (2 mm Al) fbone = 4.44	100	Surface	0.4	2.2	6	1–2	0.95 mm Pb
100 kVp (3.2 mm Al) fbone = 4.22	100	Surface	0.6	2.6	7	1–2	0.95 mm Pb
225 kVp (1.8 mm Cu) fbone = 1.46	100	Surface	1	4.1	18	2–3	1.9 mm Pb
6 MV	15	1.5	4	15.5	67	4	6.5 cm Pb
10 MV	14	2.5	5.5	18	74	5	7.0 cm Pb
18 MV	13	3–3.5	7	23	82	7	7.0 cm Pb
6 MeV	74	1.5	0.8–1.8	2.3	<1 (brem)	9*	16 mm cerrobend insert (0.6%)**
9 MeV	80	2.2	0.9–2.8	3.5	<1 (brem)	8*	16 mm cerrobend insert (1.2%)
12 MeV	84	2.8	0.6–3.7	4.7	1.6 (brem)	11	16 mm cerrobend insert (2.6%)

D_{max}, depth of maximum dose; d_{90}, depth of 90% dose; d_{50}, depth of 50% dose; Pb, lead shielding; brem, bremsstrahlung.
Approximate values, not for clinical use. Data based on 5 × 5 cm cone(ortho); 10 × 10 cm photons and electrons; for field size defined at FSD 30 cm(ortho) or 100 cm(photons) at 100 cm SSD(electrons). Estimates only, adapted from institutional data.
*3/8″ Pb rubber can be placed directly on the skin for 6–9 MeV electrons to decrease penumbra to 2–4 mm.
**Otherwise for electrons use 16 mm cerrobend or 15 mm Pb custom shielding.

the skin surface within the target. This 'stand-off' effect is a function of the inverse square law, and may cause dose variations of up to 30–40% when the irregularity is large relative to the FSD [16]. For such cases, several adjustments may considered in order to mitigate the stand-off effect: the longest available FSD should be chosen, the treatment cone should be positioned perpendicular to the surface, and a closed-end cone may be used to compress and flatten the skin surface. Finally, if the other simpler measures are inadequate, it is possible for the radiation oncologist and physicist to apply customized compensators to build up the regions of longer FSD in order to achieve dose homogeneity.

F-Factor

The 'f-factor' or f_{med} is a conversion factor between exposure in air (roentgens) to the absorbed dose with a medium (rads):

$$D_{med} = f_{med} \times X \times A$$

where D_{med} is the absorbed dose to a medium, X is exposure in air, and A is a ratio of energy fluence in the medium to air at a point of interest [16]. The f-factor is highly dependent on photon energy and the composition of the tissue medium. It is most relevant to the kV orthovoltage energy range where the photoelectric effect is predominant and energy absorption varies directly with Z^3 where Z represents the atomic number [16]. Most orthovoltage units are calibrated to a water phantom, and the relative absorbed dose in bone may increase up to fourfold for energies between 50 and 100 kV. Although

the f-factor for bone is universally included in the doctrine of radiation physics for kilovoltage techniques, the incidence of severe toxicity such as osteoradionecrosis of the skull or mandible is rare [17] and may be associated with re-treatment, high dose per fraction or field size rather than the f-factor. The irradiation of cartilaginous structures within the nose and ear appears to be safe, and is not subject to increases in absorbed dose due to similar atomic number [18–20]. In clinical practice, at the 100 kV range where the f-factor for bone is highest, the treated volumes are typically small and significant attenuation occurs as the beam traverses tumor and normal tissues. The present authors have adopted a policy that 75–100 kV orthovoltage may be considered in regions overlying the bone in selected cases where the field size is ≤3 cm in diameter, the region has not been previously irradiated, and there is no directly exposed bone or periosteum. For lesions overlying the scalp or temple, the issue of f-factor can be avoided by utilizing an electron beam.

Electron Treatment

Electron-based techniques (typically 6–12 MeV) are well-suited to the treatment of skin malignancies because of the relatively high surface dose, and the short build-up region followed by a rapid fall-off in dose with depth. The differences in percentage depth dose profiles for kV, electrons and MV therapy are shown in Figure 36.1. Electrons can penetrate deeper into tissue than orthovoltage therapy, and minor variations in source to surface

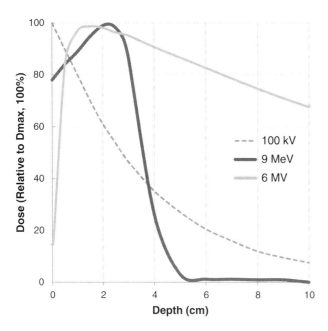

Figure 36.1 Representative percentage depth dose of kV, electron, and MV beams. Percent Depth Dose lines are approximations adapted from clinical data, based on varying field sizes 4 cm open cone for 100 kV; 6 × 6 cm applicator for 9 MeV electrons; 10 × 10 cm field for 6 MV photons.

distance (SSD) do not present a challenge to achieving dose homogeneity within the target volume. For well-delineated lesions with an easily measured thickness, a simple clinical mark-up may be sufficient, whereas CT planning is available for more complex anatomic sites where imaging of the deep structures and dosimetric verification are required. In most cases, a tissue-equivalent bolus material is required to achieve full skin dose. A number of options exist, including customized wax bolus or sheets of tissue equivalent material. The bolus material should fill air gaps, concavities or other curved surfaces in order to achieve a uniform dose. In cases where both full depth dose penetration and full skin dose are desired, a wire mesh bolus of a high-atomic number material can be utilized [21]. If air gaps and surface irregularities persist, *in-vivo* measurements of the surface dose can be used to confirm that the delivered dose is within acceptable tolerance of the planned dose.

Special Considerations for Electron Treatment

Field Size and Penumbra

A minimum electron field size is required to ensure full electron scattering conditions and account for relatively wide penumbra at a depth which can be as large as 8–10 mm. The minimum recommended electron field size for circular cone or square applicators is typically 4–5 cm;

this is in contrast to orthovoltage treatment which may be as small as 1.5 cm, with a penumbra of 2 mm.

Shielding Position

Customized shielding may be applied directly on the skin to reduce scatter and effectively decrease penumbra at the surface of the electron field to approximately 2–3 mm. This practice is typically limited to electron energies of ≤9 MeV, beyond which the size, shape, and weight of the shielding material become too cumbersome to rest directly on the patient. If a wider penumbra at the surface is acceptable, then the electron shielding/applicator may be placed within 5 cm from the skin surface to reduce electron scatter.

Surface Obliquity and Irregularities

Electron dose distributions can be severely affected by changes in surface obliquity and irregularities. When the incident angle of electrons is not perpendicular to the target surface it has been shown that, with increasing incident angle, D_{max} and the 80% depth dose curve shift toward the skin surface and that side scatter increases [16, 22]. Sudden abrupt irregularity within the treatment field will cause inhomogeneity corresponding to differences in scattering within the intervening tissue. Therefore, a tissue-equivalent bolus should be used to fill gaps and irregularities for electron treatments.

Relative Biological Effectiveness (RBE)

The Relative Biological Effectiveness (RBE) of radiotherapy is numerically defined by a ratio of doses:

$$RBE = Dx/D$$

where Dx is a reference radiation treatment (usually 220-kVp photons), and D is the dose required to achieve equivalent biological damage or outcome [16]. Differences in RBE exist due to variations in the stopping power of tissue medium and linear energy transfer mechanisms [23]. Measurement of the RBE in practice is complex, labor-intensive and highly dependent on the both the tissue type and the biological endpoint being studied [23]. For electron energies within the clinical range, the RBE compared with 220 kVp photons is estimated to be between 0.8 and 0.9 for human skin cells [24] for endpoints of erythema, desquamation, and telangiectasia.

The RBE for NMSC cells is not known, and it remains unclear whether differences in RBE between orthovoltage and electron therapy for normal skin translate into clinically significant differences in tumor control rates. Clinical results with electron therapy compared with superficial or orthovoltage treatment are mixed. Lovett *et al.* [25] reported results suggesting lower cure rates with electrons, while others have demonstrated very high local control rates in large groups of patients treated exclusively with electron therapy, ranging from 95% to

97% [26, 27]. The practice at the present authors' institution has been to utilize standardized dose fractionation regimens for all radiation modalities, but to prescribe orthovoltage treatments at the skin surface – nominal 100% dose – whereas electron treatments are typically prescribed to the 95% isodose depth at the central axis.

Megavoltage Photon Treatment

The majority of epithelial tumors encountered by the radiation oncologist can be treated effectively using orthovoltage or electron therapy. MV photon therapy may provide advantages of conformality, critical organ avoidance, and image guidance for large locally advanced tumors that may span an irregular or convex surface. In addition, MV photons may be advantageous if the regional nodes, which are typically several centimeters deep to the skin, are to be included in the target volume.

Special Consideration for Megavoltage Photon Treatment

Percent Depth Dose and Skin-Sparing
It would appear counterintuitive to apply high-energy 6–18 MV photons to the treatment of skin malignancy, where the D_{max} or depth of maximum dose ranges between 1.5 and 3.5 cm for a single direct, skin-appositional beam. In practice, a direct, skin-appositional MV photon beam is rarely used; multiple tangential beams increase the surface dose and require a thin bolus of 0.5–1.5 cm to achieve 100% skin dose.

Set-Up and Immobilization
Unlike the clinical set-ups commonly employed for orthovoltage and electron skin treatments, MV photon therapy typically requires CT simulation and immobilization. This introduces inter and intra-fraction variability, and the planning target volume (PTV) must be designed to account for those uncertainties.

Exit Dose and Organs at Risk
Advanced MV photon treatment techniques such as intensity-modulated radiation therapy (IMRT), volumetric-modulated arc therapy (VMAT), while tomotherapy may be useful in treating locally advanced skin tumors. The potential advantages must be weighed against the risks of increasingly complex beam arrangements, a larger irradiated volume, and a higher integral dose compared to orthovoltage and electron therapy [28].

Skin Brachytherapy

Brachytherapy is the oldest radiation therapy, and arguably still the most conformal. As such, it is most suited for selected clinical situations in which there is a complex target, be it superficial or deep. In this section, attention will be briefly focused on patient selection, treatment techniques, dose and fractionation, and selected results of skin brachytherapy. An example is provided of a custom surface mold applicator to treat a complex superficial target on the forearm.

Patient Selection

The highly conformal dosimetric qualities of superficial brachytherapy allow for a very uniform distribution of dose to clinical targets that are simultaneously superficial but complex in contour and shape. Clinical targets on the face, scalp, hands, feet, and extremities allow definitive and curative treatment without disfiguring or disabling surgical exonerative procedures. Added to this are the excellent physical characteristics of isotope-based brachytherapy, especially the rapid fall-off of dose away from the superficial target, and the ability to protect deeper and radiosensitive structures from radiation dose. As this is possible, a greater degree of hypofractionation may be possible, with the added benefits of a greater cell kill, a shorter overall treatment time, and lower cost.

Treatment Techniques and Applicators

As the spectrum of presentation of skins cancers can range from tiny to broadly diffuse, the availability of applicators to treat single, tiny superficial lesions, as well as custom surface mold applicators to treat the more diffuse tumors, is key. The most common utilization is with squamous cell and basal cell tumors. High-dose rate (HDR) applicators for radionuclide-based brachytherapy using cup-shaped applicators such as the Valencia (a bell-shaped applicator with a flattening filter) and Leipzig (simple bell-shaped) applicators are often appropriate for smaller-sized lesions. There is also an increasing deployment of electronically generated low-energy sources (ELS) which has sometimes been characterized as electronic brachytherapy (even though no radionuclide was involved). Many versions are available, including bell-like applicators and small-aperture contact orthovoltage units. The lack of shielding and authorized user (AU) requirements have caused significant deployment in clinics without radiation oncology standards and expertise, as well as a significant peak in overutilization.

As these various techniques only penetrate a little, this modality should be used on depths of tumor penetration up to 4 mm. This can be determined either at pathology or with ultrasound, CT, or even MRI. The presence of a greater depth of invasion, perineural invasion, scleroderma, lymph vascular invasion are counterindications to superficial brachytherapy. However for deeper lesions a superficial interstitial technique may be adequate, either alone or in combination with EBRT.

For larger lesions and lesions which present a highly complex contour, these smaller applicators are usually impracticable and often inappropriate. Also, as the curvature of a superficial clinical target increases, the ability of electron beam therapy to cover uniformly decreases. At times, there can be matched electron fields but even these have to trade off hot versus cold matches at surface and at depth, together with a significant dose gradient at the field edges. Thus, for complex superficial clinical targets the most conformal therapy is custom surface mold HDR brachytherapy. This technique allows the combination of the penetration depth of the iridium-192 source, with the computer-based graphics optimization of HDR – dose-painting for the clinical target and organs at risk (OAR). These custom surface applicators also allow treatment in proximity to very sensitive structures, such as the eyes, by the added deployment of custom shielding. Commonly used are many variations of thermoplastic mold with the incorporation of a number of catheters, most often in a premade applicator such as Freiburg (Elekta, Stockholm, Sweden) or HAM (Eckhert and Ziegler, New York, USA) applicators (Figures 36.2–36.4). Unlike the simpler forms described above, these applicators and clinical targets require complex image-based treatment planning. Many variations on the basic themes of treatment planning all include the fact that there is no need to contour the skin *per se*, or even to create a clinical target volume (CTV). Rather, it is better

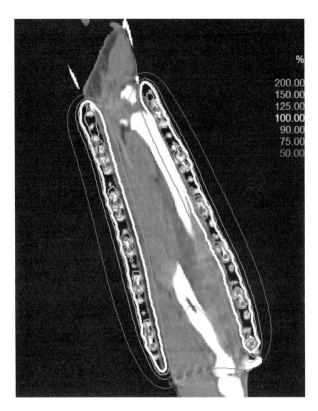

Figure 36.3 The Freiburg applicator with dummy wires in channels is tightly wrapped onto the clinical target with an elastic bandage. For a color version of this figure, see the color plate section.

to mark out on the skin with radiopaque marker wire the gross target area and the clinical margin (e.g., 2 cm). The 100% isodose is set at 3 mm depth, but this can be modified based on thicker tumor depths, to a point. Another pearl is to make sure that the 125% isodose does not touch down on the skin. Much clinical judgment is needed here; however, the dose distribution across the complex target at 3 mm should be homogeneous.

Brachytherapy Dose, Fractionation, and Results

The lack of a large amount of prospective data demonstrates a wide variety of dose and fractionation, but also acceptable results with excellent local control, and minimal late toxicity. The details of recent studies that included more than 100 patients are provided in Table 36.3.

In conclusion, skin brachytherapy covers both the use of various small lesion techniques, as well as the larger complex lesion techniques, and is most adaptable for the wide range of skin cancers, and selected non-cancerous clinical situations such as keloids. Remarkable for such a common cancer site is the paucity of published literature, and essentially little to no prospective and randomized

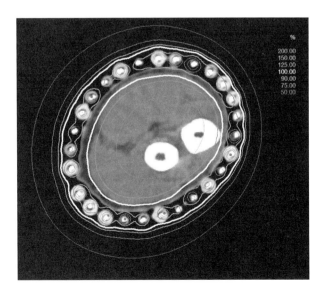

Figure 36.2 Axial (upper panel) and sagittal (lower panel) circumferential homogeneous distribution of 100% isodose (yellow) at 3 mm in tissue with sparing of deep structures and avoidance of 125% isodose from skin in a refractory cutaneous T-cell lymphoma lesion. For a color version of this figure, see the color plate section.

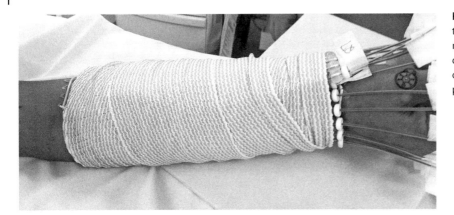

Figure 36.4 Freiburg applicator wrapped to the left forearm. The clinical target and margin are demarcated with radiopaque copper wire on the right forearm. For a color version of this figure, see the color plate section.

data. The deployment of simpler techniques in a non-radiation oncology clinical setting risks a lower quality of patient care and safety for all. There is a pressing and growing need for these techniques to be studied prospectively, with established clinical guidelines, acceptable toxicities, and collaborations among dermatology clinics and radiation oncology clinics, which are best qualified to deliver curative radiation therapy.

Radiation Dose

Curative external beam radiation doses for NMSC range from 60 to 70 Gy using standard fractionation schedules of 1.8–2 Gy per fraction, for five days per week. For many patients with small to moderate-sized tumors (≤3 cm), a hypofractionated schedule may be preferable due to a shorter treatment duration while maintaining a high local control rate and similar acute and late toxicity profile. Varying fractionation regimens have been reported in the literature with similar, high cure rates for BCC and SCC. The patient's general medical condition and ability to attend multiple treatments; tumor location and cosmetic implications, size of the tumor and treatment fields should all be considered. Some common external beam dose/fractionation regimens and common indications for their use with estimates of BED for acute and late responding tissues are summarized in Table 36.2.

Postoperative Adjuvant Radiation

The use of postoperative, adjuvant radiotherapy for non-melanoma skin cancers has not been well investigated in a prospective, randomized study. Positive margins,

Table 36.2 Reported dose fractionation schedules for treatment of skin cancer.

Dose/No. of fractions	Field size	Common clinical indications	BED (α/β = 3 Gy)	BED (α/β = 10 Gy)
24 Gy/3 fractions	Varies	Palliative regimen – treatment on days 0, 7, 21		
35 Gy/5 fractions	≤3 cm	Elderly, poor performance status or no cosmetic concerns	116.67	59.5
40–45 Gy/10 fractions	≤4–5 cm	Small to moderate-size scalp lesions	93.3*	56*
50–55 Gy/20 fractions	≤8 cm	BCC of nose, well patients, cosmesis is of concern	91.67**	62.5**
50 Gy/25 fractions	Any field size	SCC in-situ or adjuvant XRT for focally positive margins	83.3	60
60–66 Gy in 30–33 fractions	Any field size	High risk postoperative, extensive margin involvement	100***	72***
70 Gy/35 fractions	Any field size	Unresectable, locally advanced disease, T3–T4, PNI, LVI	116.67	84

Gy, Gray; PNI, perineural invasion; LVI, lymphovascular invasion; BED, biologically effective dose.
BED calculations are based on the linear quadratic model with no modifications for treatment time. Not applied to single-fraction or once-weekly regimen. α/β ratio for non-melanoma skin cancer is not known.
For BED calculations: *40 Gy/10 fractions used; **50 Gy/20 fractions used; ***60 Gy/30 fractions used.

perineural invasion (PNI), tumor size and thickness, and degree of differentiation are previously described risk factors for local recurrence after surgical excision [29].

A prospective study of 615 patients with SCC of the skin, treated surgically and with negative margins, identified two risk factors for local recurrence on multivariate analysis: thickness and desmoplasia [3]. Risk factors for metastasis included thickness, desmoplasia, immunosuppression, large size, and location (tumors involving the ear were at higher risk). Perineural invasion was not one of the risk factors defined a priori to be assessed, but "…findings of perineural and perivascular invasion were always associated with desmoplasia." [3].

In a systematic review of high-risk SCC of the skin, 2449 cases were identified from previously published data. Among these patients, 91 received adjuvant radiotherapy, and local control rates were similar between the surgery-alone versus adjuvant radiotherapy groups (7% versus 12%, p = 0.10). The authors suggested that the patients selected for adjuvant XRT may have had high-risk features such as positive margins [30]. The postoperative radiotherapy dose typically ranges from 45 to 66 Gy in 1.8–2 Gy daily fractions; the dose is determined individually, based on pathological risk factors as well as the irradiated volume and location.

Radiation Planning

Despite the shift towards image-guided radiation planning and treatment for most tumor sites, most NMSC may be treated successfully using a simple clinical mark-up and depth–dose charts, without the addition of CT-based simulation and planning.

Gross Tumor Volume (GTV)

The GTV is defined as "…the gross palpable or visible/demonstrable extent and location of malignant growth…" by the International Commission on Radiation Units and Measurements document ICRU 50 [31]. For skin cancer, the GTV can often be delineated with a fine felt-tip marking pen under good lighting. The entire tumor is identified by visual examination and palpation, and often includes a subtle sclerotic plaque and/or erythema at the periphery. Diagnostic CT and/or MRI are required to delineate the GTV in locally advanced cases if there is any suspicion of deep extension into bone, cartilage or muscle, or peri-neural invasion. Whether NMSCs located in regions overlying the embryonic fusion plates demonstrate an increased depth of invasion and a higher risk of recurrence is undetermined, and a point of some controversy [32, 33]; the analysis of patients who developed local recurrence did not identify these anatomic locations (pre/post-auricular, nasolabial fold, inner canthus, philtrum) to be independent prognostic factors for recurrence [3, 30], while the updated TNM staging classification system for NMSC does specify anatomic locations of the ear and hair-bearing lip to be at higher risk [34].

CTV (Clinical Target Volume)

This volume represents "…a tissue volume that contains a demonstrable GTV and/or subclinical microscopic malignant disease, which has to be eliminated." At the present authors' institution, a prospective, surgico-pathological study was carried out by Choo *et al.* to measure the microscopic extent of disease beyond the gross tumor identified by physical examination [35]. The GTV was assessed and delineated by a skin radiation oncologist prior to surgical excision. The microscopic resection margins were assessed based on frozen section. After negative margins were achieved, the distance between the GTV outlined and the microscopic tumor extent was measured. For the 71 lesions assessed, the mean microscopic extent beyond GTV was 5.2 mm (range: 1–15 mm); a margin of 10 mm was required to provide a 95% chance of obtaining clear resection. Tumors included for the study typically had demonstrated one or more high-risk features such as size >2 cm, sclerosing or morpheaform subtype, recurrent tumors, or poorly defined borders. A further update of 159 lesions in total suggested that in order to provide a ≥95% chance of covering microscopic disease CTV margins of 10 mm for BCC <2 cm, 11 mm for SCC <2 cm, and 14 mm for SCC >2 cm, although realistically these margins may be difficult to achieve after accounting for PTV and penumbra [36]. In contrast, Wolf and Zitelli assessed the microscopic extent of disease in previously untreated, well-demarcated BCC after treatment with Moh's surgery [37]. A minimum margin of 4 mm was recommended to eradicate >95% of cases. Based on these data, the CTV margin will vary based on tumor features:

- A CTV margin of 5–10 mm for small, well-demarcated BCCs.
- A CTV margin of 8–15 mm for SCCs, sclerosing or morpheaform BCCs, or larger tumors with poorly defined borders.

The CTV does not encompass nodal regions for BCCs. At the time of writing of this chapter, to the authors' knowledge, no data are available that strongly support or refute the use of elective nodal irradiation for SCC of the skin. In high-risk cases, such as T2–T4 disease with other adverse features (recurrence, high grade, perineural invasion, lymphovascular invasion [LVI], etc.) and where the draining lymphatics are reasonably predictable and in close proximity to the primary site, diagnostic imaging should be considered and in the absence of macroscopic disease, a nodal CTV may be considered on a case-by-case basis.

Planning Target Volume (PTV)

The PTV is defined as "…a geometrical concept.. defined to select appropriate beam sizes and beam arrangements taking into consideration the net effect of all the possible geometrical variations, in order to ensure that the prescribed dose is actually absorbed in the CTV" [31]. For orthovoltage and electron treatments using a simple clinical set-up with daily visual checks, the interfractional and intra-fractional variations are expected to be small. In practice, the PTV margin may be included or combined with penumbra, 'PTV + penumbra' to clinically define the distance of the field edge from CTV for those clinical set-ups. As demonstrated in Table 36.1, the penumbra distance varies with radiation modality, energy, field size, and proximity of shielding from the skin:

- For kilovoltage therapy the combined 'PTV + penumbra' ranges from 2 to 3 mm.
- For electrons, 'PTV + penumbra' is approximately 9–12 mm.
- For MV photon plans which require CT simulation, the PTV margin should conform to institutional data and is considered separately from penumbra.

Postoperative, Adjuvant Radiotherapy Planning

CTV definition in postoperative skin cases is a clinical challenge, with little evidence to guide volume delineation. For positive margins, if further surgical excision is not feasible, the current practice has been to treat the entire postoperative bed with a further 10–15 mm expansion into untreated tissue. Skin grafts and flaps may be at risk and often require consultation with the treating surgeon to determine areas at highest risk. PNI is associated with increased risk of locoregional recurrence [29, 38]. Mendenhall *et al.* reported on NMSC of the head and neck with PNI, and observed differences in local control rates between incidental PNI on pathology compared with clinically evident PNI and recommend treatment of the entire course of the nerve – to the base of skull in cases of positive PNI margins or named nerve involvement [29].

Radiation Treatment Planning for Common Anatomic Sites

Scalp

CT simulation and planning are important when planning scalp irradiation to minimize radiation dose to the brain, to estimate tumor thickness, and to assess for bone invasion. Most small to moderate-sized scalp lesions (<4 cm) may be treated with direct electron therapy. Flat, thin lesions can be encompassed by 6–9 MeV electrons with 1 cm tissue-equivalent bolus or a beam-spoiling mesh to achieve full skin dose. Custom shielding may be applied on the skin surface if it is flat and the set-up is stable; otherwise, the shielding is placed in the electron applicator, as close to the skin surface as possible to reduce lateral scatter. Larger scalp lesions ≥4 cm or spanning a convex region of the scalp require more complex radiation planning. IMRT or tomotherapy using a thermoplastic immobilization device have demonstrated superior target coverage and conformity compared with mixed photon/electron plan and HDR [39]. When using these techniques for locally advanced scalp lesions, bolus material should be designed at the time of CT simulation, to ensure accurate planning and reproducible set-up.

Nose

Direct orthovoltage is preferred for simplicity of clinical set-up and the depth–dose profile which achieves 100% skin dose without any beam modifiers. Most small to moderate-sized lesions (typically up to 2–2.5 cm maximum) located on the tip of nose or nasal ala can be successfully treated using this technique. A closed-end cone or applicator may be useful to flatten the skin surface and eliminate minor surface irregularities or differences in SSD. Lead shielding may be placed in the nostril to protect the medial/contralateral nasal mucosa from exit dose.

When the skin lesion spans across midline on the dorsum and cannot be encompassed by orthovoltage, alternative treatment techniques should be considered. For these more advanced nasal skin cancer cases a lateral parallel-opposed pair photon technique or IMRT may be used to treat the entire nose, with a custom wax block built to compensate for missing tissue and improve target coverage and dose homogeneity. A tissue-equivalent bolus is also used to fill air gaps created by the nostrils. Direct electrons with embedded eye shields may also be used for tumors located very high on the bridge of the nose, where POP photon fields would be too close to the optic structures.

Eyelid

The stage classification for lesions of the eyelid differs from all other non-eyelid tumors, reflecting the generally smaller tumor sizes that invade this small, thin structure [34]. Skin cancer of the eyelids or medial and lateral canthus represent a clinical challenge due to the adjacent optic structures, which are at risk of radiation-related injury. The lens, anterior chamber, conjunctiva, lacrimal gland and retina are all potential organs at risk with severe radiation toxicities such as cataract, acute angle glaucoma, dry eye syndrome, retinopathy previously reported [40, 41]. In addition, conjunctivitis, ectropion, and nasolacrimal duct stenosis/epiphora may occur. To minimize the risk of serious injury to the optic structures, internal eye shields should be applied. A topical anesthetic and lubricant are applied to the eye prior to insertion of the eye shields at each treatment. The patient must be educated regarding eye protection (patch or gauze, with eye closed) from irritants and foreign objects for the duration of the local anesthetic after each application. The composition and thickness of internal shields vary; most commercially available products utilize acrylic or gold coating to decrease backscatter, and have a range of sizes to match patient anatomy.

Orthovoltage is preferred to electrons due to a more rapid dose drop-off with depth, and thinner, more easily applied shielding. Dosimetric studies have demonstrated inadequate shielding when electron energies exceed 6–8 MeV with higher doses to the optic structures compared with orthovoltage therapy [42, 43]. In addition to internal eye shields, an external lead shield may be applied to customize the irradiated field and further protect critical structures at risk.

Ear

Skin tumors involving the ear have a higher propensity for locoregional recurrence than other anatomic locations, which is reflected in the 'high-risk' designation within the TNM skin cancer staging classification system [34].

Radiation and treatment planning for primary lesions of the ear are highly variable. Orthovoltage may be utilized for small lesions involving the pinna, helix, or antihelix. Since the thickness of the ear is typically less than 1 cm, shielding can be applied both deep to the ear, shaped to the post-auricular crease, and also on top of the ear such that the target lesion is effectively enclosed or 'sandwiched' between two layers of lead shielding.

Larger lesions extending into the external auditory canal or eroding through cartilage onto the pre-/post-auricular skin likely require CT simulation with a wire to delineate gross disease and a custom bolus to fill any air gaps within the ear and for sufficient build-up for electron or MV photon therapy. A common set-up for these more advanced lesions of the ear and postoperative treatment also involves filling the external auditory canal with a custom wax plug, filling the concha bowl/ear to level. The ear is gently pressed to self-bolus the post-auricular region, after which a large tissue-equivalent bolus is built over the entire region. A thermoplastic mask is helpful for immobilization and also the reproducible placement of the tissue bolus.

Toxicity of Skin Radiotherapy

Normal Tissue Tolerance and Radiation-Induced Skin Toxicity

Although radiation-induced skin toxicity is one of the most frequently observed side effects of radiotherapy, there is a paucity of prospective, quantitative data regarding the tissue tolerance and models for predicting acute and late skin toxicity. In addition, the prevention and optimal management of radiation-induced skin toxicity remains controversial, with wide variations in practice.

Emami *et al.*, in a seminal review of normal tissue tolerance, predicted dose associated with a 5% risk of skin ulceration/necrosis at five years (TD 5/5) for skin, based on equivalent square sizes of irradiated skin [44]. The estimated TD 5/5 for 10 cm^2, 30 cm^2, and 100 cm^2 were 70 Gy, 60 Gy, and 55 Gy, respectively. For a 50% risk of radiation ulceration/necrosis (TD 50/5), the tolerance dose was estimated to be 70 Gy to a 100 cm^2 size region. The more recent Quantitative Analysis of Normal Tissue Effects in the Clinic (QUANTEC) [45] report for normal tissue tolerance does not include a model for skin-related toxicity, and the severity of radiation skin effects continues to be difficult to predict for individual patients. Hayter *et al.* observed a 13% risk of necrosis in 128 patients treated with radiotherapy for NMSC of the pinna, and of those patients two (1.6%) required surgery [46]. Fraction size >6 Gy and treatment times of less than five days were the only factors that were significantly associated with necrosis. Similarly, when Silva *et al.* analyzed the incidence of Grade 4 late toxicity in patients treated for NMSC of the pinna [47], 19 of 313 patients (6.1%) developed Grade 4 toxicity that included chronic ulceration or necrosis. Six patients (1.9%) required surgical intervention. There were no incidents of Grade 4 toxicity in patients treated with 2–2.5 Gy per fraction, despite larger field sizes in this group. The authors identified several factors on univariate analysis which were associated with an increased risk of Grade 4 toxicity, including T-stage, field size, and fraction size >4 Gy. A retrospective review of 1005 patients treated with a single, high-dose radiation treatment of 18–22.5 Gy found rates of skin necrosis consistent with those in previous studies; in this case, 60 patients (6.0%) developed skin necrosis that typically healed with conservative management, while 10 patients (1.0%) developed skin necrosis requiring surgical repair [48].

The risk of radiation skin toxicity associated with the treatment of NMSC must be individualized, to account for patient, treatment and tumor characteristics:

- *Radiation treatment:* Total dose, high dose per fraction and field size are factors which influence the risk of severe acute and late toxicity.

- *Patient characteristics*: Elderly patients with comorbidities including diabetes, immune suppression, peripheral vascular disease or peripheral neuropathy are generally at higher risk of wound healing and complications.
- *Anatomic location*: Skin tumors located on the lower extremities pre-tibial region where circulation may be compromised are at high risk of chronic ulceration and wound healing difficulties when treated with radiotherapy [49, 50]. Other anatomic issues include 'self-bolusing' regions such as the inframammary fold, axilla and groin, or irregular surfaces that may result in dose inhomogeneity.
- *Dose inhomogeneity*: Clinical set-up and CT simulation are performed with the use of bolus and beam modifiers in order to achieve a uniform dose throughout the PTV. Inhomogeneity may result in lower tumor control or increasing skin toxicity. In a randomized study of breast radiotherapy utilizing IMRT versus conventional tangents, Pignol *et al*. demonstrated higher rates of Grade 3 skin toxicity associated with measures of dose inhomogeneity [51].

Prevention and Management of Radiation-Induced Skin Toxicity

Two systematic reviews of the literature have failed to identify a clearly superior regimen for the prevention and/or management of radiation-induced dermatitis, desquamation, and late toxicity [52,53]. The reviewers found that various topical corticosteroids may decrease the rate of acute radiation dermatitis (four randomized control trials), whereas studies involving non-steroidal creams for prevention and treatment used varying products, with the majority demonstrating no significant difference compared to control arms. Several more recent randomized controlled studies of breast cancer patients have demonstrated the benefits of steroidal creams as well as silicone-based dressings in decreasing radiation dermatitis in breast cancer patients, but these are not yet proven safe and effective for skin malignancies [54, 56]. With current evidence it remains difficult to develop specific consensus guidelines for the management of radiation-induced skin toxicity, especially in cutaneous malignancies where the radiation target includes the organ at risk.

Other Toxicity Due to Radiotherapy for Skin Cancer

In addition to acute and late skin toxicity, radiation oncologists must also consider the risks to underlying organs adjacent to the irradiated tumor. Most often, these tumors are located in the head and neck region and treatment will be dependent on the primary anatomic location and radiation technique used. The brain, optic structures, cochlea, mandible, and parotid and lacrimal glands have quantitative normal tissue tolerance dose levels that must be considered prior to radiotherapy for NMSC.

The treatment of primary head and neck malignancies (predominantly pharynx/larynx) with radiation is known to increase the risk of stroke and carotid stenosis [57,58]. Similar levels of risk are likely to be associated with the radiotherapy treatment of locally advanced NMSC when the regional lymph nodes and carotid arteries are within the treatment volume.

Finally, the increased risk of malignancy associated with radiotherapy must be considered when determining treatments. Population-based studies that have demonstrated an increased risk of second malignant neoplasms associated with radiotherapy, including relatively younger patients with lymphoma and cancers of the breast, cervix, testes and prostate [59]. In general, the risk of second malignancy appears to increase with younger age and higher radiation dose. Therefore, in very young patients surgical and ablative techniques should be strongly considered in order to avoid the risk of this rare but potentially life-threatening sequelae of radiotherapy.

Radiation Treatment Results

The data in Table 36.3 summarize results from skin brachytherapy studies that included more than 100 patients. The results of the two randomized studies that included radiotherapy for NMSC, as well as some of the larger published series of BCC and/or SCC treated with commonly employed dose-fractionation regimens, are summarized in Tables 36.4 and 36.5. The reported local control or tumor cure rates were greater than 90% in the majority of studies, with the exception of two studies that exclusively examined tumors located on the ear, and one study which utilized 55–60 kV contact therapy for almost all tumors, including T3–T4 disease [20, 46, 47].

Radiotherapy for Malignant Melanoma

The primary management of melanoma consists of wide surgical excision and management of the nodal basins by sentinel node biopsy or complete lymph node dissection. In general, adjuvant radiotherapy to the primary site is not indicated following wide local excision, but should be considered for desmoplastic melanoma, especially if other risk factors are present such as head and neck location, close margins or deep tumor [60, 61]. Advances in targeted immunotherapies have demonstrated improved outcomes for some patients and are shifting the treatment paradigm [62, 63].

Table 36.3 Outcomes of brachytherapy treatment of non-melanoma skin cancer.

Brachytherapy technique	Tumor location	Dose/fractionation	No. of patients	Outcomes	Study/Reference
Custom mold applicator Iridium-192	Facial	60–65 Gy in 33–36 fractions	136	99% local control at 5 years	Guix *et al.*, 2000 [84]
Custom mold applicator Cesium-137	Nose	24 Gy over 48 h	370	97% local control at 2 years	Debois *et al.*, 1994 [85]
Electronic brachytherapy	Various	40 Gy in 8 fractions	122	100% local control at 10 months	Bhatnagar *et al.*, 2013 [86]
Leipzig applicator Iridium-192	Various	30–40 Gy in 3–10 fractions	520	91% local control at 10 years	Kohler-Brock *et al.*, 1999 [87]
Leipzig applicator Iridium-192	Head and neck	36 Gy in 12 fractions	200	98% local control at 66 months	Gauden *et al.*, 2013 [88]

Adjuvant Lymph Node Irradiation for Melanoma

In a landmark study of adjuvant lymph node radiotherapy versus observation, Henderson and colleagues demonstrated a significant decrease in lymph node relapses with treatment [64]. This multicenter, randomized study included patients who had melanoma with a palpable lymph node treated with lymphadenectomy and were at high risk of recurrence (based on the lymph node region and number of nodes involved). Patients were randomized to regional lymph node irradiation of 48 Gy in 20 fractions, or observation. After a median follow-up of 73 months, the lymph node relapse rate was 36% in the observation group and 21% in the adjuvant radiotherapy group (HR 0.52, p = 0.023). The toxicity profile was acceptable with a 20% incidence of grade 3–4 toxicity predominantly of pain or fibrosis of the skin and subcutaneous tissues. There was no difference in overall survival or relapse-free survival, which led the authors to suggest that adjuvant nodal radiotherapy is useful for regional

Table 36.4 Outcomes of external beam radiotherapy for non-melanoma skin cancer.

Total dose (Gy)	No. of fractions	No. of tumors	Radiation treatment modality	Outcomes	Study/Reference
Prospective randomized studies involving radiotherapy for basal cell carcinoma of the skin					
40–70	Variable	174 surgery; 173 XRT	Brachytherapy (*n* = 95)*; superficial (*n* = 58); or kV (*n* = 20)	92.5% local control; (99.3% surgery group); 4-year f/u	Avril *et al.*, 1997 [15]
35–37.5	5 to 10	44 cryotx; 49 XRT	130 kV	96% local control (61% for cryotx); 2-year f/u	Hall *et al.*, 1986 [9]
Studies evaluating specific dose/fractionation schedule					
18–22.5	1	1005	45–100 kV	90% - 5-year DFS; f/u 6 months to 10 years	Chan *et al.*, 2007 [48]
30.6	3	675	45–100 kV	96% local control; min. f/u 2 years	Abbatucci *et al.*, 1988 [83]
44	10	434	Electrons 4–12 MeV		
54	18			97% local control; median f/u 42.8 months	Van Hezewijk *et al.*, 2010 [27]

Gy, Gray; f/u, follow-up; cryotx, cryotherapy; DFS, disease-free survival; XRT, x-radiotherapy.
The majority of tumors were stage T1–T2N0 and located on the face or elsewhere in the head and neck region.
*Study included some patients treated with skin brachytherapy.

Table 36.5 Outcomes of radiotherapy for non-melanoma skin cancer by anatomic location.

Total dose (Gy)	No. of fractions	Tumor site	No. of tumors	Outcomes	Study/Reference
Studies examining specific anatomic location of tumor					
30.6–70	3 to 35	Nose, nasal vestibule	1676	94% local control, median f/u > 5 years	Mazeron *et al.*, 1988 [89]
30–75	6 to 15	Nose, nasal vestibule	671	88% 5-year cure rate; mean f/u 38 months	Caccialanza *et al.*, 2009 [20]
20–60	1 to 30	Eyelid	1166	95% 5-year local control	Fitzpatrick *et al.*, 1984 [90]
45–70	Variable	Pinna of the ear	111	78% 5-year cure rate; mean f/u 29 months	Caccialanza *et al.*, 2005 [19]
20–60	Variable	Pinna of the ear	313	79% 5-year local control	Silva *et al.*, 2000 [47]
17.5–64	Variable	Pinna of the ear	128	93% 5-year local control	Hayter *et al.*, 1996 [46]
30–60	3 to 30	Lip (subset of series); 99% were SCC	250	94% 5-year local control T1–T2; (62% for T3–T4)	Petrovich *et al.*, 1987 [91]
Other published series, variable anatomic site and dose fractionation					
30–70	3 to 30	Head and neck (excluding lip subset)	646	99% 5-year local control T1; 92% for T2; 60% T3–T4	Petrovich *et al.*, 1987 [91]
45–70	Variable	Not specified	1267	95% local control BCC; 90% SCC; average f/u 77 months	Schulte *et al.* 2005 [92]

The majority of tumors were <5 cm in size; radiation treatment modalities were predominantly kV and electrons.

control, but enrollment in adjuvant systemic therapy trials or surveillance following lymphadenectomy may also be considered [64].

Looking forward, it is conceivable that the goal of radiotherapy in melanoma will be not only locoregional control but also to enhance immunotherapies through abscopal effects. The idea that radiotherapy can induce tumor inhibition in areas far from the treated site has garnered renewed interest in the setting of novel immunotherapies [65, 66]. Pre-clinical and retrospective data suggest a potential for hypofractionated radiotherapy to improve treatment, and early clinical trials are under way to evaluate this innovative approach.

Radiotherapy for Merkel Cell Carcinoma

Merkel cell cancer (MCC) of the skin is a neuroendocrine malignancy characterized by small round blue cells on hematoxylin and eosin staining and an immunohistochemical profile that is positive for CK20 and neuroendocrine markers (synaptophysin, chromogranin A) and typically negative for TTF-1 and CK7. These tumors typically grow quickly and have a high propensity to develop 'in-transit' or satellite nodules en route to regional lymph nodes and distant metastatic sites. The National Cancer Institute (NCI) reports that Merkel cell tumors have a higher mortality rate than malignant melanoma [1]. The initial treatment for these uncommon tumors is

wide local excision with sentinel lymph node biopsy, with completion of nodal dissection as required. Radiotherapy plays a critical role in the management of this challenging and aggressive clinical entity. Although limited prospective data are available, adjuvant radiotherapy should be strongly considered for the primary site and regional lymph nodes in all cases, preferably in the setting of a multidisciplinary team that includes surgical, medical, and radiation oncologists.

Adjuvant Treatment to the Primary Site

To the present authors' knowledge there have been no randomized studies of adjuvant radiotherapy to the primary site for MCC. Lewis *et al.* [67] reported on a large meta-analysis of 132 studies including 1254 patients with a single primary site of MCC who had primary surgery, and approximately one-third of those had adjuvant radiotherapy. Significant decreases in both local (HR = 0.27, $p < 0.001$) and regional (HR = 0.34, $p < 0.001$) recurrence rates were found with the use of adjuvant radiotherapy. Similarly, Mojica *et al.* [68] reviewed patients from the Surveillance Epidemiological and End Results (SEER) database and found similar results; 1487 patients with MCC were included and 40% underwent adjuvant XRT. Despite having a higher incidence of lymph node involvement at diagnosis, patients treated with XRT had a longer overall survival (median 63 versus 45 months, $p = 0.0002$).

Current evidence suggests that almost all patients with MCC treated with surgery alone are at moderate to high risk of local recurrence, and stand to benefit from adjuvant XRT to the primary site. Some studies suggest that MCC with small tumor size and wide surgical margins might be treated with surgery alone [69], but this is an uncommon scenario and it is unclear whether the risk is low enough to warrant no radiotherapy.

Adjuvant XRT to Regional Lymph Nodes

For patients who have lymph node-positive disease, adjuvant XRT should be delivered to the postoperative bed and adjacent nodal basins. Lymph node dissection alone is associated with a high risk of regional recurrences reported in some studies to be 26–37% [69, 70], whereas with surgery and adjuvant XRT the regional recurrence rates are significantly lower at approximately 6–13% [71, 72].

Prophylactic regional nodal irradiation should also be given in cases where the nodes cannot be assessed by sentinel lymph node biopsy or dissection. Jouary *et al.* [73] initiated a randomized study of prophylactic nodal irradiation versus observation for patients with stage I MCC. Although the study was not completed due to increasing use of sentinel node biopsies, results from 83 patients enrolled showed a reduction in regional recurrence from 16.7% in the observation arm compared to 0% in the prophylactic nodal XRT group (p = 0.007) [73].

Finally, for patients who have sentinel lymph node biopsy and pathologically node-negative MCC, adjuvant lymph node irradiation of the axilla and groin can be avoided for primaries located on the limbs. In the head and neck region, cutaneous lymphatic drainage may be unpredictable, aberrant, or include in-transit lesions [74, 75] resulting in false-negative rates with sentinel lymph node biopsy rate of approximately 20% [76]. Therefore, adjuvant nodal XRT must still be considered in cases of head and neck MCC with a negative sentinel lymph node biopsy. The present authors' approach in this challenging setting has been to include at a minimum the adjacent lymphatic drainage sites within 5 cm of the primary skin site, and to consider more extensive nodal irradiation on an individual case-by-case basis.

Chemotherapy

Although the role of platinum-based chemotherapy in the management of MCC is not currently well defined, current knowledge of small-cell carcinoma of the lung as well as the propensity of MCC to spread to distant sites suggests an important role for systemic therapy. In a retrospective, population-level cohort study, Chen *et al.* analyzed 4815 patients with MCC [77]. Compared to surgery alone, overall survival was improved significantly with the addition of adjuvant XRT (HR = 0.80), and even further in patients who underwent adjuvant chemoradiotherapy (HR = 0.62) [77]. Patients who are medically fit for chemotherapy should undergo consultation with the medical oncology team to discuss potential benefits and risks of treatment.

Primary Radiotherapy/Chemotherapy for MCC

In patients with MCC who are unable to have surgery, radiation alone or in combination with chemotherapy may be considered for primary curative treatment for this small-cell tumor. Veness *et al.* reported on 43 patients with a median age of 79 treated with XRT alone for MCC [78]. The in-field control rate was 75%, with most recurrences being distant. Similarly, a prospective study of concurrent chemoradiotherapy by Poulsen *et al.* included 15 patients who did not undergo surgery. The locoregional control rate was 71% at three years [79]. Other studies support the notion that primary radiotherapy is effective with locoregional control rates higher than 70% and the majority of recurrences being at distant metastatic sites [80, 81].

Radiation Target Volumes in MCC

Target volumes for MCC must be determined on an individual case-by-case basis. Local recurrences just beyond the high-dose region are reported [71, 82], suggesting the importance of wide margins beyond the primary GTV in order to encompass in-transit lymphatics and/or satellite skin metastases. Ideally, patients should be seen by the radiation oncologist at the initial presentation such that the exact location of the tumor is documented and available for postoperative planning. If feasible, a CTV margin of 5 cm beyond the primary tumor site or postoperative bed is used with normal anatomic barriers such as bone being excluded from the CTV. Using these generous margins will allow the treatment to encompass in-transit lymphatics surrounding the primary tumor site. Bolus should be used to achieve full dose to the skin surface.

Perineural invasion is known to be a risk factor for local recurrence of SCC of the skin [38]. By the same principle, MCC of the head and neck with involvement of a named nerve or clinical neurological symptoms should be considered high risk, and treatment targeted to include the involved nerves back to their origin/ganglion at the base of skull.

When regional nodal irradiation is planned, the involved region with a minimum of one echelon distal and proximal should be treated. In addition, all of the intervening skin and lymphatic pathways between the primary site and regional nodes should be included in the treatment volumes.

Radiation Dose for MCC

MCC tumors typically respond quickly and sometimes quite dramatically to radiotherapy with relatively low in-field recurrence rates. This apparent radiosensitivity allows the radiation oncology team to target the extensive volumes described above, to a moderate dose which can be tolerated by most patients. There are no prospective studies which evaluate the optimal radiation dose for MCC. Foote *et al.* [82] evaluated the dose–volume relationship in 112 MCC patients treated with XRT. The authors recommended that doses of ≥50 Gy be used for microscopic disease, whereas ≥55 Gy was recommended for macroscopic disease, citing improvement in locoregional control with increasing doses [83]. To the present authors' knowledge, there is no evidence that altered fractionation regimens are advantageous in the setting of MCC, and at their practice adjuvant (microscopic) XRT doses of 50–56 Gy are typically used. Depending on the tumor size, location and the use of chemotherapy, the macroscopic tumor dose varies between 60 and 70 Gy.

Conclusions

Radiotherapy is an effective treatment for NMSCs, and is associated with very high rates of tumor cure. With melanoma, where distant metastases present the greatest threat to patients, the best evidence for radiotherapy is in the setting of adjuvant nodal treatments to decrease locoregional risk. Merkel cell tumors are highly radiosensitive, and treatment to the primary and nodal sites should be considered in all cases and determined on an individual basis.

For the radiation oncologist, skin cancer is an interesting and challenging disease site. Treatment decisions are highly dependent on clinical assessment and knowledge of basic radiation physics of various radiation modalities. Where the expertise and resources are available, skin brachytherapy provides high conformality and excellent local control. Some special considerations in the practice of skin radiation oncology, such as f-factor, the RBE of electrons, and embryological fusion plate locations are discussed widely but not strongly correlated with clinical evidence. Acute and late toxicities are generally well tolerated and the risk of serious or severe side effects is low. Finally, it is interesting to note that, despite the high incidence of skin cancer, there are very few prospective studies examining the optimal use of radiation treatment for these patients. Further studies are required to better understand skin cancer radiobiology, normal tissue tolerance, adjuvant radiotherapy, and the optimal treatment of patients with locally advanced disease.

References

1 National Cancer Institute at National Institutes of Health Website. Available at: http://www.cancer.gov/cancertopics/types/skin. Accessed on 09/20/2015.

2 International Union Against Cancer (UICC) (2009) *TNM Classification of Malignant Tumours*, 7th edition. Wiley-Blackwell.

3 Brantsch, K.D., *et al.* (2008) Analysis of risk factors determining prognosis of cutaneous squamous-cell carcinoma: a prospective study. *Lancet Oncol.*, **9**, 713–720.

4 Kwon, S., Dong, Z.M., Wu, P.C. (2011) Sentinel lymph node biopsy for high-risk cutaneous squamous cell carcinoma: clinical experience and review of literature. *World J. Surg. Oncol.*, **9**, 80.

5 Mosterd, K. *et al.* (2008) Surgical excision versus Mohs' micrographic surgery for primary and recurrent basal-cell carcinoma of the face: a prospective randomised controlled trial with 5-years' follow-up. *Lancet Oncol.*, **9**, 1149–1156.

6 DeVita, V., Rosenberg, S., Lawrence, T. (2005) *Cancer: Principles and Practice of Oncology*, Lippincott Williams & Wilkins.

7 Madan, V., Lear, J.T., Szeimies, R.M. (2010) Non-melanoma skin cancer. *Lancet*, **375**, 673–685.

8 Silverman, M.K., Kopf, A.W., Grin, C.M., Bart, R.S., Levenstein, M.J. (1991) Recurrence rates of treated basal cell carcinomas. Part 2: Curettage-electrodesiccation. *J. Dermatol. Surg. Oncol.*, **17**, 720–726.

9 Hall, V.L., *et al.* (1986) Treatment of basal-cell carcinoma: comparison of radiotherapy and cryotherapy. *Clin. Radiol.*, **37**, 33–34.

10 Stebbins, W.G., Hanke, C.W. (2011) MAL-PDT for difficult to treat nonmelanoma skin cancer. *Dermatol. Ther.*, **24**, 82–93.

11 Arits, A.H., Mosterd, K., Essers, B.A., *et al.* (2013) Photodynamic therapy versus topical imiquimod versus topical fluorouracil for treatment of superficial basal-cell carcinoma: a single blind, non-inferiority, randomised controlled trial. *Lancet Oncol.*, **14** (7), 647–654.

12 Bath-Hextall, F.J., Perkins, W., Bong, J., Williams, H.C. (2007) Interventions for basal cell carcinoma of the skin. *Cochrane. Database. Syst. Rev.* CD003412.

13 Bath-Hextall, F., Ozolins, M., Armstrong, S.J., *et al.* (2014) Surgery versus Imiquimod for Nodular Superficial basal cell carcinoma (SINS) study group. Surgical excision versus imiquimod 5% cream for

nodular and superficial basal-cell carcinoma (SINS): a multicentre, non-inferiority, randomised controlled trial. *Lancet Oncol.*, **15** (1), 96–105.

14 Sekulic, A., Migden, M.R., Oro, A.E., *et al.* (2012) Efficacy and safety of vismodegib in advanced basal-cell carcinoma. *N. Engl. J. Med.*, **366** (23), 2171–2179.

15 Avril, M.F. *et al.* (1997) Basal cell carcinoma of the face: surgery or radiotherapy? Results of a randomized study. *Br. J. Cancer*, **76**, 100–106.

16 Khan, F.M. (2003) *The Physics of Radiation Therapy*. Lippincott Williams & Wilkins, Baltimore, MD, USA.

17 Nguyen, M.T., Billington, A., Habal, M.B. (2011) Osteoradionecrosis of the skull after radiation therapy for invasive carcinoma. *J. Craniofac. Surg.*, **22**, 1677–1681.

18 Atherton, P., Townley, J., Glaholm, J. (1993) Cartilage: the 'F'-factor fallacy. *Clin. Oncol. (R. Coll. Radiol.)*, **5**, 391–392.

19 Caccialanza, M., Piccinno, R., Kolesnikova, L., Gnecchi, L. (2005) Radiotherapy of skin carcinomas of the pinna: a study of 115 lesions in 108 patients. *Int. J. Dermatol.*, **44**, 513–517.

20 Caccialanza, M., Piccinno, R., Percivalle, S., Rozza, M. (2009) Radiotherapy of carcinomas of the skin overlying the cartilage of the nose: our experience in 671 lesions. *J. Eur. Acad. Dermatol. Venereol.*, **23**, 1044–1049.

21 Alasti, H., Galbraith, D.M. (1995) Depth dose flattening of electron beams using a wire mesh bolus. *Med. Phys.*, **22** (10), 1675–1683.

22 Ekstrand, K.E., Dixon, R.L. (1982) The problem of obliquely incident beams in electron-beam treatment planning. *Med. Phys.*, **9**, 276–278.

23 Nikjoo, H., Lindborg, L. (2010) RBE of low energy electrons and photons. *Phys. Med. Biol.*, **55**, R65–R109.

24 Turesson, I., Thames, H.D. (1989) Repair capacity and kinetics of human skin during fractionated radiotherapy: erythema, desquamation, and telangiectasia after 3 and 5 years' follow-up. *Radiother. Oncol.*, **15**, 169–188.

25 Lovett, R.D., Perez, C.A., Shapiro, S.J., Garcia, D.M. (1990) External irradiation of epithelial skin cancer. *Int. J. Radiat. Oncol. Biol. Phys.*, **19**, 235–242.

26 Griep, C., Davelaar, J., Scholten, A.N., Chin, A., Leer, J.W. (1995) Electron beam therapy is not inferior to superficial x-ray therapy in the treatment of skin carcinoma. *Int. J. Radiat. Oncol. Biol. Phys.*, **32**, 1347–1350.

27 van Hezewijk, M., *et al.* (2010) Efficacy of a hypofractionated schedule in electron beam radiotherapy for epithelial skin cancer: Analysis of 434 cases. *Radiother. Oncol.*, **95**, 245–249.

28 Hall, E.J. (2006) Intensity-modulated radiation therapy, protons, and the risk of second cancers. *Int. J. Radiat. Oncol. Biol. Phys.*, **65**, 1–7.

29 Mendenhall, W.M., *et al.* (2007) Skin cancer of the head and neck with perineural invasion. *Am. J. Clin. Oncol.*, **30**, 93–96.

30 Jambusaria-Pahlajani, A., *et al.* (2009) Surgical monotherapy versus surgery plus adjuvant radiotherapy in high-risk cutaneous squamous cell carcinoma: a systematic review of outcomes. *Dermatol. Surg.*, **35**, 574–585.

31 ICRU – International Commission on Radiation Units and Measurements (1993) Prescribing, Recording, and Reporting Photon Beam Therapy (Report 50), Bethesda, MD, USA.

32 Wentzell, J.M., Robinson, J.K. (1990) Embryologic fusion planes and the spread of cutaneous carcinoma: a review and reassessment. *J. Dermatol. Surg. Oncol.*, **16**, 1000–1006.

33 Granstrom, G., Aldenborg, F., Jeppsson, P.H. (1986) Influence of embryonal fusion lines for recurrence of basal cell carcinomas in the head and neck. *Otolaryngol. Head Neck Surg.*, **95**, 76–82.

34 Brierley, J.D., Gospodarowicz, M.K., Wittekind, C. (eds) (2009) *TNM Classification of Malignant Tumours*, 7th edition. Wiley-Blackwell.

35 Choo, R., *et al.* (2005) What is the microscopic tumor extent beyond clinically delineated gross tumor boundary in nonmelanoma skin cancers? *Int. J. Radiat. Oncol. Biol. Phys.*, **62**, 1096–1099.

36 Khan, L., Choo, R., Breen, D., *et al.* (2012) Recommendations for CTV margins in radiotherapy planning for non melanoma skin cancer. *Radiother. Oncol.*, **104** (2), 263–266.

37 Wolf, D.J., Zitelli, J.A. (1987) Surgical margins for basal cell carcinoma. *Arch. Dermatol.*, **123**, 340–344.

38 Gluck, I., *et al.* (2009) Skin cancer of the head and neck with perineural invasion: defining the clinical target volumes based on the pattern of failure. *Int. J. Radiat. Oncol. Biol. Phys.*, **74**, 38–46.

39 Wojcicka, J.B., Lasher, D.E., McAfee, S.S., Fortier, G.A. (2009) Dosimetric comparison of three different treatment techniques in extensive scalp lesion irradiation. *Radiother. Oncol.*, **91**, 255–260.

40 Parsons, J.T., Bova, F.J., Mendenhall, W.M., Million, R.R., Fitzgerald, C.R. (1996) Response of the normal eye to high dose radiotherapy. *Oncology (Williston. Park)*, **10**, 837–847.

41 Mayo, C., *et al.* (2010) Radiation dose-volume effects of optic nerves and chiasm. *Int. J. Radiat. Oncol. Biol. Phys.*, **76**, S28–S35.

42 Amdur, R.J., *et al.* (1992) Radiation therapy for skin cancer near the eye: kilovoltage x-rays versus electrons. *Int. J. Radiat. Oncol. Biol. Phys.*, **23**, 769–779.

43 Shiu, A.S., *et al.* (1996) Dosimetric evaluation of lead and tungsten eye shields in electron beam treatment. *Int. J. Radiat. Oncol. Biol. Phys.*, **35**, 599–604.

44 Emami, B., *et al.* (1991) Tolerance of normal tissue to therapeutic irradiation. *Int. J. Radiat. Oncol. Biol. Phys.*, **21**, 109–122.

45 Marks, L.B., Ten Haken, R.K., Martel, M.K. (2010) Guest editor's introduction to QUANTEC: a user's guide. *Int. J. Radiat. Oncol. Biol. Phys.*, **76** (3 Suppl.), S1–S2.

46 Hayter, C.R., Lee, K.H., Groome, P.A., Brundage, M.D. (1996) Necrosis following radiotherapy for carcinoma of the pinna. *Int. J. Radiat. Oncol. Biol. Phys.*, **36**, 1033–1037.

47 Silva, J.J., Tsang, R.W., Panzarella, T., Levin, W., Wells, W. (2000) Results of radiotherapy for epithelial skin cancer of the pinna: the Princess Margaret Hospital experience, 1982–1993. *Int. J. Radiat. Oncol. Biol. Phys.*, **47**, 451–459.

48 Chan, S., Dhadda, A.S., Swindell, R. (2007) Single fraction radiotherapy for small superficial carcinoma of the skin. *Clin. Oncol. (R. Coll. Radiol.)*, **19**, 256–259.

49 Dupree, M.T., Kiteley, R.A., Weismantle, K., Panos, R., Johnstone, P.A. (2001) Radiation therapy for Bowen's disease: lessons for lesions of the lower extremity. *J. Am. Acad. Dermatol.*, **45**, 401–404.

50 Cox, N.H., Dyson, P. (1995) Wound healing on the lower leg after radiotherapy or cryotherapy of Bowen's disease and other malignant skin lesions. *Br. J. Dermatol.*, **133**, 60–65.

51 Pignol, J.P., *et al.* (2008) A multicenter randomized trial of breast intensity-modulated radiation therapy to reduce acute radiation dermatitis. *J. Clin. Oncol.*, **26**, 2085–2092.

52 Salvo, N., *et al.* (2010) Prophylaxis and management of acute radiation-induced skin reactions: a systematic review of the literature. *Curr. Oncol.*, **17**, 94–112.

53 Kumar, S., Juresic, E., Barton, M., Shafiq, J. (2010) Management of skin toxicity during radiation therapy: a review of the evidence. *J. Med. Imaging Radiat. Oncol.*, **54**, 264–279.

54 Herst, P.M., Bennett, N.C., Sutherland, A.E., Peszynski, R.I., Paterson, D.B., Jasperse, M.L. (2014) Prophylactic use of Mepitel Film prevents radiation-induced moist desquamation in an intra-patient randomised controlled clinical trial of 78 breast cancer patients. *Radiother. Oncol.*, **110** (1), 137–143.

55 Hindley, A., Zain, Z., Wood, L., *et al.* (2014) Mometasone furoate cream reduces acute radiation dermatitis in patients receiving breast radiation therapy: results of a randomized trial. *Int. J. Radiat. Oncol. Biol. Phys.*, **90** (4), 748–755.

56 Ulff, E., Maroti, M., Serup, J., Falkmer, U. (2013) A potent steroid cream is superior to emollients in reducing acute radiation dermatitis in breast cancer patients treated with adjuvant radiotherapy. A randomised study of betamethasone versus two moisturizing creams. *Radiother. Oncol.*, **108** (2), 287–292.

57 Smith, G.L., *et al.* (2008) Cerebrovascular disease risk in older head and neck cancer patients after radiotherapy. *J. Clin. Oncol.*, **26**, 5119–5125.

58 Scott, A.S., Parr, L.A., Johnstone, P.A. (2009) Risk of cerebrovascular events after neck and supraclavicular radiotherapy: a systematic review. *Radiother. Oncol.*, **90**, 163–165.

59 Travis, L.B., *et al.* (2012) Second malignant neoplasms and cardiovascular disease following radiotherapy. *J. Natl Cancer Inst.*, **104**, 357–370.

60 Strom, T., Caudell, J.J., Han, D., *et al.* (2014) Radiotherapy influences local control in patients with desmoplastic melanoma. *Cancer*, **120**, 1369–1378.

61 Guadagnolo, B.A., Prieto, V., Weber, R., *et al.* (2014) The role of adjuvant radiotherapy in the local management of desmoplastic melanoma. *Cancer*, **120**, 1361–1368.

62 Larkin, J., Chiarion-Sileni, V., Gonzalez, R., *et al.* (2015) Combined Nivolumab and Ipilimumab or Monotherapy in Untreated Melanoma. *N. Engl. J. Med.*, **373** (1), 23–34.

63 Hodi, F.S., O'Day, S.J., McDermott, D.F., *et al.* (2010) Improved survival with ipilimumab in patients with metastatic melanoma. *N. Engl. J. Med.*, **363** (8), 711–723.

64 Henderson, M.A., Burmeister, B.H., Ainslie, J., *et al.* (2015) Adjuvant lymph-node field radiotherapy versus observation only in patients with melanoma at high risk of further lymph-node field relapse after lymphadenectomy (ANZMTG 01.02/TROG 02.01): 6-year follow-up of a phase 3, randomised controlled trial. *Lancet Oncol.*, **16** (9),1049–1060.

65 Postow, M.A., Callahan, M.K., Barker, C.A., *et al.* (2012) Immunologic correlates of the abscopal effect in a patient with melanoma. *N. Engl. J. Med.*, **366** (10), 925–931.

66 Reynders, K., Illidge, T., Siva, S., Chang, J.Y., De Ruysscher, D. (2015) The abscopal effect of local radiotherapy: using immunotherapy to make a rare event clinically relevant. *Cancer Treat. Rev.*, **41** (6), 503–510.

67 Lewis, K.G., Weinstock, M.A., Weaver, A.L., Otley, C.C. (2006) Adjuvant local irradiation for Merkel cell carcinoma. *Arch. Dermatol.*, **142** (6), 693–700.

68 Mojica, P., Smith, D., Ellenhorn, J.D.I. (2007) Adjuvant radiation therapy is associated with improved survival in Merkel cell carcinoma of the skin. *J. Clin. Oncol.*, **25** (9), 1043–1047.

69 Allen, P.J., Bowne, W.B., Jaques, D.P., Brennan, M.F., Busam, K., Coit, D.G. (2005) Merkel cell carcinoma: prognosis and treatment of patients from a single institution. *J. Clin. Oncol.*, **23** (10), 2300–2309.

70 Veness, M.J., Perera, L., McCourt, J., Shannon, J., Hughes, T.M., Morgan, G.J., Gebski, V. (2005) Merkel cell carcinoma: improved outcome with adjuvant radiotherapy. *Aust. N. Z. J. Surg.*, **75** (5), 275–281.

71 Lok, B., Khan, S., Mutter, R., *et al.* (2012) Selective radiotherapy for the treatment of head and neck Merkel cell carcinoma. *Cancer*, **118** (16), 3937–3944.

72 Veness, M.J. (2005) Merkel cell carcinoma: improved outcome with the addition of adjuvant therapy. *J. Clin. Oncol.*, **23** (28), 7235–7236.

73 Jouary, T., Leyral, C., Dreno, B., *et al.* (2012) Adjuvant prophylactic regional radiotherapy versus observation in stage I Merkel cell carcinoma: a multicentric prospective randomized study. *Ann. Oncol.*, **23** (4), 1074–1080.

74 Klop, W.M.C., Veenstra, H.J., Vermeeren, L., Nieweg, O. E., Balm, A.J.M, Lohuis, P.J.F.M. (2011) Assessment of lymphatic drainage patterns and implications for the extent of neck dissection in head and neck melanoma patients. *J. Surg. Oncol.*, **103** (8), 756–760.

75 Lin, D., Franc, B.L., Kashani-Sabet, M., Singer, M.I. (2006) Lymphatic drainage patterns of head and neck cutaneous melanoma observed on lymphoscintigraphy and sentinel lymph node biopsy. *Head Neck*, **28** (3), 249–255.

76 de Rosa, N., Lyman, G.H., Silbermins, D., *et al.* (2011) Sentinel node biopsy for head and neck melanoma: a systematic review. *Otolaryngol. Head Neck Surg.*, **145** (3), 375–382.

77 Chen, M.M., Roman, S.A., Sosa, J.A., Judson, L. (2015) The role of adjuvant therapy in the management of head and neck Merkel cell carcinoma: an analysis of 4815 patients. *JAMA Otolaryngol. Head Neck Surg.*, **141** (2), 137–141.

78 Veness, M.J., Morgan, G.J., Gebski, V. (2005) Adjuvant locoregional radiotherapy as best practice in patients with Merkel cell carcinoma of the head and neck. *Head Neck*, **27** (3), 208–216.

79 Poulsen, M., Rischin, D., Walpole, E., *et al.* (2003) High-risk Merkel cell carcinoma of the skin treated with synchronous carboplatin/etoposide and radiation: a trans-Tasman Radiation Oncology Group study-TROG 96:07. *J. Clin. Oncol.*, **21** (23), 4371–4376.

80 Fang, L.C., Lemos, B., Douglas, J., Iyer, J., Nghiem, P. (2010) Radiation monotherapy as regional treatment for lymph node-positive Merkel cell carcinoma. *Cancer*, **116** (7), 1783–1790.

81 Pape, E., Rezvoy, N., Penel, N., *et al.* (2011) Radiotherapy alone for Merkel cell carcinoma: a comparative and retrospective study of 25 patients. *J. Am. Acad. Dermatol.*, **65** (5), 983–990.

82 Foote, M., Harvey, J., Porceddu, S., *et al.* (2010) Effect of radiotherapy dose and volume on relapse in Merkel cell cancer of the skin. *Int. J. Radiat. Oncol. Biol. Phys.*, **77** (3), 677–684.

83 Abbatucci, J.S., Boulier, N., Laforge, T., Lozier, J.C. (1989) Radiation therapy of skin carcinomas: results of a hypofractionated irradiation schedule in 675 cases followed more than 2 years. *Radiother. Oncol.*, **14**, 113–119.

84 Guix, B., Finestres, F., Tello, J., *et al.* (2000) Treatment of skin carcinomas of the face by high-dose-rate brachytherapy and custom-made surface molds. *Int. J. Radiat. Oncol. Biol. Phys.*, **47** (1), 95–102.

85 Debois, J.M. (1994) Cesium-137 brachytherapy for epithelioma of the skin of the nose: experience with 370 patients. *J. Belge. Radiol.*, **77** (1), 1–4.

86 Bhatnagar, A. (2013) Nonmelanoma skin cancer treated with electronic brachytherapy: Results at 1 year. *Brachytherapy*, **12** (2), 134–140.

87 Köhler-Brock, A., Prager, W., Pohlmann, S., Kunze, S. [The indications for and results of HDR afterloading therapy in diseases of the skin and mucosa with standardized surface applicators (the Leipzig applicator)]. *Strahlenther. Onkol.*, **175** (4), 170–174.

88 Gauden, R., Pracy, M., Avery, A.M., Hodgetts, I., Gauden, S. (2013) HDR brachytherapy for superficial non-melanoma skin cancers. *J. Med. Imaging Radiat. Oncol.*, **57** (2), 212–217.

89 Mazeron, J.J., *et al.* (1988) Radiation therapy of carcinomas of the skin of nose and nasal vestibule: a report of 1676 cases by the Groupe Europeen de Curietherapie. *Radiother. Oncol.*, **13**, 165–173.

90 Fitzpatrick, P.J., Thompson, G.A., Easterbrook, W.M., Gallie, B.L., Payne, D.G. (1984) Basal and squamous cell carcinoma of the eyelids and their treatment by radiotherapy. *Int. J. Radiat. Oncol. Biol. Phys.*, **10**, 449–454.

91 Petrovich, Z., Parker, R.G., Luxton, G., Kuisk, H., Jepson, J. (1987) Carcinoma of the lip and selected sites of head and neck skin. A clinical study of 896 patients. *Radiother. Oncol.*, **8**, 11–17.

92 Schulte, K.W., *et al.* Soft x-ray therapy for cutaneous basal cell and squamous cell carcinomas. *J. Am. Acad. Dermatol.*, **53**, 993–1001.

37

Cancer of the Breast

Jonathan B. Strauss, Monica Morrow and William Small Jr

Introduction

The aim of the present chapter is to serve as a primer on the treatment of breast cancer with radiotherapy. As space constraints necessitate brevity, the chapter is focused on the results of randomized trials. Clear guidelines for standard practice are stated where available. Only statistically significant differences between treatment arms are presented in the text unless otherwise stated.

Epidemiology

Breast cancer is the most common malignancy of women in the United States (excluding non-melanoma skin cancers). In the US in 2017, an estimated 252 710 women will be diagnosed with invasive breast cancer, and 63 410 women will be diagnosed with *in situ* breast cancer [1]. In the US, breast cancer will account for 29% of all cancer diagnoses in women, and will yield the second highest total of cancer-related deaths at 40 610, representing 14% of all cancer deaths in women. In addition, an estimated 2470 men will be diagnosed with breast cancer, comprising approximately 1% of all cases.

Anatomy

The breast, or mammary gland, is an apocrine gland of the female that produces milk. It is composed primarily of fat in which are embedded glandular milk-producing lobules. The lobules are connected by a network of ducts that coalesce at the nipple. Glandular breast tissue extends anteriorly to the dermis and posteriorly to the pectoralis fascia. Suspensory ligaments of the breast, or Cooper's ligaments, extend from the clavipectoral fascia to the dermis.

The lymphatic drainage of the breast is primarily to the axillary, supraclavicular (SCV) and internal mammary (IM) nodal chains. In traditional nomenclature, the axilla is composed of three anatomic divisions: level I extends laterally and inferiorly to the pectoralis minor muscle; level II lies beneath this muscle (and includes the interpectoral, or Rotter's nodes); and level III extends medially and superiorly to the pectoralis minor muscle and is alternatively referred to as the infraclavicular fossa [2]. The IM lymph nodes are found along the IM artery and vein at the lateral edge of the sternum. The majority of IM nodes are found in the first three intercostal spaces between the first and fourth ribs.

Staging

The current breast cancer staging system in widespread use is the American Joint Committee on Cancer (AJCC) TNM staging system. The 2017 (8th edition) edition staging system is shown in Figure 37.1 [3].

Pathology

Carcinoma *in situ*

Carcinoma *in situ* of the breast, or non-invasive breast cancer, is a term that denotes a clonal proliferation of cells that do not penetrate the basement membrane. It is an umbrella category that includes three established subtypes: Paget's disease; lobular carcinoma *in situ* (LCIS), and ductal carcinoma *in situ* (DCIS). The incidence of carcinoma *in situ* has been rising, mostly attributable to an increase in mammographic screening and subsequent biopsies [4].

Paget's Disease

Paget's disease of the breast, first elucidated by Sir James Paget, is characterized by the presence of malignant

Clinical Radiation Oncology: Indications, Techniques, and Results, Third Edition. Edited by William Small Jr.

Definition of Primary Tumor (T) – Clinical and Pathological

T Category	T Criteria
TX	Primary tumor cannot be assessed
T0	No evidence of primary tumor
Tis(DCIS)*	Ductal carcinoma in situ
Tis(Paget)	Paget disease of the nipple NOT associated with invasive carcinoma and/or carcinoma in situ in the underlying breast parenchyma. Carcinomas in the breast parenchyma associated with Paget disease are categorized based on the size and characteristics of the parenchymal disease, although the presence of Paget should be noted
T1	Tumor ≤20 mm in greatest dimension
T1mi	Tumor ≤1 mm in greatest dimension
T1a	Tumor >1 mm but ≤5 mm in greatest dimension
T1b	Tumor >5 mm but ≤10 mm in greatest dimension
T1c	Tumor >10 mm but ≤20 mm in greatest dimension
T2	Tumor >20 mm but ≤50 mm in greatest dimension
T3	Tumor >50 mm in greatest dimension
T4	Tumor of any size with direct extension to the chest wall and/or to the skin (ulceration or macroscopic nodules); invasion of the dermis alone is not T4
T4a	Extension to the chest wall; invasion or adherence to pectoralis muscle in the absence of invasion of chest wall structures does not qualify as T4
T4b	Ulceration and/or ipsilateral macroscopic satellite nodules and/or edema (including peau d'orange) of the skin that does not meet the criteria for inflammatory carcinoma
T4c	Both T4a and T4b are present
T4d	Inflammatory carcinoma

*Lobular carcinoma in situ (LCIS) is a benign entity and is removed from TNM staging

Definition of Regional Lymph Nodes – Clinical

cN Category	cN Criteria
cNX*	Regional lymph nodes cannot be assessed (e.g., previously removed)
cN0	No regional lymph node metastases (by imaging or clinical examination)
cN1	Metastases to movable ipsilateral Level I, II axillary lymph node(s)
cN1mi**	Micrometastases (approximately 200 cells, larger than 0.2 mm, but noe larger than 2.0 mm)
cN2	Metastases in ipsilateral Level I, II axillary lymph nodes that are clinically fixed or matted; or in ipsilateral internal mammary nodes in the absence of axillary lymph node metastases
cN2a	Metastases in ipsilateral Level 1, II axillary lymph nodes fixed to one another (matted) or to other structures
cN2b	Metastases only in ipsilateral internal mammary nodes in the absence of axillary lymph node metastases
cN3	Metastases in ipsilateral infraclavicular (Level III axillary) lymph node(s) with or without Level I, II axillary lymph node involvement; or in ipsilateral internal mammary lymph node(s) with Level I, II axillary lymph node metastases; or metastases in ipsilateral supraclavicular lymph node(s) with or without axillary or internal mammary lymph node involvement.
cN3a	Metastases in ipsilateral infraclavicular lymph node(s)
cN3b	Metastases in ipsilateral internal mammary lymph node(s) and axillary lymph node(s)
cN3c	Metastases in ipsilateral supraclavicular lymph node(s)

Note: (sn) and (f) suffixes should be added to the N category to denote confirmation of metastasis by sentinel node biopsy or FNA/core needle biopsy respectively.
*The cNX category is used sparingly in cases where regional lymph nodes have previously been surgically removed or where there is no documentation of physical examination of the axilla.
**cN1mi is rarely used but may be appropriate in cases where sentinel node biopsy is performed before tumor resection, most likely to occur in cases treated with neoadjuvant therapy.

Definition of Regional Lymph Nodes – Pathological

pN Category	pN Criteria
pNX	Regional lymph nodes cannot be assessed (e.g., not removed for pathological study or previously removed)
pN0	No regional lymph node metastasis identified or ITCs only
pN0(+)	ITCs only (malignant cell clusters no larger than 0.2 mm) in regional lymph node(s)
pN0(mo1+)	Positive molecular findings by reverse transcriptase polymerase chain reaction (RT-PCR); no ITCs detected
pN1	Micrometastases; or metastases in 1-3 axillary lymph nodes; and/or clinically negative internal mammary nodes with micrometastases or macrometastases by sentinel lymph node biopsy
pN1mi	Micrometastases (approximately 200 cells, larger than 0.2 mm, but none larger than 2.0 mm)
pN1a	Metastases in 1-3 axillary lymph nodes, at least one metastasis larger than 2.0 mm.
pN1b	Metastases in ipsilateral internal mammary sentinel nodes, excluding ITCs
pN1c	pN1a and pN1b combined
pN2	Metastases in 4-9 axillary lymph nodes; or positive ipsilateral internal mammary lymph nodes by imaging in the absence of axillary lymph node metastases
pN2a	Metastases in 4-9 axillary lymph nodes (at least one tumor deposit larger than 2.0 mm)
pN2b	Metastases in clinically detected internal mammary lymph nodes with or without microscopic confirmation; with pathologically negative axillary nodes
pN3	Metastases in 10 or more axillary lymph nodes; or in infraclavicular (Level III axillary) lymph nodes; or positive ipsilateral internal mammary lymph nodes by imaging in the presence of one or more positive Level I, II axillary Lymph nodes; or in more than three axillary lymph nodes and micrometastases or macrometastases by sentinel lymph node biopsy in clinically negative ipsilateral internal mammary lympho nodes; or in ipsilateral supraclavicular lymph nodes
pN3a	Metastases in 10 or more axillary lymph nodes (at least one tumor deposit larger than 2.0 mm); or metastases to the infraclavicular (Level III axillary lymph) nodes
pN3b	pN1a or pN2a in the presence of cN2b (positive internal mammary nodes by imaging); or pN2a in the presence of pN1b
pN3c	Metastases in ipsilateral supraclavicular lymph nodes

Note: (sn) and (f) suffixes should be added to the N category to denote confirmation of metastasis by sentinel node biopsy or FNA/core needle biopsy respectively with NO further resection of nodes.

Definition of Distant Metastasis (M)

M category	M Criteria
M0	No clinical or radiographic evidence of distant metastases*
cM0(i+)	No clinical or radiographic evidence of distant metastases in the presence of tumor cells or deposits no larger than 0.2 mm detected microscopically or by molecular techniques in circulating blood, bone marrow, or other nonregional nodal tissue in a patient without symptoms or signs of metastases
M1	Distant metastases detected by clinical and radiographic means (cM) and/or histologically proven metastases larger han 0.2 mm (pM).

*Note that imaging studies are not required to assign the cM0 category.

Note: Within the U.S., the AJCC mandates the use of the Prognostic Stage Group system when biomarker tests are available. This system is too elaborate for inclusion in the text due to space constraints. Please see the AJCC Cancer Staging Manual, 8th edition, for more detail.

Figure 37.1 American Joint Committee on Cancer (AJCC) TNM staging system for breast cancer (8th edition). *Source*: AJCC Cancer Staging Manual, Eighth Edition (2017), Springer, New York, Inc.

epithelial breast cancer cells within the epidermis. It presents clinically as a pruritic, erythematous, eczematous, crusting rash over the nipple and areola. This disease entity appears to represent epidermotropic behavior of cells from an underlying breast malignancy [5]. A focus of intraparenchymal breast malignancy – either invasive carcinoma or DCIS – can be identified in the vast majority of cases of Paget's disease of the breast, in which case the disease is staged based on the underlying lesion [6, 7].

Lobular Carcinoma *in situ*

LCIS is characterized microscopically by the presence of a discohesive clonal proliferation of epithelial cells filling the acinar space. On molecular analysis, LCIS cells are typically estrogen receptor- and progesterone receptor-positive, exhibit the loss of the E-cadherin gene (*CDH1*) expression and rarely show Her-2/Neu amplification [8, 9]. The protein product of the *CDH1* gene is a cellular adhesion molecule, and its absence may explain the classic morphology of this disease entity, in which the cells infiltrate in individual rows. Classic LCIS is rarely detectable via mammography as it is not typically associated with calcifications. Similarly, it does not form a palpable mass. Instead, its detection most often represents an incidental finding on tissue biopsy or excision. Classically, LCIS is thought to represent a marker for a higher risk of developing invasive breast cancer. LCIS is not typically considered a premalignant lesion in its own right, although some data exist to suggest that it may be a non-obligate precursor lesion [10]. Women with known LCIS are at approximately eightfold the risk of the general population of developing an invasive breast cancer in the future [11]. An elevated risk of breast cancer is found for both the ipsilateral and contralateral breasts [12].

A subset of LCIS with distinctive histopathologic features, termed pleomorphic LCIS, comprises a small minority of cases. This entity is characterized by the presence of large, pleomorphic and dyscohesive cells with eccentric nuclei and, often, comedo necrosis [13]. Although no clear consensus exists, very limited evidence suggests that pleomorphic LCIS may follow a more aggressive clinical course and represent a true precursor lesion that can progress into an invasive cancer [14].

Ductal Carcinoma *in situ*

DCIS represents a spectrum of disease entities sharing the characteristics of clonal proliferation of breast epithelial cells contained within the basement membrane of the duct. Although controversy exists, DCIS is thought to be a non-obligate precursor of invasive carcinoma. DCIS is an umbrella category that includes several histologic subtypes based on their predominant microscopic growth pattern: comedo, solid, micropapillary, papillary, and cribriform [15]. The comedo subtype appears

to carry a higher risk of local recurrence than other subtypes when radiation is not given, and has a shorter time to recurrence when radiation is used [16]. DCIS rarely presents as a palpable mass; instead, it is often associated with microcalcifications and is typically identified on mammography. The incidence of DCIS has been climbing over the past three decades, likely due to the advent of radiographic screening [4].

Invasive Ductal Carcinoma

Invasive ductal carcinomas (IDCs) comprise the vast majority of all invasive breast carcinomas. The nomenclature 'ductal' is used in reference to the cytologic features of the malignancy, and is not a claim on its cell of origin. IDC includes the standard ductal subtype as well as special histologic subtypes: medullary, mucinous, and tubular. Medullary carcinomas are characterized by pathognomonic histologic features: a syncytial growth pattern; stromal infiltration by lymphoplasmacytic infiltrate; and sparse necrosis [17]. Mucinous carcinoma is defined by the presence of extracellular mucin admixed with tumor cells [18]. Tubular carcinomas exhibit ovoid tubules or glands with a single layer of epithelial cells. These cells are typically well-differentiated and of low histologic grade [19]. The presence of any of these special histologic subtypes appears to confer a superior prognosis as compared to other invasive carcinomas [17, 20].

Invasive Lobular Carcinoma

Invasive lobular carcinoma (ILC) comprises 5–10% of all invasive breast carcinomas [21]. ILC is characterized by small uniform malignant cells that appear in a single-file pattern [22]. The invasive lobular phenotype appears to be related to the loss of expression of the E-cadherin adhesion molecule [23]. Given these histological characteristics, on physical examination ILC is often associated not with a mass but as an area of thickening or induration. Some series suggest that ILC may be more likely to be multifocal [24].

Intact-Breast Radiotherapy

Background

Breast-conserving therapy (BCT) consists of breast-conserving surgery followed by radiotherapy. BCT is one of the most thoroughly studied therapies in oncology, and is a standard of care in the treatment of eligible patients. Preservation of the breast offers an improved quality of life as compared to mastectomy [25, 26]. The following section is applicable to BCT for both DCIS and early-stage invasive breast cancer.

Imaging

The work-up of breast cancer should certainly include mammography and ultrasound of the tumor site. The role of whole-breast ultrasound and magnetic resonance imaging (MRI) is controversial and evolving. MRI may offer increased sensitivity in detecting mammographically occult lesions; however, a meta-analysis of the impact of MRI on surgical outcomes such as margin status and unexpected conversion to mastectomy showed that, after age adjustment, although MRI triples the rate of initial mastectomy it does not reduce the incidence of positive margins or unplanned mastectomy [27]. The details of this work-up are beyond the scope of this chapter. The utility of mammography performed after lumpectomy to ensure the removal of all suspicious abnormalities is not yet clear. Some series show a very low yield of mammography in this setting [28]. By contradistinction, other studies have suggested a higher yield for post-lumpectomy mammography [29]. A large series from Yale found a lower rate of in-breast tumor recurrence (IBTR) in those patients with documented removal of all calcifications [30]. The present authors' institutional practice has been to obtain post-lumpectomy mammograms for all women with radiographically detected calcifications on preoperative imaging.

Eligibility Criteria

Both breast-conserving surgery and radiotherapy are (typically) obligate components of BCT. Therefore, eligibility for BCT is usually contingent upon a patient's ability to receive both treatments. Exclusion criteria for BCT are summarized in Table 37.1. Exclusion criteria for radiotherapy can include prior radiotherapy to the breast, pregnancy, active collagen vascular disease (CVD) and ataxia-telangiectasia. Prior irradiation of the affected breast precludes the use of radiotherapy and is considered an absolute contraindication to BCT. Of note, RTOG 1014, a Phase II trial evaluating partial breast

Table 37.1 Contraindications to breast-conserving therapy.

Absolute contraindications	Relative contraindications
Prior breast radiotherapy	Active lupus or scleroderma
Pregnancy	Large tumor-to-breast ratio
Ataxia-telangiectasia	Deleterious *BRCA* mutation
Diffuse malignant calcifications	Microscopic focally positive margin
Persistent positive margins	
Widespread disease throughout breast	

re-irradiation, may lead to some alteration of this iron-clad rule in the future. The exquisite radiosensitivity of the human fetus mandates that pregnant women not undergo radiotherapy until after delivery [31, 32]. If this would create an unacceptable delay in treatment, then BCT cannot be accomplished. Historically, active CVD has been thought to predispose for greater radiotherapy-related skin toxicity. The largest retrospective series available suggests that this effect may be limited to late toxicity in non-rheumatoid CVD, most notably scleroderma [33–35]. Other series have found contradictory results. Uncertainty remains over the influence of CVD on late toxicity of radiotherapy [36]. Exclusion criteria for undergoing successful breast-conserving surgery include: diffuse malignant appearing calcifications throughout the breast; an inability to achieve a negative margin due to tumor extent; and very large tumor size – especially a large tumor in relation to a small breast. However, large unicentric tumors can often be downsized with neoadjuvant chemotherapy in patients desiring BCT.

Several series have shown that age is a consistent prognostic factor for IBTR [37–39], and this remains true after controlling for other known prognostic factors. Therefore, it might be concluded that BCT is contraindicated in very young women (variably defined, but often meaning those aged <35 years). Yet, emerging data show that young women also have a higher risk of locoregional recurrence (LRR) after mastectomy, which suggests that mastectomy alone may not be a better alternative. A series from the MD Anderson Cancer Center (MDACC) reported on LRR in a population of 652 women aged <35 years [40]. In women with stage I disease, there was no difference in LRR between BCT and mastectomy, but in women with stage II disease a multivariate analysis showed only grade 3 disease, the omission of chemotherapy, and the receipt of mastectomy predicted for a higher rate of LRR. A Dutch series of 1453 women aged <40 years yielded very similar results: the 10-year overall survival was equivalent between mastectomy and BCT for node-negative women, but favored BCT for women with N1 disease [41]. Given these data, and in light of the plentitude of randomized data supporting the equivalence of BCT and mastectomy with regards to survival, BCT remains an acceptable standard of care for young women.

BRCA mutation carriers present a particular challenge to BCT. Some series have found a higher rate of metachronous contralateral breast cancer, but no increase in ipsilateral recurrence, after BCT in *BRCA* mutation carriers [42, 43]. In one large series of women with *BRCA* mutations undergoing BCT, the 10-year rate of IBTR was 13.6%, whereas the 10-year rate of metachronous contralateral breast cancer was 37.6% [42]. Other series have found that both ipsilateral and contralateral breast cancers are more common, in equal proportion [43–46]. In summary, women with deleterious *BRCA* mutations appear to have satisfactory tumor control after BCT, but have a significant risk of developing a metachronous primary breast cancer. This risk is modified by age of onset of the initial cancer, oophorectomy, and adjuvant endocrine therapy, and these factors should be considered when deciding if BCT or bilateral mastectomy is an appropriate approach.

Surgery

A description of the technical details of breast surgery is beyond the scope of this chapter, but a brief definition of terms may be helpful. Breast-conserving surgery is a term that encompasses any surgical procedure that removes the malignancy (ideally with negative margins) and preserves the remainder of the breast. This includes quadrantectomy, in which a quadrant of the breast tissue is removed along with the overlying skin and underlying fascia, as well as lumpectomy, tylectomy, or partial mastectomy in which the tumor and variable amounts of normal breast parenchyma are removed.

Limited axillary dissection denotes the removal of levels I and II of the axilla, whereas complete dissection denotes removal of levels I, II, and III. The latter is usually reserved for patients with a large number of grossly positive nodes intraoperatively. Axillary dissection as a staging procedure has been supplanted by the sentinel lymph node biopsy (SLNB), a procedure that involves the injection of a radiotracer and/or dye into the breast in order to identify, and remove, the first echelon of draining lymph nodes. The SLNB reduces the risk of upper-extremity lymph edema and dysfunction and improves quality of life as compared to the axillary dissection [47–49]. Randomized trials comparing axillary dissection for all women versus SLNB followed by axillary dissection only for those women found to be node-positive have shown equivalent regional control, disease-free survival, and overall survival between the two approaches [50–52]. More recently, the ACOSOG Z0011 trial has shown equivalent regional control, disease-free survival and overall survival for SLNB alone as compared to completion axillary lymph node dissection for clinically node-negative women undergoing breast-conserving

surgery with one or two positive sentinel nodes [53, 54]. Of note, all women in this study received whole-breast radiotherapy in the supine position, which likely included level 1 of the axilla in the radiotherapy fields.

BCT for Ductal Carcinoma *In Situ*

Local Treatment

Historically, mastectomy was the traditional treatment for ductal carcinoma *in situ* (DCIS). This therapy is very successful with recurrence rates of only 1–2% [55]. In DCIS, BCT has never been compared to mastectomy in a randomized trial, nor is such a study likely to be performed. Instead, multiple studies in invasive cancer have shown the equivalence of BCT and mastectomy with regard to survival (see section on BCT for early-stage breast cancer for details), and these results have been extrapolated to DCIS. Additionally, large series with long follow-up have confirmed very low cause-specific mortality for women treated with BCT for DCIS. For these reasons, BCT has emerged as a standard treatment for DCIS despite the absence of randomized trials establishing equivalence to mastectomy.

Intact-Breast Radiotherapy

The role of radiotherapy after excision for DCIS in unselected women has been evaluated in four randomized trials [56–60]. In each trial, women with DCIS treated with breast-conserving surgery were randomized to receive either radiotherapy or observation. Relatively few of these women received tamoxifen. The results of these trials are summarized in Table 37.2. In summary, radiotherapy after breast-conserving surgery for DCIS yields a relative reduction in the risk of an IBTR of 50–60%. The individual data from all four randomized trials were pooled in a meta-analysis that included 3729 women. The use of radiotherapy reduced the risk of an IBTR at 10 years by 15.2% (12.9% versus 28.1%) [61]. A subset of patients that derived no benefit from radiotherapy was not identified. No survival advantage has been established by prospective studies for the addition of radiotherapy, although none of the available trials have

Table 37.2 Randomized trials comparing breast-conserving surgery for DCIS with and without radiotherapy (RT).

Study/Reference(s)	No. of patients	Follow-up (years)	I-IBTR (RT, no RT)	D-IBTR (RT, no RT)	All IBTR (RT, no RT)
NSABP B17 [56]	813	15	9%, 19%	9%, 16%	
UK/ANZ [57]	1030	10	3%, 9%	4%, 10%	7%, 19%
EORTC 10853 [58, 59]	1010	15	10%, 16%	8%, 15%	18%, 31%
SweDCIS [60]	1046	20	HR 0.87 for RT	HR 0.33 for RT	20%,32%

EORTC, European Organization for Research and Treatment of Cancer; D-IBTR, DCIS in-breast tumor recurrence; I-IBTR, invasive in-breast tumor recurrence; NSABP, National Surgical Adjuvant Breast and Bowel Project; UK/ANZ, United Kingdom, Australia and New Zealand.

had sufficient statistical power to make firm conclusions. It is possible that a small survival advantage for the use of intact-breast radiotherapy for DCIS may exist given the reduction in invasive recurrences [62]. A recent SEER analysis found a small reduction in breast cancer mortality associated with the use of RT in higher risk DCIS but not lower risk DCIS using patient age, tumor size and histologic grade in a prognostic index [63].

Endocrine Therapy

In the NSABP B-24 study, enrolled women with DCIS were treated with breast-conserving surgery followed by radiotherapy and then randomized to receive tamoxifen or placebo over five years [56]. Of note, estrogen receptor (ER) and progesterone receptor (PR) assessment was not an eligibility criterion. The addition of tamoxifen reduced the 15-year cumulative incidence of invasive breast recurrence from 10% to 8.5%, while the 15-year cumulative incidence of contralateral breast events (*in situ* or invasive) was reduced from 10.8% to 7.3%. This dataset was subsequently re-analyzed after central laboratory review had confirmed ER and PR status in 732 patients (41% of the original population) [64]. In women with ER-positive DCIS, tamoxifen reduced the rate of any subsequent breast cancer at 10 years (HR 0.49), but no benefit was seen in women with ER-negative DCIS.

The UK/ANZ trial enrolled women in a trial with a quasi 2 × 2 factorial design, randomizing them to radiotherapy, tamoxifen, both, or neither [57]. Some women were enrolled in only one of the two randomizations per institutional preference. In this trial, tamoxifen had no effect on invasive IBTR but reduced the risk of *in-situ* IBTR (HR 0.7) and reduced contralateral breast events (HR 0.44). The randomized data concerning tamoxifen in BCT for DCIS are summarized in Table 37.3. New data have emerged regarding the role of aromatase inhibitors (AIs) in the treatment of DCIS. NSABP B-35 and IBIS-II trial each randomized postmenopausal women with ER- or PR-positive DCIS undergoing breast-conserving therapy to 5 years of either tamoxifen or anastrazole. In NSABP B-35, there were fewer breast cancer events in the anastrazole arm (HR 0.73), although on subset analysis this effect appeared to be limited to women under the age of 60 [65]. Although the anastrazole arm

had numerically fewer breast events in the IBIS-II trial, it did not reach statistical significance [66]. On subset analysis, there were significantly fewer subsequent ER-positive events in the anastazole arm (HR 0.55). In both trials, the rates of adverse events were similar between the arms, but the type of events differ between agents. Both tamoxifen and anastrazole appear to be effective for postmenopausal women with ER-positive DCIS and consideration should be given to the side effect profile when choosing an endocrine agent.

Prognostic Factors

As established in the randomized trials discussed above, radiotherapy after breast-conserving surgery for DCIS yields a relative reduction in the risk of an IBTR of 50–60%. However, the absolute value of this risk reduction depends, in part, on the baseline risk of IBTR. Several series have evaluated the prognostic value of various clinical and pathologic features. A summary of the findings of large series is available in Table 37.4.

Age

Subset analysis of pooled data from NSABP B-17 and B-24 found that age under 45 years was associated with an elevated risk of IBTR (HR 2.14) [56]. Similarly, the European Organization for Research and Treatment of Cancer (EORTC) 10853 found a higher risk of IBTR in women aged under 40 years (HR 1.89) [58]. A multi-institution series with long follow-up of 1003 women found that age over 50 years strongly predicted for a lower rate of IBTR [67].

Grade

The SweDCIS trial and EORTC 10853, as well as several meta-analyses, have found an association between high nuclear grade and a higher risk of IBTR [58, 60]. Of note, grade appears to be more prognostic in the absence of radiotherapy. Additionally, the time course of recurrence of low-grade DCIS appears to be more protracted than high-grade disease. The difference in recurrence rates of low- and high-grade DCIS may decrease over time.

Method of Detection

Subset analyses of randomized trials were consistent in showing that clinical detection (as opposed to

Table 37.3 Randomized trials comparing breast-conserving therapy for DCIS with and without tamoxifen.

Study/Reference	No. of patients	Follow-up (years)	I-IBTR (Tam, no Tam)	D-IBTR (Tam, no Tam)	All IBTR (Tam, no Tam)
NSABP B24 [56]	1804	10	5%, 7%	6%, 7%	
UK/ANZ [57]	1576	10	7%, 7%*	9%, 12%	16%, 20%

D-IBTR, DCIS in-breast tumor recurrence; I-IBTR, invasive in-breast tumor recurrence; NSABP, National Surgical Adjuvant Breast and Bowel Project; UK/ANZ, United Kingdom, Australia and New Zealand; Tam, Tamoxifen.
*Not statistically different.

Table 37.4 Adverse prognostic factors for IBTR after breast-conserving surgery for DCIS.

Study/Reference	Factor(s) of higher risk of IBTR
NSABP [56]	Age <45 years, clinical presentation, comedo necrosis (in absence of RT), (+) margin
EORTC 10853 [58]	Age ≤40 years, grade 2–3, uncertain margins, clinical presentation
SweDCIS [60]	Grade 3, necrosis
Solin *et al.* [67]	Age <50 years, (+) margin
Wang *et al.* (Review) [72]	Comedo necrosis, multifocality, (+) margin, clinical presentation, grade 3, large size
Boyages *et al.* (Review) [55]	Grade 3, comedo subtype, close or (+) margin
Dunne *et al.* (Review) [73]	Close or (+) margin, young age, # of excisions, year of surgery, margin status, family history [68]

RT, radiotherapy.

radiographic detection) was associated with a higher risk of IBTR [56, 58]. A very large single institution series from MSKCC replicated this finding [68]. The underlying reason for this association is unknown but may be related to the stromal response that yields a palpable mass in the setting of DCIS.

Gene Profiling

The assessment of IBTR risk after excision alone for DCIS using only clinical and pathologic features is limited. The incorporation of gene profiling data offers the possibility of improved prognostication. Early data using the Oncotype DX assay on a subset of patients from ECOG 5194 suggests the utility of this recurrence score in predicting the risk of an invasive IBTR [69]. In this highly selected group of women with DCIS, not receiving RT, the Oncotype Dx DCIS assay offered modest additional prognostic information in addition to well-established clinical variables. A similar analysis was performed on a larger and less selected population-based cohort from Ontario, Canada [70]. In this seres, the Oncotype Dx DCIS score again added modest prognostic information in addition to multiple clinical variables including size, multifocality, age, and histologic subtype. The questionable cost-effectiveness of this additional prognostic information may be one obstacle to widespread adoption of this test [71]. The ECOG-ACRIN E4112 trial will evaluate the feasibility of omitting radiotherapy in women with a low-risk DCIS Oncotype score (<39).

Surgical Margin Status

Data from NSABP B-24, which allowed positive surgical margins, suggest that a positive margin status is associated with a higher risk of IBTR in women not receiving tamoxifen. The finding that close or positive margins are associated with a higher risk of IBTR has been replicated in several multi-institution reviews and meta-analyses [56, 67, 72, 73]. A meta-analysis identified 4660 patients treated with breast-conserving surgery and radiotherapy in published trials and found that margin-negativity was associated with a lower risk of IBTR compared to the presence of a positive margin (OR 0.36), while margins of 2 mm or more were superior to margins of <2 mm (OR 0.53) [73]. There did not appear to be any advantage for margins greater than 2 mm. This is reflected in the most current ASTRO-ASCO guidelines regarding margin status in DCIS, in which a preference is expressed for 2 mm clear margins, but the routine practice re-excision to achieve margins wider than 2 mm is discouraged [74].

Excision Alone

Many attempts have been made to identify subgroups of patients with DCIS at sufficiently low risk of IBTR that radiotherapy can be safely omitted. In most cases, the use of traditional patient and tumor characteristics has been relatively unsuccessful at identifying a very low-risk group. In a meta-analysis of randomized trials, women with negative margins and small, low-grade tumors had an absolute 10-year reduction in IBTR of 18% with the addition of radiotherapy [61].

A single-institution prospective series conducted by Dana Farber enrolled women with grade 1 or 2 DCIS, measuring 2.5 cm or smaller, with clear margins of at least 1 cm, treated with breast-conserving surgery alone without tamoxifen or radiotherapy [75]. Although the initial accrual goal was 200, the number of local recurrences exceeded stopping rules after 157 patients were enrolled. In total, 13 patients had a local recurrence for a five-year rate of IBTR of 12.5%. Of note, a subset of patients with a minor component of high grade DCIS accounted for a high proportion of these early recurrences. A multi-institution prospective single-arm trial, ECOG 5194, enrolled women with grade 1 or 2 DCIS measuring 2.5 cm or smaller, as well as women with grade 3 DCIS measuring 1 cm or smaller [76]. To be eligible, the women were treated with breast-conserving surgery with clear margins measuring 3 mm or greater. The women enrolled on this study comprised a very favorable subset of patients. In both groups, the median age was approximately 60 years, median tumor size was 5–6 mm, and margins were wider than 1 cm in half of the patients. Approximately 30% of women in both groups indicated an intention to take tamoxifen over a five-year period. The five-year rate of IBTR was 6.1% in the grade 1 or 2 group, and 15.3% in the grade 3 group. At seven years the IBTR rates were 10.5% and 18%, respectively. Although the IBTR rate in the grade 1–2 group was favorable, a longer follow-up is needed to confirm these results. In some series with longer follow-up, the rate of IBTR in women with low- to intermediate-grade DCIS climbed steadily over time, ultimately nearing parity with high-grade disease [77].

RTOG 98-04 enrolled women with favorable DCIS as defined similarly to the grade 1–2 group in ECOG 5194. The study was closed early due to poor accrual, but preliminary data have been published [78]. Of a planned 1790 patients, 636 were randomized to receive either 50 Gy in 25 fractions to the breast or no radiotherapy. Tamoxifen was used in 62% of women. At seven years, the rates of IBTR were 0.9% in the radiotherapy arm and 6.7% in the observation arm. In sum, RT after excision of DCIS always reduces the risk of IBTR including the risk of invasive cancer recurrence. However, some women are at very low baseline risk for recurrence, rendering the benefit of RT very small. For these women, a discussion of patient preference concerning the pros and cons of RT is advisable.

Hypofractionation

In most trials, DCIS was treated with 50 Gy to the whole breast in 2-Gy fractions. Although women with an *in situ* component were allowed in the large randomized trials of hypofractionation, those with pure DCIS were excluded. The use of hypofractionated radiotherapy in DCIS has been evaluated in a retrospective series from the Princess Margaret Hospital, with early results suggesting equivalence between whole-breast radiotherapy delivered using a standard or hypofractionated regimens [79]. This question is currently the subject of a randomized trial from the Trans-Tasman Radiation Oncology Group (TROG) [80].

Boost

The role of a lumpectomy bed boost in DCIS has not been evaluated in a randomized trial as of yet. Some clinicians advocate for a boost, extrapolating from trials in the setting of invasive disease (see section on BCT for early-stage breast cancer). A multicenter retrospective series included 373 women with DCIS, aged 45 years and younger, treated with breast-conserving surgery [81]. The addition of a boost to whole-breast radiotherapy resulted in a significant reduction in IBTR. By contrast, an unpublished review of NSABP B-24 evaluated the impact of boost (assigned in a non-randomized fashion)

on IBRT and found no reduction in IBTR after controlling for other known prognostic factors [82]. The utility of a boost for DCIS is still uncertain. However, two currently accruing trials – the French BONBIS trial and a TROG trial – are addressing this question in a randomized format [80, 83].

Salvage

Overall, breast-cancer specific survival in DCIS is extremely high. Even after IBTR, salvage offers favorable long-term outcomes. A multi-institution series of 90 women with local ($n = 85$) or regional ($n = 5$) recurrence after BCT for DCIS reported a10-year rate of freedom from distant metastases of 91% [84]. Invasive IBTR and nodal recurrences were adverse prognostic factors. In a pooled analysis of women treated on NSABP B17 and B24, the cumulative probability of a breast-cancer related death at 10 years after IBTR was 10.4% for invasive recurrence, and 2.7% for *in situ* recurrence [56].

Section Summary

- DCIS can be treated with BCT with excellent long-term breast cancer-specific mortality.
- Radiotherapy reduces the relative risk of IBTR by 50–60%.
- No survival advantage for radiotherapy in the setting of DCIS has been identified, but available trials were not powered for this endpoint.
- Young age, and, likely, high nuclear grade are associated with higher rates of IBTR.
- Surgery that achieves negative margins and the use of radiotherapy are both associated with lower risks of IBTR.
- All patients exhibit a local control benefit from RT, although some subsets of women are at low baseline risk of recurrence.
- The role of hypofractionated whole-breast radiotherapy and the benefit of a boost have not yet been elucidated in the treatment of DCIS.
- Endocrine therapy provides an additional reduction in the rate of IBTR in ER-positive DCIS and reduces the risk of contralateral breast cancer.

BCT for Early-Stage Breast Cancer

Support for BCT

Decades ago, mastectomy was the standard of care for early-stage breast cancer. Starting in the early 1970s, several trials began to enroll patients and randomize them to mastectomy versus breast-conserving surgery followed by radiotherapy (Table 37.5). Most of these trials now

Table 37.5 Randomized trials comparing breast-conserving therapy (BCT) and radiotherapy (RT) to mastectomy without RT.

Trial/Reference	No. of patients	Tumor size (cm)	Follow-up (years)	Stage	Systemic Tx	OS (BCT versus Mast)[†]
Milan I [85]	701	≤2	20	I	CMF	58%, 59%
IGR [86]	179	≤2	22	I	None	RR 0.7*
NSABP B-06 [87]	1217	≤4	20.7	I–II	Mel/F	46%, 47%
NCI [88]	237	≤5	25.7	I–II	AC	38%, 44%
EORTC 10801 [89]	868	≤5	22.1	I–II	CMF	39%, 45%
DBCG-82TM [90]	793	T1–T3	19.6	I–III	CMF or Tam	58%, 51%

IGR, Institut Gustave-Roussy; NSABP, National Surgical Adjuvant Breast and Bowel Project; NCI, National Cancer Institute; EORTC, European Organization for Research and Treatment of Cancer; DBCG, Danish Breast Cancer Cooperative Group; CMF, cytoxan, methotrexate, 5-fluorouracil; Mast, mastectomy; Mel/F, melphalan, 5-fluorouracil; AC, adriamycin, cytoxan; Tam, tamoxifen.
[†]None reached statistical significance.
*RR = 0.7 in favor of BCT (not statistically significant).

have more than 20 years' follow-up and all confirm that BCT yields long-term overall survival (OS) equivalent to mastectomy [85–90]. These results have been confirmed in a meta-analysis of randomized trials [91]. In summary, these findings have clearly established BCT as a standard of care for early-stage breast cancer.

Role of Intact-Breast Radiotherapy

The contribution of radiotherapy to outcomes in BCT has been studied in great detail. Several large trials have enrolled women with stage I and II breast cancer treated with breast-conserving surgery and randomized them to radiotherapy versus observation [87, 92–98] (Table 37.6). The type of limited surgery, inclusion criteria, and systemic therapy regimens varied widely. Consistently, the omission of radiotherapy resulted in a dramatic increase in the rate of IBTR. In every trial, the difference in local recurrence between the radiotherapy and observation arms persists over time with decades of follow-up. The largest of these trials with long follow-up is NSABP B-06, which enrolled women with primary tumors ≤4 cm in size and randomized them to one of three treatment arms: mastectomy, lumpectomy alone, or lumpectomy

and radiotherapy [87]. All women underwent axillary dissection, and those with positive nodes received chemotherapy. The rate of IBTR after a 20-year follow-up was 39% in the lumpectomy-alone arm versus 14% in the lumpectomy and radiotherapy arm.

No single trial established a benefit in OS for intact-breast radiotherapy. A meta-analysis of the Early Breast Cancer Trialists' Collaborative Group (EBCTCG) evaluated individual patient data for 10 801 women enrolled in 17 randomized trials of BCT [99]. In the population as a whole at 15 years of follow-up, radiotherapy reduced the risk of any recurrence from 35% to 19%, the risk of breast cancer death by 4%, and the risk of all-cause mortality by 3%. The finding that intact-breast radiotherapy improves OS provides the most compelling argument for its inclusion as an integral component of BCT in early-stage breast cancer.

Omission of Radiotherapy in Select Groups

The trials summarized in Table 37.6 enrolled relatively unselected women. The question of whether these results apply equally to women at low risk for IBTR has been the subject of considerable study. Several trials have enrolled

Table 37.6 Randomized trials comparing breast-conserving surgery with and without radiotherapy (RT) in relatively unselected patients.

Trial/Reference	No. of patients	Tumor size (cm)	Follow-up (years)	Systemic Tx	LRR (w/ versus w/o RT)
NSABP B-06 [87]	1137	≤4	20.7	Mel/F	14%, 39%
Uppsala-Orebro [92]	381	≤2	10	None	9%, 24%
Milan III [93]	579	<2.5	10	CMF, Tam	6%, 24%
Scottish [94]	585	≤4	5.7	CMF, Tam	6%, 25%
British [95]	400	≤5	13.7	CMF, Tam	29%, 50%
OCOG [96]	837	≤4	7.6	None	11%, 35%
Swedish [97]	1187	Stage I–II	5	Mixed	4%, 14%
Finnish [98]	152	<2	12.1	None	12%, 27%

NSABP, National Surgical Adjuvant Breast and Bowel Project; OCOG, Ontario Clinical Oncology Group; CMF, cytoxan, methotrexate, 5-fluorouracil; Mel/F, melphalan, 5-fluorouracil; Tam, tamoxifen.

Table 37.7 Randomized trials comparing breast-conserving surgery with and without radiotherapy (RT) in highly selected patients.

Trial/Reference(s)	No. of patients	Tumor size (cm)	Follow-up (years)	Age (years)	Systemic tx	LRR (w/ versus w/o RT)
NSABP B-21 [100]	668	≤1	8	Any	Tam	3%, 17%
Ontario [101]	769	≤5	5	≥50	Tam	1%, 8%
CALGB 9343 [102, 103]	636	≤2	10.5	≥70	Tam	2%, 8%
GBCSG-V [104]	347	≤2	9.9	45–75	Tam (2×2 design)	RR 0.36*
BASO II [105]	1158	<2	10.2	<70	Tam (2×2 design)	8%, 22%† 2%, 8%‡
ABCSG [106]	869	<3	5	PM	Tam or AI	0.4%, 5.1%
PRIME II [107]	658	≤3	5	≥65	Tam or AI	1.8%, 5.6%#

ABCSG: Austrian Breast and Colorectal Study Group; CALGB, Cancer and Leukemia Group B; GBCSG, German Breast Cancer Study Group; BASO, British Association of Surgical Oncology; PM, Postmenopausal; Tam, Tamoxifen.
*RR = 0.36 in favor of RT without Tam versus no RT without Tam.
†RT without Tam versus no RT without Tam.
‡RT with Tam versus no RT with Tam.
#Rates of LR and RR were summed for this total.

women thought to be at low risk for recurrence, typically restricting eligibility to women with older age and smaller tumor size who received tamoxifen [100–107] (Table 37.7). Most of these trials have failed to indentify a subset of women at sufficiently low risk for recurrence that omission of radiotherapy is acceptable. NSABP B-21 enrolled node-negative women with tumors ≤1 cm excised by lumpectomy with negative margins [100]. The majority of tumors were hormone receptor-positive, and 80% of the women were aged ≥50 years. Women were randomized to one of three treatment arms: tamoxifen alone; radiotherapy alone; or both radiotherapy and tamoxifen. The eight-year risks of IBTR were 16.5%, 9.3%, and 2.8%, respectively. Thus, even highly selected women with small tumors receiving tamoxifen exhibited an eight-year IBTR rate exceeding 16% in the absence of radiotherapy.

By contrast, a CALGB study restricted enrollment to women ages >70 years with ER-positive tumors measuring 2 cm or smaller [102, 103]. All participants received tamoxifen and were randomized to intact-breast radiotherapy versus observation. At the 10-year follow-up, the risk of IBTR was 9% (LRR of 10%) without radiotherapy versus 2% with radiotherapy. At the last follow-up, 53% of the participating women had died and only 6% of those deaths were from breast cancer. Given the relatively low rate of IBTR, coupled with the high risk of death from comorbid conditions, omission of radiotherapy in this highly select group may be reasonable. Eligible women should engage in a conversation regarding the risks and benefits of this approach.

Risk Factors for IBTR

Several patient and tumor-related factors are associated with the risk of IBTR. Some of these risk factors are well established; others have contradictory evidence concerning their prognostic value. The risk factors for

IBTR after BCT for early-stage breast cancer are summarized in Table 37.8.

Margin Status

The presence of a positive margin is a consistent marker for an elevated risk of IBTR [108–111]. For this reason, current clinical practice involves orientation of the surgical specimen and careful histologic evaluation to assess microscopically involved margins. In most cases, re-excision of a positive margin is standard practice. However, there is not clear evidence that widely free margins are associated with a lower risk of local recurrence than negative margin as defined by no tumor on ink. A meta-analysis of 14 571 patients adjusted for use of a radiation boost and endocrine therapy showed no difference in outcome based on margins of 1 mm or less compared to more widely clear margins [112]. A similar meta-analysis of study-level data adjusted for covariates found that while a positive (as compared to negative) margins status was associated with a higher risk of local recurrence (OR = 2.44), there was no clear effect for a reduction in the odds of local recurrence for increasing margin distance [113]. While selected patients may benefit from more widely clear margins, the use of arbitrary margin width definitions promotes unnecessary re-excision surgery. New consensus guidelines on margin

Table 37.8 Adverse prognostic factors for IBTR after breast-conserving surgery for early-stage breast cancer.

Clearly prognostic	Probably prognostic	Possibly prognostic
Margin status	Tumor size	Nodal status
Histologic grade	Biological subtype	LVI
Patient age	Gene profile	EIC
Systemic therapy		Lobular histology

LVI, Lymphovascular invasion; EIC, Extensive intraductal component.

status for breast-conserving surgery from SSO_ASTRO support 'no ink on tumor' as the standard adequate margin in invasive cancer [114].

Grade

Grade is less well established as a prognostic factor, though some evidence of the influence of grade on IBTR is found in the EORTC study of the role of a boost [115]. On multivariate analysis, the presence of high-grade disease yielded a hazard ratio of IBTR of 1.67.

Age

As stated above, several series have established young age as a clear risk factor for IBTR, as well as for the development of a metachronous contralateral breast primary [37–39, 115].

Size

Some support exists for the influence of tumor size in IBTR. Notably, a multivariate analysis of two European trials found that tumors >2 cm had a relative risk for IBTR of 2.88 as compared to tumors 1 cm or smaller [37].

Systemic Therapy

The use of endocrine therapy reduces the risk of IBTR for hormone receptor-positive tumors [104, 105]. The EBCTCG meta-analysis found that the use of tamoxifen reduced the risk of local recurrence in hormone receptor-positive disease by approximately one-half (RR = 0.47) [116]. Similarly, the use of systemic chemotherapy also reduces LRR. The same EBCTCG meta-analysis found that polychemotherapy regimens reduced the risk of local recurrence by approximately one-third. Further, more intensive chemotherapy appears to yield an even greater reduction in local recurrence. CALGB 9344 randomized women to receive adriamycin and cytoxan with or without sequential taxol. A post-hoc evaluation of this randomized trial found that women treated with BCT experienced a five-year risk of LRR of 12.9% in the adriamycin and cytoxan arm, as compared to 6.1% in the adriamycin, cytoxan, and taxol arm [117]. This advantage in IBTR was seen despite the additional delay between surgery and radiotherapy necessitated by chemotherapy delivery. The addition of trastuzumab to chemotherapy further reduces LR (HR = 0.47) in women with amplification of the Her-2/Neu receptor [118].

Biological Subtype

Biologic subtype – clinically approximated by ER, PR, and her-2/neu (Her-2) – is an emerging factor that has both prognostic value for the risk of IBTR and predictive value for the efficacy of radiotherapy. The descriptive nomenclature of biological subtypes is complex and in flux. In a simplified version, the gene expression profile that segregates to 'luminal A' is associated with ER positivity, Her-2 negativity, and low to intermediate histologic grade; 'luminal B' is associated with ER positivity and high-grade; 'basal-like' with ER, PR, and Her-2 negativity (triple negative) and high-grade, and 'Her-2' with Her-2 amplification, ER negativity, and high grade [119].

A series from Harvard of 1223 women treated with BCT found the risk of IBTR at five years to be 4.4% in triple-negative tumors, 9% in ER/PR-negative and H2N-positive tumors, and 0.2% in ER- or PR-positive tumors [120]. A series of women treated with BCT from the British Columbia Cancer Agency found that women with ER/PR negativity and H2N over-expression (treated before the trastuzumab era), as well as those with triple-negative status, had higher risk of LRR as compared with those for ER/PR-positive tumors [121]. However, this pattern of increased local recurrence in patients with triple-negative cancers and those overexpressing HER2 and not receiving trastuzumab is also seen after treatment with mastectomy, indicating that biologic subtype is not a selection factor for BCT versus mastectomy. Hormone receptor negativity is not only associated with a higher baseline risk of recurrence, but also a proportionately smaller reduction in LR in response to radiotherapy. The smaller relative reduction in risk of LR for radiotherapy was seen in the most recent EBCTCG meta-analysis [99]. This finding mirrors a retrospective analysis from the Danish Breast Cancer Cooperative Group (DBCG) [122], in which the relative reduction in LRR was smaller for ER/PR-negative tumors (both H2N over-expressed and triple-negative) as compared to ER/PR-positive tumors. Whether this effect persists in the era of modern systemic therapies, including taxanes and targeted therapies (e.g., traztuzumab), which may exhibit synergy with radiotherapy, is not clear.

Gene Profile

The Oncotype Dx is a multi-gene array that assesses a panel of 21 genes within a tumor to assign a recurrence score that predicts the risk of distant recurrence in women with ER-positive, node-negative breast cancer treated with tamoxifen. The association between recurrence score and LRR was assessed in a retrospective review of NSABP B-14 and B-20 [123]. The 10-year LRR risks in women with low, intermediate, and high recurrence scores were 4%, 7%, and 16%, respectively. The use of appropriate systemic therapy in the high-risk group (tamoxifen plus chemotherapy) was effective in reducing LRR. Several other institutional series using different gene-expression arrays have reported significant prognostic value with regard to LRR [124–126].

Other Factors

Other factors, such as nodal positivity, the presence of lymphovascular invasion, an extensive intraductal component, or a tumor of lobular histology, may prognosticate a higher risk of IBRT, although available data are conflicting.

Tumor Bed Boost

As established above, whole-breast radiotherapy to approximately 50 Gy dramatically reduces, but does not eliminate, the risk of IBTR. Conceptually, one can consider dose escalation to further reduce the risk of recurrence, but the whole-breast dose is has not been increased due to potential toxicities. Large series have shown that the majority of IBTRs after BCT appear near the tumor bed [87, 92, 93]. Given this pattern of recurrence, the value of a tumor bed boost, or more targeted escalation of dose, has been evaluated in randomized trials.

A trial from Lyon, France, enrolled 1024 women with tumors ≤3 cm treated with breast-conserving surgery followed by intact-breast radiotherapy to 50 Gy in 20 fractions [127]. Participants were randomized to receive an additional 10 Gy boost versus no further radiotherapy. The addition of a boost reduced the risk of a local recurrence at five years from 4.5% to 3.6%, but was associated with an increase in the risk of grade 1 and 2 telangiectasia.

An EORTC trial enrolled 5318 women with stage I or II breast cancer who were treated with margin-negative surgery and whole-breast radiotherapy to 50 Gy in 25 fractions [128, 129]. Participants were randomized to receive an additional 16 Gy boost versus no further radiotherapy. The 10-year LR rate was reduced from 10.2% to 6.2% by addition of the boost, but this improvement in LR came at the cost of severe fibrosis, which was increased from 1.6% to 4.4%. Although a benefit in LR was noted in every age group, the boost yielded a larger absolute benefit in women aged ≤40 years. A post-hoc analysis review found that the benefit of a boost was also quite large in women with high-grade histology (18.9% versus 8.6%) [115]. The EORTC launched a parallel trial for those with tumors excised with positive margins, and randomized them to a boost of 10 Gy versus 26 Gy [130]. The 10-year local recurrence risk was numerically reduced from 17.5% to 10.8% by the larger boost, but this difference did not reach statistical significance. The rate of severe fibrosis was larger in the 26-Gy arm.

Nodal Radiotherapy

Classically, the treatment of invasive breast cancer included an axillary lymph node dissection. This procedure provides prognostic information, guides management decisions (most notably, concerning the use of systemic therapy), and removes a potential reservoir of disease. In a meta-analysis, axillary dissection

improved OS, with the caveat that most of the trials included in this analysis omitted systemic therapy and radiotherapy [131]. As discussed above, in modern practice, management of the clinically node-negative axilla begins with SLNB. Regional nodal irradiation (RNI) can be used instead of, or as an adjunct to, surgical dissection of the axilla. The therapeutic options and techniques will be discussed in brief.

Axillary/SCV Radiotherapy After Surgery

Traditionally, after a level I and II axillary dissection, radiotherapy to the undissected axillary apex (level III) and the SCV fossa is clearly indicated if metastases are present in four or more lymph nodes. The full axilla (levels I–III) can be included in the radiotherapy field if risk factors for residual disease are found, such as fixed or matted nodes, gross extracapsular extension (ECE) or inflammatory breast cancer. Otherwise, exclusion of the dissected axilla from the radiotherapy field is preferred in order to reduce toxicity. Although radiation of the SCV fossa is routine, the design of the radiotherapy field(s) varies greatly across institutions. Relatively little information is available on the patterns of failure in this area to guide field design. An anatomic map is available from the M.D. Anderson Cancer Center, which merges the location of 52 identified involved SCV nodes from breast cancer onto a single image set [132]. The locations of SCV failure suggest that coverage may be inadequate at the medial and posterior extent of the traditional SCV field.

In the setting of one to three positive nodes identified on axillary dissection, there is controversy over the necessity of RNI. Several retrospective series have evaluated the risk of nodal recurrences in this patient population. Most of these series have found a relatively low risk of nodal recurrence, although young age, high-grade histology, ER/PR negativity, LVI, and ECE may predispose for a higher risk [133–136].

The NCIC MA-20 trial enrolled high-risk node-negative or node-positive women treated with BCT with axillary dissection, and randomized them to whole-breast radiotherapy or whole-breast radiotherapy plus RNI to the axillary apex, SCV fossa, and upper three intercostal spaces of the internal mammary chain [137]. The dissected axilla was included if fewer than 10 nodes were dissected or more than three nodes were involved. Of the 1832 women enrolled, 85% had one to three positive nodes and 10% were node-negative. The vast majority of the women on this trial received systemic therapy; combination chemotherapy was administered to 91%, and endocrine therapy to 76%. The addition of RNI to whole-breast radiotherapy improved the 10-year rates of LRR (95.2% versus 92.2%), and improved DFS (82% versus 77%) and dDFS (86.3% versus 82.4%). There was no significant difference in OS (82.8% versus 81.8%), although in the prespecified subset of ER-negative patients there was an improvement in OS (81.3% versus 73.9%). RNI was associated with increases in both lymphedema (8.5% versus 4.5%) and pneumonitis (1.2% versus 0.2%). There was no difference in the rates of cardiac morbidity or mortality, or non-breast cancer death.

The EORTC 22922/10925 trial performed a similar randomization for women with stage I–III breast cancer [138]. A total of 4004 patients with either node-positive breast cancer (56%) or a medially located tumor (44%) was treated with mastectomy or breast-conserving surgery; all underwent axillary dissection. The vast majority of patients received adjuvant systemic therapy (node-positive 99%, node-negative 66%), receiving radiotherapy to the breast or chest wall as per institution standards, and were then randomized to RNI (50 Gy to the IM chain and SCV fossa) versus no nodal radiotherapy. RNI was associated with an improved 10-year DFS (72.1% versus 69.1%, HR = 0.89) and 10-year dDFS (78% versus 75%), and reduced breast cancer mortality (12.5% versus 14.4%). The difference in 10-year OS (82.3% versus 80.7%) did not achieve statistical significance (p = 0.06). The benefit of treatment was independent of all stratification factors, although there appeared to be a larger benefit in women who received both chemotherapy and endocrine therapy. There was no evidence of increased non-breast cancer death or second cancers. RNI was associated with an increase in the risk of pulmonary fibrosis (4.4% versus 1.7%).

Axillary Radiotherapy versus Surgery

Given the morbidity associated with axillary dissection, the efficacy of radiotherapy used in lieu of surgery has been, and continues to be, a subject of study. The foundational breast cancer trial NSABP B-04 enrolled 1079 women with clinically negative axillary nodes, and randomized them to one of three arms: total mastectomy alone with delayed axillary dissection for nodal recurrence; radical mastectomy (including axillary nodal dissection); or total mastectomy and radiotherapy to the chest wall and draining lymphatics [139]. The rates of regional recurrence as the site of first failure were 6%, 4%, and 4%, respectively, and with 25 years of follow-up no survival differences were observed. Although the rate of nodal involvement in the axillary dissection arm was 40%, only 18.6% of the women in the total mastectomy arm ultimately presented with clinically apparent axillary nodal disease, even in this pre-adjuvant therapy era study. The Institut Curie enrolled 658 women with clinically negative nodes and tumors <3 cm who were treated with breast-conserving surgery, and randomized them to axillary dissection versus axillary radiotherapy [140]. At 15-years, the rate of axillary recurrence was 1% versus 3% in favor of the axillary dissection arm, although no difference in survival was found.

Radiotherapy after SLNB

After a positive SLNB, the traditional practice has been to proceed to an axillary dissection. In this case, surgical clearance of the axilla rarely contributes to decisions concerning systemic therapy, but is instead solely intended to aid in the control of axillary disease. The ability of radiotherapy to control axillary disease in lieu of surgery after SLNB is a topic of considerable study. The ACOSOG Z0011 trial enrolled women undergoing breast-conserving surgery and SLNB with one or two positive axillary nodes, and randomized them to either axillary node dissection or no further surgery [53, 54]. All women received intact breast radiotherapy in the supine position, and the trial protocol prohibited the use of a separate nodal field. There was no difference in regional recurrence, DFS or OS between the two arms. Additionally, the risk of regional nodal recurrence was very low in both arms. After trial completion, an attempt was made to ascertain the extent of radiotherapy nodal coverage in treated patients [141]. Of the 605 patients with a completed radiotherapy form, 89% received the mandated whole-breast radiotherapy, and 15% received a supraclavicular field. Of 142 patients for whom in-depth radiotherapy data are available, 51% received 'high tangent' fields, defined as having a superior border within 2 cm of the humeral head.

The EORTC AMAROS trial 10981/22023 enrolled 4823 women with clinical T1-2N0 breast cancer, and those women with positive SLNB (n = 1425) were randomized to axillary dissection versus axillary radiotherapy [142]. The five-year rate of axillary recurrence was 0.43% in the axillary dissection arm, and 1.19% in the axillary radiotherapy arm. There was no difference in DFS or OS between the arms. The rates of clinical signs of lymphedema at one year and five years were higher after axillary dissection (28% and 23%) than after axillary radiotherapy (15% and 11%). A post-hoc analysis suggested that fewer patients in the axillary dissection group reported difficulties in moving the ipsilateral arm.

Internal Mammary Radiotherapy

Early surgical series found a relatively high rate of involvement of the internal mammary (IM) nodes, especially in patients with multiple positive axillary nodes and tumors located in the medial aspect of the breast [143, 144]. The IM chain within the upper three intercostal spaces is considered to be at highest risk of nodal involvement. The relevance of these series to patients in the modern era, in which the majority have mammographically detected early stage cancers, is not clear. The interest in radiotherapy to the IM chain is due largely to the robust survival advantage seen in trials of post-mastectomy radiotherapy that included the IM chain in addition to the chest wall, axilla, and SCV fossa [145–148]. The contribution to the survival benefit seen in those studies that was attributable to treating the IM nodal chain is not clear.

A single randomized trial has evaluated the role of radiotherapy to the IM nodes [149]. Women with tumors in the medial breast and any nodal status, and those with tumors in the outer breast and positive axillary nodes, were enrolled. Participants were treated with mastectomy and randomized to receive radiotherapy to the chest wall, axilla, and SCV fossa, with or without radiotherapy to the IM nodes in the upper five intercostal spaces. The study was powered to detect a 10% difference in 10-year OS. Preliminary data showed a 10-year OS of 62.6% in the arm with radiotherapy to the IM nodes versus 59.6% in the arm without radiotherapy to the IM nodes (p = 0.88). Whether the absence of a difference reflects a lack of benefit or inadequate statistical power of this trial is unclear. Recommendations regarding IM nodal radiotherapy remain controversial. If performed, techniques to minimize normal tissue dose are important.

Timing of Radiotherapy

Chemotherapy and radiotherapy each have been established as important adjunctive treatments in breast cancer. The optimal timing and sequence of these treatments have been the subject of study.

Concurrent Chemoradiotherapy

The ARCOSEIN trial enrolled women with stage I or II breast cancer treated with breast-conserving surgery and randomized them to concurrent versus sequential chemotherapy (mitoxantrone, 5-FU, cyclophosphamide) and radiotherapy [150]. There were no differences in outcomes between these arms with the exception that, in women with node-positive disease, the five-year LRR-free survival favored concurrent chemoradiotherapy (97% versus 91%). Physician ratings of cosmetic outcome were worse for women in the concurrent arm, although patient ratings were not different [151].

A French trial enrolled 638 women with node-positive breast cancer treated with breast-conserving surgery and axillary dissection, and randomized them to concurrent radiotherapy and chemotherapy (mitoxantrone, 5-FU, cyclophosphamide) or sequential chemotherapy (epirubicin, 5-FU, cyclophosphamide) followed by radiotherapy [152]. The concurrent arm yielded a reduction in LRR (3% versus 9%) at the cost of increase acute toxicity. There were no differences in DFS or OS.

The Sequencing of Chemotherapy and Radiotherapy in Adjuvant breast Cancer (SECRAB) study enrolled 2296 women treated with either breast-conserving surgery or mastectomy, and randomized them to synchronous (interdigitated) or sequential chemotherapy (either cyclophosphamide, methotrexate, 5-fluorouracil

[CMF] or anthracycline-CMF) and radiotherapy [153]. Final results are not yet available, but the initial rates of five-year LR were 2.8% versus 5.1% in the concurrent versus sequential arms, respectively. Acute skin toxicity was worse in the concurrent arm. In summary, the concurrent administration of chemotherapy and radiotherapy appears to improve locoregional control at the expense of increased skin toxicity. Currently, sequential administration of chemotherapy and radiotherapy is standard. After publication of the results of the SECRAB trial, it is possible that subsets of patients at higher risk of LRR who derive sufficient benefit from concurrent chemoradiotherapy will be identified.

Sequential Chemotherapy and Radiotherapy

A trial from Harvard enrolled 244 patients with stage I or II breast cancer and randomized them to receive CMF chemotherapy before or after radiotherapy. At the five-year follow-up, the rate of LR as first failure was higher in the chemotherapy-first arm, while the rate of distant recurrence as first failure was higher in the radiotherapy-first arm [154]. At longer follow-up, no clear difference between the arms persisted [155]. In part due to the early results of this trial, in current practice chemotherapy is typically administered prior to radiotherapy.

Delay Between Surgery and Radiotherapy

No randomized data exist to describe the optimal interval between surgery and radiotherapy. Many retrospective series have attempted to tease out the effect of treatment delay on local control. A meta-analysis that included only 'high-quality' trials (those that controlled for confounding prognostic factors) found that the risk of LR increased by a ratio of 1.11 for each month of delay [156]. A SEER-Medicare database analysis examined the outcomes of 18 050 women aged over 65 years with stage 0–II breast cancer that were treated with breast-conserving surgery and radiotherapy without chemotherapy [157]. The HR of LR was 1.005 per day of delay between surgery and radiotherapy. A delay of more than six weeks was associated with a HR of LR of 1.19, as compared to an interval of six weeks or less. Given these data, it is advisable to initiate radiotherapy relatively soon after surgery once wound healing is complete. Currently, scant data are available concerning the effect of radiotherapy delay when sequenced after adjuvant chemotherapy, although caution suggests minimizing this interval as well.

Hypofractionated Whole-Breast Radiotherapy

Whole-breast radiotherapy using standard fractionation involves a total dose of 45–50.4 Gy delivered in 1.8- to 2.0-Gy daily fractions. This treatment course takes approximately five weeks, can be logistically challenging for patients, and is associated with considerable expense.

Table 37.9 Randomized trials comparing whole-breast radiotherapy (RT) using standard versus hypofractionated regimens.

Trial/Reference(s)	No. of patients	Follow-up (years)	Frequency of chemotherapy (%)	Fractionation schemes (Gy/Gy per fraction)	LRR (%)
Hôpital Necker [337]	230	≥4	21	45/1.8	5
				23/5.75	7
Royal Marsden [338]	1410	10	14	50/2	12.1
				39/3	14.8
				42.9/3.3	9.6
START A [158, 159]	2236	10	36	50/2	7.4
				39/3	8.8
				41.6/3.2	6.3
START B [160, 159]	2215	10	22	50/2	5.5
				40.05/2.67	4.3
Canadian [162]	1234	10	11	50/2	6.7
				42.56/2.66	6.2

START, Standardization of Breast Radiotherapy.

Hypofractionation, in which a larger daily dose is administered in fewer treatment days, can reduce the logistical burdens and expense of radiotherapy. This course can be administered in an accelerated fashion, in which the total treatment duration is reduced, or without acceleration, in which treatments are administered fewer than five times per week and the total treatment duration is unchanged. Several randomized trials have evaluated the outcomes of hypofractionation in whole-breast radiotherapy (Table 37.9).

The START A trial enrolled 2236 women with early-stage breast cancer, most of whom underwent breast-conserving surgery (85%), and randomized them to radiotherapy with either 50 Gy in 25 fractions, 41.6 Gy in 13 fractions over five weeks, or 39 Gy in 13 fractions over five weeks [158]. The 10-year rates of LRR were similar at 7.4%, 6.3%, and 8.8%, respectively [159]. The rate of late change in breast appearance at 10 years was lowest in the 39-Gy arm. The START B trial enrolled 2215 women, most of whom underwent breast-conserving surgery (92%), and randomized them to either 50 Gy in 25 fractions over five weeks or an accelerated hypofractionated schedule of 40.05 Gy in 15 fractions over three weeks [160]). The 10-year rates of LRR were 5.5% and 4.3%, respectively, and were not statistically different [159]. Taken together, patient reports of adverse effects at five years were fewer for the 39-Gy arm in START A and the 40-Gy arm in START B than for the 50-Gy control arm or the 41.6-Gy arm of START A [161].

A Canadian trial enrolled 1234 women with early-stage breast cancer treated with breast-conserving surgery, and randomized them to receive whole-breast radiotherapy using standard fractionation (50 Gy in 25 fractions) versus accelerated hypofractionation (42.5 Gy in 16 fractions) [162]. Women with central axis separation >25 cm were not eligible, given concerns over dose inhomogeneity. The 10-year rate of LR was not statistically different between arms (6.7% versus 6.2%, respectively), and nor was the rate of good to excellent cosmetic outcome. No boost was employed in either arm. Of note, a subset analysis found the risk of recurrence in women with high-grade disease to be greater in the hypofractionation arm. The implications of this finding are unclear, given the risk of a type I error inherent in this analysis. The finding of an interaction between grade and fractionation regimen was not replicated in larger analyses from the START or Royal Marsden trials [163].

The UK FAST TRIAL enrolled women with early-stage breast cancer over the age of 50 years, and randomized them to one of three arms: 50 Gy in 25 daily fractions over five weeks; 30 Gy in five weekly fractions; or 28.5 Gy in five weekly fractions [164]. At the three-year follow-up the rates of physician-assessed moderate to marked adverse effects were 9.5%, 17.3%, and 11.1%, respectively. The difference between the 30-Gy arm and the other two arms was statistically significant.

There are notable caveats to the implementation of hypofractionated radiotherapy. Most patients in the trials described above underwent breast-conserving surgery, did not receive chemotherapy, were aged over 50 years, did not receive a boost, and were treated with relatively homogeneous breast doses. No patients on the above referenced trials had DCIS alone, although many patients had an *in-situ* component of the tumor. An ASTRO consensus panel issued guidelines concerning the use of hypofractionated radiotherapy, suggesting that for the time being it be limited to women aged over 50 years with invasive cancer, stage T1–T2, not receiving chemotherapy, and with dose inhomogeneity limited to ±107% of the prescription dose [165]. For patients not receiving a boost, the Canadian study fractionation regimen of 42.5 Gy was favored. Concern still lingers about late toxicities (e.g., cardiac toxicity) that have not yet had an opportunity to become fully manifest.

Partial Breast Radiotherapy

As discussed above, most in-breast failures occur in or near the operative bed [87, 92, 93]. Therefore, it may be possible to limit the delivery of radiotherapy to the tissue at high risk for harboring residual cancer cells. When radiotherapy is delivered to only a portion of the breast, it is possible to use large fractions; this technique is termed accelerated partial breast irradiation (APBI). Such irradiation may be delivered with 3D conformal radiotherapy, balloon brachytherapy, or multi-catheter interstitial brachytherapy. APBI promises to reduce the logistical challenges of breast radiotherapy considerably. A few small trials have evaluated the efficacy of APBI by randomizing women to whole-breast radiotherapy versus APBI after breast-conserving surgery. The results of these trials are summarized in Table 37.10. The largest of the trials that have provided data is the GEC ESTRO trial, in which 551 women with DCIS or invase cancer smaller than 3 cm, N0/N1mi were randomized to either whole breast RT with a boost or interstitial multicatheter brachytherapy [171]. At 5 years, the APBI arm was non-inferior to the whole breast RT arm with regard to local control, overall survival, and cosmesis. The largest non-randomized series evaluating the effectiveness of APBI using brachytherapy was a retrospective population-based cohort study of 92 735 women aged ≥67 years who underwent BCT; of these women, 6952 received APBI [166]. The rate of subsequent mastectomy was higher in women treated with APBI with brachytherapy than those treated with whole-breast radiotherapy (HR = 2.2). Additionally, the rate of both infectious and non-infectious complications appeared higher in the brachytherapy group.

Until the results of large randomized trials become available, a consensus panel convened by ASTRO has provided guidance on the suitability of individual patients for APBI [167]. The recommendations of this panel are summarized in Table 37.11. Some, but not all, retrospective reports have confirmed a higher rate of IBTR in women in the cautionary and unsuitable groups as compared to the suitable group [168, 169]. It remains to be seen whether this classification system identifies poor candidates for APBI, or simply women at somewhat higher risk of IBTR regardless of the type of RT.

A Phase III cooperative group trial, NSABP B-39/RTOG 0413, is currently open to accrual with the goal of recruiting 4300 patients [170]. This trial randomizes patients to whole-breast radiotherapy versus APBI delivered with one of three modalities selected by the enrolling institution. The RAPID/Ontario Clinical Oncology Group trial, which has completed accrual, randomized 2135 women to whole-breast radiotherapy to APBI using 3D-CRT to 38.5 Gy in 10 fractions [172]. Although no efficacy data are available, preliminary data on cosmetic outcome report an increased rate in adverse cosmetic outcome at three years for the APBI arm as compared to whole-breast radiotherapy (35% versus 17%) [171]. The final results of these trials, when available, may help to define subsets of patients for whom APBI is an appropriate alternative to whole-breast radiotherapy.

Intraoperative Radiotherapy

Intraoperative radiotherapy (IORT) is an extension of APBI, in which a course of radiotherapy is delivered in a single fraction at the time of breast-conserving surgery.

Table 37.10 Randomized trials comparing whole-breast radiotherapy (RT) to APBI.

Trial/Reference	No. of patients	Follow-up (years)	Randomization	IBTR (%)
Christie Hospital [340]	708	8	WB: 40 Gy/15 fx	13
			APBI: 8–14 MeV e-	25
YBCG [341]	174	8	WB: 40 Gy/15 fx	4
			APBI: 55 Gy/20 fx (EBRT)	12
Hungarian [342]	258	5.5	WB: 50 Gy/25 fx	3.4
			APBI: 50 Gy/25 fx (EBRT) or Interstitial 36.4 Gy/7 fx	4.7
University of Florence [343]	520	5	WB: 50 Gy/25 + 10 Gy Boost	1.5
			APBI: 30 Gy/6 fx (EBRT)	1.5
GEC ESTRO [171]	551	5	WB: 50 Gy/25 + 10 Gy Boost	1.4
			Interstitial 32 Gy/8 fx	0.9

YBCG, Yorkshire Breast Cancer Group; APBI, Accelerated Partial Breast Irradiation; WB, Whole Breast; EBRT, External Beam Radiotherapy.
Bold font denotes statistical significance.

Table 37.11 Patient groups defined by the ASTRO Consensus Statement of APBI.

Parameter	Suitable*	Cautionary†	Unsuitable‡
Age (years)	≥60	50–59	<50
Tumor size (cm)	≤2	2.1–3.0	>3
T-stage	T1	T0, T2	T3, T4
Margins	Negative by ≥0.2 cm	Close (<0.32 cm)	Positive
Histology	IDC or favorable subtype, no EIC	ILC or pure DCIS or EIC	
LVI	No	Limited/Focal	Extensive
ER status	Positive	Negative	
Focality/Centricity	Clinically unifocal		Clinically multifocal
N-stage	pN0 (i-, i+)		pN1–3
Nodal surgery	SLNB, ALND		None
Neoadjuvant therapy	None		Used
BRCA 1/2 status	No mutations		Mutation present

ASTRO, American Society for Radiation Oncology; APBI, Accelerated Partial Breast Irradiation; IDC, Invasive Ductal Carcinoma; ILC, Invasive Lobular Carcinoma; DCIS, Ductal Carcinoma In-Situ; SLNB, Sentinel Lymph Node Biopsy; ALND, Axillary Lymph Node Dissection.
*All criteria in this column must be met to place this patient in the 'Suitable' group.
†Any criterion in this column places the patient in a 'Cautionary' group.
‡Any criterion in this column places the patient in an 'Unsuitable' group.

The TARGIT-A trial enrolled 3451 women, and randomized them to either whole-breast EBRT or a strategy of IORT with postoperative whole-breast EBRT delivered if adverse features were identified on final pathology [173]. IORT was delivered with 50 kV photons to a dose of 20 Gy prescribed to the surface of the applicator. Using this approach, the tissue at 1 cm depth receives approximately 5 Gy. Notably, 15% of the patients in the IORT arm (22% of those treated at the time of surgery) received whole-breast EBRT. The indications for EBRT were (to some extent) institution-dependent and included: involved axillary node(s), LVI, high-grade, positive margin, lobular histology and the presence of an extensive intraductal component (EIC). In the TARGIT-A trial, the five-year risk of IBRT was 3.3% in the IORT (± EBRT) arm versus 1.3% in the EBRT arm. When the post-pathology stratum was eliminated, the five-year IBTR rate of the pre-pathology stratum in the IORT (± EBRT) arm approached the EBRT arm (2.1% versus 1.1%). These early results are encouraging, though only a very short follow-up is available. The low dose used and the small volume of tissue irradiated in the TARGIT-A trial are somewhat at odds with conventional understanding of radiobiology, and suggest that longer follow-up should be obtained prior to considering IORT to be a standard substitute for whole-breast radiotherapy [174].

The ELIOT trial randomized women to either whole-breast radiotherapy or intraoperative radiotherapy using 3–12 MeV electrons delivering a dose of 21 Gy prescribed to the 90% isodose line. Initial results have been published; five-year local recurrence rates were 4.4% versus 0.4%, favoring the whole-breast radiotherapy arm [175].

The higher rate of IBTR in the IORT arm may be related to patient selection. On subset analysis of the IORT arm, the high-risk stratum (defined post-hoc as size between 2 and 2.5 cm, high histologic grade, four or more nodes positive, or ER negativity) had a five-year rate of IBTR of 11.3%, while the remainder of patients had a five-year rate of IBTR of 1.5%. Fewer skin side effects were noted in women in the IORT arm. The incidence of CT-detected pulmonary fibrosis was lower in women in the IORT arm [176].

Neoadjuvant Chemotherapy

Neoadjuvant chemotherapy can be used for the purpose of downsizing tumors in order to make them amenable to BCT. In NSABP B-18, women who required mastectomy at initial presentation and received adriamycin and cyclophosphamide preoperatively had a 27% rate of conversion to breast-conserving surgery [177]. Women who were converted to breast-conserving surgery experienced a higher rate of IBTR at nine years than those who were candidates for lumpectomy prior to chemotherapy (14.5% versus 6.9%). This difference may be due to pre-surgical downsizing, or to confounding prognostic factors that differ between these two groups. As such, tumor reduction using neoadjuvant chemotherapy in order to render women with large tumors eligible for BCT remains a reasonable strategy. A clip should be placed in the tumor at the time of biopsy so that localization of the operative bed can be confirmed, especially in the case of a complete response.

Table 37.12 Classical borders of whole-breast irradiation with patient in the supine position.

Border	Description
Inferior	2 cm inferior to the inframammary fold
Superior	The inferior edge of the medial head of the clavicle, at least 1 cm above the superior margin of the breast
Lateral	The midaxillary line, at least 1 cm lateral to the edge of the breast
Medial	The midsternum, as long as the IM nodes are not included
Anterior	2 cm of flash anterior to the breast
Posterior	A non-divergent edge connecting the medial and lateral borders at central axis

IM, internal mammary.

Intact-Breast Radiotherapy Techniques

Supine Position

In the supine position, the patient is immobilized with the ipsilateral arm, or both arms, above the head. The classic field borders are described in Table 37.12. The posterior edge of the tangent beams should be non-divergent, using either a half-beam technique or appropriate gantry rotation in order to reduce lung dose. With the use of CT simulation, deviation from the classic clinical boundaries may be warranted. Notably, a heart block, if distant from the operative bed, is acceptable and does not appear to increase the rate of IBTR [178]. Supine positioning provides adequate coverage of the whole breast, but by necessity irradiates an underlying sliver of lung and occasionally a sliver of heart (if left-sided). The supine position is also associated with dose inhomogeneity within the breast, although this is much reduced with modern techniques such as the use of multiple beam segments. Dose inhomogeneity is more problematic in women with large breasts.

Prone Position

In the prone position, the breast falls away from the chest wall and its separation narrows. Multiple dosimetric comparisons have shown that whole-breast irradiation in the prone position reduces dose to the ipsilateral lung [179–182]. Available data are conflicting regarding the benefit of prone positioning on heart dose as compared to supine positioning; some series suggest a benefit for prone positioning while others do not [179, 182, 183]. This may be because the heart also displaces anteriorly in the prone position [184]. As a result, the effect of prone positioning on heart dose appears to vary by individual patient anatomy, as well as by field design. The prone position appears to reduce dose to the axilla and may not be ideal when nodal coverage is required [185]. Additionally, random set-up error appears to be higher in the prone position and may necessitate the use of a larger planned target volume expansion for targeted techniques [186]. Clinical data support satisfactory oncologic outcomes with radiotherapy delivered in the prone position. With a five-year follow-up, a series of 245 women treated in the prone position at MSKCC showed low rates of IBTR, comparable to irradiation in the supine position [187].

Nodal Irradiation (Three-Field)

Nodal radiotherapy is typically performed with the patient in the supine position. The low axilla is, at least in part, included in standard breast tangents, given the close apposition of the axillary lymph nodes and the tail of breast [188]. The upper axilla and SCV fossa are classically included in a 'third field.' The exact details of technique vary by institution. Many institutions employ a mono-isocentric match with a half beam block approach, creating a perfect geometric match between the chest wall and the nodal field(s) without couch or collimator rotations (Figure 37.2) [189]. At the present authors' institution, an anterior nodal field is used at an oblique angle of approximately 5-15°. The lateral border of this field is determined by the volume at risk. After an axillary dissection, and in the absence of high-risk factors for residual disease in the dissected axilla, the dissected axilla are excluded from the radiotherapy field. In this case, placement of the lateral border is guided by the CT contours but is typically between the coracoid process and the humeral head (Figure 37.3). In the absence of an axillary dissection, or in the presence of significant risk for residual disease, the lateral border extends beyond the humeral head to encompass the full axilla (Figure 37.4). In the event that dosimetric coverage appears inadequate using an anterior oblique field only, a posterior axillary boost or an opposed oblique field can be added (Figure 37.5).

Forward-Planned IMRT

Classically, breast radiotherapy was delivered with opposed tangential open fields without wedging. Given that the breast is non-uniform in contour, the thinner portion of the breast towards the nipple received an undesirably high dose of radiation (a 'hot spot') and the thicker portion of the breast, towards the chest wall, received an undesirably low dose of radiation (a 'cold spot'). This distribution is improved with the use of wedges that compensate for the irregular contour of the breast. Wedges compensate well for the non-uniform contour at the center plane of the breast, but cannot correct for the 3-D non-uniformity towards the superior

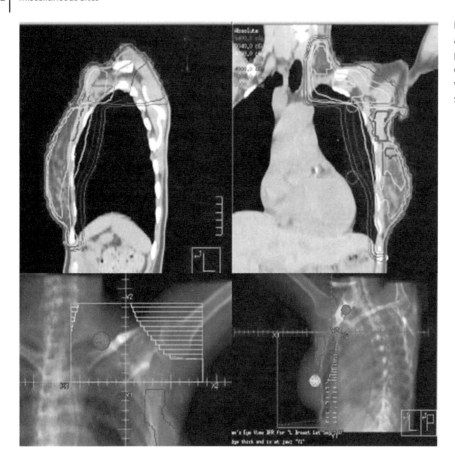

Figure 37.2 A mono-isocentric match with a half beam block approach, creating a perfect geometric match between the chest wall and the nodal field. For a color version of this figure, see the color plate section.

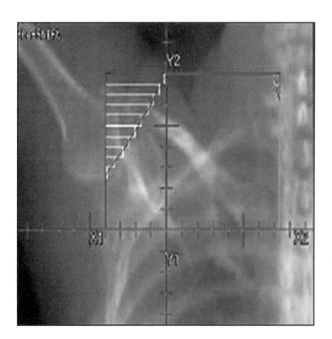

Figure 37.3 A nodal field encompassing the supraclavicular fossa and undissected axillary apex (defined on CT contour using clips). For a color version of this figure, see the color plate section.

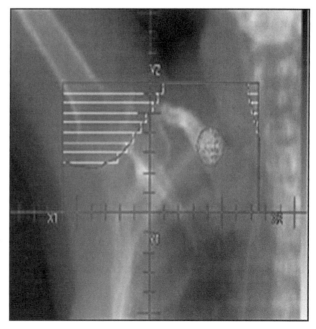

Figure 37.4 A nodal field encompassing the supraclavicular fossa and full axilla. For a color version of this figure, see the color plate section.

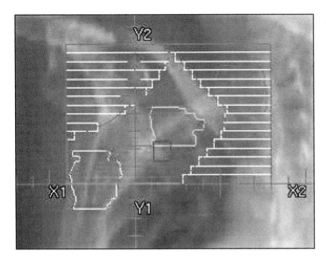

Figure 37.5 A posterior axillary boost (PAB) encompassing the lateral axilla for improved dosimetric coverage. For a color version of this figure, see the color plate section.

and interior poles of the breast. Forward-planned IMRT (f-IMRT) uses multiple beam segments, and is similar in principle to wedges in three dimensions. This approach clearly improves the dose homogeneity of whole-breast radiotherapy.

Three randomized trials have assessed the impact of f-IMRT on radiotherapy toxicity and breast cosmesis. Two Canadian centers enrolled 358 women and randomized them to receive whole-breast radiotherapy using either standard radiotherapy or f-IMRT [190]. The use of f-IMRT improved the dose distribution and, as a result, reduced the rate of acute moist desquamation (47.8% versus 31.2%). A trial from the Royal Marsden included 306 women at high risk for toxicity, and enrolled them in a similar randomization [191]. The five-year photographic evaluation revealed a change in breast appearance in 58% of women randomized to standard radiotherapy as compared to 40% in the f-IMRT arm. Fewer women in the f-IMRT arm developed breast induration. The University of Cambridge performed a single-center trial in which standard breast radiotherapy plans were analyzed for dose inhomogeneity. In total, 814 patients with >2 cm^3 volume that received >107% of the prescribed dose were randomized to standard breast radiotherapy or f-IMRT [192]. Women who received standard radiotherapy were more likely to develop telangiectasia (OR = 1.68) as assessed on two-year photographic follow-up. The f-IMRT technique is gradually becoming a standard in breast radiotherapy [193].

Local Recurrence/Salvage

LRR after BCT augurs a poor prognosis. OS after IBTR is superior to that of a regional nodal recurrence. A combined analysis of NSABP trials of women with node-negative disease treated with BCT found five-year OS of 76.6% after an IBTR, and 34.9% after a regional nodal recurrence [194]. ER negativity and short disease-free interval were additional poor prognostic factors in the setting of LRR. A similar NSABP analysis of women with node-positive disease treated with BCT found five-year OS of 59.9% after an IBTR, and 24.1% after a regional nodal recurrence [195]. The standard local treatment of an IBTR is mastectomy. Repeat breast conservation with re-irradiation of the breast is currently the subject of clinical investigation in RTOG 1014 but should be considered experimental.

Summary Guidelines

- BCT yields long-term survival equivalent to mastectomy and is a standard treatment in early-stage breast cancer.
- Intact-breast radiotherapy after lumpectomy reduces IBTR by 65–70%, all recurrences by almost half, and improves breast cancer-specific survival and overall survival.
- Most attempts to find subsets of women for which intact-breast radiotherapy can be safely omitted have not been successful.
- Women aged over 70 years with small hormone receptor-positive tumors who receive tamoxifen experience a reduction in IBTR from radiotherapy, but have a sufficiently low risk for recurrence that omission of radiotherapy is reasonable.
- Several risk factors for IBTR have been consistently identified, most notably: young age, positive margins, omission of systemic therapy, and high histologic grade.
- While margin positivity is associated with a higher risk of IBTR, there is no established benefit for increasing the width of negative margins.
- Emerging data suggest that biologic subtype and genetic profile add additional prognostic information concerning IBTR.
- The use of a boost after whole-breast radiotherapy yields a further reduction in the risk of IBTR at the cost of a small decline in cosmetic outcome.
- The absolute benefit of the boost is largest in young women and those with high-grade histology.
- The axillary apex and SCV fossa should be irradiated in women with four or more positive axillary lymph nodes after dissection.
- The role of RNI in the setting of one to three positive axillary nodes is currently being refined; randomized data support the use of nodal radiotherapy in these patients, given that it improves dDFS and reduces breast cancer mortality.

- The benefit of IM nodal radiotherapy currently unclear, but it was included in all trials of nodal radiotherapy.
- In conventional sequencing, chemotherapy precedes radiotherapy; the role of concurrent chemoradiotherapy in high-risk subsets is promising but not yet clearly defined.
- In the absence of systemic therapy, a long delay between surgery and radiotherapy may lead to a small increase in the risk of IBTR.
- Conventional radiotherapy involves treating the whole breast to 45–50 Gy using 1.8- to 2-Gy fractions.
- Hypofractionation is becoming established as a viable option with the caveats that very long-term follow-up is not yet available and few patients enrolled on randomized trials received chemotherapy or a boost.
- APBI and IORT are potentially emerging as viable alternatives to whole-breast radiotherapy, although long-term confirmatory data from randomized trials are not yet available.
- LRR after BCT is associated with unfavorable long-term outcomes.

Post-Mastectomy Radiotherapy

Rationale

Total mastectomy, in combination with sentinel lymph node biopsy or axillary dissection, is an excellent locoregional therapy for early-stage breast cancer, yielding very low rates of LRR. However, the incidence of LRR rises for those patients with certain risk factors, most notably lymph node positivity. For many of these patients, post-mastectomy radiotherapy (PMRT) is an appropriate adjunct to further reduce the risk of recurrent disease.

Meta-Analyses

The use of PMRT has generated considerable controversy over the past few decades. Early randomized trials yielded conflicting results as to its value, most likely due to the heterogeneity of inclusion criteria, systemic therapy, surgical practice, and radiation technique. A meta-analysis of these early trials established a clear reduction in LRR and an improvement in disease-specific survival with the use of PMRT [196]. These benefits were offset by treatment-related toxicity (notably cardiac death) resulting in the absence of an advantage in OS. When analysis was restricted to those trials employing modern techniques and standard fractionation, an advantage in OS was seen [197]. Similarly, a separate meta-analysis found a 6.4% improvement in 10-year OS for trials that employed a biologically equivalent dose of 40–60 Gy in 2 Gy fractions and treated an appropriate target volume, but no survival benefit in the absence of these factors

[198]. A meta-analysis that included only those trials in which systemic therapy was used in both arms also found a survival advantage for the addition of PMRT [199].

In the most thorough analysis currently available, the EBCTCG included data on 8500 women treated with mastectomy with or without radiotherapy [200]. The authors found improvements in five-year LRR of 17%, a 15-year disease-specific mortality of 5.4%, and OS of 4.4% in favor of radiotherapy. The trialists posited that a 4% reduction in LRR at five years translated into a 1% reduction in breast cancer mortality at 15 years. In this formulation, the absolute risk of LRR is an important determinant of the benefit of PMRT.

Randomized Trials

Three large relatively modern randomized trials of PMRT provide the clearest picture of the benefits of the approach. The DBCG 82b trial included 1708 premenopausal women with stage II or III breast cancer treated with modified-radical mastectomy (MRM) followed by adjuvant chemotherapy with cyclophosphamide, methotrexate, and flurouracil (CMF) [201]. Participants were then randomized to receive radiotherapy or not. Radiotherapy fields included the chest wall, axilla, supraclavicular fossa and ipsilateral internal mammary chain. Radiotherapy yielded a reduction in 10-year LLR from 32% to 9%, an improved 10-year DFS from 34% to 48%, and an improved OS from 45% to 54%. An identical benefit in OS was seen for women with one to three positive lymph nodes, and those with four or more positive lymph nodes. Of note, the modal patient in this trial was stage T2N1.

The DBCG 82c trial represented a sister trial that included 1375 postmenopausal women with stage II or III breast cancer [145]. Women on this trial underwent MRM, received a single year of adjuvant tamoxifen, and were randomized to radiotherapy, or not. The 10-year risk of LRR was reduced to 8% from 35%, the 10-year DFS was improved from 24% to 36%, and the 10-year OS was improved from 36% to 45%. An identical benefit in OS was seen for women with one to three positive lymph nodes and those with four or more positive lymph nodes. The combined data from trials 82b and 82c were updated at an 18-year follow-up [146]. The 18-year rate of LRR was 14% in the radiotherapy arm versus 49% in the non-radiotherapy arm. The rate distant metastatic disease was 53% in the radiotherapy arm but 64% in the non-radiotherapy arm.

The British Columbia Cancer Agency enrolled 318 premenopausal women with node-positive breast cancer treated with MRM and CMF chemotherapy, and randomized them to radiotherapy or not [147]. The radiotherapy fields included the chest wall, axilla, supraclavicular fossa and bilateral internal mammary chains. Radiotherapy improved the 15-year DFS from

33% to 50%, but a benefit in 15-year OS did not reach statistical significance. An identical benefit in distant metastasis-free survival was seen for women with one to three positive lymph nodes and those with four or more positive lymph nodes. In an updated analysis, the 20-year OS was 37% in the non-radiotherapy arm versus 47% in the radiotherapy arm and did reach significance [148].

These seminal trials demonstrated an impressive survival advantage for the use of PMRT in all lymph node-positive women. However, the results of these trials have been criticized for methodological shortcomings. The axillary dissections in these trials were limited; in the DBCG 82b and 82c trials a median of seven lymph nodes were removed, and in the British Columbia trial a median of 11 were removed. In the US, a level I and II axillary dissection typically yields 15 or more lymph nodes. A less-complete axillary dissection may both under-stage patients by missing some involved axillary nodes, and may leave a reservoir of disease in the axilla. Additionally, the systemic therapies used in these trials (CMF or tamoxifen) are less efficacious than modern regimens that include anthracyclines, taxanes, and targeted agents. For these reasons, the trials described above may have overestimated the risk of LRR – especially in the subset of women with one to three positive lymph nodes – and, therefore, may have overestimated the benefit of PMRT. As evidence for this hypothesis, several non-randomized series that included women with more thorough surgery found considerably lower rates of LRR in women with one to three positive lymph nodes [202–205]. These series are summarized in Table 37.13. Other explanations for the discrepancy between the rates of LRR in the DBCG trials and non-randomized series include: differences in scoring LRR (e.g., isolated LRR only versus all LRR); variation in prognostic factors for LRR between populations; diversity of follow-up interval and technique; and disparities in the type of statistical analyses performed [202].

PMRT in One to Three Positive Nodes

Recent re-analyses of the DBCG trials shed some light on the value of PMRT women with one to three positive nodes. The DBCG 82b and 82c data were re-analyzed, and only those 1152 patients with eight or more lymph nodes dissected were included [206]. Again, patients with four or more positive nodes experienced a larger absolute reduction in LRR from PMRT than did patients with one to three positive nodes (41% versus 23%), but they displayed an equivalent benefit in OS (9%). This analysis supports the benefit of PMRT in women with one to three positive nodes and refutes the notion that a reduction in LRR leads to a proportional benefit in OS. Instead, it appears that the relationship between LRR and OS may be modified by the competing risk of metastatic disease. This point is highlighted by a subsequent re-analysis of the DBCG data in which 1000 women for whom tumor markers were available were divided into three prognostic groups for the risk of LRR [207]. Although the good prognosis group experienced the smallest absolute reduction in LRR from PMRT, it had the largest benefit in OS.

The most recent meta-analysis by the EBCTCG identified 1314 women with one to three positive nodes treated with mastectomy and axillary dissection and randomized to post-mastectomy radiotherapy or observation [208]. Radiotherapy reduced the 10-year rate of any recurrence from 45.7% to 34.2% (RR = 0.68) and 20-year breast cancer mortality from 50.2% to 42.3% (RR = 0.80). A subsequent analysis included only the 1133 of these women who also received systemic therapy (chemotherapy or tamoxifen) and yielded similar results.

Several large retrospective series from sources such as the EORTC, as well as the Surveillance Epidemiology and End Results (SEER) registries, also suggest that a survival advantage exists for PMRT in women with one to three positive nodes [40, 209–211]. Other series suggest that

Table 37.13 10-year rate of LRR in patients treated with mastectomy and systemic therapy without radiotherapy (RT).

Study/Reference	No. of patients	10-year LRR rate (%)		
		Combined	1–3+ nodes	>3+ nodes
British Columbia [250]	318	25		
DBCG 82b [201]	1708	32		
DBCG 82c [145]	1375	35		
ECOG [202]	2016		13	29
MDACC [203]	1031		13	25
NSABP [204]	5758		13	27
IBCSG [205]	4072		17	31

DBCG, Danish Breast Cancer Cooperative Group; ECOG, Eastern Cooperative Oncology Group; MDACC, MD Anderson Cancer Center; NSABP, National Surgical Adjuvant Breast and Bowel Project; IBSCG, International Breast Cancer Study Group.

Table 37.14 Adverse prognostic factors for LRR after mastectomy in women with one to three positive lymph nodes.

Study/Reference	Adverse prognostic factor(s) for LRR
MDACC [212]	Invasion of skin or nipple, pectoral fascia invasion, close or positive margins
MDACC [213]	Tumor size $\geq$4 cm, ECE $\geq$2 mm, <10 lymph nodes sampled
BCCA [214]	Nodal ratio $\geq$20%,
BCCA [215]	Age <45 years, nodal ratio >25%, medial tumor location, ER-negative
Taipei [344]	Age <40 years, T2, ER negativity, LVI
NSABP [204]	Age <50 years, T2
ECOG [202]	Premenopausal status, $\leq$5 lymph nodes examined
IBCSG [216]	Grade 3, LVI, T2
Ankara [217]	Age $\leq$35 years, nodal ratio >15%, LVI

MDACC, MD Anderson Cancer Center; BCCA, British Columbia Cancer Agency; ECE, Extracapsular extension; LVI, Lymphovascular invasion.

certain pathologic features, in combination with the finding of one to three positive lymph nodes, identify subsets of women at sufficient risk of recurrence to merit PMRT [202, 204, 212–217]. The findings of these series are summarized in Table 37.14. The ongoing MRC/EORTC SUPREMO Trial, which is enrolling women with N1 or high-risk N0 disease after mastectomy and randomizing them to PMRT versus observation, may shed light on this controversy [218].

PMRT in Node-Negative Disease

An EBCTCG meta-analysis found a low risk of LRR in women with node-negative breast cancer after MRM, which was reduced further by PMRT (6% versus 2%) [200]. Similarly, a retrospective study of 313 women with T3 node-negative tumors treated on NSABP trials with mastectomy and systemic therapy without PMRT found the 10-year cumulative incidence of any LRR to be 10% [214]. This relatively low risk of LRR may be insufficient

to justify PMRT for most women, but individual subsets of patients appear to be at higher risk.

A series of 70 patients with T3N0 breast cancer treated with mastectomy and systemic therapy without PMRT found that the presence of LVI correlated with a higher risk of LRR [220]. Several retrospective series have evaluated prognostic factors for LRR in women with T1–T2 node-negative breast cancer treated with mastectomy without radiotherapy [221–223]. Consistently, young age, high grade, LVI and T2 tumor stage were prognostic for LRR. A systematic review in node-negative women after mastectomy found the following risk factors for LRR: LVI, grade 3 histology, T2 or T3 tumor, close margin and age less than 50 years [224]. In the presence of two or more of these factors, the risk of LRR exceeded 15%. Prospective validation that these criteria reliably identify a subset of node-negative women at high enough risk of LRR to justify the routine use of PMRT is lacking. The prognostic factors that appear to predispose for a higher risk of LRR in women with node-negative breast cancer after MRM are summarized in Table 37.15.

Triple-negative breast cancer may represent a biologic subtype at higher risk for LRR. A retrospective comparison of women with T1–T2 node-negative, triple-negative breast cancer treated with lumpectomy and radiotherapy or MRM without radiotherapy found that the receipt of MRM was the sole predictor of LRR [225]. A recent Chinese trial enrolled 681 women with triple-negative breast cancer (86% of whom where node-negative) who were treated with MRM and adjuvant CMF chemotherapy and randomized them to PMRT or observation [226]. PMRT improved five-year OS from 78.7% to 90.4%.

Close/Positive Margin

The presence of a close or positive margin is often considered to be an indication to use PMRT. No randomized data exist to clarify this point. A retrospective series from Fox Chase suggests that only women aged <50 years with a margin <5 mm have an elevated risk of recurrence [227]. Retrospective data from the British Columbia Cancer Agency found the risk of LRR was high in women with

Table 37.15 Adverse prognostic factors for LRR after mastectomy in women with node-negative disease.

Study/Reference	Stage	No. of patients	Adverse prognostic factor(s) for LRR
MGH [221]	T1–T2	1136	LVI, T2, Close or positive margin, age $\leq$50 years, omission of systemic therapy
BCCA [222]	T1–T2	1505	Grade 3, LVI, T2, omission of systemic therapy
Ankara [223]	T1–T2	502	Age $\leq$40 years: T2, LVI
			Age >40 years: Tumor size >3 cm, LVI, grade 3
MGH/MDACC/Yale [220]	T3	70	LVI
Kent – Review [224]	T1–T3		LVI, Grade 3, T2 or T3, Close margin, Age <50 years

MGH, Massachusetts General Hospital; BCCA, British Columbia Cancer Agency; MDACC, MD Anderson Cancer Center; LVI, Lymphovascular invasion.

a positive margin and at least one of the following risk factors: age <50 years, T2 tumor, grade 3 histology, or LVI [228].

Neoadjuvant Chemotherapy

Decisions concerning PMRT have traditionally been made based on pathologic findings from the mastectomy specimen. The use of neoadjuvant chemotherapy is increasingly common. When neoadjuvant chemotherapy is used, it alters the pathologic findings, clouding the decision regarding PMRT. The use of neoadjuvant chemotherapy does yield the additional information of tumor response to treatment. Data from NSABP B-18 and B-27 demonstrated that those patients exhibiting a pathologic complete response have superior OS as compared to those who do not; however, it is not yet clear how the response to neoadjuvant chemotherapy information should influence radiotherapy decisions [229]. A retrospective review of pooled data from B-18 and B-27 suggests that after neoadjuvant chemotherapy and mastectomy, independent predictors for LRR include clinical tumor size and nodal status before chemotherapy, as well as the absence of a pathologic complete response in the breast or nodal beds [230]. In these series, the presence of a pathologic complete response in the breast and nodes is associated with a very low risk of LRR and suggests that therapeutic reduction, including omission of nodal irradiation or PMRT, may be appropriate. By contrast, early data from a pooled analysis of the Gepar trials found significantly worse outcomes after omission of RT even for women who exhibited a pathologic complete response [231].

Most of the data concerning the use of PMRT after neoadjuvant chemotherapy are retrospective in nature. Data from the MDACC suggest that patients with clinical stage III or stage T3N0 breast cancers exhibit a high risk of LRR and benefit from PMRT [232–234]. This remains true even for those patients with a pathologic complete response to chemotherapy. In one series, women with clinical stage III disease that exhibited a pathologic complete response to neoadjuvant chemotherapy still had a 33% risk of 10-year LRR if PMRT was omitted, but a 7% risk after receipt of PMRT [233]. Similarly, women with clinical T3N0 disease had a 24% risk of five-year LRR without PMRT, but a 4% risk with PMRT [234]. The presence of skin or nipple involvement, SCV nodal disease, extracapsular extension and ER negativity also predict for a higher risk of LRR after neoadjuvant chemotherapy [235]. Current consensus opinion holds that both pre-chemotherapy clinical stage as well as post-chemotherapy pathologic stage are independent prognostic factors, and should be taken into consideration when making radiotherapy decisions [236]. Additional data are needed to further characterize the role of PMRT in this setting. The currently accruing NSABP B-51 trial is evaluating the value of RT after pathologic complete response to neoadjuvant chemotherapy and will hopefully bring clarity to these areas of uncertainty.

Inflammatory Breast Cancer

Inflammatory breast cancer (IBC) is a clinical diagnosis characterized by the rapid onset and spread of erythema, warmth, and edema throughout the breast. A discrete breast mass may not be palpable because the breast is diffusely infiltrated with tumor. The frequent pathologic correlate of this constellation of signs is the finding of tumor emboli in the dermal lymphatics, although this finding is neither necessary nor sufficient for assigning the clinical diagnosis. Dermal lymphatic invasion, if present, may be an independent poor prognostic factor [237]. The rarity of IBC – in the modern era it may comprise only 1% of all breast cancers – accounts for the absence of randomized trials [238]. Based on non-randomized data, the accepted standard treatment for this disease is aggressive multimodality therapy starting with neoadjuvant chemotherapy followed by mastectomy and PMRT [239]. Mastectomy should not be performed unless the inflammatory skin changes resolve completely with chemotherapy. The addition of taxanes to the chemotherapy regimen and the use of daily bolus during radiotherapy, among other modern improvements, appear to provide superior local control as compared to historical series. A series from MSKCC using multimodality therapy including taxanes and PMRT with daily bolus, reported a five-year LRC of 87% [240]. A report from the University of Florida suggests that dose escalation beyond 60 Gy may improve outcomes [241]. A series from M.D. Anderson Cancer Center reported on the use of twice-daily radiotherapy with dose escalation; the chest wall and draining lymphatics were treated to 51 Gy in 1.5-Gy fractions followed by a 15 Gy chest wall boost [242]. In this regimen, bolus was used during half of the treatments. With this regimen, the five- and 10-year rates of LRC were 84.3% and 77%, respectively, and significantly improved from their historical experience with standard fractionation. Despite these advances, IBC augurs a considerably poorer outlook as compared to other locally advanced breast cancers [243]. Favorable prognostic factors for IBC include tumor less than 4 cm, age over 55 years, and ER positivity [241, 244].

Salvage after LRR

The value of PMRT in preventing LRR is highlighted by the relatively dire prognosis of LRR after mastectomy. In a pooled analysis of DBCG 82b and 82c, 535 of the 3083 patients experienced solitary LRR as a site of first failure [245]. The five-year probability of developing distant metastatic disease was 73%, regardless of initial randomization assignment. Women with infraclavicular or supraclavicular failures exhibited worse outcomes (10-year OS of 15%) as compared to those with failures in the chest wall or low axilla. A series from the MDACC recorded the outcomes of 140 patients with LRR after mastectomy [246]. Those patients with a nodal recurrence in the SCV fossa had a 10-year DFS of 12% versus 40% for those with a chest wall recurrence only. A series of 145 patients with LRR after mastectomy from the University of Würzburg found a 10-year metastasis-free survival of 36% [247]. This series identified a favorable subgroup of patients as women aged over 50 years with a solitary chest wall or axillary recurrence and a disease-free interval more than one year. A Taiwanese series of 115 women with LRR after mastectomy found high grade, ER negativity, a short disease-free interval, nodal positivity, and less comprehensive treatment to be negative prognostic variables [248].

The treatment of LRR after mastectomy should include multimodality consultation. Although outcomes are poor, long-term disease-free survival is achievable for a subset of patients. The excision of gross disease from the chest wall or axilla is associated with improved outcomes [249, 250]. In a previously unirradiated patient, comprehensive radiotherapy to the chest wall and draining lymphatics is likely indicated. A boost to residual gross disease, if present, is advisable while respecting normal tissue tolerance. Re-irradiation of the SCV fossa is not typically feasible given the tolerance of the brachial plexus, but chest wall re-irradiation is indicated in some circumstances. Several series suggest that chest wall re-irradiation is relatively well tolerated and provides durable local control for many patients [249–252]. A multi-institutional series of breast and chest wall re-irradiation for recurrent breast cancer found an overall complete response rate of 57% [248]. Some series support an improvement in the rate of complete response with the addition of hyperthermia [249, 252].

Reconstruction

Many women desire reconstruction of the breast after mastectomy. This can be accomplished at the time of mastectomy (immediate) or after the mastectomy in a separate procedure (delayed). Reconstruction can be performed with autologous tissue transferred from an adjacent site in one of several techniques: latissimus dorsi flap, transverse rectus abdominus musculocutaneous (TRAM) flap or a deep inferior epigastic perforator artery (DIEP) flap. Not all women have a body habitus that is amenable to autologous techniques. Alternatively, reconstruction can be performed with an expander that is inflated to expand a tissue envelope; the expander is subsequently replaced with a permanent implant. In some cases, a full-size permanent implant can

be placed at the time of mastectomy. There are advantages and disadvantages to each surgical approach and to immediate versus delayed timing. Ideally, these decisions are made in a multidisciplinary fashion and account for patient preferences.

Immediate reconstruction techniques eliminate the window of time during which the patient is left without a breast, allow skin preservation that helps to minimize scars, and avoid the need for a second major operative procedure and recovery. They also allow women who require PMRT but do not qualify for (or would not accept) autologous procedures to receive breast reconstruction. However, PMRT delivered to a reconstructed breast can create fibrosis and encapsulation that lead to the impairment of cosmetic outcome as well as raising the risk of complication necessitating implant removal [253]. A comprehensive review of the literature estimated the rate of complications in woman who underwent an implant-based reconstruction followed by PMRT at over 40% and the extrusion rate at 15% [254]. Other reviews suggest even higher rates of toxicity when minor complications are also considered [255]. The use of acellular dermal matrix may amerliorate, but not eliminate, this risk [256]. Certain subsets of patients, including those over 55, the obese, and active smokers appear to be at higher risk for complications [257]. Consideration should be given to the optimal reconstruction decisions in women with more that one of these risk factors. Additionally, the presence of an inflated expander can create difficulties for the radiation oncologist. In dosimetric studies, the presence of an inflated expander frequently compromises either target coverage or normal tissue sparing (especially lung and heart) or both [258, 259]. This difficulty may be overcome, to some extent, with the use of IMRT although this greater conformality of the high isodose lines is typicallyy accompanied by an increase in the spread of low dose across the thorax [260]. The clinical outcomes may not be adversely affected if a multidisciplinary approach is taken. In one large series, women treated with PMRT in the presence of deflated expanders did not appear to have increased rates of LRR [261]. Although the presence of metal in the expander port does perturb the radiotherapy dose in adjacent tissues, the magnitude of this effect is relatively small [262–264]. In women with a very high risk of LRR, such as IBC, it is usually preferable to avoid immediate reconstruction.

If autologous reconstruction and PMRT are both planned, delayed reconstruction may be preferable. It appears that TRAM flap reconstruction delayed until after PMRT results in a lower rate of late complications and superior aesthetic appearance as compared to immediate TRAM flap reconstruction [265, 266]. Cigarette use is an independent risk factor for the development of tissue necrosis, and smoking cessation should be stressed prior to surgery [267].

Techniques

Techniques for the delivery of PMRT have evolved over time, and multiple acceptable approaches are currently in practice. A comparison of seven techniques for the irradiation of the chest wall and the IM chain in left-sided breast cancer from the University of Michigan found that no single technique was consistently superior with regard to coverage of the target regions and sparing of the lung and heart [268]. In this analysis, the partially-wide tangent (PWT) technique emerged as the favored balance in most cases. The DBCG performed a similar comparison and reached a similar conclusion, favoring the PWT technique [269]. When using IMRT, a tangential beamlet approach appears to reduce normal tissue exposure but maintain target coverage as compared to other field designs [270]. The MDACC has described a photon-electron match technique that uses higher-energy electrons in the upper medial aspect of the chest wall to encompass the IM nodes and a lower energy electron field in the lower medial aspect of the chest wall to spare the heart [271].

The preference at the present authors' institution in the administration of PMRT is to begin with CT simulation. First, the chest wall (and IM chain if desired) is treated with either PWT (Figure 37.6) or a medial electron strip matched to shallow lateral tangents (Figure 37.7) after dosimetric comparison and selection on an individual basis. When using PWT a 1 cm bolus every other day or daily for inflammatory cancers. When using a photon-electron match the junction then feathered at least once to smooth out dose inhomogeneity at the interface between fields. With either chest wall technique, is a mono-isocentric match to the nodal field is employed. The details of this monoisocentric technique and classic field borders have been described previously (see section on BCT for early-stage breast cancer). A boost might then be administered to the mastectomy incision with a 2–3 cm margin using *en face* electrons with daily bolus. Deep-inspiration breath hold (DIBH) has shown significant promise in reducing dose to the heart and left anterior descending artery. The authors favor its use when treating the left breast in the supine position, especially when the internal mammary chain is to be included in the RT field.

Standard Guidelines

Several collaborative bodies have issued guidelines on the use of PMRT [272–275]. In summary, the guidelines strongly support the use of PMRT in women with T4 tumors, T3 tumors and any involved nodes, and those with T1–T2 and four or more involved nodes. For women with T1–T2 tumors and one to three involved nodes, controversy persists despite strong empirical evidence in support of PMRT. A conversation with the patient concerning the risks and benefits of PMRT is indicated. Consideration of other risk factors for LRR in the setting of one to three involved nodes may be warranted. A dose of 50–50.4 Gy by 1.8–2 Gy fractions is standard. When PMRT is delivered, the chest wall – and most notably the mastectomy incision – should be included. Bolus should be used for at least a portion of treatment when using linear accelerators with photon energies greater than 4 mV. The use of a boost to the incision or chest wall is optional. The SCV fossa and undissected axilla should be included in all women with a significant risk of additional nodal involvement. Inclusion of the dissected axilla is typically unnecessary given the low risk of recurrence in this area unless other risk factors are present. The value of irradiation of the IM chain is uncertain. Careful sparing of the heart using CT planning is strongly advised so as to avoid an increase in late cardiac events.

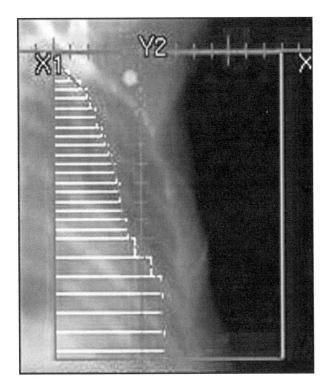

Figure 37.6 A partially-wide tangent (PWT) field encompassing the internal mammary nodes in the superior aspect of the field. For a color version of this figure, see the color plate section.

Summary Guidelines

- In node-positive patients, PMRT reduces the risk of LRR by approximately 75%, and significantly improves breast cancer-specific survival and overall survival.
- In recent randomized trials and on meta-analysis, the survival benefit of PMRT in women with one to three positive nodes was equivalent to that seen for women with four or more positive nodes.

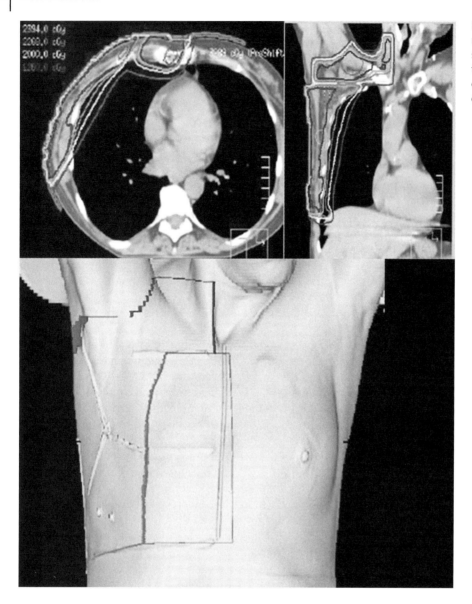

Figure 37.7 Post-mastectomy radiotherapy using a medial electron strip matched to a shallow photon tangent for chest wall coverage. For a color version of this figure, see the color plate section.

- Risk factors for LRR after mastectomy in the setting of one to three positive nodes include: young age, high-grade histology, ECE, LVI, and high nodal ratio.
- A low rate of LRR is seen for most women with node-negative tumors after mastectomy, although some patients with high-risk factors may have sufficient likelihood of recurrence to benefit from PMRT.
- LRR after mastectomy is associated with a high risk of subsequent development of metastatic disease.
- The clinical finding of inflammatory breast cancer augurs a poor prognosis, and comprehensive PMRT should follow neoadjuvant chemotherapy and mastectomy.
- Consideration should be given to the use of daily bolus or dose-escalation in the treatment of inflammatory breast cancer.
- Decisions regarding reconstruction in the setting of PMRT require multidisciplinary input and coordination.

Sequelae of Radiotherapy

Cosmetic Outcomes

There is no universally accepted system for evaluating cosmetic outcome after BCT. Evaluation schemas have included clinician's overall impression, clinician's ratings of cosmetic endpoints (e.g., telangiectasia, fibrosis, symmetry and hyperpigmentation), patient-reported ratings, and digital photographs reviewed by a panel of physicians not involved in the care of the patient. Cosmetic outcomes are influenced by all aspects of treatment as well as patient-related factors such as breast size, tumor size, and tumor location. Surgical technique has considerable influence on cosmetic outcome. The volume of breast tissue resected strongly influences cosmetic outcome [276, 277]. The cosmetic impairment associated with surgery may be ameliorated by the use of oncoplastic techniques [278].

Radiotherapy also contributes to a decline in cosmetic outcome. Radiotherapy can cause hyperpigmentation, telangiectasia, fibrosis, and breast retraction. The latter effect appears to be more common and pronounced in women with large or pendulous breasts [279]. A small separation between the medial and lateral field borders has associated with better cosmetic outcome after radiotherapy, likely due to a more homogeneous dose distribution throughout the breast [280, 281]. This finding has been validated by trials evaluating f-IMRT; the use of this technique to improve homogeneity reduces rates of moist desquamation, telangiectasia, and late cosmetic change [190–192]. The effect of radiotherapy on cosmetic change is dose-dependent. Whole-breast doses in excess of 50 Gy have been found to yield inferior cosmetic outcomes [276]. Similarly, dose escalation to part of the breast using a boost has been associated with telangiectasia and fibrosis [127, 128].

Systemic therapy has an impact on cosmetic outcome. Several reports have found that the addition of sequential adjuvant chemotherapy to BCT worsens cosmetic outcome [282–284]. In randomized trials of sequential versus concurrent chemotherapy and radiotherapy, there appears to be a greater degree of skin toxicity and cosmetic compromise in the concurrent arms [150, 152]. The impact of hormonal therapy on cosmetic outcome is less clear, and existing data are conflicting [282, 285, 286].

Late cosmetic outcomes stabilize after a few years and then remain constant [287]. For the most part, the severity of fibrosis and telangiectasia does not worsen after three to five years [287]. Few options exist to improve cosmetic outcomes after treatment is complete. Both, pulsed dye laser and hyfrecator have been used successfully to reduce telangiectasia resulting from breast radiotherapy [288, 289]. The use of vitamin E and pentoxifylline to reduce fibrosis has been studied, with mixed results [290–292]. If this regimen is to be used, a long course of treatment (more than three years) may be necessary [293].

Lymphedema/Upper-Extremity Function

The absolute risks of lymphedema vary greatly between studies, likely representing differences in surgical and hyfrecator technique, variability in the threshold change in arm circumference for diagnosis of lymphedema, and the length of follow-up. The risk of lymphedema of the upper extremity appears to rise along with the intensity of therapy to the draining lymphatics. An axillary dissection yields considerably higher rates of lymphedema than a SLNB [47–49]. In NSABP B-32, the rate of arm circumference difference exceeding 10% was 14% in the axillary dissection arm versus 8% in the SLNB arm. The addition of nodal hyfrecator increases the rate of lymphedema over axillary surgery alone [294, 295]. The reported rates of lymphedema after axillary dissection and nodal hyfrecator range from 9% to 38% [294, 295]. Tangential breast hyfrecator does not appear to increase the rate of lymphedema [295]. In the setting of nodal radiotherapy, the inclusion of the full axilla and the addition of a posterior axillary boost appear to increase the risk of lymphedema over irradiation of the SCV fossa and axillary apex alone [296]. Other high-risk factors include obesity and the use of systemic chemotherapy [296, 297]. These data suggest that, if clinically appropriate, an axillary dissection should be avoided. If an axillary dissection is indicated, then the dissected axilla should be omitted from the radiotherapy field as long as high-risk factors are not present. If feasible, an attempt should be made to spare a strip of skin at the superior aspect of the shoulder to preserve collateral lymphatic drainage. Lymphedema, when it occurs, tends to be chronic and treatment options are limited. The use of compression garments, exercise and manual drainage can be considered. The value of manual drainage has not been supported in a randomized trial [298].

Pulmonary Toxicity

Breast radiotherapy can induce both radiographic pulmonary changes such as an infiltrate or fibrosis, as well as the clinical syndrome of pneumonitis. Radiation pneumonitis is characterized by the appearance of cough, shortness of breath, and/or low-grade fever beginning weeks to months after the completion of therapy. The risk of radiation pneumonitis is clearly associated with the volume of lung irradiated [299, 300]. Classically, this was estimated by the central lung distance; presently it can also be calculated using dosimetric parameters. The percent volume of the ipsilateral lung receiving 20 Gy (V_{20}) may be the most valuable of these parameters [301]. As would be expected, the addition of a nodal radiotherapy field, which includes the apex of the lung, increases the risk of pneumonitis [302]. Early data from the EORTC 22922/10925 trial show that the three-year risk of lung toxicity increases from 1.3% to 4.3% with the addition of nodal radiotherapy [303]. The use of systemic corticosteroids can be considered if clinical symptoms are significant.

Cardiac Disease

The effect of radiotherapy on cardiac function is well documented. The possible late cardiac sequelae include ischemic heart disease, pericarditis, pericardial fibrosis, and valvular disease [304]. Ischemic heart disease is by far the most common adverse cardiac event following breast radiotherapy. The area of coronary artery disease induced by radiotherapy, as seen on angiography, correlates directly to the radiotherapy field [305]. During breast or chest wall radiotherapy, the apex of the heart can be included in the tangential fields. As a result, the mid and distal left anterior descending artery is at risk for accelerated atherosclerosis. The dose and volume of heart irradiated is correlated to the risk of cardiac injury. The inclusion of more than 5% of the left ventricle in radiotherapy fields is associated with a higher risk of perfusion deficits and motion abnormalities [306].

The dose-dependence of radiation-induced cardiac toxicity is shown most clearly by data from Sweden and Denmark in which treatment and clinical data for 2168 women treated with radiotherapy for breast cancer between 1958 and 2001 were reviewed [307]. The average mean heart dose (estimate) was 4.9 Gy. The rate of major coronary events [307] increased linearly with mean heart dose by 7.4% per Gy. There was no apparent threshold and the increased risk began within the first five years after radiotherapy.

Data from the EBCTCG have demonstrated a relative increase in the risk of cardiac death of 27% for the addition of radiotherapy to breast surgery [200]. This magnitude of cardiac toxicity may be a result of older radiotherapy techniques which delivered a higher dose to a larger volume of the heart. Data from the SEER registry show the hazard of death from ischemic heart disease for women with left-sided breast radiotherapy (as compared to right-sided) declined by 6% per year every year after 1979 [308]. Thus, modern techniques may be reducing the iatrogenic cardiac toxicity of radiotherapy and improving the therapeutic ratio. In a SEER analysis of patients treated from 1986 to 1993, no increased risk of cardiac morbidity at 15 years was seen for left-sided breast radiotherapy [309].

The introduction of heart block, prone positioning and deep inspiration breath-hold (DIBH) techniques hold the promise to further reduce cardiac irradiation. A cardiac block is the simplest technique for cardiac sparing, consisting of extension of the block or MLCs to exclude the heart from the tangent fields. This is typically restricted to women with low-risk cancers in whom the lumpectomy bed is located far from the heart. Early clinical data show no reduction in in-breast control with this technique [178]. DIBH describes a technique in which the patient inhales deeply, filling the lungs with air, increasing intrathoracic pressure, and moving the heart in both the posterior and inferior (caudal) directions. This motion results in displacement of the heart out of the radiotherapy field and consequent reduction in cardiac dose. The magnitude of this dosimetric improvement varies between studies with most series suggesting that heart dose is at least halved [310]. Early clinical data suggest that this dosimetric advantage translates into clinical benefits. In a series of 32 patients treated with RT to the breast and regional nodes (including the IM chain) at deep inspiration, pre- and post-RT perfusion scans were equivalent [311]. Unlike prior series in which perfusion

deficits were evident within the irradiated heart, exclusion of the heart from the RT field prevented these changes. DIBH can be accomplished with a variety of techniques including spirometry, optical guidance, RPM, a laser guide system, and others. The UK HeartSpare study found that a voluntary DIBH technique was equivalent to active breathing control with regard to positional reproducibility and cardiac sparing but was preferred by patients [312].

While DIBH achieves cardiac sparing by displacing the heart away from the breast, the prone position uses gravity to pull the breast away from the chest wall. Dosimetric analyses consistently show that the prone position reduces dose to the ipsilateral lung. The effect of prone positioning on cardiac dose is more variable since the heart is also subject to gravity and can move towards the chest wall, however, most series show a reduction in mean dose to the heart and left anterior descending artery [313]. High quality dosimetric comparisons of cardiac and pulmonary doses between DIBH and the prone position find DIBH superior in cardiac parameters, the prone position superior in lung sparing, and both techniques significantly better than supine free-breathing [314, 315]. Efforts have been made to combine the benefits of these two techniques using prone DIBH. Early clinical series show that DIBH in the prone position results in retraction of the heart from the chest wall and, consequently, optimal heart and lung sparing using this combination [316, 317]. It is not yet clear how the combination of radiotherapy and cardiotoxic systemic therapies such as anthracyclines and trastuzumab will affect long-term cardiac function, although early data suggest low rates of cardiac morbidity for this combination [318].

Brachial Plexopathy

Brachial plexopathy presents as numbness, pain, paresthesias or weakness of the affected upper extremity. This is an uncommon radiotherapy-associated toxicity in the modern era. Given its rarity, cancer recurrence must be ruled out as a cause prior to assigning a diagnosis of radiation-induced brachial plexopathy. The use of an aggressive hypofractionated regimen in combination with match-line overlap has been associated with a higher risk of injury. In a Swedish series, 77 women received approximately 57 Gy over 16–17 fractions to the brachial plexus [319]. At last follow-up, 11 of the 12 living patients had paralysis of the treated arm. In this cohort, the severity and frequency of brachial plexopathy increased over decades, underscoring the insidious nature of this side effect. Similarly, a series from Germany of 140 women who received approximately 52 Gy to the brachial plexus at 2.6 Gy per fraction found an annual rate of brachial plexopathy of grade 1 or higher of 2.9% [320]. This rate was essentially constant over 20 years of follow-up. Historically, the risk of brachial plexopathy has been much lower when standard fractionation was used as compared to hypofractionation [321]. It is unclear if this effect would persist if the total dose were reduced appropriately.

A modern single-institution series from Harvard found a rate of brachial plexopathy after 50 Gy in standard fractions of 0.4% without chemotherapy, and 3.4% with chemotherapy [322]. The rate of brachial plexopathy was lower if the prescribed dose did not exceed 50 Gy than if it exceeded 50 Gy (1.3% versus 5.6%). No standard treatment exists for brachial plexopathy; occupational therapy, medical therapy or transcutaneous electrical nerve stimulation can be considered.

Radiation-Induced Malignancy

The use of radiotherapy for breast cancer leads to a small but measurable elevation in the risk of developing a future malignancy, most notably an ipsilateral lung cancer or in-field sarcoma. The magnitude of this risk is small; in a large SEER analysis, radiotherapy resulted in five excess cancers per 1000 treated patients by 15 years after diagnosis [323].

A small excess in the rate of contralateral breast cancer (RR = 1.09) has been identified after radiotherapy [324]. This risk declines with increasing patient age and more recent year of treatment. The elevation in incidence of contralateral breast cancers may be attributable, in part, to older techniques in which backscatter dose was generated by the use of a physical wedge in the medial tangent field. The use of multiple beam segments reduces the contralateral breast dose by two-thirds as compared to a physical wedge [325].

Data from several large series have demonstrated a higher risk of lung cancer after breast irradiation [326, 327]. A SEER registry analysis found the lung cancer mortality ratio (ipsilateral versus contralateral) to be 1.17 at 10 years and 2.71 at 15 years after breast radiotherapy [325]. In several series the elevation in lung cancer risk appears to be almost entirely limited to smokers (former or current) as compared to non-smokers [328, 329].

A SEER registry analysis found a small elevation in the risk of soft-tissue sarcoma after breast irradiation, from 22 to 31 per 100 000 person–years (HR = 1.5) [331]. The prone position, which offers a dramatic reduction in lung dose, may also reduce the risk of an RT-induced lung cancer [330]. An elevated risk was noted for both malignant fibrous histiocytomas (HR = 2.5) and angiosarcomas (HR = 7.6). The hazard for diagnosis of a sarcoma peaked at 10 years before reaching non-radiotherapy hazard at 23 years. The median latency period between radiotherapy and the diagnosis of an angiosarcoma appears to be shorter than for other solid tumors, and has been reported in the range of five to seven years in some series [332, 333]. Due to the rarity of these tumors, the relationship between dose and risk of sarcoma development is unclear. Some studies suggest that there is a plateau beyond which an increasing dose does not increase the risk of tumor induction; other data support a linear-quadratic relationship without an adjustment for cell killing at high doses [334, 335]. The extent to which other treatments modify the risk of malignancy induction is also unclear. The addition of chemotherapy may increase the risk of sarcoma development after breast radiotherapy [336]. The risk of sarcoma induction may be elevated after BCT as compared to mastectomy with PMRT [331]. Similarly, angiosarcoma induction may be more common after a lymph node dissection as compared to no nodal surgery [331].

Summary

- Cosmetic outcome after BCT is dependent on patient factors, tumor characteristics, surgical factors, and radiotherapy parameters.
- Overall, cosmetic outcomes after BCT are typically quite good, and cosmetic decline stabilizes within a few years after treatment.
- Dose inhomogeneity within the breast, whole-breast dose escalation above 50 Gy, the use of a boost, and receipt of chemotherapy are associated with somewhat poorer cosmetic outcomes.
- The risk of lymphedema rises along with the intensity of therapy to the draining lymphatics; axillary dissection increases the risk of lymphedema over SLNB, and nodal radiotherapy after axillary dissection further increases this risk.
- Radiation pneumonitis is uncommon after breast radiotherapy, and its risk is correlated to the volume of lung irradiated.
- Cardiac toxicity from radiotherapy is related to the dose delivered and volume of heart irradiated.
- Modern 3D-CT simulation and conformal radiotherapy delivery, if used appropriately, allow far superior cardiac-sparing than older techniques.
- Population registries suggest that cardiac toxicity has been declining substantially in more recent years.
- Brachial plexopathy is a rare late side effect after nodal radiotherapy.
- The use of standard fraction size (1.8–2 Gy), limitation of the prescription dose to 50 Gy or less, avoidance of field overlap, and careful CT planning minimize the risk of brachial plexopathy.
- Radiation-induced malignancy is a rare late effect after breast radiotherapy.
- Breast radiotherapy raises the rate of ipsilateral lung cancers; this effect is seen primarily in smokers.
- Breast radiotherapy elevates the risk of a sarcoma, especially an in-field angiosarcoma, although the absolute risk of this toxicity is extremely small.

References

1 Siegel, R., Miller, K., Jemal, A. (2017) Cancer Statistics 2017. *CA Cancer J. Clin.*, **67**, 7–30.

2 Berg, J.W. (1955) The significance of axillary node levels in the study of breast carcinoma. *Cancer*, **8** (4), 776–778.

3 Amin, M.B. (2017) AJCC Cancer Staging Manual, 8th edition. Springer.

4 Kerlikowske, K. (2010) Epidemiology of ductal carcinoma in situ. *J. Natl Cancer Inst. Monogr.*, **2010** (41), 139–141.

5 Fu, W., Lobocki, C.A., Silverberg, B.K., Chelladurai, M., Young, S.C. (2001) Molecular markers in Paget disease of the breast. *J. Surg. Oncol.*, **77** (3), 171–178.

6 Chen, C.Y., Sun, L.M., Anderson, B.O. (2006) Paget disease of the breast: changing patterns of incidence, clinical presentation, and treatment in the U.S. *Cancer*, **107** (7), 1448–1458.

7 Bijker, N., Rutgers, E.J., Duchateau, L., *et al.* (2001) Breast-conserving therapy for Paget disease of the nipple: a prospective European Organization for Research and Treatment of Cancer study of 61 patients. *Cancer*, **91** (3), 472–477.

8 Moshin, S.K., O'Connell, P., Allred, D.C., Libby, A.L. (2005) Biomarker profile and genetic abnormalities in lobular carcinoma in situ. *Breast Cancer Res. Treat.*, **90** (3), 249–256.

9 Chen, Y.Y., Hwang, E.S., Roy, R., *et al.* (2009) Genetic and phenotypic characteristics of pleomorphic lobular carcinoma in situ of the breast. *Am. J. Surg. Pathol.*, **33** (11), 1683–1694.

10 Page, D.L., Schuyler, P.A., Dupont, W.D., *et al.* (2003) Atypical lobular hyperplasia as an unilateral predictor of breast cancer risk: a retrospective cohort study. *Lancet*, **361** (9352), 125–129.

11 Page, D.L., Kidd, T.E., Jr, Dupont, W.D., Simpson, J.F., Rogers, L.W. (1991) Lobular neoplasia of the breast: higher risk for subsequent invasive cancer predicted by more extensive disease. *Hum. Pathol.*, **22** (12), 1232–1239.

12 Chuba, P.J., Hamre, M.R., Yap, J., *et al.* (2005) Bilateral risk for subsequent breast cancer after lobular carcinoma-in-situ: analysis of surveillance, epidemiology, and end results data. *J. Clin. Oncol.*, **23** (24), 5534–5541.

13 Sneige, N., Wang, J., Baker, B.A., Krishnamurthy, S., Middleton, L.P. (2002) Clinical, histopathologic, and biologic features of pleomorphic lobular (ductal-lobular) carcinoma in situ of the breast: a report of 24 cases. *Mod. Pathol.*, **15** (10), 1044–1050.

14 Reis-Filho, J.S., Simpson, P.T., Jones, C. (2005) Pleomorphic lobular carcinoma of the breast: role of comprehensive molecular pathology in characterization of an entity. *J. Pathol.*, **207** (1), 1–13.

15 Allred, D.C. (2010) Ductal carcinoma in situ: terminology, classification and natural history. *J. Natl Cancer Inst. Monogr.*, **2010** (41), 134–138.

16 Schnitt, S.J. (2010) Local outcomes in ductal carcinoma in situ based on patient and tumor characteristics. *J. Natl Cancer Inst. Monogr.*, **2010** (41), 158–161.

17 Pedersen, L., Zedeler, K., Holck, S., Schiodt, T., Mouridsen, H.T. (1995) Medullary carcinoma of the breast. Prevalence and prognostic importance of classical risk factors in breast cancer. *Eur. J. Cancer*, **31A** (13-14), 2289–2295.

18 Chinyama, C.N., Davies, J.D. (1996) Mammary mucinous lesions: congeners, prevalence and important pathological associations. *Histopathology*, **29** (6), 533–539.

19 Tremblay, G. (1974) Elastosis in tubular carcinoma of the breast. *Arch. Pathol.*, **98** (5), 302–307.

20 Cabral, A.H., Recine, M., Paramo, J.C., McPhee, M., Poppiti, R., Mesko, T.W. (2003) Tubular carcinoma of the breast: an institutional experience and review of the literature. *Breast J.*, **9** (4), 298–301.

21 Rosen, P.P. (1979) The pathological classification of human mammary carcinoma: past, present and future. *Ann. Clin. Lab. Sci.*, **9** (2), 144–156.

22 Dixon, J.M., Anderson, T.J., Page, D.L., Lee, D., Duffy, S.W. (1982) Infiltrating lobular carcinoma of the breast. *Histopathology*, **6** (2), 149–161.

23 Moll, R., Mitze, M., Frixen, U.H., Birchmeier, W. (1993) Differential loss of E-cadherin expression in infiltrating ductal and lobular breast carcinomas. *Am. J. Pathol.*, **143** (6), 1731–1742.

24 Dedes, K.J., Fink, D. (2008) Clinical presentation and surgical management of invasive lobular carcinoma of the breast. *Breast Dis.*, **30**, 31–37.

25 Arndt, V., Stegmaier, C., Ziegler, H., Brenner, H. (2008) Quality of life over 5 years in women with breast cancer after breast-conserving therapy versus mastectomy: a population-based study. *J. Cancer Res. Clin. Oncol.*, **134** (12), 1311–1318.

26 Ganz, K.L, Stanton, A.L., *et al.* (2004) Quality of life at the end of primary treatment of breast cancer first results from the moving beyond cancer randomized trial. *J. Natl Cancer Inst.*, **96** (5), 376–387.

27 Houssami, N., Turner, R., Morrow, M. (2013) Preoperative magnetic resonance imaging in breast cancer: meta-analysis of surgical outcomes. *Ann. Surg.*, **257** (2), 249–255.

28 Grann, A., Abdou, J.C., Dragman, N., Goodman, R. (2004) The value of postexcision preradiation mammography in patients with early-stage breast cancer. *Am J. Clin. Oncol.*, **27** (3), 285–288.

29 Aref, A., Youssef, E., Washington, T., *et al.* (2000) The value of postlumpectomy mammogram in the

management of breast cancer patients presenting with suspicious microcalcifications. *Cancer J. Sci. Am.*, **6** (1), 25–27.

30 Lally, B.E., Haffty, B.G., Moran, M.S., Colasanto, J.M., Higgins, S.A. (2005) Management of suspicious or indeterminate calcifications and impact on local control. *Cancer*, **103** (11), 2236–2240.

31 Mazonakis, M., Varveris, H., Damilakis, J., Theoharopoulos, N., Gourtsoyiannis, N. (2003) Radiation dose to conceptus resulting from tangential breast irradiation. *Int. J. Radiat. Oncol. Biol. Phys.*, **55** (2), 386–391.

32 De Santis, M., Di Gianantonio, E., Straface, G. (2005) Ionizing radiations in pregnancy and teratogenesis: A review of literature. *Reprod. Toxicol.*, **20** (3), 323–329.

33 Lin, A., Abu-Isa, E., Griffith, K.A., Ben-Josef, E. (2008) Toxicity of radiotherapy in patients with collagen vascular disease. *Cancer*, **113** (3), 648–653.

34 Morris, M.M., Powell, S.N. (1997) Irradiation in the setting of collagen vascular disease: acute and late complications. *J. Clin. Oncol.*, **15** (7), 2728–2735.

35 Chen, A.M., Obedian, E., Haffty, B.G. (2001) Breast-conserving therapy in the setting of collagen vascular disease. *Cancer J.*, **7** (6), 480–491.

36 Wo, J., Taghian, A. (2007) Radiotherapy in setting of collagen vascular disease. *Int. J. Radiat. Oncol. Biol. Phys.*, **69** (5), 1347–1353.

37 Voogd, A.C., Nielsen, M., Peterse, J.L., *et al.* (2001) Difference in risk factors for local and distant recurrence after breast-conserving therapy or mastectomy for stage I and II breast cancer: pooled results of two large European randomized trials. *J. Clin. Oncol.*, **19** (6), 1688–1697.

38 Arvold, N.D., Taghian, A.G., Niemierko, A., *et al.* (2011) Age, breast cancer subtype approximation, and local recurrence after breast-conserving therapy. *J. Clin. Oncol.*, **29** (29), 3885–3891.

39 Veronesi, U., Cascinelli, N., Mariani, L., *et al.* (2002) Twenty-year follow-up of a randomized study comparing breast-conserving surgery with radical mastectomy for early breast cancer. *N. Engl. J. Med.*, **347** (16), 1227–1232.

40 Beadle, B.M., Woodward, W.A., Tucker, S.L., *et al.* (2009) Ten-year recurrence rates in young women with breast cancer by locoregional treatment approach. *Int. J. Radiat. Oncol. Biol. Phys.*, **73** (3), 734–744.

41 Bantema-Joppe, E.J., de Munck, L., Visser, O., *et al.* (2011) Early-stage young breast cancer patients: impact of local regional treatment on survival. *Int. J. Radiat. Oncol. Biol. Phys.*, **81** (4), e553–e559.

42 Robson, M., Svahn, T., McCormick, B., *et al.* (2005) Appropriateness of breast-conserving treatment of breast carcinoma in women with germline mutations in BRCA1 or BRCA2: a clinic-based series. *Cancer*, **103** (1), 44–51.

43 Kriova, Y.M., Stoppa-Lyonnet, D., Savignoni, A., *et al.* (2005) Risk of breast cancer recurrence and contralateral breast cancer in relation to BRCA1 and BRCA2 mutation status following breast-conserving surgery and radiotherapy. *Eur. J. Cancer*, **41** (15), 2304–2311.

44 Garcia-Etienne, C.A., Barile, M., Gentilini, O.D., *et al.* (2009) Breast-conserving surgery in BRCA1/2 mutation carriers: are we approaching an answer? *Ann. Surg. Oncol.*, **16** (12), 3380–3387.

45 Haffty, B.G., Harrold, E., Khan, A.J., *et al.* (2002) Outcome of conservatively managed early-onset breast cancer by BRCA1/2 status. *Lancet*, **359** (9316), 1471–1477.

46 Robson, M., Levin, D., Federici, M., *et al.* (1999) Breast conservation therapy for invasive breast cancer in Ashkenazi women with BRCA gene founder mutations. *J. Natl Cancer Inst.*, **91** (24), 2112–2117.

47 Gill, G., SNAC Trial Group of the Royal Australasian College of Surgeons (RACS) and NHMRC Clinical Trials Centre (2009) Sentinel-lymph-node-based management or routine axillar clearance? One-year outcomes of sentinel node biopsy versus axillary clearance (SNAC): a randomized controlled surgical trial. *Ann. Surg. Oncol.*, **16** (2), 266–275.

48 Land, S.R., Kopec, J.A., Julian, T.B., *et al.* (2010) Patient-reported outcomes in sentinel node-negative adjuvant breast cancer patients receiving sentinel-node biopsy or axillary dissection: National Surgical Adjuvant Breast and Bowel Project phase III protocol B-32. *J. Clin. Oncol.*, **28** (25), 3929–3936.

49 Ashikaga, T., Krag, D.N., Land, S.R., *et al.* (2010) Morbidity results from the NSABP B-32 trial comparing sentinel lymph node dissection versus axillary dissection. *J. Surg. Oncol.*, **102** (2), 111–118.

50 Krag, D.N., Anderson, S.J., Julian, T.B., *et al.* (2010) Sentinel-lymph-node resection compared with conventional axillary-lymph-node dissection in clinically node-negative patients with breast cancer: overall survival findings from the NSABP B-32 randomised phase 3 trial. *Lancet Oncol.*, **11** (10), 927–933.

51 Veronesi, U., Viale, G., Paganelli, G., *et al.* (2010) Sentinel lymph node biopsy in breast cancer: ten-year results of a randomized controlled study. *Ann. Surg.*, **251** (4), 595–600.

52 Canavese, G., Catturich, A., Vecchio, C., *et al.* (2009) Sentinel node biopsy compared with complete axillary dissection for staging early breast cancer with clinically negative lymph nodes: results of randomized trial. *Ann. Oncol.*, **20** (6), 1001–1007.

53 Guiliano, A.E., Hunt, K.K., Ballman, K.V., *et al.* (2011) Axillary dissection vs no axillary dissection in women with invasive breast cancer and sentinel node metastasis: a randomized clinical trial. *JAMA*, **305** (6), 569–575.

54 Guiliano, A.E., McCall, L., Beitsch, P., *et al.* (2010) Locoregional recurrence after sentinel lymph node dissection with or without axillary dissection in patients with sentinel lymph node metastases: the American College of Surgeons Oncology Group Z0011 randomized trial. *Ann. Surg.*, **252** (3), 426–432.

55 Boyages, J., Delaney, G., Taylor, R. (1999) Predictors of local recurrence after treatment of ductal carcinoma in situ: a meta-analysis. *Cancer*, **85** (3), 616–628.

56 Wapnir, I.L., Dignam, J.J., Fisher, B., *et al.* (2011) Long-term outcomes of invasive ipsilateral breast tumor recurrence after lumpectomy in NSABP B-17 and B-24 randomized clinical trials for DCIS. *J. Natl Cancer Inst.*, **103** (6), 478–488.

57 Cuzick, J., Sestak, I., Pinder, S.E., *et al.* (2011) Effect of tamoxifen and radiotherapy in women with locally excised ductal carcinoma in situ: long-term results from the UK/ANZ DCIS trial. *Lancet Oncol.*, **12** (1) 21–29.

58 EORTC Breast Cancer Cooperative Group, EORTC Radiotherapy Group, Bijker, N., *et al.* (2006) Breast-conserving treatment with or without radiotherapy in ductal carcinoma-in-situ: ten-year results of European Organization for Research and Treatment of Cancer randomized phase III trial 10853 – a study by the EORTC Breast Cancer Cooperative Group and EORTC Radiotherapy Group. *J. Clin. Oncol.*, **24** (21), 3381–3387.

59 Donker, M., Litiere, S., Werutsky, G., *et al.* (2013) Breast-conserving treatment with or without radiotherapy in ductal carcinoma in situ: 15-year recurrent rates and outcome after a recurrence, from the EORTC 10853 randomized phase III trial. *J. Clin. Oncol.*, **31** (32), 4054–4059.

60 Warnberg, F., Garmo, H., Emdin, S., *et al.* (2014) Effect of radiotherapy after breast-conserving surgery for ductal carcinoma in situ: 20 years follow-up in the randomized SweDCIS Trial. *J. Clin. Oncol.*, **32** (32), 3613–3618.

61 Early Breast Cancer Trialists' Collaborative Group (EBCTCG), Correa, C., McGale, P., *et al.* (2010) Overview of the randomized trials of radiotherapy in ductal carcinoma in situ of the breast. *J. Natl Cancer Inst. Monogr.*, **2010** (41), 162–177.

62 Buchholz, T.A., Haffty, B.G., Harris, J.R. (2007) Should all patients undergoing breast conserving therapy for DCIS receive radiation therapy? Yes. Radiation therapy, an important component of breast conserving treatment for patients with ductal carcinoma in situ of the breast. *J. Surg. Oncol.*, **95** (8), 610–613.

63 Sagara, Y., Freedman, R., Vaz-Luis, I., *et al.* (2016) Patient Prognostic Score and Associations With Survival Improvement Offered by Radiotherapy After Breast-Conserving Surgery for Ductal Carcinoma In Situ: A Population-Based Longitudinal Cohort Study. *J. Clin. Oncol.*, **34** (11), 1190–1196.

64 Allred, D.C., Anderson, S.J., Paik, S., *et al.* (2012) Adjuvant tamoxifen reduces subsequent breast cancer in women with estrogen receptor-positive ductal carcinoma in situ: a study based on NSABP protocol B-24. *J. Clin. Oncol.*, **30** (12), 1268–1273.

65 Margolese, R.G., Cecchini, R.S., Julian, T.B., *et al.* (0000) Anastrazole versus tamoxifen in postmenopausal women with ductal carcinoma in situ undergoing lumpectomy plus radiotherapy (NSABP B-35): a randomised, double-blind, phase 3 clinical trial. *Lancet*, **387** (10021), 849–856.

66 Forbes, J.F., Sestak, I., Howell, A., *et al.* (0000) Anastrazole versus tamoxifen for the prevention of locoregional and contralateral breast cancer in postmenopausal women with locally excised ductal carcinoma in situ (IBIS-II DCIS): a double-blind, randomised controlled trial. *Lancet*, **387** (10021), 866–873.

67 Solin, L.J., Fourquet, A., Vicini, F.A., *et al.* (2005) Long-term outcome after breast-conservation treatment with radiation for mammographically detected ductal carcinoma in situ of the breast. *Cancer*, **103** (6), 1137–1146.

68 Van Zee, K.J., Subhedar, P., Olcese, C., *et al.* (2015) Relationship Between Margin Width and Recurrence of Ductal Carcinoma In Situ: Analysis of 2996 Women Treated With Breast-conserving Surgery for 30 Years. *Ann. Surg. Oncol.*, **262** (4), 623–631.

69 Solin, L.J., Gray, R., Baehner, F.L., *et al.* (2013) A multigene expression assay to predict local recurrence risk for ductal carcinoma in situ of the breast. *J. Natl Cancer Inst.*, **105** (10), 701–710.

70 Rakovitch, E., Nofech-Mozes, S., Hannah, W. (2015) A population-based validation study of the DCIS Score predicting recurrence risk in individuals treated by breast-conserving surgery alone. *Breast Cancer Res. Treat.*, **152** (2), 389–398.

71 Raldow, A., Sher, D., Chen, A., *et al.* (2016) Cost Effectiveness of the Oncotype DX DCIS Score for Guiding Treatment of Patients With Ductal Carcinoma In Situ. *J. Clin. Oncol.*, **34** (33), 3963–3968.

72 Wang, S.Y., Shamliyan, T., Virnig, B.A., Kane, R. (2011) Tumor characteristics as predictors of local recurrence after treatment of ductal carcinoma in situ: a meta-analysis. *Breast Cancer Res. Treat.*, **127** (1), 1–14.

73 Dunne, C., Burke, J.P., Morrow, M., Kell, M.R. (2009) Effect of margin status on local recurrence after breast conservation and radiation therapy for ductal carcinoma in situ. *J. Clin. Oncol.*, **27** (10), 1615–1620.

74 Morrow, M., Van Zee, K.J., Solin, L.J., *et al.* (2016) Society of Surgical Oncology-American Society for Radiation Oncology-American Society of Clinical Oncology Consensus Guideline on Margins for Breast-Conserving Surgery With Whole-Breast

Irradiation in Ductal Carcinoma In Situ. *J. Clin. Oncol.* 2016 Aug 15., Epub ahead of print.

75 Wong, J.S., Kaelin, C.M., Troyan, S.L., *et al.* (2006) Prospective study of wide excision alone for ductal carcinoma in situ of the breast. *J. Clin. Oncol.*, **24** (7), 1031–1036.

76 Hughes, L.L., Wang, M., Page, D.L., *et al.* (2009) Local excision alone without irradiation for ductal carcinoma in situ of the breast: a trial of the Eastern Cooperative Oncology Group. *J. Clin. Oncol.*, **27** (32), 5319–5324.

77 Solin, L.J., Kurtz, J., Fourquet, A., *et al.* (1996) Fifteen-year results of breast-conserving surgery and definitive breast irradiation for the treatment of ductal carcinoma in situ of the breast. *J. Clin. Oncol.*, **14** (3), 754–763.

78 McCormick, B., Winter, K., Hudis, C., *et al.* (2015) RTOG 9804: A prospective randomized trial for good risk ductal carcinoma in situ (DCIS) comparing radiotherapy to observation. *J. Clin. Oncol.*, **33** (7), 709–715.

79 Williamson, D., Dinniwell, R., Fung, S., Pintilie, M., Done, S.J., Fyles, A.W. (2010) Local control with conventional and hypofractionated adjuvant radiotherapy after breast-conserving surgery for ductal carcinoma in-situ. *Radiother. Oncol.*, **95** (3), 317–320.

80 NCT00470236 [cited 6 January 2013]. Available at: http://clinicaltrials.gov/show/NCT00470236.

81 Omlin, A., Amichetti, M., Azria, D., *et al.* (2006) Boost radiotherapy in young women with ductal carcinoma in situ: a multicentre, retrospective study of the Rare Cancer Network. *Lancet Oncol.*, **7** (8), 652–656.

82 Julian, T.B., Land, S.R., Wang, Y., *et al.* (2008) Is boost therapy necessary in the treatment of DCIS. *J. Clin. Oncol.*, **26** (Suppl.), abstract 537.

83 Azria, D., Cowen, D., De La Lande, B., *et al.* (2011) Phase III randomized French multicentric study to evaluate the impact of a localized 16 Gy boost after conservative surgery and a 50-Gy whole-breast irradiation breast ductal carcinoma in situ (the BONBIS trial). *Cancer Res.*, **71** (24 Suppl.), OT2-06-01–OT2-06-01.

84 Solin, L.J., Fourquet, A., Vicini, F.A., *et al.* (2005) Salvage treatment for local or local-regional recurrence after initial breast conservation treatment with radiation for ductal carcinoma in situ. *Eur. J. Cancer*, **41** (12), 1715–1723.

85 Veronesi, U., Cascinelli, N., Mariani, L., *et al.* (2002) Twenty-year follow-up of a randomized study comparing breast-conserving surgery with radical mastectomy for early breast cancer. *N. Engl. J. Med.*, **347** (16), 1227–1232.

86 Arriagada, R., Le, M.G., Guinebretiere, J.M., Dunant, A., Rochard, F., Tursz, T. (2003) Late local recurrences in a randomised trial comparing conservative

treatment with total mastectomy in early breast cancer patients. *Ann. Oncol.*, **14** (11), 1617–1622.

87 Fisher, B., Anderson, S., Bryant, J., *et al.* (2002) Twenty-year follow-up of a randomized trial comparing total mastectomy, lumpectomy, and lumpectomy plus irradiation for the treatment of invasive breast cancer. *N. Engl. J. Med.*, **347** (16), 1233–1241.

88 Simone, N.L., Dan, T., Shih, J., *et al.* (2012) Twenty-five year results of the national cancer institute randomized breast conservation trial. *Breast Cancer Res. Treat.*, **132** (1), 197–203.

89 Litiere, S., Werutsky, G., Fentiman, I.S., *et al.* (2012) Breast conserving therapy versus mastectomy for stage I–II breast cancer: 20 year follow-up of the EORTC 10901 phase 3 randomised trial. *Lancet Oncol.*, **13** (4), 412–419.

90 Blichert-Toft, M., Nielsen, M., During, M., *et al.* (2008) Long-term results of breast conserving surgery vs. mastectomy for early stage invasive breast cancer: 20-year follow-up of the Danish randomized DBCG-82TM protocol. *Acta Oncol.*, **47** (4), 672–681.

91 Early Breast Cancer Trialists' Collaborative Group (1995) Effects of radiotherapy and surgery in early breast cancer. An overview of the randomized trials. *N. Engl. J. Med.*, **333** (22), 1444–1455.

92 Liljegren, G., Holmberg, L., Bergh, J., *et al.* (1999) 10-year results after sector resection with or without postoperative radiotherapy for stage I breast cancer: a randomized trial. *J. Clin. Oncol.*, **17** (8), 2326–2333.

93 Veronesi, U., Marubini, E., Mariani, L., *et al.* (2001) Radiotherapy after breast-conserving surgery in small breast carcinoma: long-term results of a randomized trial. *Ann. Oncol.*, **12** (7), 997–1003.

94 Forrest, A.P., Stewart, H.J., Everington, D., *et al.* (1996) Randomised controlled trial of conservation therapy for breast cancer: 6-year analysis of the Scottish trial. Scottish Cancer Trials Breast Group. *Lancet*, **348** (9029), 708–713.

95 Ford, H.T., Coombes, R.C., Gazet, J.C., *et al.* (2006) Long-term follow-up of a randomized trial designed to determine the need for irradiation following conservative surgery for the treatment of invasive breast cancer. *Ann Oncol.*, **17** (3), 401–408.

96 Clark, R.M., Whelan, T., Levine, M., *et al.* (1996) Randomized clinical trial of breast irradiation following lumpectomy and axillary dissection for node-negative breast cancer: an update. Ontario Clinical Oncology Group. *J. Natl Cancer Inst.*, **88** (22), 1659–1664.

97 Malmstrom, P., Holmberg, L., Anderson, H., *et al.* (2003) Breast conservation surgery, with and without radiotherapy, in women with lymph node-negative breast cancer: a randomised clinical trial in a population with access to public mammography screening. *Eur. J. Cancer*, **39** (12), 1690–1697.

98 Holli, K., Hietanen, P., Saaristo, R., Huhtala, H., Hakama, M., Joensuu, H. (2009) Radiotherapy after segmental resection of breast cancer with favorable prognostic features: 12-year follow-up results of a randomized trial. *J. Clin. Oncol.*, **27** (6), 927–932.

99 Early Breast Cancer Trialists' Collaborative Group (EBCTCG), Darby, S., McGale, P., *et al.* (2011) Effect of radiotherapy after breast-conserving surgery on 10-year recurrence and 15-year breast cancer death: meta-analysis of individual patient data for 10,801 women in 17 randomised trials. *Lancet*, **378** (9804), 1707–1716.

100 Fisher, B., Bryant, J., Dignam, J.J., *et al.* (2002) Tamoxifen, radiation therapy, or both for prevention of ipsilateral breast tumor recurrence after lumpectomy in women with invasive breast cancers of one centimeter or less. *J. Clin. Oncol.*, **20** (20), 4141–4149.

101 Fyles, A.W., McCready, D.R., Manchul, L.A., *et al.* (2004) Tamoxifen with or without breast irradiation in women 50 years of age or older with early breast cancer. *N. Engl. J. Med.*, **351** (10), 963–970.

102 Hughes, K.S., Schnaper, L.A., Berry, D., *et al.* (2004) Lumpectomy plus tamoxifen with or without irradiation in women 70 years of age or older with early breast cancer. *N. Engl. J. Med.*, **351** (10), 971–977.

103 Hughes, K.S., Schnaper, L.A., Bellon, J.R., *et al.* (2013) Lumpectomy plus tamoxifen with or without irradiation in women age 70 years or older with early breast cancer: long-term follow-up of CALGB 9343. *J. Clin. Oncol.*, **31** (19), 2382–2387.

104 Winzer, K.J., Sauerbrei, W., Braun, M., *et al.* (2010) Radiation therapy and tamoxifen after breast-conserving surgery: updated results of a 2×2 randomised clinical trial in patients with low risk of recurrence. *Eur. J. Cancer*, **46** (1), 95–101.

105 Blamey, R.W., Bates, T., Chetty, U., *et al.* (2013) Radiotherapy or tamoxifen after conserving surgery for breast cancers of excellent prognosis: British Association of Surgical Oncology (BASO) II trial. *Eur. J. Cancer*, **49** (10), 2294–2302.

106 Potter, R., Gnant, M., Kwasny, W., *et al.* (2007) Lumpectomy plus tamoxifen or anastrozole with or without whole breast irradiation in women with favorable early breast cancer. *Int. J. Radiat. Oncol. Biol. Phys.*, **68** (2), 334–340.

107 Kunkler, I.H., Williams, L.J., Jack, W.J.L., *et al.* (2015) Breast-conserving surgery with or without irradiation in women aged 65 years or older with early breast cancer (PRIME II): a randomized controlled trial. *Lancet Oncol.*, **16** (3), 266–273.

108 Renton, S.C., Gazet, J.C., Ford, H.T., Corbishley, C., Sutcliffe, R. (1996) The importance of the resection margin in conservative surgery for breast cancer. *Eur. J. Surg. Oncol.*, **22** (1), 17–22.

109 Freedman, G., Fowble, B., Hanlon, A., *et al.* (1999) Patients with early stage invasive cancer with close or positive margins treated with conservative surgery and radiation have an increased risk of breast recurrence that is delayed by adjuvant systemic therapy. *Int. J. Radiat. Oncol. Biol. Phys.*, **44** (5), 1005–1015.

110 Wazer, D.E., Jabro, G., Ruthazer, R., *et al.* (1999) Extent of margin positivity as a predictor for local recurrence after breast conserving irradiation. *Radiat. Oncol. Investig.*, **7** (2), 111–117.

111 Obedian, E., Haffty, B.G. (2000) Negative margin status improves local control in conservatively managed breast cancer patients. *Cancer J. Sci. Am.*, **6** (1), 28–33.

112 Houssami, N., Macaskill, P., Marinovich, M.L., *et al.* (2010) Meta-analysis of the impact of surgical margins on local recurrence in women with early-stage invasive breast cancer treated with breast-conserving therapy. *Eur. J. Cancer*, **46** (18), 3219–3232.

113 Houssami, N., Macaskill, P., Luke Marinovich, M. (2014) The association of surgical margins and local recurrence in women with early-stage invasive breast cancer treated with breast-conserving therapy: a meta-analysis. *Ann. Surg. Oncol.*, **21** (3), 717–730.

114 Moran, M.S., Schnitt, S.J., Giuliano, A.E., *et al.* (2014) Society of Surgical Oncology-American Society for Radiation Oncology guideline on margins for breast-conserving surgery with whole-breast irradiation in stages I and II invasive breast cancer. *J. Clin. Oncol.*, **32** (14), 1507–1515.

115 Jones, H.A., Antonini, N., Hart, A.A., *et al.* (2009) Impact of pathological characteristics on local relapse after breast-conserving therapy: a subgroup analysis of the EORTC boost versus no boost trial. *J. Clin. Oncol.*, **27** (30), 4939–4947.

116 Early Breast Cancer Trialists' Collaborative Group (2005) Effects of chemotherapy and hormonal therapy for early breast cancer on recurrence and 15-year survival: an overview of the randomised trials. *Lancet*, **365** (9472), 1687–1717.

117 Sartor, C.I., Peterson, B.L., Woolf, S., *et al.* (2005) Effect of addition of adjuvant paclitaxel on radiotherapy delivery and locoregional control of node-positive breast cancer: cancer and leukemia group B 9344. *J. Clin. Oncol.*, **23** (1), 30–40.

118 Romond, E.H., Perez, E.A., Bryant, J., *et al.* (2005) Trastuzumab plus adjuvant chemotherapy for operable HER2-positive breast cancer. *N. Engl. J. Med.*, **353** (16), 1673–1684.

119 Cancer Genome Atlas Network (2012) Comprehensive molecular portraits of human breast tumours. *Nature*, **490** (7418), 61–70.

120 Hattangadi-Gluth, J.A., Wo, J.Y., Nguyen, P.L., *et al.* (2012) Basal subtype of invasive breast cancer is associated with a higher risk of true recurrence after

conventional breast-conserving therapy. *Int. J. Radiat. Oncol. Biol. Phys.*, **82** (3), 1185–1191.

121 Voduc, K.D., Cheang, M.C., Tyldesley, S., Gelmon, K., Nielsen, T.O., Kennecke, H. (2010) Breast cancer subtypes and the risk of local and regional relapse. *J. Clin. Oncol.*, **28** (10), 1684–1691.

122 Kyndi, M., Sorensen, F.B., Knudsen, H., *et al.* (2008) Estrogen receptor, progesterone receptor, HER-2, and response to postmastectomy radiotherapy in high-risk breast cancer: the Danish Breast Cancer Cooperative Group. *J. Clin. Oncol.*, **26** (9), 1419–1426.

123 Mamounas, E.P., Tang, G., Fisher, B., *et al.* (2010) Association between the 21-gene recurrence score assay and risk of locoregional recurrence in node-negative estrogen receptor-positive breast cancer: results from NSABP B-14 and NSABP B-20. *J. Clin. Oncol.*, **28** (10), 1677–1683.

124 Nimeus-Malmstrom, E., Krogh, M., Malmstrom, P., *et al.* (2008) Gene expression profiling in primary breast cancer distinguishes patients developing local recurrence after breast-conservation surgery, with or without postoperative radiotherapy. *Breast Cancer Res.*, **10** (2), R34.

125 Kreike, B., Halfwerk, H., Armstron, N., *et al.* (2009) Local recurrence after breast-conserving therapy in relation to gene expression patterns in a large series of patients. *Clin. Cancer Res.*, **15** (12), 4181–4190.

126 Nuyten, D.S., Kreike, B., Hart, A.A., *et al.* (2006) Predicting a local recurrence after breast-conserving therapy by gene expression profiling. *Breast Cancer Res.*, **8** (5), R62.

127 Romestaing, P., Lehingue, Y., Carrie, C., *et al.* (1997) Role of a 10-Gy boost in the conservative treatment of early breast cancer: results of a randomized clinical trial in Lyon, France. *J. Clin. Oncol.*, **15** (3), 963–968.

128 Bartelink, H., Horiot, J.C., Poortmans, P., *et al.* (2001) Recurrence rates after treatment of breast cancer with standard radiotherapy with or without additional radiation. *N. Engl. J. Med.*, **345** (19), 1378–1387.

129 Bartelink, H., Horiot, J.C., Poortmans, P.M., *et al.* (2007) Impact of a higher radiation dose on local control and survival in breast-conserving therapy of early breast cancer: 10-year results of the randomized boost versus no boost EORTC 22881-10882 trial. *J. Clin. Oncol.*, **25** (22), 3259–3265.

130 Poortmans, P.M., Collette, L., Horiot, J.C., *et al.* (2009) Impact of the boost dose of 10 Gy versus 26 Gy in patients with early stage breast cancer after a microscopically incomplete lumpectomy: 10-year results of the randomised EORTC boost trial. *Radiother. Oncol.*, **90** (1), 80–85.

131 Orr, R.K. (1999) The impact of prophylactic axillary node dissection on breast cancer survival–a Bayesian meta-analysis. *Ann. Surg. Oncol.*, **6** (1), 109–116.

132 Reed, V.K., Cavalcanti, J.L., Strom, E.A., *et al.* (2008) Risk of subclinical micrometastatic disease in the supraclavicular nodal bed according to the anatomic distribution in patients with advanced breast cancer. *Int. J. Radiat. Oncol. Biol. Phys.*, **71** (2), 435–440.

133 Reddy, S.G., Kiel, K.D. (2007) Supraclavicular nodal failure in patients with one to three positive axillary lymph nodes treated with breast conserving surgery and breast irradiation, without supraclavicular node radiation. *Breast J.*, **13** (1), 12–18.

134 Yu, J.I., Park, W., Huh, S.J., *et al.* (2010) Determining which patients require irradiation of the supraclavicular nodal area after surgery for N1 breast cancer. *Int. J. Radiat. Oncol. Biol. Phys.*, **78** (4), 1135–1141.

135 Truong, P.T., Jones, S.O., Kader, H.A., *et al.* (2009) Patients with t1 to t2 breast cancer with one to three positive nodes have higher local and regional recurrence risks compared with node-negative patients after breast-conserving surgery and whole-breast radiotherapy. *Int. J. Radiat. Oncol. Biol. Phys.*, **73** (2), 357–364.

136 Wo, J.Y., Taghian, A.G., Nguyen, P.L., *et al.* (2010) The association between biological subtype and isolated regional nodal failure after breast-conserving therapy. *Int. J. Radiat. Oncol. Biol. Phys.*, **77** (1), 188–196.

137 Whelan, T.J., Olivotto, I., Parulekar, W.R., *et al.* (2015) Regional nodal irradiation in early-stage breast cancer. *N. Engl. J. Med.*, **373**, 306–316.

138 Poortmans, P., Collette, S., Kirkove, C., *et al.* (2015) Internal mammary and medial supraclavicular irradiation in breast cancer. *N. Engl. J. Med.*, **373**, 317–327.

139 Fisher, B., Jeong, J.H., Anderson, S., Bryant, J., Fisher, E.R., Wolmark, N. (2002) Twenty-five-year follow-up of a randomized trial comparing radical mastectomy, total mastectomy, and total mastectomy followed by irradiation. *N. Engl. J. Med.*, **347** (8), 567–575.

140 Louis-Sylvestre, C., Clough, K., Asselain, B., *et al.* (2004) Axillary treatment in conservative management of operable breast cancer: dissection or radiotherapy? Results of a randomized study with 15 years of follow-up. *J. Clin. Oncol.*, **22** (1), 97–101.

141 Jagsi, R., Ballman, K., Chadha, M., *et al.* (2014) Radiation field design in the ACOSOG Z0011 (Alliance) trial. *J. Clin. Oncol.*, **32** (32), 3600–3606.

142 Donker, M., van Tienhoven, G., Straver, M.E., *et al.* (2014) Radiotherapy or surgery of the axilla after a positive sentinel node in breast cancer (EORTC 10981-22023 AMAROS): a randomised, multicentre, open-label, phase 3 non-inferiority trial. *Lancet Oncol.*, **15**, 1303–1310.

143 Livingston, S.F., Arlen, M. (1974) The extended extrapleural radical mastectomy: its role in the

treatment of carcinoma of the breast. *Ann. Surg.*, **179** (3), 260–265.

144 Urban, J.A., Marjani, M.A. (1971) Significance of internal mammary lymph node metastases in breast cancer. *Am. J. Roentgenol. Radium Ther. Nucl. Med.*, **111** (1), 130–136.

145 Overgaard, M., Jensen, M.B., Overgaard, J., *et al.* (1999) Postoperative radiotherapy in high-risk postmenopausal breast-cancer patients given adjuvant tamoxifen: Danish Breast Cancer Cooperative Group DBCG 82c randomised trial. *Lancet*, **353** (9165), 1641–1648.

146 Danish Breast Cancer Cooperative Group, Nielsen, H.M., Overgaard, M., Grau, C., Jensen, A.R., Overgaard, J. (2006) Study of failure pattern among high-risk breast cancer patients with or without postmastectomy radiotherapy in addition to adjuvant systemic therapy: long-term results from the Danish Breast Cancer Cooperative Group DBCG 82 b and c randomized studies. *J. Clin. Oncol.*, **24** (15), 2268–2275.

147 Ragaz, J., Jackson, S.M., Le, N., *et al.* (1997) Adjuvant radiotherapy and chemotherapy in node-positive premenopausal women with breast cancer. *N. Engl. J. Med.*, **337** (14), 956–962.

148 Ragaz, J., Oivotto, I.A., Spinelli, J.J., *et al.* (2005) Locoregional radiation therapy in patients with high-risk breast cancer receiving adjuvant chemotherapy: 20-year results of the British Columbia randomized trial. *J. Natl Cancer Inst.*, **97** (2), 116–126.

149 Romestaing, P., Belot, A., Hennequin, C., *et al.* (2009) Ten-year results of a randomized trial of internal mammary chain irradiation after mastectomy. *Int. J. Radiat. Oncol. Biol. Phys.*, **75** (3, Suppl.), S1.

150 Toledano, A., Azria, D., Garaud, P., *et al.* (2007) Phase III trial of concurrent or sequential adjuvant chemoradiotherapy after conservative surgery for early-stage breast cancer: final results of the ARCOSEIN trial. *J. Clin. Oncol.*, **25** (4), 405–410.

151 Toledano, A.H., Bollet, M.A., Fourquet, A., *et al.* (2007) Does concurrent radiochemotherapy affect cosmetic results in the adjuvant setting after breast-conserving surgery? Results of the ARCOSEIN multicenter, Phase III study: patients' and doctors' views. *Int. J. Radiat. Oncol. Biol. Phys.*, **68** (1), 66–72.

152 Rouesse, J., de la Lande, B., Bertheault-Cvitkovic, F., *et al.* (2006) A phase III randomized trial comparing adjuvant concomitant chemoradiotherapy versus standard adjuvant chemotherapy followed by radiotherapy in operable node-positive breast cancer: final results. *Int. J. Radiat. Oncol. Biol. Phys.*, **64** (4), 1072–1080.

153 Fernando, I.N. Bowden, S.J., Buckley, L., *et al.* (2011) SECRAB: The optimal sequencing of adjuvant chemotherapy (CT) and radiotherapy (RT) in early breast cancer (EBC), results of a UK multicentre prospective randomised trial. Abstract presented at European Multidisciplinary Cancer Conference of the European Cancer Organization (ECCO), 25 September. Abstract S4-4.

154 Recht, A., Come, S.E., Henderson, I.C., *et al.* (1996) The sequencing of chemotherapy and radiation therapy after conservative surgery for early-stage breast cancer. *N. Engl. J. Med.*, **334** (21), 1356–1361.

155 Bellon, J.R., Come, S.E., Gelman, R.S., *et al.* (2005) Sequencing of chemotherapy and radiation therapy in early-stage breast cancer: updated results of a prospective randomized trial. *J. Clin. Oncol.*, **23** (9), 1934–1940.

156 Chen, Z., King, W., Pearcey, R., Kerba, M., Mackillop, W.J. (2008) The relationship between waiting time for radiotherapy and clinical outcomes: a systematic review of the literature. *Radiother. Oncol.*, **87** (1), 3–16.

157 Punglia, R.S., Saito, A.M., Neville, B.A., Earle, C.C., Weeks, J.C. (2010) Impact of interval from breast conserving surgery to radiotherapy on local recurrence in older women with breast cancer: retrospective cohort analysis. *Br. Med. J.*, **340**, c845.

158 START Trialists' Group, Bentzen, S.M., Agrawal, R.K., *et al.* (2008) The UK Standardisation of Breast Radiotherapy (START) Trial A of radiotherapy hypofractionation for treatment of early breast cancer: a randomised trial. *Lancet Oncol.*, **9** (4), 331–341.

159 Haviland, J.S., Owen, J.R., Dewar, J.A., *et al.* (2013) The UK Standardisation of Breast Radiotherapy (START) trials of radiotherapy hypofractionation for treatment of early breast cancer: 10-year follow-up results of two randomized controlled trials. *Lancet Oncol.*, **14** (11), 1086–1094.

160 START Trialists' Group, Bentzen, S.M., Agrawal, R.K., *et al.* (2008) The UK Standardisation of Breast Radiotherapy (START) Trial B of radiotherapy hypofractionation for treatment of early breast cancer: a randomised trial. *Lancet Oncol.*, **371** (9618), 1098–1107.

161 Hopwood, P., Haviland, J.S., Sumo, G., *et al.* (2010) Comparison of patient-reported breast, arm, and shoulder symptoms and body image after radiotherapy for early breast cancer: 5-year follow-up in the randomised Standardisation of Breast Radiotherapy (START) trials. *Lancet Oncol.*, **11** (3), 231–240.

162 Whelan, T.J., Pignol, J.P., Levine, M.N., *et al.* (2010) Long-term results of hypofractionated radiation therapy for breast cancer. *N. Engl. J. Med.*, **362** (6), 513–520.

163 Haviland, J.S., Tarnold, J.R., Bentzen, S.M. (2010) Hypofractionated radiotherapy for breast cancer. *N. Engl. J. Med.*, **362** (19), 1843.

164 FAST Trialists group, Agrawal, R.K., Alhasso, A., *et al.* (2011) First results of the randomised UK FAST

TRIAL of radiotherapy hypofractionation for treatment of early breast cancer (CRUKE/04/015). *Radiother. Oncol.*, **100** (1), 93–100.

165 Smith, B.D., Bentzen, S.M., Correa, C.R., *et al.* (2011) Fractionation for whole breast irradiation: an American Society for Radiation Oncology (ASTRO) evidence-based guideline. *Int. J. Radiat. Oncol. Biol. Phys.*, **81** (1), 59–68.

166 Smith, G.L., Xu, Y., Buchholz, T.A., *et al.* (2012) Association between treatment with brachytherapy vs whole-breast irradiation and subsequent mastectomy, complications, and survival among older women with invasive breast cancer. *JAMA*, **307** (17), 1827–1837.

167 Smith, B.D., Arthur, D.W., Buchholz, T.A., *et al.* (2009) Accelerated partial breast irradiation consensus statement from the American Society for Radiation Oncology (ASTRO). *Int. J. Radiat. Oncol. Biol. Phys.*, **74** (4), 987–1001.

168 Leonardi, M.C., Maisonneuve, P., Mastropasqua, M.G., *et al.* (2012) How do the ASTRO consensus statement guidelines for the application of accelerated partial breast irradiation fit intraoperative radiotherapy? A retrospective analysis of patients treated at the European Institute of Oncology. *Int. J. Radiat. Oncol. Biol. Phys.*, **83** (3), 806–813.

169 Shaitelman, S.F., Vicini, F.A., Beitsch, P., Haffty, B., Keisch, M., Lyden, M. (2010) Five-year outcome of patients classified using the American Society for Radiation Oncology consensus statement guidelines for the application of accelerated partial breast irradiation: an analysis of patients treated on the American Society of Breast Surgeons MammoSite Registry Trial. *Cancer*, **116** (20), 4677–4685.

170 NSABP B-39, RTOG 0413 (2006) A randomized Phase III study of conventional whole breast irradiation versus partial breast irradiation for women with stage 0, I, or II breast cancer. *Clin. Adv. Hematol. Oncol.*, **4** (10), 719–721.

171 Strnad, V., Ott, O.J., Hildebrandt, G., *et al.* (0000) 5-year results of accelerated partial breast irradiation using sole interstitial multicatheter brachytherapy versus whole-breast irradiation with boost after breast-conserving surgery for low-risk invasive and in-situ carcinoma of the female breast: a randomised, phase 3, non-inferiority trial. *Lancet*, **387** (10015), 229–238.

172 Olivotto, I., Whelan, T.J., Parpia, S., *et al.* (2013) Interim cosmetic and toxicity results from RAPID: a randomized trial of accelerated partial breast irradiation using three-dimensional conformal external beam radiation therapy. *J. Clin. Oncol.*, **31** (32), 4038–4045.

173 Vaidya, J.S., Wenz, F., Bulsara, M., *et al.* (2014) Risk-adapted targeted intraoperative radiotherapy versus whole-breast radiotherapy for breast cancer: 5-year results for local control and overall survival from the TARGIT-A randomised trial. *Lancet*, **383** (9917), 603–613.

174 Khan, A.J., Arthur, D.W., Dale, R.G., Haffty, B.G., Vicini, F.A. (2012) Ultra-short courses of adjuvant breast radiotherapy: promised land or primrose path. *Int. J. Radiat. Oncol. Biol. Phys.*, **82** (2), 499–501.

175 Veronesi, U., Orecchia, R., Maisonneuve, P., *et al.* (2013) Intraoperative radiotherapy versus external radiotherapy for early breast cancer (ELIOT): a randomized controlled equivalence trial. *Lancet Oncol.*, **14** (13), 1269–1277.

176 Rampinelli, C., Bellomi, M., Ivaldi, G.B., *et al.* (2011) Assessment of pulmonary fibrosis after radiotherapy (RT) in breast conserving surgery: comparison between conventional external beam RT (EBRT) and intraoperative RT with electrons (ELIOT). *Technol. Cancer Res. Treat.*, **10** (4), 323–329.

177 Fisher, B., Bryant, J., Wolmark, N., *et al.* (1998) Effect of preoperative chemotherapy on the outcome of women with operable breast cancer. *J. Clin. Oncol.*, **16** (8), 2672–2685.

178 Raj, K.A., Evans, E.S., Prosnitz, R.G., *et al.* (2006) Is there an increased risk of local recurrence under the heart block in patients with left-sided breast cancer? *Cancer J.*, **12** (4), 309–317.

179 Griem, K.L., Fetherston, P., Kuznetsova, M., Foster, G.S., Shott, S., Chu, J. (2003) Three-dimensional photon dosimetry: a comparison of treatment of the intact breast in the supine and prone position. *Int. J. Radiat. Oncol. Biol. Phys.*, **57** (3), 891–899.

180 Gielda, B.T., Strauss, J.B., Marsh, J.C., Turian, J.V., Griem, K.L. (2011) A dosimetric comparison between the supine and prone positions for three-field intact breast radiotherapy. *Am J. Clin. Oncol.*, **34** (3), 223–230.

181 Sethi, R.A., No, H.S., Jozsef, G., Ko, J.P., Formenti, S.C. (2012) Comparison of three-dimensional versus intensity-modulated radiotherapy techniques to treat breast and axillary level III and supraclavicular nodes in a prone versus supine position. *Radiother. Oncol.*, **102** (1), 74–81.

182 Varga, Z., Hideghety, K., Mezo, T., Nikolenyi, A., Thurzo, L., Kahan, Z. (2009) Individual positioning: a comparative study of adjuvant breast radiotherapy in the prone versus supine position. *Int. J. Radiat. Oncol. Biol. Phys.*, **75** (1), 94–100.

183 Kirby, A.M., Evans, P.M., Donovan, E.M., Convery, H.M., Haviland, J.S., Yarnold, J.R. (2010) Prone versus supine positioning for whole and partial-breast radiotherapy: a comparison of non-target tissue dosimetry. *Radiother. Oncol.*, **96** (2), 178–184.

184 Chino, J.P., Marks, L.B. (2008) Prone positioning causes the heart to be displaced anteriorly within the thorax: implications for breast cancer treatment. *Int. J. Radiat. Oncol. Biol. Phys.*, **70** (3), 916–920.

185 Alonso-Basanta, M., Ko, J., Babcock, M., Dewyngaert, J.K., Formenti, S.C. (2009) Coverage of axillary lymph nodes in supine vs. prone breast radiotherapy. *Int. J. Radiat. Oncol. Biol. Phys.*, **73** (3), 745–751.

186 Kirby, A.M., Evans, P.M., Helyer, S.J., Donovan, E.M., Convery, H.M., Yarnold, J.R. (2011) A randomised trial of supine versus prone breast radiotherapy (SuPr study): comparing set-up errors and respiratory motion. *Radiother. Oncol.*, **100** (2), 221–226.

187 Stegman, L.D., Beal, K.P., Hunt, M.A., Fornier, M.N., McCormick, B. (2007) Long-term clinical outcomes of whole-breast irradiation delivered in the prone position. *Int. J. Radiat. Oncol. Biol. Phys.*, **68** (1), 73–81.

188 Reed, D.R., Lindsley, S.K., Mann, G.N., *et al.* (2005) Axillary lymph node dose with tangential breast irradiation. *Int. J. Radiat. Oncol. Biol. Phys.*, **61** (2), 358–364.

189 Hartsell, W.F., Kelly, C.A., Schneider, L., Wang, X.Y., Chu, J.C. (1994) A single isocenter three-field breast irradiation technique using an empiric simulation and asymmetric collimator. *Med. Dosim.*, **19** (3), 169–173.

190 Pignol, J.P., Olivotto, I., Rakovitch, E., *et al.* (2008) A multicenter randomized trial of breast intensity-modulated radiation therapy to reduce acute radiation dermatitis. *J. Clin. Oncol.*, **26** (13), 2085–2092.

191 Donovan, E., Bleakley, N., Denholm, E., *et al.* (2007) Randomised trial of standard 2D radiotherapy (RT) versus intensity modulated radiotherapy (IMRT) in patients prescribed breast radiotherapy. *Radiother. Oncol.*, **82** (3), 254–264.

192 Barnett, G.C., Wilkinson, J.S., Moody, A.M., *et al.* (2012) Randomized controlled trial of forward-planned intensity modulated radiotherapy for early breast cancer: interim results at 2 years. *Int. J. Radiat. Oncol. Biol. Phys.*, **82** (2), 715–723.

193 Haffty, B.G., Buchholz, T.A., McCormick, B. (2008) Should intensity-modulated radiation therapy be the standard of care in the conservatively managed breast cancer patient? *J. Clin. Oncol.*, **26** (13), 2072–2074.

194 Anderson, S.J., Wapnir, I., Dignam, J.J., *et al.* (2009) Prognosis after ipsilateral breast tumor recurrence and locoregional recurrences in patients treated by breast-conserving therapy in five National Surgical Adjuvant Breast and Bowel Project protocols of node-negative breast cancer. *J. Clin. Oncol.*, **27** (15), 2466–2473.

195 Wapnir, I.L., Anderson, S.J., Mamounas, E.P., *et al.* (2006) Prognosis after ipsilateral breast tumor recurrence and locoregional recurrences in five National Surgical Adjuvant Breast and Bowel Project node-positive adjuvant breast cancer trials. *J. Clin. Oncol.*, **24** (13), 2028–2037.

196 Cuzick, J., Stewart, H., Rutqvist, L., *et al.* (1994) Cause-specific mortality in long-term survivors of breast cancer who participated in trials of radiotherapy. *J. Clin. Oncol.*, **12** (3), 447–453.

197 Van de Steene, J., Soete, G., Storme, G. (2000) Adjuvant radiotherapy for breast cancer significantly improves overall survival: the missing link. *Radiother. Oncol.*, **55** (3), 263–272.

198 Gebski, V., Lagleva, M., Keech, A., Simes, J., Langlands, A.O. (2006) Survival effects of postmastectomy adjuvant radiation therapy using biologically equivalent doses: a clinical perspective. *J. Natl Cancer Inst.*, **98** (1), 26–38.

199 Whelan, T.J., Julian, J., Wright, J., Jadad, A.R., Levine, M.L. (2000) Does locoregional radiation therapy improve survival in breast cancer? A meta-analysis. *J. Clin. Oncol.*, **18** (6), 1220–1229.

200 Clarke, M., Collins, R., Darby, S., *et al.* (2005) Effects of radiotherapy and of differences in the extent of surgery for early breast cancer on local recurrence and 15-year survival: an overview of the randomised trials. *Lancet*, **366** (9503), 2087–2106.

201 Overgaard, M., Hansen, P.S., Overgaard, J., *et al.* (1997) Postoperative radiotherapy in high-risk premenopausal women with breast cancer who receive adjuvant chemotherapy. Danish Breast Cancer Cooperative Group 82b Trial. *N. Engl. J. Med.*, **337** (14), 949–955.

202 Recht, A., Gray, R., Davidson, N.E., *et al.* (1999) Locoregional failure 10 years after mastectomy and adjuvant chemotherapy with or without tamoxifen without irradiation: experience of the Eastern Cooperative Oncology Group. *J. Clin. Oncol.*, **17** (6), 1689–1700.

203 Katz, A., Strom, E.A., Buchholz, T.A., *et al.* (2000) Locoregional recurrence patterns after mastectomy and doxorubicin-based chemotherapy: implications for postoperative irradiation. *J. Clin. Oncol.*, **18** (15), 2817–2827.

204 Taghian, A., Jeong, J.H., Mamounas, E., *et al.* (2004) Patterns of locoregional failure in patients with operable breast cancer treatment by mastectomy and adjuvant chemotherapy with or without radiotherapy: results from five National Surgical Adjuvant Breast and Bowel Project randomized trials. *J. Clin. Oncol.*, **22** (21), 4247–4254.

205 Karlsson, P., Cole, B.F., Price, K.N., *et al.* (2007) The role of the number of uninvolved lymph nodes in predicting locoregional recurrence in breast cancer. *J. Clin. Oncol.*, **25** (15), 2019–2026.

206 Overgaard, M., Nielsen, H.M., Overgaard, J. (2007) Is the benefit of postmastectomy irradiation limited to patients with four or more positive nodes, as recommended in international consensus reports? A subgroup analysis of the DBCG 82 b&c randomized trials. *Radiother. Oncol.*, **82** (3), 247–253.

207 Kyndi, M., Overgaard, M., Nielsen, H.M., Sorensen, F.B., Knudsen, H., Overgaard, J. (2009) High local

recurrence risk is not associated with large survival reduction after postmastectomy radiotherapy in high-risk breast cancer: a subgroup analysis of DBCG 82 b&c. *Radiother. Oncol.*, **90** (1), 74–79.

208 Early Breast Cancer Trialists' Collaborative Group (2014) Effect of radiotherapy after mastectomy and axillary surgery on 10-year recurrence and 20-year breast cancer mortality: meta-analysis of individual patient data for 8135 women in 22 randomised trials. *Lancet*, **383** (9935), 2127–2135.

209 van der Hage, J.A., Putter, H., Bonnema, J., *et al.* (2003) Impact of locoregional treatment on the early-stage breast cancer patients: a retrospective analysis. *Eur. J. Cancer*, **39** (15), 2192–2199.

210 Voordeckers, M., Vinh-Hung, V., Lamote, J., Bretz, A., Storme, G. (2009) Survival benefit with radiation therapy in node-positive breast carcinoma patients. *Strahlenther. Onkol.*, **185** (10), 656–662.

211 Buchholz, T.A., Woodward, W.A., Duan, Z., *et al.* (2008) Radiation use and long-term survival in breast cancer patients with T1, T2 primary tumors and one to three positive axillary lymph nodes. *Int. J. Radiat. Oncol. Biol. Phys.*, **71** (4), 1022–1027.

212 Katz, A., Strom, E.A., Buchholz, T.A., *et al.* (2001) The influence of pathologic tumor characteristics on locoregional recurrence rates following mastectomy. *Int. J. Radiat. Oncol. Biol. Phys.*, **50** (3), 735–742.

213 Katz, A., Strom, E.A., Buchholz, T.A., *et al.* (2000) Locoregional recurrence patterns after mastectomy and doxorubicin-based chemotherapy: implications for postoperative irradiation. *J. Clin. Oncol.*, **18** (15), 2817–2827.

214 Truong, P.T., Woodward, W.A., Thames, H.D., Ragaz, J., Olivotto, I.A., Buchholz, T.A. (2007) The ratio of positive to excised nodes identifies high-risk subsets and reduces inter-institutional differences in locoregional recurrence risk estimate in breast cancer patients with 1-3 positive nodes: an analysis of prospective data from British Columbia and the M. D. Anderson Cancer Center. *Int. J. Radiat. Oncol. Biol. Phys.*, **68** (1), 59–65.

215 Troung, P.T., Olivotto, I.A., Kader, H.A., Panades, M., Speers, C.H., Berthelet, E. (2005) Selecting breast cancer patients with T1–T2 tumors and one to three positive axillary nodes at high postmastectomy locoregional recurrence risk for adjuvant radiotherapy. *Int. J. Radiat. Oncol. Biol. Phys.*, **61** (5), 1337–1347.

216 Wallgren, A., Bonetti, M., Gelber, R.D., *et al.* (2003) Risk factors for locoregional recurrence among breast cancer patients: results from International Breast Cancer Study Group Trials I through VII. *J. Clin. Oncol.*, **21** (7), 1205–1213.

217 Yildirim, E., Berberoglu, U. (2007) Local recurrence in breast carcinoma patients with T(1–2) and 1–3

positive nodes: indications for radiotherapy. *Eur. J. Surg. Oncol.*, **33** (1), 28–32.

218 Kunkler, I.H., Canney, P., van Tienhoven, G., Russell, N.S., MRC/EORTC (BIG 2-04) SUPREMO Trial Management Group (2008) Elucidating the role of chest wall irradiation in 'intermediate-risk' breast cancer: the MRC/EORTC SUPREMO trial. *Clin. Oncol. (R. Coll. Radiol.)*, **20** (1), 31–34.

219 Taghian, A.G., Jeong, J.H., Mamounas, E.P., *et al.* (2006) Low locoregional recurrence rate among node-negative breast cancer patients with tumors 5 cm or larger treated by mastectomy, with or without adjuvant systemic therapy and without radiotherapy: results from five national surgical adjuvant breast and bowel project randomized clinical trials. *J. Clin. Oncol.*, **24** (24), 3927–3932.

220 Floyd, S.R., Buchholz, T.A., Haffty, B.G., *et al.* (2006) Low local recurrence rate without postmastectomy radiation in node-negative breast cancer patients with tumors 5 cm and larger. *Int. J. Radiat. Oncol. Biol. Phys.*, **66** (2), 358–364.

221 Abi-Raad, R., Boutrus, R., Wang, R., *et al.* (2011) Patterns and risk factors of locoregional recurrence in T1-T2 node negative breast cancer patients treated with mastectomy: implications for postmastectomy radiotherapy. *Int. J. Radiat. Oncol. Biol. Phys.*, **81** (3), e151–e157.

222 Truong, P.T., Lesperance, M., Culhaci, A., Kader, H.A., Speers, C.H., Olivotto, I.A. (2005) Patient subsets with T1–T2, node-negative breast cancer at high locoregional recurrence risk after mastectomy. *Int. J. Radiat. Oncol. Biol. Phys.*, **62** (1), 175–182.

223 Yildirim, E., Berberoglu, U. (2007) Can a subgroup of node-negative breast carcinoma patients with T1-2 tumor who may benefit from postmastectomy radiotherapy be identified? *Int. J. Radiat. Oncol. Biol. Phys.*, **68** (4), 1024–1029.

224 Rowell, N.P. (2009) Radiotherapy to the chest wall following mastectomy for node-negative breast cancer: a systematic review. *Radiother. Oncol.*, **91** (1), 23–32.

225 Abdulkarim, B.S., Cuartero, J., Hanson, J., Deschenes, J., Lesniak, D., Sabri, S. (2011) Increased risk of locoregional recurrence for women with T1-2N0 triple-negative breast cancer treated with modified radical mastectomy without adjuvant radiation therapy compared with breast-conserving therapy. *J. Clin. Oncol.*, **29** (21), 2852–2858.

226 Wang, J., Shi, M., Ling, R., *et al.* (2011) Adjuvant chemotherapy and radiotherapy in triple-negative breast carcinoma: a prospective randomized controlled multi-center trial. *Radiother. Oncol.*, **100** (2), 200–204.

227 Freedman, G.M., Fowble, B.L., Hanlon, A.L., *et al.* (1998) A close or positive margin after mastectomy is not an indication for chest wall irradiation except in

women aged fifty or younger. *Int. J. Radiat. Oncol. Biol. Phys.*, **41** (3), 599–605.

228 Truong, P.T., Olivotto, I.A., Speers, C.H., Wai, E.S., Berthelet, E., Kader, H.A. (2004) A positive margin is not always an indication for radiotherapy after mastectomy in early breast cancer. *Int. J. Radiat. Oncol. Biol. Phys.*, **58** (3), 797–804.

229 Rastogi, P., Anderson, S.J., Bear, H.D., *et al.* (2008) Preoperative chemotherapy: updates of National Surgical Adjuvant Breast and Bowel Project Protocols B-18 and B-27. *J. Clin. Oncol.*, **26** (5), 778–785.

230 Mamounas, E.P., Anderson, S.J., Bear, H.D., *et al.* (2012) Predictors of locoregional recurrence after neoadjuvant chemotherapy: results from combined analysis of national surgical adjuvant breast and bowel project NSABP B-18 and B-27. *J. Clin. Oncol.*, **30** (32), 3960–3966.

231 Krug, D., Lederer, B., Debus, J., *et al.* (2015) Relationship of omission of adjuvant radiotherapy to outcomes of logoregional control and disease-free survival in patients with or without PCR after neoadjuvant chemotherapy for breast cancer: A meta-analysis on 3481 patients from the Gepar-trials. *J. Clin. Oncol.*, **33** (suppl; abstr 1008).

232 Huang, E.H., Tucker, S.L., Strom, E.A., *et al.* (2004) Postmastectomy radiation improves local-regional control and survival for selected patients with locally advanced breast cancer treated with neoadjuvant chemotherapy and mastectomy. *J. Clin. Oncol.*, **22** (23), 4691–4699.

233 McGuire, S.E., Gonzalez-Angulo, A.M., Huang, E.H., *et al.* (2007) Postmastectomy radiation improves the outcome of patients with locally advanced breast cancer who achieve a pathologic complete response to neoadjuvant chemotherapy. *Int. J. Radiat. Oncol. Biol. Phys.*, **68** (4), 1004–1009.

234 Nagar, H., Mittendorf, E.A., Strom, E.A., *et al.* (2011) Local-regional recurrence with and without radiation therapy after neoadjuvant chemotherapy and mastectomy for clinically staged T3N0 breast cancer. *Int. J. Radiat. Oncol. Biol. Phys.*, **81** (3), 782–787.

235 Huang, E.H., Tucker, S.L., Strom, E.A., *et al.* (2005) Predictors of locoregional recurrence in patients with locally advanced breast cancer treated with neoadjuvant chemotherapy, mastectomy, and radiotherapy. *Int. J. Radiat. Oncol. Biol. Phys.*, **62** (2), 351–357.

236 Buchholz, T.A., Lehman, C.D., Harris, J.R., *et al.* (2008) Statement of the science concerning locoregional treatments after preoperative chemotherapy for breast cancer: a National Cancer Institute conference. *J. Clin. Oncol.*, **26** (5), 791–797.

237 Abramowitz, M.C., Li, T., Morrow, M., *et al.* (2009) Dermal lymphatic invasion and inflammatory breast cancer are independent predictors of outcome after postmastectomy radiation. *Am J. Clin. Oncol.*, **32** (1), 30–33.

238 Wingo, P.A., Jamison, P.M., Young, J.L., Garguillo, P. (2004) Population-based statistics for women diagnosed with inflammatory breast cancer (United States). *Cancer Causes Control*, **15** (3), 321–328.

239 Dawood, S., Merajver, S.D., Viens, P., *et al.* (2011) International expert panel on inflammatory breast cancer: consensus statement for standardized diagnosis and treatment. *Ann. Oncol.*, **22** (3), 515–523.

240 Damast, S., Ho, A.Y., Montgomery, L., *et al.* (2010) Locoregional outcomes of inflammatory breast cancer patients treated with standard fractionation radiation and daily skin bolus in the taxane era. *Int. J. Radiat. Oncol. Biol. Phys.*, **77** (4), 1105–1112.

241 Liauw, S.L., Benda, R.K., Morris, C.G., Mendenhall, N.P. (2004) Inflammatory breast carcinoma: outcomes with trimodality therapy for nonmetastatic disease. *Cancer*, **100** (5), 920–928.

242 Liao, Z., Strom, E.A., Buzdar, A.U., *et al.* (2000) Locoregional irradiation for inflammatory breast cancer: effectiveness of dose escalation in decreasing recurrence. *Int. J. Radiat. Oncol. Biol. Phys.*, **47** (5), 1191–1200.

243 Dawood, S., Ueno, N.T., Valero, V., *et al.* (2011) Difference in survival among women with stage III inflammatory and noninflammatory locally advanced breast cancer appear early: a large population-based study. *Cancer*, **117** (9), 1819–1826.

244 Sutherland, S., Ashley, S., Walsh, G., Smith, I.E., Johnston, S.R. (2010) Inflammatory breast cancer–The Royal Marsden Hospital experience: a review of 155 patients treated from 1990 to 2007. *Cancer*, **116** (11 Suppl.), 2815–2820.

245 Nielsen, H.M., Overgaard, M., Grau, C., Jensen, A.R., Overgaard, J. (2006) Loco-regional recurrence after mastectomy in high-risk breast cancer–risk and prognosis. An analysis of patients from the DBCG 82 b&c randomization trials. *Radiother. Oncol.*, **79** (2), 147–155.

246 Reddy, J.P., Levy, L., Oh, J.L., *et al.* (2011) Long-term outcomes in patients with isolated supraclavicular nodal recurrences after mastectomy and doxorubicin-based chemotherapy for breast cancer. *Int. J. Radiat. Oncol. Biol. Phys.*, **80** (5), 1453–1457.

247 Willner, J., Kiricuta, I.C., Kolbl, O. (1997) Locoregional recurrence of breast cancer following mastectomy: always a fatal event? Results of univariate and multivariate analysis. *Int. J. Radiat. Oncol. Biol. Phys.*, **37** (4), 853–863.

248 Kuo, S.H., Huang, C.S., Kuo, W.H., Cheng, A.L., Chang, K.J., Chia-Hsien Cheng, J. (2008) Comprehensive locoregional treatment and systemic therapy for postmastectomy isolated locoregional

recurrence. *Int. J. Radiat. Oncol. Biol. Phys.*, **72** (5), 1456–1464.

249 Wahl, A.O., Rademaker, A., Kiel, K.D., *et al.* (2008) Multi-institutional review of repeat irradiation of the chest wall and breast for recurrent breast cancer. *Int. J. Radiat. Oncol. Biol. Phys.*, **70** (2), 477–484.

250 Würschmidt, F., Dahle, J., Petersen, C., *et al.* (2008) Reirradiation of recurrent breast cancer with and without concurrent chemotherapy. *Radiat. Oncol.*, **3**, 28.

251 Harkenrider, M.M., Wilson, M.R., Dragun, A.E. (2011) Reirradiation as a component of the multidisciplinary management of locally recurrent breast cancer. *Clin. Breast Cancer*, **11** (3), 171–176.

252 Van Der Zee, J., De Bruijne, M., Mens, J.W., *et al.* (2010) Reirradiation combined with hyperthermia in breast cancer recurrences: overview of experience in Erasmus MC. *Int. J. Hyperthemia*, **26** (7), 638–648.

253 Krueger, E.A., Wilkins, E.G., Strawderman, M., *et al.* (2001) Complications and patient satisfaction following expander/implant breast reconstruction with and without radiotherapy. *Int. J. Radiat. Oncol. Biol. Phys.*, **49** (3), 713–721.

254 Kronowitz, S.J., Robb, G.L. (2009) Radiation therapy and breast reconstruction: a critical review of the literature. *Plast. Reconstr. Surg.*, **124** (2), 395–408.

255 Momoh, A., Ahmed, R., Kelley, B., *et al.* (2014) A systematic review of complications of implant-based breast reconstruction with prereconstruction and postreconstruction radiotherapy. *Ann. Surg. Oncol.*, **21** (1), 118–124.

256 Valdata, L., Cattaneo, A., Pellegatta, I., *et al.* (2014) Acellular Dermal Matrices and Radiotherapy in Breast Reconstruction: A Systematic Review and Meta-Analysis of the Literature. *Plast. Surg. Int.*, Volume 2014, Article ID 472604.

257 Fischer, J.P., Nelson, J.A., Serletti, J.M., *et al.* (2013) Peri-operative risk factors associated with early tissue expander (TE) loss following immediate breast reconstruction (IBR): a review of 9305 patients from the 2005–2010 ACS-NSQIP datasets. *J. Plast. Reconstr. Aesthet. Surg.*, **66** (11), 1504–1512.

258 Motwani, S.B., Strom, E.A., Schechter, N.R., *et al.* (2006) The impact of immediate breast reconstruction on the technical delivery of postmastectomy radiotherapy. *Int. J. Radiat. Oncol. Biol. Phys.*, **66** (1), 76–82.

259 Schechter, N.R., Strom, E.A., Perkins, G.H., *et al.* (2005) Immediate breast reconstruction can impact postmastectomy irradiation. *Am J. Clin. Oncol.*, **28** (5), 485–494.

260 Koutcher, L., Ballangrud, A., Cordeiro, P.G., *et al.* (2010) Postmastectomy intensity modulated radiation therapy following immediate expander-

implant reconstruction. *Radiother. Oncol.*, **94** (3), 319–323.

261 Kronowitz, S.J., Lam, C., Terefe, W., *et al.* (2011) A multidisciplinary protocol for planned skin-preserving delayed breast reconstruction for patients with locally advanced breast cancer requiring postmastectomy radiation therapy: 3-year follow-up. *Plast. Reconstr. Surg.*, **127** (6), 2154–2166.

262 Moni, J., Graves-Ditman, M., Cederna, P., *et al.* (2004) Dosimetry around metallic ports in tissue expanders in patients receiving postmastectomy radiation therapy: an ex-vivo evaluation. *Med. Dosim.*, **29** (1), 49–54.

263 Damast, S., Beal, K., Ballangrud, A., *et al.* (2006) Do metallic ports in tissue expanders affect postmastectomy radiation delivery? *Int. J. Radiat. Oncol. Biol. Phys.*, **66** (1), 305–310.

264 Chatzigiannis, C., Lymperopoulou, G., Sandilos, P., *et al.* (2011) Dose perturbation in the radiotherapy of breast cancer patients implanted with the Magna-Site: a Monte Carlo study. *J. Appl. Clin. Med. Phys.*, **12** (2), 3295.

265 Tran, N.V., Chang, D.W., Gupta, A., Kroll, S.S., Robb, G.L. (2001) Comparison of immediate and delayed free TRAM flap breast reconstruction in patients receiving postmastectomy radiation therapy. *Plast. Reconstr. Surg.*, **108** (1), 78–82.

266 Spear, S.L., Ducic, I., Low, M., Cuoco, F. (2005) The effect of radiation on pedicled TRAM flap breast reconstruction: outcomes and implications. *Plast. Reconstr. Surg.*, **115** (1), 84–95.

267 Chang, D.W., Reece, G.P., Wang, B., *et al.* (2000) Effect of smoking on complications in patients undergoing free TRAM flap breast reconstruction. *Plast. Reconstr. Surg.*, **105** (7), 2374–2380.

268 Pierce, L.J., Butler, J.B., Martel, M.K., *et al.* (2002) Postmastectomy radiotherapy of the chest wall: dosimetric comparison of common techniques. *Int. J. Radiat. Oncol. Biol. Phys.*, **52** (5), 1220–1230.

269 Thomsen, M.S., Berg, M., Nielsen, H.M., *et al.* (2008) Post-mastectomy radiotherapy in Denmark: from 2D to 3D treatment planning guidelines of The Danish Breast Cancer Cooperative Group. *Acta Oncol.*, **47** (4), 654–661.

270 Jagsi, R., Moran, J., Marsh, R., Masi, K., Griffith, K.A., Pierce, L.J. (2010) Evaluation of four techniques using intensity-modulated radiation therapy for comprehensive locoregional irradiation of breast cancer. *Int. J. Radiat. Oncol. Biol. Phys.*, **78** (5), 1594–1603.

271 Oh, J.L., Buchholz, T.A. (2009) Internal mammary node radiation: a proposed technique to spare cardiac toxicity. *J. Clin. Oncol.*, **27** (31), e172–e173.

272 Harris, J.R., Halpin-Murphy, P., McNeese, M., Mendenhall, N.P., Morrow, M., Robert, J.N. (1999)

Consensus Statement on postmastectomy radiation therapy. *Int. J. Radiat. Oncol. Biol. Phys.*, **44** (5), 989–990.

273 Recht, A., Edge, S.B., Solin, L.J., *et al.* (2001) Postmastectomy radiotherapy: clinical practice guidelines of the American Society of Clinical Oncology. *J. Clin. Oncol.*, **19** (5), 1539–1569.

274 Taylor, M.E., Haffty, B.G., Rabinovitch, R., *et al.* (2009) ACR appropriateness criteria on postmastectomy radiotherapy expert panel on radiation oncology-breast. *Int. J. Radiat. Oncol. Biol. Phys.*, **73** (4), 997–1002.

275 Carlson, R.W., Allred, D.C., Anderson, B.O., *et al.* (2009) Breast cancer. Clinical practice guidelines in oncology. *J. Natl Compr. Cancer Network*, **7** (2), 122–192.

276 Taylor, M.E., Perez, C.A., Halverson, K.J., *et al.* (1995) Factors influencing cosmetic results after conservation therapy for breast cancer. *Int. J. Radiat. Oncol. Biol. Phys.*, **31** (4), 753–764.

277 Olivotto, I.A., Rose, M.S., Osteen, R.T., *et al.* (1989) Late cosmetic outcome after conservative surgery and radiotherapy: analysis of causes of cosmetic failure. *Int. J. Radiat. Oncol. Biol. Phys.*, **17** (4), 747–753.

278 Chan, S.W., Cheung, P.S., Lam, S.H. (2010) Cosmetic outcome and percentage of breast volume excision in oncoplastic breast conserving surgery. *World J. Surg.*, **34** (7), 1447–1452.

279 Gray, J.R., McCormick, B., Cox, L., Yahalom, J. (1991) Primary breast irradiation in large-breasted or heavy women: analysis of cosmetic outcome. *Int. J. Radiat. Oncol. Biol. Phys.*, **21** (2), 347–354.

280 Deutsch, M., Flickinger, J.C. (2003) Patient characteristics and treatment factors affecting cosmesis following lumpectomy and breast irradiation. *Am J. Clin. Oncol.*, **26** (4), 350–353.

281 Moody, A.M., Mayles, W.P., Bliss, J.M., *et al.* (1994) The influence of breast size on late radiation effects and association with radiotherapy dose inhomogeneity. *Radiother. Oncol.*, **33** (2), 106–112.

282 Johansen, J., Overgaard, J., Overgaard, M. (2007) Effect of adjuvant systemic treatment on cosmetic outcome and late normal-tissue reactions after breast conservation. *Acta Oncol.*, **46** (4), 525–533.

283 Budrukkar, A.N., Sarin, R., Shrivastava, S.K., Deshpande, D.D., Dinshaw, K.A. (2007) Cosmesis, late sequelae and local control after breast-conserving therapy: influence of type of tumor bed boost and adjuvant chemotherapy. *Clin. Oncol. (R. Coll. Radiol.)*, **19** (8), 596–603.

284 Rose, M.A., Olivotto, I., Cady, B., *et al.* (1989) Conservative surgery and radiation therapy for early breast cancer. Long-term cosmetic results. *Arch. Surg.*, **124** (2), 153–157.

285 Wazer, D.E., Morr, J., Erban, J.K., Schmid, C.H., Ruthazer, R., Schmidt-Ullrich, R.K. (1997) The effect of postradiation treatment with tamoxifen on local control and cosmetic outcome in the conservatively treated breast. *Cancer*, **80** (4), 732–740.

286 Markiewicz, D.A., Schultz, D.J., Haas, J.A., *et al.* (1996) The effects of sequence and type of chemotherapy and radiation therapy on cosmesis and complications after breast conservation therapy. *Int. J. Radiat. Oncol. Biol. Phys.*, **35** (4), 661–668.

287 Bentzen, S.M., Thames, H.D., Overgaard, M. (1989) Latent-time estimation for late cutaneous and subcutaneous radiation reactions in a single-follow-up clinical study. *Radiother. Oncol.*, **15** (3), 267–274.

288 Lanigan, S.W., Joannides, T. (2003) Pulsed dye laser treatment of telangiectasia after radiotherapy for carcinoma of the breast. *Br. J. Dermatol.*, **148** (1), 77–79.

289 Rowland Payne, C.M., Somaiah, N., Neal, A.J., Glees, J.P. (2005) The hyfrecator: a treatment for radiation induced telangiectasia in breast cancer patients. *Br. J. Radiol.*, **78** (926), 143–146.

290 Gothard, L., Cornes, P., Earl, J., *et al.* (2004) Double-blind placebo-controlled randomised trial of vitamin E and pentoxifylline in patients with chronic arm lymphedema and fibrosis after surgery and radiotherapy for breast cancer. *Radiother. Oncol.*, **73** (2), 133–139.

291 Magnusson, M., Hoglund, P., Johansson, K., *et al.* (2009) Pentoxifylline and vitamin E treatment for prevention of radiation-induced side-effects in women with breast cancer: a phase two, double-blind, placebo-controlled randomised clinical trial (Ptx-5). *Eur. J. Cancer*, **45** (14), 2488–2495.

292 Delanian, S., Porcher, R., Balla-Mekias, S., Lefaix, J.L. (2003) Randomized, placebo-controlled trial of combined pentoxifylline and tocopherol for regression of superficial radiation-induced fibrosis. *J. Clin. Oncol.*, **21** (13), 2545–2550.

293 Delanian, S., Porcher, R., Rudant, J., Lefaix, J.L. (2005) Kinetics of response to long-term treatment combining pentoxifylline and tocopherol in patients with superficial radiation-induced fibrosis. *J. Clin. Oncol.*, **23** (34), 8570–8579.

294 Kissin, M.W., Querci della Rovere, G., Easton, D., Westbury, G. (1986) Risk of lymphoedema following the treatment of breast cancer. *Br. J. Surg.*, **73** (7), 580–584.

295 Coen, J.J., Taghian, A.G., Kachnic, L.A., Assasd, S.I., Powell, S.N. (2003) Risk of lymphedema after regional nodal irradiation with breast conservation therapy. *Int. J. Radiat. Oncol. Biol. Phys.*, **55** (5), 1209–1215.

296 Hayes, S.B., Freedman, G.M., Li, T., Anderson, P.R., Ross, E. (2008) Does axillary boost increase lymphedema compared with supraclavicular radiation alone after breast conservation? *Int. J. Radiat. Oncol. Biol. Phys.*, **72** (5), 1449–1455.

297 Norman, S.A., Localio, A.R., Kallan, M.J., *et al.* (2010) Risk factors for lymphedema after breast cancer treatment. *Cancer Epidemiol. Biomarkers Prev.*, **19** (11), 2743–2746.

298 Devoogdt, N., Christiaens, M.R., Geraerts, I., *et al.* (2011) Effect of manual lymph drainage in addition to guidelines and exercise therapy on arm lymphoedema related to breast cancer: randomised controlled trial. *Br. Med. J.*, **343**, d5326.

299 Kuno, A., Osaki, K., Kawanaka, T., Furutani, S., Ikushima, H., Nishitani, H. (2009) Risk factors for radiation pneumonitis caused by whole breast irradiation following breast-conserving surgery. *J. Med. Invest.*, **56** (3-4), 99–110.

300 Lind, P.A., Wennberg, B., Gagliardi, G., Fornander, T. (2001) Pulmonary complications following different radiotherapy techniques for breast cancer, and the association to irradiated lung volume and dose. *Breast Cancer Res. Treat.*, **68** (3), 199–210.

301 Lind, P.A., Wennberg, B., Gagliardi, G., *et al.* (2006) ROC curves and evaluation of radiation-induced pulmonary toxicity in breast cancer. *Int. J. Radiat. Oncol. Biol. Phys.*, **64** (3), 765–770.

302 Lingos, T.I., Recht, A., Vicini, F., Abner, A., Silver, B., Harris, J.R. (1991) Radiation pneumonitis in breast cancer patients treated with conservative surgery and radiation therapy. *Int. J. Radiat. Oncol. Biol. Phys.*, **21** (2), 355–360.

303 Matzinger, O., Heimsoth, I., Poortmans, P., *et al.* (2010) Toxicity at three years with and without irradiation of the internal mammary and medial supraclavicular lymph node chain in stage I to III breast cancer (EORTC trial 22922/10925). *Acta Oncol.*, **49** (1), 24–34.

304 McGale, P., Darby, S.C., Hall, P., *et al.* (2011) Incidence of heart disease in 35,000 women treated with radiotherapy for breast cancer in Denmark and Sweden. *Radiother. Oncol.*, **100** (2), 167–175.

305 Nilsson, G., Holmberg, L., Garmo, H., *et al.* (2012) Distribution of coronary artery stenosis after radiation for breast cancer. *J. Clin. Oncol.*, **30** (4), 380–386.

306 Marks, L.B., Yu, X., Prosnitz, R.G., *et al.* (2005) The incidence and functional consequences of RT-associated cardiac perfusion defects. *Int. J. Radiat. Oncol. Biol. Phys.*, **63** (1), 214–223.

307 Darby, S.C., Ewertz, M., McGale, P., *et al.* (2013) Risk of ischemic heart disease in women after radiotherapy for breast cancer. *N. Engl. J. Med.*, **368** (11), 987–998.

308 Giordano, S.H., Kuo, Y.F., Freeman, J.L., Buchholz, T.A., Hortobagyi, G.N., Goodwin, J.S. (2005) Risk of cardiac death after adjuvant radiotherapy for breast cancer. *J. Natl Cancer Inst.*, **97** (6), 419–424.

309 Patt, D.A., Goodwin, J.S., Kuo, Y.F., *et al.* (2005) Cardiac morbidity of adjuvant radiotherapy for breast cancer. *J. Clin. Oncol.*, **23** (30), 7475–7482.

310 Bergom, C., Currey, A., Tai, A., Strauss, J.B. (2016) Deep Inspiration Breath Hold. *Radiation Therapy Techniques and Treatment Planning for Breast Cancer.* Springer.

311 Chung, E., Corbett, J.R., Moran, J.M., *et al.* (2013) Is there a dose-response relationship for heart disease with low-dose radiation therapy? *Int. J. Radiat. Oncol. Biol. Phys.*, **85** (4), 959–964.

312 Bartlett, F.R., Colgan, R.M., Carr, K., *et al.* (2013) The UK HeartSpare Study: randomised evaluation of voluntary deep-inspiratory breath-hold in women undergoing breast radiotherapy. *Radiother. Oncol.*, **108** (2), 242–247.

313 Mulliez, T., Veldeman, L., van Greveling, A., *et al.* (2013) Hypofractionated whole breast irradiation for patients with large breasts: A randomized trial comparing prone and supine positions. *Radiother. Oncol.*, **108** (2), 203–208.

314 Bartlett, F., Colgan, R., Donovan, E., *et al.* (2015) The UK HeartSpare Study (Stage IB): Randomised comparison of a voluntary breath-hold technique and prone radiotherapy after breast conserving surgery. *Radiother. Oncol.*, **114**, 66–72.

315 Verhoeven, K., Sweldens, C., Petillion, S., *et al.* (0000) Breathing adapted radiation therapy in comparison with prone position to reduce the doses to the heart, left anterior descending coronary artery, and contralateral breast in whole breast radiation therapy. *Pract. Radiat. Oncol.*, **4** (2), 123–129.

316 Mulliez, T., Van de Velde, J., Veldeman, L., *et al.* (2015) Deep inspiration breath hold in the prone position retracts the heart from the breast and internal mammary lymph node region. *Radiother. and Oncol.*, **117**, 473–476.

317 Mulliez, T., Veldeman, L., Speleers, B., *et al.* (0000) Heart dose reduction by prone deep inspiration breath hold in left-sided breast irradiation. *Radiother. and Oncol.*, **114**, 79–84

318 Halyard, M.Y., Pisansky, T.M., Dueck, A.C., *et al.* (2009) Radiotherapy and adjuvant trastuzumab in operable breast cancer: tolerability and adverse event data from the NCCTG Phase II trial N9831. *J. Clin. Oncol.*, **27** (16), 2638–2644.

319 Johansson, S., Svensson, H., Larsson, L.G., Denekamp, J. (2000) Brachial plexopathy after postoperative radiotherapy of breast cancer patients–a long-term follow-up. *Acta Oncol.*, **39** (3), 373–382.

320 Bajrovic, A., Rades, D., Fehlauer, F., *et al.* (2004) Is there a life-long risk of brachial plexopathy after radiotherapy of supraclavicular lymph nodes in breast cancer patients? *Radiother. Oncol.*, **71** (3), 297–301.

321 Powell, S., Cooke, J., Parsons, C. (1990) Radiation-induced brachial plexus injury: follow-up of two different fractionation schedules. *Radiother. Oncol.*, **18** (3), 213–220.

322 Pierce, S.M., Recht, A., Lingos, T.I., *et al.* (1992) Long-term radiation complications following conservative surgery (CS) and radiation therapy (RT) in patients with early stage breast cancer. *Int. J. Radiat. Oncol. Biol. Phys.*, **23** (5), 915–923.

323 Berrington de Gonzalez, A., Curtis, R.E., Kry, S.F., *et al.* (2011) Proportion of second cancers attributable to radiotherapy treatment in adults: a cohort study in the US SEER cancer registries. *Lancet Oncol.*, **12** (4), 353–360.

324 Berrington de Gonzalez, A., Curtis, R.E., Gilbert, E., *et al.* (2010) Second solid cancers after radiotherapy for breast cancer in SEER cancer registries. *Br. J. Cancer*, **102** (1), 220–226.

325 Williams, T.M., Moran, J.M., Hsu, S.H., *et al.* (2012) Contralateral breast dose after whole-breast irradiation: an analysis by treatment technique. *Int. J. Radiat. Oncol. Biol. Phys.*, **82** (5), 2079–2085.

326 Deutsch, M., Land, S.R., Begovic, M., Wieand, H.S., Wolmark, N., Fisher, B. (2003) The incidence of lung carcinoma after surgery for breast carcinoma with and without postoperative radiotherapy. Results of National Surgical Adjuvant Breast and Bowel Project (NSABP) clinical trials B-04 and B-06. *Cancer*, **98** (7), 1362–1368.

327 Darby, S.C., McGale, P., Taylor, C.W., Peto, R. (2005) Long-term mortality from heart disease and lung cancer after radiotherapy for early breast cancer: prospective cohort study of about 300,000 women in US SEER cancer registries. *Lancet Oncol.*, **6** (8), 557–565.

328 Kaufman, E.L., Jacobson, J.S., Hershman, D.L., Desai, M., Neugut, A.I. (2008) Effect of breast cancer radiotherapy and cigarette smoking on risk of second primary lung cancer. *J. Clin. Oncol.*, **26** (3), 392–398.

329 Ford, M.B., Sigurdson, A.J., Petrulis, E.S., *et al.* (2003) Effects of smoking and radiotherapy on lung carcinoma in breast carcinoma survivors. *Cancer*, **98** (7), 1457–1464.

330 Ng, J., Shuryak, I., Xu, Y., *et al.* (2012) Predicting the risk of secondary lung malignancies associated with whole-breast radiation therapy. *Int. J. Radiat. Oncol. Biol. Phys.*, **83** (4), 1101–1106.

331 Mery, C.M., George, S., Bertagnolli, M.M., Raut, C.P. (2009) Secondary sarcomas after radiotherapy for breast cancer: sustained risk and poor survival. *Cancer*, **115** (18), 4055–4063.

332 Scow, J.S., Reynolds, C.A., Degnim, A.C., Petersen, I.A., Jakub, J.W., Boughey, J.C. (2010) Primary and secondary angiosarcoma of the breast: the Mayo Clinic experience. *J. Surg. Oncol.*, **101** (5), 401–407.

333 Hodgson, N.C., Bowen-Wells, C., Moffat, F., Franceschi, D., Avisar, E. (2007) Angiosarcomas of the breast: a review of 70 cases. *Am J. Clin. Oncol.*, **30** (6), 570–573.

334 Rubino, C., Shamsaldin, A., Le, M.G., *et al.* (2005) Radiation dose and risk of soft tissue and bone sarcoma after breast cancer treatment. *Breast Cancer Res. Treat.*, **89** (3), 277–288.

335 Karlsson, P., Holmberg, E., Samuelsson, A., Johansson, K.A., Wallgren, A. (1998) Soft tissue sarcoma after treatment for breast cancer – a Swedish population-based study. *Eur. J. Cancer*, **34** (13), 2068–2075.

336 Virtanen, A., Pukkala, E., Auvinen, A. (2007) Angiosarcoma after radiotherapy: a cohort study of 332,163 Finish cancer patients. *Br. J. Cancer*, **97** (1), 115–117.

337 Ringberg, A., Nordgren, H., Thorstensson, S., *et al.* (2007) Histopathological risk factors for ipsilateral breast events after breast conserving treatment for ductal carcinoma in situ of the breast–results from the Swedish randomised trial. *Eur. J. Cancer*, **43** (2), 291–298.

338 Naillet, F., Housset, M., Maylin, C., *et al.* (1990) The use of a specific hypofractionated radiation therapy regimen versus classical fractionation in the treatment of breast cancer: a randomized study of 230 patients. *Int. J. Radiat. Oncol. Biol. Phys.*, **19** (5), 1131–1133.

339 Owen, J.R., Ashton, A., Bliss, J.M., *et al.* (2006) Effect of radiotherapy fraction size on tumor control in patients with early-stage breast cancer after local tumour excision: long-term results of a randomised trial. *Lancet Oncol.*, **7** (6), 467–471.

340 Magee, B., Swindell, R., Harris, M., Banerjee, S.S. (1996) Prognostic factors for breast recurrence after conservative breast surgery and radiotherapy: results from a randomised trial. *Radiother. Oncol.*, **39** (3), 223–227.

341 Dodwell, D.J., Dyker, K., Brown, J., *et al.* (2005) A randomised study of whole-breast vs tumour-bed irradiation after local excision and axillary dissection for early breast cancer. *Clin. Oncol. (R. Coll. Radiol.)*, **17** (8), 618–622.

342 Polgar, C., Fodor, J., Major, T., *et al.* (2007) Breast-conserving treatment with partial or whole breast irradiation for low-risk invasive breast carcinoma–5-year results of a randomized trial. *Int. J. Radiat. Oncol. Biol. Phys.*, **69** (3), 694–702.

343 University of Florence, Livi, L., Meattini, I., Marrazzo, L., *et al.* (2015) Accelerated partial breast irradiation using intensity-modulated radiotherapy versus whole breast irradiation: 5-year survival analysis of a phase 3 randomised controlled trial. *Eur. J. Cancer*, **51**, 451–563.

344 Cheng, J.C., Chen, C.M., Liu, M.C., *et al.* (2002) Locoregional failure of postmastectomy patients with 1-3 positive axillary lymph nodes without adjuvant radiotherapy. *Int. J. Radiat. Oncol. Biol. Phys.*, **52** (4), 980–988.

38

Soft-Tissue Sarcomas

Jonathan B. Ashman and Kaled M. Alektiar

Introduction

Sarcomas are a relatively rare and heterogeneous group of mesenchymal malignancies that comprise less than 1% of all cancer diagnoses. Approximately 12 390 new cases of soft-tissue sarcoma (STS) and an additional 3260 cases of primary bone tumors are estimated in 2017 [1]. The incidence is slightly greater in men than women (1.2:1). There are about 50 histologic subtypes of sarcoma, but three-fourths are undifferentiated/unclassified sarcoma (formerly malignant fibrous histiocytoma; MFH), liposarcoma, leiomyosarcoma, synovial sarcoma, and malignant peripheral nerve sheath tumor (MPNST) [2]. Although certain sarcoma subtypes may have a normal differentiated counterpart, such as liposarcoma and normal fat, the malignant cells most likely arise from multipotent mesenchymal stem cells [3]. For example, most synovial sarcomas occur in organs such as the lung, heart, or kidney, and not within joints. Approximately one-half of sarcomas arise from the extremities or trunk, and another 15% from the abdomen or retroperitoneum [4]. The median age of diagnosis is 65 years, but certain subtypes are typically found in pediatric and young adult populations. Most cases of sarcoma are spontaneous, but environmental exposures such as ionizing radiation or chemicals can sometimes contribute to tumor development. Lymphedema, typically after treatment for breast cancer, is a risk factor for angiosarcoma. The human herpes 8 virus and Epstein–Barr virus have been associated with the development of Kaposi sarcoma and smooth muscle tumors in immunodeficient patients, respectively.

Genetics of Sarcoma

Sarcomas are generally divided between STS and primary bone tumors by location and histopathology. However, with recent advances in genomics, classification based on molecular features has proven to be more informative. The majority of sarcomas arise *de novo*, but familial genetic syndromes such as Li–Fraumeni and neurofibromatosis 1 carry an increased risk of sarcoma. From the genetic perspective, sarcomas can be divided into two broad categories [5,6]. First, there are tumors that display specific genetic alterations and maintain diploid or simple karyotypes. Characteristic genetic changes include either fusion genes with reciprocal translocations or specific point mutations. Synovial sarcoma containing the t(X, 18) translocation and myxoid liposarcoma containing the t(12,16) translocation are well-described examples of the former. The activating point mutations in the c-*KIT* gene in gastrointestinal stromal tumor (GIST) are an example of the latter. It has been estimated that approximately one-fourth of sarcomas contain these balanced and simple genetic alterations [7]. The second category encompasses sarcomas with complex genetic alterations and complex karyotypes but without displaying a specific pattern. Included in this group are undifferentiated/unclassified (previously designated MFH), pleomorphic liposarcoma, and leiomyosarcoma.

Functional genomics such as gene expression profiling has begun to differentiate sarcomas by genetic subtype, even among genetically complex sarcomas such as pleomorphic sarcoma and leiomyosarcoma [8,9]. Although limited by the availability of tissue in this relatively rare cancer, these techniques can produce comprehensive datasets of genomic signaling pathway alterations and signaling pathways critical to sarcoma development [10]. This progress has allowed the establishment of a basic taxonomy of sarcoma linking together lineage and prognosis [11]. It is hoped that this greater understanding will lead to therapeutic advances through the identification of potential target development. The development of animal models will be key in translating these basic science discoveries into deliverable therapeutics [12]. For example, mouse models have recently been described which recapitulate rhabdomyosarcoma, undifferentiated pleomorphic sarcoma, and malignant peripheral nerve sheath-like tumors [13,14].

Soft-Tissue Sarcoma of the Extremities

Diagnosis and Staging

The diagnosis of and treatment of extremity sarcoma can be complex, with multiple potential options. A suggested algorithm is presented in Figure 38.1. The involvement of a multidisciplinary team with sub-specialty experience is recommended as early as possible in the evaluation when a sarcoma is considered within a differential diagnosis. Most cases of extremity sarcoma present with a painless mass. A recent injury is often associated with the discovery of the mass, but this is typically a coincidental

relationship. The physical examination is central to both diagnosis and surgical planning; it allows for direct tumor evaluation, for the assessment of any tumor-related functional deficits, and for consideration of the patient's overall performance status. Signs of malignancy include a painful mass presenting deep to the fascia, larger than 5 cm, and increasing in size. If a mass is associated with all four of these signs, the chance of diagnosing malignant sarcoma is 86% [15].

In addition to the physical examination, imaging is critical for diagnosis and treatment planning. Ultrasound has been prospectively demonstrated to be an effective tool to triage benign from malignant masses [16]. Plain imaging can be useful to assess for intratumoral calcifications and relationship to adjacent bones. However, magnetic resonance imaging (MRI) is the primary modality for evaluating sarcomas because of the multiplanar capability and superior contrast resolution (Figure 38.2). MRI provides limited but imprecise

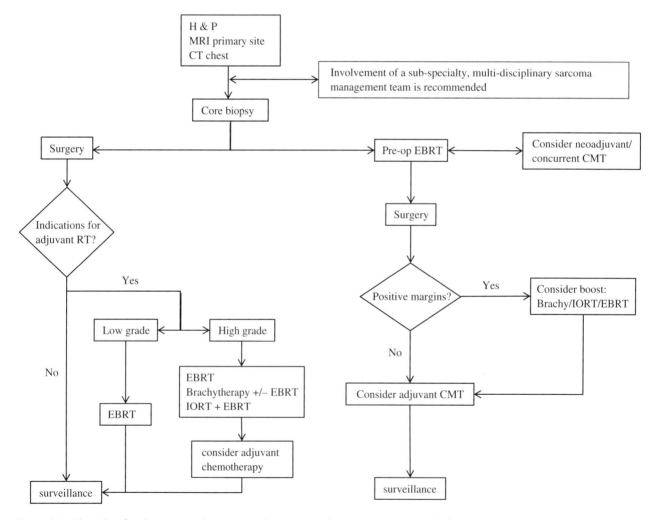

Figure 38.1 Algorithm for diagnosis and treatment of extremity soft-tissue sarcoma eligible for limb-sparing surgery. H&P, history and physical; RT, radiation therapy; EBRT, external beam radiation therapy; brachy, brachytherapy; IORT, intraoperative radiation therapy; CMT, chemotherapy.

Figure 38.2 Popliteal fossa soft-tissue sarcoma.

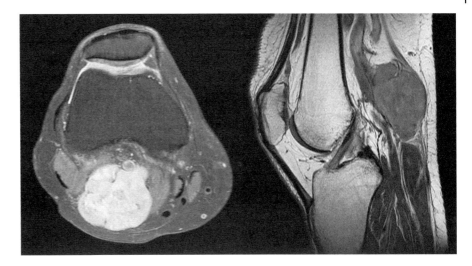

information regarding the histology of the tumor mass, and it predicts the correct histologic diagnosis in only 25–40% of cases [5]. Computed tomography (CT) can also provide important anatomic information, especially in the evaluation of bone architecture adjacent to tumors. CT is also standard to evaluate for metastatic disease in the chest. The role of positron emission tomography (PET) is less well defined [17]. PET may be useful in differentiating between low- and high-grade tumors, and it also may detect lymph node or sites of distant metastases. After neoadjuvant therapy, PET may provide a measure of tumor response. However, some centers have found limited value in adding PET to the diagnostic evaluation [18].

Tissue biopsy must be carefully planned and optimally is performed at a sarcoma specialty center. Up to 10% of patients may have changes in treatment or outcome because of a poorly executed biopsy, and the rate is significantly lower at specialty centers [19]. Open surgical biopsy, core-needle biopsy, or fine-needle aspiration are all acceptable techniques [20]. Classic teaching required a surgical, incisional biopsy because it yielded the highest accuracy. However, with the advantage of efficiency and low cost, a core-needle biopsy has become the standard. A core-needle biopsy has been demonstrated in one study to result in 93% sensitivity, 100% specificity, and 95% accuracy, which compares favorably to incisional biopsy [21]. If surgical biopsy is required, it is critical that the incision be orientated such that it can be fully excised at the time of the subsequent definitive surgical procedure [22].

Similar to other cancer sites, the American Joint Committee on Cancer (AJCC) stages sarcoma using the tumor, node, and metastasis (TNM) system. The primary tumor stage is divided by size (T1 ≤5 cm, T2 >5 cm) and depth (T1a/T2a superficial, T1b/T2b deep). However, unlike most other cancer sites, histologic grade is

an integral component of the sarcoma staging system. Any low-grade tumor regardless of size or depth remains stage I, while intermediate-grade tumors of any size or depth or small high-grade tumors constitute stage II. Stage III includes both high-grade tumors >5 cm and node-positive disease. The staging system does provide strong prognostic information, with long-term survival ranging between 90% for early stage to 40% for stage III tumors >10 cm [5].

Treatment of the Primary Site

Surgery remains central for the treatment of limited disease with curative intent. Limb-preservation strategies have been developed to achieve cure while also improving the quality of life compared to amputation. In order to prospectively examine the outcomes of limb-preservation treatment, a Phase III trial was conducted at the National Cancer Institute (NCI) randomizing patients to either amputation or limb-sparing surgery (LSS) followed by external beam radiation therapy (EBRT). While the five-year local control for the limb-preservation arm was only 80% compared to 100% for the amputation arm (P = 0.06), this difference did not compromise disease-free survival (DFS) or overall survival (OS) [23]. Following this study, LSS combined with radiation rapidly became the standard of care.

A second NCI trial examined the benefit of adjuvant radiation after LSS [24]. Patients were randomized to LSS alone or LSS plus adjuvant EBRT, and all patients with high-grade disease also received chemotherapy. Radiation therapy significantly improved local control with no benefit in OS. The effect of radiation therapy was especially apparent for patients with high-grade disease with 10-year actuarial local control rates of 100% in patients treated with radiation compared to 78% with surgery alone (P = 0.003). A significant difference in local control was also found among all patients with low-grade disease. Also examining the role of adjuvant radiation after surgery, investigators at Memorial Sloan Kettering Cancer Center (MSKCC) conducted a Phase III trial randomizing patients either to LSS alone or to LSS plus adjuvant brachytherapy [25–27]. Improvement in local control was observed in patients with high-grade sarcoma who received adjuvant brachytherapy with no improvement in OS. No benefit to brachytherapy was observed in patients with low-grade disease [28].

Despite the advantages demonstrated to adjuvant radiation, surgery alone is adequate treatment for selected patients [29–31]. Pisters *et al.* reported a prospective study on 74 patients with small (<5 cm) extremity or trunk STS who underwent an oncologic complete gross resection with negative microscopic margin (R0) and were then observed without adjuvant therapy [32]. With a median follow-up of 75 months, the cumulative five- and 10-year rates of local recurrence were 7.9% and 10.6%, respectively. These favorable results suggested that observation after surgery is a consideration in a select group of patients with small STS and R0 resection. In contrast, a small series from the Mayo Clinic reported on 34 patients treated with surgery alone and observed a suboptimal local control rate of 60% among patients with high-grade disease [33]. Therefore, while surgery alone may be adequate for some patients, careful multidisciplinary decision-making is required to determine the appropriate use of radiation therapy. At MSKCC, a nomogram was developed to try to determine the risk of local recurrence after oncologic limb-sparing surgery in primary non-metastatic extremity STS [34]. Such a tool can help the treating physicians as well as patients in deciding whether to pursue adjuvant radiation or not, based on the predicted risk of local recurrence after surgery alone (Figure 38.3).

Many patients will have initial surgical procedures performed at non-specialty centers for presumed benign disease. After the diagnosis of sarcoma, a referral will be made to a specialty center for further management. Re-excision of the site is typically indicated to achieve adequate margins. Goodlad *et al.* [35] examined the pathologic re-excision specimens from 95 cases of primary sarcoma who underwent a second procedure after initial surgery was presumed to have inadequate margins. Incomplete excision was confirmed in 56% of cases, and almost one-third had macroscopically visible residual tumor. A similar study from Princess Margaret Hospital (PMH) examined re-excision in 65 patients and identified residual disease in 35% [36]. Considering that it was not possible to predict prior to re-excision which patient harbored residual disease, re-excision should be standard treatment after unplanned primary surgery. Even after re-excision, outcomes may be inferior to appropriate up-front treatment. In the PMH report, a relatively

high rate of positive margins (39%) at re-excision also translated into a higher recurrence rate of 22% among the group of patients with residual disease [36]. Therefore, unplanned excision should be avoided when sarcoma is a potential differential diagnosis. While many patients who undergo re-excision are found to have residual disease, some show no evidence of residual disease at all. This subset of patients with pathologically negative re-excision is considered at very low risk of local recurrence. In a study from MSKCC, 200 such patients with primary extremity STS were observed after negative re-exicision without additional therapy [37]. With a median follow-up of 82 months, the overall five-year local recurrence rate was 9%, but that rate varied significantly (p <0.01) based on age and stage; it was 4% for stage I/II and age <50 years, 12% for either age >50 years or stage III, and 31% for those with stage III and aged >50 years.

Much of the evidence demonstrating the benefit of radiation therapy utilized treatment in postoperative setting. However, preoperative irradiation had very early proponents [38]. The relative merits of preoperative versus postoperative radiation continue to be debated. Suit *et al.* [39] outlined the benefits of a preoperative approach: smaller treatment volumes; lower total doses; opportunities to improve multidisciplinary care; potential tumor response leading to less-extensive and more complete surgery; less risk for tumor seeding at surgery; no delay in radiation initiation; and the opportunity for intraoperative radiation therapy (IORT) [39]. An advantage to postoperative radiation is the opportunity for the surgeon and the pathologist to examine tumor unaltered by neoadjuvant therapy. In addition, proceeding without delay to surgery was noted to be a psychological advantage for some patients. The major disadvantage with regard to preoperative radiation has been the potential for increased surgical wound complications.

To prospectively address the question of radiation timing, a multicenter Phase III randomized trial was performed by the National Cancer Institute of Canada (NCIC) comparing preoperative to postoperative radiation [40]. Patients were stratified by tumor size (≤10 cm versus >10 cm) and randomized to 50 Gy preoperative EBRT or 66–70 Gy postoperative EBRT. Patients in the preoperative arm with positive margins at surgery were given a postoperative boost. In both groups, surgery and radiation were separated by three to six weeks. The primary endpoint was the rate of significant wound complications, which was doubled in the preoperative arm compared to the postoperative arm (35% versus 17%; p = 0.01). No differences were observed in local, regional, or distant recurrence. A borderline significant OS advantage in favor of preoperative therapy was likely due to an excess in non-sarcoma deaths in the postoperative arm. Often, patients are concerned about the delay in

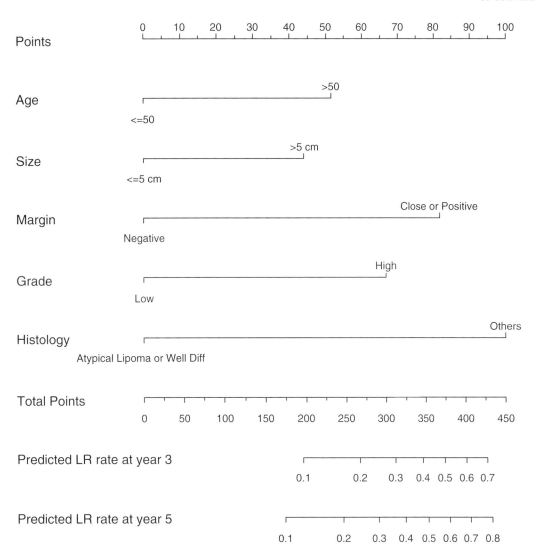

Figure 38.3 Nomogram for predicting risk of local recurrence at three and five years in primary soft-tissue sarcoma (STS) of the extremity after surgery alone.

institing surgery when preoperative radiation is being considered. The fact that the NCIC trial showed that OS with preoperative radiotherapy was equivalent, if not slightly better than postoperative radiotherapy, is an important point to highlight to alleviate their concerns.

Chemotherapy

Chemotherapy has been used both in neoadjuvant or adjuvant curative therapy and also in the palliative therapy of metastatic disease. The randomized NCI trials that defined the strategy of LSS followed by postoperative radiation also utilized adjuvant chemotherapy [23,24]. Indeed, after treatment with either amputation or LSS and radiation, the initial trial randomized a second cohort of patients with high-grade disease to receive adjuvant chemotherapy or not, and reported a significant

benefit in both DFS and OS to chemotherapy [23]. However, multiple other trials failed to show a significant benefit to chemotherapy delivered adjuvantly after curative surgery. A meta-analysis did find significant improvements in local control and DFS, but a significant benefit in OS could not be demonstrated [41]. An update of this meta-analysis confirmed these findings with respect to the use of regimens containing single-agent doxorubicin [42]. In contrast, an OS advantage was observed in trials using the combination of doxorubicin and ifosfamide (HR = 0.56; 95% CI 0.36–0.85; p = 0.01).

Experience with neoadjuvant chemoradiation in extremity sarcoma has been reported by several groups. Eilber and colleagues published a regimen of intra-arterial doxorubicin infused over 24 h for three days prior to radiation, followed by surgery [43]. Other single agents that have been studied with preoperative radiation include ifosfamide and gemcitabine [44,45]. Multi-agent chemotherapy regimens given preoperatively with radiation included MAID (mesna, doxorubicin, ifosfamide and dacarbazine) or IMAP/MAP (ifosfamide, mitomycin, doxorubicin, and cisplatin) [46–48]. These strategies have shown promising results. Local control rates at five years have been reported as 92%, and limb-preservation rates as high as 100% [44,46]. In addition, multiple studies have reported five-year OS rates of up to 70% [49–52]. Toxicities of neoadjuvant chemotherapy and radiation typically include wound complications and long bone fracture [53]. A retrospective study from the Mayo Clinic compared the outcomes of patients treated with surgery alone, preoperative radiation, or combined preoperative chemotherapy and radiation [54]. Patients with tumors >5 cm appeared to benefit from a neoadjuvant strategy, but a benefit to the addition of chemotherapy with radiation was not observed. Both neoadjuvant strategies resulted in increased wound complications compared to surgery alone. Several additional single-institution retrospective studies have been reported recently demonstrating favorable outcomes with neoadjuvant therapy regimens including chemotherapy [55–57]. In the report by Bedi *et al.* [55], chemotherapy was independently associated with improved distant metastasis-free survival.

Outcomes

The overall prognosis for patients with extremity sarcoma has changed little over the past several decades despite many improvements in therapy. When analyzing the details of 1261 patients treated at MSKCC by five-year cohorts of 1982–1986, 1987–1991, 1992–1996, and 1997–2001, Weitz *et al.* reported five-year disease-specific survival rates of 78%, 79%, 79%, and 85%, respectively (p = NS) [58]. For high-risk patients with large, high-grade, and deep tumors, the five-year disease-specific survival for each time cohort was 50%, 45%, 52%, 65%, respectively (p = NS). Multiple prognostic factors were found to be predictive of outcome, but the time period of treatment was not significant. For example, factors predictive of local recurrence included age >50 years, recurrent disease at presentation, tumor size >10 cm, and positive surgical margins. Factors predictive of decreased disease-specific survival included age >50 years, recurrent disease at presentation, tumor size, deep tumors, high-grade, and leiomyosarcoma histology. An earlier study from MSKCC had previously identified many of these factors as important prognostic indicators of outcomes, with grade and size consistently being found to be among the strongest risk factors [59]. Positive resection margins have also been reported in some studies as a risk factor for both local recurrence and disease-specific survival [60,61].

The histologic subtype can provide important prognostic information. Coindre *et al.* [62] utilized the French Federation of Cancer Centers (FNCLCC) database to analyze the risk of metastasis in 1205 patients according to individual histology. Grade was the strongest predictor of metastasis in MFH, synovial sarcoma, unclassified or 'other' sarcomas, and these combined represented 62% of the patient population. Among patients with MFH, the five-year metastasis-free survival rate with grade 1, 2, and 3 tumors was 90%, 77%, and 48%, respectively (p = 3×10^{-9}). The histologic subtype was the strongest prognostic factor for metastasis in the case of liposarcoma, but grade remained an independent predictor on multivariate analysis. For leiomyosarcoma, multiple factors including grade, size, bone, and neurovascular involvement all were independent predictors of metastasis. Pisters *et al.* [59] reported significantly worse disease-specific survival with malignant peripheral nerve tumor and leiomyosarcoma. Subtypes associated with lymph node involvement, such as epithelioid sarcoma, synovial sarcoma, rhabdomyosarcoma and clear-cell sarcoma, may also have lower rates of disease-specific survival [60,61].

Another consistent prognostic factor for poor outcome is older age. Singer *et al.* [60] showed that older age modeled as a continuous variable was an independent predictor of decreased OS. Identifying a cut-point of 64 years, Zagars *et al.* [61] observed older age to be a poor prognostic factor for both local control and disease-specific survival. A recent multicenter study has retrospectively analyzed over 2000 patients from prospective databases in order to examine the impact of older age [63]. While older patients more commonly present with high-risk disease, older age remained an independent predictor of both increased local recurrence and metastasis on multivariate analysis.

Once a patient has metastatic disease, the median survival is approximately one year [64]. The lungs are the most common first site of metastasis. The strongest predictor of survival after the diagnosis of metastatic disease is whether resection can be performed of all metastatic sites (HR 2.3; 95% CI 1.2–3.7) [64]. Negative prognostic factors included the presence of local recurrence in addition to metastasis, disease-free interval of less than one year, and age >50 years. In an analysis of patients specifically with lung metastases, complete resection was the strongest predictor of outcome, with a median survival of 33.5 months compared to 16.5 months after incomplete resection and 11.2 months with no resection (p <0.001) [65]. The presence of unilateral or bilateral metastases was not predictive of outcome. On multivariate analysis, the hazard ratio for complete resection was 0.51 (95% CI 0.43–0.63; p <0.0001). Interestingly, both liposarcoma and MPNST were both identified as additional independent negative prognostic factors. More recently, stereotactic body radiotherapy (SBRT) has emerged as a useful non-invasive treatment approach for pulmonary metastasis. Dhakal and colleagues have reported the largest experience thus far using SBRT to treatment pulmonary metastases exclusively from sarcoma [66]. Among 52 patients treated typically with 50 Gy in five fractions, local control was 82% at three years and median OS was 2.1 years.

Nomograms have been clinically useful tools to predict outcomes based on the interactions of these prognostic factors. Using the MSKCC prospective database, the first nomogram was developed by Kattan *et al.* to predict 12-year sarcoma-specific death [67]. Variables included were size, depth, site, histology, and age. The nomogram then was externally validated using the independent, prospective University of California at Los Angeles database [68]. An additional external validation using an Italian database extended the nomogram to accommodate the three-tiered FNCLCC pathologic grading system [69]. Using similar prognostic variables and a competing risks model, the MSKCC group produced another nomogram to predict for sarcoma-specific death in patients with recurrent disease [70]. A third nomogram was also produced from the MSKCC database specific for the liposarcoma histologic subtype [71]. This nomogram accounted for additional variables such as disease site (extremity, truncal or retroperitoneal), gender, presentation status, subtype variant, margin status, and tumor burden. Nomograms have not been the only prognostic models defined for sarcoma. The Swedish 'SIN-system' defined groups at either low or high risk for developing metastatic disease based on three factors: size >10 cm; vascular invasion; and microscopic necrosis [72,73]. Recently, this model was extended to include the new risk factor of infiltrative growth pattern to create the 'SING-system' [73].

Radiation Therapy Techniques

Radiation techniques for sarcoma continue to evolve from two-dimensional (2-D) planning to three-dimensional (3-D) CT-guided conformal planning and, more recently, to intensity-modulated radiotherapy (IMRT). However, regardless of the technique an understanding of the patterns of tumor spread and the tissues at risk is required to appropriately design a radiotherapy plan. Since sarcomas tend to spread within compartments, classical teaching had been to allow a 5-cm margin in the longitudinal dimension and a 2-cm margin in the circumferential dimension for initial fields followed a cone-down boost. These margins are customized for tissue planes the tumor would not be expected to breech. Volumes are smaller for preoperative radiation because of the presence of a defined gross target volume (GTV). In contrast, without a GTV, postoperative volumes are larger because the entire surgical bed with margin must be encompassed. In addition, the surgical scar and drain sites are typically included within initial postoperative treatments fields. MRI fused to the planning CT scan is critical for GTV definition. The addition of intravenous contrast for the planning CT often can be very beneficial for tumor delineation; especially if no planning MRI is available (e.g., the patient has a pacemaker). The clinical target volume (CTV) and the planning target volume (PTV) are expanded around the GTV to account for microscopic disease spread and set-up error, respectively.

With the widespread adoption of image-guided therapy and volumetric treatment planning, the issue of target definition required updating from the 2-D treatment planning era. A panel of sarcoma radiation oncologists first evaluated how much variability existed in the definition of the GTV and CTV [74]. The encouraging results demonstrated almost perfect agreement among the experts on the definition of the GTV for both upper- and lower-extremity targets, and of the CTV for the lower-extremity target. Increased variation was identified in the case of the CTV definition for the upper-extremity target, but overall agreement still remained substantial. The same panel also published their consensus recommendations for 3 cm longitudinal expansion and 1.5 cm radial expansion (not confined by fascial plane, bone, or skin) from the GTV to create the CTV [75].

The question of PTV margins has also been addressed in the era of image-guided radiotherapy (IGRT). The RTOG recently published the results of a Phase II trial using the consensus CTV guidelines discussed above with a 5-mm CTV to PTV margin combined with IGRT [76]. No marginal failures were identified, and the study met its primary endpoint to reduce late toxicities. Dickie *et al.* [77] examined inter- and intra-fractional motion in preoperative, lower-extremity sarcoma using cone beam CT. These authors concluded that a uniform 5 mm PTV margin was appropriate for the delivery of IMRT for lower-extremity tumors. At MSKCC, an expansion margin of 1 cm from CTV to PTV is used. The expansion from GTV to CTV is 4 cm in the long axis and 1 cm radially, excluding adjacent bone (Figure 38.4).

Regional lymph nodes are uncommonly involved in most cases of sarcoma and are also rarely the site of an isolated first recurrence. For example, Behranwala *et al.* [78] reported the experience from the Royal Marsden Hospital that only 3.4% of over 2000 patients developed regional nodal metastasis, and regional nodal disease was the site of first recurrence in only 1.5% of patients. Therefore, radiotherapy fields should not typically be expanded to cover regional node. Attention should be given to regional nodes for certain histologic subtypes such as epithelioid sarcoma, angiosarcoma, and clear-cell sarcoma. Therapeutic or prophylactic coverage of nodal

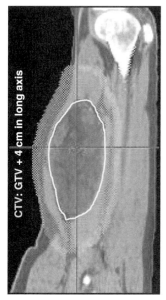

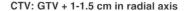

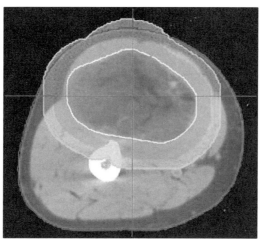

PTV: CTV plus 1 cm margin in all directions

Figure 38.4 Clinical target volume (CTV; orange), planned target volume (PTV; cyan) expansions from gross tumor volume (GTV; yellow). For a color version of this figure, see the color plate section.

regions may be appropriate in such selected cases of these tumor types. However, these subtypes also are among the most likely to develop distant metastatic disease, especially once nodal disease is established. Sarcoma of the head and neck, especially rhabdomyosarcoma, may be a setting where prophylactic coverage of draining regional nodes should be considered.

The standard dose of postoperative radiation has been between 60 and 66 Gy. In patients with negative resection margins, Mundt *et al.* [79] observed increased local failure with postoperative doses <60 Gy but no additional benefit for doses ≥64 Gy. In patients with high-grade sarcoma and positive margins after LSS, a significant benefit in local control has been demonstrated for adjuvant radiation compared to LSS alone [80]. In a study including multiple sites of sarcoma with positive surgical margins, DeLaney *et al.* demonstrated a benefit of adjuvant EBRT with an overall LC rate of 76% [81]. Extremity sarcoma was the site with the highest rate of local control of 82% at five years. Higher doses may be indicated when resection margins are positive or uncertain. Zagars and Ballo [82] found that doses ≥64 Gy were an independent prognostic factor for improved local control in high-risk patients such as positive or uncertain margin and locally recurrent presentation. The standard dose of preoperative radiation is 50 Gy, typically delivered in 25 fractions of 2 Gy each. The major complication after preoperative therapy is poor wound healing. Therefore, one hypothesis would be that lower doses of preoperative therapy combined with a boost could decrease wound complications while still maintaining adequate local control. Devisetty *et al.* [83] retrospectively

identified 42 patients who had been treated with a median preoperative dose of 20 Gy and then given a boost either with postoperative EBRT, brachytherapy, or IORT. However, despite the lower doses the wound complication rate remained at 36%. Given the higher risk of long-term complications, the utility of a postoperative boost after preoperative EBRT has been questioned. An analysis of patients treated with preoperative EBRT at PMH did not find a statistically significant difference in LR with or without an EBRT boost [84]. A more recent study also failed to show a significant difference in local control in patients with positive margins after preoperative EBRT who received no boost, IORT, brachytherapy, or an EBRT boost [85]. However, firm conclusions are difficult to draw from this small retrospective study, which reported on 67 patients and only 10 of these received no boost.

Much of the experience with multi-catheter interstitial brachytherapy has been with low-dose rate (LDR) implants. Brachytherapy can be used as the only modality of adjuvant therapy for high-grade STS, as per the MSKCC Phase III trial [28,86]. Alternatively, brachytherapy can be delivered as a boost after preoperative radiation, which has been the preferred technique at Mayo Clinic [87]. When LDR brachytherapy is used as a single modality, the dose is typically 45 Gy, and this is reduced to approximately 20 Gy when given as an boost after 50 Gy EBRT. The technique requires that afterloading catheters be placed approximately 1 cm apart with approximately 2 cm of margin around the surgical bed, with more margin considered in the longitudinal dimensions compared to the medial and lateral dimensions. At MSKCC, the catheters are oriented in the longitudinal direction and secured with absorbable sutures. The distal end of the catheters could be buried in the wound with only a single end protruding for source afterloading. The technique preferred at the Mayo Clinic orients the catheters transversely, with both ends exiting the wound. This technique requires more catheters to cover the length of the wound, but the loading length of each catheter is smaller and no anchoring is required within the wound. In each technique, a drain is placed in the wound and should remain in place throughout the planning and delivery of the treatment. Dosimetry can be performed using 2-D techniques, although CT-based planning has been implemented widely. The Ir-192 ribbons should not be loaded before day 5 after surgery. Investigators at MSKCC observed increased wound complications when loading at earlier time-points [88]. The use of brachytherapy is limited by the geometry of the tumor bed. For example, resections in the groin and the axilla may leave a wound that is difficult to obtain adequate catheter distribution. Brachytherapy can also be performed using high-dose rate (HDR) techniques [89,90]. Total doses have varied depending on the use of EBRT and the margin status, but the use of 4 Gy per fraction is typical. The American Brachytherapy Society published their recommendations for sarcoma brachytherapy in 2013 [91].

After preoperative EBRT, single-fraction IORT represents an alternative boost technique compared to either additional postoperative EBRT or brachytherapy. The delivery of intraoperative electrons has been facilitated by the development of mobile, dedicated electron linear accelerator units. HDR brachytherapy typically utilizes a super-flab, multi-channel planar applicator with an HDR delivery machine located in a shielded operating room. The two techniques each have relative advantages and disadvantages, but institutions have reported good results with both [92–98].

More recent interest in sarcoma radiotherapy has focused on the use of IMRT. Dosimetric studies have demonstrated the benefit of IMRT compared to 3-D conformal techniques in producing superior dose distributions. IMRT techniques reduced the volume of femur receiving high doses, which could translate into less long-term morbidity from fracture [99,100]. Hong *et al.* [99] also reported fewer hot spots in the skin with IMRT planning, which could reduce wound complications after preoperative therapy. One concern about the adoption of IMRT with highly conformal dose distributions has been the possibility of increased local recurrences. The early experience from MSKCC reported favorable toxicity profiles without obviously compromising local control [101,102]. A retrospective cohort comparison between patients treated with either adjuvant brachytherapy or IMRT actually observed better local control in the IMRT group [103]. Similar comparison between IMRT and conventional EBRT demonstrated better local control in favor of IMRT despite an imbalance of higher-risk features within the IMRT cohort [104]. Currently at MSKCC, IMRT is the radiation modality of choice for extremity STS.

Complications and Functional Outcome

The NCIC trial showed a significant increase in the rate of wound complications (35% versus 17%; p = 0.01) for preoperative compared to postoperative radiotherapy. The increased risk was observed almost exclusively in patients with lower-extremity tumors. Multivariate analysis showed that tumor site (lower versus upper extremity) was the strongest independent predictor of wound complication in addition to radiation sequence and tumor size [105]. This finding was confirmed by others [106]. Reassuringly, since patients receiving preoperative therapy may need tissue transfer procedures more frequently, Davidge *et al.* [107] did not find that flap reconstruction was an independent predictor of long-term functional outcome. In addition, in patients who require both flap reconstruction and then postoperative radiation, the tissue transfers appeared to tolerate adjuvant radiation without significantly increased wound healing complications [108]. Working towards decreasing wound complications in lower-extremity STS, Griffin *et al.* [109] contoured the volume of planned skin flaps as a defined organ-at-risk. It was then demonstrated that more conformal plans producing greater skin flap sparing could be generated using IMRT compared to 3-D or conventional techniques [109]. Although the rate of wound complications was 30% using this technique, compared to 43% in the NCIC trial, the difference was not statistically significant. The need for tissue transfer to achieve wound closure was less, however [105]. Data from MSKCC showed that patients treated with IMRT, had less grade ≥2 skin desquamation (32% versus 49%, p = 0.002) and required less treatment interruption (p <0.001) than those treated with conventional EBRT [104].

The choice of preoperative or postoperative therapy, chemotherapy, and radiation technique are some of the factors impacting long-term functional outcomes and quality of life. In the NCIC trial, the rates of grade ≥2 late toxicity were higher (albeit not statistically significant) in the postoperative arm compared to preoperative radiotherapy arm; fibrosis (48.2% versus 31.5%), edema (23.2% versus 15.1%), and joint stiffness (23.2% versus 17.8%). The Musculoskeletal Tumor Society Rating Scale (MSTS) is a physician-reported tool, while the Toronto Extremity Salvage Score (TESS) is a patient-reported outcome measure [110,111]. Multiple factors contribute to long-term functional outcomes as measured by the TESS and the MSTS instruments, such as large tumor size, bone resection, motor nerve resection, and complications [112]. Patients treated with postoperative radiation compared to preoperative radiation on the Phase III randomized trial did have better function and quality of life six weeks after surgery [113]. However, longer-term follow-up over the next two years did not demonstrate a persistent difference. When controlling for treatment arm, other typical factors such as lower-extremity site, large tumor size, and nerve sacrifice were predictive of decreased function. Although patients with wound complications did have lower MSTS and TESS scores over the first two years, these near-term consequences of preoperative therapy were balanced against the long-term morbidity of increased late fibrosis in patients treated postoperatively [113,114]. Patients who experienced fibrosis, joint stiffness, or edema were found to have significantly lower MSTS and TESS function scores. The larger field-sizes used in postoperative treatment were a predictor of late morbidity [114].

In addition to fibrosis, fracture represents another significant delayed complication. Factors contributing to an increased risk of fracture include older age, female gender, higher radiation dose, thigh location, tissue compartment, and periosteal stripping [115,116]. Dickie *et al.* [117] reported multiple dose–volume parameters associated with a risk of lower-extremity fracture. Subsequently, a nomogram was developed to predict the risk of femur fracture [116]. Because postoperative radiation requires higher radiation doses to larger volumes, one of the conclusions from these analyses would be a preference for preoperative therapy to reduce long-term morbidity and improve function and quality of life. This is especially true for upper-extremity STS where the risk of wound complications from preoperative radiotherapy is minimal.

Retroperitoneal Sarcomas

Sarcomas arising from the retroperitoneum, abdomen, or pelvis constitute only 15% of all soft-tissue tumor cases [118]. In contrast to the diversity of histologies found with extremity sarcoma, two-thirds of retroperitoneal sarcoma (RPS) are either liposarcoma or leiomyosarcoma. Because of the tumor location and lack of early symptoms, patients with RPS typically present with large tumors. Although the principles of treatment with surgery and radiation therapy are similar to extremity sarcoma, the close proximity of bowel and other visceral organs makes the treatment of RPS more challenging. Local failure is a frequent cause of morbidity and mortality for patient with RPS, and late recurrence is common. The early experience with RPS at MSKCC reported a 5% per year recurrence rate and, among those patients who were disease-free at postoperative year 5, there

remained a 40% risk of recurrence by postoperative year 10 [119]. The only independent predictor for OS was complete surgical resection. This finding has led to the development of aggressive up-front surgical approaches including *en bloc* multi-organ resection as needed to achieve at least gross total tumor resection. For example, Bonvalot *et al.* [120] reported their series of 249 patients treated with aggressive surgery alone where they achieved 93% complete macroscopic resection. A median of two *en bloc* organs were resected, but 47% of patients had at least three organs resected. The observed five-year rates of OS were 65%, local recurrence was 22%, and distant metastasis was 24%. A multivariate analysis identified compartmental resection as one of the strongest independent predictors of abdominal control compared to standard resections (three-year recurrence rate 10% versus 50%) [121]. Additional predictors of local recurrence and OS included high-grade disease, tumor rupture, positive margins, and low-volume treatment centers. The original MSKCC nomogram included retroperitoneal location as a risk factor, but most of the patients included in the analysis had extremity tumors [67]. Recently, a RPS-specific nomogram has been published [122].

The role of radiation in the treatment of RPS has not been as clearly defined as in extremity sarcoma. Because of the radiosensitivity of the bowel, typical postoperative doses greater than 60 Gy are not achievable in the abdomen without significant toxicity. Preoperative EBRT is often facilitated by a clearly defined target volume and by the displacement of bowel outside of the high-dose field by the tumor itself. In contrast, postoperative EBRT is complicated by poorly defined fields containing large volumes of bowel. Initial experience with EBRT was mostly postoperative, and early reports from MSKCC did suggest a significant decrease in local recurrence in patients treated with surgery and radiation compared to surgery alone [119]. However, additional data on the benefit of postoperative EBRT has been conflicting, and a recent analysis of the Surveillance, Epidemiology, and End Results (SEER) database could not find a significant OS benefit in patients treated with postoperative EBRT compared to surgery alone [123]. Ballo *et al.* [124] reviewed both their institutional experience and the relevant literature, and concluded that routine postoperative EBRT should be discouraged in favor of preoperative EBRT.

IORT has been extensively explored in the treatment of RPS. The NCI conducted a small, randomized Phase III trial with 35 surgically resected RPS patients [125]. Patients were randomized to 20 Gy IORT combined with 35–40 Gy 'low-dose' postoperative EBRT, or to 50–55 Gy 'high-dose' postoperative EBRT without IORT. There were no differences observed in terms of DFS or OS between the two arms. However, the patients in the IORT arm experienced decreased local failure. Local recurrence was observed in 16/20 (80%) of patients in the EBRT-alone arm compared to 6/15 (40%) of patients in the IORT arm (p <0.05). At the time of death, all 16 patients in the EBRT-alone arm had local in-field recurrence compared to only three of 10 patients in the IORT arm (p <0.001). In addition, patients in the EBRT-alone arm experienced significantly more acute and chronic enteritis compared to the IORT group, while those treated with IORT developed moderate to severe neuropathy more frequently than the EBRT-alone patients. Overall, there was little benefit, but significant toxicity was observed when using EBRT alone as well as an improved therapeutic ratio by combining IORT and EBRT. Multiple single-institution studies using either intraoperative electrons or HDR brachytherapy have supported the use of IORT combined with EBRT as adjuvant therapy with surgery [126–132]. When Pawlik *et al.* [133] reported the combined results of two prospective trials using preoperative therapy EBRT, approximately two-thirds of grossly resected patients received a boost with either IORT or brachytherapy, and the five-year local control and OS were 60% and 61%, respectively. An interim analysis has been reported of an ongoing single-center prospective Phase I/II study using preoperative IMRT followed by surgery and IORT [134]. Local control and OS at three and five years were 74%.

RPS is a disease site in which sophisticated radiation techniques might significantly impact outcome. IMRT can reduce dose to critical normal tissues such as bowel, kidney, and liver [135]. IMRT also allows for a simultaneous integrated boost dose to be delivered to areas of predicted close surgical margins. Using this technique, Tzeng *et al.* [136] reported initial results on 16 consecutive patients and observed a two-year local control rate of 80%. RPS may be a disease site optimally treated with protons instead of photons. Compared to photons, protons have reduced entrance dose and no exit dose. Yoon *et al.* [137] reported the early experience at MGH combining proton beam radiotherapy with IMRT and IORT in which they observed only a 10% local recurrence rate at median follow-up of 33 months. The present authors' current approach to RPS favors preoperative IMRT combined with surgery and IORT.

Desmoid Tumors

Desmoid tumors (aggressive fibromatosis) are locally aggressive tumors without metastatic potential. Treatment can include observation, systemic therapy, surgery alone, EBRT alone, or a combination of surgery and EBRT. With optimal multimodality therapy, five-year control rates have improved with time from 70% to 80% overall [138]. A systematic review of the literature has

suggested that surgery alone results in inferior tumor control compared to patients treated with either surgery plus adjuvant EBRT or EBRT alone [139]. However, not all single-institution series clearly demonstrate a benefit for adjuvant radiotherapy [140]. Increasing tumor size and age <30 years, but not surgical margin status, were independent, significant predictors of increased local recurrence [141]. In addition, a radiation dose >56 Gy was associated with increased complications but no additional increase in tumor control; therefore, moderate doses of EBRT were recommended. Recently, Salas *et al.* [142] identified three independent poor prognostic factors for progression-free survival: age <37 years; tumor size >7 cm; and extra-abdominal location. Based on the presence of none or one factor, two factors, or all three factors, three prognostic groups were defined with 10-year progression-free survival rates of approximately 50%, 30%, and 10%.

Primary Tumors of Bone

Primary bone tumors include Ewing sarcoma, osteosarcoma, chordoma, and chondrosarcoma. Ewing sarcoma is highly sensitive to chemotherapy, and local tumor control is achieved with surgery, EBRT, or a combination of both. Surgery is the primary treatment for chordoma and chondrosarcoma. These tumors are sensitive to radiation, but require high doses that can be challenging to deliver while respecting adjacent normal tissue tolerance. Specialized techniques such as proton beam therapy have demonstrated improved control rates. The treatment of osteosarcoma includes surgery combined with preoperative and postoperative chemotherapy [143]. Although osteosarcoma has also been considered to be a relatively radioresistant tumor, multiple reports over the past decade have demonstrated favorable long-term tumor control with radiation therapy when adequate surgery is not possible [144–147]. A recent retrospective review of the MGH database reported a five-year local control rate of 72% after treatment to a mean dose of 68.4 Gy using protons or a proton/photon mix [148].

Conclusions

Sarcomas of the soft tissue and bone are a heterogeneous group of tumors. Progress in the understanding and treatment of these diseases is likely to be accomplished through continued research into genetic expression patterns. Because of the relative rarity of these tumors, their comprehensive diagnosis and treatment is optimally delivered at specialty centers with a dedicated, multidisciplinary team.

References

1 Siegel, R., Miller, K., Jemal, A. (2017) Cancer treatment and survivor statistics, 2017. *CA: A Cancer Journal for Clinicians*, **67** (1), 7–30.

2 Fletcher, C.D., Hogendoorn, P., Mertens, F., Bridge, J. (2013) WHO Classification of Tumours of Soft Tissue and Bone, 4th edition. IARC Press, Lyon, France.

3 Mohseny, A.B., Hogendoorn, P.C. (2011) Concise review: Mesenchymal tumors: When stem cells go mad. *Stem Cells*, **29** (3), 397–403.

4 Brennan, M.F., Singer, S., Maki, R.G., O'Sullivan, B. (2008) Sarcomas of the soft tissue and bone, in *Cancer: Principles and Practice of Oncology*, 8th edition (eds V.T. DeVita, T.S. Lawrence, S.A. Rosenberg), Lippincott, Philadelphia, pp. 1741–1794.

5 Borden, E.C., Baker, L.H., Bell, R.S., *et al.* (2003) Soft tissue sarcomas of adults: State of the translational science. *Clin. Cancer Res.*, **9** (6), 1941–1956.

6 Helman, L.J., Meltzer, P. (2003) Mechanisms of sarcoma development. *Nat. Rev.*, **3** (9), 685–694.

7 Mitelman, F. (2000) Recurrent chromosome aberrations in cancer. *Mutat. Res.*, **462** (2-3), 247–253.

8 Segal, N.H., Pavlidis, P., Antonescu, C.R., *et al.* (2003) Classification and subtype prediction of adult soft tissue sarcoma by functional genomics. *Am. J. Pathol.*, **163** (2), 691–700.

9 West, R.B. (2010) Expression profiling in soft tissue sarcomas with emphasis on synovial sarcoma, gastrointestinal stromal tumor, and leiomyosarcoma. *Adv. Anat. Pathol.*, **17** (5), 366–373.

10 Barretina, J., Taylor, B.S., Banerji, S., *et al.* (2010) Subtype-specific genomic alterations define new targets for soft-tissue sarcoma therapy. *Nat. Genet.*, **42** (8), 715–721.

11 Taylor, B.S., Barretina, J., Maki, R.G., Antonescu, C.R., Singer, S., Ladanyi, M. (2011) Advances in sarcoma genomics and new therapeutic targets. *Nat. Rev.*, **11** (8), 541–557.

12 Dodd, R.D., Mito, J.K., Kirsch, D.G. (2010) Animal models of soft-tissue sarcoma. *Dis. Models Mech.*, **3** (9-10), 557–566.

13 Blum, J.M., Ano, L., Li, Z., *et al.* (2013) Distinct and overlapping sarcoma subtypes initiated from muscle stem and progenitor cells. *Cell Rep.*, **5** (4), 933–940.

14 Dodd, R.D., Mito, J.K., Eward, W.C., *et al.* (2013) NF1 deletion generates multiple subtypes of soft-tissue sarcoma that respond to MEK inhibition. *Mol. Cancer Ther.*, **12** (9), 1906–1917.

15 Johnson, C.J., Pynsent, P.B., Grimer, R.J. (2001) Clinical features of soft tissue sarcomas. *Ann. R. Coll. Surg. Engl.*, **83** (3), 203–205.

16 Lakkaraju, A., Sinha, R., Garikipati, R., Edward, S., Robinson, P. (2009) Ultrasound for initial evaluation and triage of clinically suspicious soft-tissue masses. *Clin. Radiol.*, **64** (6), 615–621.

17 Benz, M.R., Tchekmedyian, N., Eilber, F.C., Federman, N., Czernin, J., Tap, W.D. (2009) Utilization of positron emission tomography in the management of patients with sarcoma. *Curr. Opin. Oncol.*, **21** (4), 345–351.

18 Roberge, D., Hickeson, M., Charest, M., Turcotte, R.E. (2010) Initial McGill experience with fluorodeoxyglucose PET/CT staging of soft-tissue sarcoma. *Curr. Oncol.*, **17** (6), 18–22.

19 Mankin, H.J., Mankin, C.J., Simon, M.A. (1996) The hazards of the biopsy, revisited. Members of the Musculoskeletal Tumor Society. *J. Bone Joint Surg.*, **78** (5), 656–663.

20 Rougraff, B.T., Aboulafia, A., Biermann, J.S., Healey, J. (2009) Biopsy of soft tissue masses: Evidence-based medicine for the musculoskeletal tumor society. *Clin. Orthopaed. Rel. Res.*, **467** (11), 2783–2791.

21 Heslin, M.J., Lewis, J.J., Woodruff, J.M., Brennan, M.F. (1997) Core needle biopsy for diagnosis of extremity soft tissue sarcoma. *Ann. Surg. Oncol.*, **4** (5), 425–431.

22 Cheng, E.Y. (2005) Surgical management of sarcomas. *Hematol. Oncol. Clin. North Am.*, **19** (3), 451–470.

23 Rosenberg, S.A., Tepper, J., Glatstein, E., *et al.* (1982) The treatment of soft-tissue sarcomas of the extremities: Prospective randomized evaluations of (1) limb-sparing surgery plus radiation therapy compared with amputation and (2) the role of adjuvant chemotherapy. *Ann. Surg.*, **196** (3), 305–315.

24 Yang, J.C., Chang, A.E., Baker, A.R., *et al.* (1998) Randomized prospective study of the benefit of adjuvant radiation therapy in the treatment of soft tissue sarcomas of the extremity. *J. Clin. Oncol.*, **16** (1), 197–203.

25 Brennan, M.F., Hilaris, B., Shiu, M.H., Lane, J., Magill, G., Friedrich, C., Hajdu, S.I. (1987) Local recurrence in adult soft-tissue sarcoma. A randomized trial of brachytherapy. *Arch. Surg.*, **122** (11), 1289–1293.

26 Harrison, L.B., Franzese, F., Gaynor, J.J., Brennan, M.F. (1993) Long-term results of a prospective randomized trial of adjuvant brachytherapy in the management of completely resected soft tissue sarcomas of the extremity and superficial trunk. *Int. J. Radiat. Oncol. Biol. Phys.*, **27** (2), 259–265.

27 Pisters, P.W., Harrison, L.B., Leung, D.H., Woodruff, J.M., Casper, E.S., Brennan, M.F. (1996) Long-term results of a prospective randomized trial of adjuvant brachytherapy in soft tissue sarcoma. *J. Clin. Oncol.*, **14** (3), 859–868.

28 Pisters, P.W., Harrison, L.B., Woodruff, J.M., Gaynor, J.J., Brennan, M.F. (1994) A prospective randomized trial of adjuvant brachytherapy in the management of low-grade soft tissue sarcomas of the extremity and superficial trunk. *J. Clin. Oncol.*, **12** (6), 1150–1155.

29 Rydholm, A., Gustafson, P., Rooser, B., *et al.* (1991) Limb-sparing surgery without radiotherapy based on anatomic location of soft tissue sarcoma. *J. Clin. Oncol.*, **9** (10), 1757–1765.

30 Baldini, E.H., Goldberg, J., Jenner, C., Manola, J.B., Demetri, G.D., Fletcher, C.D., Singer, S (1999) Long-term outcomes after function-sparing surgery without radiotherapy for soft tissue sarcoma of the extremities and trunk. *J. Clin. Oncol.*, **17** (10), 3252–325.

31 Alektiar, K.M., Leung, D., Zelefsky, M.J., Brennan, M.F. (2002) Adjuvant radiation for stage II-b soft tissue sarcoma of the extremity. *J. Clin. Oncol.*, **20** (6), 1643–1650.

32 Pisters, P.W., Pollock, R.E., Lewis, V.O., *et al.* (2007) Long-term results of prospective trial of surgery alone with selective use of radiation for patients with T1 extremity and trunk soft tissue sarcomas. *Ann. Surg.*, **246** (4), 675–681.

33 Fabrizio, P.L., Stafford, S.L., Pritchard, D.J. (2000) Extremity soft-tissue sarcomas selectively treated with surgery alone. *Int. J. Radiat. Oncol. Biol. Phys.*, **48** (1), 227–232.

34 Cahlon, O., Brennan, M.F., Jia, X., Qin, L.X., Singer, S., Alektiar, K.M. (2012) A postoperative nomogram for local recurrence risk in extremity soft tissue sarcomas after limb-sparing surgery without adjuvant radiation. *Ann. Surg.*, **255** (2), 343–347.

35 Goodlad, J.R., Fletcher, C.D., Smith, M.A. (1996) Surgical resection of primary soft-tissue sarcoma. Incidence of residual tumour in 95 patients needing re-excision after local resection. *J. Bone Joint Surg.*, **78** (4), 658–661.

36 Noria, S., Davis, A., Kandel, R., Levesque, J., O'Sullivan, B., Wunder, J., Bell, R. (1996) Residual disease following unplanned excision of soft-tissue sarcoma of an extremity. *J. Bone Joint Surg.*, **78** (5), 650–655.

37 Cahlon, O., Spierer, M., Brennan, M.F., Singer, S., Alektiar, K.M. (2008) Long-term outcomes in extremity soft tissue sarcoma after a pathologically negative re-resection and without radiotherapy. *Cancer*, **112** (12), 2774–2779.

38 McNeer, G.P., Cantin, J., Chu, F., Nickson, J.J. (1968) Effectiveness of radiation therapy in the management of sarcoma of the soft somatic tissues. *Cancer*, **22** (2), 391–397.

39 Suit, H.D., Mankin, H.J., Wood, W.C., Proppe, K.H. (1985) Preoperative, intraoperative, and postoperative radiation in the treatment of primary soft tissue sarcoma. *Cancer*, **55** (11), 2659–2667.

40 O'Sullivan, B., Davis, A.M., Turcotte, R., *et al.* (2002) Preoperative versus postoperative radiotherapy in soft-tissue sarcoma of the limbs: A randomised trial. *Lancet*, **359** (9325), 2235–2241.

41 Sarcoma Meta-Analysis Collaboration (1997) Adjuvant chemotherapy for localised resectable soft-tissue sarcoma of adults: Meta-analysis of individual data. *Lancet*, **350** (9092), 1647–1654.

42 Pervaiz, N., Colterjohn, N., Farrokhyar, F., Tozer, R., Figueredo, A., Ghert, M. (2008) A systematic meta-analysis of randomized controlled trials of adjuvant chemotherapy for localized resectable soft-tissue sarcoma. *Cancer*, **113** (3), 573–581.

43 Eilber, F.R., Morton, D.L., Eckardt, J., Grant, T., Weisenburger, T. (1984) Limb salvage for skeletal and soft tissue sarcomas. Multidisciplinary preoperative therapy. *Cancer*, **53** (12), 2579–2584.

44 Pisters, P.W., Ballo, M., Bekele, N., *et al.* (2004) Phase I trial using toxicity severity weights for dose finding of gemcitabine combined with radiation therapy and subsequent surgery for patients with extremity and trunk soft tissue sarcomas. *J. Clin. Oncol.*, **22** (14s), 9008.

45 Cormier, J.N., Patel, S.R., Herzog, C.E., *et al.* (2001) Concurrent ifosfamide-based chemotherapy and irradiation. Analysis of treatment-related toxicity in 43 patients with sarcoma. *Cancer*, **92** (6), 1550–1555.

46 DeLaney, T.F., Spiro, I.J., Suit, H.D., *et al.* (2003) Neoadjuvant chemotherapy and radiotherapy for large extremity soft-tissue sarcomas. *Int. J. Radiat. Oncol. Biol. Phys.*, **56** (4), 1117–1127.

47 Kraybill, W.G., Harris, J., Spiro, I.J., *et al.* (2006) Phase II study of neoadjuvant chemotherapy and radiation therapy in the management of high-risk, high-grade, soft tissue sarcomas of the extremities and body wall: Radiation Therapy Oncology Group trial 9514. *J. Clin. Oncol.*, **24** (4), 619–625.

48 Edmonson, J.H., Petersen, I.A., Shives, T.C., *et al.* (2002) Chemotherapy, irradiation, and surgery for function-preserving therapy of primary extremity soft tissue sarcomas: Initial treatment with ifosfamide, mitomycin, doxorubicin, and cisplatin plus granulocyte macrophage-colony-stimulating factor. *Cancer*, **94** (3), 786–792.

49 Soulen, M.C., Weissmann, J.R., Sullivan, K.L., *et al.* (1992) Intraarterial chemotherapy with limb-sparing resection of large soft-tissue sarcomas of the extremities. *J. Vasc. Interv. Radiol.*, **3** (4), 659–663.

50 Wanebo, H.J., Temple, W.J., Popp, M.B., Constable, W., Aron, B., Cunningham, S.L. (1995) Preoperative regional therapy for extremity sarcoma. A tricenter update. *Cancer*, **75** (9), 2299–2306.

51 Levine, E.A., Trippon, M., Das Gupta, T.K. (1993) Preoperative multimodality treatment for soft tissue sarcomas. *Cancer*, **71** (11), 3685–3689.

52 Rossi, C.R., Vecchiato, A., Foletto, M., *et al.* (1994) Phase II study on neoadjuvant hyperthermic-antiblastic perfusion with doxorubicin in patients with intermediate or high grade limb sarcomas. *Cancer*, **73** (8), 2140–2146.

53 Pisters, P.W., Ballo, M.T., Patel, S.R. (2002) Preoperative chemoradiation treatment strategies for localized sarcoma. *Ann. Surg. Oncol.*, **9** (6), 535–542.

54 Curtis, K.K., Ashman, J.B., Beauchamp, C.P., *et al.* (2011) Neoadjuvant chemoradiation compared to neoadjuvant radiation alone and surgery alone for stage II and III soft tissue sarcoma of the extremities. *Radiat. Oncol.*, **6**, 91.

55 Bedi, M., King, D.M., Shivakoti, M., *et al.* (2013) Prognostic variables in patients with primary soft tissue sarcoma of the extremity and trunk treated with neoadjuvant radiotherapy or neoadjuvant sequential chemoradiotherapy. *Radiat. Oncol.*, **8**, 60–66.

56 Look Hong, N.J., Hornicek, F.J., Harmon, D.C., *et al.* (2013) Neoadjuvant chemoradiotherapy for patients with high risk extremity and truncal sarcomas; a 10-year single institution retrospective study. *Eur. J. Cancer*, **49**, 875–883.

57 Raval, R.R., Frassica, D., Thornton, K., *et al.* (2014) Evaluating the role of interdigitated neoadjuvant chemotherapy and radiation in the management of high-grade soft-tissue sarcoma: the Johns Hopkins experience. *Am. J. Clin. Oncol.* E-pub ahead of print.

58 Weitz, J., Antonescu, C.R., Brennan, M.F. (2003) Localized extremity soft tissue sarcoma: Improved knowledge with unchanged survival over time. *J. Clin. Oncol.*, **21** (14), 2719–2725.

59 Pisters, P.W., Leung, D.H., Woodruff, J., Shi, W., Brennan, M.F. (1996) Analysis of prognostic factors in 1,041 patients with localized soft tissue sarcomas of the extremities. *J. Clin. Oncol.*, **14** (5), 1679–1689.

60 Singer, S., Corson, J.M., Gonin, R., Labow, B., Eberlein, T.J. (1994) Prognostic factors predictive of survival and local recurrence for extremity soft tissue sarcoma. *Ann. Surg.*, **219** (2), 165–173.

61 Zagars, G.K., Ballo, M.T., Pisters, P.W., Pollock, R.E., Patel, S.R., Benjamin, R.S., Evans, H.L. (2003) Prognostic factors for patients with localized soft-tissue sarcoma treated with conservation surgery and radiation therapy: An analysis of 1225 patients. *Cancer*, **97** (10), 2530–2543.

62 Coindre, J.M., Terrier, P., Guillou, L., *et al.* (2001) Predictive value of grade for metastasis development in the main histologic types of adult soft tissue sarcomas: A study of 1240 patients from the French Federation of Cancer Centers Sarcoma Group. *Cancer*, **91** (10), 1914–1926.

63 Biau, D.J., Ferguson, P.C., Turcotte, R.E., *et al.* (2011) Adverse effect of older age on the recurrence of soft tissue sarcoma of the extremities and trunk. *J. Clin. Oncol.*, **29** (30), 4029–4035.

64 Billingsley, K.G., Lewis, J.J., Leung, D.H., Casper, E.S., Woodruff, J.M., Brennan, M.F. (1999) Multifactorial analysis of the survival of patients with distant metastasis arising from primary extremity sarcoma. *Cancer*, **85** (2), 389–395.

65 Billingsley, K.G., Burt, M.E., Jara, E., Ginsberg, R.J., Woodruff, J.M., Leung, D.H., Brennan, M.F. (1999) Pulmonary metastases from soft tissue sarcoma: Analysis of patterns of diseases and postmetastasis survival. *Ann. Surg.*, **229** (5), 602–610; discussion 602–612.

66 Dhakal, S., Corbin, K.S., Milano, M.T., Phillip, A., Sahasrabudhe, D., Jones, C., Constine, L.S. (2012) Sterotactic body radiotherapy for pulmonary metastases from soft-tissue sarcomas: excellent local lesion control and improved patient survival. *Int. J. Radiat. Oncol. Biol. Phys.*, **82** (2), 940–945.

67 Kattan, M.W., Leung, D.H., Brennan, M.F. (2002) Postoperative nomogram for 12-year sarcoma-specific death. *J. Clin. Oncol.*, **20** (3), 791–796.

68 Eilber, F.C., Brennan, M.F., Eilber, F.R., Dry, S.M., Singer, S., Kattan, M.W. (2004) Validation of the postoperative nomogram for 12-year sarcoma-specific mortality. *Cancer*, **101** (10), 2270–2275.

69 Mariani, L., Miceli, R., Kattan, M.W., *et al.* (2005) Validation and adaptation of a nomogram for predicting the survival of patients with extremity soft tissue sarcoma using a three-grade system. *Cancer*, **103** (2), 402–408.

70 Kattan, M.W., Heller, G., Brennan, M.F. (2003) A competing-risks nomogram for sarcoma-specific death following local recurrence. *Statist. Med.*, **22** (22), 3515–3525.

71 Dalal, K.M., Kattan, M.W., Antonescu, C.R., Brennan, M.F., Singer, S. (2006) Subtype specific prognostic nomogram for patients with primary liposarcoma of the retroperitoneum, extremity, or trunk. *Ann. Surg.*, **244** (3), 381–391.

72 Gustafson, P., Akerman, M., Alvegard, T.A., Coindre, J.M., Fletcher, C.D., Rydholm, A., Willen, H. (2003) Prognostic information in soft tissue sarcoma using tumour size, vascular invasion and microscopic tumour necrosis – the SIN-system. *Eur. J. Cancer*, **39** (11), 1568–1576.

73 Carneiro, A., Bendahl, P.O., Engellau, J., *et al.* (2011) A prognostic model for soft tissue sarcoma of the extremities and trunk wall based on size, vascular invasion, necrosis, and growth pattern. *Cancer*, **117** (6), 1279–1287.

74 Wang, D., Bosch, W., Kirsch, D.G., *et al.* (2011) Variation in the gross tumor volume and clinical target

volume for preoperative radiotherapy of primary large high-grade soft tissue sarcoma of the extremity among RTOG Sarcoma Radiation Oncologists. *Int. J. Radiat. Oncol. Biol. Phys.*, **81** (5), e775–e780.

75 Wang, D., Bosch, W., Roberge, D., *et al.* (2011) RTOG Sarcoma Radiation Oncologists reach consensus on gross tumor volume and clinical target volume on computed tomographic images for preoperative radiotherapy of primary soft tissue sarcoma of extremity in radiation therapy oncology group studies. *Int. J. Radiat. Oncol. Biol. Phys.*, **81** (4), e525–e528.

76 Wang, D., Zhang, Q., Eisenberg, B.L., *et al.* (2015) Significant reduction of late toxicities in patients with extremity sarcoma treated with image-guided radiation therapy to a reduced target volume: results of Radiation Therapy Oncology Group RTOG-0630 trial. *J. Clin. Oncol.*, **33** (20), 2231–2238.

77 Dickie, C.I., Parent, A.L., Chung, P.W., *et al.* (2010) Measuring interfractional and intrafractional motion with cone beam computed tomography and an optical localization system for lower extremity soft tissue sarcoma patients treated with preoperative intensity-modulated radiation therapy. *Int. J. Radiat. Oncol. Biol. Phys.*, **78** (5), 1437–1444.

78 Behranwala, K.A., A'Hern, R., Al-Muderis, O., Thomas, J.M. (2004) Prognosis of lymph node metastasis in soft tissue sarcoma. *Ann. Surg. Oncol.*, **11** (7), 714–719.

79 Mundt, A.J., Awan, A., Sibley, G.S., *et al.* (1995) Conservative surgery and adjuvant radiation therapy in the management of adult soft tissue sarcoma of the extremities: Clinical and radiobiological results. *Int. J. Radiat. Oncol. Biol. Phys.*, **32** (4), 977–985.

80 Alektiar, K.M., Velasco, J., Zelefsky, M.J., Woodruff, J.M., Lewis, J.J., Brennan, M.F. (2000) Adjuvant radiotherapy for margin-positive high-grade soft tissue sarcoma of the extremity. *Int. J. Radiat. Oncol. Biol. Phys.*, **48** (4), 1051–1058.

81 DeLaney, T.F., Kepka, L., Goldberg, S.I., *et al.* (2007) Radiation therapy for control of soft-tissue sarcomas resected with positive margins. *Int. J. Radiat. Oncol. Biol. Phys.*, **67** (5), 1460–1469.

82 Zagars, G.K., Ballo, M.T. (2003) Significance of dose in postoperative radiotherapy for soft tissue sarcoma. *Int. J. Radiat. Oncol. Biol. Phys.*, **56** (2), 473–481.

83 Devisetty, K., Kobayashi, W., Suit, H.D., *et al.* (2011) Low-dose neoadjuvant external beam radiation therapy for soft tissue sarcoma. *Int. J. Radiat. Oncol. Biol. Phys.*, **80** (3), 779–786.

84 Al Yami, A., Griffin, A.M., Ferguson, P.C., *et al.* (2010) Positive surgical margins in soft tissue sarcoma treated with preoperative radiation: Is a postoperative boost necessary? *Int. J. Radiat. Oncol. Biol. Phys.*, **77** (4), 1191–1197.

85 Pan, E., Goldberg, S.I., Chen, Y.-L., *et al.* (2014) Role of post-operative radiation boost for soft tissue sarcomas with positive margins following pre-operative radiation and surgery. *J. Surg. Oncol.*, **110**, 817–822.

86 Alektiar, K.M., Leung, D., Zelefsky, M.J., Healey, J.H., Brennan, M.F. (2002) Adjuvant brachytherapy for primary high-grade soft tissue sarcoma of the extremity. *Ann. Surg. Oncol.*, **9** (1), 48–56.

87 Schray, M.F., Gunderson, L.L., Sim, F.H., Pritchard, D.J., Shives, T.C., Yeakel, P.D. (1990) Soft tissue sarcoma. Integration of brachytherapy, resection, and external irradiation. *Cancer*, **66** (3), 451–456.

88 Ormsby, M.V., Hilaris, B.S., Nori, D., Brennan, M.F. (1989) Wound complications of adjuvant radiation therapy in patients with soft-tissue sarcomas. *Ann. Surg.*, **210** (1), 93–99.

89 Pohar, S., Haq, R., Liu, L., Koniarczyk, M., Hahn, S., Damron, T., Aronowitz, J.N. (2007) Adjuvant high-dose-rate and low-dose-rate brachytherapy with external beam radiation in soft tissue sarcoma: A comparison of outcomes. *Brachytherapy*, **6** (1), 53–57.

90 Martinez-Monge, R., San Julian, M., Amillo, S., *et al.* (2005) Perioperative high-dose-rate brachytherapy in soft tissue sarcomas of the extremity and superficial trunk in adults: Initial results of a pilot study. *Brachytherapy*, **4** (4), 264–270.

91 Holloway, C.L., Delaney, T.F., Alektiar, K.M., Devlin, P.M., O'Farrell, D.A., Demanes, D.J. (2013) American Brachytherapy Society (ABS) consensus statement for sarcoma brachytherapy. *Brachytherapy*, **12** (3), 179–190.

92 Kretzler, A., Molls, M., Gradinger, R., Lukas, P., Steinau, H.U., Wurschmidt, F. (2004) Intraoperative radiotherapy of soft tissue sarcoma of the extremity. *Strahlenther. Onkol.*, **180** (6), 365–370.

93 Azinovic, I., Martinez Monge, R., Javier Aristu, J., *et al.* (2003) Intraoperative radiotherapy electron boost followed by moderate doses of external beam radiotherapy in resected soft-tissue sarcoma of the extremities. *Radiother. Oncol.*, **67** (3), 331–337.

94 Niewald, M., Fleckenstein, J., Licht, N., Bleuzen, C., Ruebe, C. (2009) Intraoperative radiotherapy (IORT) combined with external beam radiotherapy (EBRT) for soft-tissue sarcomas – a retrospective evaluation of the homburg experience in the years 1995–2007. *Radiat. Oncol.*, **4**, 32.

95 Tran, Q.N., Kim, A.C., Gottschalk, A.R., *et al.* (2006) Clinical outcomes of intraoperative radiation therapy for extremity sarcomas. *Sarcoma*, **2006** (1), 91671.

96 Haddock, M.G., Petersen, I.A., Pritchard, D., Gunderson, L.L. (1997) IORT in the management of extremity and limb girdle soft tissue sarcomas. *Front. Radiat. Ther. Oncol.*, **31**, 151–152.

97 Goodman, K.A., Wolden, S.L., LaQuaglia, M.P., Alektiar, K., D'Souza, D., Zelefsky, M.J. (2003)

Intraoperative high-dose-rate brachytherapy for pediatric solid tumors: A 10-year experience. *Brachytherapy*, **2** (3), 139–146.

98 Nag, S., Hu, K.S. (2003) Intraoperative high-dose-rate brachytherapy. *Surg. Oncol. Clin. North Am.*, **12** (4), 1079–1097.

99 Hong, L., Alektiar, K.M., Hunt, M., Venkatraman, E., Leibel, S.A. (2004) Intensity-modulated radiotherapy for soft tissue sarcoma of the thigh. *Int. J. Radiat. Oncol. Biol. Phys.*, **59** (3), 752–759.

100 Stewart, A.J., Lee, Y.K., Saran, F.H. (2009) Comparison of conventional radiotherapy and intensity-modulated radiotherapy for post-operative radiotherapy for primary extremity soft tissue sarcoma. *Radiother. Oncol.*, **93** (1), 125–130.

101 Alektiar, K.M., Hong, L., Brennan, M.F., Della-Biancia, C., Singer, S. (2007) Intensity modulated radiation therapy for primary soft tissue sarcoma of the extremity: Preliminary results. *Int. J. Radiat. Oncol. Biol. Phys.*, **68** (2), 458–464.

102 Alektiar, K.M., Brennan, M.F., Healey, J.H., Singer, S. (2008) Impact of intensity-modulated radiation therapy on local control in primary soft-tissue sarcoma of the extremity. *J. Clin. Oncol.*, **26** (20), 3440–3444.

103 Alektiar, K.M., Brennan, M.F., Singer, S. (2011) Local control comparison of adjuvant brachytherapy to intensity-modulated radiotherapy in primary high-grade sarcoma of the extremity. *Cancer*, **117** (14), 3229–3234.

104 Folkert, M.R., Singer, S., Brennan, M.F., *et al.* (2014) Comparison of local recurrence with conventional and intensity-modulated radiation therapy for primary soft-tissue sarcomas of the extremity. *J. Clin. Oncol.*, **32** (29), 3236–3241.

105 O'Sullivan, B., Griffin, A.M., Dickie, C.I., *et al.* (2013) Phase 2 study of preoperative image-guided intensity-modulated radiation therapy to reduce wound and combined modality morbidities in lower extremity soft tissue sarcoma. *Cancer*, **119** (10), 1878–1884.

106 Alektiar, K.M., Brennan, M.F., Singer, S. (2005) Influence of site on the therapeutic ratio of adjuvant radiotherapy in soft-tissue sarcoma of the extremity. *Int. J. Radiat. Oncol. Biol. Phys.*, **63** (1), 202–208.

107 Davidge, K.M., Wunder, J., Tomlinson, G., Wong, R., Lipa, J., Davis, A.M. (2010) Function and health status outcomes following soft tissue reconstruction for limb preservation in extremity soft tissue sarcoma. *Ann. Surg. Oncol.*, **17** (4), 1052–1062.

108 Spierer, M.M., Alektiar, K.M., Zelefsky, M.J., Brennan, M.F., Cordiero, P.G. (2003) Tolerance of tissue transfers to adjuvant radiation therapy in primary soft tissue sarcoma of the extremity. *Int. J. Radiat. Oncol. Biol. Phys.*, **56** (4), 1112–1116.

109 Griffin, A.M., Euler, C.I., Sharpe, M.B., *et al.* (2007) Radiation planning comparison for superficial tissue avoidance in radiotherapy for soft tissue sarcoma of the lower extremity. *Int. J. Radiat. Oncol. Biol. Phys.*, **67** (3), 847–856.

110 Davis, A.M., Wright, J.G., Williams, J.I., Bombardier, C., Griffin, A., Bell, R.S. (1996) Development of a measure of physical function for patients with bone and soft tissue sarcoma. *Qual. Life Res.*, **5** (5), 508–516.

111 Enneking, W.F., Dunham, W., Gebhardt, M.C., Malawar, M., Pritchard, D.J. (1993) A system for the functional evaluation of reconstructive procedures after surgical treatment of tumors of the musculoskeletal system. *Clin. Orthopaed. Relat. Res.*, (286), 241–246.

112 Davis, A.M., Sennik, S., Griffin, A.M., Wunder, J.S., O'Sullivan, B., Catton, C.N., Bell, R.S. (2000) Predictors of functional outcomes following limb salvage surgery for lower-extremity soft tissue sarcoma. *J. Surg. Oncol.*, **73** (4), 206–211.

113 Davis, A.M., O'Sullivan, B., Bell, R.S., *et al.* (2002) Function and health status outcomes in a randomized trial comparing preoperative and postoperative radiotherapy in extremity soft tissue sarcoma. *J. Clin. Oncol.*, **20** (22), 4472–4477.

114 Davis, A.M., O'Sullivan, B., Turcotte, R., *et al.* (2005) Late radiation morbidity following randomization to preoperative versus postoperative radiotherapy in extremity soft tissue sarcoma. *Radiother. Oncol.*, **75** (1), 48–53.

115 Holt, G.E., Griffin, A.M., Pintilie, M., Wunder, J.S., Catton, C., O'Sullivan, B., Bell, R.S. (2005) Fractures following radiotherapy and limb-salvage surgery for lower extremity soft-tissue sarcomas. A comparison of high-dose and low-dose radiotherapy. *J. Bone Joint Surg.*, **87** (2), 315–319.

116 Gortzak, Y., Lockwood, G.A., Mahendra, A., *et al.* (2010) Prediction of pathologic fracture risk of the femur after combined modality treatment of soft tissue sarcoma of the thigh. *Cancer*, **116** (6), 1553–1559.

117 Dickie, C.I., Parent, A.L., Griffin, A.M., *et al.* (2009) Bone fractures following external beam radiotherapy and limb-preservation surgery for lower extremity soft tissue sarcoma: Relationship to irradiated bone length, volume, tumor location and dose. *Int. J. Radiat. Oncol. Biol. Phys.*, **75** (4), 1119–1124.

118 Bartlett, E., Yoon, S.S. (2011) Current treatment for the local control of retroperitoneal sarcomas. *J. Am. Coll. Surg.*, **213** (3), 436–446.

119 Heslin, M.J., Lewis, J.J., Nadler, E., *et al.* (1997) Prognostic factors associated with long-term survival for retroperitoneal sarcoma: Implications for management. *J. Clin. Oncol.*, **15** (8), 2832–2839.

120 Bonvalot, S., Miceli, R., Berselli, M., *et al.* (2010) Aggressive surgery in retroperitoneal soft tissue sarcoma carried out at high-volume centers is safe and is associated with improved local control. *Ann. Surg. Oncol.*, **17** (6), 1507–1514.

121 Bonvalot, S., Rivoire, M., Castaing, M., Stoeckle, E., Le Cesne, A., Blay, J.Y., Laplanche, A. (2009) Primary retroperitoneal sarcomas: A multivariate analysis of surgical factors associated with local control. *J. Clin. Oncol.*, **27** (1), 31–37.

122 Ardoino, I., Miceli, R., Berselli, M., *et al.* (2010) Histology-specific nomogram for primary retroperitoneal soft tissue sarcoma. *Cancer*, **116** (10), 2429–2436.

123 Tseng, W.H., Martinez, S.R., Do, L., Tamurian, R.M., Borys, D., Canter, R.J. (2011) Lack of survival benefit following adjuvant radiation in patients with retroperitoneal sarcoma: A SEER analysis. *J. Surg. Res.*, **168** (2), e173–e180.

124 Ballo, M.T., Zagars, G.K., Pollock, R.E., *et al.* (2007) Retroperitoneal soft tissue sarcoma: An analysis of radiation and surgical treatment. *Int. J. Radiat. Oncol. Biol. Phys.*, **67** (1), 158–163.

125 Sindelar, W.F., Kinsella, T.J., Chen, P.W., *et al.* (1993) Intraoperative radiotherapy in retroperitoneal sarcomas. Final results of a prospective, randomized, clinical trial. *Arch. Surg.*, **128** (4), 402–410.

126 Petersen, I.A., Haddock, M.G., Donohue, J.H., *et al.* (2002) Use of intraoperative electron beam radiotherapy in the management of retroperitoneal soft tissue sarcomas. *Int. J. Radiat. Oncol. Biol. Phys.*, **52** (2), 469–475.

127 Krempien, R., Roeder, F., Oertel, S., *et al.* (2006) Intraoperative electron-beam therapy for primary and recurrent retroperitoneal soft-tissue sarcoma. *Int. J. Radiat. Oncol. Biol. Phys.*, **65** (3), 773–779.

128 Dziewirski, W., Rutkowski, P., Nowecki, Z.I., *et al.* (2006) Surgery combined with intraoperative brachytherapy in the treatment of retroperitoneal sarcomas. *Ann. Surg. Oncol.*, **13** (2), 245–252.

129 Willett, C.G., Suit, H.D., Tepper, J.E., Mankin, H.J., Convery, K., Rosenberg, A.L., Wood, W.C. (1991) Intraoperative electron beam radiation therapy for retroperitoneal soft tissue sarcoma. *Cancer*, **68** (2), 278–283.

130 Alektiar, K.M., Hu, K., Anderson, L., Brennan, M.F., Harrison, L.B. (2000) High-dose-rate intraoperative radiation therapy (HDR-IORT) for retroperitoneal sarcomas. *Int. J. Radiat. Oncol. Biol. Phys.*, **47** (1), 157–163.

131 Pierie, J.P., Betensky, R.A., Choudry, U., Willett, C.G., Souba, W.W., Ott, M.J. (2006) Outcomes in a series of 103 retroperitoneal sarcomas. *Eur. J. Surg. Oncol.*, **32** (10), 1235–1241.

132 Gieschen, H.L., Spiro, I.J., Suit, H.D., Ott, M.J., Rattner, D.W., Ancukiewicz, M., Willett, C.G. (2001) Long-term results of intraoperative electron beam radiotherapy for primary and recurrent retroperitoneal soft tissue sarcoma. *Int. J. Radiat. Oncol. Biol. Phys.*, **50** (1), 127–131.

133 Pawlik, T.M., Pisters, P.W., Mikula, L., *et al.* (2006) Long-term results of two prospective trials of preoperative external beam radiotherapy for localized intermediate- or high-grade retroperitoneal soft tissue sarcoma. *Ann. Surg. Oncol.*, **13** (4), 508–517.

134 Roeder, F., Ulrich, A., Habl, G., *et al.* (2014) Clinical phase I/II trial to investigate pre-operative dose-escalated intensity-modulated radiation therapy (IMRT) and intraoperative radiation therapy (IORT) in patients with retroperitoneal soft tissue sarcoma: interim analysis. *BMC Cancer*, **14**, 617.

135 Koshy, M., Landry, J.C., Lawson, J.D., *et al.* (2003) Intensity modulated radiation therapy for retroperitoneal sarcoma: A case for dose escalation and organ at risk toxicity reduction. *Sarcoma*, **7** (3-4), 137–148.

136 Tzeng, C.W., Fiveash, J.B., Popple, R.A., *et al.* (2006) Preoperative radiation therapy with selective dose escalation to the margin at risk for retroperitoneal sarcoma. *Cancer*, **107** (2), 371–379.

137 Yoon, S.S., Chen, Y.L., Kirsch, D.G., *et al.* (2010) Proton-beam, intensity-modulated, and/or intraoperative electron radiation therapy combined with aggressive anterior surgical resection for retroperitoneal sarcomas. *Ann. Surg. Oncol.*, **17** (6), 1515–1529.

138 Lev, D., Kotilingam, D., Wei, C., *et al.* (2007) Optimizing treatment of desmoid tumors. *J. Clin. Oncol.*, **25** (13), 1785–1791.

139 Nuyttens, J.J., Rust, P.F., Thomas, C.R., Jr, Turrisi, A.T., 3rd (2000) Surgery versus radiation therapy for patients with aggressive fibromatosis or desmoid tumors: A comparative review of 22 articles. *Cancer*, **88** (7), 1517–1523.

140 Gluck, I., Griffith, K.A., Biermann, J.S., Feng, F.Y., Lucas, D.R., Ben-Josef, E. (2011) Role of radiotherapy in the management of desmoid tumors. *Int. J. Radiat. Oncol. Biol. Phys.*, **80** (3), 787–792.

141 Guadagnolo, B.A., Zagars, G.K., Ballo, M.T. (2008) Long-term outcomes for desmoid tumors treated with radiation therapy. *Int. J. Radiat. Oncol. Biol. Phys.*, **71** (2), 441–447.

142 Salas, S., Dufresne, A., Bui, B., *et al.* (2011) Prognostic factors influencing progression-free survival determined from a series of sporadic desmoid tumors: A wait-and-see policy according to tumor presentation. *J. Clin. Oncol.*, **29** (26), 3553–3558.

143 Ritter, J., Bielack, S.S. (2010) Osteosarcoma. *Ann. Oncol.*, **21** (Suppl. 7), 320–325.

144 Machak, G.N., Tkachev, S.I., Solovyev, Y.N., *et al.* (2003) Neoadjuvant chemotherapy and local radiotherapy for high-grade osteosarcoma of the extremities. *Mayo Clin. Proc.*, **78** (2), 147–155.

145 Ozaki, T., Flege, S., Kevric, M., *et al.* (2003) Osteosarcoma of the pelvis: Experience of the cooperative osteosarcoma study group. *J. Clin. Oncol.*, **21** (2), 334–341.

146 DeLaney, T.F., Park, L., Goldberg, S.I., Hug, E.B., Liebsch, N.J., Munzenrider, J.E., Suit, H.D. (2005) Radiotherapy for local control of osteosarcoma. *Int. J. Radiat. Oncol. Biol. Phys.*, **61** (2), 492–498.

147 Hundsdoerfer, P., Albrecht, M., Ruhl, U., Fengler, R., Kulozik, A.E., Henze, G. (2009) Long-term outcome after polychemotherapy and intensive local radiation therapy of high-grade osteosarcoma. *Eur. J. Cancer*, **45** (14), 2447–2451.

148 Ciernik, I.F., Niemierko, A., Harmon, D.C., *et al.* (2011) Proton-based radiotherapy for unresectable or incompletely resected osteosarcoma. *Cancer*, **117** (19), 4522–4530.

39

Tumors of the Central Nervous System

Phillip J. Gray, Jay S. Loeffler and Helen A. Shih

Epidemiology

Individual central nervous system (CNS) tumor types are relatively uncommon with the exception of disease metastatic from other sites. In 2017 it is estimated that, in the United States, a combined 23 800 primary CNS tumors will be diagnosed, resulting in 16 700 deaths [1]. In general, however, the epidemiology, incidence and prevalence of individual CNS tumors are poorly understood. The reasons for this are multifactorial but include an under-reporting of metastatic brain disease and poor recording of 'benign' entities such as meningioma, pituitary adenoma and low-grade gliomas before the year 2000. Data from the Surveillance Epidemiology and End Results (SEER) database shows an incidence rate for invasive CNS tumors of 7.7 per 100 000 in men and 5.4 per 100 000 in women. CNS tumors are more common in whites than in blacks (incidence in men 8.4 per 100 000 versus 4.7 per 100,000 and 6 per 100 000 versus 3.7 per 100 000 in women).

Approximately 13% of cases occur in the pediatric population (under age 20 years) with incidence highest in the fourth and fifth decades of life with a median age at diagnosis of 57 years. The age-adjusted death rate from CNS tumors has remained steady during the period between 1975 and 2010 at around 4–5 per 100 000 for all races and sexes [2].

Although these differences in age, sex and ethnic distribution of primary brain tumors suggest that some types have distinct causes, many of these causes remain unidentified. There are several genetic syndromes known to carry an increased risk of developing a benign or malignant brain tumor. One of the best studied of these is neurofibromatosis type-1 (NF-1), an autosomal dominant disorder resulting from defective production of the protein neurofibromin coded on chromosome 17. Patients with NF-1 have a very high incidence of intracranial and extracranial Schwann cell tumors, and 15% will also go on to develop low-grade optic pathway gliomas, cerebellar astrocytomas, pilocytic astrocytomas of the third ventricle or high-grade gliomas [3]. Neurofibromatosis type-2 (NF-2) is a much less common disorder which typically manifests with vestibular schwannomas (often and pathognomonic when bilateral), spinal cord ependymomas, meningiomas and schwannomas of other cranial nerves. Other hereditary syndromes include Li–Fraumeni syndrome, an autosomal dominant syndrome resulting from a germline mutation in p53. While more commonly associated with osteosarcoma and breast cancer, an increase in gliomas is also seen in this population. Turcot syndrome is an inherited syndrome characterized by multiple adenomatous colon polyps that is also associated with astrocytomas and medulloblastoma, while Gorlin's syndrome (nevoid basal cell carcinoma syndrome) is associated with an increased risk of medulloblastoma and meningioma [4, 5]. Retinoblastoma and paraganglioma can also arise from inherited genetic defects.

Environmental factors associated with the development of benign and malignant CNS tumors have been extensively studied. Several chemical agents have been implicated in the development of such tumors, though evidence remains weak [6]. Ionizing radiation is a well-described induction agent. Cases of glioma, meningioma, schwannoma and sarcoma of the CNS have been reported in patients who underwent alopecia-producing low-dose irradiation (1.5 Gy) to the scalp in childhood for the treatment of tinea capitis [7]. It has been estimated that the risk of second tumor formation following irradiation of the CNS is between 1% and 3% at 20 years

Clinical Radiation Oncology: Indications, Techniques, and Results, Third Edition. Edited by William Small Jr.
© 2017 John Wiley & Sons, Inc. Published 2017 by John Wiley & Sons, Inc.

after therapy [8]. The dose and volume of CNS irradiated are important parameters associated with second tumor formation. Discussion of this risk is vital when imparting information to patients, especially children and young adults about their risks. Moreover, it represents an added incentive to reduce the irradiated volume by using conformal techniques or advanced technology, such as particle therapy. Exposure to electromagnetic fields and CNS trauma are other potential factors which have been studied, but no convincing data have yet been provided to support these as valid risk factors. The use of cellular telephones has become commonplace in the United States and beyond, and there has been some concern that electromagnetic radiation from cellular phone use could increase the risk of CNS tumors. A large Danish cohort study showed no increased risk over 3.8 million person–years, and these data are supported by other recent studies [9–11].

Diagnosis

Neuroimaging

The diagnosis of intracranial and spinal tumors requires sophisticated neuroimaging. Computed tomography (CT) and magnetic resonance imaging (MRI) are routine diagnostic tests used for patients suspected of harboring a brain tumor. Angiography is rarely used in modern imaging but may still play a role for large vascular benign tumors such as paragangliomas and arteriovenous malformations as part of surgical planning or preoperative embolization. CT is superior to MRI in detecting calcifications in tumors such as oligodendrogliomas, meningiomas and craniopharyngiomas, and is also more useful for detecting bony abnormalities of the calvarium or vertebral column. It is, however, less ideal for the analysis of soft tissues and is limited by artifacts caused by high-Z materials such as dental prostheses. As such, MRI is the technique of choice for the imaging of CNS tumors. The most useful MRI sequences include T1- and T2-weighted images. T2-weighted fluid attenuated inversion recovery (FLAIR) images are the most useful for full visualization of tumor-associated edema. T1-weighted imaging with gadolinium contrast provides the single most useful sequence for many tumors, particularly extra-axial processes such as schwannomas and meningiomas. A combination of all of the above sequences in axial, sagittal and coronal planes is often sufficient for determining a particular tumor's type, grade, and extent. Assuming that a patient has sufficient renal function to allow their use, both CT and MRI contrast agents greatly aid in this process. Essentially all glioblastomas, meningiomas, schwannomas, ependymomas, lymphomas, medulloblastomas, germinomas and craniopharyngiomas exhibit brisk but often heterogeneous enhancement. The majority of low-grade gliomas and approximately 50% of anaplastic gliomas will not exhibit contrast enhancement.

In the evaluation of intramedullary and extramedullary spinal cord lesions, MRI is the diagnostic study of choice. Full spinal imaging is also particularly important in the evaluation of CNS tumors with a high propensity to spread throughout the neuraxis such as medulloblastoma, or whenever there is clinical concern for multifocal disease such as in the case of leptomeningeal carcinomatosis. Spinal MRI imaging has largely supplanted CT myelography except in the case of patients unable to tolerate MRI or those with absolute contraindications such as implanted pacemakers or other ferromagnetic foreign objects. MRI is vital in radiotherapy treatment planning because of the ability to delineate the extent of tumor-associated edema or to visualize particularly small targets. CT-MRI fusion should be routinely employed as part of stereotactic, intensity-modulated radiotherapy (IMRT), proton, or other highly conformal radiotherapy planning. Following high-dose radiotherapy treatment, routine MRI or CT imaging are often inadequate in differentiating tumor recurrence from radiation injury. Functional MRI, MR spectroscopy and positron-emission tomography (PET) imaging are sometimes used to aid in this differentiation but are still considered investigational [12–14].

Surgery

It is impossible to discuss neuro-oncology without at least a brief discussion of the role of surgery. Surgery remains the most important initial therapy for most patients with brain tumors amenable to resection. Advances in image-guided surgery have made operative approaches in even the most remote areas of the CNS possible and reasonably safe. Functional mapping during surgery, stereotactic navigation systems and intraoperative MRI-guided surgery have become commonplace in large hospital centers throughout the United States. The goal of any brain tumor surgery is to obtain a complete curative resection of the tumor without the need for adjuvant therapy. This is possible for many tumor types such as convexity meningiomas, pituitary microadenomas, pilocytic astrocytomas, central neurocytomas and gangliogliomas. If surgical cure is not possible (such as for malignant gliomas) tumor debulking and reduction of mass effect allows for adjuvant therapy to be provided and is often associated with improved outcomes [15]. Another benefit of surgical resection is to provide enough tissue for accurate histopathologic analysis. This has become even more important in recent years with the emergence of predictive and prognostic biomarkers for many diseases.

Approach to Management of CNS Tumors

The remainder of this chapter will focus on the management of individual adult CNS malignancies. It is impossible in the space allotted to review all possible topics, and so this chapter will focus on the most common diseases seen in consultation by radiation oncologists. A discussion of tumor types more commonly seen in the pediatric population (such as medulloblastoma, intracranial ependymoma, pilocytic astrocytoma and germ cell tumors) can be found in the chapter on pediatric tumors.

Low-Grade Glioma

Low-grade or well-differentiated gliomas constitute a heterogeneous group of intracranial and spinal tumors that occur primarily in children and young adults. Around 2000 cases of low-grade glioma are diagnosed per year in the United States [4, 16]. Grading of such neuroglial tumors is based on the World Health Organization (WHO) grading system. Differentiation, pleomorphism, hyperchromasia, degree of cellularity, mitotic index, necrosis and vascular proliferation are all used to determine the particular grade and thus diagnosis of a tumor. Low-grade gliomas are defined as WHO grades I to II/IV.

The present understanding of the clinical behavior of these tumors has increased through recent molecular and genetic analyses. One of the most important factors for prognosis is tumor proliferation rate, which is often measured using Ki-67 staining. A labeling index of below 1% is a very good prognostic factor and is perhaps even a better predictor of survival than clinical grade. Montine *et al.* previously investigated the role of Ki-67 proliferation index and found the median value in 11 tumors to be 2.1%. In their study, this labeling index directly correlated with survival, with 100% of patients with an index under 3% alive at the last follow-up (16–60 months), while only 25% of those over this cut-off were alive (follow-up 0.5 to 117 months) [17]. This cut-off of 3% is used by many centers to direct decisions regarding the timing of adjuvant therapy. Despite this, Ki-67 does not appear to predict which patients will benefit from immediate postoperative radiotherapy [18]. 1p/19q loss and mutations in isocitrate dehydrogenase are also useful prognostic markers for low-grade glioma, and are discussed in more detail below.

Seizure is the most common presenting symptom in patients with low-grade glioma. Patients presenting with seizure and no other neurologic symptoms have a better prognosis than patients presenting with mental status changes or other focal neurologic deficits [19, 20]. The most important prognostic factor in patients with low-grade glioma is age at diagnosis. Several studies have demonstrated older age as a poor prognostic factor, and a cut-off of 40 years of age is often used [21–23]. Other important negative prognostic factors include astrocytic histology, tumor size ≥6 cm, tumors which cross midline, and a persistence of neurologic deficits following resection. These factors can be combined to define low-risk (0–2 factors) and high-risk (3–5 factors) subgroups. In a combined analysis of two randomized trials, in patients using this definition of low-risk disease, the median overall survival was 7.8 years versus 3.7 years for the high-risk group [21].

The role for immediate postoperative radiation therapy is less clear. The European Organization for the Research and Treatment of Cancer (EORTC) 22845 trial is the largest to investigate the role of postoperative radiotherapy in low-grade glioma [24]. This trial included 314 patients aged 16–65 years with supratentorial low-grade astrocytoma, oligoastrocytoma, or oligodendroglioma. Small, completely resected pilocytic astrocytomas, optic nerve gliomas, brainstem gliomas, third ventricle gliomas, and infratentorial gliomas were excluded. All patients underwent maximal debulking surgery at diagnosis. Patients were then randomized to early radiotherapy (54 Gy in 1.8-Gy daily fractions) or radiotherapy at the time of clinical and/or radiographic progression. Patients were followed with contrast-enhanced CT every four months. At a median follow-up of 7.8 years, up-front radiotherapy improved the five-year progression-free survival (PFS) (55% versus 35%, p < 0.0001) but not the five-year overall survival (OS) (68.4% versus 65.7%, p = 0.872). During the study period, 70% of patient tumors transformed to high-grade histology, though this was not affected by the timing of radiotherapy. Radiotherapy did improve seizure control in those who received it up-front, but a full quality of life analysis was not performed and so it is unclear how radiotherapy affected other measures. In general, however, this trial suggests that salvage radiotherapy is just as effective as up-front radiotherapy, and so appropriately-selected patients can be safely observed following tumor resection.

In patients for whom radiotherapy is recommended, the results of two randomized Phase III trials are available to inform the decision of treatment dose. The EORTC 22844 trial was the first to be published on this topic [25]. This trial randomized 379 patients following resection or biopsy alone to receive either 45 Gy in five weeks or 59.4 Gy over six-and-a-half weeks. With a median follow-up of 74 months there was no significant difference in OS between the arms (58% for low-dose and 59% for high-dose). PFS was also similar (47% for low-dose and 50% for high-dose). Tumor size, performance status, extent of surgery and histologic subtype (increasing astrocytic component being worse) were all independent predictors of survival. In a separate quality of life study, those who received high-dose radiotherapy tended to report lower levels of functioning and more symptom burden following completion of radiotherapy [26].

The second trial to address this question was an Intergroup trial conducted by the North Central Cancer Treatment Group (NCCTG), the Radiation Therapy Oncology Group (RTOG) and the Eastern Cooperative Oncology Group (ECOG). This trial included 203 adult patients with low-grade astrocytoma, oligodendroglioma, or mixed oligoastrocytoma [27]. Patients were randomized to receive 50.4 Gy in 28 fractions or 64.8 Gy in 36 fractions. At a median follow-up of 6.4 years, the dose of radiation delivered was not associated with five-year OS (72% for low-dose versus 64% for high-dose, p = 0.48) or time-to-progression. Grade 3–5 radionecrosis was more common in the high-dose arm than in the low-dose arm (5% versus 2.5%). Age, tumor size, and astrocytic histology again correlated with survival. Despite the increased toxicity seen in the trial, cognitive outcomes were similar between the arms [28, 29].

Given these data, the decision of when to proceed with radiotherapy should be made after a careful review of the individual patient's risk factors, clinical status, and following a frank discussion of the risks and potential benefits of therapy. Once the decision is made to proceed with therapy, conformal radiotherapy techniques (including IMRT) are strongly encouraged to reduce the dose to uninvolved brain tissue. Most practitioners favor doses of 50.4–54 Gy in 1.8-Gy daily fractions.

The role of chemotherapy as an initial treatment for patients with low-grade glioma is currently becoming apparent with the maturation of prospective data. RTOG 9802 investigated the role of PCV (procarbazine, lomustine, vincristine) chemotherapy in patients treated with radiotherapy. This trial randomized 251 patients with high-risk disease (defined as age ≥40 years or sub-total resection) to postoperative radiation alone (54 Gy in 30 fractions) or radiotherapy plus six cycles of PCV. The initial publication of results at a median follow-up of 5.9 years demonstrated no difference in five-year OS between the arms (63% for radiotherapy alone versus 72% for radiotherapy + PCV, p = 0.13), but a statistical trend for a PFS benefit for the addition of PCV (five-year PFS 46% versus 63%, p = 0.06). A recent update in abstract form with a median follow-up of 11.9 years demonstrated both a median survival time benefit (13.3 versus 7.8 years, p = 0.03) and PFS benefit (10.4 versus 4.0 years, p = 0.002) [30]. The agent temozolomide (TMZ) has become commonplace in the management of brain tumor patients, has been used for patients with recurrent low-grade gliomas, and is under investigation for its potential role as an up-front treatment integrated for low-grade gliomas. The RTOG 0424 study recently reported results from a single-arm prospective trial of low-grade glioma patients felt to be at high risk for progression based on the eligibility criteria of three or more risk factors of age ≥40 years, astrocytoma histology, bilateral hemispheric involvement, tumor size ≥6 cm preoperatively, or having a preoperative neurological function status >1 [31]. There were 129 evaluable patients treated with concurrent radiation (54 Gy) and concurrent and adjuvant TMZ (adjuvant cycles repeated every four weeks with a maximum of 12 cycles) with a median follow-up of 4.1 years. The three-year OS was 73.1% and three-year PFS 59.2%; both values were comparatively favorable to historical controls, especially considering their perceived higher risk for early disease progression.

Chemotherapy alone as an initial approach for the subset of low-grade oligodendrogliomas has also been investigated [32–34]. Early data from the EORTC 22033-26033 trial has recently been presented in abstract form [35]. This trial randomized 477 patients with progressive low-grade glioma to radiation therapy (50.4 Gy in 28 fractions) or up-front TMZ. While no clear difference in PFS or OS was seen, there was a suggestion of inferior PFS with TMZ in 1p-intact patients while 1p-deleted patients had a trend towards better survival with TMZ. Additional maturation of these data is required before final conclusions can be drawn.

More so today than ever before, the prognostic and predictive value of classifying gliomas by molecular status has taken a central role in the evaluation of patients, including those that have been traditionally classified as low-grade gliomas. Recent assessment of 293 lower-grade glioma genomic mutations or alterations have deduced the combination of the isocitrate dehydrogenase gene (*IDH*), 1p/19q, and *TP53* as being most predictive of the tumor behavior, with the classical indolent progression characteristic of low-grade gliomas most consistently seen with tumors harboring *IDH* mutations [36].

High-Grade Glioma

Common high-grade gliomas include anaplastic astrocytoma (AA), anaplastic oligodendroglioma (AO), anaplastic oligoastrocytoma (AOA) and glioblastoma (GBM). These tumors represent the majority of primary CNS tumors in adults, and occur 10 times more frequently in adults than in children. GBM is estimated to comprise 82% of high-grade gliomas [16]. Surgery is the initial therapy of choice for high-grade glioma. Maximal surgical resection allows for a rapid reduction of mass effect and also allows for adjuvant therapies to be delivered with reduced acute side effects and need for escalating doses of corticosteroids to counteract brain edema. More extensive surgical resection has been shown to improve outcomes in several retrospective analyses [15, 37, 38]. If resection cannot be safely performed due to tumor location or comorbid illness, a biopsy is still required in order to provide an accurate diagnosis, except in circumstances where the tumor is limited to an area where biopsy would almost certainly result in severe neurologic deficits (such as the brainstem). It is especially important to differentiate a primary brain tumor from a solitary metastatic deposit which may appear very similar on MRI imaging, and also to rule out infection or other disease processes.

In addition to the extent of surgical resection, other prognostic factors include patient age, performance status, and baseline neurologic function [15, 38–40]. In recent years, a number of prognostic biomarkers have also emerged which correlate closely with outcome. Most commonly found in tumors with oligodendroglial components (AO and AOA), chromosome 1p/19q loss of heterozygosity is associated with superior treatment response and survival [41–43]. In both grade III and grade IV tumors, O^6-methylguanine methyltransferase (MGMT) has been identified as a particularly important prognostic marker. Silencing of this gene by promoter methylation is associated with improved survival [44]. The value of this prognostic marker has gained even more recognition with the introduction of the alkylating agent TMZ, the use of which has become the standard of care in many malignant gliomas. MGMT is able to remove alkylation damage caused by TMZ at the O^6 site which correlates with improved treatment response. Despite this, patients without gene methylation still derive some benefit from the drug, though it is less pronounced than in those with promoter methylation [44]. This may in part be due to drug-induced methylation of other sites such as the guanine N^7 position. In recent genomic analyses, mutations in IDH1 and IDH2 have emerged as powerful predictors of survival in patients with malignant gliomas, and correlate with lower-grade tumors, younger patients, a prerequisite to 1p/19q loss, and additional differences in molecular mutational profile [45–47]. Exploratory analyses of the roles of these and other biomarkers are a subject of intense ongoing research and increasingly the classification of gliomas that dictate care of these patients is guided by the tumor mutation profile.

For nearly all patients with GBM, radiotherapy is recommended following maximal surgical resection. Despite the aggressive nature of GBM, adjuvant radiotherapy has been shown to more than double the median OS compared to supportive care alone [48, 49]. Radiotherapy should typically start no earlier than two weeks following surgery to allow for adequate wound healing. MRI-CT fusion for treatment planning is now considered standard of care [50]. Historically, whole-brain irradiation was offered for GBM, but studies have shown no significant improvement with this technique versus more focal irradiation [51, 52]. A typical approach involves treating T2 hyperintense areas plus a 1–2 cm margin to

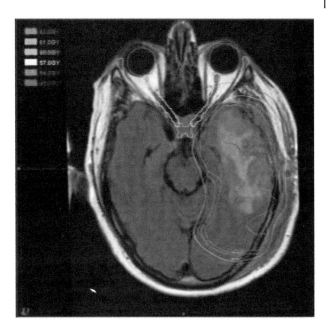

Figure 39.1 Case of a glioblastoma patient treated with IMRT using five fields prescribed to 60 Gy. The high-dose GTV is in red, CTV is in pink. The plan is overlaid on the fused FLAIR MRI image. For a color version of this figure, see the color plate section.

encompass potential microscopic disease extension to a dose of 45 or 50 Gy, followed by a boost to the enhancing tumor on T1-post contrast imaging to a dose of 60 Gy using standard fractionation (Figure 39.1). 3D conformal or IMRT planning can be utilized depending on tumor size and location.

For elderly patients and those with poor performance status, such long courses of radiotherapy may not be tolerable, and in fact single-modality treatment is often offered. Radiotherapy alone has been shown to still confer a significant survival advantage over supportive care alone, with minimal additional toxicity [53]. One randomized trial of 60 Gy in 30 fractions versus 40 Gy in 15 fractions identified no significant difference in outcome for patient 60 years of age or older [54]. Even more compelling has been the Nordic trail that prospectively randomized patients over age 60 years to six monthly cycles of temozolomide versus 60 Gy in 30 fractions versus hypofractionated 34 Gy in 10 fractions [55]. Among patients age 60–70 years there was no difference in OS; however, among patients aged >70 years there was superior OS for either TMZ or hypofractionated radiation over the standard 60 Gy course of radiotherapy. The option of administering TMZ alone versus standard 60 Gy alone was also supported in the prospective randomized NOA-08 trial [56]. Additionally, this study was paramount for affirming the superior role of chemotherapy alone specifically for the patients harboring MGMT promoter hypermethylation.

Given the radioresistant nature of malignant gliomas, significant effort has been spent on investigating the role of dose-escalation with stereotactic radiosurgery or particle therapy. To date, there has been little convincing evidence that dose escalation with these techniques provides any significant benefit for patients [57–59]. Further studies investigating unique techniques such as carbon ion therapy and boron neutron capture are ongoing [60–64].

Perhaps the most significant change in the approach to the treatment of GBM in recent years is the introduction of the alkylating agent TMZ. In their landmark trial published in 2005, Stupp *et al.* showed that the addition of concomitant and adjuvant TMZ to radiation for patients with GBM improved median survival time from 12.1 to 14.6 months and improved two-year OS from 10% to 26% [65]. Further analysis of their data indicated a survival advantage in all subgroups, though it is important to note that patients aged >70 years were excluded [66]. As previously discussed, MGMT promoter methylation was the strongest predictor of outcome conferring a median survival time of 23.4 months versus 12.6 months for those without promoter methylation. Despite the significant benefit of TMZ, early radiotherapy remains the mainstay of adjuvant therapy. A recent small trial of induction TMZ showed inferior results compared to the standard combined approach [67]. An exception may be in elderly patients with GBM, for which there is emerging data that TMZ alone does not confer inferior results compared to standard or hypofractionated radiotherapy regimens [56].

The management of anaplastic (grade III) gliomas is generally inferred from the evidence and approach to the management of GBM. There are, however, several trials which focus on this subgroup. Before the advent of TMZ, the combination of procarbazine, lomustine and vincristine (PCV) was commonly prescribed. The RTOG 9402 randomized 291 patients with AO or AOA to four cycles of induction PCV followed by radiotherapy (59.4 Gy) or radiotherapy alone [66, 67]. The results revealed that among patients with 1p/19q co-deletion, the addition of chemotherapy resulted in significantly improved median survival (14.7 versus 7.3 years, p = 0.03), thus suggesting an ongoing role for chemotherapy in the management of this patient subset. The EORTC 26951 similarly reported on 368 patients with AO and AOA who were randomized to radiotherapy versus radiotherapy plus adjuvant PCV. At a median follow-up of 140 months, the median survival time for the 1p/19q co-deleted group receiving radiation and PCV has not yet been reached, whereas it was 112 months in the radiation-alone group [68]. The PFS was significantly extended with the use of chemotherapy, with median values of 157 versus 50 months for the combined modality and radiation-alone groups, respectively. At most

centers, PCV chemotherapy has been abandoned due to increased toxicity relative to TMZ. A trial that randomized patients with all forms of anaplastic glioma to up-front radiotherapy versus PCV versus TMZ demonstrated no significant difference in OS or PFs between the arms [45]. It is important to note, however, that 78% of patients who received chemotherapy received salvage radiotherapy, and 48% of those receiving radiotherapy received salvage chemotherapy. As such, these results suggest only that treatment sequencing has no effect on outcome.

Similarly, as stated with the low-grade glioma molecular alterations, all gliomas are increasingly recognized to be better classified and defined based on these factors. The traditional distinction by WHO classification becomes decreasingly relevant, and these factors are being strongly weighed as the next WHO classification system is underway. Recently available data have suggested that WHO grade 2 and 3 gliomas can be far better reclassified by consideration of the three tumor markers of *TERT* promoter mutation, *IDH* mutation, and 1p/19q codeletion to define distinct patient populations with markedly different survival patterns [69].

Primary CNS Lymphoma

Primary CNS lymphoma (PCNSL) is defined as a non-Hodgkin lymphoma that is confined to the craniospinal axis, without evidence of systemic involvement. It should not be confused with systemic lymphoma with spread to the CNS, which is managed differently. The incidence of PCNSL has increased 10-fold during the past 30 years. While some of this increase has been attributed to the increasing prevalence of HIV in the United States, a striking increase has also been seen in immunocompetent patients [70]. However, it appears that during the last decade the incidence is no longer increasing. Incidence for patients with HIV relates to HIV stage and CD4 count. Multiple prognostic factors for PCNSL have been identified including older age, poor performance status, elevated lactate dehydrogenase (LDH), elevated CNS protein levels, and involvement of deep brain areas. Depending on the number of risk factors present, median survival can vary from over five years to less than one year [71–73].

Treatment for PCNSL historically consisted of whole-brain radiotherapy, but outcomes were dismal despite initial high response rates [74]. During the 1990s, the RTOG investigated the use of pre-irradiation multi-agent chemotherapy including high-dose methotrexate (MTX). This study showed a significant benefit to the addition of chemotherapy, though the toxicity rate was high, especially in older patients [75]. Several centers have also reported encouraging results using MTX-based regimens with radiotherapy delayed until progression [76–78]. Memorial Sloan Kettering has recently published their experience using a regimen consisting of induction chemotherapy including MTX and rituximab followed by reduced-dose whole-brain radiotherapy (23.4 Gy) for those with a complete response, and standard dose (45 Gy) for those with a partial response [79]. With a median follow-up of three years the authors of this study reported a two-year OS rate of 67% and a PFS rate of 57%, which compares favorably with historical controls. This approach remains controversial, however, with many centers treating PCNSL with chemotherapy alone with radiotherapy reserved for palliation of recurrent disease. In patients who fail primary chemotherapy, radiotherapy produces a nine-month median survival [80]. Intrathecal chemotherapy is a possible consideration in patients with multifocal disease [81].

Meningioma

Meningiomas account for approximately 15–20% of primary brain tumors in the US, and are the most common benign CNS tumor [82]. Spinal meningiomas are rare, representing only 10–12% of all meningiomas. The incidence of meningioma increases with age, peaking around age 70 years, with tumors twice as common in females. This fact is at least partially attributable to the presence of hormone receptors such as the progesterone receptor on the tumor cell surface in many cases [83]. Indeed, the use of hormone replacement therapy is associated with an increased risk of meningioma development [84]. Other risk factors include NF-2 and prior radiation therapy.

On CT and MRI scans, meningiomas typically appear as well-defined, extra-axial masses that displace normal brain. They are isointense on T1 imaging and show strong enhancement with intravenous contrast. Meningiomas are classified according to the WHO grading criteria updated in 2000 [85]. Grade I or benign meningiomas comprise 70–90% of cases and >80% of patients will remain disease-free with appropriate treatment. Grade II or atypical meningiomas account for 15–25% of cases and are seven- to eightfold more likely to recur within five years. Only 1–2% of meningiomas are classified as anaplastic or malignant (WHO grade III) and are associated with a very poor prognosis, despite aggressive treatment.

Not all meningiomas require therapeutic intervention, and in fact many are diagnosed incidentally and never become symptomatic. For those tumors that cause symptoms or are at high risk of causing symptoms, complete surgical resection is curative in the vast majority of patients with benign meningiomas, though this is not possible in 20–30% of cases [86]. Completeness of resection is typically graded on the Simpson scale, where grade I represents complete resection including removal of underlying bone and dura, grade II represents complete tumor removal with coagulation of the dural attachment, grade III represents complete tumor removal without resection or coagulation of the dura, and grade IV represents subtotal resection [87]. Ten-year recurrence rates vary from 9% for a Simpson grade I resection to 40% for a grade IV. In the setting of unresectable lesions, partially resected lesions or recurrent lesions, radiotherapy is often employed. The benefit of the addition of radiation to partially resected meningiomas was demonstrated in multiple trials during the 1980s [88–90]. In one large retrospective series, Goldsmith *et al.* showed that the addition of radiotherapy to partially resected meningiomas was safe and effective with doses in the range of 54 to 60 Gy [91]. More recent series have demonstrated excellent long-term local control rates in excess of 90% at five years, with minimal long-term morbidity [92, 93].

In addition to fractionated radiation techniques used for treating meningiomas, stereotactic radiosurgery (SRS) is an alternative for small lesions safely amenable to the technique. SRS has the benefit of reducing treatment time while still delivering curative doses of radiotherapy even in areas abutting sensitive normal structures. Several centers have published their experiences using SRS with typical single-fraction doses ranging from 12 to 20 Gy [94–96]. Local control rates in these and other series range from 75% to 100% at five to ten years. Toxicity is typically low but increases with tumor size and dose. As such, fractionated therapy is usually indicated for larger tumors or those located in close proximity to radiation-sensitive tissues. Proton therapy can also provide improved tumor coverage and reduced dose to normal structures in certain locations (Figure 39.2).

Pituitary Tumors

Tumors of the pituitary gland are generally benign and are associated with a wide range of endocrine manifestations and clinical syndromes. As a group they come to medical attention in three principal ways: (i) as a mass lesion sometimes causing increased intracranial pressure; (ii) with effects on the optic apparatus (classically compression of the optic chiasm though upward growth leading to bitemporal hemianopsia or other visual disturbances); and (iii) by alteration of one or more endocrine signaling pathways with associated clinical symptoms. Given the recent increase in the use of CT and MRI imaging throughout the US, many adenomas are also discovered incidentally.

Neuroendocrine abnormalities are typically associated with tumors arising from the anterior pituitary, which is derived from Rathke's pouch. Such tumors comprise about 80% of adult pituitary adenomas and

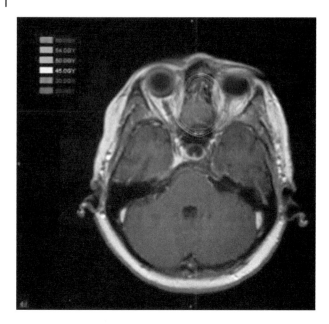

Figure 39.2 Case of a meningioma patient treated with fractionated proton therapy. The GTV is shown in red. For a color version of this figure, see the color plate section.

can produce at least six different hormones: prolactin, corticotropin, follicle-stimulating hormone, luteinizing hormone, growth hormone, and thyroid-stimulating hormone. About one-third of pituitary tumors are classified as non-functioning adenomas which secrete no detectable levels of pituitary hormones.

Since the 1970s the standard surgical approach for the resection of pituitary adenomas has been transsphenoidal, which replaced the more dangerous frontotemporal craniotomy approach [97,98]. This procedure offers the opportunity for decompression and also sampling of tissue for detailed pathologic analysis. Surgical cure rates with this approach using modern techniques approach 90% [99]. Despite this, tumors involving the cavernous sinus, clivus or suprasellar region are rarely cured surgically, and so adjuvant treatment modalities such as external beam radiotherapy (EBRT) must be considered. Patients may also be considered for radiation therapy when medical therapies such as bromocriptine, cabergoline or octreotide fail to control endocrine abnormalities.

When radiotherapy is indicated, several techniques can be employed, including 3D conformal, IMRT, and stereotactic radiotherapy. Fractionated radiotherapy with doses of 45–50.4 Gy in 1.8 Gy daily fractions is reasonable for non-functioning adenomas, while functioning adenomas are typically treated with doses of 50.4–54 Gy [100]. When SRS is utilized a dose of 15–18 Gy is appropriate for non-functioning tumors, while 20 Gy should be employed for functioning tumors, with many practitioners using even higher doses up to 30 Gy

routinely [101, 102]. Fractionated radiotherapy is associated with a substantially lower risk of optic pathway injury compared to SRS [103,104]. Such toxicity is wholly dependent on the dose received by the optic apparatus, and as such SRS remains appropriate in carefully selected cases with benefit of not only patient convenience but also faster biochemical response. Particle therapy is also emerging as a useful tool for treating pituitary adenoma, given its ability to reduce dose to nearby normal structures and reduce the overall volume of irradiated tissue [105, 106]. The latter is particularly important given that most patients will enjoy a normal lifespan after treatment putting them at risk for radiation-associated second malignancies.

It must be remembered that in the case of functioning tumors, the normalization of hormones may take several years and that patients will often need to continue on medical therapy until this occurs. Secondary pituitary dysfunction requiring hormonal replacement develops in over 20% of patients within five years of completing pituitary radiotherapy, and in the majority of patients with longer follow up [100]. As such, these patients require careful endocrinological follow-up, particularly younger patients who may need growth hormone replacement as well as counseling regarding fertility issues.

Arteriovenous Malformation

Intracranial arteriovenous malformations (AVMs) are rare vascular abnormalities consisting of abnormally large arteries and veins which communicate directly instead of across a capillary bed. Because of this aberrant arrangement, the draining veins for such abnormalities are subject to abnormally high hydrodynamic stress. This results in an annual bleeding risk of 2–4% per year [107]. Such events are often catastrophic, with up to a 30% mortality rate after the first bleed. Large size, deep location and venous drainage pattern are all associated with increased risk of bleeding [108–110]. Spontaneous bleeding is the most common presentation; seizure, headache and focal neurologic deficits are also seen.

The therapeutic goal for AVMs is to prevent future bleeding while minimizing therapy-associated side effects given the expected otherwise normal lifespan of these patients. Surgical resection or embolization are preferred if feasible. For more deep-seated lesions or based on the lesion's vasculature, radiotherapy (specifically SRS) is an effective alternative for non-surgical candidates. Fractionated radiotherapy produces inferior results [111, 112]. Depending on the size and location of the nidus, single doses of between 15 and 25 Gy are typically used. Such therapy is thought to unleash a cytokine cascade resulting in endothelial proliferation and leading to eventual obliteration of the vessels and collapse of the vascular abnormality. Obliteration rates in most series vary between 60% and 85% and are dose-dependent [113–116]. Complete obliteration after radiotherapy can take several years, and a significant risk of re-bleeding remains during this latency period [117]. It has been clearly shown that radiosurgery does *not* increase the hemorrhage rate during the latency period from treatment to obliteration.

Vestibular Schwannoma

Vestibular schwannomas, also known as acoustic neuromas, are benign tumors derived from myelin-producing Schwann cells which develop along the vestibular nerve. They are always unilateral except in patients with NF-2 (where the presence of bilateral lesions is pathognomonic). While accounting for less than 8% of intracranial tumors they represent 80–90% of tumors arising in the cerebellopontine angle. Up to 95% of patients will present with hearing loss which is associated with tinnitus in two-thirds of patients. Mild disequilibrium is also a common presenting symptom. Facial pain and paralysis are less common and typically associated with larger lesions.

For small, minimally symptomatic tumors, close observation is a viable option, especially in older patients. A recent large Japanese study, however, suggested that >50% of tumors will progress within three years [118]. Surgical resection is often possible but preserves hearing in less than 50% of cases and is associated with a higher risk of facial nerve paralysis compared to radiotherapy [119–121]. SRS and fractionated radiotherapy are now widely accepted as a safe and effective primary treatments, with local control rates approaching 100% in several series [122–125]. Single-fraction doses of 12–14 Gy are used in most series while fractionated dose schedules are more variable, ranging from 25 Gy in five fractions to 54 Gy in 30 fractions. Some data are available to suggest that fractionated regimens reduce the risk of hearing loss, but this remains controversial [126, 127].

Brain Metastases

Brain metastases are a common complication of metastatic cancer and far outnumber primary brain tumors. Radiation therapy has been the mainstay of treatment for such patients for over 50 years. The role of radiotherapy has been greatly influenced by improved brain imaging techniques able to identify progressively smaller lesions. Radiotherapy for brain metastases achieves both palliation and improvement of overall survival for many patients.

Patients with brain metastases may present with any combination of symptoms related to local compression or cerebral edema. Corticosteroids are an important initial treatment for patients presenting with neurologic compromise. For those with significant tumor mass effect-related symptoms for whom up-front radiotherapy is recommended, steroid therapy should be initiated and, depending on the risk of herniation, may need to be given for 24–48 h prior to initiating radiation treatment. The American Association of Neurologic Surgeons recommends a dose of 4–8 mg of dexamethasone per day for those with mild symptoms, and 16 mg per day for those with more severe symptoms [128]. Seizure prophylaxis is not necessary unless there has been documented seizure-like activity [129]. Prognostic factors for patients with brain metastases include performance status, age, and extent of extracranial disease. RTOG recursive partitioning analysis (RPA) class is often used as a rough guide for predicting patient outcome [130]. For patients with a Karnofsky performance score of <70 (RPA class III) aggressive therapy is unlikely to greatly prolong survival. Prognostic factors often vary depending on the primary site of disease, and a more disease-specific graded prognostic assessment index allows for more accurate prediction of patient outcomes [131].

The use of whole-brain radiotherapy (WBRT) was first shown to be superior to corticosteroids alone during the early 1970s [132]. Numerous studies on dose and fractionation have been conducted, but with no clear benefits of any one regimen emerging. In general, a dose of 30 Gy in 10 fractions is considered standard. Doses of 35–37.5 Gy at 2.5 Gy per fraction is also widely used. A daily fraction size of more than 3 Gy may lead to unacceptable late toxicity, particularly in terms of cognitive function, though the impact of higher dose per fraction in the subset of patients with an extremely short projected lifespan is likely clinically insignificant [133]. The concurrent administration of multiple chemotherapeutic agents during the delivery of WBRT has been tested in multiple trials, but results have overall been negative to date and have suggested an increase in toxicity [134–138]. Many malignancies are actively benefiting from new molecularly based targeted therapies and immunotherapy, some of which provide some CNS activity and the opportunity to delay use of radiation therapy for the diagnosis of brain metastases. Such therapies include erlotinib and crizotinib in patients with sensitive non-small-cell lung cancers, ipilimumab or BRAF/MEK inhibitors for patients with melanoma, and lapatinib and other agents acting on the HER2 pathway in patients with breast cancer [139].

The potential benefit of adding surgical resection to WBRT for patients with single metastases was first postulated during the 1980s when retrospective data suggested a potential improvement in outcomes. Three subsequent randomized trials were conducted, two of which showed a clear survival benefit for the addition of surgery [140–142]. Several of these studies suggested, however, that the benefit of surgery was limited to patients with controlled extracranial disease and good performance status. Surgical resection alone with omission of WBRT was also examined during this period. In this study, Patchell *et al.* demonstrated that the omission of postoperative WBRT resulted in increased rates of recurrence and increased neurologic death [143]. However, there no overall survival benefit was seen in this study. These results would later be confirmed in a more recent EORTC trial [144].

Stereotactic radiosurgery is also an important tool for the treatment of brain metastases. In radiosurgery, multiple highly collimated beams of radiation are stereotactically directed towards a radiographically discrete treatment site. The hallmark of all stereotactic radiation techniques is the rapid dose fall-off at the edges of the treatment volume. The biological and physical characteristics of metastases (radiographically discrete, small, spherical, non-invasive) make them ideal targets for radiosurgery, which was first employed as an adjunct to WBRT. RTOG 9508 was a large randomized trial which sought to investigate the potential benefit of the addition of SRS to patients treated with WBRT. In this trial of 331 patients, the addition of SRS to WBRT improved local control and provided a significant survival benefit for patients with a single intracranial metastasis [145].

In an effort to avoid the toxicity typically associated with WBRT, many centers evolved to using SRS alone in patients with brain metastases after retrospective data suggested similar outcomes for these patients compared to those treated with WBRT [146]. Three randomized trials of SRS alone versus SRS + WBRT have now been published [144,147,148]. In each of these studies the addition of whole-brain irradiation did not improve survival or time to loss of functional independence, despite its impact on recurrence-free survival. As such, for patients with limited brain metastases, SRS appears to be an acceptable primary treatment reserving WBRT for later multifocal dissemination, should it occur.

Radiosurgery can be a particularly useful tool for treating recurrent lesions in patients who have already undergone WBRT. Unfortunately, some patients will present with recurrent lesions at multiple sites, making SRS less feasible, and in these situations repeat WBRT may be recommended. In a recent publication on the use of repeat WBRT, treatment with doses of 14–30 Gy resulted in complete or partial resolution of symptoms in 80% of patients [149]. For those patients with controlled extracranial disease, median survival approached 20 months. Most patients experienced mild to moderate toxicity, but rates of severe late toxicity were very low. The use of repeat WBRT should be limited to those with a good performance status and in whom more than six months has elapsed since the first course of therapy.

Primary Spinal Tumors

Primary spinal tumors represent about 10–15% of all primary tumors in the CNS. Intradural, extramedullary tumors include meningiomas, neurilemmomas, chordomas, and epidermoids. These lesions, with the exception of chordomas, are usually controlled with surgery alone and rarely require postoperative radiotherapy. Intramedullary tumors include ependymomas, astrocytomas, oligodendrogliomas, and hemangioblastomas. These tumors are often not cured with surgery alone and as such often require postoperative radiotherapy. Due to the sensitivity of the spinal cord to radiation therapy, doses of 45–50 Gy are typically employed [150].

Spinal cord ependymoma is a relatively rare tumor which, unlike its counterpart in the brain, is more common in adults than children, with a mean presentation age of 40 years [151, 152]. These tumors are typically low grade and patients can present with insidious symptoms years before final diagnosis. Myxopapillary ependymomas in particular typically occur in the lumbosacral region near the filum terminale. Gross total resection is preferred and can lead to long-term local control without adjuvant therapy, though it is only possible in approximately 50% of patients. For those who undergo a subtotal resection the addition of adjuvant radiotherapy can lead to local control rates of 90–100% [153, 154]. Unfortunately, this tumor has the propensity to recur elsewhere in the CNS over time.

Malignant Spinal Cord Compression

Malignant spinal cord compression (MSCC) from metastatic lesions in the spine has the potential for devastating neurologic compromise, and is estimated to affect 5–10% of patients with cancer [4]. Most epidural tumors causing spinal cord compression arise from metastatic foci in the vertebral body which invade directly into the spinal extradural space. As such, the bulk of the tumor is often anterior to the spinal cord. The most common primary tumor types are those that commonly spread to bone, including lung, breast and prostate cancers as well as from direct extension from bone involvement by myeloma or lymphoma.

The successful treatment of MSCC depends on early recognition. Symptoms may occur acutely or insidiously. Four symptoms characterize malignant spinal cord compression: pain; weakness; sensory deficits; and autonomic dysfunction (especially loss of bowel and bladder control). Almost all patients experience pain as an initial symptom. This pain is often close to the site of the compression, though radicular pain is more common with cervical and lumbosacral lesions. Pain from MSCC is often worse in the recumbent position. Weakness is rarely the primary presenting symptom but is common by the time the diagnosis is made. About 50% of patients will also have sensory deficits consisting of numbness or paresthesias. Metastases to the conus medullaris or cauda equina can cause saddle anesthesia in addition to loss of bowel and bladder control.

Standard treatment options include surgical resection and/or radiotherapy. Several scoring systems have been developed to aid the treating physician in determining which option may be of greatest benefit to the patient [155–157]. These systems take into account tumor type, interval since diagnosis, extent of metastases, and severity of motor deficits at the time of presentation. In general, those patients with severe deficits present for increasing number of days are less likely to achieve neurological recovery from either surgery or radiotherapy.

Surgical decompression is almost always accomplished by means of wide laminectomy in the region of the tumor mass. Since many tumors causing cord compression arise anterior to the spinal cord, this posterior approach rarely results in complete removal of the tumor. As such, postoperative radiotherapy is almost always recommended following surgical resection. A recent randomized trial has investigated the role for surgery with postoperative radiotherapy compared to up-front radiotherapy alone [158]. In this trial, the addition of surgery resulted in a significantly improved ambulatory ability (94% versus 74%) and duration of treatment response. It is important to note, however, that this trial took 10 years to accrue 101 patients, and so its generalizability is questionable. A recent retrospective analysis revealed minimal differences in outcomes between primary surgery and radiotherapy when patients were carefully matched for 11 prognostic factors [159].

Historically, radiation treatment fields include the upper and lower extent of the compression with a margin of one vertebral body above and below. However, as with brain tumors, the extent of irradiated volume is determined using contrast-enhanced MRI. Numerous trials have been performed to identify the most optimal treatment dose for patients with MSCC. Most of these have shown no difference in functional outcomes for single-fraction regimens (typically 8 Gy) versus multifraction regimens [160–163]. Despite this, patients with a good prognosis may benefit from increased PFS associated with longer regimens, and those with myeloma also appear to benefit from longer courses [164].

Decompressive surgery should be the first recommended intervention when a patient experiences recurrent spinal cord compression in a previously irradiated area. Unfortunately, many previously irradiated patients may not be considered appropriate candidates for surgical intervention. In this setting, re-irradiation must be considered despite the risk of radiation myelopathy. Retrospective studies have identified several risk factors for the development of radiation myelopathy, including the time from the first course of radiation, timing of deficits and cumulative radiation dose received by the cord. In general, re-irradiation appears safe if the cumulative biologically effective dose (BED) can be kept below 120, though outcomes for these patients are still poor [165, 166]. Stereotactic body radiotherapy (SBRT) is another option that is increasingly employed either up-front or for salvage of recurrent lesions and often managed jointly with spine surgeons to optimize decompression followed immediately by SBRT [167–170]. Spinal SBRT has gained a significantly prominent role in the management of oligometastatic disease with at least equivalent, if not superior, results to traditional fractionated radiation [171]. Multiple clinical research studies investigating this technique are ongoing.

Conclusions

The management of CNS tumors is complex. Given the diversity of tumor types and clinical presentations, a careful understanding of the appropriate approaches for each tumor and the management of potential side effects of treatment is vital. Patients with CNS tumors are often best managed with a dedicated team consisting of radiation oncologists, neurosurgeons and neuro-oncologists, amongst others. This multidisciplinary approach can help ensure that the best possible care is delivered to patients in an ever-changing landscape of novel biomarkers, new treatment technologies, and emerging adjuvant therapies.

References

1 Siegel, R.L., Miller, K.D., Jemal, A. (2017) Cancer statistics, 2017. *CA: A Cancer Journal for Clinicians*, **67** (1), 7–30.

2 Surveillance, Epidemiology, and End Results (SEER) Program Populations. 1969–2010. Available at: www.seer.cancer.gov, January 2014.

3 Black, P.M., Loeffler, J.S. (2005) *Cancer of the Nervous System*, 2nd edition. Lippincott Williams & Wilkins, Philadelphia.

4 DeVita, V.T., Lawrence, T.S., Rosenberg, S.A. (2011) *DeVita, Hellman, and Rosenberg's Cancer: Principles & Practice of Oncology*, 9th edition. Wolters

Kluwer Health/Lippincott Williams & Wilkins, Philadelphia.

5 Evans, D.G., Farndon, P.A., Burnell, L.D., Gattamaneni, H.R., Birch, J.M. (1991) The incidence of Gorlin syndrome in 173 consecutive cases of medulloblastoma. *Br. J. Cancer*, **64** (5), 959–961.

6 Ohgaki, H., Kleihues, P. (2005) Epidemiology and etiology of gliomas. *Acta Neuropathol.*, **109** (1), 93–108.

7 Ron, E., Modan, B., Boice, J.D., Jr., *et al.* (1988) Tumors of the brain and nervous system after radiotherapy in childhood. *N. Engl. J. Med.*, **319** (16), 1033–1039.

8 Brada, M., Ford, D., Ashley, S., *et al.* (1992) Risk of second brain tumour after conservative surgery and radiotherapy for pituitary adenoma. *Br. Med. J.*, **304** (6838), 1343–1346.

9 Frei, P., Poulsen, A.H., Johansen, C., Olsen, J.H., Steding-Jessen, M., Schuz, J. (2011) Use of mobile phones and risk of brain tumours: update of Danish cohort study. *Br. Med. J.*, **343**, d6387.

10 Aydin, D., Feychting, M., Schuz, J., *et al.* (2011) Mobile phone use and brain tumors in children and adolescents: a multicenter case-control study. *J. Natl Cancer Inst.*, **103** (16), 1264–1276.

11 Inskip, P.D., Hoover, R.N., Devesa, S.S. (2010) Brain cancer incidence trends in relation to cellular telephone use in the United States. *NeuroOncology*, **12** (11), 1147–1151.

12 Tan, H., Chen, L., Guan, Y., Lin, X. (2011) Comparison of MRI, F-18 FDG, and 11C-choline PET/CT for their potentials in differentiating brain tumor recurrence from brain tumor necrosis following radiotherapy. *Clin. Nucl. Med.*, **36** (11), 978–981.

13 Zeng, Q.S., Li, C.F., Liu, H., Zhen, J.H., Feng, D.C. (2007) Distinction between recurrent glioma and radiation injury using magnetic resonance spectroscopy in combination with diffusion-weighted imaging. *Int. J. Radiat. Oncol. Biol. Phys.*, **68** (1), 151–158.

14 Xiangsong, Z., Weian, C. (2007) Differentiation of recurrent astrocytoma from radiation necrosis: a pilot study with ^{13}N-NH$_3$ PET. *J. Neurooncol.*, **82** (3), 305–311.

15 Mirimanoff, R.O., Gorlia, T., Mason, W., *et al.* (2006) Radiotherapy and temozolomide for newly diagnosed glioblastoma: recursive partitioning analysis of the EORTC 26981/22981-NCIC CE3 phase III randomized trial. *J. Clin. Oncol.*, **24** (16), 2563–2569.

16 Gunderson, L.L., Tepper, J.E. (2007) *Clinical Radiation Oncology*, 2nd edition. Elsevier Churchill Livingstone, Philadelphia, PA.

17 Montine, T.J., Vandersteenhoven, J.J., Aguzzi, A., *et al.* (1994) Prognostic significance of Ki-67 proliferation index in supratentorial fibrillary astrocytic neoplasms. *Neurosurgery*, **34** (4), 674–678; discussion 678–679.

18 Fisher, B.J., Naumova, E., Leighton, C.C., *et al.* (2002) Ki-67: a prognostic factor for low-grade glioma? *Int. J. Radiat. Oncol. Biol. Phys.*, **52** (4), 996–1001.

19 McCormack, B.M., Miller, D.C., Budzilovich, G.N., Voorhees, G.J., Ransohoff, J. (1992) Treatment and survival of low-grade astrocytoma in adults – 1977–1988. *Neurosurgery*, **31** (4), 636–642; discussion 642.

20 North, C.A., North, R.B., Epstein, J.A., Piantadosi, S., Wharam, M.D. (1990) Low-grade cerebral astrocytomas. Survival and quality of life after radiation therapy. *Cancer*, **66** (1), 6–14.

21 Pignatti, F., van den Bent, M., Curran, D., *et al.* (2002) Prognostic factors for survival in adult patients with cerebral low-grade glioma. *J. Clin. Oncol.*, **20** (8), 2076–2084.

22 Leighton, C., Fisher, B., Bauman, G., *et al.* (1997) Supratentorial low-grade glioma in adults: an analysis of prognostic factors and timing of radiation. *J. Clin. Oncol.*, **15** (4), 1294–1301.

23 Medbery, C.A., 3rd, Straus, K.L., Steinberg, S.M., Cotelingam, J.D., Fisher, W.S. (1988) Low-grade astrocytomas: treatment results and prognostic variables. *Int. J. Radiat. Oncol. Biol. Phys.*, **15** (4), 837–841.

24 van den Bent, M.J., Afra, D., de Witte, O., *et al.* (2005) Long-term efficacy of early versus delayed radiotherapy for low-grade astrocytoma and oligodendroglioma in adults: the EORTC 22845 randomised trial. *Lancet*, **366** (9490), 985–990.

25 Karim, A.B., Maat, B., Hatlevoll, R., *et al.* (1996) A randomized trial on dose–response in radiation therapy of low-grade cerebral glioma: European Organization for Research and Treatment of Cancer (EORTC) Study 22844. *Int. J. Radiat. Oncol. Biol. Phys.*, **36** (3), 549–556.

26 Kiebert, G.M., Curran, D., Aaronson, N.K., *et al.* (1998) Quality of life after radiation therapy of cerebral low-grade gliomas of the adult: results of a randomised phase III trial on dose response (EORTC trial 22844). EORTC Radiotherapy Co-operative Group. *Eur. J. Cancer*, **34** (12), 1902–1909.

27 Shaw, E., Arusell, R., Scheithauer, B., *et al.* (2002) Prospective randomized trial of low- versus high-dose radiation therapy in adults with supratentorial low-grade glioma: initial report of a North Central Cancer Treatment Group/Radiation Therapy Oncology Group/Eastern Cooperative Oncology Group study. *J. Clin. Oncol.*, **20** (9), 2267–2276.

28 Laack, N.N., Brown, P.D., Ivnik, R.J., *et al.* (2005) Cognitive function after radiotherapy for supratentorial low-grade glioma: a North Central Cancer Treatment Group prospective study. *Int. J. Clin. Oncol. Biol. Phys.*, **63** (4), 1175–1183.

29 Brown, P.D., Buckner, J.C., O'Fallon, J.R., *et al.* (2003) Effects of radiotherapy on cognitive function in patients with low-grade glioma measured by the Folstein mini-mental state examination. *J. Clin. Oncol.*, **21** (13), 2519–2524.

30 Shaw, E.G., Wang, M., Coons, S.W., *et al.* (2012) Randomized trial of radaition therapy plus procarbazine, lomustine, and vincritine chemotherapy for supratentorial adult low-grade glioma: initial results of RTOG 9802. *J. Clin. Oncol.*, **30** (25), 3065–3070.

31 Fisher, B.J., Hu, C., Macdonald, D.R., *et al.* (2015) Phase 2 study of temozolomide-based chemoradiation therapy for high-risk low-grade gliomas: preliminary results of Radiation Therapy Oncology Group 0424. *Int. J. Clin. Oncol. Biol. Phys.*, **91** (3), 497–504.

32 Pace, A., Vidiri, A., Galie, E., *et al.* (2003) Temozolomide chemotherapy for progressive low-grade glioma: clinical benefits and radiological response. *Ann. Oncol.*, **14** (12), 1722–1726.

33 Brada, M., Viviers, L., Abson, C., *et al.* (2003) Phase II study of primary temozolomide chemotherapy in patients with WHO grade II gliomas. *Ann. Oncol.*, **14** (12), 1715–1721.

34 Quinn, J.A., Reardon, D.A., Friedman, A.H., *et al.* (2003) Phase II trial of temozolomide in patients with progressive low-grade glioma. *J. Clin. Oncol.*, **21** (4), 646–651.

35 Baumert, B.G., Mason, W.P., Ryan, G., *et al.* (2013) Temozolomide chemotherapy versus radiotherapy in molecularly characterized (1p loss) low-grade glioma: A randomized phase III intergroup study by the EORTC/NCIC-CTG/TROG/MRC-CTU (EORTC 22033-26033). *J. Clin. Oncol.*, **31** (Suppl.), abstract 2007.

36 Cancer Genome Atlas Research Network, Brat, D.J., Verhaak, R.G., *et al.* (2015) Comprehensive, integrative genomic analysis of diffuse lower-grade gliomas. *N. Engl. J. Med.*, **372** (26), 2481–2498.

37 Lacroix, M., Abi-Said, D., Fourney, D.R., *et al.* (2001) A multivariate analysis of 416 patients with glioblastoma multiforme: prognosis, extent of resection, and survival. *J. Neurosurg.*, **95** (2), 190–198.

38 Curran, W.J., Jr., Scott, C.B., Horton, J., *et al.* (1993) Recursive partitioning analysis of prognostic factors in three Radiation Therapy Oncology Group malignant glioma trials. *J. Natl Cancer Inst.*, **85** (9), 704–710.

39 Gorlia, T., van den Bent, M.J., Hegi, M.E., *et al.* (2008) Nomograms for predicting survival of patients with newly diagnosed glioblastoma: prognostic factor analysis of EORTC and NCIC trial 26981-22981/CE.3. *Lancet Oncol.*, **9** (1), 29–38.

40 Scott, C.B., Scarantino, C., Urtasun, R., *et al.* (1998) Validation and predictive power of Radiation Therapy Oncology Group (RTOG) recursive partitioning analysis classes for malignant glioma patients: a report using RTOG 90-06. *Int. J. Clin. Oncol. Biol. Phys.*, **40** (1), 51–55.

41 Cairncross, J.G., Ueki, K., Zlatescu, M.C., *et al.* (1998) Specific genetic predictors of chemotherapeutic response and survival in patients with anaplastic oligodendrogliomas. *J. Natl Cancer Inst.*, **90** (19), 1473–1479.

42 Bello, M.J., Leone, P.E., Vaquero, J., *et al.* (1995) Allelic loss at 1p and 19q frequently occurs in association and may represent early oncogenic events in oligodendroglial tumors. *Int. J. Cancer*, **64** (3), 207–210.

43 von Deimling, A., Bender, B., Jahnke, R., *et al.* (1994) Loci associated with malignant progression in astrocytomas: a candidate on chromosome 19q. *Cancer Res.*, **54** (6), 1397–1401.

44 Hegi, M.E., Diserens, A.C., Gorlia, T., *et al.* (2005) MGMT gene silencing and benefit from temozolomide in glioblastoma. *N. Engl. J. Med.*, **352** (10), 997–1003.

45 Wick, W., Hartmann, C., Engel, C., *et al.* (2009) NOA-04 randomized phase III trial of sequential radiochemotherapy of anaplastic glioma with procarbazine, lomustine, and vincristine or temozolomide. *J. Clin. Oncol.*, **27** (35), 5874–5880.

46 Yan, H., Parsons, D.W., Jin, G., *et al.* (2009) IDH1 and IDH2 mutations in gliomas. *N. Engl. J. Med.*, **360** (8), 765–773.

47 Parsons, D.W., Jones, S., Zhang, X., *et al.* (2008) An integrated genomic analysis of human glioblastoma multiforme. *Science*, **321** (5897), 1807–1812.

48 Kristiansen, K., Hagen, S., Kollevold, T., *et al.* (1981) Combined modality therapy of operated astrocytomas grade III and IV. Confirmation of the value of postoperative irradiation and lack of potentiation of bleomycin on survival time: a prospective multicenter trial of the Scandinavian Glioblastoma Study Group. *Cancer*, **47** (4), 649–652.

49 Walker, M.D., Alexander, E., Jr., Hunt, W.E., *et al.* (1978) Evaluation of BCNU and/or radiotherapy in the treatment of anaplastic gliomas. A cooperative clinical trial. *J. Neurosurg.*, **49** (3), 333–343.

50 Thornton, A.F., Jr., Sandler, H.M., Ten Haken, R.K., *et al.* (1992) The clinical utility of magnetic resonance imaging in 3-dimensional treatment planning of brain neoplasms. *Int. J. Clin. Oncol. Biol. Phys.*, **24** (4), 767–775.

51 Garden, A.S., Maor, M.H., Yung, W.K., *et al.* (1991) Outcome and patterns of failure following limited-volume irradiation for malignant astrocytomas. *Radiother. Oncol.*, **20** (2), 99–110.

52 Shapiro, W.R., Green, S.B., Burger, P.C., *et al.* (1989) Randomized trial of three chemotherapy regimens and two radiotherapy regimens and two radiotherapy regimens in postoperative treatment of malignant glioma. Brain Tumor Cooperative Group Trial 8001. *J. Neurosurg.*, **71** (1), 1–9.

53 Keime-Guibert, F., Chinot, O., Taillandier, L., *et al.* (2007) Radiotherapy for glioblastoma in the elderly. *N. Engl. J. Med.*, **356** (15), 1527–1535.

54 Roa, W., Brasher, P.M., Bauman, G., *et al.* (2004) Abbreviated course of radiation therapy in older patients with glioblastoma multiforme: a prospective randomized clinical trial. *J. Clin. Oncol.*, **22** (9), 1583–1588.

55 Malmstrom, A., Gronberg, B.H., Marosi, C., *et al.* (2012) Temozolomide versus standard 6-week radiotherapy versus hypofractionated radiotherapy in patients older than 60 years with glioblastoma: the Nordic randomised, phase 3 trial. *Lancet Oncol.*, **13** (9), 916–926.

56 Wick, W., Platten, M., Meisner, C., *et al.* (2012) Temozolomide chemotherapy alone versus radiotherapy alone for malignant astrocytoma in the elderly: the NOA-08 randomised, phase 3 trial. *Lancet Oncol.*, **13** (7), 707–715.

57 Tsao, M.N., Mehta, M.P., Whelan, T.J., *et al.* (2005) The American Society for Therapeutic Radiology and Oncology (ASTRO) evidence-based review of the role of radiosurgery for malignant glioma. *Int. J. Clin. Oncol. Biol. Phys.*, **63** (1), 47–55.

58 Souhami, L., Seiferheld, W., Brachman, D., *et al.* (2004) Randomized comparison of stereotactic radiosurgery followed by conventional radiotherapy with carmustine to conventional radiotherapy with carmustine for patients with glioblastoma multiforme: report of Radiation Therapy Oncology Group 93-05 protocol. *Int. J. Clin. Oncol. Biol. Phys.*, **60** (3), 853–860.

59 Fitzek, M.M., Thornton, A.F., Rabinov, J.D., *et al.* (1999) Accelerated fractionated proton/photon irradiation to 90 cobalt gray equivalent for glioblastoma multiforme: results of a phase II prospective trial. *J. Neurosurg.*, **91** (2), 251–260.

60 Mizumoto, M., Tsuboi, K., Igaki, H., *et al.* (2010) Phase I/II trial of hyperfractionated concomitant boost proton radiotherapy for supratentorial glioblastoma multiforme. *Int. J. Clin. Oncol. Biol. Phys.*, **77** (1), 98–105.

61 Mizoe, J.E., Tsujii, H., Hasegawa, A., *et al.* (2007) Phase I/II clinical trial of carbon ion radiotherapy for malignant gliomas: combined X-ray radiotherapy, chemotherapy, and carbon ion radiotherapy. *Int. J. Clin. Oncol. Biol. Phys.*, **69** (2), 390–396.

62 Miyatake, S.I., Kawabata, S., Hiramatsu, R., Furuse, M., Kuroiwa, T., Suzuki, M. (2014) Boron neutron capture therapy with bevacizumab may prolong the survival of recurrent malignant glioma patients: four cases. *Radiat. Oncol.*, **9** (1), 6.

63 Barth, R.F., Vicente, M.G., Harling, O.K., *et al.* (2012) Current status of boron neutron capture therapy of high grade gliomas and recurrent head and neck cancer. *Radiat. Oncol.*, **7**, 146.

64 Kankaanranta, L., Seppala, T., Koivunoro, H., *et al.* (2011) L-boronophenylalanine-mediated boron neutron capture therapy for malignant glioma progressing after external beam radiation therapy: a Phase I study. *Int. J. Clin. Oncol. Biol. Phys.*, **80** (2), 369–376.

65 Stupp, R., Mason, W.P., van den Bent, M.J., *et al.* (2005) Radiotherapy plus concomitant and adjuvant temozolomide for glioblastoma. *N. Engl. J. Med.*, **352** (10), 987–996.

66 Stupp, R., Hegi, M.E., Mason, W.P., *et al.* (2009) Effects of radiotherapy with concomitant and adjuvant temozolomide versus radiotherapy alone on survival in glioblastoma in a randomised phase III study: 5-year analysis of the EORTC-NCIC trial. *Lancet Oncol.*, **10** (5), 459–466.

67 Chinot, O.L., Barrie, M., Fuentes, S., *et al.* (2007) Correlation between O6-methylguanine-DNA methyltransferase and survival in inoperable newly diagnosed glioblastoma patients treated with neoadjuvant temozolomide. *J. Clin. Oncol.*, **25** (12), 1470–1475.

68 van den Bent, M.J., Brandes, A.A., Taphoorn, M.J., *et al.* (2013) Adjuvant procarbazine, lomustine, and vincristine chemotherapy in newly diagnosed anaplastic oligodendroglioma: long-term follow-up of EORTC brain tumor group study 26951. *J. Clin. Oncol.*, **31** (3), 344–350.

69 Eckel-Passow, J.E., Lachance, D.H., Molinaro, A.M., *et al.* (2015) Glioma groups based on 1p/19q, IDH, and TERT promoter mutations in tumors. *N. Engl. J. Med.*, **372** (26), 2499–2508.

70 Olson, J.E., Janney, C.A., Rao, R.D., *et al.* (2002) The continuing increase in the incidence of primary central nervous system non-Hodgkin lymphoma: a surveillance, epidemiology, and end results analysis. *Cancer*, **95** (7), 1504–1510.

71 Abrey, L.E., Ben-Porat, L., Panageas, K.S., *et al.* (2006) Primary central nervous system lymphoma: the Memorial Sloan-Kettering Cancer Center prognostic model. *J. Clin. Oncol.*, **24** (36), 5711–5715.

72 Ferreri, A.J., Blay, J.Y., Reni, M., *et al.* (2003) Prognostic scoring system for primary CNS lymphomas: the International Extranodal Lymphoma Study Group experience. *J. Clin. Oncol.*, **21** (2), 266–272.

73 Blay, J.Y., Lasset, C., Carrie, C., *et al.* (1993) Multivariate analysis of prognostic factors in patients with non HIV-related primary cerebral lymphoma. A proposal for a prognostic scoring. *Br. J. Cancer*, **67** (5), 1136–1141.

74 Nelson, D.F., Martz, K.L., Bonner, H., *et al.* (1992) Non-Hodgkin's lymphoma of the brain: can high dose, large volume radiation therapy improve survival? Report on a prospective trial by the Radiation Therapy Oncology Group (RTOG): RTOG 8315. *Int. J. Clin. Oncol. Biol. Phys.*, **23** (1), 9–17.

75 Milburn, J. (1976) Shared management expertise spells survival for the small. *Hospitals*, **50** (4), 52–54.

76 Angelov, L., Doolittle, N.D., Kraemer, D.F., *et al.* (2009) Blood–brain barrier disruption and intra-arterial methotrexate-based therapy for newly diagnosed primary CNS lymphoma: a multi-institutional experience. *J. Clin. Oncol.*, **27** (21), 3503–3509.

77 Jahnke, K., Korfel, A., Martus, P., *et al.* (2005) High-dose methotrexate toxicity in elderly patients with primary central nervous system lymphoma. *Ann. Oncol.*, **16** (3), 445–449.

78 Pels, H., Schmidt-Wolf, I.G., Glasmacher, A., *et al.* (2003) Primary central nervous system lymphoma: results of a pilot and phase II study of systemic and intraventricular chemotherapy with deferred radiotherapy. *J. Clin. Oncol.*, **21** (24), 4489–4495.

79 Shah, G.D., Yahalom, J., Correa, D.D., *et al.* (2007) Combined immunochemotherapy with reduced whole-brain radiotherapy for newly diagnosed primary CNS lymphoma. *J. Clin. Oncol.*, **25** (30), 4730–4735.

80 Nguyen, P.L., Chakravarti, A., Finkelstein, D.M., Hochberg, F.H., Batchelor, T.T., Loeffler, J.S. (2005) Results of whole-brain radiation as salvage of methotrexate failure for immunocompetent patients with primary CNS lymphoma. *J. Clin. Oncol.*, **23** (7), 1507–1513.

81 Korfel, A., Schlegel, U. (2013) Diagnosis and treatment of primary CNS lymphoma. *Nat. Rev. Neurol.*, **9** (6), 317–327.

82 Whittle, I.R., Smith, C., Navoo, P., Collie, D. (2004) Meningiomas. *Lancet*, **363** (9420), 1535–1543.

83 Donnell, M.S., Meyer, G.A., Donegan, W.L. (1979) Estrogen-receptor protein in intracranial meningiomas. *J. Neurosurg.*, **50** (4), 499–502.

84 Blitshteyn, S., Crook, J.E., Jaeckle, K.A. (2008) Is there an association between meningioma and hormone replacement therapy? *J. Clin. Oncol.*, **26** (2), 279–282.

85 Kleihues, P., Louis, D.N., Scheithauer, B.W., *et al.* (2002) The WHO classification of tumors of the nervous system. *J. Neuropathol. Exp. Neurol.*, **61** (3), 215–225; discussion 226–219.

86 Mirimanoff, R.O., Dosoretz, D.E., Linggood, R.M., Ojemann, R.G., Martuza, R.L. (1985) Meningioma: analysis of recurrence and progression following neurosurgical resection. *J. Neurosurg.*, **62** (1), 18–24.

87 Simpson, D. (1957) The recurrence of intracranial meningiomas after surgical treatment. *J. Neurol. Neurosurg. Psychiatry*, **20** (1), 22–39.

88 Miralbell, R., Linggood, R.M., de la Monte, S., Convery, K., Munzenrider, J.E., Mirimanoff, R.O. (1992) The role of radiotherapy in the treatment of subtotally resected benign meningiomas. *J. Neurooncol.*, **13** (2), 157–164.

89 Taylor, B.W., Jr., Marcus, R.B., Jr., Friedman, W.A., Ballinger, W.E., Jr., Million, R.R. (1988) The meningioma controversy: postoperative radiation therapy. *Int. J. Clin. Oncol. Biol. Phys.*, **15** (2), 299–304.

90 Barbaro, N.M., Gutin, P.H., Wilson, C.B., Sheline, G.E., Boldrey, E.B., Wara, W.M. (1987) Radiation therapy in the treatment of partially resected meningiomas. *Neurosurgery*, **20** (4), 525–528.

91 Goldsmith, B.J., Wara, W.M., Wilson, C.B., Larson, D.A. (1994) Postoperative irradiation for subtotally resected meningiomas. A retrospective analysis of 140 patients treated from 1967 to 1990. *J. Neurosurg.*, **80** (2), 195–201.

92 Solda, F., Wharram, B., De Ieso, P.B., Bonner, J., Ashley, S., Brada, M. (2013) Long-term efficacy of fractionated radiotherapy for benign meningiomas. *Radiother. Oncol.*, **109** (2) 330–334.

93 Combs, S.E., Adeberg, S., Dittmar, J.O., *et al.* (2013) Skull base meningiomas: Long-term results and patient self-reported outcome in 507 patients treated with fractionated stereotactic radiotherapy (FSRT) or intensity modulated radiotherapy (IMRT). *Radiother. Oncol.*, **106** (2), 186–191.

94 Kollova, A., Liscak, R., Novotny, J., Jr., Vladyka, V., Simonova, G., Janouskova, L. (2007) Gamma Knife surgery for benign meningioma. *J. Neurosurg.*, **107** (2), 325–336.

95 Pollock, B.E., Stafford, S.L., Utter, A., Giannini, C., Schreiner, S.A. (2003) Stereotactic radiosurgery provides equivalent tumor control to Simpson Grade 1 resection for patients with small- to medium-size meningiomas. *Int. J. Clin. Oncol. Biol. Phys.*, **55** (4), 1000–1005.

96 Kondziolka, D., Levy, E.I., Niranjan, A., Flickinger, J.C., Lunsford, L.D. (1999) Long-term outcomes after meningioma radiosurgery: physician and patient perspectives. *J. Neurosurg.*, **91** (1), 44–50.

97 Mortini, P., Losa, M., Barzaghi, R., Boari, N., Giovanelli, M. (2005) Results of transsphenoidal surgery in a large series of patients with pituitary adenoma. *Neurosurgery*, **56** (6), 1222–1233; discussion 1233.

98 Jane, J.A., Jr., Thapar, K., Kaptain, G.J., Maartens, N., Laws, E.R., Jr. (2002) Pituitary surgery: transsphenoidal approach. *Neurosurgery*, **51** (2), 435–442; discussion 442–444.

99 Swearingen, B., Biller, B.M., Barker, F.G., II, *et al.* (1999) Long-term mortality after transsphenoidal surgery for Cushing disease. *Ann. Intern. Med.*, **130** (10), 821–824.

100 Loeffler, J.S., Shih, H.A. (2011) Radiation therapy in the management of pituitary adenomas. *J. Clin. Endocrinol. Metab.*, **96** (7), 1992–2003.

101 Sheehan, J.P., Pouratian, N., Steiner, L., Laws, E.R., Vance, M.L. (2011) Gamma Knife surgery for pituitary adenomas: factors related to radiological and endocrine outcomes. *J. Neurosurg.*, **114** (2), 303–309.

102 Castinetti, F., Nagai, M., Dufour, H., *et al.* (2007) Gamma knife radiosurgery is a successful adjunctive treatment in Cushing's disease. *Eur. J. Endocrinol.*, **156** (1), 91–98.

103 Erridge, S.C., Conkey, D.S., Stockton, D., *et al.* (2009) Radiotherapy for pituitary adenomas: long-term efficacy and toxicity. *Radiother. Oncol.*, **93** (3), 597–601.

104 Brada, M., Rajan, B., Traish, D., *et al.* (1993) The long-term efficacy of conservative surgery and radiotherapy in the control of pituitary adenomas. *Clin. Endocrinol. (Oxf.)*, **38** (6), 571–578.

105 Ronson, B.B., Schulte, R.W., Han, K.P., Loredo, L.N., Slater, J.M., Slater, J.D. (2006) Fractionated proton beam irradiation of pituitary adenomas. *Int. J. Clin. Oncol. Biol. Phys.*, **64** (2), 425–434.

106 Wattson, D.A., Tanguturi, S.K., Spiegel, D.Y., *et al.* (2014) Outcomes of proton therapy for patients with functional pituitary adenomas. *Int. J. Clin. Oncol. Biol. Phys.*, **90** (3), 532–539.

107 Ondra, S.L., Troupp, H., George, E.D., Schwab, K. (1990) The natural history of symptomatic arteriovenous malformations of the brain: a 24-year follow-up assessment. *J. Neurosurg.*, **73** (3), 387–391.

108 Stefani, M.A., Porter, P.J., terBrugge, K.G., Montanera, W., Willinsky, R.A., Wallace, M.C. (2002) Large and deep brain arteriovenous malformations are associated with risk of future hemorrhage. *Stroke*, **33** (5), 1220–1224.

109 Stefani, M.A., Porter, P.J., terBrugge, K.G., Montanera, W., Willinsky, R.A., Wallace, M.C. (2002) Angioarchitectural factors present in brain arteriovenous malformations associated with hemorrhagic presentation. *Stroke*, **33** (4), 920–924.

110 Spetzler, R.F., Martin, N.A. (1986) A proposed grading system for arteriovenous malformations. *J. Neurosurg.*, **65** (4), 476–483.

111 Karlsson, B., Lindqvist, M., Blomgren, H., *et al.* (2005) Long-term results after fractionated radiation therapy for large brain arteriovenous malformations. *Neurosurgery*, **57** (1), 42–48; discussion 48–49.

112 Laing, R.W., Childs, J., Brada, M. (1992) Failure of conventionally fractionated radiotherapy to decrease the risk of hemorrhage in inoperable arteriovenous malformations. *Neurosurgery*, **30** (6), 872–875; discussion 875–876.

113 Schlienger, M., Atlan, D., Lefkopoulos, D., *et al.* (2000) Linac radiosurgery for cerebral arteriovenous malformations: results in 169 patients. *Int. J. Clin. Oncol. Biol. Phys.*, **46** (5), 1135–1142.

114 Flickinger, J.C., Pollock, B.E., Kondziolka, D., Lunsford, L.D. (1996) A dose–response analysis of arteriovenous malformation obliteration after radiosurgery. *Int. J. Clin. Oncol. Biol. Phys.*, **36** (4), 873–879.

115 Friedman, W.A., Bova, F.J., Mendenhall, W.M. (1995) Linear accelerator radiosurgery for arteriovenous malformations: the relationship of size to outcome. *J. Neurosurg.*, **82** (2), 180–189.

116 Engenhart, R., Wowra, B., Debus, J., *et al.* (1994) The role of high-dose, single-fraction irradiation in small and large intracranial arteriovenous malformations. *Int. J. Clin. Oncol. Biol. Phys.*, **30** (3), 521–529.

117 Maruyama, K., Kawahara, N., Shin, M., *et al.* (2005) The risk of hemorrhage after radiosurgery for cerebral arteriovenous malformations. *N. Engl. J. Med.*, **352** (2), 146–153.

118 Yamakami, I., Uchino, Y., Kobayashi, E., Yamaura, A. (2003) Conservative management, gamma-knife radiosurgery, and microsurgery for acoustic neurinomas: a systematic review of outcome and risk of three therapeutic options. *Neurol. Res.*, **25** (7), 682–690.

119 Karpinos, M., The, B.S., Zeck, O., *et al.* (2002) Treatment of acoustic neuroma: stereotactic radiosurgery versus microsurgery. *Int. J. Clin. Oncol. Biol. Phys.*, **54** (5), 1410–1421.

120 Regis, J., Pellet, W., Delsanti, C., *et al.* (2002) Functional outcome after gamma knife surgery or microsurgery for vestibular schwannomas. *J. Neurosurg.*, **97** (5), 1091–1100.

121 Samii, M., Matthies, C. (1997) Management of 1000 vestibular schwannomas (acoustic neuromas): surgical management and results with an emphasis on complications and how to avoid them. *Neurosurgery*, **40** (1), 11–21; discussion 21–23.

122 Andrews, D.W., Werner-Wasik, M., Den, R.B., *et al.* (2009) Toward dose optimization for fractionated stereotactic radiotherapy for acoustic neuromas: comparison of two dose cohorts. *Int. J. Clin. Oncol. Biol. Phys.*, **74** (2), 419–426.

123 Chopra, R., Kondziolka, D., Niranjan, A., Lunsford, L.D., Flickinger, J.C. (2007) Long-term follow-up of acoustic schwannoma radiosurgery with marginal tumor doses of 12 to 13 Gy. *Int. J. Clin. Oncol. Biol. Phys.*, **68** (3), 845–851.

124 Chan, A.W., Black, P., Ojemann, R.G., *et al.* (2005) Stereotactic radiotherapy for vestibular schwannomas:

favorable outcome with minimal toxicity. *Neurosurgery*, **57** (1), 60–70; discussion 60–70.

125 Fuss, M., Debus, J., Lohr, F., *et al.* (2000) Conventionally fractionated stereotactic radiotherapy (FSRT) for acoustic neuromas. *Int. J. Clin. Oncol. Biol. Phys.*, **48** (5), 1381–1387.

126 Meijer, O.W., Vandertop, W.P., Baayen, J.C., Slotman, B.J. (2003) Single-fraction versus fractionated linac-based stereotactic radiosurgery for vestibular schwannoma: a single-institution study. *Int. J. Clin. Oncol. Biol. Phys.*, **56** (5), 1390–1396.

127 Andrews, D.W., Suarez, O., Goldman, H.W., *et al.* (2001) Stereotactic radiosurgery and fractionated stereotactic radiotherapy for the treatment of acoustic schwannomas: comparative observations of 125 patients treated at one institution. *Int. J. Clin. Oncol. Biol. Phys.*, **50** (5), 1265–1278.

128 Ryken, T.C., McDermott, M., Robinson, P.D., *et al.* (2010) The role of steroids in the management of brain metastases: a systematic review and evidence-based clinical practice guideline. *J. Neurooncol.*, **96** (1), 103–114.

129 Mikkelsen, T., Paleologos, N.A., Robinson, P.D., *et al.* (2010) The role of prophylactic anticonvulsants in the management of brain metastases: a systematic review and evidence-based clinical practice guideline. *J. Neurooncol.*, **96** (1), 97–102.

130 Gaspar, L., Scott, C., Rotman, M., *et al.* (1997) Recursive partitioning analysis (RPA) of prognostic factors in three Radiation Therapy Oncology Group (RTOG) brain metastases trials. *Int. J. Clin. Oncol. Biol. Phys.*, **37** (4), 745–751.

131 Sperduto, P.W., Kased, N., Roberge, D., *et al.* (2012) Summary report on the graded prognostic assessment: an accurate and facile diagnosis-specific tool to estimate survival for patients with brain metastases. *J. Clin. Oncol.*, **30** (4), 419–425.

132 Horton, J., Baxter, D.H., Olson, K.B. (1971) The management of metastases to the brain by irradiation and corticosteroids. *Am. J. Roentgenol. Radium Ther. Nucl. Med.*, **111** (2), 334–336.

133 DeAngelis, L.M., Delattre, J.Y., Posner, J.B. (1989) Radiation-induced dementia in patients cured of brain metastases. *Neurology*, **39** (6), 789–796.

134 Liu, R., Wang, X., Ma, B., Yang, K., Zhang, Q., Tian, J. (2010) Concomitant or adjuvant temozolomide with whole-brain irradiation for brain metastases: a meta-analysis. *Anticancer Drugs*, **21** (1), 120–128.

135 Neuhaus, T., Ko, Y., Muller, R.P., *et al.* (2009) A phase III trial of topotecan and whole brain radiation therapy for patients with CNS-metastases due to lung cancer. *Br. J. Cancer*, **100** (2), 291–297.

136 Knisely, J.P., Berkey, B., Chakravarti, A., *et al.* (2008) A phase III study of conventional radiation therapy plus thalidomide versus conventional radiation therapy for

multiple brain metastases (RTOG 0118). *Int. J. Clin. Oncol. Biol. Phys.*, **71** (1), 79–86.

137 Mehta, M.P., Rodrigus, P., Terhaard, C.H., *et al.* (2003) Survival and neurologic outcomes in a randomized trial of motexafin gadolinium and whole-brain radiation therapy in brain metastases. *J. Clin. Oncol.*, **21** (13), 2529–2536.

138 Phillips, T.L., Scott, C.B., Leibel, S.A., Rotman, M., Weigensberg, I.J. (1995) Results of a randomized comparison of radiotherapy and bromodeoxyuridine with radiotherapy alone for brain metastases: report of RTOG trial 89-05. *Int. J. Clin. Oncol. Biol. Phys.*, **33** (2), 339–348.

139 Soffietti, R., Trevisan, E., Ruda, R. (2012) Targeted therapy in brain metastasis. *Curr. Opin. Oncol.*, **24** (6), 679–686.

140 Mintz, A.H., Kestle, J., Rathbone, M.P., *et al.* (1996) A randomized trial to assess the efficacy of surgery in addition to radiotherapy in patients with a single cerebral metastasis. *Cancer*, **78** (7), 1470–1476.

141 Noordijk, E.M., Vecht, C.J., Haaxma-Reiche, H., *et al.* (1994) The choice of treatment of single brain metastasis should be based on extracranial tumor activity and age. *Int. J. Clin. Oncol. Biol. Phys.*, **29** (4), 711–717.

142 Patchell, R.A., Tibbs, P.A., Walsh, J.W., *et al.* (1990) A randomized trial of surgery in the treatment of single metastases to the brain. *N. Engl. J. Med.*, **322** (8), 494–500.

143 Patchell, R.A., Tibbs, P.A., Regine, W.F., *et al.* (1998) Postoperative radiotherapy in the treatment of single metastases to the brain: a randomized trial. *JAMA*, **280** (17), 1485–1489.

144 Kocher, M., Soffietti, R., Abacioglu, U., *et al.* (2011) Adjuvant whole-brain radiotherapy versus observation after radiosurgery or surgical resection of one to three cerebral metastases: results of the EORTC 22952-26001 study. *J. Clin. Oncol.*, **29** (2), 134–141.

145 Andrews, D.W., Scott, C.B., Sperduto, P.W., *et al.* (2004) Whole-brain radiation therapy with or without stereotactic radiosurgery boost for patients with one to three brain metastases: phase III results of the RTOG 9508 randomised trial. *Lancet*, **363** (9422), 1665–1672.

146 Pirzkall, A., Debus, J., Lohr, F., *et al.* (1998) Radiosurgery alone or in combination with whole-brain radiotherapy for brain metastases. *J. Clin. Oncol.*, **16** (11), 3563–3569.

147 Chang, E.L., Wefel, J.S., Hess, K.R., *et al.* (2009) Neurocognition in patients with brain metastases treated with radiosurgery or radiosurgery plus whole-brain irradiation: a randomised controlled trial. *Lancet Oncol.*, **10** (11), 1037–1044.

148 Aoyama, H., Shirato, H., Tago, M., *et al.* (2006) Stereotactic radiosurgery plus whole-brain radiation

therapy vs stereotactic radiosurgery alone for treatment of brain metastases: a randomized controlled trial. *JAMA*, **295** (21), 2483–2491.

149 Son, C.H., Jimenez, R., Niemierko, A., Loeffler, J.S., Oh, K.S., Shih, H.A. (2012) Outcomes after whole brain reirradiation in patients with brain metastases. *Int. J. Clin. Oncol. Biol. Phys.*, **82** (2), e167–e172.

150 Marks, L.B., Yorke, E.D., Jackson, A., *et al.* (2010) Use of normal tissue complication probability models in the clinic. *Int. J. Clin. Oncol. Biol. Phys.*, **76** (3 Suppl.), S10–S19.

151 Hanbali, F., Fourney, D.R., Marmor, E., *et al.* (2002) Spinal cord ependymoma: radical surgical resection and outcome. *Neurosurgery*, **51** (5), 1162–1172; discussion 1172–1174.

152 Whitaker, S.J., Bessell, E.M., Ashley, S.E., Bloom, H.J., Bell, B.A., Brada, M. (1991) Postoperative radiotherapy in the management of spinal cord ependymoma. *J. Neurosurg.*, **74** (5), 720–728.

153 McLaughlin, M.P., Marcus, R.B., Jr., Buatti, J.M., *et al.* (1998) Ependymoma: results, prognostic factors and treatment recommendations. *Int. J. Clin. Oncol. Biol. Phys.*, **40** (4), 845–850.

154 Wen, B.C., Hussey, D.H., Hitchon, P.W., *et al.* (1991) The role of radiation therapy in the management of ependymomas of the spinal cord. *Int. J. Clin. Oncol. Biol. Phys.*, **20** (4), 781–786.

155 Rades, D., Douglas, S., Huttenlocher, S., *et al.* (2011) Validation of a score predicting post-treatment ambulatory status after radiotherapy for metastatic spinal cord compression. *Int. J. Clin. Oncol. Biol. Phys.*, **79** (5), 1503–1506.

156 Rades, D., Rudat, V., Veninga, T., *et al.* (2008) A score predicting posttreatment ambulatory status in patients irradiated for metastatic spinal cord compression. *Int. J. Clin. Oncol. Biol. Phys.*, **72** (3), 905–908.

157 Rades, D., Heidenreich, F., Karstens, J.H. (2002) Final results of a prospective study of the prognostic value of the time to develop motor deficits before irradiation in metastatic spinal cord compression. *Int. J. Clin. Oncol. Biol. Phys.*, **53** (4), 975–979.

158 Patchell, R.A., Tibbs, P.A., Regine, W.F., *et al.* (2005) Direct decompressive surgical resection in the treatment of spinal cord compression caused by metastatic cancer: a randomised trial. *Lancet*, **366** (9486), 643–648.

159 Rades, D., Huttenlocher, S., Dunst, J., *et al.* (2010) Matched pair analysis comparing surgery followed by radiotherapy and radiotherapy alone for metastatic spinal cord compression. *J. Clin. Oncol.*, **28** (22), 3597–3604.

160 Rades, D., Lange, M., Veninga, T., *et al.* (2009) Preliminary results of spinal cord compression recurrence evaluation (score-1) study comparing short-course versus long-course radiotherapy for local control of malignant epidural spinal cord compression. *Int. J. Clin. Oncol. Biol. Phys.*, **73** (1), 228–234.

161 Rades, D., Stalpers, L.J., Schulte, R., *et al.* (2006) Defining the appropriate radiotherapy regimen for metastatic spinal cord compression in non-small cell lung cancer patients. *Eur. J. Cancer*, **42** (8), 1052–1056.

162 Rades, D., Stalpers, L.J., Veninga, T., *et al.* (2005) Evaluation of five radiation schedules and prognostic factors for metastatic spinal cord compression. *J. Clin. Oncol.*, **23** (15), 3366–3375.

163 Rades, D., Stalpers, L.J., Hulshof, M.C., *et al.* (2005) Comparison of 1 × 8 Gy and 10 × 3 Gy for functional outcome in patients with metastatic spinal cord compression. *Int. J. Clin. Oncol. Biol. Phys.*, **62** (2), 514–518.

164 Rades, D., Hoskin, P.J., Stalpers, L.J., *et al.* (2006) Short-course radiotherapy is not optimal for spinal cord compression due to myeloma. *Int. J. Clin. Oncol. Biol. Phys.*, **64** (5), 1452–1457.

165 Rades, D., Rudat, V., Veninga, T., Stalpers, L.J., Hoskin, P.J., Schild, S.E. (2008) Prognostic factors for functional outcome and survival after reirradiation for in-field recurrences of metastatic spinal cord compression. *Cancer*, **113** (5), 1090–1096.

166 Mahan, S.L., Ramsey, C.R., Scaperoth, D.D., Chase, D.J., Byrne, T.E. (2005) Evaluation of image-guided helical tomotherapy for the retreatment of spinal metastasis. *Int. J. Clin. Oncol. Biol. Phys.*, **63** (5), 1576–1583.

167 Wang, X.S., Rhines, L.D., Shiu, A.S., *et al.* (2012) Stereotactic body radiation therapy for management of spinal metastases in patients without spinal cord compression: a phase 1–2 trial. *Lancet Oncol.*, **13** (4), 395–402.

168 Chang, E.L., Shiu, A.S., Mendel, E., *et al.* (2007) Phase I/II study of stereotactic body radiotherapy for spinal metastasis and its pattern of failure. *J. Neurosurg. Spine*, **7** (2), 151–160.

169 Gerszten, P.C., Burton, S.A., Ozhasoglu, C., Welch, W.C. (2007) Radiosurgery for spinal metastases: clinical experience in 500 cases from a single institution. *Spine (Phila. Pa, 1976)*, **32** (2), 193–199.

170 Yamada, Y., Lovelock, D.M., Yenice, K.M., *et al.* (2005) Multifractionated image-guided and stereotactic intensity-modulated radiotherapy of paraspinal tumors: a preliminary report. *Int. J. Clin. Oncol. Biol. Phys.*, **62** (1), 53–61.

171 Alongi, F., Arcangeli, S., Filippi, A.R., Ricardi, U., Scorsetti, M. (2012) Review and uses of stereotactic body radiation therapy for oligometastases. *Oncologist*, **17** (8), 1100–1107.

40

The Lymphomas

Caitlin Costello, Loren K. Mell and Parag Sanghvi

A Brief History of Lymphoma

Thomas Hodgkin was born in Pentonville, Middlesex, England on 17th August 1798. As a physician at Guy's Hospital in London, he wrote *On Some Morbid Appearances of the Absorbent Glands and Spleen*, which first appeared in 1832. The initial description of the disease by Marcello Malpighi (1666), however, preceded his by more than a century. Samuel Wilks, also a physician at Guy's Hospital, further characterized the disease in 1856, and named the disease after Hodgkin.

The first description of therapy for lymphoma is credited to Sir William Osler in 1894, who mentions treatment with 'Fowler's solution,' an arsenic-containing alkylating compound, in his *Textbook of Medicine*. This was followed a year later by Roentgen's discovery of x-rays. William A. Pusey at the University of Illinois, Chicago, was the first to record the use of ionizing radiation to treat lymphoma, in 1902. That same year, Dorothy Reed first described the peculiar cells that are now considered pathognomonic for Hodgkin disease, also independently discovered by Sternberg in 1898. The exposure of troops to mustard gas during World Wars I and II gave rise to the discovery of alkylating agents as hematopoietic suppressants, and their subsequent development as therapeutics by Goodman and Gilman in 1943.

The development of megavoltage irradiation and multi-agent chemotherapy with vinca alkaloids, anthracyclines, and dacarbazine from the 1950s to the 1970s revolutionized therapy for lymphomas, and has given rise to the dominant treatment paradigms in use today. During the past 40 years modern imaging modalities and targeted therapies have emerged, along with a deeper understanding of the causes and classification of this diverse disease.

Epidemiology

Lymphoma is the eighth most common cancer worldwide. Non-Hodgkin lymphoma (NHL) is at least five-fold more common than Hodgkin lymphoma (HL). In 2017, an estimated 72 240 people in the United States will be diagnosed with NHL, and there will be approximately 20 140 deaths due to the disease [1]. Corresponding estimates for HL are 8260 new cases and 1070 deaths. Both NHL and HL are more prevalent in men. Their incidence is highest in more developed nations, and the age-adjusted incidence of both NHL and HL rises with age. The peak age-adjusted incidence of NHL is above 65, and almost half of patients are between the ages of 65 and 84 years at diagnosis. In contrast, while the peak age-adjusted incidence of HL is also above 65 years, the most common age at presentation is 20–34 years.

Infectious diseases are the most common and well-established risk factors for lymphomas. Epstein–Barr virus (EBV) is a putative cause of HL, based on observations that elevated levels of antibodies directed at EBV antigens have been detected in serum of HL patients [2], and EBV genomes have been detected in Reed–Sternberg cells [3]. The causal relationship between EBV and Burkitt's lymphoma is perhaps more well established, based on the presence of EBV DNA and a high prevalence of clonal EBV found in Burkitt's lymphoma cells [4, 5]. EBV has also been associated with central nervous system (CNS) lymphoma [6]. *Helicobacter pylori* is a cause of mucosa-associated lymphoid tissue (MALT) lymphoma, while human T-cell lymphotropic virus (HTLV-1) causes adult T-cell lymphoma/leukemia.

Though the proximal cause of the majority of lymphomas is unknown, characteristic genetic translocations can be found in many lymphomas, such as follicular

Clinical Radiation Oncology: Indications, Techniques, and Results, Third Edition. Edited by William Small Jr.

lymphoma (t(14;18)(q32;q21)), Burkitt's lymphoma (t(8;14)), mantle cell lymphoma (t(11;14)), and MALT lymphoma (t(11;18)). For example, the t(14;18) rearrangement leads to an uncontrolled expression of the bcl-2 oncogene, by transposing the bcl-2 gene on chromosome 18 next to the heavy-chain immunoglobulin (Ig) gene on chromosome 14 [7]. Similarly, the t(11;14) rearrangement transposes the bcl-1 oncogene [8], and the t(8;14) rearrangement transposes the c-myc oncogene at the same heavy chain Ig locus [9]. The t(11;18)(q21;q21) translocation generates a fusion product, c-IAP2/MALT1 that activates the NF-κB transcription pathway, leading to malignant transformation [10, 11].

Histopathologic Classification

The classification of lymphoproliferative disorders has evolved as a result of an increasing understanding of the biology of these diseases. The *WHO Classification of Tumors of Hematopoietic and Lymphoid Tissue* recognizes B-cell and T-cell/NK-cell neoplasms, and HL in its revised 2008 edition [12]. Based on the earlier Revised European-American Lymphoma (REAL) classification system, the integration of morphologic, immunophenotypic, molecular genetic, and clinical features has allowed for further re-definition of these lymphoid neoplasms [13].

Hodgkin Lymphoma

Biological and clinical studies conducted in the past 30 years have shown that Hodgkin lymphomas are comprised of two disease entities: nodular lymphocyte predominant Hodgkin lymphoma (NLPHL) and classical Hodgkin lymphoma (CHL) [14, 15]. The histologic finding associated with HL is the Reed–Sternberg cell, a large cell with abundant slightly basophilic cytoplasm and at least two nuclear lobes or nuclei, giving the appearance of 'owl's eyes.' Reed–Sternberg cells represent a minority of the cellular infiltrate, ranging in frequency from 1% to 10%, admixed with a rich inflammatory background, which varies amongst the classical HL subtypes. Polymerase chain reaction (PCR) analysis of single cells reveals that HL comprises a monoclonal population of B cells, likely derived from germinal centers [16]. An excisional biopsy is recommended for the initial diagnosis of a suspected lymphoma, and a diagnosis can be made by immunophenotyping of cell-surface markers. The classic phenotype of the Reed–Sternberg cell is CD15+, CD30+, and CD45- [17, 18].

Classical HL can be further divided into specific subtypes, with nodular sclerosis being the most common subtype in Western populations (Table 40.1). Nodular

Table 40.1 Subtypes of Hodgkin lymphoma.

Classical Hodgkin lymphoma
- Nodular sclerosis
- Mixed cellularity
- Lymphocyte-rich
- Lymphocyte-depleted

Nodular lymphocyte-predominant Hodgkin lymphoma

lymphocyte-predominant HL is differentiated from classic HL based on distinct pathologic and clinical features. The neoplastic cells in NLPHL are known as lymphocyte-predominant cells, or the so-called 'popcorn cells,' based on the characteristic appearance of the often-folded or multilobated nuclei. These cells differ immunophenotypically by expression of B-cell markers such as CD20, CD79a, BCL6, and CD45, but not CD15 and CD30 [19–21]. A nodular pattern is typical by morphology, and clonally rearranged immunoglobulin genes can be found at the molecular level [22]. Immunophenotyping is essential to differentiate subtypes of HL.

Non-Hodgkin Lymphoma

Non-Hodgkin lymphomas (NHLs) are a biologically and clinically heterogeneous group of lymphoproliferative disorders. Each lymphoma subtype represents the clonal expansion of the development of a specific lymphocyte lineage or sub-lineage, such as B-cell, T-cell, NK-cell, or rarely, histocytic/dendritic-cell origin. The natural history, prognosis and therapeutic approach for each depend on the specific subtype of lymphoma and the clinical stage, such that the diagnosis and accurate staging are quintessential to optimal management.

The Fourth Edition of the WHO Classification of Tumors of Hematopoietic and Lymphoid Tissues has greatly enhanced the earlier REAL classification to integrate morphologic, immunophenotypic, molecular genetic, and clinical features to define individual entities [12, 13]. NHLs are divided into precursor and mature B- or T/NK-cell categories (Table 40.2). More than 90% of NHLs seen in Western countries are of mature B-cell origin, with diffuse large B-cell (DLBCL) and follicular lymphoma being the most common subtypes. The incidence of NHL is lower among Asian populations, in whom T-cell neoplasms are more frequent. For clinical purposes, however, the NHLs are more broadly separated into indolent or aggressive categories. While localized indolent lymphomas may be potentially curable with localized radiotherapy [23–26], advanced indolent lymphomas are generally incurable with the standard therapeutic approaches, and tend to have a chronic course with repeated relapses and progression.

Table 40.2 Classification of non-Hodgkin lymphoma.

B-cell lymphomas	T-cell lymphomas
Precursor B-cell	**Precursor T-cell neoplasm**
• B-lymphoblastic leukemia/lymphoma, NOS	• T-lymphoblastic leukemia/lymphoma
Mature B-cell neoplasms	**Mature T-cell neoplasms**
Very aggressive lymphomas	*Aggressive lymphomas*
• Burkitt's lymphoma/B-cell acute leukemia	• T-cell prolymphocytic leukemia
Aggressive lymphomas	• Aggressive NK-cell leukemia
• Diffuse large B-cell lymphoma	• Peripheral T-cell lymphoma, NOS
• Primary DLBCL of the CNS	• Angioimmunoblastic T-cell lymphoma
• Primary cutaneous DLBCL, leg type	• Anaplastic large-cell lymphoma, ALK$^+$
• EBV-positive DLBCL of the elderly	• Anaplastic large-cell lymphoma, ALK$^-$
• Primary mediastinal large B-cell lymphoma	• Extranodal NK/T-cell lymphoma, nasal type
• Intravascular large B-cell lymphoma	• Enteropathy-type T-cell lymphoma
• Lymphomatoid granulomatosis	• Hepatosplenic T-cell lymphoma
• ALK-positive large B-cell lymphoma	• Subcutaneous panniculitis-like T-cell lymphoma
• Plasmablastic lymphoma	• Adult T-cell leukemia/lymphoma
• HHV-8-associated multi-centricentric Castleman disease	• Primary cutaneous T-cell lymphoma
• Primary effusion lymphoma	
Borderline cases	
• B-cell lymphoma, with features indeterminate between DLBCL and Burkitt's lymphoma	
• Mantle cell lymphoma	
Indolent B-cell lymphomas	**Indolent T-cell lymphomas**
• Follicular lymphoma	• T-cell large granular lymphocytic leukemia
• Primary cutaneous follicle center lymphoma	• Chronic lymphoproliferative disorders of NK cells
• Extranodal marginal zone lymphoma of mucosa-associated lymphoid tissue (MALT)	• Mycosis fungoides
• Nodal marginal zone lymphoma	• Sezary syndrome
• Splenic marginal zone lymphoma	• Primary cutaneous CD30+ T cell lymphoproliferative disorder
• Splenic B-cell lymphoma/leukemia, unclassifiable	• Primary cutaneous CD4+ small/medium T-cell lymphoma
• Lymphoplasmacytic lymphoma	
• Heavy chain disease	
• Plasma cell neoplasms	
• CLL/SLL	
• B-cell prolymphocytic leukemia	
• Hairy cell leukemia	

The median survival of these NHLs is usually eight to 10 years, but commonly exceeds 15–20 years [27–29]. Aggressive lymphomas are potentially curable with combination chemotherapy, and more often have an acute presentation and more rapid progression than indolent lymphomas [30, 31].

Staging and Risk Stratification

Staging procedures define the anatomic extent of the disease and include a careful physical examination for lymphadenopathy and organomegaly, and computed tomography (CT) scans of the neck, chest, abdomen, and pelvis. Bone marrow aspiration and biopsy are routinely performed but may not be needed if a positron-emission tomography (PET) scan shows homogenous activity in the marrow. 18-Fluoro-deoxy-glucose positron-emission tomography (^{18}F-FDG-PET), with or without CT, has excellent sensitivity and is useful both in diagnosis and for assessing response to treatment. Staging laparotomy, splenectomy, and bipedal lymphangiograms are no longer performed in HL management.

The Ann Arbor Staging System (Table 40.3) has commonly been used to describe the disease extent in HL [32]. Patients are further stratified as to the absence (A) or presence (B) of systemic symptoms, and the presence of bulky disease (X), as defined by a node or nodal mass

Table 40.3 Ann Arbor staging system.

Stage	Definition
I	Involvement of a single lymph node or of a single extranodal* organ or site (IE).
II	Involvement of two or more lymph node regions on the same side of the diaphragm, or localized involvement of an extranodal site or organ (IIE) and one or more lymph node regions on the same side of the diaphragm.
III	Involvement of lymph node regions on both sides of the diaphragm, which may also be accompanied by localized involvement of an extranodal organ or site (IIIE) or spleen (IIIS) or both (IIISE).
IV	Diffuse or disseminated involvement of one or more distant extranodal organs with or without associated lymph node involvement. Fever >38.0 °C, night sweats, and/or weight loss >10% of body weight during the six months preceding diagnosis are defined as systemic (B) symptoms.

greater than 6.5 cm in diameter, or greater than one-third the internal transverse diameter of the thorax. This staging system represents a means to simplify the complex process by which HL spreads and disseminates via a contiguous process to adjacent lymph nodes via connecting lymphatic channels.

Hodgkin Lymphoma

Once a stage has been determined, patients can be categorized into early-stage (I–II) or advanced-stage (III–IV) disease. These prognostic groups allow for the identification of a group of patients at high risk for first relapse and who might benefit from more intensive initial therapy. The identification of several clinical features has allowed for further stratification of patients with early-stage disease into favorable or unfavorable prognostic groups. This stratification has led to the reduction of chemotherapy and radiation therapy, particularly in patients with favorable early-stage disease.

The European Organization for the Research and Treatment of Cancer (EORTC) clinical trials, along with trials from the Princess Margaret Hospital and the German Hodgkin's Study Group (GHSG), have contributed to a better understanding of specific prognostic factors associated with clinical stage I–II disease [33–36]. These trials stratified patients with early-stage disease into favorable or unfavorable prognostic groups based on the presence or absence of several clinical features (Table 40.4) [37]. These factors can help to predict prognosis, but also aid in determining clinical management.

The heterogeneity of clinical outcomes seen in patients with advanced-stage (III–IV) disease demonstrates that advanced-stage disease has a variable prognosis. The International Prognostic Score (IPS) was developed as a means to incorporate clinical features to further stratify advanced-stage disease and estimate five-year freedom from progression and rates of overall survival (OS) (Table 40.5) [38].

Table 40.4 Adverse prognostic factors in Hodgkin lymphoma.

Early-stage	Advanced-stage (IPS)
Includes any one of the following factors:	One point for each:
Bulky adenopathy*	Serum albumin <4 g dl^{-1}
Involvement of four or more lymphnode regions**	Hemoglobin <10.5 g dl^{-1}
	Male gender
Age >50 years at diagnosis**	Age >45 years
B symptoms + ESR	Stage IV disease
>30 mm h^{-1}	White blood count
	$\geq 15\,000$ mm^{-3}
Absence of B symptoms +	Absolute lymphocyte count
ESR >50 mm h^{-1}	<600 mm^{-3} and/or $<8\%$
	of total white cell count

*Defined as a ratio of the maximum width of the mass and the maximum intrathoracic diameter greater than 0.33, or any single node or nodal mass ≥ 10 cm in diameter
**The German Hodgkin's Study Group trials did not define age as an adverse factor, and involvement of three or more lymph node regions is an adverse factor.
IPS, International Prognostic Score; ESR, erythrocyte sedimentation rate.

Table 40.5 International prognostic score for Hodgkin lymphoma.

Score	5-year FFP (%)	5-year OS (%)
0	84	89
1	77	90
2	67	81
3	60	78
4	51	61
5 or more	42	56

FFP, freedom from progression; OS, overall survival.

Non-Hodgkin Lymphoma

Staging procedures in NHLs define the anatomic extent of disease. The diagnostic work-up employs the use of a careful physical examination for the presence of lymphadenopathy and organomegaly; CT scans of the neck, chest, abdomen and pelvis; and a PET scan. In most instances, if a PET-CT scan displays a homogenous pattern of marrow uptake, a bone marrow biopsy is not required. If there are multifocal skeletal PET-CT lesions, marrow involvement may be assumed. CT or magnetic resonance imaging (MRI) of the brain and evaluation of the cerebrospinal fluid are indicated in patients with Burkitt or lymphoblastic lymphomas, and are frequently included in the evaluation of patients with aggressive histology lymphoma involving the bone marrow, paraspinal or sinonasal regions, or testis. The Ann Arbor staging system, commonly used for HL, has several limitations when applied to NHL because of the known hematogenous spread of disease and involvement of non-contiguous lymph node sites. In order to fully incorporate additional relevant prognostic features of NHL, prognostic models have been developed for the most common NHLs, that is, DLBCL, follicular, and mantle cell lymphoma.

The International Prognostic Index (IPI) is the most widely used clinical prognostic model used to stratify patients with aggressive NHLs [39]. This model uses common risk factors as a means to estimate the prognosis in patients with NHL (Table 40.6). As the majority of indolent lymphomas tend to fall into low-risk or low–intermediate-risk categories, a new index was developed specifically for follicular lymphoma called the Follicular Lymphoma International Prognostic Index (FLIPI) as a means to better stratify patients by risk [40]. The FLIPI incorporates more than five nodal sites and a hemoglobin level <10 g l^{-1} into the IPI system to better distribute patients with follicular lymphoma into good, intermediate-, or poor-risk categories. More recently, a prognostic index for mantle cell lymphoma (MCL),

Table 40.6 International prognostic index (IPI) for non-Hodgkin lymphoma.

Risk group	Risk factors*	Distribution of cases (%)	CR (%)	5-year OS (%)
Low	0–1	35	87	73
Low–Intermediate	2	27	67	51
High–Intermediate	3	22	55	43
High	4–5	16	44	26

*IPI risk factors are: age >60 years, LDH > normal, PS ≥ 2, stage III or IV, and more than one extranodal site.
CR, complete response; LDH, lactate dehydrogenase; OS, overall survival; PS, performance status.

the MCL International Prognostic Index (MIPI) has also been designed to facilitate risk-adapted treatment decisions in advanced-stage MCL [41].

Treatment of Hodgkin Lymphoma

Classical Hodgkin Lymphoma

Early-Stage, Favorable Risk

Favorable-risk HL patients have stage I–II disease in the absence of all unfavorable risk factors. These risk factors include: B symptoms, bulky mediastinal or greater than 10 cm disease, an erythrocyte sedimentation rate ≥50 mm h^{-1}, or more than three nodal sites of disease. The prognosis of patients with favorable early-stage HL is excellent, with a five-year OS of 95% [42]. The challenge thus remains to maintain high cure rates and minimize long-term toxicities of therapy, particularly given the young age of presentation of many patients with HL. With the exclusion of the historic staging laparotomy from current management, chemotherapy has become increasingly incorporated into the treatment of early-stage HL. Based on studies of chemotherapy in advanced HL, systemic treatment including doxorubicin, bleomycin, vinblastine and dacarbazine (ABVD) emerged as an ideal option for the treatment of early-stage HL due to its overall high efficacy and low toxicity [43–46].

The standard approach to the treatment of early-stage disease includes combined-modality therapy with short-course chemotherapy and involved site radiotherapy (ISRT). During the past three years, ISRT has replaced involved field radiotherapy (IFRT) in the radiotherapeutic management of all lymphomas. ISRT is defined as treating only the initially involved nodes and extra-nodal sites as defined by pretreatment evaluation (physical examination, imaging) with appropriate margins accounting for differences in anatomic positioning between images obtained at the time of diagnosis and at the time of treatment planning. The guiding principle behind ISRT is to decrease the size of treatment fields and to limit the dose to all adjacent uninvolved normal tissues as much as possible, with the goal of decreasing long-term side effects. This necessitates going beyond the traditional two-dimensional (2-D) anterior-posterior/posterior-anterior (AP/PA) fields historically used in the lymphoma and employing advanced treatment planning techniques that include but are not limited to fluence editing, intensity-modulated radiotherapy (IMRT), volumetric arc therapy (VMAT) or proton radiotherapy when appropriate, combined with appropriate motion management techniques such as respiratory gating and four-dimensional (4-D) treatment

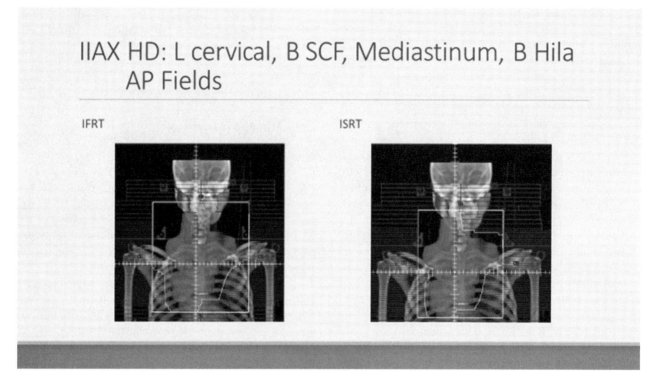

Figure 40.1 Stage IIAX nodular sclerosing Hodgkin's lymphoma. Left: IFRT (AP block). Right: ISRT (AP block). For a color version of this figure, see the color plate section.

planning and image-guided radiotherapy at treatment delivery (Figure 40.1).

An important caveat in early-stage disease is to further risk-stratify patients into those with favorable disease and those with unfavorable disease. In patients with favorable disease who fulfill the strict criteria of GSHG 10, it is feasible to de-intensify their therapy to two cycles of ABVD followed by ISRT to 20 Gy. In this trial, early-stage favorable patients with up to two sites of involvement, non-bulky disease and no B symptoms were randomized favorable risk early-stage patients to receive two versus Four cycles of ABVD and 20 versus 30 Gy IFRT [47]. With a median follow-up of 7.5 years, there were no significant differences between two versus four cycles of ABVD or 20 Gy versus 30 Gy in terms of five-year OS (97.1% versus 96.6%), freedom from treatment failure (93.0% versus 91.1%), or PFS (93.5% versus 91.2%).

Favorable patients who do not meet the criteria are recommended to be treated with four cycles of ABVD followed by ISRT to 20–30 Gy as long as they have a complete response by PET (Deauville score 1–3).

An alternate strategy in the early-stage favorable patients is to use the Stanford V regimen for eight weeks. ISRT to 30 Gy is incorporated as part of this regimen, which is based on the Stanford G4 study in which patients with early-stage non-bulky I/IIA patients were treated with eight weeks of the Stanford V regimen, followed by 30 Gy IFRT. At a median follow-up of 10.6 years,

the estimated 10-year freedom from progression and disease-free survival (DFS) was 94% and 99%, respectively, with an OS of 94% [48]. It is important to note that in this trial almost 50% of the patients would have been considered unfavorable by GHSG criteria, and approximately 38% had unfavorable features by EORTC criteria.

There are also multiple recent trials, including the UK RAPID NCRI trial and EORTC H10F, that have evaluated omitting radiotherapy in select early-stage favorable patients. In the UK RAPID trial, patients with early-stage favorable disease were treated with three cycles of ABVD. They were then restaged with a PET-CT. Those patients with either Deauville 1 or 2 score were then randomized to either IFRT or observation. At a median follow-up of 45.7 months, the estimated three-year PFS (in the intent-to-treat analysis) was 94.6% for those treated with IFRT compared to 90.8% for those who were observed. However, when accounting for as-treated patients, the three-year PFS was 97.1% in patients receiving radiotherapy compared to 90.7% for those receiving no further therapy. There was no difference in OS between the two groups. It was concluded that radiotherapy could be omitted in carefully selected favorable risk patients with a modest and acceptable decrease in their PFS [49].

The EORTC is currently conducting trials incorporating interim PET in the treatment paradigm. In the H10F trial, patients with early-stage favorable disease were treated with two cycles of ABVD, followed by re-staging

PET-CT. Patients in the standard arm then were to receive one additional cycle of ABVD followed by 30 Gy INRT, regardless of the response on PET. Patients in the experimental arm were assigned to two cycles of ABVD, and no further radiation if the interim PET was negative. If the interim PET was positive, however, the patients were switched to a more intensive chemotherapy regimen of two cycles of BEACOPP followed by INRT to 30 Gy. However, at interim analysis the experimental arm of PET-negative patients receiving two cycles of ABVD and no radiotherapy was closed due to an unexpectedly one-year PFS (94.9% versus 100% in the standard arm) [50].

Similarly, in the companion H10U trial, patients with unfavorable early-stage disease were treated with two cycles of ABVD followed by an interim PET. In the standard arm, patients received two additional cycles of ABVD followed by 30 Gy INRT, regardless of PET response. In the experimental arm, patients with a complete response on PET were treated with four additional cycles of ABVD (for a total of six cycles) and no radiation. The patients with a positive PET were switched to two cycles of escalated BEACOPP, followed by 30 Gy INRT. Again, at interim analysis there was a decrease in the one-year PFS in the no-radiation arm when compared to the standard arm (94.7% versus 97.3%). Subsequently, the no-radiation arms were closed in both HD10F and H10U trials. It was felt that omitting radiotherapy in early PET responders in stage I/II patients is associated with an increased risk of early relapse [50].

Hence, in the modern era of PET-based assessment of treatment response, as well as extremely conformal radiotherapy with ISRT, questions remain as to whether adjuvant radiation is needed in the early-stage favorable patients. Both, the UK RAPID trial and the interim results of the EORTC H10 trials showed that there is a decrease in PFS even in early responders when radiotherapy is omitted. However, it is important to note that, due to excellent salvage options, the ultimate OS is extremely favorable for this group of patients. Therefore, this treatment decision needs to be individualized for patients, taking into account the location of the disease, the potential risks of salvage therapy, and the risk of late toxicities from both radiation and chemotherapy. Patients with bulky disease, older patients, as well as those with an interim positive PET, are most likely to benefit from combined modality therapy.

Early-Stage, Unfavorable Risk

Stage I–II patients with bulky disease, B symptoms, and/or multiple involved nodal sites are classified as having unfavorable risk. Bulky disease is defined as having either: (i) a mediastinal mass with maximum width more than threefold the maximum intrathoracic diameter; or (ii) a conglomerate of lymph nodes measuring greater than 6.5 cm. Other unfavorable prognostic factors include an erythrocyte sedimentation rate $\geq$50 mm h^{-1}, or having more than one extranodal site involved. These patients are typically managed with more intensive combined modality therapy using chemotherapy and ISRT.

Multiple randomized trials have helped clarify standards for the treatment of early-stage unfavorable HL. The NCIC/ECOG trial found a significant difference in five-year freedom from disease progression (95% versus 88%), favoring combined modality therapy for stage IA–IIA patients with unfavorable risk factors [42]. Overall survival, however, was not significantly different. The EORTC-GELA H8-U study [51], which compared four versus six cycles of MOPP-ABV and IFRT versus STNI, found no significant differences in outcome. Therefore, four cycles of chemotherapy plus IFRT was recommended to be standard for this risk group.

In terms of comparing chemotherapy regimens, the EORTC H7 trial [52] found that MOPP-ABV was superior to EBVP, whereas the United Kingdom and German HD11 [53] studies found no advantage for Stanford V versus ABVD or BEACOPP versus ABVD, respectively. In comparing radiotherapy techniques, the German HD8 trial found no significant difference in OS or freedom from treatment failure when comparing IFRT versus EFRT in unfavorable HL patients receiving COPP-ABVD [54]. The German HD11 study [53] found that, in the setting of four cycles of ABVD, five-year freedom from treatment failure was superior with 30 Gy compared to 20 Gy. The five-year PFS in the best arm of the German HD11 study was 87.2%. More recently, the German HD14 study evaluated ABVD × four cycles followed by 30 Gy IFRT to a hybrid chemotherapy regimen of two cycles of ABVD and two cycles of escalated BEACOPP, followed by 30 Gy IFRT. This intensification of chemotherapy in the experimental arm resulted in an improved five-year freedom from treatment failure (FFTF) of 94.8% versus 87.7% [55].

The current generation of GHSG and EORTC trials in Europe have incorporated a hybrid chemotherapy approach with ABVD and BEACOPP. The latter is either incorporated into the treatment paradigm up-front or added when the early interim PET after two cycles of ABVD shows persistent disease. In the US, the strategy has been to increase the number of cycles of ABVD from four to six.

Therefore, current options for the management of early-stage unfavorable disease include four cycles of ABVD followed by 30 Gy ISRT, six cycles of ABVD followed by 30 Gy ISRT, Stanford V regimen × 12 weeks followed by 30 Gy ISRT, or a hybrid two cycles of ABVD and two cycles of BEACOPP followed by 30 Gy ISRT. Newer trials such as the EORTC H10U, which incorporate an interim PET after two cycles of chemotherapy, will help answer whether treatment intensification is needed

Table 40.7 Chemotherapy regimens for Hodgkin lymphoma.

ABVD – 1 cycle every four weeks
Doxorubicin – 25 mg m^{-2} IV days 1, 15
Bleomycin – 10 IU m^{-2} IV days 1, 15
Vinblastine – 6 mg m^{-2} IV days 1, 15
Dacarabazine – 375 mg m^{-2} IV days 1, 15

MOPP – 1 cycle given every 4 weeks for six cycles
Mechlorethamine – 6 mg m^{-2} IV, days 1, 8
Vincristine – 1.4 mg m^{-2} IV, days 1, 8
Procarbazine – 100 mg m^{-2} PO, days 1-14
Prednisone – 40 mg m^{-2} PO, days 1-14

MOPP/ABVD
MOPP and ABVD alternated every 28 days

MOPP/ABV hybrid
MOPP and ABV alternating within each treatment cycle

Stanford V (12-week regimen) 1 cycle given every 4 weeks for 3 cycles
Mechlorethamine – 6 mg m^{-2} IV, day 1
Doxorubicin – 25 mg m^{-2} IV, days 1, 15
Vinblastine – 6 mg m^{-2} IV, days 1, 15
Vincristine – 1.4 mg m^{-2} IV, days 8, 22
Bleomycin – 5 mg m^{-2} IV, days 8, 22
Etoposide – 60 mg m^{-2} IV, days 15, 16
Prednisone – 40 mg PO every other day × 10 weeks, then taper weeks 10–12
Plus irradiation 36 Gy to initial sites of disease ≥5 cm

BEACOPP – 1 cycle every 3 weeks
Bleomycin – 10 IU m^{-2} IV day 8
Etoposide – 100 mg m^{-2}/day IV, days 1-3
Doxorubicin – 25 mg m^{-2} IV, day 1
Cyclophosphamide – 650 mg m^{-2} IV, day 1
Vincristine – 1.4 mg m^{-2} IV, day 8
Procarbazine – 100 mg m^{-2} PO, days 1–7
Prednisone – 40 mg m^{-2}, days 1–7
Plus irradiation to initial sites of disease

IV, intravenous; PO, per os (oral).

for all early-stage unfavorable patients or can be limited to those who have persistent disease after the initial two cycles of chemotherapy.

Advanced Stage

Patients with B-symptoms, bulky disease, or stage III or IV disease require more intensive and extended chemotherapy (Table 40.7). Combined-modality therapy is an effective treatment option for patients with large mediastinal masses. The original regimen successfully used to treat HL was MOPP, with a response rate of 84% and a 66% DFS of more than 10 years from the end of treatment [45]. However, MOPP was found to be associated with a loss of fertility and myelodysplasia (MDS), in addition to other long-term toxicities and has fallen out of favor.

Ultimately, several studies showed that multidrug regimens, including alternating or hybrid regimens, in patients with advanced HL were more toxic and resulted in poorer outcomes than in those patients treated with ABVD [44–46]. ABVD has since become the standard treatment option for patients with advanced-stage HL, although Stanford V and BEACOPP are also used (Table 40.7). A risk-adapted approach using BEACOPP to treat advanced-stage disease with high-risk features with an IPS score of four or more has more recently been implemented in clinical practice.

The EORTC conducted a randomized trial to assess the role of radiotherapy in patients with advanced HL treated with MOPP-ABV [56]. Patients with a complete response to chemotherapy were randomized to 24 Gy IFRT versus no further therapy. All patients with a less-than-complete response received 30 Gy IFRT. For complete responders, there was no significant difference in event-free survival or OS with radiotherapy. The five-year event-free survival and OS in partial responders were 79% and 87%, respectively. Therefore, the role of adjuvant radiotherapy in advanced HL is reserved for consolidating bulky or poorly responding sites of disease.

Response Assessment

The Deauville five-point scale is an internationally recommended scale for routine and clinical trials using FDG-PET-CT in the initial staging, and the assessment of treatment response in Hodgkin lymphoma and certain subtypes of non-Hodgkin lymphoma. This scale is based on a visual interpretation of FDG-uptake, using two reference points of the individual patient which have demonstrated relatively constant uptake on serial imaging, namely the mediastinum and the liver. The scale ranges from 1 to 5, whereby each FDG-avid lesion is rated independently, providing a score to discriminate between positive and negative test results (Figure 40.2) [57].

Post-Treatment Assessment and Surveillance

In order to assess treatment response, a PET-CT is recommended one month after finishing chemotherapy

Deauville Criteria

- Score 1 no uptake
- Score 2 uptake ≤ mediastinum
- Score 3 uptake > mediastinum but ≤ liver
- Score 4 uptake > liver at any site
- Score 5 uptake > liver and new sites of disease
- *Score X: new areas of uptake unlikely to be related to lymphoma*

Figure 40.2 Deauville criteria.

in those patients who do not receive radiotherapy, or at three to six months after completion of radiotherapy in those who do receive it. A bone marrow biopsy is also repeated after treatment in those patients who had bone marrow involvement at the initial diagnosis, or in those with persistently abnormal blood counts. A tissue biopsy is required to establish the presence or absence of active disease in unusual or highly suspicious lesions detected by PET-CT in cases of progressive disease or relapse before proceeding with further salvage therapy. The follow-up schedule is individualized, depending on the clinical circumstances, including the patient's age, stage of disease, and initial treatment modality used.

Long-term morbidity has been of great concern, as patients cured of their disease during the 1970s and 1980s developed a high rate of late toxicity and death from causes other than HL. The historical use of large-volume radiation therapy was eventually associated with significant delayed toxicities among long-term survivors which included second cancers, heart disease, and endocrine dysfunction. Improvements in radiotherapy and the evolution of combined radiotherapy and chemotherapy have shown substantial reductions in the incidence of late effects. Multiple series have been conducted in pediatric Hodgkin patients demonstrating the risk of delayed cardiac complications to be correlated to cumulative dose of anthracyclines, sex of the patient, age at treatment, as well as the volume of the heart in the radiation portal and the mean heart dose [58].

Secondary malignancies are the leading cause of morbidity and mortality among long-term survivors of HL, primarily related to radiation therapy. There is an 18.5-fold increased risk when compared with the general population, with a cumulative incidence of 11% at 20 years and 26% at 30 years [59]. Chemotherapy-related myelodysplasia and acute myelogenous leukemia occur within 10 years of treatment, and are more likely to be caused by alkylating chemotherapeutic agents. The risk of this has decreased overall however, as the use of MOPP and BEACOPP have fallen out of favor.

Secondary solid tumors are frequently attributed to prior radiation, the majority of which occur within or on the border of the prior radiation field. These commonly include breast, lung, gastrointestinal or thyroid carcinomas, and bone or soft-tissue sarcomas. Cardiovascular disease is common in those who undergo mediastinal irradiation and anthracycline-based chemotherapy [60–62]. Both of these toxicities appear to be related to the patient age at the treatment, and the volume of tissue in the radiation volume. Hence, with ISRT considerable care is taken to limit the radiation to involved sites of disease only, and to maximize sparing of the heart. A baseline stress test or echocardiogram at 10 years after treatment, in addition to blood pressure monitoring, is generally recommended. Pulmonary toxicity, a well-documented

consequence of bleomycin use, is of particular concern in older patients with a prior history of pulmonary irradiation or lung disease [63, 64]. Abnormal thyroid function – most commonly hypothyroidism – is reported in long-term survivors who received neck or upper mediastinal irradiation [65]. Thyroid function tests are recommended annually, particularly in those patients who received radiotherapy to the neck.

Relapsed/Refractory Disease

The approach to patients with relapsed HL depends on the primary therapy and duration of initial remission. Those patients treated with irradiation alone for early-stage disease are generally chemotherapy-sensitive at relapse, and 50–80% will achieve long-term DFS with standard chemotherapy. The majority of patients, however, will have received chemotherapy as part of their initial therapy. Poor prognostic signs in patients who relapse includes: relapse within 12 months of treatment; advanced stage; relapse in extranodal sites; relapse in previously irradiated sites; and the presence of B-symptoms. Patients with these risk factors or those who relapse less than 12 months after completion of initial chemotherapy should be considered for high-dose chemotherapy with autologous stem cell rescue (HDT/ASCT).

Further cytoreduction is often appropriate for patients with relapsed/refractory disease. Brentuximab vedotin, a CD30-directed antibody–drug conjugate, has demonstrated activity in patients with relapsed or refractory CD30-positive lymphomas [66]. A Phase II multicenter study of patients with relapsed or refractory HL after HDT/ASCT showed that brentuximab vedotin could induce objective responses and complete responses in 75% and 34% of patients, respectively, with a median follow-up of nine months [67]. These data ultimately led to approval by the FDA for its use in the treatment of patients with HL after failure of HDT/ASCT or at least two prior chemotherapy regimens, regardless of eligibility for HDT/ASCT.

Several retrospective studies have investigated the role of radiotherapy in the setting of HDT/ASCT. Generally, most have found higher rates of locoregional control and DFS, without a definite impact on survival [60]. Although radiotherapy is not commonly used in the setting of relapsed/refractory HL, ISRT with 30–36 Gy may be used prior to transplantation in order to consolidate large or poorly responsive sites of disease.

Hematopoietic Stem Cell Transplantation

For patients with HL whose disease is refractory to primary therapy, or which relapses shortly after an initial response (<12 months), follow-up standard-dose chemotherapy is unlikely to be beneficial. HDT/ASCT has shown significant improvement in event-free survival, PFS, and freedom from treatment failure, when compared to conventional chemotherapy, although without any difference in OS [69, 70]. Patients receive a salvage regimen of chemotherapy prior to HDT/ASCT, and ultimately undergo transplantation with HDT regimens such as carmustine, etoposide, cytarabine and melphalan (BEAM) or cyclophosphamide, carmustine, and etoposide (CBV).

The Phase III randomized, placebo-controlled AETHERA trial evaluated the use of brentuximab vedotin as consolidation in the post-HDT/ASCT setting. The results demonstrated an improvement in median PFS of 42.9 months in treated patients compared to 24.1 months in the placebo group. There was no difference in OS between the two groups [71].

Studies have also evaluated the benefit of HDT/ASCT in first remission for patients with high-risk disease. Although a slightly lower risk of relapse was seen in the HDT/ASCT arm than in those randomized to receive standard chemotherapy, there was no difference in OS, suggesting that standard-dose chemotherapy is appropriate for high-risk patients.

Nodular Lymphocyte-Predominant Hodgkin Lymphoma

In contrast to classical HL, NLPHL has a more indolent course, characterized by late relapses. It most often presents as early-stage disease with favorable risk factors, and has a slightly better prognosis than classical HL [72, 73]. The favored treatment approach for early-stage non-bulky disease is ISRT alone, whereas combined modality treatment is used in advanced or unfavorable disease where ISRT appears to be equally efficacious compared to more intensive treatments [15, 74]. In the setting of advanced disease, chemotherapy (e.g., ABVD, R-CHOP, R-CVP), with consolidative radiotherapy to bulky sites, is recommended. As the majority of NLPHL expresses CD20, rituximab could also be considered, particularly for advanced disease [75].

Gray Zone Lymphoma

During recent years there has been recognition of tumors that demonstrate features intermediate between classical HL and DLBCL, and appear closely related to primary mediastinal large B-cell lymphoma [76]. These so-called 'gray zone' lymphomas stain strongly for CD20 and CD15 in a case otherwise resembling large B-cell lymphomas. They present more often in men and younger patients, and the clinical course may be refractory to standard therapies for HL, sometimes requiring chemotherapy regimens more commonly used in aggressive B-cell lymphomas [77].

Treatment of Non-Hodgkin Lymphoma

The approach to the treatment of NHL varies greatly among the subtypes, and this can include observation, radiation, or intensive chemotherapy. Observation is frequently recommended for indolent lymphomas, particularly in asymptomatic elderly patients. Radiation therapy, commonly employed alone or as part of a combined-modality therapy for the cure of localized disease, can also be used for palliation or local control of advanced incurable lymphoma. More intensive chemotherapy regimens are required for management of advanced low-grade, intermediate-grade, and aggressive lymphomas.

Indolent B-Cell Lymphomas

The most common subtype of indolent B-cell lymphoma is follicular lymphoma, which accounts for 20% of all lymphomas. Other subtypes include marginal zone lymphomas, including extranodal marginal zone lymphomas (previously referred to as MALT lymphomas), lymphoplasmacytic lymphoma, and CLL/SLL. These low-grade lymphomas follow an indolent course, permitting prolonged survivals, but are virtually incurable. The diverse therapeutic options for indolent lymphomas have become increasingly complex, such that the therapeutic goals and treatment algorithm must be carefully considered and discussed with the patient at diagnosis.

Follicular Lymphoma
Follicular lymphoma (FL) is derived from germinal center B cells, and is graded based on the number of centroblasts per high-power field: grade 1 (0–5); grade 2 (6–15); and grade 3 (>15). The tumor cells are classically CD20+, CD10+, BCL6+, BCL2+, and CD5-. The genetic hallmark of FL is characterized by a t(14;18)(q32;q21), resulting in constitutive overexpression of the bcl-2 protein, which impairs the normal germinal center apoptotic program [78, 79]. A number of variants of FL have been identified and include primary intestinal FL, extranodal FL, or primary cutaneous follicular center lymphoma.

Clinically, FL is often characterized by an indolent course, and many patients remain asymptomatic despite extended disease, such that many patients are frequently diagnosed at advanced stages III and IV [80]. For the 15–25% of FL patients diagnosed with localized, early-stage low-grade FL, the standard management is ISRT alone, due to the high radiosensitivity and potential for cure [81]. This strategy has resulted in a 10-year overall survival of 60–80%, with a median survival of approximately 15 years [25,82]. However, the majority of patients with stage I disease in the US do not receive radiation therapy [83]. Long-term data from Stanford indicates that deferred therapy is a reasonable option for selected patients, particularly those with asymptomatic disease.

Among a series of 43 patients with a median follow-up of 86 months, 63% remained untreated at a median of six years, and the 10-year OS was 85% [84].

In 2014, Hoskin and colleagues reported the results of a UK randomized trial (FORT) evaluating two different dose regimens in the management of indolent lymphomas [85]. Patients were randomized to either 24 Gy in 12 fractions versus 4 Gy in two fractions in this trial. Approximately half of the patients had FL, and 60% had early-stage disease. It showed that patients who received the more protracted regimen had a higher rate of any response (91% versus 48%) and a higher likelihood of a complete response (67% versus 48%).

An alternative approach includes the use of multi-modality therapy with chemotherapy and ISRT, although no randomized studies demonstrate an added benefit of chemotherapy in early-stage indolent NHL. The use of chemotherapy or immunotherapy alone may be appropriate for patients with stage II disease, particularly for disease located in the case that radiation therapy would be expected to result in significant morbidity. Ultimately, observation is a reasonable initial alternative if radiotherapy is not pursued, particularly in asymptomatic patients with non-threatening disease. Prospective randomized trials are comparing the different treatment options including rituximab followed by radiotherapy, immunochemotherapy followed by radiotherapy, or single-agent rituximab evaluating a variety of different administration schedules [86–89].

Conventional therapies are not generally considered curative for the 70–85% of patients who present with advanced-stage FL. Although lengthy remissions are frequently achievable, repeated relapses and eventual progression are the norm. Standard treatment therefore focuses on the palliation of symptoms and improvement in quality of life. Asymptomatic patients can generally be observed initially, as no clear survival benefit has been seen in initiating chemotherapy in these patients with non-threatening disease, and prospective randomized studies demonstrated that cytostatic therapy could be safely delayed until treatment became necessary without any negative impact on the patients' outcome [90,91]. However, an increasing number of therapeutic options have become available for the management of both initial disease and progression or relapse.

A variety of combination chemotherapy options have been considered for the treatment of advanced-stage FL, with the combination of rituximab with cyclophosphamide, doxorubicin, vincristine, and prednisone (CHOP) being the standard of care (Table 40.8). Prospective, randomized studies have uniformly demonstrated a significant increase in response rates, PFS and particularly OS when comparing rituximab-chemotherapy with chemotherapy alone [92–94]. Modern R-chemotherapeutic regimens have resulted in

overall response rates of more than 90%, with complete responses in the range of 20% to 60% with subsequent periods of median PFS exceeding four to five years.

Randomized prospective studies, including the PRIMA study, have also suggested a beneficial effect of rituximab maintenance in patients with untreated and relapsed FL, after treatment with initial chemotherapy. A benefit of rituximab maintenance was seen across all ages and the Follicular Lymphoma International Prognostic Index (FLIPI) risk groups, and leads to a further increase in the rate of compete responses at the end of the two-year maintenance [89–92]. Rituximab maintenance following successful initial R-chemotherapy is broadly considered a standard for first-line therapy of patients with advanced-stage FL, although increased expense and toxicity remain important considerations with this strategy.

With regards to immunotherapy, radioimmunoconjugates (e.g., ibritumomab tiuxetan, tositumomab) have also demonstrated efficacy in relapsed or refractory FL [99]. This strategy is a viable option for patients with minimal bone marrow involvement and non-bulky disease. Several prospective trials have investigated the use of these agents in previously untreated patients receiving chemotherapy without rituximab, but no difference has been seen in outcomes when compared to immunochemotherapeutic approaches [100].

Future approaches to the treatment of FL includes: new monoclonal CD20 antibodies; other B-lineage antigen-directed antibodies such as CD22 or bispecific T-cell-engaging antibodies targeting CD19 and CD3, such as blinatumomab; drugs targeting oncogeneic pathways, such as the PI3K/Akt/mTOR pathway; Bcl 2 inhibitors; and immunomodulatory drugs such as lenalidomide.

Tumor Vaccine Strategies

Each B cell expresses a unique immunoglobulin molecule that expresses a specific recombination gene sequence known as the idiotype. The clonal proliferation of lymphocytes in lymphomas presents a unique idiotype for each patient. This observation led to studies exploring the active immunization of patients against their own tumor idiotype. Early testing of this approach in follicular lymphoma suggested that the development of an anti-idiotype response could be beneficial, but Phase III studies produced mixed results [101, 102]. Long-term data however may show a role for active immunization in the post-transplant setting of immune reconstitution for patients who undergo ASCT [103].

Marginal Zone Lymphomas

The WHO classification separates marginal zone B-cell lymphomas (MZL) into three distinct diseases that have been classically categorized together because they appear to arise from post-germinal center marginal zone B cells:

Table 40.8 Chemotherapy combinations used in the treatment of non-Hodgkin lymphomas.

Newly diagnosed patients	Relapsed and refractory patients
CHOP – every 3 weeks, 6–8 cycles Cyclophosphamide – 750 mg m² IV, day 1 Doxorubicin – 50 mg m² IV, day 1 Vincristine – 1.4 mg m² IV, day 1 Prednisone – 100 mg m² PO, days 1–5 +/– Rituximab – 375 mg m² IV, day 1	*ICE* – every 2 weeks, 3 cycles Ifosfamide – 5000 mg m² IV, day 2 Carboplatin – AUC 5 IV, day 2 Etoposide – 100 mg m² IV, days 1–3 ± Rituximab – 375 mg m² IV, day 1
CVP – every 3 weeks, 6–8 cycles Cyclophosphamide – 750 mg m² IV, day 1 Vincristine – 1.4 mg m² IV, day 1 Prednisone – 40 mg m² PO, days 1–5 ±-Rituximab – 375 mg m² IV, day 1	*DHAP* – every 3–4 weeks, 3–4 cycles Dexamethasone – 40 mg PO, days 1–4 Cytarabine – 2000 mg m² IV, day 2 Cisplatin – 100 mg m² IV, day 1
Rituximab – 375 mg m² IV weekly × 4 weeks *Can be repeated as maintenance therapy every 2 or 6 months*	*GDP* – every 3 weeks, 3–4 cycles Dexamethasone – 20–40 mg PO, days 1–3 Gemcitabine – 1000 mg m² IV, days 1, 8 Cisplatin – 25 mg m² IV, days 1–3 ± Rituximab – 375 mg m² IV, day 1
Hyper-CVAD/MTX-Ara-C Cycle 1, 3, 5, 7 (3–4 weeks/cycle) Cyclophosphamide 300 mg m² IV q12 h × 6 doses days 1–3 Cisplatin – 25 mg m² IV, days 1–4 Doxorubicin 50 mg m² IV, day 4 Dexamethasone 40 mg m² PO days 1–4, 11–14	*ESHAP* – every 3–4 weeks, 6–8 cycles Etoposide – 40 mg m² IV, days 1–4 Methylprednisolone – 500 mg IV, days 1–5 Cytarabine – 2000 mg m² IV, day 5 Vincristine 2 mg m² IV, days 4, 11
EPOCH – every 3 weeks, 6–8 cycles Etoposide – 50 mg m², days 1–4 Vincristine – 0.4 mg m² IV, days 1–4 Doxorubicin – 10 mg m² IV, days 1–4 Cyclophosphamide – 750 mg m² IV, day 5 Prednisone – 60 mg m² PO, days 1–5 ± Rituximab – 375 mg m² IV, day 1	*EPOCH* – every 3 weeks, 6–8 cycles Etoposide – 50 mg m² IV, days 1–4 Vincristine – 0.4 mg m² IV, days 1–4 Doxorubicin – 10 mg m² IV, days 1–4 Cyclophosphamide – 750 mg m² IV, day 5 Prednisone – 60 mg m² PO, days 1–5 ± Rituximab – 375 mg m² IV, day 1
Hyper-CVAD/MTX-Ara-C Cycle 2, 4, 6, 8 (3–4 weeks/cycle) Methotrexate 1 g m⁻² IV, day 1 Cytarabine 3 g m⁻² IV q12 h × 4 doses, days 2–3 Leucovorin 50 mg IV q6 h, day 2 until MTX level <0.05 μM	*GemOx* – 1 cycle every 2 weeks × 8 cycles Gemcitabine – 1000 mg m² IV, day 2 Oxaliplatin – 100 mg m² IV, day 2 ± Rituximab – 375 mg m² IV, day 1

extranodal MZL of mucosa-associated lymphoid tissue (MALT); nodal MZL; and splenic MZL with or without villous lymphocytes. These disorders are characterized by an infiltrate of centrocyte-like small-cleaved cells, monocytoid B cells, or small lymphocytes, and may exhibit an expanded marginal zone surrounding lymphoid follicles. They share a common immunophenotype with CD20 expression but a lack of CD5 or CD10 expression, which helps to distinguish MZL from other indolent lymphomas.

Extranodal Lymphoma

MALT lymphomas account for 50–70% of all MZLs. They primarily occur in mucosal sites, commonly in gastric or intestinal sites as well as some non-mucosal sites including the lung, salivary gland, periorbital or soft tissue, skin, and thyroid. The typical presentation is an isolated mass in any of these sites, or an ulcerative lesion in the stomach. Clinically, they behave as an indolent lymphoma. MALT lymphomas are characterized by t(11;18)(q21;q21) translocations in approximately 40% of cases, and present as somatically mutated IGHV genes. Increasing evidence suggests that extranodal MZL may be related to chronic immune stimulation, often due to bacterial or autoimmune stimuli. A common example of this includes the association of *H. pylori* infection in the majority of gastric MALT lymphoma cases, thought to arise as a result of chronic stimulation of the B and T cells in the stomach by *H. pylori*. Initial treatment of early-stage *H. pylori*-positive lymphomas includes *H. pylori* eradication therapy. Patients without evidence of *H. pylori* infection that demonstrate the t(11;18) translocation are typically treated with primary radiotherapy, as this has been highly effective in producing disease-free survival or PFS rates of >80% at five and 10 years [104, 105].

Non-gastric MALT lymphomas usually have an indolent course, and treatment approaches depend largely on the stage and site of primary involvement. Patients with limited stage (I–II) disease are typically treated with locoregional radiotherapy alone with 24–30 Gy, with expected control rates exceeding 90%. More than one-third of patients with non-gastric MALT will have advanced disease at the time of diagnosis, for which immunotherapy or chemoimmunotherapy can be used in a similar fashion to FL.

Nodal Marginal Zone Lymphoma

Nodal MZL is a primary nodal lymphoma with features identical to lymph nodes involved by extranodal MALT, but without evidence of extranodal or splenic disease, or t(11;18) karyotypic changes. It accounts for nearly 10% of patients with MZL. There is no general consensus regarding the treatment of nodal MZL, and most data derives from retrospective studies and extrapolation from other common indolent lymphomas. Treatment generally follows guidelines for FL and MZL, and is chosen based on the extent of disease and comorbidities of the patient.

Splenic Marginal Zone Lymphoma

Splenic MZLs are rare and tend to occur in the elderly. Patients commonly present with splenomegaly in the absence of peripheral node involvement. Evaluation commonly reveals mesenteric or hepatic involvement, and the bone marrow and blood are typically involved. Patients with splenic MZL demonstrate an indolent course, with a median survival of approximately 10 years. Most patients with SMZL can initially be managed with a 'wait-and-see' strategy, and treatment is directed at those with symptomatic massive splenomegaly or cytopenias. Historically, splenectomy has been the preferred treatment option for symptomatic patients or in the case of cytopenias not felt to be related to bone marrow infiltration. Alternatively, single-agent rituximab can result in the disappearance of splenomegaly and normalization of absolute lymphocyte counts in more than 90% of patients. As some cases have been associated with hepatitis C infection, similar responses have been seen with clearance of the virus alone.

Chronic Lymphocytic Leukemia/Small Lymphocytic Lymphoma

B-cell chronic lymphocytic leukemia (CLL) is a lymphoproliferative disorder manifested by a clonal expansion of mature, monomorphic, small B lymphocytes. The disease is identical to small lymphocytic lymphoma (SLL) but is distinguished by whether the leukemic or nodal components of the disease predominate, respectively. The clinical course of this malignant disease can be quite variable due to the diverse complications that are associated with it. The immunophenotype expresses CD 5, CD19, CD20

and CD23, whereas FMC7, CD10 and cyclin D1 are negative. Cytogenetic abnormalities are common in approximately 80% of CLL cases with the use of fluorescence in-situ hybridization (FISH). A deletion in chromosome 13 at band q14 is the most common abnormality, followed by a deletion in chromosome 11 at q22-23. Karyotypic abnormalities have been shown to be of prognostic value as an isolated finding of del13q is associated with a favorable prognosis, whereas the presence of del(17p13.1) or del(11q22.3) confers a poor prognosis with regards to disease course and overall survival [106, 107].

Observation continues to be the mainstay for patients with early-stage CLL. Patients with stage I or stage II SLL can be treated with primary radiotherapy, producing 10-year freedom from relapse rates of 80% and 62%, respectively. For patients with symptomatic CLL or advanced SLL, systemic therapy is indicated. Whereas alkylating agents had historically been used for therapy, combination chemoimmunotherapy regimens have become much more widely implemented. The use of single-agent chlorambucil was traditionally used as it produced symptomatic improvement but only a 3–5% complete response rate without a survival advantage. This therapy is still used for elderly patients due to its tolerability. Fludarabine has gained the widest use, with complete response rates of 15–30%. Ultimately, modern treatment options include purine analogs (fludarabine, pentostatin), alkylating agents (chlorambucil, bendamustine), monoclonal antibodies (rituximab, alemtuzumab), or a combination of these agents. The combination of fludarabine, cyclophosphamide and rituximab in previously untreated patients has produced high overall response and complete response rates of 95% and 70%, respectively, and is commonly used as first-line therapy for appropriate patients [108, 109]. The introduction of novel therapies in the first-line and relapsed settings has extended treatment options to frail or chemo-ineligible patients. New anti-CD20 antibodies such as obinutuzumab and ofatumumab, the anti-CD52 monoclonal antibody alemtuzumab, and also ibrutinib (an irreversible inhibitor of BTK) have all been introduced as options in the front line setting [110–113].

Lymphoplasmacytic Lymphoma

Lymphoplasmacytic lymphoma is an indolent neoplasm of small B lymphocytes, plasmacytoid lymphocytes, and plasma cells. Symptoms may be due to tumor infiltration in the marrow, spleen, liver or lymph nodes, circulating IgM macroglobulin, and tissue deposition of IgM or other proteins. The consequences of such include: hyperviscosity; cryoglobulinemia; cold agglutinin hemolytic anemia; neuropathy; glomerular disease; amyloid; or coagulopathies. The approach to treatment is similar to that of other indolent lymphomas. More recently, bortezomib and ibrutinib have both been approved as additional treatment options.

Aggressive B-Cell Lymphomas

Aggressive B-cell lymphomas commonly present with acute symptoms and are frequently curable, but are associated with short survival times in the absence of achieving a complete response with therapy. Diffuse large B-cell lymphoma (DLBCL) is the most common subtype of aggressive NHL, constituting 25–30% of all NHLs. These tumors commonly present with both nodal and extranodal involvement.

Diffuse Large B-Cell Lymphoma

DLBCL comprises a heterogeneous group of tumors with distinct molecular features. The immunophenotype commonly expressed CD20 and CD19, although it may also express CD10, BCL6, and IRF4/MUM1. Two distinct molecular subtypes – germinal center origin (GCB) and activated B-cell origin (ABC) based on gene expression profiles – have emerged. These two subtypes have distinct prognostic implications and will be important in developing risk-adapted treatment strategies in the future. The germinal center subtype resembles a normal germinal center B cell GCB and frequently demonstrates t(14;18) translocations. These GCB DLBCLs have a more favorable prognosis with current treatment options. The activated B-cell ABC group is most likely derived from a post-germinal center B cell, and has a gene expression profile that resembles an activated B cell. It is associated with a poorer prognosis.

The initial treatment of DLBCL is dependent on the histologic subtype, stage, risk factors (e.g., bulky and/or extranodal disease) and performance status (see Table 40.6). Patients with favorable risk have stage IA–IIA non-bulky disease, and are generally treated with combined-modality therapy consisting of abbreviated systemic chemotherapy, rituximab, and IFRT. The SWOG study randomized patients with localized intermediate and high-grade NHL to eight cycles of CHOP versus three cycles of CHOP plus IFRT. At five years, OS was significantly better in the arm receiving three cycles of CHOP plus IFRT (82% versus 72%) [114]. With a longer follow-up, however, differences in relapse-free survival and OS were non-significant, due to late relapses and lymphoma deaths in the arm receiving three cycles of CHOP and IFRT [115]. Further analysis showed that in patients with an IPI score of 0–1 who received IFRT, the five-year OS was 82% versus 71% in patients with IPI score 2, and 48% in those with IPI score 3. Hence, the loss of significance in PFS and OS in the trial at longer follow-up was likely due to delayed failures in the higher-IPI score patients.

The ECOG study randomized early-stage NHL patients following eight cycles of CHOP to 30 Gy IFRT versus no further therapy [116]. Disease-free survival at six years was improved in the arm receiving IFRT (73% versus 56%), but no survival difference was observed. GELA ran a similar trial in patients aged >60 years who were randomized following four cycles of CHOP to IFRT versus no further therapy [117]. The MabThera International Trial showed that the addition of rituximab to six cycles of CHOP (R-CHOP) increased both the six-year event-free survival (74% versus 56%) and OS (90% versus 80%) [118]. No significant difference in OS or DFS was observed with the addition of IFRT.

In 2014, the results of the RICOVER-60, a prospective trial evaluating six versus eight cycles of CHOP-14 with or without eight administrations of rituximab in elderly patients aged >60 years were published [119]. The best arm of this trial entailed patients receiving six cycles of R-CHOP-14 + two additional doses of rituximab. A cohort of these patients received adjuvant radiotherapy to sites of initial bulky (>7.5 cm) or extralymphatic disease. A total of 36 Gy was given in 18 fractions. The patients were then compared to a cohort who received the same chemotherapy regimen without adjuvant radiotherapy. Patients who received consolidation radiotherapy to sites of bulky disease had a statistically significant improvement in both PFS and OS.

The ongoing UNFOLDER trial evaluates the role of radiotherapy in the rituximab era [120]. Patients aged 18–60 years with early-stage disease (either IPI score 0 with bulky disease or IPI score 1) have been randomized to either R-CHOP-21 or R-CHOP-14 × six cycles, with or without radiotherapy. The interim results of this trial were presented in 2013. The three-year event-free survival was noted as 81% in patients who received radiotherapy versus 65% in those who did not receive radiotherapy. Hence, the no radiation arm was prematurely closed. The final results of this trial are pending.

Typically, radiation doses of 36 Gy have been used in the setting of complete response to chemotherapy. However, based on the recently published randomized trial by Lowry and colleagues in 2011, patients with intermediate-grade lymphoma were randomized to 30 Gy versus 40 45 Gy [121]. The majority of these patients had DLBCL and had received prior chemotherapy, with radiation used as consolidation therapy. There was no difference in PFS or OS between the two arms. Hence, 30 Gy after a complete response is reasonable.

Based on the results of these studies, the current standard approach for early-stage DLBCL involves R-CHOP × six cycles followed by ISRT. In patients with an IPI score of 0 or 1, a reduction in the chemotherapy to three or four cycles of R-CHOP can be considered.

The treatment of advanced-stage DLBCL primarily involves immunochemotherapy. With this approach, long-term DFS is approximately 40% [122]. Multiple regimens have been compared to CHOP, including: low-dose methotrexate with leucavorin rescue, bleomycin, doxorubicin, cyclophosphamide, vincristine, and dexamethasone (m-BACOD); prednisone, doxorubicin, cyclophosphamide, and etoposide, followed by cytarabine, bleomycin, vincristine, and methotrexate with leucavorin rescue (ProMACE-CytaBOM); and methotrexate with leucavorin rescue, doxorubicin, cyclophosphamide, vincristine, prednisone, and bleomycin (MACOP-B). These regimens showed promise, but ultimately CHOP has been found to yield equivalent outcomes with less toxicity [122, 123]. Rituximab has been shown as a means to sensitize otherwise resistant lymphoma cells to chemotherapy agents *in vitro*. In a randomized trial, R-CHOP was found to improve complete response rates, event-free survival, and OS compared to CHOP alone, making R-CHOP the current standard of care [124]. The optimal number of cycles of CHOP remains unclear. In practice, the number of cycles can either be defined independent of response, or based on response. Common practice includes six to eight cycles of R-CHOP. Maintenance rituximab does not appear to improve survival among patients who have completed initial therapy with R-CHOP [125]. Patients with relapse should receive a second-line chemotherapy regimen such as ICE, DHAP, EPOCH, or ESHAP, followed by high-dose therapy with autologous stem cell rescue if chemotherapy-sensitive disease is demonstrated. ISRT with 30–40 Gy may be considered to consolidate active or bulky sites prior to transplant [126].

Primary Mediastinal Large B-Cell Lymphoma

Primary mediastinal large B-cell lymphoma (PMLBCL) is a specific subtype of DLBCL that was distinguished based on unique clinicopathologic characteristics. Patients are typically female, with a median age of 35 years, and present with a bulky anterior mediastinal mass. Distant spread, including bone marrow involvement, is uncommon at diagnosis. Histologically, PMLBCL is molecularly distinct from typical DLBCL but shares many molecular features with HL. Most patients with PMLBCL have BCL6 mutations along with somatic mutations in the IGVH, suggesting late-stage germinal center differentiation [127]. Treatment has historically been similar to that for DLBCL, with R-CHOP chemotherapy considered the standard therapy. More recently, it has been observed that adequate tumor control is frequently not achieved with standard immunochemotherapy, necessitating routine mediastinal radiotherapy [128, 129]. Unfortunately, involved radiotherapy without gating techniques has frequently been associated with serious late side effects and progressive disease in up to 20% of patients [130]. It is important to bear in mind, however, that these late effects have been demonstrated in patients who have either received EFRT or IFRT without modern respiratory gating or treatment planning techniques. More aggressive chemotherapy has been associated with improved outcomes, and dose-adjusted EPOCH-R has become the standard of care for PMLBCL as a strategy to obviate the need for radiotherapy. This is based on the findings of a Phase II single-arm study in which 51 patients with PMDLBCL were treated with six cycles of DA-EPOCH*-R without any radiotherapy. With a five-year median follow-up, the event-free survival was 93% and the OS was 97%. It was felt that radiotherapy could be safely omitted in these patients [131].

Burkitt Lymphoma

Burkitt lymphoma is a highly aggressive B cell neoplasm, with a rapid doubling time, acute onset, and progression of symptoms. It is characterized by the translocation and deregulation of the c-*myc* gene on chromosome 8. Most Burkitt lymphomas seen in the US are sporadic variants that may show evidence of Epstein–Barr virus infection in a minority of patients. Patients typically present with a bulky abdominal mass, and B-symptoms. Extranodal and bone marrow involvement occur in up to 70% of patients. CNS dissemination, usually manifesting as leptomeningeal involvement, may be present in up to 40% of patients. Therapy for Burkitt lymphoma must be initiated quickly due its aggressive clinical course, and prophylaxis against tumor lysis syndrome is essential due to rapid tumor cell death which can be associated with high morbidity and mortality.

Multi-agent chemotherapy, including high-dose alkylating agents with CNS prophylaxis, is the predominant treatment strategy. Many regimens employ ALL-like therapy (cyclophosphamide, vincristine, doxorubicin, and dexamethasone with or without rituximab, alternating with high-dose methotrexate and cytarabine [hyper-CVAD]) followed by high-dose chemotherapy and ASCT. Alternative approaches have used cyclophosphamide, vincristine, doxorubicin, and high-dose methotrexate (CODOX-M) with ifosfamide, cytarabine, etoposide, and intrathecal methotrexate (IVAC). Cranial radiotherapy historically has been administered to select patients, but presently there is no standard role for radiotherapy in the treatment of Burkitt lymphoma, even for localized disease.

B-Cell Lymphoma, Unclassifiable with Features Intermediate Between Diffuse Large B-Cell Lymphoma and Burkitt Lymphoma

B-cell lymphomas with features intermediate between DLBCL and Burkitt lymphoma are aggressive lymphomas that have morphological and genetic of both DLBCL and Burkitt lymphoma. An important subset of this aggressive large B-cell lymphoma includes the 'double-hit' lymphomas, with MYC and BCL2 and/or

BCL6 rearrangements identified based on cytogenetic testing. Immunohistochemical staining of MYC and BCL2 can also distinguish these 'double-expressor' lymphomas. The implication of these very aggressive neoplasms is that they do not respond well to therapy and are associated with a very poor prognosis [132, 133]. The appropriate treatment regimen for this subtype of lymphoma remains unclear, however. The current trend is to substitute R-CHOP with more intensive chemotherapy regimens such as R-DA*-EPOCH, followed by adjuvant ISRT.

Mantle Cell Lymphoma

Mantle cell lymphoma (MCL), although frequently discussed with indolent forms of NHL, more often behaves similarly to that of an aggressive lymphoma. Most patients present with advanced-stage disease with lymphadenopathy as the common presentation, while extranodal disease is seen in approximately 25% of cases. Common sites of involvement include lymph nodes, spleen, Waldeyer's ring, bone marrow, blood and extranodal sites such as the gastrointestinal tract. Virtually all MCLs carry t(11;14)(q13;q32) on karyotypic analysis or FISH, and the immunophenotype is typically CD5+, FMC+, and CD43+, but CD10-. Nuclear staining for cyclin D1 (BCL-1) is present in more than 90% of cases.

The majority of patients require treatment of MCL at the time of diagnosis. Combination chemotherapy remains the main treatment modality, as there is little role for surgery and radiation therapy is reserved for palliation. Two strategies are commonly employed for the treatment of MCL: conventional chemoimmunotherapy (R-CHOP or R-CVP) followed by autologous SCT; or intensive chemoimmunotherapy (R-hyper-CVAD). These approaches have not been directly compared prospectively, but non-randomized trials have suggested longer median OS rates with a more aggressive treatment approach, but associated with a higher incidence of treatment-related toxicities [134, 135].

T-Cell Lymphomas

Peripheral T-Cell Lymphomas

Peripheral T-cell lymphomas (PTCLs) are a heterogeneous group of mature T-cell tumors arising from post-thymic T cells at various stages of differentiation. They represent approximately 12% of all NHL in Western populations. The Prognostic Index for PTCL incorporates age, LDH, performance status, and bone marrow involvement. PTCLs are highly aggressive and resistant to standard chemotherapeutic options, conferring a poorer prognosis than B-cell neoplasms. Five-year survival rates may be as high as 75% among patients with a low risk score on the IPI, though such low-risk patients are uncommon. The five-year survival rates after combination chemotherapy are 21% and 6% for the more common patient with high intermediate or high IPI scores, respectively. CHOP has historically been used as primary therapy for PTCL, but with five-year PFS rates ranging from 18% to 36% [136]. The poor outcomes with conventional chemotherapy has generated interest in more aggressive treatment strategies, including the addition of etoposide to CHOP, ASCT, or radiation therapy as consolidation.

Anaplastic large-cell lymphomas, recently distinguished by the presence or absence of t(2;5)(p23;35), resulting in a fusion gene and expression of ALK, confers a favorable prognosis with standard CHOP therapy. A fraction of patients with angioimmunoblastic T-cell lymphoma can be treated with steroids or combination chemotherapy and can frequently achieve a complete response, although relapse is frequent.

Extranodal NK/T-cell lymphomas, nasal type, have a varied racial and geographic distribution, with the majority of cases occurring in East Asia. Most cases arise in the nasal region and associated structures, although identical tumors can also occur at extranasal sites, such as the skin, gastrointestinal tract, soft tissue, and testis. Patients with localized disease can be treated effectively with radiation therapy, with or without consolidation chemotherapy. The radiation field should encompass all involved areas and should preferably be given concurrently with chemotherapy. If concurrent chemoradiation is not appropriate for a patient, radiation should be administered prior to chemotherapy. Combined-modality treatment includes concurrent radiotherapy (50.4 Gy in 28 fractions or higher) and weekly cisplatin, followed by three cycles of etoposide, ifosfamide, cisplatin and dexamethasone (VIPD) or dexamethasone, etoposide, ifosfamide, and carboplatin (DeVIC) [137]. Patients with disseminated extranodal NK/T-cell lymphomas undergo treatment with combination chemotherapy including L-asparaginase rather than CHOP chemotherapy, with the consideration of CNS prophylaxis with intrathecal or high-dose systemic methotrexate.

Lymphoblastic Lymphoma

Highly aggressive precursor lymphoid neoplasms are those that are comprised of immature B or T cells, with precursor T lymphoblastic leukemia/lymphomas (precursor T-ALL) consisting of immature lymphoblasts committed to the T-cell lineage that may arise with the thymus or bone marrow. Patients are typically younger males in their teens to early twenties who present with lymphadenopathy and commonly have a bulky, anterior mediastinal mass associated with pleural effusions. These masses can produce complications such as superior vena cava syndrome, tracheal obstruction, and pericardial effusions with or without tamponade. Treatment has followed the basic strategy of induction, consolidation-intensification, CNS prophylaxis, and maintenance therapy that has been used successfully in pediatric ALL.

Precursor T-ALL has a more favorable outcome than B-lineage ALL, likely due to the younger patient age and lack of distinctive adverse cytogenetic abnormalities. The majority of adults (75–90%) will achieve remission, but relapses are common and the five-year OS remains at 30–40%.

Central Nervous System Lymphomas

Historically, radiotherapy was the exclusive treatment for patients with primary CNS lymphoma (PCNSL). However, the high rates of neurotoxicity with radiotherapy has led to the evaluation of chemoimmunotherapy, and high-dose methotrexate and rituximab play a central role in the management of primary CNS lymphomas [138]. Detailed discussion of the management of CNS lymphoma, however, is beyond the scope of this chapter; the reader is referred to the chapter on CNS tumors.

Cutaneous B- and T-Cell Lymphomas

Primary cutaneous lymphomas (PCLs) are non-Hodgkin lymphomas that present in the skin with no evidence of extracutaneous disease at the time of disease. PCL must be distinguished from nodal or systemic malignant lymphomas that secondarily involve the skin. PCLs are distinguished by the T or B cell of origin, with cutaneous B-cell lymphomas representing 25–30% and cutaneous T-cell lymphoma representing 75–80% of all lesions.

There are three main types of cutaneous B-cell lymphomas; these include primary cutaneous marginal zone lymphoma (PC-MZL), primary cutaneous follicle center cell lymphoma (PC-FCL), and primary cutaneous diffuse large B-cell lymphoma, leg type (PC-DLBCL). PC-FCL is the most common type, accounting for 50–60% of cases, and is most common in the head and neck region. Early-stage disease PC-FCL and PC-MZL are primarily treated with primary ISRT to doses of 24–30 Gy, with excellent long-term local control rates, while systemic therapy is reserved for more advanced-stage disease. Single-agent rituximab monotherapy has been used in early-stage patients with excellent initial complete response rates of 85% or higher; however, approximately one-third of these patients eventually suffer a local relapse [139]. In contrast, PC-DLBCL leg-type accounts for approximately 15% of cutaneous B-cell lymphomas and has a five-year OS in the region of 40%. While the cutaneous lesions do respond to radiotherapy alone, there is a high propensity for both local relapse and distant dissemination. Hence, in early-stage disease the patients are managed with combined-modality therapy with up-front anthracycline-based chemotherapy (often R-CHOP), followed by ISRT [140].

T-cell lymphomas account for approximately 75% of all other cutaneous lymphomas. Mycosis fungoides is the most common cutaneous T-cell lymphoma, with approximately 70% of those cases. For early-stage localized disease, skin-directed therapies such as topical steroids, PUVA, narrow-band UVB and topical cytostatic agents can be used. Radiotherapy can be also used to treat local lesions, with excellent control and palliation of symptoms. For patients with either generalized skin disease or more advanced stage with either nodal, visceral or blood involvement, systemic therapy is recommended. Total skin electron radiation (TSEBT) has been shown to be effective in patients with early-stage disease with more generalized skin involvement. TSEBT is generally performed using the Stanford technique, and doses in the range of 30–36 Gy were used with excellent response rates in the region of 95% and complete response rates of 85–87.5% [141]. More recently, there has been increasing evidence that lower doses of TSEBT may be effective, particularly as *Mycosis fungoides* is typically a chronic disease with eventual systemic involvement. Several series have shown that doses of 10–24 Gy provide equivalent overall response rates to more protracted regimens without any impact on PFS or OS [142, 143].

Peripheral T-cell lymphomas (PTCL) are a heterogeneous group of NHL which account for approximately 10% of NHLs. A comprehensive review of these diseases is beyond the scope of this chapter. Anaplastic large-cell lymphoma (ALCL) is a CD30-expressing subtype of PTCL. There are three distinct subtypes of ALCL: systemic ALK-1-positive ALCL, systemic ALK-1-negative ALCL, and primary cutaneous ALCL. In general, ALK-positive ALCL has a more favorable prognosis than ALK-negative ALCL. Both types are treated with multi-agent chemotherapy regimens. Primary cutaneous ALCL is generally ALK1-negative and has a more indolent course than the systemic variants, though there is higher propensity for local recurrences. Early-stage solitary or grouped lesions are treated with primary ISRT to doses of 30–40 Gy. Multifocal lesions or cutaneous disease with regional nodal involvement should be treated with up-front chemotherapy with consolidation ISRT when appropriate.

Treatment of Special Populations

Pediatrics

Hodgkin Lymphoma

Hodgkin lymphoma represents 5% of childhood cancers, and is uncommon before the age of 10 years. Of the histologic subtypes, nodular sclerosis is the most common (40–70% of patients), followed by mixed cellularity in 30%, and lymphocyte-predominant in 1–15%. Few risk factors have been identified for the development of HL. The treatment of HL in pediatric patients has evolved because of the long-term side effects associated with high-dose radiation therapy that had been used in the past, including the development of second malignancies, growth impairment of bones and soft tissues, cardiomyopathy, and sterility. In an effort to reduce these side effects, standard chemotherapy regimens used in adults with HL have also been used in pediatric patients. Treatment of HL depends on the extent of disease, as classified by the Ann Arbor Staging system (see Table 40.3) as used with adults. Children with early-stage HL are usually treated with combination chemotherapy, followed by involved field radiation with five-year survival rates exceeding 90%. Patients with advanced-stage HL undergo more intensive combination chemotherapy plus involved field radiation, with five-year survival rates approaching 87–93%. Patients who relapse after initial treatment will frequently respond to subsequent treatment options, including chemotherapy, irradiation, and stem cell transplantation. The long-term follow-up of pediatric HL is essential, where late complications must be anticipated, monitored, and treated.

The Children's Oncology Group randomized patients under age 21 who had achieved an initial complete response after risk-adapted combination chemotherapy to receive low-dose IFRT (21 Gy in 12 fractions) or no further treatment [144]. Patients who received low-dose IFRT showed an improved event-free survival at three years (93% versus 85%), but there was no significant difference in survival. This suggested a possible advantage to multi-modality therapy with the use of low-IFRT as a means to reduce the incidence of late effects of standard-dose radiotherapy.

The current generation of COG trials has risk-stratified patients into low-, intermediate- and high-risk groups. These trials have incorporated early PET (usually after the first or second cycle) in the treatment paradigm. In the low-risk group study (COG AHOD 0431), all patients received three cycles of AVCP [145] and also underwent a re-staging PET after the first cycle. Patients who had a complete response after three cycles were observed, and patients who had a partial response after three cycles underwent consolidative radiotherapy to 21 Gy. The two-year event-free survival rate was 84%, and the two-year OS was 100% for all patients. The two-year event-free survival in patients who had a complete response after three cycles (and did not receive radiotherapy) was 80%, and in those who had a partial response who received adjuvant radiotherapy was 88% (p = 0.11). However, there was a dramatic difference in the two-year event-free survival of complete response patients when stratified based on the early PET after the first cycle of chemotherapy. Those who were PET-negative had an event-free survival of 87%, while those who were still PET-positive had an event-free survival of 65% (p = 0.005). Based on the two-year interim results, complete response patients who were either PET+ or equivocal after the first cycle of chemotherapy were called back for adjuvant radiotherapy if they were within one year of completing chemotherapy.

In the intermediate-risk patients, the COG AHOD 0031 trial evaluated risk-adapted therapy based on early response [146]. All patients received two cycles of ABVE-PE and were then assessed for response based on CT. Patients showed either a rapid early response (RER, defined as >60% reduction in the product of perpendicular diameters (PPD) of each lesion on CT imaging) or were slow early responders. Patients with a RER then went on to receive two additional cycles of chemotherapy followed by additional imaging using a CT and either a PET or gallium scan. A complete response was defined as 80% or greater reduction in PPD of each lesion on CT and either a negative PET or gallium scan. The RER patients with a complete response were then randomized to either adjuvant radiotherapy (IFRT, 21 Gy) or observation. The RER patients with less than a complete response went on to receive adjuvant radiotherapy (IFRT, 21 Gy). The SER patients, after the initial two cycles of chemotherapy, were randomized to either two additional cycles of ABVE-PE followed by adjuvant IFRT, or to a more intensive chemotherapy with two additional cycles of ABVE-PE and DECA followed by adjuvant IFRT. All SER patients also received either PET or gallium scans upon conclusion of all chemotherapy. The four year event-free survival for all patients was 85.0%, and the four-year OS was 97.8%. In the RER patients, the event-free survival for those who received adjuvant radiotherapy was 87.9%, and for those who did not receive radiotherapy was 84.3% (p = 0.07). There was a statistically significant difference in event-free survival between the RER and SER patients (86.7% versus 77.4%, p < 0.001). The difference in OS between the two groups was of a much smaller magnitude, reflecting excellent salvage options in those who relapsed (98.5% versus 95.3%, p < 0.001). There was no difference in event-free survival in the SER patients, regardless of the chemotherapy regimen (DECA versus no DECA, 79.3% versus 75.2%). However, there was a significant difference in event-free survival for patients who remained PET+ at the end of chemotherapy (54.6% versus 70.7%, p = 0.05).

Thus, early assessment of response with PET either after the first or second cycle appears to be prognostic in children with either low-risk or intermediate-risk disease. While radiotherapy improves disease control in all patients, it can be safely omitted in patients who are rapid early responders to chemotherapy.

Non-Hodgkin Lymphoma

NHLs comprise 8% of cancers in children. There is an increased incidence in patients with congenital or acquired immunodeficiency states. Approximately one-third of pediatric NHLs are comprised of Burkitt lymphomas, lymphoblastic lymphomas (primarily T-cell) account for 30%, and large-cell lymphomas of multiple lineages account for 25–30%. Childhood NHLs are staged using the Murphy staging system, and therapy depends on the stage. Stage I–II Burkitt or large-cell lymphomas can be cured with CHOP-like chemotherapy in 90% of pediatric patients, whereas only 70% of those with stage I or II lymphoblastic lymphoma are cured. Advanced-stage III or IV lymphomas require more intensive chemotherapy regimens, but cure can be achieved in approximately 80% of patients. CNS chemoprophylaxis with intrathecal medication is an essential component of all subtypes of advanced-stage NHLs in children. Some regimens may include the use of low-dose (12–18 Gy) cranial irradiation as part of CNS prophylaxis for patients with advanced lymphoblastic lymphomas.

Link *et al.* [147] randomized children and young adults aged <21 years with early-stage NHL to receive IFRT versus no therapy, after all had received induction and continuation chemotherapy. A second consecutive trial randomly assigned patients to induction chemotherapy followed by continuation chemotherapy versus no further therapy. Long-term survival was approximately 90%, and there was no advantage in outcomes with the addition of IFRT or continuation chemotherapy. The conclusion from this study was that a nine-week course of multi-agent chemotherapy is sufficient therapy for most children and young adults with early-stage NHL.

Immunosuppressed Patients

Immunodeficiency-Associated Lymphoproliferative Disorders

Congenital or acquired immunodeficiency states are associated with an increased risk of lymphoproliferative disorders. These disorders can be broadly categorized as: (i) primary immunodeficiency disorders; (ii) HIV infection; (iii) post solid organ or marrow transplantation with iatrogenic immunosuppression; and (iv) methotrexate- or other iatrogenic-related immunosuppression for autoimmune disease. The lymphomas associated with these disorders are heterogeneous and may be either HL or NHL.

Primary Immunodeficiency Disorders

Lymphoproliferative disorders associated with primary immunodeficiencies are most commonly seen in children. These disorders include Wiskott–Aldrich syndrome, ataxia-telangiectasia, common variable or severe combined immunodeficiency, X-linked lymphoproliferative disorder, Nijmegan breakage syndrome, hyper-IgM syndrome, and autoimmune lymphoproliferative syndrome. The lymphomas that occur do not differ morphologically compared to immunocompetent hosts, and DLBCL is the most frequent type seen. These malignancies respond poorly to standard chemotherapy, and

treatment depends on the underlying disorder and the specific lymphoma subtype. Allogeneic transplantation has been successfully used in some patients. As these lymphoproliferative disorders are commonly associated with EBV infection, novel immunotherapeutic or pharmacologic strategies targeting EBV are being explored.

Human Immunodeficiency Virus (HIV)

HIV-associated lymphomas are typically monoclonal, B-cell aggressive subtypes, usually DLBCL or Burkitt lymphoma. Approximately 25–40% of HIV-positive patients will develop a malignancy, with approximately 10% developing NHL, conferring a more than 400-fold overall risk of developing NHL. The development of NHL is considered an AIDS-defining malignancy, and there are three general categories of AIDS-related NHL that can be seen, based on location: systemic NHL; primary CNS lymphoma; and primary effusion lymphoma. Approximately two-thirds of cases are EBV-associated, and many carry c-*MYC* oncogene translocations. Primary effusion lymphoma presents in HIV-positive patients with ascites or pleural effusions, but may also involve soft tissue or visceral masses. It is associated with human herpes virus-8 (HHV-8) and generally confers a poor prognosis. HL also occurs in HIV-positive patients, but with less frequency and is usually the mixed cellularity of lymphocyte-depleted subtypes. Therapy for HIV-associated lymphomas requires the concurrent treatment with highly active antiretroviral therapy and chemotherapy. Options for chemotherapy include both full-dose and dose-modified combination regimens, usually with growth factor support, and can lead to durable remissions.

Post-Transplantation Lymphoproliferative Disorders

Post-transplantation lymphoproliferative disorders (PTLDs) occur as a consequence of chronic immunosuppression in recipients of solid organ, bone marrow, or stem cell allografts. PTLDs are mostly large-cell lymphomas, the great majority of which are of the B-cell type, as T- or NK-cell types are extremely uncommon. PTLDs are comprised of a spectrum of disorders ranging from EBV-positive infectious mononucleosis to polymorphic PTLD or monomorphic PTLD that can be either EBV-positive or EBV-negative. The risk of lymphoma is directly related to the degree of immunosuppression, and may arise within the first six months of transplantation, or have a later onset several years later. EBV-positive PTLD most commonly occurs within the first six months post-transplantation. More than 90% of PTCLs in solid organ recipients are of host origin, whereas most PTLDs in bone marrow allograft recipients are of donor origin. A minority of patients will respond to a reduction in intensity of immunosuppression alone, although the majority will require systemic therapy as well. Unfortunately, the prognosis of these

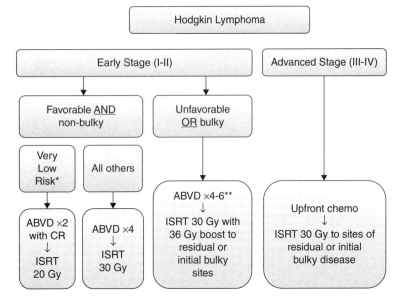

Figure 40.3 Treatment algorithm for Hodgkin lymphoma.

*GSHG HD10 trial included patients with only 1-2 sites, no bulky, no B sxs.
** Can also do a hybrid of ABVD × 2 and esc BEACOPP × 2

patients is poor due to both inadequate response and poor tolerance of chemotherapy.

Radiotherapy Techniques

Involved-Site Radiotherapy

Involved-node radiotherapy (INRT) and involved-site radiotherapy (ISRT) have largely replaced the conventional IFRT over the past five years. The International Lymphoma Radiation Oncology Group has published detailed target definition and dose guidelines for Hodgkin's lymphoma and non-Hodgkin's lymphoma [148, 149]. The guiding principle behind both ISRT and INRT is to treat the originally involved sites of disease with modern and focused radiotherapy aimed at minimizing normal tissue exposure (see Figures 40.3 and 40.4). As long-term control rates improve with effective curative regimens, there is an increasing need to minimize dose to normal tissues to lower the likelihood and severity of late side effects. Also, there is recognition that in the era of improved systemic therapy, effective chemotherapy manages microscopic disease and most

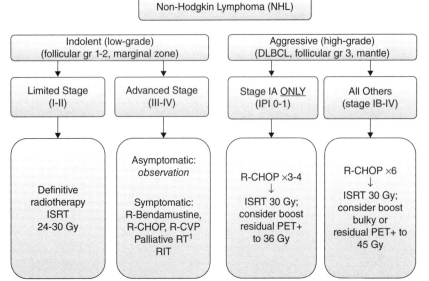

Figure 40.4 Treatment algorithm for non-Hodgkin lymphoma.

[1]Hoskin, PJ., Kirkwood AA, Popova, B, et al. 4 Gy versus 24 Gy radiotherapy for patients with indolent lymphoma (FORT): a randomized phase 3 non-inferiority trial. *Lancet Oncol 2014*, 15 (4): 457–463.

recurrences in HL and NHL are local in the sites of initial involvement. Radiation is extremely effective at reducing local failures.

Simulation and Treatment Planning

Simulation

Three-dimensional (3-D) simulation with either a CT simulator, PET-CT simulator or MRI simulator is essential for treatment planning. If the initial diagnostic PET or CT scans have been acquired prior to simulation, careful electronic fusion is required. Since diagnostic imaging is often acquired in a different patient position, deformable fusion is recommended when available. Intravenous contrast can be very useful for rendering target volumes for 3-D planning, and is helpful for delineating nodal stations and differentiating nodes from vessels and muscles. Four-dimensional CT imaging should be considered to delineate an internal target volume (ITV) in situations where respiratory motion is of concern. Additional motion-management strategies such as deep inspiration breath-hold should be considered to maximize cardiac and pulmonary sparing. Customized immobilization is recommended to achieve reproducible positioning and to limit intra-fraction motion.

Contouring

- *Prechemotherapy or presurgery gross tumor volume (GTV)*: The initial gross nodal and extra-nodal disease should be contoured on the treatment planning CT. This is typically performed on the pre-chemotherapy diagnostic CT or PET that has been fused with the simulation CT.
- *No chemotherapy or post-chemotherapy GTV*: The primary imaging of the untreated lesions or residual disease post-chemotherapy should be contoured on the simulation CT.
- *Clinical tumor volume (CTV) determination*: The CTV entails the original pre-treatment GTV. However, normal surrounding structures such as lungs, vessels, muscles and kidneys can be excluded as long as they were clearly uninvolved based on clinical judgment. As per the ILROG guidelines, there should be careful consideration of the quality and accuracy of diagnostic imaging and fusion with the simulation CT, concerns for changes in volume since diagnostic imaging, spread patterns of disease, potential subclinical involvement and adjacent organ constraints. The pre-chemotherapy GTV is often deformed in the left-to-right and anterior-to-posterior dimension to match the post-chemotherapy anatomy on the simulation CT. It remains important to maintain the superior-inferior margins of the original extent of pre-chemotherapy disease.

Internal Target Volume (ITV)

The ITV is defined in the ICRU Report 62 as the CTV plus margin taking into account uncertainties in size, shape, and position of the CTV within the patient. The ITV is of particular importance in location with significant motion with respiration (chest, abdomen). A 4-D CT simulation is often very helpful in assessing motion and obtaining ITV margins. If a 4-D CT is not available, an ITV margin of 1.5–2 cm in the superior-inferior position should be considered in the chest and abdomen.

CT simulation with deep inspiration breath-hold is also helpful in patients with mediastinal nodal involvement as it allows for better cardiac and pulmonary sparing.

Planned Treatment Volume (PTV)

The PTV is an additional margin around the CTV or ITV and takes into account set-up uncertainties in patient positioning and the alignment of beams during treatment planning and treatment delivery. The exact extent of this margin should be determined based on immobilization, treatment planning, and the extent of image guidance for set-up and motion management during delivery.

Organs at Risk

Critical normal organs at risk (OAR) entailed within the volume of irradiation should be contoured on the simulation CT. A dose–volume histogram (DVH) should be calculated by the planner and evaluated by the clinician.

Treatment Techniques

The treating radiation oncologist makes a clinical judgment as to which treatment technique is appropriate for an individual patient. This should be based on consideration of various factors including the anatomic site of disease, the age of the patient, the gender of the patient, comorbidities, organs at risk, prior radiotherapy, and respiratory motion.

In some situations, conventional radiotherapy with AP and PA beam arrangement is appropriate if it results in the smallest volume of normal tissue being irradiated. In other situations, more conformal techniques such as IMRT, volumetric-modulated arc therapy (VMAT) and helical arc therapy (tomotherapy) may be indicated as they may offer significantly better sparing of critical structures.

Motion-management strategies such as DIBH or 4D-CT to generate an ITV is recommended to account for tumor motion and sparing of normal surrounding tissues as needed (Figure 40.5).

Free breathing vs. Deep Inspiration Breath Hold
Lungs

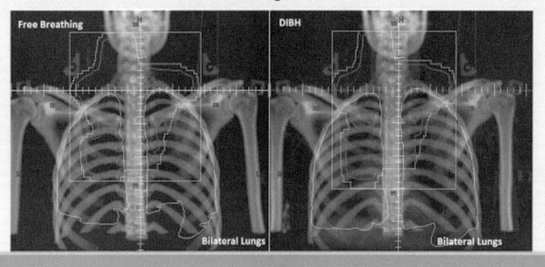

(a)

Free breathing vs. Deep Inspiration Breath Hold
Heart

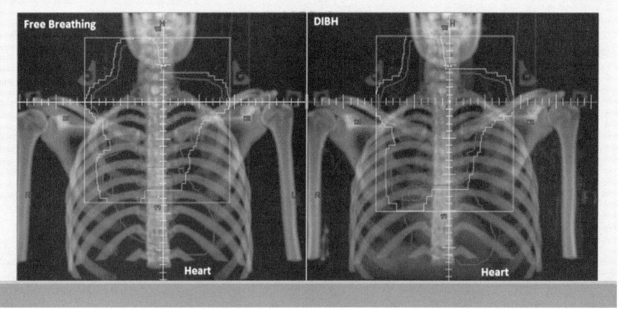

(b)

Figure 40.5 (a) Comparison of free-breathing versus deep-inspiration breath-hold. Pulmonary-sparing figure. (b) Comparison of free-breathing versus deep inspiration breath-hold. Cardiac sparing. For a color version of this figure, see the color plate section.

Dose Considerations

Hodgkin Lymphoma

Combined Modality Therapy

- Early-stage favorable non-bulky disease as per GSHG 10 requirements (stage IA–IIA): 20 Gy (two cycles of ABVD) or 30 Gy (Stanford V).
- Early-stage favorable non-bulky disease: 30 Gy.
- Early-stage unfavorable or bulky disease: 30 Gy.
- Incomplete response after chemotherapy: 30 Gy to initial sites of disease with a 6–10 Gy boost to post-chemotherapy PET avid disease.

Radiotherapy Alone

Classic HL: If no chemotherapy planned, consider IFRT or EFRT:

- Uninvolved regions: 25–30 Gy.
- Involved Regions: 36 Gy.

NLPHL:

- Stage IA/IIA non-bulky: 30 Gy ISRT with more generous superior/inferior margins of 3–5 cm. Can consider a boost of an additional 6 Gy to sites of gross disease.

Non-Hodgkin Lymphoma

DLBCL:

- Consolidation after chemotherapy complete response: 30–36 Gy.
- Complimentary after chemotherapy partial response: Pre-chemotherapy involved sites to 30–36 Gy followed by boost to post-chemotherapy residual disease to 40–50 Gy.
- Radiotherapy alone: 40–55 Gy.
- In combination with SCT, 20–36 Gy depending on sites of disease and prior radiotherapy exposure.

Follicular Lymphoma:

- Early-stage, definitive therapy 24–30 Gy.
- Advanced disease, palliative 4 Gy.

Marginal Zone Lymphoma:

- Gastric: 30 Gy.
- Extranodal 24–30 Gy.
- Nodal: 24–30 Gy.

NK/T-cell lymphoma:

- Combined modality: 45–60 Gy.
- Radiotherapy alone: 50–65 Gy.

Cutaneous lymphomas:

- Primary cutaneous follicle center or marginal zone lymphoma: 24-30 Gy.
- Primary cutaneous DLBCL, leg type: 30–36 Gy.
- Primary cutaneous anaplastic large cell lymphoma: 30–36 Gy.
- Mycosis fungoides:
  - Local therapy for individual lesions: 8–30 Gy.
  - Total skin electron beam therapy (TSEBT): 10–24 Gy.

Total Body Irradiation

Total body irradiation (TBI) doses of 12–14 Gy in six to eight fractions twice daily may be used for patients in need of myeloablative conditioning for ASCT. Single-fraction non-myeloablative TBI regimens of 2 Gy are occasionally implemented in elderly patients. For a detailed description of varying TBI techniques, the reader is referred to Chapter 00.

Unsealed Sources (Radioimmunotherapy)

Radioimmunotherapy (^{90}Y-ibritumomab tiuxetan or ^{131}I-tositumomab) is commonly used to treat advanced low-grade NHL, particularly FL. Studies of radioimmunotherapy have found it to be beneficial as first-line therapy or as consolidative therapy for patients with advanced FL [150]. Tositumomab therapy can be given as a 1-h intravenous infusion of 450 mg tositumomab, followed by a 20-min infusion of 35 mg of tositumomab labeled with 5 mCi of ^{131}I. A second infusion is given 7–14 days later, of 450 mg tositumomab over 1 h followed by 35 mg tositumomab labeled with ^{131}I, with activity calculated to deliver a total body dose of 75 cGy. ^{90}Y-ibritumomab therapy can be administered with rituximab 250 mg m^{-2} on days 1 and 8, followed by ^{111}In-ibritumomab tiuxetan 185 MBq for imaging/dosimetry studies. ^{90}Y-ibritumomab is given in doses of 14.8 MBq kg^{-1} (not to exceed a total dose of 1184 MBq) as a slow intravenous push over 10 min on day 8.

Conclusions

Lymphomas are an extraordinarily complex and diverse set of tumors with a broad spectrum of treatment approaches. Randomized trials have helped define the optimal therapeutic strategies for common lymphomas such as classical HL and DLBCL. The fact that, each year more than 200 000 people die from lymphoma underscores the need for a continuous advancement in understanding the prevention and management of these conditions.

References

1 Siegel, R.L., Miller, K.D., Jemal, A. (2017) Cancer Statistics, 2017. *CA Cancer J. Clin.*, **67**, 7–30.

2 Rocchi, G., Tosato, G., Papa, G., Ragona, G. (1975) Antibodies to Epstein–Barr virus-associated nuclear antigen and to other viral and non-viral antigens in Hodgkin's disease. *Int. J. Cancer*, **16**, 323–328.

3 Weiss, L.M., Movahed, L.A., Warnke, R.A., Sklar, J. (1989) Detection of Epstein–Barr viral genomes in Reed–Sternberg cells of Hodgkin's disease. *N. Engl. J. Med.*, **320**, 502–506.

4 Nonoyama, M., Huang, C.H., Pagano, J.S., Klein, G., Singh, S. (1973) DNA of Epstein–Barr virus detected in tissue of Burkitt's lymphoma and nasopharyngeal carcinoma. *Proc. Natl Acad. Sci. USA*, **70**, 3265–3268.

5 Thorley-Lawson, D.A., Gross, A. (2004) Persistence of the Epstein–Barr virus and the origins of associated lymphomas. *N. Engl. J. Med.*, **350**, 1328–1337.

6 Hochberg, F.H., Miller, G., Schooley, R.T., Hirsch, M.S., Feorino, P., Henle, W. (1983) Central-nervous-system lymphoma related to Epstein–Barr virus. *N. Engl. J. Med.*, **309**, 745–748.

7 Tsujimoto, Y., Finger, L.R., Yunis, J., Nowell, P.C., Croce, C.M. (1984) *Science*, **226**, 1097–1099.

8 Williams, M.E., Meeker, T.C., Swerdlow, S.H. (1991) Rearrangement of the chromosome 11 bcl-1 locus in centrocytic lymphoma: Analysis with multiple breakpoint proves. *Blood*, **78**, 493.

9 Cory, S. (1986) Activation of cellular oncogenes in hematopoietic cells by chromosome translocation. *Adv. Cancer Res.*, **47**, 189–234.

10 Dierlamm, J., Baens, M., Wlodarska, I., *et al.* (1999) The apoptosis inhibitor gene API2 and a novel 18q gene, MLT, are recurrently rearranged in the t(11;18)(q21;q21) associated with mucosa-associated lymphoid tissue lymphomas. *Blood*, **93** (11), 3601–3609.

11 Garrison, J.B., Samuel, T., Reed, J.C. (2009) TRAF2-binding BIR1 domain of c-IAP2/MALT1 fusion protein is essential for activation of NK-kappaB. *Oncogene*, **28** (13), 1584–1593.

12 Swerdlow, S.H., Harris, N.L., *et al.* (2008) *WHO Classification of Tumours of Haematopoietic and Lymphoid Tissues*. IARC Press, Lyon, France.

13 Harris, N.L., Jaffe, E.S., Stein, H., *et al.* (1994) A revised European-American classification of malignant lymphoid neoplasms: a proposal from the International Lymphoma Study Group. *Blood*, **84**, 1361–1392.

14 Anagnostopoulos, I., Hansmann, M.L., Franssila, K., *et al.* (2000) European Task Force on Lymphoma project on lymphocyte predominance Hodgkin disease: histologic and immunohistologic analysis of submitted cases reveals 2 types of Hodgkin disease with a nodular growth pattern and abundant lymphocytes. *Blood*, **96**, 1889–1899.

15 Nogova, L., Reineke, T., Brillant, C., *et al.* (2008) Lymphocyte-predominant and classical Hodgkin's lymphoma: a comprehensive analysis from the German Hodgkin Study Group. *J. Clin. Oncol.*, **26**, 434–439.

16 Foss, H.D., Reusch, R., Demel, G., *et al.* (1999) Frequent expression of the B-cell-specific activator protein in Reed–Sternberg cells of classical Hodgkin's disease provides further evidence of its B-cell origin. *Blood*, **94**, 3108–3113.

17 Stein, H., Mason, D.Y., Gerdes, J., *et al.* (1985) The expression of the Hodgkin's disease associated antigen Ki-1 in reactive and neoplastic lymphoid tissue: evidence that Reed–Sternberg cells and histiocytic malignancies are derived from activated lymphoid cells. *Blood*, **66**, 848–858.

18 Stein, H., Uchanska-Ziegler, B., Gerdes, J., *et al.* (1982) Hodgkin and Sternberg–Reed cells contain antigens specific to late cells of granulopoiesis. *Int. J. Cancer*, **29**, 283–290.

19 Coles, F.B., Cartun, R.W., Pastuszak, W.T. (1988) Hodgkin's disease, lymphocyte-predominant type: immunoreactivity with B-cell antibodies. *Mod. Pathol.*, **1**, 274–278.

20 Pinkus, G.S., Said, J.W. (1985) Hodgkin's disease, lymphocyte predominance type, nodular – a distinct entity? Unique staining profile for L*H variants of Reed–Sternberg cells defined by monoclonal antibodies to leukocyte common antigen, granulocyte-specific antigen, and B-cell-specific antigen. *Am. J. Pathol.*, **118**, 1–6.

21 Poppema, S. (1980) The diversity of the immunohistological staining pattern of Sternberg–Reed cells. *J. Histochem. Cytochem.*, **28**, 788–791.

22 Marafioti, T., Hummel, M., Anagnostopoulos, I., *et al.* (1997) Origin of nodular lymphocyte-predominant Hodgkin's disease from a clonal expansion of highly mutated germinal-center B cells. *N. Engl. J. Med.*, **337**, 453–458.

23 Hoppe, R.T., Advani, R.H., Ai, W.Z., *et al.* (2011) Hodgkin lymphoma. *J. Natl Compr. Cancer Networks*, **9**, 1020–1058.

24 Straus, D.J., Portlock, C.S., Qin, J., *et al.* (2004) Results of a prospective randomized clinical trial of doxorubicin, bleomycin, vinblastine, and dacarbazine (ABVD) followed by radiation therapy (RT) versus ABVD alone for stages I, II, and IIIA nonbulky Hodgkin disease. *Blood*, **104**, 3483–3489.

25 MacManus, M., Hoppe, R.T. (1996) Is radiotherapy curative for stage I and II low-grade follicular lymphoma? Results of a long-term follow-up study of patients treated at Stanford University. *J. Clin. Oncol.*, **14**, 1282–1290.

26 Petersen, P.M., Gospodarowicz, M., Tsang, R., *et al.* (2004) Long-term outcome in stage I and II follicular lymphoma following treatment with involved field radiation therapy alone. *J. Clin. Oncol.*, **22**, 563.

27 Miller T.P., Dahlberg S. (1993) Treatment of diffuse large-cell lymphoma: a summary of outcomes for patients treated by Southwest Oncology Group. *Cancer. Treat Res.*, **16**, 53–63.

28 Zimmermann M., Oehler C., Zwahlen D., *et al.* (2016) Radiotherapy for Non-Hodgkin's Lymphoma: still standard practice and not an outdated treatment option. *Radiation Oncology*, **11**, 1–10.

29 Kahl B.S., Yang D.T. (2016). Follicular lymphoma: evolving therapeutic strategies. *Blood*, **127**, 2055–2063.

30 Magrath, I.T., Janus, C., Edwards, B.K., *et al.* (1984) An effective therapy for both undifferentiated (including Burkitt's) lymphomas and lymphoblastic lymphomas in children and young adults. *Blood*, **63**, 1102–1111.

31 McClure, R.F., Remstein, E.D., Macon, W.R., *et al.* (2005) Adult B-cell lymphomas with Burkitt-like morphology are phenotypically and genotypically heterogeneous with aggressive clinical behavior. *Am. J. Surg. Pathol.*, **29**, 1652–1660.

32 Carbone, P., Kaplan, H., Musshoff, K., Smithers, D., Tubiana, M. (1971) Report of the committee on Hodgkin's disease staging classification. *Cancer Res.*, **31**, 1860–1861.

33 Gospodarowicz, M.K., Sutcliffe, S.B., Clark, R.M., *et al.* (1992) Analysis of supradiaphragmatic clinical stage I and II Hodgkin's disease treated with radiation alone. *Int. J. Radiat. Oncol. Biol. Phys.*, **22**, 85965.

34 Henry-Amar, M., Friedman, S., Hayat, M., *et al.* (1991) Erythrocyte sedimentation rate predicts early relapse and survival in early-stage Hodgkin disease. The EORTC Lymphoma Cooperative Group. *Ann. Intern. Med.*, **114**, 361–365.

35 Tubiana, M., Henry-Amar, M., Carde, P., *et al.* (1989) Toward comprehensive management tailored to prognostic factors of patients with clinical stages I and II in Hodgkin's disease. The EORTC Lymphoma Group controlled clinical trials: 1964–1987. *Blood*, **73**, 47–56.

36 Duhmke, E., Diehl, V., Loeffler, M., *et al.* (1996) Randomized trial with early-stage Hodgkin's disease testing 30 Gy vs. 40 Gy extended field radiotherapy alone. *Int. J. Radiat. Oncol. Biol. Phys.*, **36**, 305–310.

37 Cosset, J.M., Henry-Amar, M., Meerwaldt, J.H., *et al.* (1992) The EORTC trials for limited stage Hodgkin's disease. The EORTC Lymphoma Cooperative Group. *Eur. J. Cancer*, **28A**, 1847–1850.

38 Hasenclever, D., Diehl, V. (1998) A prognostic score for advanced Hodgkin's disease. International Prognostic Factors Project on Advanced Hodgkin's Disease. *N. Engl. J. Med.*, **339**, 1506–1514.

39 Shipp, M., Harrington, D., Anderson, J., *et al.* (1993) A predictive model for aggressive non-Hodgkin's lymphoma. The International Non-Hodgkin's Lymphoma Prognostic Factors Project. *N. Engl. J. Med.*, **329**, 987–994.

40 Solal-Celigny, P., Roy, P., Colombat, P., *et al.* (2004) Follicular lymphoma international prognostic index. *Blood*, **104**, 1258–1265.

41 Hoster, E., Dreyling, M., Klapper, W., *et al.* (2008) A new prognostic index (MIPI) for patients with advanced-stage mantle cell lymphoma. *Blood*, **111**, 558–565.

42 Meyer, R.M., Gospodarowicz, M.K., Connors, J.M., *et al.* (2005) Randomized comparison of ABVD chemotherapy with a strategy that includes radiation therapy in patients with limited-stage Hodgkin's lymphoma: National Cancer Institute of Canada Clinical Trials Group and the Eastern Cooperative Oncology Group. *J. Clin. Oncol.*, **23**, 4634–4642.

43 Connors, J.M. (2005) State-of-the-art therapeutics: Hodgkin's lymphoma. *J. Clin. Oncol.*, **23**, 6400–6408.

44 Macdonald, D.A., Connors, J.M. (2007) New strategies for the treatment of early stages of Hodgkin's lymphoma. *Hematol. Oncol. Clin. North Am.*, **21**, 871–880.

45 Santoro, A., Bonadonna, G., Valagussa, P., *et al.* (1987) Long-term results of combined chemotherapy-radiotherapy approach in Hodgkin's disease: superiority of ABVD plus radiotherapy versus MOPP plus radiotherapy. *J. Clin. Oncol.*, **5**, 27–37.

46 Engert, A., Franklin, J., Eich, H.T., *et al.* (2007) Two cycles of doxorubicin, bleomycin, vinblastine, and dacarbazine plus extended-field radiotherapy is superior to radiotherapy alone in early favorable Hodgkin's lymphoma: final results of the GHSG HD7 trial. *J. Clin. Oncol.*, **25**, 3495–3502.

47 Engert, A., Plutschow, A., Eich, H., *et al.* (2010) Reduced treatment intensity in patients with early stage Hodgkin's lymphoma. *N. Engl. J. Med.*, **363**, 640–652.

48 Advani, R.H., Hoppe, R.T., Horning, S.J., *et al.* (2013) Efficacy of abbreviated Stanford V chemotherapy and involved-field radiotherapy in early-stage Hodgkin lymphoma: mature results of G4 trial. *Ann. Oncol.*, **24** (4), 1044–1048.

49 Radford, J., Illidge, T., Barrington, S., *et al.* (2015) Results of a trial of PET-directed therapy for early-stage Hodgkin's lymphoma. *N. Engl. J. Med.*, **372** (17), 1598–1607.

50 Raemaekers, J., Andre, M., Fortpeid, C., *et al.* (2014) Omitting radiotherapy in early positron emission tomography negative Stage I/II Hodgkin lymphoma is associated with an increased risk of relapse. *J. Clin. Oncol.*, **32** (12), 1188–1193.

51 Ferme, C., Eghbali, H., Henry-Amar, M., *et al.* (2007) Chemotherapy plus involved field radiation in early-stage Hodgkin's disease. *N. Engl. J. Med.*, **357** (19), 1916–1927.

52 Noordijk, E., Carde, P., Henry-Amar, M., *et al.* (2006) Combined modality therapy for clinical stage I or II Hodgkin's lymphoma: Long term results of the European Organization for Research and Treatment of Cancer H7 Randomized Controlled Trials. *J. Clin. Oncol.*, **24** (19), 3128–3135.

53 Eich, H., Diehl, V., Engert, A., *et al.* (2011) Intensified chemotherapy and dose-reduced involved-field radiotherapy in patients with early unfavorable Hodgkin's lymphoma: Final analysis of the German Hodgkin Study Group HD11 trial. *J. Clin. Oncol.*, **28** (27), 4199–4206.

54 Engert, A., Schiller, P., Diehl, V., *et al.* (2003) Involved field radiotherapy is equally effective and less toxic compared to extended field radiotherapy in patients with early stage unfavorable Hodgkin's lymphoma: results of the HD8 trial of the German Hodgkin's Lymphoma Study Group. *J. Clin. Oncol.*, **21** (19), 3601–3608.

55 von Tresckow, B., *et al.* (2012) Dose-intensification in early unfavorable Hodgkin's lymphoma: final analysis of the German Hodgkin Study Group HD14 trial. *J. Clin. Oncol.*, **30**, 907–913.

56 Aleman, B., Raemaekers, J., Henry-Amar, M., *et al.* (2003) Involved field radiotherapy for advanced Hodgkin's lymphoma. *N. Engl. J. Med.*, **348** (24), 2396–2406.

57 Meignan, M., Gallamini, A., Itti, E., *et al.* (2012) Report on the Third International Workshop on Interim Positron Emission Tomography in Lymphoma held in Menton, France, 26–27 September 2011 and Menton 2011 consensus. *Leuk. Lymphoma*, **53** (10), 1876–1881.

58 Armstrong, G., Oeffinger, K., Chen, Y., *et al.* (2013) Modifiable risk factors and major cardiac events among adult survivors of childhood cancer. *J. Clin. Oncol.*, **31**, 3673–3680.

59 Bhatia, S., Yasui, Y., Robison, L.L., *et al.* (2003) High risk of subsequent neoplasms continues with extended follow-up of childhood Hodgkin's disease: report from the Late Effects Study Group. *J. Clin. Oncol.*, **21**, 4386–4394.

60 Meacham, L.J., Chow, E.J., Ness, K.K., *et al.* (2010) Cardiovascular risk factors in adult survivors of pediatric cancer – a report from the childhood cancer survivor study. *Cancer Epidemiol. Biomarkers Prev.*, **19**, 170–181.

61 Hequet, O., Le, Q.H., Moullet, I., *et al.* (2004) Subclinical late cardiomyopathy after doxorubicin therapy for lymphoma in adults. *J. Clin. Oncol.*, **22**, 1864–1871.

62 Hull, M.C., Morris, C.G., Pepine, C.J. *et al.* (2003) Valvular dysfunction and carotid, subclavian and coronary artery disease in survivors of Hodgkin lymphoma treated with radiation therapy. *J. Am. Med. Assoc.*, **290**, 2831–2837.

63 Sleijfer, S. (2001) Bleomycin-induced pneumonitis. *Chest*, **120**, 617–624.

64 Allen, S.C., Riddell, G.S., Butchart, E.G. (1981) Bleomycin therapy and anaesthesia: the possible hazards of oxygen administration to patients after treatment with bleomycin. *Anaesthesia*, **36**, 60–63.

65 Jereczek-Fossa, B.A., Alterio, D., Jassem, J., *et al.* (2004) Radiotherapy-induced thyroid disorders. *Cancer Treat. Rev.*, **30**, 369–384.

66 Younes, A., Bartlett, N.L., Leonard, J.P., *et al.* (2010) Brentuximab vedotin (SGN-35) for relapsed CD30-positive lymphomas. *N. Engl. J. Med.*, **363**, 1812–1821.

67 Younes, A., Gopal, A.K., Smith, S.E., *et al.* (2012) Results of a pivotal phase II study of brentuximab vedotin for patients with relapsed or refractory Hodgkin's lymphoma. *J. Clin. Oncol.*, **30**, 2183–2189.

68 Kahn, S., Flowers, C., Xu, Z., Esiashvili, N. (2011) Does the addition of involved field radiotherapy to high-dose chemotherapy and stem cell transplantation improve outcomes for patients with relapsed/refractory Hodgkin lymphoma? *Int. J. Radiat. Oncol. Biol. Phys.*, **81**, 175–180.

69 Linch, D.C., Winfield, D., Goldstone, A.H., *et al.* (1993) Dose intensification with autologous bone-marrow transplantation in relapsed and resistant Hodgkin's disease: results of a BNLI randomised trial. *Lancet*, **341**, 1051–1054.

70 Schmitz, N., Pfistner, B., Sextro, M., *et al.* (2002) Aggressive conventional chemotherapy compared with high-dose chemotherapy with autologous haemopoietic stem-cell transplantation for relapsed chemosensitive Hodgkin's disease: a randomised trial. *Lancet*, **359**, 2065–2071.

71 Moskowitz, C.H., Nademanee, A., Masszi, T., *et al.* (2015) Brentuximab vedotin as consolidation therapy after autologous stem-cell transplantation in patients with Hodgkin's lymphoma at risk of relapse or progression (AETHERA): a randomized, double-blind, placebo-controlled, phase 3 trial. *Lancet*, **385**, 1853–1862.

72 Anagnostopolous, I., Hansmann, M.L., Franssila, K., *et al.* (2000) European Task Force on Lymphoma

project on lymphocyte predominance Hodgkin disease: histologic and immunohistologic analysis of submitted cases reveals 2 types of Hodgkin disease with a nodular growth pattern and abundant lymphocytes. *Blood*, **96**, 1889–1899.

73 Shimabukuro-Vornhagean, A., Haverkamp, H., Enert, A., *et al.* (2005) Lymphocyte-rich classical Hodgkin's lymphoma: clinical presentation and treatment outcome in 100 patients treated within German Hodgkin's Study Group trials. *J. Clin. Oncol.*, **23**, 5739–5745.

74 Wilder, R.B., Schlembach, P.J., Jones, D., *et al.* (2002) European Organization for Research and Treatment of Cancer and Groupe d'Etude des Lymphomes de l'Adulte very favorable and favorable, lymphocyte-predominant Hodgkin disease. *Cancer*, **94**, 1731–1738.

75 Schulz, H., Rehwald, U., Morschhauser, F., *et al.* (2008) Rituximab in relapsed lymphocyte-predominant Hodgkin lymphoma: long-term results of a phase 2 trial by the German Hodgkin Lymphoma Study Group (GHSG). *Blood*, **111**, 109–111.

76 Eberle, F.C., Salaverria, I., Steidl, C., *et al.* (2011) Gray zone lymphoma: chromosomal aberrations with immunophenotypic and clinical correlations. *Mod. Pathol.*, **24** (12), 1586–1597.

77 Wilson, W.H., Pittaluga, S., Nicolae, A., *et al.* (2014) A prospective study of mediastinal gray-zone lymphoma. *Blood*, **124** (10), 1563–1569.

78 Kridel, R., Sehn, L.H., Gascoyne, R.D. (2012) Pathogenesis of follicular lymphoma. *J. Clin. Invest.*, **122**, 3424–3431.

79 Stevenson, F.K., Stevenson, G.T. (2012) Follicular lymphoma and the immune system: from pathogenesis to antibody therapy. *Blood*, **119**, 3659–3667.

80 Anonymous (1997) A clinical evaluation of the International Lymphoma Study Group classification of non-Hodgkin's lymphoma. The Non-Hodgkin's Lymphoma Classification Project. *Blood*, **89**, 3909–3918.

81 Ghielmini, M., Vitolo, U., Kimbe, E., *et al.* (2013) ESMO guidelines consensus conference on malignant lymphoma 2011 part 1: diffuse large B-cell lymphoma (DLBCL), follicular lymphoma (FL) and chronic lymphocytic leukemia (CLL). *Ann. Oncol.*, **24**, 561–576.

82 Guadagnolo, B.A., Li, S., Neuberg, D., *et al.* (2006) Long-term outcome and mortality trends in early-stage, grade 1-2 follicular lymphoma treated with radiation therapy. *Int. J. Radiat. Oncol. Biol. Phys.*, **64**, 928–934.

83 Friedberg, J.W., Taylor, M.D., Cerhan, J.R., *et al.* (2009) Follicular lymphoma in the United States: first report of the national LymphoCare study. *J. Clin. Oncol.*, **27** (8), 1202–1208.

84 Advani, R., Rosenberg, S.A., Horning, S.J. (2004) Stage I and II follicular non-Hodgkin's lymphoma: long-term follow-up of no initial therapy. *J. Clin. Oncol.*, **22**, 1454–1459.

85 Hoskin, P., Kirkwood, A., Syndikus, I. *et al.* (2014) 4 Gy vs. 24 Gy radiotherapy for patients with indolent lymphoma (FORT): a randomized phase 3 non-inferiority trial. *Lancet Oncol.*, **15**, 457–463.

86 Ruella, M., Filippi, A., Di Russo, A., *et al.* (2011) Rituximab followed by involved field radiotherapy (IF-RT) in stage I-II follicular lymphoma (FL): long term results. *Blood* (ASH annual meeting abstracts), **118**, a3699.

87 Herfarth, K., Engelhard, M., Borchmann, P., *et al.* (2012) Treatment of early stage nodal follicular lymphoma using involved-field radiotherapy and rituximab: preliminary results of the MIR trial (phase II study of the German Low Grade Lymphoma Study Group (GLSG)). *Blood* (ASH annual meeting abstracts), **120**, a1634.

88 Martinelli, G., Schmitz, S.F., Utiger, U., *et al.* (2010) Long-term follow up of patients with follicular lymphoma receiving single-agent rituximab at two different schedules in trial SAKK 35/98. *J. Clin. Oncol.*, **28**, 4480–4484.

89 Colombat, P., Brousse, N., Salles, G., *et al.* (2012) Rituximab induction immunotherapy for first-line low-tumor-burden follicular lymphoma: survival analyses with 7-year follow up. *Ann. Oncol.*, **23**, 2380–2385.

90 Brice, P., Bastion, Y., Lepage, E., *et al.* (1997) Comparison in low-tumor-burden follicular lymphomas between an initial no-treatment policy, prednimustine, or interferon alfa: a randomized study from the Groupe d'Etude des Lymphomes Folliculaires. Groupe d'Etude des Lymphomes de l'Adulte. *J. Clin. Oncol.*, **15**, 1110–1117.

91 Ardeshna, K.M., Smith, P., Norton, A., *et al.* (2003) Long term effect of a watch and wait policy versus immediate systemic treatment for asymptomatic advanced-stage non-Hodgkin lymphoma: a randomized controlled trial. *Lancet*, **362**, 516–522.

92 Hiddemann, W., Kneba, M., Dreyling, M., *et al.* (2005) Frontline therapy with rituximab added to the combination of cyclophosphamide, doxorubicin, vincristine, and prednisone (CHOP) significantly improves the outcome for patients with advanced-stage follicular lymphoma compared with therapy with CHOP alone: results of a prospective randomized study of the German Low-Grade Lymphoma Study Group. *Blood*, **106**, 3725–3732.

93 Marcus, R., Imrie, K., Belcha, A., *et al.* (2005) CVP chemotherapy plus rituximab compared with CVP as first-line treatment for advanced follicular lymphoma. *Blood*, **105**, 1417–1423.

94 Herold, M., Haas, A., Srock, S., *et al.* (2007) Rituximab added to first-line mitoxantrone, chlorambucil, and prednisolone chemotherapy followed by interferon maintenance prolongs survival in patients with advanced follicular lymphoma: an East German Study Group Hematology and Oncology Study. *J. Clin. Oncol.*, **25**, 1986–1992.

95 Hainsworth, J.D., Litchy, S., Burris, H.A., III., *et al.* (2002) Rituximab as first-line and maintenance therapy for patients with indolent non-Hodgkin's lymphoma. *J. Clin. Oncol.*, **20**, 4261–4267.

96 Ghielmini, M., Schmitz, S.F., Cogliatti, S.B., Pichert, G., *et al.* (2004) Prolonged treatment with rituximab in patients with follicular lymphoma significantly increases event-free survival and response duration compared with the standard weekly x 4 schedule. *Blood*, **103**, 4416–4423.

97 Van Oers, M.H., Klasa, R., Marcus, R.E., *et al.* (2006) Rituximab maintenance improves clinical outcome of relapsed/resistant follicular non-Hodgkin lymphoma in patients both with and without rituximab during induction: results of a prospective randomized phase 3 intergroup trial. *Blood*, **108**, 3295–3301.

98 Salles, G., Seymour, J.F., Offner, F., *et al.* (2011) Rituximab maintenance for 2 years in patients with high tumour burden follicular lymphoma responding to rituximab plus chemotherapy (PRIMA): a phase 3, randomized controlled trial. *Lancet*, **377**, 42–51.

99 Morschhauser, F., Radford, J., Van Hoof, A., *et al.* (2008) Phase III trial of consolidation therapy with yttrium-90-ibritumomab tiuxetan compared with no additional therapy after first remission in advanced follicular lymphoma. *J. Clin. Oncol.*, **26**, 5156–5164.

100 Press, O.W., Unger, J.M., Rimsza, L.M., *et al.* (2013) Phase III randomized intergroup trial of CHOP plus rituximab compared with CHOP chemotherapy plus (131) iodine-tositumomab for previously untreated follicular non-Hodgkin lymphoma: SWOG S0016. *J. Clin. Oncol.*, **31**, 314–320.

101 Freedman, A., Neelapu, S.S., Nichols, C., *et al.* (2009) Placebo-controlled phase III trial of patient-specific immunotherapy with mitumprotimut-T and granulocyte-macrophage colony-stimulating factor after rituximab in patients with follicular lymphoma. *J. Clin. Oncol.*, **27**, 3036–3043.

102 Levy, R., Robertson, M.J., Leonard, J., Vose, J.M., Denney, D. (2008) Results of a phase 3 trial evaluating safety and efficacy of specific immunotherapy, recombinant idiotype (ID) conjugated to KLH (ID-KLH) with GM-CSF, compared to non-specific immunotherapy, KLH with GM-CSF, in patients with follicular non-Hodgkin lymphoma (abstr.) *Ann. Oncol.*, **19**, 057.

103 Holman, P.R., Costello, C., Demagalhaes-Silverman, M., Corringham, S., Castro, J., Ball, E.D. (2012) Idiotype immunization following high-dose therapy and autologous stem cell transplantation for non-Hodgkin lymphoma. *Biol. Blood Marrow Transplant.*, **18** (2), 257–264.

104 Tomita, N., Kodaira, T., Tachibana, H., Nakamura, T., Mizoguchi, N., Takada, A. (2009) Favorable outcomes of radiotherapy for early-stage mucosa-associated lymphoid tissue lymphoma. *Radiother. Oncol.*, **90** (2), 231–235.

105 Tsai, H.K., Li, S., Ng, A.K., Silver, B., Stevenson, M.A., Mauch, P.M. (2007) Role of radiation therapy in the treatment of stage I/II mucosa-associated lymphoid tissue lymphoma. *Ann. Oncol.*, **18**, 672–678.

106 Cordone, I., Masi, S., Mauro, F.R., *et al.* (1998) p53 expression in B-cell chronic lymphocytic leukemia: a marker of disease progression and poor prognosis. *Blood*, **91**, 4342–4349.

107 Dohner, H., Stilgenbauer, S., Benner, A., *et al.* (2000) Genomic aberrations and survival in chronic lymphocytic leukemia. *N. Engl. J. Med.*, **343**, 1910–1916.

108 Keating, M.J., O'Brien, S., Albitar, M., *et al.* (2005) Early results of a chemoimmunotherapy regimen of fludarabine, cyclophosphamide, and rituximab as initial therapy for chronic lymphocytic leukemia. *J. Clin. Oncol.*, **23** (18), 4079–4088.

109 Tam, C.S., O'Brien, S., Wierda, W., *et al.* (2010) Long-term results of the fludarabine, cyclophosphamide, rituximab regimen as initial therapy of chronic lymphocytic leukemia: a randomized, open-lab, phase 3 trial. *Lancet*, **376** (9747), 1164–1174.

110 Goede, V., Fischer, K., Engelke, A., *et al.* (2015) Obinutuzumab as frontline treatment of chronic lymphocytic leukemia: updated results of the CLL11 study. *Leukemia*, **29**, 1602–1604.

111 Hillmen, P., Robak, T., Janssens, A., *et al.* (2013) Ofatumumab + chlorambucil versus chlorambucil alone in patients with untreated chronic lymphocytic leukemia (CLL): results of the phase III study complement 1 (OMB110911). *Blood*, **122** (21), 528a.

112 Pettitt, A.R., Jackson, R., Carruthers, S., *et al.* (2012) Alemtuzumab in combination with methylprednisolone is a highly effective induction regimen for patients with chronic lymphocytic leukemia and deletion of TP53: final results of the National Cancer Research Institute CLL206 trial. *J. Clin. Oncol.*, **30** (14), 1647–1655.

113 O'Brien, S., Furman, R.R., Coutre, S.E., *et al.* (2014) Ibrutinib as initial therapy for elderly patients with

chronic lymphocytic leukemia or small lymphocytic lymphoma: an open-label multicenter, phase 1b/2 trial. *Lancet Oncol.*, **15** (1), 48–58.

114 Miller, T.P., Dahlberg, S., Cassady, J.R., *et al.* (1998) Chemotherapy alone compared with chemotherapy plus radiotherapy for localized intermediate- and high-grade non-Hodgkin's lymphoma. *N. Engl. J. Med.*, **339**, 21–26.

115 Miller, T., Leblanc, M., Spier, C., *et al.* (2001) CHOP alone compared to CHOP plus radiotherapy for early stage aggressive non-Hodgkin's lymphomas: update of the Southwest Oncology Group (SWOG) randomized trial (abstr.) *Blood*, **98**, 724a.

116 Horning, S.J., Weller, E., Kim, K., *et al.* (2004) Chemotherapy with or without radiotherapy in limited-stage diffuse aggressive non-Hodgkin's lymphoma: Eastern Cooperative Oncology Group study 1484. *J. Clin. Oncol.*, **22**, 3032–3038.

117 Bonnet, C., Fillet, G., Mounier, N., *et al.* (2007) CHOP alone compared with CHOP plus radiotherapy for localized aggressive lymphoma in elderly patients: a study by the Groupe d'Etude des Lymphomes de l'Adulte. *J. Clin. Oncol.*, **25**, 787–792.

118 Pfreundschuh, M., Kuhnt, E., Trümper, L., *et al.* (2011) CHOP-like chemotherapy with or without rituximab in young patients with good-prognosis diffuse large-B-cell lymphoma: 6-year results of an open-label randomised study of the MabThera International Trial (MInT) Group. *Lancet Oncol.*, **12**, 1013–1022.

119 Held, G., Murawski, N., Pfreundschuh, M., *et al.* (2014) Role of radiotherapy to bulky disease in elderly patients with aggressive B-cell lymphoma. *J. Clin. Oncol.*, **32**, 1112–1118.

120 German High-Grade Non-Hodgkin's Lymphoma Study Group: Rituximab and combination chemotherapy with or without radiation therapy in treating patients with B-cell non-Hodgkin's lymphoma. Available at: https://clinicaltrials.gov/show/NCT00278408.

121 Lowry, L., *et al.* (2011) Reduced dose radiotherapy for local control in non-Hodgkin lymphoma: a randomized trial. *Radiother. Oncol.*, **100**, 86–92.

122 Fisher, R.I., Gaynor, E.R., Dahlberg, S., *et al.* (1993) Comparison of a standard regimen (CHOP) with three intensive chemotherapy regimens for advanced non-Hodgkin's lymphoma. *N. Engl. J. Med.*, **328**, 1002–1006.

123 Vitolo U, Bertini M, Meneghini V *et al.* (1992) MACOP-B treatment in diffuse large-cell lymphoma: identification of prognostic groups in an Italian multicenter study. *J. Clin. Oncol.*, **10**, 219–27.

124 Coiffier, B., Lepage, E., Briere, J., *et al.* (2002) CHOP chemotherapy plus rituximab compared with CHOP alone in elderly patients with diffuse large-B-cell lymphoma. *N. Engl. J. Med.*, **346**, 235–242.

125 Morrison, V., Weller, E., Habermann, T.M. (2007) Maintenance rituximab compared to observation after R-CHOP or CHOP in older patients with diffuse large B-cell lymphoma: an intergroup E4494/C9793 update (abstr.) *J. Clin. Oncol.*, **25**, 8011a.

126 Mundt, A.J., Williams, S.F., Hallahan, D. (1997) High dose chemotherapy and stem cell rescue for aggressive non-Hodgkin's lymphoma: pattern of failure and implications for involved-field radiotherapy. *Int. J. Radiat. Oncol. Biol. Phys.*, **39**, 617–625.

127 Pileri, S.A., Gaidano, G., Zinzani, P.L., *et al.* (2003) Primary mediastinal B-cell lymphoma: high frequency of BCL-6 mutations and consistent expression of the transcription factors OCT-2, BOB.1, and PU.1 in the absence of immunoglobulins. *Am. J. Pathol.*, **162**, 243–253.

128 Zinzani, P.L., Martelli, M., Bertini, M., *et al.* (2002) Induction chemotherapy strategies for primary mediastinal large B-cell lymphoma with sclerosis: a retrospective multinational study on 426 previously untreated patients. *Haematologica*, **87**, 1258–1264.

129 Zinzani, P.L., Martelli, M., Magagnoli, M., *et al.* (1999) Treatment and clinical management of primary mediastinal large B-cell lymphoma with sclerosis: MaCOP-B regimen and mediastinal radiotherapy monitored by (67)Gallium scan in 50 patients. *Blood*, **94**, 3289–3293.

130 Reiger, M., Osterborg, A., Pettengell, R., *et al.* (2011) Primary mediastinal B-cell lymphoma treated with CHOP-like chemotherapy with or without rituximab: results of the MabThera International Trial Group Study. *Ann. Oncol.*, **22**, 664–670.

131 Dunleavy, K., Pittaluga, S., Maeda, L.S., *et al.* (2013) Dose-adjusted EPOCH-rituximab therapy in primary mediastinal B-cell lymphoma. *N. Engl. J. Med.*, **368**, 1408–1416.

132 Gebauer, N., Bernard, V., Gebauer, W., *et al.* (2015) TP53 mutations are frequent events in double-hit B-cell lymphomas with MYC and BCL2 but not MYC and BCL6 translocations. *Leuk. Lymphoma*, **56** (1), 179–185.

133 Vaidya, R., Witzig, T.E. (2014) Prognostic factors for diffuse large B-cell lymphoma in the R(X)CHOP era. *Ann. Oncol.*, **25** (11), 2124–2133.

134 Martin, P., Chadburn, A., Christos, P., *et al.* (2008) Intensive treatment strategies may not provide superior outcomes in mantle cell lymphoma: overall survival exceeding 7 years with standard therapies. *Ann. Oncol.*, **19**, 1327–1330.

135 Till, B.G., Gooley, T.A., Crawford, N., *et al.* (2008) Effect of remission status and induction chemotherapy regimen on outcome of autologous stem cell transplantation for mantle cell lymphoma. *Leuk. Lymphoma*, **49**, 1062–1073.

136 Savage, K.J., Chhanabhai, M., Gascoyne, R.D., *et al.* (2004) Characterization of peripheral T-cell lymphomas in a single North American institution by the WHO classification. *Ann. Oncol.*, **15** (10), 1467–1475.

137 Yamaguchi, M., Tobinai, K., Oshimi, K., *et al.* (2009) Phase I/II Study of concurrent chemoradiotherapy for localized nasal natural killer/T-cell lymphoma: Japanese Clinical Oncology Group Study JCOG 0211. *J. Clin. Oncol.*, **27** (33), 5594–5600.

138 Batchelor, T., Carson, K., O'Neill, A., *et al.* (2003) Treatment of primary CNS lymphoma with methotrexate and deferred radiotherapy: a report of NABTT 96-07. *J. Clin. Oncol.*, **21** (6), 1044–1049.

139 Valencak J., Weihsengruber F., Raderer M., *et al.* (2009) Rituximab monotherapy for primary cutaneous B cell lymphoma; response and follow-up in 16 patients. *Ann. Oncol.* **20**, 326–330.

140 Grange, F., *et al.* (2007) Primary cutaneous diffuse large B cell lymphoma, leg type: clinicopathologic features and prognostic analysis in 60 cases. *Arch. Dermatol.*, **143**, 1144–1150.

141 Ysebaert, L., *et al.* (2004) Ultimate results of radiation therapy for T1-T2 mycosis fungoides. *Int. J. Radiat. Oncol. Biol. Phys.*, **58**, 1128–1134.

142 Harrison. C., *et al.* (2011) Revisiting low dose total skin electron beam therapy in mycosis fungoides. *Int. J. Radiat. Oncol. Biol. Phys.*, **81**, e651–e657.

143 Kamstrup, M.R., *et al.* (2012) Low-dose total skin electron beam therapy as a debulking agent for cutaneous T cell lymphoma: an open-label prospective phase II study. *Br. J. Dermatol.*, **166**, 399–404.

144 Nachman, J.B., Sposto, R., Herzog, P., *et al.* (2002) Randomized comparison of low-dose involved-field radiotherapy and no radiotherapy for children with Hodgkin's disease who achieve a complete response to chemotherapy. *J. Clin. Oncol.*, **20**, 3765–3771.

145 Keller F.G., Nachman J, Schwartz C., *et al.* (2010) *Blood.* **116**, 767.

146 Friedman, D.L., Chen, L., Schwartz, C.L., *et al.* (2014) Dose-intensive response-based chemotherapy and radiation therapy for children and adolescents with newly diagnosed intermediate-risk Hodgkin lymphoma: A report from the Children's Oncology Group Study AHOD0031. *J. Clin. Oncol.*, **32** (32), 3651–3658.

147 Link, M.P., Shuster, J.J., Donaldson, S.S., Berard, C.W., Murphy, S.B. (1997) Treatment of children and young adults with early-stage non-Hodgkin's lymphoma. *N. Engl. J. Med.*, **337**, 1259–1266.

148 Illidge T., Specht L., Wirth A., *et al.* (2014) Modern radiation therapy for nodal non-Hodgkin's lymphoma – Target definition and dose guidelines from International Lymphoma Radiation Oncology Group. *Int. J. Radiat. Oncol. Biol. Phys.*, **89**, 49–58.

149 Specht, L., *et al.* (2014) Modern radiotherapy for Hodgkin lymphoma – field and dose guidelines from the International Lymphoma Radiation Oncology Group. *Int. J. Radiat. Oncol. Biol. Phys.*, **89**, 854–862.

150 Kaminski, M.S., Tuck, M., Estes, J., *et al.* (2005) 131I-tositumomab therapy as initial treatment for follicular lymphoma. *N. Engl. J. Med.*, **352**, 441–449.

41

Pediatric Tumors

Shannon M. MacDonald, Torunn I. Yock, Nancy J. Tarbell and Tamara Z. Vern-Gross

Cancer in Childhood: A Special Situation

A childhood diagnosis of cancer often carries multiple layers of complexity for the patient and the family or caretakers. Children are generally unable to make treatment decisions on their own, and families may be equally overwhelmed by the responsibility of caring for and making difficult decisions regarding their child. Pediatric oncologists are responsible not only for the care of the child but also for ensuring that parents understand thoroughly the prognosis, management, options, and consequences of cancer therapies. Although prognosis is often favorable, cure does not come without cost. Over two-thirds of pediatric cancer survivors will experience at least one late toxicity from their treatment, and by the age of 50 years over half of childhood cancer survivors will endure a severe, disabling, and/or potentially fatal health condition [1, 2]. Treatment-related late side effects include chronic medical problems that can impair quality of life and result in substantial expenses to families, insurers, and society. For these reasons, the management of childhood cancer warrants special attention. A multidisciplinary team consisting of a pediatric medical oncologist, a pediatric surgeon, pediatric radiation oncologist, nurses, child life therapist, social worker, nutritionist, physical therapist, and pharmacists ensures the best possible delivery of care, which is focused on cure and maintaining optimal quality of life, while minimizing treatment-related complications. Following cancer treatment, pediatric patients require lifelong care and surveillance for potential late side effects of therapy.

Epidemiology of Childhood Cancers

It is estimated that, in the United States, a total of 10 270 children up to the age of 14 years will be diagnosed with cancer in 2017, and that 1190 children will die of cancer

[3]. Cancer is the second leading cause of death for children following accidents. Advances in therapy have led to marked improvements in survival over the past several decades, with a combined five-year survival for all childhood cancers from 63% in the mid-1970s to 83% today [4]. Pediatric cancers are a highly heterogeneous group of malignancies, with variable prognoses and treatments. The incidences of the major categories of pediatric cancers as a percentage of all childhood malignancies are shown in Figure 41.1.

CNS Malignancies

Tumors of the brain and central nervous system (CNS) represent the most common childhood malignancy, followed by leukemia, with an annual incidence of 5.57 per 100 000 population [5], and are the most common pediatric malignancies requiring radiation therapy. Pediatric brain tumors differ from adult brain tumors in terms of location, histology, and outcome [6] Symptoms are highly dependent on tumor location, and often include headache, nausea, vomiting, and/or seizures. Most patients will have a neurological deficit on physical examination. Imaging of the brain with computed tomography (CT) or magnetic resonance imaging (MRI) is typically the first step in diagnosis, and MRI allows for a better visualization of most tumors. Surgery to relieve symptoms and obtain tissue for a pathological diagnosis is indicated, unless there is either a high risk of injury or there is a pathognomonic radiographic diagnosis. Metastatic work-up, treatment, and prognosis are all dependent on diagnosis.

Medulloblastoma/Embryonal Tumors

Medulloblastoma, an embryonal tumor located in the cerebellum, is a relatively common pediatric brain tumor,

Clinical Radiation Oncology: Indications, Techniques, and Results, Third Edition. Edited by William Small Jr.
© 2017 John Wiley & Sons, Inc. Published 2017 by John Wiley & Sons, Inc.

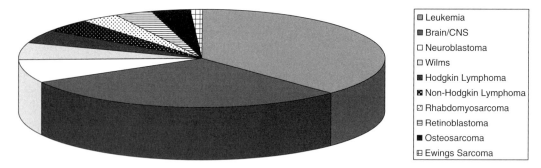

Figure 41.1 Incidence of major categories of childhood malignancies. Adapted from *American Cancer Society Cancer Facts and Figures 2017* [3].

with approximately 540 cases diagnosed per year in the United States. Children are generally young at diagnosis, with a median age at onset of five to six years, but range from infants to adults [7]. Boys are frequently affected more than girls. Medulloblastomas often present within the midline cerebellar vermis, growing and filling the fourth ventricle. As a result, symptoms occur related to increased intracranial pressure resulting from the tumor obstructing the cerebral spinal fluid (CSF) flow through the sylvian aqueduct and fourth ventricle. Adolescents and young adults may present with more lateralized tumors, and are more likely to have dysmetria and ataxia. Postoperatively, these children may develop posterior fossa syndrome, which includes symptoms of difficulty in swallowing, truncal ataxia, mutism, and rarely respiratory failure. Treatment with radiotherapy should proceed, as this is self-limiting and supportive services should be initiated.

Medulloblastoma is associated with a relatively high risk of CNS dissemination at presentation, reported at 11–43%; thus, appropriate postoperative staging is necessary prior to the initiation of treatment [8]. Postoperative imaging of the brain to assess extent of the resection within 24–48 hours is ideal. To complete staging, a gadolinium-enhanced spinal MRI approximately 10–14 days after surgery to rule out metastatic involvement, and a lumbar puncture for CSF cytology should be obtained. At present, disease extent is categorized as either standard-risk or high-risk, with standard-risk defined as non-metastatic disease in children at least three years of age with ≤ 1.5 cm^2 of residual disease following surgery. High-risk is defined as all others (<3 years old, >1.5 cm^2, or metastatic). Although not included in this stratification, anaplastic histology has been shown to carry an inferior prognosis compared to classic medulloblastoma and patients with anaplastic histology, but otherwise standard-risk diseases are considered for therapy and protocols for high-risk disease [9].

Classically, medulloblastoma is a primitive (embryonal) tumor of the cerebellum, originating from presumed undifferentiated progenitor medulloblasts within

the granular layer of the cerebellum. They are densely cellular tumors composed predominantly of small, round blue cells with many histological variants (e.g., desmoplastic/nodular, large cell, medulloblastoma with extensive nodularity, anaplastic), and now genetic (molecular) groups [10]. According to an international consensus statement published in 2012, there are four major subgroups of medulloblastoma, and only recently have these been linked to prognosis: (i) the WNT pathway subgroup, which is especially favorable; (ii) the SHH pathway subgroup, which is of good prognosis; (iii) the group 3 subgroup, which connotes the worst prognosis and is more likely to have C-myc amplification and frequently M+; and (iv) the group 4 subgroup, which has variable to poor prognosis and M+ [11, 12]. Molecular characteristics are starting to be incorporated into risk stratification for this disease on protocol, since recent research has indicated that prognosis may be more dependent on molecular correlations [13].

For patients with standard-risk disease receiving craniospinal irradiation (CSI) and chemotherapy, cure rates exceed 80% [14]. The Children's Oncology Group (COG) protocol, ACNS0331, raised the question of whether reducing the CSI dose of radiotherapy from 23.4 Gy to 18 Gy in children aged <8 years would maintain an event-free survival and overall survival (OS) in order to decrease radiation side effects, as these children are at highest risk of late toxicity [15]. Similar objectives were evaluated with reduced involved field boost compared to whole posterior fossa. In this trial, survival rates following reduced involved field boost were comparable to standard treatment volumes for the primary tumor site, with five-year OS estimates of 84.1% and 85.2%, respectively. Reduced CSI dose was associated with higher events and lower five-year survival estimates (78.1% versus 85.9%, respectively) [16]. Medulloblastoma standard treatment continues to involve irradiation to the entire craniospinal axis to a dose of 23.4 Gy, usually with concurrent vincristine, followed by additional radiation to the tumor bed, plus a margin (involved field) for an additional 30.6 Gy to bring the total dose to this region to

54 Gy [14]. For the involved field boost, the gross tumor volume (GTV) is based on pre- and post-gadolinium contrast T_1 signal changes. The preoperative extent should be taken into account, as well as any shift following surgery, and all sequences (T2, T2FLAIR, T1 pre- and post-gadolinium) should be reviewed as these tumors are often heterogeneously enhancing. The GTV includes the postoperative resection cavity, any area with which the preoperative tumor was in contact, and any residual enhancing tumor mass. The clinical target volume (CTV) is typically delineated as a 1.5 cm margin expansion around the GTV, accounting for bone or tentorial boundaries. A final planning target volume (PTV) margin of 0.3–0.5 cm around the CTV is added to offset any movement or errors.

Outcomes are less favorable for patients with high-risk medulloblastoma, but five-year disease-free survival rates of 60–70% can be achieved with a higher CSI dose and more intensive chemotherapy [14, 17–19]. For children with high-risk medulloblastoma or other embryonal tumors occurring in the cerebrum (such as pineoblastoma, ependymoblastoma, and medulloepithelioma), treatment includes a CSI dose to 36 Gy followed by a boost to the posterior fossa for an additional 19.8 Gy to bring the total dose to 55.8 Gy (including tumor bed) with concurrent chemotherapy. The CNS WHO 2016 recently underwent significant changes in the classification, removing supratentorial primitive neuroectodermal tumors (SPNETs) from the diagnostic lexicon [10]. These rare tumors amplify the C19MC region on chromosome 19 (19q13.42), resulting in a diagnosis of embryonal tumor with multilayered rosettes (ETMR) C19MC-altered. In treatment planning of the whole-posterior fossa boost for high-risk medulloblastoma, the CTV should extend inferiorly from the C1 vertebral canal through the foramen magnum, and superiorly to the tentorium cerebelli. Laterally, the posterior fossa extends to the bony aspect of the occiput and temporal bones. The PTV should extend with a margin of 0.3–0.5 cm for day-to-day set-up variations. Patients with diffuse disease may require the entire spine boosted to 39.6 Gy. Gross spinal metastatic disease will require a final boost to 45 Gy. The current COG protocol, ACNS0332, is evaluating the addition of daily carboplatin concurrent with radiation and post-treatment isotretinoin. Modern techniques, including intensity-modulated radiotherapy (IMRT) and protons, can decrease the dose and/or volume of uninvolved tissues receiving radiation [20]. Early proton beam data has demonstrated a significant dosimetric advantage in the treatment of many CNS tumors without compromising target volume coverage; this has been translated into a decrease in toxicities and improved quality of life outcomes [21–23]. The whole-posterior fossa dose should not exceed 54 Gy or 54 Gy(RBE) off of protocol to limit the risk of brainstem necrosis. A mean brainstem dose of less than 52–53 Gy(RBE) has been recommended when using proton therapy [24, 25]. More prospective data is necessary to further identify the clinical benefit and successful incorporation of these therapeutic modalities.

Craniospinal radiation planning requires knowledge of general principles in both proton and/or photon planning of pediatric and adult patients. The key is to establish immobilization and reproducibility of the treatment set-up at the time of CT simulation. An alpha cradle system or a vacuum bag can often provide assistance with accuracy when aligning fields and junctions. Sedation and the inclusion of a child-life therapist as part of a pediatric treatment team is recommended when applicable, to improve patient/caregiver education, treatment safety and efficacy, and improvement of quality of life and treatment experience [26, 27]. Prior to any treatment planning, ensure that any plans for immobilization and/or sedation have been discussed with the pediatric team. While planning, identify all critical anatomic sites intended for treatment to full dose: cribiform plate, middle cranial fossa, margin around the calvarium in order to achieve full dose levels; spinal cord, thecal sac, gross disease, and areas at risk including the clinical tumor volume. Identification of the thecal sac should be verified with MRI registration with CT planning scan. The thecal sac is usually located at or below S2. The width of this inferior aspect of the spinal fields should extend laterally and encompass the dorsal nerve roots, providing sufficient coverage dosimetrically of the sacral foramina.

Ongoing efforts are being developed to further reduce the radiotherapeutic dose, decrease treatment fields, and/or ultimately eliminate the need for radiation therapy in select patients [28]. Molecular subtypes are being incorporated into ongoing clinical trials for both standard- and high-risk patients in order to customize and target disease-specific therapy. St. Jude Children's Research Hospital initiated a risk-directed craniospinal irradiation protocol (SJMB 12) in patients with newly diagnosed medulloblastoma/PNET, and treatment is based on WNT/SHH subgroups versus non-WNT/non-SHH subgroups. The CSI doses will range between 15 and 39.6 Gy, and patients with SHH tumors will also receive maintenance vismodegib (GDC-0449), a hedgehog antagonist [29, 30]. Similarly, COG will be applying reduced-dose 18 Gy CSI, but limited to WNT+ only patients in the new ACNS1422 protocol [31]. In an attempt to eliminate radiotherapy altogether, the NCT02212574 study is assessing the feasibility of a surgery and chemotherapy-only approach in children with the WNT+ standard-risk medulloblastoma, the goal being to reduce the toxicity of therapy. Patients will receive nine cycles of chemotherapy, including cisplatin, lomustine, vincristine, and cyclophosphamide [30, 32].

The management of children under the age of three years presents a particular challenge, when survivals range from 20% in those with high-risk features to 90% in those with favorable histology and standard-risk features [33]. Outcomes in these patients have been inferior, perhaps as a result of treatment omission, deferral as a result of parental preference, toxicity of therapy, or alteration of radiation therapy. CSI leads to unacceptable toxicities for children this young, specifically resulting in neurotoxicity and growth failure. As a result, management generally consists of maximal safe resection followed by chemotherapy in order to delay radiation therapy. Achieving a gross total resection has survival benefits, as demonstrated in BABY POG1 [34]. Radiotherapy is not mandatory and currently the role remains unclear [35]. The Head Start trials had demonstrated promising outcomes with initiation of chemotherapy followed by High Dose Chemotherapy Stem Cell Rescue (HDCSTR) with or without radiotherapy with five-year OS rates up to 60–70% [36]. The COG protocol ACNS0334 is evaluating the role for intensive chemotherapy high-dose and peripheral blood stem cell rescue results ± methotrexate, to determine if this regimen results in a higher response rate. Similarly, the Pediatric Brain Tumor Consortium (PBTC) recently closed PBTC 026, which evaluated children aged two to four years who had been diagnosed with medulloblastoma and who received induction therapy followed by consolidative (HDSCRT) and radiotherapy for M0 disease, followed by SAHA/isotretinoin [37]. Guided by histologic subgroups, ACNS1221 has eliminated all radiotherapy and is a Phase II study designed for the treatment of non-metastatic nodular desmoplastic medulloblastoma in children aged less than four years, using combination chemotherapy, completely removing radiotherapy [38]. Even in children with M+ disease, CSI may be considered but should be delayed if possible until the child is aged more than three years. Radiation volumes are often being limited to the involved field, or sometimes are even omitted [36, 39].

Atypical Teratoid/Rhabdoid Tumor

Atypical teratoid/rhabdoid tumor (AT/RT) is a highly malignant tumor of the CNS that occurs in approximately 3% of pediatric CNS tumors, previously diagnosed as other embryonal tumors including medulloblastoma, PNET, and choroid plexus tumor (CPC). It has only been recognized as a distinct entity since discovery of the tumor suppressor gene, *INI1* [40]. AT/RT is histologically identical to rhabdoid tumors diagnosed outside of the CNS, and typically occurs in very young children. Most series show a high risk of relapse, and patients historically have had a poor prognosis, dying from their disease [41]. Approximately 50–60% of tumors present within the posterior fossa; thus, patients often present with symptoms of increased ICP. Current treatment includes maximal tumor resection, high-dose chemotherapy, and early radiation therapy. Young children generally receive involved-field radiation to a dose of 50.4–54 Gy, whereas older children or those diagnosed with metastatic disease may benefit from more comprehensive CSI, which has been associated with improved outcomes [42]. The most recent ACNS 0333 study evaluated the outcomes in treatment of AT/RT with surgery, intensive chemotherapy which included HDCSCR and three-dimensional (3D) conformal therapy, and closed in February of 2014 [43]. At a medium follow-up of 24 months, event-free survival (EFS) and OS were 43% and 52%, respectively [44]. Future review of patient outcomes may identify the benefit of further CSI dose reduction/omission with the incorporation of molecular stratification, which may have a role in the treatment of these patients.

Ependymoma

Ependymomas are relatively rare brain tumors, with nearly 200 cases diagnosed in the United States per year; of these tumors, up to 40% occurred in children aged <3 years [45, 46]. Over 90% of ependymomas present as intracranial tumors, with approximately two-thirds occurring in the posterior fossa. These tumors may be radiographically similar in appearance to medulloblastoma; however, ependymomas more frequently extend through the foramen of Luschka or foramen of Magende [36, 47]. Approximately 50% of fourth ventricular lesions will grow below the foramen magnum [48]. CNS dissemination is uncommon at presentation, identified in only 10–15% of patients. Histologically, ependymomas consist of polygonal cells, comprised of ependymal rosettes which orient around blood vessels, forming perivascular pseudorosette arrangements of tumor cells [49]. Ependymomas have been subdivided into WHO Grade I tumors, which include myxopapillary ependymoma (spine presentation) and subependymoma (intracranial presentation). These tumors are associated with a favorable outcome [10]. Classic ependymomas are divided between WHO Grade II and WHO Grade III; however, the distinction between these tumors remains challenging [50, 51].

Standard treatment for both supratentorial and infratentorial ependymoma consists of maximal surgical resection followed by involved field radiation therapy [48, 52]. With this treatment, local control rates of close to 80% have been achieved [53, 54]. It is unclear if chemotherapy is of benefit for this disease, and trials attempting to use chemotherapy and omit radiation have led to dismal outcomes [55]. However, a short seven-week course of chemotherapy can be considered with intent as a bridge to a second-look surgery [56,57].

Radiation therapy is prescribed to the tumor bed (GTV) plus a margin of approximately 0.5 cm to delineate the CTV, respecting anatomic boundaries. A PTV margin of approximately 0.3–0.5 cm is added to account for set-up error and patient variability. Care must be taken to carefully delineate the tumor bed and areas that the tumor was in contact with prior to surgery; thus, both preoperative and postoperative imaging is useful during treatment planning. After registration of MR imaging, the preoperative imaging will allow visualization of what the tumor touched, while the postoperative imaging will assist with making contour shifts as a result of tissue changes and volume loss. Sagittal views will help to identify any tumor extension into the spinal canal. The prescribed dose is 54–59.4 Gy in 30 to 33 fractions to this volume. If a child has metastatic disease involving the spine on MRI, or a positive CSF, a total dose of 36 Gy CSI should be prescribed for children aged >3 years. The recently closed and current COG protocols (ACN0121 and ACNS0831) prescribed a total dose to 59.4 Gy, but ACNS0831 requires that critical structures outside of the area of highest risk are blocked for any additional dose after 54 Gy. Given the young age of these patients, it is important to use very conformal techniques to avoid the normal developing brain, cochlea, and neuroendocrine structures. The use of 3D conformal radiation therapy (CRT), IMRT, and protons has demonstrated superior sparing of nearby critical structures while maintaining excellent outcomes [54, 58]. In the recurrent setting, re-irradiation has demonstrated promising disease control, particularly utilizing standard fractionation and CSI in distant metastatic failures [59]. However, stereotactic radiosurgery (SRS) has been associated with radionecrosis, and may not be the preferred method of treatment approach [60].

Children are at risk for ototoxicity, particularly from injury to the organ of Corti and the basal areas. These risks increase with the addition of platinum-based chemotherapy. The goal is to maintain the mean less than 30–35 Gy to at least one cochlea [60]. When planning, it is important to identify the earlobes and the auditory canals, which will then lead to the internal auditory canals, all best identified on T2 MRI sequences at the end of the 7th and 8th cranial nerves. Annual audiology evaluations are recommended when the child is age-appropriate and tolerated so that early intervention can be initiated when a deficit is detected. The cochlea are best visualized on the bone window of the CT at the end of the internal auditory canal.

Despite similarities in histopathologic make-up, particularly WHO Grade II and III, the differences in biologic behavior have triggered an interest in identifying a distinct genetic and a molecular classification system [50, 51]. A recent study performed a classification for ependymomas and completed genome-wide DNA methylation profiles for 500 tumors, identifying nine distinct molecular subgroups; three in each anatomic compartment of the CNS, including the spine (SP), posterior fossa (PF), and supratentorial (ST). These molecular subgroups surpassed the current histopathological grading in terms of patient risk stratification. Extent of resection continues to be a key feature; however, an evaluation of whether specific subgroups could omit radiotherapy after complete resection is warranted. Future prospective clinical trials should be designed to include molecular risk stratification of patients to identify ways in which therapy can be modified or reduced in order to avoid late toxicities of radiotherapy.

Low-Grade Glioma

Low grade glioma (LGG), or astrocytoma, are the most common brain tumors in children, and are composed of multiple subtypes [61]. Historically, pilocytic (WHO Grade 1) and diffuse fibrillary astrocytoma (WHO Grade 2) are the two most common LGGs diagnosed in children. The cerebellum is the most frequent site of origin (15–25%), followed by the cerebrum (10–15%), deep midline structures (10–15%), optic pathway (5%), and finally the brainstem (2–4%) [60]. Two most common genetic cancer-predisposing syndromes include tuberous sclerosis (subependymal giant cell astrocytomas) and neurofibromatosis type-1 (NF-1) (pilocytic astrocytomas of the optic pathway/hypothalamus). Approximately 2–5% of low-grade astrocytomas occur in the optic pathway. About one-third of patients with tumors in this location carry the diagnosis of NF-1) [62]. Recent updates within the 2016 CNS WHO classifications, (integrating both phenotypic and genotypic markers), have added additional layers of objectivity and complexity, in turn allowing for more accurate diagnoses, prognostication, and management of disease [10]. Likewise, several mutations have been identified among pediatric LGGs, which may serve as potential therapeutic targets for the different subtypes of LGG, including BRAF oncogene mutations that activate the mitogen-activated protein kinase (MAPK) pathway as the most common [63]. Recent data have suggested significant variations in pediatric clinical outcomes based on the distributions of genetic alterations in relation to tumor pathology and location [64]. Children may present with a slow progression of symptoms over a six-month period or more before a diagnosis is successfully made [65]. The clinical presentation may differ depending on whether the tumor is within the cerebral hemispheres (seizures), thalamus (lateralizing neurologic symptoms), or midline/suprasellar structures (visual signs, endocrine abnormalities, diencephalic syndrome). Care should be taken to review all MRI sequences, as many tumors either do not enhance or have a non-enhancing component that can only be appreciated on T2 sequences. On MRI, pediatric LGGs tend to be hypointense on T1-weighted and hyper-intense on T2-weighted sequences, varying in degree following gadolinium infusion. Staging studies include postoperative MRI, ideally within 24 48 hours to best distinguish between residual tumor and postoperative disease. Tumor dissemination throughout the neuroaxis of with leptomeningeal spread is rare, but has been reported at rates of 5–18% [66, 67]. If a new diagnosis, is suspected or if the child has known disease, spinal imaging is warranted.

Depending on the age, symptoms, location of tumor and previous therapies, various tumor and patient characteristics may warrant or preclude aggressive interventions. A surgical biopsy is indicated if safe and/or maximal safe resection is recommended in order to obtain histologic and genomic information. A biopsy may be omitted if the tumor location involves eloquent brain, increasing the risk of procedural complications, and/or MRI findings that are consistent with LGG. Surgery followed by observation alone may be curative; however, a subtotal resection may also be sufficient, especially in younger children. Children with a STR have inferior PFS and may require additional therapy, including radiotherapy or chemotherapy [68]. Observation may be appropriate if the child is asymptomatic and the tumor has not progressed on serial MRIs. This is especially recommended for patients with NF-1, as tumors tend to be more indolent and these children may also suffer from learning disabilities [69]. Chemotherapy is often considered, although for the majority of patients this is only a temporizing measure. In general, chemotherapy is used for young patients, with carboplatin and vincristine often utilized in the setting of progressive disease [70]. Radiation is often the first choice for older patients, but there is no clear age cut-off. Radiation is not recommended if gross total resection (GTR) is achieved, but often plays a role in the management of tumors in locations that preclude complete resection. Treatment is indicated to alleviate symptoms, or if radiographic progression is documented. Excellent long-term outcomes have been documented following conformal radiation treatment [71]. Stereotactic radiation provides a highly conformal treatment, with excellent outcomes for small tumors [72]. During the preparation of treatment planning, all previous MRIs should be obtained at diagnosis and prior to chemotherapeutic or surgical intervention for registration to the current treatment planning scan. In doing so, complete tumor volumes can be created, including previously involved areas by the tumor 'pre-treatment', and appropriate contour shifts should be made as the volume changes over time. A radiation treatment dose of 50.4–54 Gy is recommended. The GTV includes all gross

tumor/residual and the tumor bed, while a CTV margin of 0.5 cm is recommended for well-demarcated tumors, modified depending on initial tumor involvement, areas of suspected subclinical disease, and respecting anatomic boundaries. Proton radiation may allow for decreased late side effects by reducing radiation to the uninvolved brain [73, 74]. A radiation treatment plan for a patient with a hypothalamic/optic glioma is shown in Figure 41.2. Care should be taken when treating these patients, especially with primaries that involve the optic structures. Depending on the type and location of injury, visual impairment from radiation-induced optic neuropathy (RION) can present as visual acuity loss or visual field loss (optic nerve, chiasmal, or optic pathway injury). Although the maximum dose is often reported, there is likely a dose/volume relationship and an impact of the mean dose. Fractionation with a lower dose per fraction may lower the risk of injury. Doses below 50.4 Gy at 1.8 Gy per fraction are recommended, but the risk of RION is unusual if the D_{max} is maintained <55 Gy [75, 76]. Retinopathy results in loss of visual acuity and floaters, ultimately leading to central visual loss. Doses should be kept below 45 Gy in order to minimize this risk. The lenses are the most sensitive, and cataracts may develop at single doses as low as 2–3 Gy, or fractionated doses of 12 Gy or more. Treatment volume coverage should not be compromised in order to reduce the risk of cataracts, as they can be treated with lens replacement [77].

Some current studies are evaluating BRAF duplication/MAPK pathway and BRAF V600E-targeting agents. The Pediatric Brain Tumor Consortium (NCT01089101) is evaluating the activity of selumetinib (AZD4266), which is a MEK1/2 inhibitor. Another ongoing protocol (NCT01677741) is utilizing dabrafenib, which binds to the ATP-binding domain of mutant BRAF V600E, and is being examined as a targeting agent in the management of BRAF V600E-mutant pediatric tumors [78]. Based on the results of these studies and other ongoing investigations, future studies will be necessary to examine the patient-specific role of radiotherapy and/or targeted therapies in the management of LGG.

High-Grade Glioma

Anaplastic astrocytoma and glioblastoma multiforme are much less common in children than in adults. The prognosis is still poor, but some patients do experience long-term survival from disease [79]. Extent of resection and histologic grade remain the strongest clinical prognostic factors for survival. Although single-agent temozolamide administered during and after radiotherapy demonstrated a benefit in EFS and OS in adults, COG protocol ACNS0126 failed to show a similar

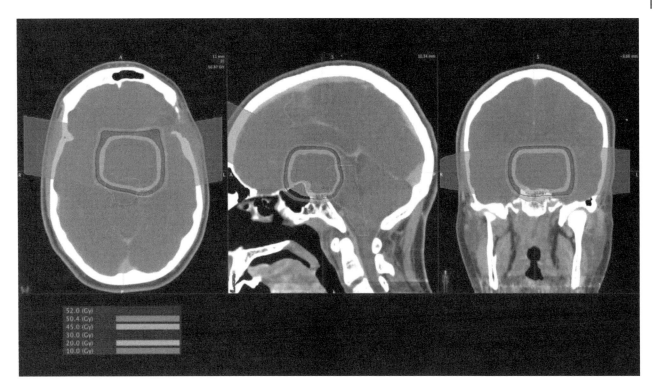

Figure 41.2 Radiation treatment plan using passively scattered protons for a low-grade glioma involving the optic chiasm/hypothalamic region. For a color version of this figure, see the color plate section.

benefit in the setting of pediatric HGG compared to traditional chemotherapeutic regimens [80,81]. ACNS0822 compared standard therapy (combined therapy, including temozolamide) with two combined-modality experimental arms that included either vorinistat or bevacizumab [82]. The study was closed early after the pre-defined endpoint of improved one-year improved EFS compared with standard therapy was not met. Because of the biologic heterogeneity of pediatric HGG, any clinical benefit of chemotherapy may have been missed and isolated to a subset of patients. The most recent COG protocol ACNS0423 evaluated radiotherapy to 54 Gy with a boost to 59.4 Gy with concurrent temozolamide with the addition of maintenance CCNU and temozolamide compared to standard temozolamide alone. EFS and OS were significantly improved compared to those treated with temozolamide alone in ACNS 0126, even in those who did not achieve a GTR [83]. However, chemotherapy alone remains a treatment option for children aged less than three years, as Head Start II and Head Start III trials recently reported promising survival outcomes of five-year EFS and OS of 44% and 63% in children aged <36 months compared to those aged 36–71 months (31% and 38%) and those aged >72 months (0% and 13%) treated with chemotherapy alone [84]. Maximal safe resection followed by radiation ± chemotherapy is standard treatment for children and adolescents diagnosed with HGG. Overall treatment target volume

and prescription includes an initial treatment volume followed by a boost volume to deliver a total dose of 54–59.4 Gy to this region. Detailed summary includes the following:

- GTV1 – Includes enhancing and non-enhancing areas of the residual tumor and/or tumor resection bed defined on both preoperative and postoperative MRI, which includes the pre- and post-contrast MR T1 and T2 abnormalities.
- CTV1 – A margin of approximately 2 cm, modified by tissue interfaces and bony anatomy.
- PTV1 – A margin of approximately 0.3–0.5 cm to CTV1 to account for set-up variability and movement.
  - Primary Site (PTV1) – 54 Gy at 1.8 Gy per fractions in 30 fractions.
- GTV2 – Includes enhancing and non-enhancing areas of the residual tumor and/or tumor resection bed defined on postoperative MRI, which includes post-contrast MR T1 abnormalities.
- CTV2 – A margin of approximately 1 cm, modified by tissue interfaces and bony anatomy.
- PTV2 – A margin of approximately 0.3–0.5 cm to CTV2 to account for set-up variability and movement.
  - Primary Site (PTV1) – 54 Gy at 1.8 Gy per fraction in three fractions.

Another highly malignant tumor is diffusely infiltrating brainstem glioma (DIPG), which accounts for approximately 70% of pediatric brainstem gliomas. The clinical presentation includes cranial nerve palsies (commonly VI and VII), long-tract signs, and ataxia. According to the 2016 CNS WHO, DIPG is also included in the newly defined category of *diffuse midline glioma*, histone H3 K27M-mutant, which could potentially provide a foundation for directed therapies in the future combined with radiotherapy [10]. These tumors typically arise in the pons or upper medulla, expanding the brainstem, and have a classic appearance on MRI of a homogeneous hypointense lesion on T1, whereas a nonenhancing T2 bright lesion. There may be evidence of exophytic growth. Biopsy is not indicated if the appearance is classic, although recently there has been a trend to perform a biopsy if feasible to obtain molecular information. Standard of care includes radiation alone based on the German Hirntumor Cooperative group study (HIT-GBM-C), as patients in the DIPG arm failed to demonstrate a benefit in EFS with the addition of intensive chemotherapy during and after radiotherapy [85].

A dose of 54–59.4 Gy is generally recommended; however, based on the most recent trial ACNS0423 demonstrating superior outcomes, a dose of 54 Gy in 30 fractions is recommended for PTV-1, followed by a boost of 5.4 Gy in three fractions for PTV2 for a total dose of 59.4 Gy [86]. These tumors respond promptly to radiation, but without any known exception they recur, usually within one year [79]. Immediately prior to radiotherapy planning, the sequences that best define the extent of disease (especially in the postoperative setting) should be registered with the planning CT, and used to identify the GTV. This often includes the MR T2 and FLAIR sequences. The GTV includes gross residual tumor and resection bed (if applicable), and considers all sites of involved tissue. An added margin of 1 cm creates the CTV, anatomically constrained by neuroanatomic structures where invasion is not likely (including bone, falx, and tentorium). A PTV of 0.3–0.5 cm is created to account for set-up error and patient movement.

Because of the clinical, biologic, and molecular heterogeneity of both pediatric HGG and DIPG, there continues to be great interest identifying subgroups using genomic and epigenomic characteristics with the goals of risk stratification and clinical application to improve patient outcomes. Most recently, subgroups of pediatric HGG have been identified based on German Cancer Research Center (DKFZ) methylation, age of onset, tumor location, median survival, oncogenic drivers, and gene expression [87].

Craniopharyngioma

Craniopharyngiomas represent approximately 5–10% of pediatric CNS brain tumors and 50% of all sellar/parasellar tumors [5, 88]. They are histologically benign tumors that arise from remnants of Rathke's pouch which ultimately differentiates into the anterior pituitary. Craniopharyngiomas are bimodal in age distribution, occurring predominantly in children between the ages of 5 and 14 years and in adults between 65 and 74 years. These are highly curable tumors; however, the complications from tumor involvement, surgical intervention, and radiotherapy can be detrimental. Clinical presentation includes increased intracranial pressure (most common), visual field deficits (bitemporal hemianopsia from inferior chiasmatic compression), behavioral/personality changes (from frontal involvement), and hormonal deficits (short stature and precocious puberty) [89,90]. Emergent symptoms should be addressed preoperatively, including low cortisol and diabetes insipidus [91]. Patients may require surgical decompression for increased ICP or visual deterioration. Once the patient is stable, evaluation should include baseline endocrine level determination and correction as needed, CT, MRI, baseline vision, hearing and neuropsychological evaluation (if age-appropriate); MRA should also be considered because of the risk for vasculopathy [92]. The classical appearance consists of a sellar/parasellar partial solid and cystic calcified mass, with decreased rates of calcification in adults [93].

Aggressive surgery to achieve gross total resection can be challenging and is often associated with major complications [94]. In the setting of incomplete resection, approximately 70% of these tumors will demonstrate progression within a few years [95, 96]. Thus, the standard approach involves limited surgery, followed by radiation, which typically achieves excellent disease control rates of 85–90% at 10 years [96–99]. The GTV includes residual solid and cystic components and the postoperative bed with a CTV margin of approximately 0.5 cm. All calcifications identified on CT imaging should also be incorporated within target volume, as these are also part of the tumor. A dose of 50.4–54 Gy is recommended. Conformal techniques should be used to decrease the dose to the surrounding temporal lobes and brain [100, 101]. These tumors typically have a cystic component that may change in volume during radiation [102]. This is especially important when treating with proton beam therapy, because of the sensitivity of protons to fluctuations in tissue density, which may require adaptive radiotherapy to ensure adequate target volume coverage and minimize the radiation dose to surrounding critical structures. Weekly MRI or CT during treatment is advised to ensure that this component of the tumor is included in the treatment volume for the entire course of therapy [103]. Changes in vision or neurocognitive status may indicate cyst expansion, which may warrant physical examination or additional imaging to rule out hydrocephalus, or possible shunt malfunction if the patient has an intracranial device.

Close lifelong follow-up in these patients is required because they remain at risk for significant neurological, cardiovascular, and psychosocial morbidity which could impact both quality and quantity of life [104]. Compared to photon therapy, proton therapy may have a role in significantly reducing additional radiation dose to critical structures [74, 105]. The ongoing RT2CR study through St Jude Children's Research Hospital and University Florida Proton Therapy Institute is a Phase II trial evaluating limited surgery and proton therapy in patients diagnosed with craniopharyngioma receiving a total dose to the tumor and postoperative bed of 54 Gy. Those patients with a successful radical resection continue on with observation alone [106]. The study endpoints are planned to evaluate CNS necrosis, vasculopathy, and permanent neurological deficits. Interim analysis at a median follow-up of 18 months (range 1–50 months) has not demonstrated any increased incidence of severe complications with passively scattered proton therapy compared to IMRT. Functional and disease outcomes are planned for evaluation at 36 months in April of 2017 [107].

Germ Cell Tumors

Germ cell tumors (GCTs) of the CNS are rare, and primarily affect the adolescent population with peak incidences in the second and third decades [108–110]. These tumors typically arise within the suprasellar region or pineal gland, but can be multifocal, occurring in approximately 5–10% of patients, and are not considered metastatic [108]. GCTs are divided into two main histologic subgroups that are highly prognostic, namely pure germinomas (GCT) and non-germinomatous germ cell tumor (NGGCT). These include embryonal carcinoma, endodermal sinus tumor, choriocarcinoma, and immature teratoma. Depending on the location of the tumor, key clinical presentations include diabetes insipidus, precocious puberty, or delayed sexual development. Patients with pineal tumors may present with ocular signs noted as Parinaud's syndrome as a result of pressure on the colliculus of the tectum; this includes an upward gaze, Argyll Robertson pupil, and convergence nystagmus. Initially, a shunt or 3rd ventriculostomy should be performed to stabilize a patient in the setting of hydrocephalus. Work-up involves MRI of the brain and spine with and without gadolinium, with thin cuts through the pineal and suprasellar regions. Serum and CSF for alpha fetal protein (AFP) and human chorionic gonadotropin-beta (hCGβ) should be obtained (with caution if there is increased intracranial pressure). Patients with a histologic confirmation of germinoma should have a normal AFP $\leq$10 ng ml^{-1} and hCGβ $\leq$100 mIU ml^{-1} in serum and/or CSF. Patients with NGGCT must have serum or CSF hCGβ >100 mIU ml^{-1} or elevation of serum or CSF AFP >10 ng ml^{-1} or above institutional norm. No biopsy is necessary of the lesion if the serum and/or CSF markers are elevated, though this remains controversial. The ongoing ACNS 1123 response-based radiation therapy protocol for patients diagnosed with GCTs requires an hCGβ $\leq$ 50 mIU ml^{-1} if no histologic confirmation is made. Pure germinoma is the most common type of GCT, and typically has the most favorable prognosis. Excellent outcomes can be achieved with radiation alone or a combination of radiation and chemotherapy [111–114].

Whole-ventricle radiotherapy (WVRT) to a dose of 24 Gy, followed by a boost to the tumor bed to total 45–50 Gy, is an accepted treatment for localized GCT. For patients with disseminated pure germinoma the prognosis is still excellent, but CSI is recommended. CSI alone to a dose of 24 Gy followed by a boost to 45 Gy is standard. With the use of pre-radiotherapy chemotherapy, the radiation dose may be reduced but the volumes should not change. This would include two to four cycles of carboplatin/etoposide or a platinum-based chemotherapy followed by 21 Gy (WVRT) followed by a boost to the primary tumor for a total dose of 30 Gy. In the setting of disseminated disease, chemotherapy would be the same, followed by 21 Gy CSI and a boost to the primary tumor for a total dose of 30 Gy. If there is a partial response, and no second-look surgery, consideration should be given to increasing the total dose to 36 Gy. Chemotherapy followed by focal radiation had been investigated, but results from the French Society of Pediatric Oncology (SFOP) showed a relapse rate in the ventricles of 14–16%, and this treatment has largely fallen out of favor since its publication [115]. The current COG protocol ACNS1223 Stratum 2 is investigating the use of pre-radiotherapy chemotherapy followed by reduced dose 18 Gy to the whole ventricles, followed by a boost to total 30 Gy.

NGGCT carries a less-favorable prognosis, with OS rates with radiation-alone being dismal, ranging from 20% to 45% [109, 115, 116]. The recent COG study, ACNS0122, delivered six cycles of induction chemotherapy (carboplatin, ifosfamide, and etoposide) followed by CSI to 36 Gy, followed by an involved-field boost to 54 Gy. Updated reports demonstrated favorable outcomes among these patients with five-year EFS and OS of 84% and 91%, respectively [116]. The current COG study ACNS 0123 attempted to evaluate whether dose and volume reduction could be safely attained, by delivering the same chemotherapy followed by WVRT to 30.6 Gy, then followed by an involved-field boost to deliver 54 Gy to the tumor bed. The whole-ventricle contour is shown in Figure 41.3. This trial has not yet been formally reported, but COG has issued a notice that this arm closed as it met predetermined stopping rules. The current recommendation is to follow the ACNS0122 regimen including 36 Gy CSI followed by an involved-field boost to 54 Gy is the current recommended radiation dose for patients diagnosed with NGGCT.

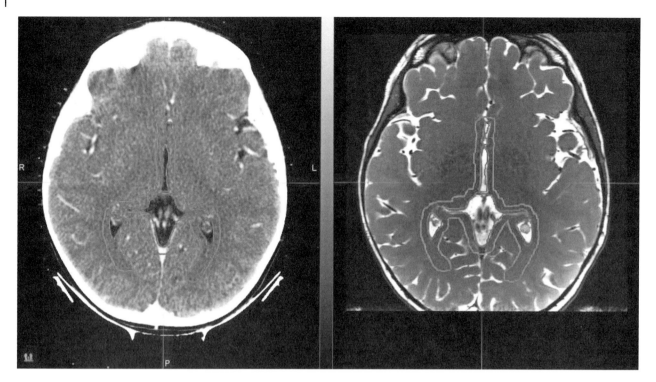

Figure 41.3 Contours for the whole-ventricle volume at the level of the pineal cistern for a patient with a germ-cell tumor. Left, CT scan. Right, T2 MRI. For a color version of this figure, see the color plate section.

When treatment planning, the whole ventricles present a challenge when contouring, and should encompass the lateral, third, and fourth ventricles, as well as the suprasellar and pineal cisterns. It is encouraged to fuse T2 MRI sequences obtained just prior to radiotherapy treatment when contouring to help delineate the CSF and ventricle volume. Details on contouring are available in the atlas at the COG and QARC websites [117]. The GTV should include any residual tumor at the time of treatment planning, tumor bed at diagnosis, any region of brain infiltration and all tissues initially involved or in contact with the tumor. Be sure to evaluate for changes in the pineal gland or infundibulum after neoadjuvant chemotherapy. The CTV margin should be 0.5 cm, limited to anatomic constraints. Of note, after the CTV is created, it should be combined with the whole ventricular CTV that is created to ensure that the involved field boost receives the full prescribed dose throughout the treatment course.

Spinal Tumors

Primary spinal cord neoplasms are rare in children, accounting for approximately 5% of CNS malignancies [118]. Most tumors are either low-grade astrocytoma or myxopapillary ependymomas. Surgical resection is the primary treatment, with radiation being reserved for situations when either complete resection is not possible

or in the setting of tumor recurrence. The prescribed dose is typically 45–54 Gy based primarily on spinal cord tolerance [119]. Grade II ependymomas of the spine that are gross totally resected do not require postoperative radiation, but Grade III anaplastic ependymomas of the spine do require such treatment. When dose escalation is required for the treatment of tumors involving the sacrum, spine, or skull base (including chordomas or chondrosarcoma), proton beam therapy should be considered after maximal safe resection is achieved for dose escalation [120]. Depending on the tumor requiring treatment, care to obtain all pre- and post-imaging for image registration at the time of treatment planning is essential.

Hematologic Malignancies

Advancements in cancer therapy have led to extraordinary improvements in both disease-specific survival and OS for children with hematologic malignancies. At this time, survival exceeds 85% for children with Hodgkin's disease (HD), non-Hodgkin's lymphoma (NHL), and acute lymphoblastic leukemia (ALL) [121]. Contemporary therapy places an emphasis on risk adaptation and an avoidance of treatment-related complications while maintaining high rates of cure. Children with hematologic malignancies are currently treated with combinations of cytotoxic chemotherapy, and sometimes with radiation. The addition of chemotherapy over the past several decades has allowed for a reduction in radiation dose and volume for those patients requiring it.

Hodgkin's Lymphoma

Hodgkin's disease accounts for 4% of childhood malignancies [3]. There is a marked male to female predominance and an age-specific incidence rates with a bimodal distribution. Most children present with painless lymphadenopathy or shortness of breath due to mediastinal disease. One-third of patients present with 'B' symptoms, which include unexplained persistent or recurrent fevers with temperature >100.4 °C, recurrent drenching night sweats in the month prior to diagnosis, and weight loss >10% of body weight during the previous six months. Diagnosis is established by excisional lymph node biopsy, which requires adequate tissue to identify the classic Reed–Sternberg cells, which are derived from neoplastic clones originating from B lymphocytes within the lymphoid germinal centers. Different cellular subtypes of HD of varying prognoses have been established: Classic Hodgkin (nodular sclerosis, mixed-cellularity, and lymphocyte-rich), nodular lymphocyte predominant, and lymphocyte-depleted. The Ann Arbor staging system (Table 41.1) is based on the extent of lymphatic and organ involvement as well as symptoms at the time of presentation. The diagnostic work-up includes a careful physical examination with attention to all lymphatic sites, symptoms of mediastinal compression, and organomegaly. Important routine laboratory parameters should be obtained: hemoglobin, erythrocyte sedimentation rate (ESR), C-reactive protein (CRP), ferritin, and

Table 41.1 The Ann Arbor staging system.

Stage I:	Involvement of single lymph node region (I) or localized involvement of a single extra-lymphatic organ or site (IE).
Stage II:	Involvement of two or more lymph node regions on the same side of the diaphragm (II) or localized contiguous involvement of a single extra-lymphatic organ or site and its regional lymph node(s) with involvement of one or more lymph node regions on the same side of the diaphragm (IIE).
Stage III:	Involvement of lymph node regions on both sides of the diaphragm (III), which may also be accompanied by localized contiguous involvement of an extra-lymphatic organ or site (IIIE), by involvement of the spleen (IIIS), or both (IIIE+S).
Stage IV:	Disseminated (multifocal) involvement of one or more extra-lymphatic organs or tissues, with or without associated lymph node involvement, or isolated extra-lymphatic organ involvement with distant (non-regional) nodal involvement.

liver function tests [122, 123]. Patients with 'B' symptoms or stage III or IV disease should have bilateral bone marrow biopsies. Imaging includes CT or positron emission tomography (PET)/CT of the neck, chest, abdomen, and pelvis. Bulk disease is defined as contiguous extra-mediastinal nodal aggregate that measures >6 cm in the longest transverse diameter on craniocaudal dimension as identified on CT, or if the patient has a mediastinal mass with a tumor diameter more than one-third the maximal thoracic diameter on an upright PA chest X-ray [124].

Radiation therapy alone was established as the first definitive treatment for HD [125]. Chemotherapy was added because of the inability to cure bulky, more advanced disease, and the impact of high dose and large volume radiation on morbidity and mortality in children, which included late effects such as abnormal musculoskeletal development, thyroid abnormalities, cardiopulmonary toxicity, and secondary cancers, ultimately leading to the investigation of chemotherapy for this disease [126–131]. Modern regimens include chemotherapy ± radiotherapy, adopting treatments based on risk and response to therapy. Many pediatric HD trials focus on tailoring chemotherapy and radiation to provide adequate disease control while minimizing late effects of treatment [122, 132–134]. Patients are generally grouped into one of three risk groups: low/lymphocyte predominant; intermediate; or high-risk groups. It is challenging to compare results between trials, even among pediatric HL study groups, because of the evolving risk stratification and treatment group allocations [135].

Low-risk patients and those with lymphocyte-predominant histology include those patients with stage IA, IIA and no bulky disease, and these are generally treated with minimal therapy. AHOD0431 was a low-risk study that evaluated early response-based treatment after three cycles of AVPC (doxorubicin/vincristine/prednisone/cyclophosphamide). Despite achieving complete response (CR) after one cycle of chemotherapy, patients with positive or equivocal initial PET had inferior event-free survival (EFS) were called back for involved field radiotherapy (IFRT) if they were within one year of completing chemotherapy. This study suggested that PET evaluation after one cycle of AV-PC may predict the need for radiotherapy in patients with low-risk disease [136]. Patients with intermediate-risk disease (generally excluding stage IA, IIA without bulk disease and stage IIIB/IVB) are evaluated and treated based on a dose response-based paradigm. Response is assessed after two and four cycles of chemotherapy. The most recent Intermediate Risk Study AHOD 0031 protocol evaluated dose-intensive therapy pediatric patients diagnosed with Hodgkin lymphoma with ABVE-PC (doxorubicin/bleomycin/vincristine/etoposide/cyclophosphamide/prednisone) and IFRT incorporating early response-based treatment. Rapid early response (RER) was defined as ≥60% reduction in the product of the perpendicular diameters (PPD) of each lesion on CT imaging. Slow early response (SER) was defined as <60% reduction in PPD in each lesion on CT imaging. A complete response was achieved if there was a ≥80% reduction in the PPD of each lesion on CT with a negative PET or gallium scan. The trial confirmed that early response assessment allowed for the omission of radiotherapy in RER patients who achieved CR, and SER patients with PET-positive disease benefited from augmentation of chemotherapy [137]. Despite excellent four-year OS rates for RERs and SERs, the four-year EFS was inferior, particularly in SERs (86.9% versus 77.4%, P < 0.001).Relapses rarely occurred in uninvolved disease sites, underscoring the current trend for minimizing radiation treatment volumes to reduce normal tissue toxicities. Because relapses occurred at initial disease sites (both bulky and non-bulky), future studies should evaluate the role of dose escalation and include sites other than bulk disease for treatment targets. Additionally, RER patients diagnosed with a combination of anemia and bulky limited-stage disease had significantly better EFS with the addition of IFRT [138]. Based on the outcomes using clinical data from AHOD0031, a predictive model was developed and validated to identify a prognostic score and identify patients who may benefit from treatment augmentation (Childhood International Prognostic Score; CHIPS) [139]: Stage 4, large mediastinal adenopathy, albumin <3.5, and fever. Patients with CHIPS of 0 or 1 achieved EFS of nearly 90%, whereas those with CHIPS of 2 or 3 had EFS of 78% and 62%, respectively.

High-risk patients include stage IIB and IVB patients and treatment is response-based, with slow responders placed on augmented regimens. Recent studies have suggested that therapy can be limited for rapid early responders, but intensified for slow early responders, ultimately leading to treatment efficacy and a reduction of toxicity. The pediatric HL CCG59704 evaluated dose-dense BEA-COPP (bleomycin, etoposide, doxorubicin, cyclophosphamide, vincristine, procarbazine, and prednisone) in high-risk patients (defined as stage IIB or IIB with bulky disease, stage IV). Response to therapy was assessed following four cycles of therapy and consolidation of chemotherapy ± IFRT resulting in a five-year EFS of 94% at a median follow-up of 6.3 years, highlighting a remarkably effective therapy for these high-risk patients [140]. Brentuximab is an antibody conjugate directed against CD30 coupled to a microtubule-disrupting agent. Favorable response rates have been identified in relapsed and refractory disease, now on the forefront of clinical trials. The most current COG AHOD1331 protocol is evaluating Brentuximab Vedotin in the treatment of newly diagnosed high-risk classical Hodgkin lymphoma [124].

General indications for radiotherapy include initial bulky disease (large mediastinal mass, nodal adenopathy >6 cm and macroscopic splenic nodules regardless of whether the patient is rapid or slow to respond to therapy), SER defined by residual avidity on fluorodeoxyglucose-(FDG)-PET following the first two cycles of chemotherapy (Deauville score 4 or 5, and patients with residual disease >2.5 cm at the end of chemotherapy). Because of varied treatment approaches internationally, greater efforts are being made to unite staging and response criteria to improve risk stratification and treatment provisions for pediatric HL through interactive forums such as the Children, Adolescent and Young Adult HL (CAYAHL) symposium and programs to share clinical experience, including the Staging Evaluation and Response Criteria Harmonization (SEARCH) [135].

Radiation volumes have been successfully reduced to the involved field defined as a region of lymph nodes including, and in close proximity to, the disease defined by diagnostic imaging [141]. There has been an interest in reducing this volume even further, and involved and extended-field radiotherapy has been replaced with involved site and at times involved nodal irradiation [142, 143]. The EORTC-GELA and International Lymphoma Radiation Oncology Group (ILROG) group have established guidelines for this treatment, and this is an active research question that aims to achieve equivalent disease control with decreased toxicity [144,145]. Early outcomes for favorable disease show excellent disease control, with no failures in the involved region outside of the treatment field [146]. Radiotherapy will consist of a total dose of 2100 cGy in 14 fractions at 150 cGy, with or without an additional boost of 900 cGy in six fractions, depending on the risk group and/or the presence of persistent FDG-PET uptake following chemotherapy.

Hodgkin lymphoma survivors are at risk for many late complications of therapy, particularly cardiac morbidities, especially when radiotherapy is given in the setting of previous anthracycline therapy [147]. Decreasing treatment volumes plays a significant role in mitigating dose–volume distribution, thus minimizing radiation exposure to the normal heart and decreasing the risk of cardiac events [148]. Secondary malignancies have remained a substantial concern in patients requiring treatment for therapy, especially with previously reported increased risks by volume of tissue treated and increased risk of breast cancer in children and adolescents following mediastinal radiotherapy [149, 150]. Breast-sparing proton beam therapy has demonstrated a potential advantage of reducing unnecessary dose in young girls with HL compared to 3D-CRT; however, prospective clinical outcomes are still needed to establish the clinical significance [142]. It is also important to note that some breast-sparing proton techniques use a posterior approach that spares breast tissue but exposes a large volume of the heart. Some centers use an anterior approach with protons that does not avoid breast tissue but minimizes the cardiac dose. Future studies in Hodgkin's lymphoma will continue to evaluate the role of involved site radiotherapy, novel therapies, and response-based radiotherapy in order to maximize treatment efficacy and continue to reduce unnecessary toxicity of therapy [124].

Non-Hodgkin's Lymphoma

Non-Hodgkin's lymphoma has a similar, but slightly greater, incidence in children [3]. With nearly 500 children diagnosed annually, it is the third most common malignancy of childhood. The median age at diagnosis is 10 years, presenting less frequently in those aged less than three years. There is a slight predilection for males over females, and Caucasians over African Americans. Populations most at risk are those with immunodeficiencies including HIV, Wiskott–Aldrich syndrome (X-linked recessive, eczema, thrombocytopenia, immune deficiency, and bloody diarrhea), ataxia-telangiectasia (autosomal dominant, neurodegenerative, poor coordination, telangiectasia, and immune weakness), and X-linked lymphoproliferative syndrome (immunodeficiency, predilection for hemophagocytic lymphohistiocytosis, fatal Epstein–Barr virus, hypogammaglobulinemia). Most pediatric NHLs are high-grade and are categorized as one of three major subtypes, mostly of B-cell origin: lymphoblastic lymphoma (29%); Burkitt's lymphoma (39%); large-cell lymphoma (27%). Two of the most common subtypes of large-cell lymphoma are anaplastic large-cell lymphoma (40–50%) and diffuse large B-cell lymphoma (30–40%). Presenting symptoms are often similar to those of HD, with the exception of Burkitt's lymphoma, which often involves the gastrointestinal tract. CNS involvement is rare at diagnosis, but may occur, and the CNS is a potential site of relapse for high-risk disease. The Ann Arbor classification is not adapted as the staging system, because these patients have greater extranodal primary sites of disease. The St Jude staging classification identifies mediastinal and extensive abdominal lesions as stage III and stage IV is limited to the bone marrow and CNS. Bone marrow involvement is more commonly seen in patients with NHL. Lymphoblastic lymphoma commonly presents in the mediastinum or head and neck, and usually has involvement of the bone marrow and peripheral blood. Although useful in the assessment of disease involvement, the role of FDG PET/CT has yet to be established in the management of these patients.

Multi-agent chemotherapy is required for all patients, and intrathecal chemotherapy as a prophylactic CNS treatment is used for many cases [151]. The use of radiation is limited to patients with CNS disease or those without complete response to chemotherapy. Total body irradiation may be required in the setting of bone marrow transplantation. Rarely, radiotherapy is indicated for the palliation of symptoms; however, this may impact on pathologic results if a primary diagnosis has not been established [152].

Leukemia

Leukemia is one of the most common pediatric malignancies, with acute lymphoblastic leukemia (ALL) being the most common leukemia. The mean age at diagnosis for ALL is four years. Chromosomal disorders that have been associated with the development of leukemia include Down's syndrome and Klinefelter syndrome. Leukemic cells accumulate within the BM cavity, ultimately replacing most of the normal hematopoietic cells. As a result, children often present with signs and symptoms of bone marrow failure and consequences of bleeding, infection, and anemia, including fever, easy bruising, hepatosplenomegaly, and lymphadenopathy, fatigue, and bone pain. Complete blood chemistry with a differential (CBC) may reveal an elevated or decreased cell count, and bone marrow aspirate or biopsy generally has diffuse involvement with leukemic cells. CNS or testicular involvement is rare at diagnosis, but the patient may present with irritability, headache, vomiting, weight gain, cranial nerve palsies, or testicular mass/enlargement. Evaluation includes a complete history and physical, laboratory studies including CBC, comprehensive metabolic panel (CMP), clotting studies, lactate dehydrogenase (LDH) and uric acid. Urine and blood cultures may identify the source of infection, especially in the setting of immunodeficiency. If there is concern for an immunodeficiency, other studies (e.g., serum immunoglobulin, varicella zoster titers, HIV test/ PPD skin test) may be indicated. In order to establish a diagnosis and complete staging, a bone marrow biopsy/aspirate and lumbar puncture for CSF are required, including a testicular ultrasound when appropriate. On evaluation of the CSF, CNS leukemia at diagnosis is defined by the following: CNS1- no blasts regardless of white blood cells (WBCs); CNS2- <5/μL WBCs positive for blasts, OR traumatic LP, >5/μL WBCs, and positive for blasts; and CN3- after traumatic LP presence of ≥5/μL WBCs and positive for blasts and/or clinical signs of CNS leukemia (such as facial nerve palsy, brain/eye involvement or hypothalamic syndrome). A chest X-ray and echocardiogram are indicated prior to initiation of therapy and/or to rule out a mediastinal mass.

Historically, patients had been stratified into: low-risk (B-cell ALL in children aged 1–10 years, WBC <50 × 10^9); standard risk (<1 or >10 years of age, B-cell ALL with WBC >50 × 10^9, T-cell lineage and t(1; 19)/ E2A-PBX1 fusion); and high-risk (t9; 22/BRC-ABL fusion (Ph+ ALL), which would guide therapy, including enrollment on protocols that would involve radiotherapy.

Improved outcomes of children diagnosed with ALL can be ascribed to modified combinations of modern chemotherapy regimens and risk-directed therapy based on response to induction chemotherapy and clinical/biological features (e.g., MLL rearrangement BCR-ABL1, hypodiploidy, chromosome trisomy, 11q23 rearrangement, MRC UKALL X, etc.), which consists of multi-agent chemotherapy that are delivered in phases of induction, consolidation, delayed intensification, and maintenance, with or without the addition of radiotherapy [153–158]. Greater than 80% of children diagnosed with ALL are cured with contemporary chemotherapeutic regimens, with a predicted increase to approximately 90–95% in pediatric subsets with favorable prognostic features [159–162]. The prognosis is influenced by response to therapy, and patients may be treated more intensively, particularly if they have a poor response to induction chemotherapy. In the past, radiation played a major role in the prevention of CNS relapse, but due to more effective chemotherapeutic agents, radiation is now reserved for patients with a high risk of CNS relapse. Currently, radiotherapy is recommended for patients with T-cell ALL with high-risk features, CNS3 disease (>5 WBC l^{-1} or blasts in the CSF) at the time of diagnosis, CNS relapse, or other high-risk disease with poor response to induction chemotherapy. Cranial irradiation (CRI) to a dose of 12–18 Gy in 8–10 fractions at 1.5–1.8 Gy per daily fraction is recommended [160,163]. Very high-risk T-ALL patients who are CNS 1 or 2 who receive prophylactic CRI are usually treated to a dose of 12 Gy in eight fractions at 1.5 Gy per daily fraction.

Radiotherapy is delivered during the first four weeks of maintenance of therapy. The goal of CRI is to cover the meninges and any area of potential access to the CNS; this includes the cribriform plate, posterior retina, posterior half-globe of the eye, the exit of cranial nerves III, IV, V, VI, and the inferior extent of the meninges. The treatment field extends to the C1–C2 interspace and the lower limit of the temporal fossa at the skull base. The shielding blocks should cover the anterior halves of the eyes and protect the nose and mouth. Radiation is delivered using a parallel-opposed technique. Radiation may also be indicated for testicular involvement that is refractory to chemotherapy, or in disease relapse involving the testicles. The recommended dose for testicular radiation for ALL is 20–24 Gy [164]. The key points are to place the patient in the supine frog-leg position so that the testes/scrotum are included within the PTV. To minimize toxicity, the testes should be supported posteriorly to avoid dose to the perineum, and the penis should be secured to the skin overlying the pubic symphysis, out of the radiation field. Beware of the cremasteric reflex, which could remove the testicle (s) from the treatment field. The prescription point is near the center of the PTV, with 90% of the dose prescribed to the posterior aspect of the testes delivered using an en-face technique.

Occasionally, supplemental cranial and testicular irradiation is indicated in the setting of total body irradiation (TBI). For example, patients diagnosed with B-ALL who develop relapse involving the bone marrow, CNS, or a combination of the sites, may require TBI as a conditioning regimen for patients undergoing HSCT, as in the current AALL1331 Phase III Risk-Stratified randomized Phase III testing of blinatumomab in first relapse of childhood B-lymphoblastic leukemia [165]. Supplemental cranial irradiation is necessary for HSCT patients who present with CNS leukemia at the time of relapse, and will be delivered prior to TBI; doses and timing of supplement irradiation may vary on the risk and protocol. Generally, TBI is administered at 12 Gy over three to four consecutive days at 1–5–2 Gy twice daily. The mid-plan dose rate should remain between 6 and 15 cGy per minute. High-dose chemotherapy and single fraction regimens (2 Gy × 1) are also currently being evaluated. Several treatment positions are possible for TBI treatments, including seated, standing, lateral decubitus, supine and prone, depending on patient factors and institutional capabilities. When planning and at treatment, the patient should be maintained within the entire treatment volume and 90% isodose line. Furthermore, efforts should be made so that total lung volume is maintained at <800 cGy.

Children and adolescents treated for, and who are survivors of, leukemia require long-term medical surveillance for late effects and recurrence of disease, as they are at risk for challenging lifestyle adaptations and health-related comorbidities [166]. Long-term complications include neurocognitive deficits (sleep disturbance, fatigue, depression, cognitive impairment/decreased IQ), behavioral disorders, somnolence syndrome, leukoencephalopathy, endocrinopathies, obesity, cardiac toxicity, sterility, and secondary malignancies [167]. The 30-year cumulative incidence of secondary malignant neoplasm in survivors of childhood ALL was reported at 15% by the Childhood Cancer Survivor Study (CCSS), approximately 4.4-fold increased risk; non-malignant skin cancer (40%), meningioma (20%), glial tumors (8%), breast cancer (3%), soft-tissue sarcoma (3%), and other tumors (26%) [168]. The SJLIFE cohort reported on ALL survivors that they had a higher risk of metabolic syndrome (hypertension, low high-density lipoprotein, obesity, and insulin resistance), thereby identifying an association between older age and previous CRI and the development of metabolic syndrome [169].

New efforts are being made to determine underlying genomic risk factors and association with adverse effects based on treatment regimens. Various inherited genomic variations that contribute to ALL toxicity have been identified, including methotrexate-induced leukoencephalopathy, several genes affiliated with osteonecrosis, and several others predominantly associated with chemotherapy-related toxicity [170–172]. Together, ongoing and future collaborative group studies will further define clinical, biologic and genomic prognostic risk factors of children and adolescents diagnosed with leukemia in order to intensify or minimize therapy to optimize personalized treatment outcomes and further reduce the risk of treatment-related toxicity [173].

Neuroblastoma

Neuroblastoma is the most common solid non-CNS malignancy of childhood, representing 8–10% of all pediatric cancers; approximately 650 cases are diagnosed each year in the United States [3]. Children are typically very young at diagnosis, with the majority of cases being diagnosed before the age of four years. Neuroblastoma is notable for its heterogeneity in behavior, with some cases showing spontaneous regression and others demonstrating dismal outcomes. Neuroblastoma arises from primitive adrenergic neuroblasts located in the adrenal glands or paraspinal ganglia. The International Pathology Classification (INPC) is the currently accepted pathologic classification system, as it incorporated morphological changes that occur with age in order to provide prognostic information [174]. Anaplastic lymphoma kinase (ALK) mutations are identified in approximately 14% of children, who are found to be at high risk with an inferior prognosis [175]. Crizotinib is a tyrosine kinase inhibitor of *ALK* and *ROS1* genes, and will be incorporated into the next Phase II COG high-risk neuroblastoma protocol ANBL1531. Similarly, 20% of children have *MYCN* amplifications, also noted to be associated with inferior outcomes. Children with a high telomerase activity, which is present in 30% of cases, tend to have worse EFS and OS [176]. The most common presentation is a palpable abdominal mass, often with manifestations of abdominal organ compression. Over 50% of children will have metastases at diagnosis involving the bone, liver, lymph nodes, and skin. Bone metastases may also cause pain or a refusal to walk. Skin metastases that occur in infants may present with clinical manifestations of blue skin lesions that blanch with pressure due to the release of vasoactive catecholamines (this is referred to as the 'blueberry muffin' sign). Also, it is not uncommon to see systemic symptoms such fever, weight loss, sweating, flushing, abdominal pain, failure to thrive, and generalized weakness. Paraneoplastic syndromes include opsoclonus-myoclonus truncal ataxia syndrome, attributed to antibody formation to neurons, and diarrhea from vasoactive intestinal polypeptide (VIP) secretion.

The work-up for suspected neuroblastoma is generally initiated after a complete history and physical examination is completed, evaluating for hypertension, and examination of the abdomen, eyes, skin, ataxia, and so forth. Imaging is initially directed to the area of concern.

If an abdominal mass is present, ultrasound is often used as the initial imaging modality. CT and/or MRI should be performed to evaluate the primary lesion. If feasible, it may be of benefit to obtain both studies at the initial diagnosis to best evaluate the initial extent of disease and to determine the best imaging modality for subsequent studies. Adrenal neuroblastoma can often be radiographically distinguished from Wilm's tumor by the presence of calcifications (much more common in neuroblastoma) and an absence of renal parenchymal distortion. Baseline bilateral posterior iliac bone marrow biopsies and bone scan (with ^{99m}Tc-diphosphonate) and/or MIBG scan (using ^{123}I-MIBG) should be obtained. Baseline CBC, CMP, and urinary catecholamines (vanillylmandelic acid and homovanillic acid levels are elevated in 90% of patients) should be obtained. PET/CT should be considered for patients with MIBG-negative disease. Pathology (biopsy or surgical resection if feasible) is necessary for diagnosis unless urinary catecholamines are elevated. Pathology does provide additional prognostic information. If surgery is performed initially, post-surgical imaging should be obtained to determine the extent of resection. Baseline imaging of the chest (chest radiography or preferably chest CT) and CT imaging of the abdomen and pelvis to rule out metastatic disease is recommended. If the patient receives chemotherapy prior to surgery, a post-chemotherapy, pre-surgical MRI and/or CT scan of the area of primary disease is necessary as this volume is generally the target for radiation therapy.

Currently, staging is based on the extent of disease and extent of surgical resection. The International Neuroblastoma Staging System is shown in Table 41.2. Additional prognostic factors include age at diagnosis, *MYCN* amplification, histology (favorable/unfavorable), and DNA ploidy. Because these prognostic factors have such an impact on patient outcome and potentially management decisions, the next Phase III COG protocol will utilize the International Neuroblastoma Risk Groups Staging System (INRGSS) (see Table 41.3). This system will provide a comparison of patient outcomes based on pretreatment characteristics worldwide, incorporating age, histological status, differentiation, DNA ploidy, *MYCN*, and the 11q aberration [177, 178]. Children aged under 12 months are considered to have more favorable outcomes. Recent studies have indicated that this age cut-off can be extended to 18 months for children with favorable histology [179]. The Children's Oncology Group stratifies neuroblastoma into low-, intermediate-, and high-risk groups based on the amalgamation of these prognostic factors. Radiation therapy is recommended for children with intermediate-risk disease who progress through chemotherapy, those who have persistent disease following all treatment, and for children with high-risk neuroblastoma. Chemotherapy, myeloablative chemotherapy with stem cell rescue, and anti-G2

Table 41.2 International Neuroblastoma Staging System (INSS).

Stage 1	Localized tumor with complete gross excision, with or without microscopic residual disease; representative ipsilateral lymph nodes negative for tumor microscopically (nodes attached to and removed with the primary tumor may be positive).
Stage 2A	Localized tumor with incomplete gross resection; representative ipsilateral non-adherent lymph nodes negative for tumor microscopically.
Stage 2B	Localized tumor with or without complete gross excision, with ipsilateral non adherent lymph nodes positive for tumor; enlarged contralateral lymph nodes must be negative microscopically.
Stage 3	Unresectable unilateral tumor infiltrating across the midline, with or without regional lymph node involvement; or localized unilateral tumor with contralateral regional lymph node involvement; or midline tumor with bilateral extension by infiltration (unresectable) or by lymph node involvement.
Stage 4	Any primary tumor with dissemination to distant lymph nodes, bone, bone marrow, liver, skin, and/or other organs (except as defined for Stage 4S).
Stage 4S	Localized primary tumor (as defined for Stage 1, 2A or 2B) with dissemination limited to skin, liver, and/or bone marrow (limited to infants aged <1 year).

antibody with interleukin (IL)-2 may be used [180, 181]. ANBL0032 was a Phase III randomized protocol that was stopped early because of improved OS and EFS secondary to the addition of immunotherapy [181]. Current treatment for high-risk disease consists of multi-modality therapy, including five to six cycles of induction chemotherapy, and second-look surgery, consolidation therapy (myeloablative chemotherapy followed by autologous stem cell transplant; ASCT). ABNL 0532, a randomized trial for high-risk patients, recently reported improved outcomes for the use of a tandem consolidation of thiotepa/cyclophosphamide followed by carboplatin/etoposide/melphalan (CEM) that were superior compared to single CEM consolidation. The three-year EFS following tandem myeloablative therapy was significantly improved at 63.2% compared with a single myeloablative therapy (48.6%; p = 0.0064), meeting the protocol-defined end point for improvement in EFS. The three-year OS following tandem myeloablative therapy versus single myeloablative therapy was 73.5% and 68.8%, respectively (p = 0.2207). Tandem transplant is now considered standard for all patients. Transplant is then followed by site-based radiotherapy at 28–40 days post transplant (if the child has recovered sufficiently) to both primary and metastatic sites of disease. Radiation

Table 41.3 International Neuroblastoma Risk Groups Staging System (INRGSS).

Stage L1	Localized tumor not involving vital structures as defined by the list of image-defined risk factors and confined to one body component.
Stage L2	Locoregional tumor with presence of one or more image-defined risk factors (IDRFs):
	• **Neck**: Tumor encasing carotid and/or vertebral artery and/or internal jugular vein; tumor extending to base of skull; tumor compressing the trachea.
	• **Cervico-thoracic junction**: Tumor encasing brachial plexus roots; tumor encasing subclavian vessels and/or vertebral and/or carotid artery; tumor compressing the trachea.
	• **Thorax**: Tumor encasing the aorta and/or major branches; tumor compressing the trachea and/or principal bronchi; lower mediastinal tumor, infiltrating the costo-vertebral junction between T9 and T12.
	• **Thoraco-abdominal**: Tumor encasing the aorta and/or vena cava.
	• **Abdomen/pelvis**: Tumor infiltrating the porta hepatis and/or the hepatoduodenal ligament; tumor encasing branches of the superior mesenteric artery at the mesenteric root; tumor encasing the origin of the coeliac axis, and/or of the superior mesenteric artery; tumor invading one or both renal pedicles; tumor encasing the aorta and/or vena cava; tumor encasing the iliac vessels; pelvic tumor crossing the sciatic notch.
	• **Intraspinal tumor extension whatever the location provided that**: More than one-third of the spinal canal in the axial plane is invaded and/or the perimedullary leptomeningeal spaces are not visible and/or the spinal cord signal is abnormal.
	• **Infiltration of adjacent organs/structures**: Pericardium, diaphragm, kidney, liver, duodeno-pancreatic block, and mesentery.
	• **Conditions to be recorded, but not considered IDRFs**: Multifocal primary tumors; pleural effusion, with or without malignant cells; ascites, with or without malignant cell
Stage M	Distant metastatic disease (except stage MS).
Stage MS	Metastatic disease in children aged younger than 18 months with metastases confined to skin, liver, and/or bone marrow.

Adapted from Refs [177, 178].

treatment is followed by a course of maintenance therapy consisting of immunological agents and cis-retinoic acid. Even with induction chemotherapy, surgery, and high-dose chemotherapy followed by stem cell transplant, relapse rates are high and most recurrences are local without radiotherapy. For this reason, radiation therapy is recommended to the post-induction chemotherapy tumor bed, regardless of the extent of resection. The standard dose of radiotherapy recommended to this volume is 21.6 Gy at 1.8 Gy per fraction in the setting of gross total resection. The GTV includes the tumor remaining prior to surgical resection and the post-induction therapy; thus, all imaging is important for treatment planning to be registered to the CT planning scan in order to create the GTV. A 1.5 cm marginal expansion creates the CTV, accounting for anatomic barriers and tissue/organ shifts. A 0.5 cm PTV margin around the CTV accounts for patient movement and set-up error. For children with residual disease following surgery, a total dose of 36 Gy is recommended, but is broken down in two separate treatment volumes. The initial target volume (GTV1/CTV1/PTV1) is treated to a dose of 21.6 Gy. The GTV1 is defined by the tumor remaining prior to surgical resection and post-induction therapy. The CTV1 includes the GTV1 with an additional 1.5 cm margin in all directions, modified to account for anatomic boundaries and/or shifts in organs. An additional 0.5 cm margin is expanded to create the PTV1. The boost volume (GTV2/CTV2/PTV2) is treated to a final dose of 14.4 Gy for a cumulative dose of 36 Gy. GTV2 includes gross residual disease present following the incomplete resection. A margin of 1.5 cm generates the CTV2. Finally, a margin of 0.5 cm to produce the PTV2 accounts for patient set-up error. Emergent radiation is required in some scenarios for neuroblastoma. Hepatomegaly causing respiratory compromise may require emergent radiation and is treated to a total dose of 4.5 Gy at 1.5 Gy per daily fraction. It is not necessary to treat the entire liver, and avoidance of the ovaries or other radiosensitive structures may be considered. In the setting of cord compression in children aged less than three years, 9 Gy at 1.8 Gy per fraction is delivered; however, in children aged over three years a dose of 21.6 Gy at 1.8 Gy per fraction is prescribed.

Although the radiation dose required to control neuroblastoma is low, these children are typically very young and treatment volumes may be large. Complications of therapy include scoliosis, which can occur in approximately 25% of patients, especially when doses over 18 Gy are delivered to the vertebral bodies. Care should be taken to evenly dose the vertebral bodies when using advanced techniques such as proton therapy or IMRT. Patients require annual audiologic evaluation secondary to hearing loss as a result of platinum agents. Children are also at risk of ovarian dysfunction, hypothyroidism, diabetes (>10 Gy to the tail of the pancreas), and may require lifelong hormonal supplementation and/or fertility counseling [182].

Advanced radiation techniques such as IMRT, intraoperative radiation and proton radiation should be considered, particularly with high-risk patients in order to decrease the dose to normal tissues. To help facilitate this, additional radiotherapy changes within the COG Protocol ANBL1531 include further CTV1 margin reduction from 1.5 cm to 1 cm. When possible, the use of proton beam therapy should be considered in patients diagnosed with neuroblastoma, since there is a potential for significant sparing of the lung, kidney(s), vertebral bodies, bowel, stomach, liver, and soft tissue compared to traditional radiotherapeutic techniques, including 3D conformal therapy and IMRT [183].

Important treatment techniques should be considered. For instance, posterior beams should be used when treating proton beams when directed at retroperitoneal tumors, because bowel filling and intermittent gas can create dose uncertainty and uncertainty with the use of anterior and/or lateral fields. Although still controversial, consideration should be given to encompassing the entire vertebral body in pre-pubertal patients in order to ensure a homogeneous dose distribution and to decrease the risk of scoliosis. The use of protons to treat a large paraspinal neuroblastoma is shown in Figure 41.4.

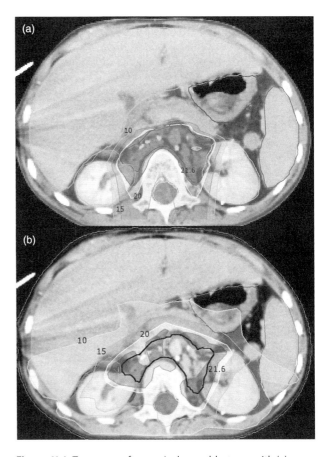

Figure 41.4 Treatment of paraspinal neuroblastoma with (a) scanned proton beam treatment and (b) IMRT (Individual isodose lines indicate dose in Gy). For a color version of this figure, see the color plate section.

Wilms Tumor and Other Renal Malignancies

Wilms tumor is the most common abdominal malignancy in children, representing 5% of childhood malignancies in the United States, with approximately 650 new cases per year in North America. Most children are diagnosed under the age of five years, with a slight predilection for African Americans [3]. Children generally present with a painless abdominal mass and, in contrast to neuroblastoma, aside from the mass, these children are usually otherwise well. However, one-third of patients have anorexia, malaise, vomiting, and/or hematuria.

Wilms tumor is thought to be an embryonal malignancy arising from the remnants of an immature kidney. The cause is unknown, but it may arise sporadically or from hereditary origins. Characteristic syndromes and genetic foci have been associated with the risk of developing Wilms tumors, including WAGR (Wilms tumor, Aniridia, Genitourinary anomalies, and Retardation), Beckwith–Wiedmann syndrome (hemihypertrophy, ear creases, macroglossia, macrosomia, midline abdominal wall defects, hypoglycemia), and Denys–Drash syndrome (pseudohermaphroditism, mesangial sclerosis, renal failure). Furthermore, a loss of heterozygosity at chromosomes 1p and 16q, and *WT1* mutations and 11p15 loss have been associated with Wilms tumor, predictors for relapse and markers for adverse prognosis. Classically, Wilms tumor consists of three cell components: tubular, blastemal, and stromal. Wilms tumor histology is categorized as favorable histology (FH), focal anaplasia (FA), or diffuse anaplasia (DA), with anaplastic subtypes considered unfavorable histologies (UH). Rhabdoid tumor of the kidney (RTK) and clear-cell sarcoma of the kidney (CCSK) were categorized as UH Wilms tumor in the past, but these are now considered distinct entities of childhood renal cancer [184].

The work-up for suspected Wilms tumor typically starts with an abdominal ultrasound, followed by a CT scan of the abdomen and pelvis, to better characterize the abdominal mass and the extent of local disease and assess for contralateral kidney involvement. Chest CT and/or chest X-radiography is performed to evaluate for lung metastases. A bone scan, skeletal survey, and MRI of the brain should be performed if pathology reveals rhabdoid tumor of the kidney, as 10–15% of these patients may have CNS involvement of the cerebellum or pineal region. As CCSK tends to metastasize to the bone and brain, a bone scan, bone marrow biopsy and MRI of the brain are indicated when diagnosed. A biopsy of the tumor is reserved for unresectable primaries or in children diagnosed with bilateral disease [185]. In bilateral Wilms tumor, an initial biopsy is allowed to facilitate a nephron-sparing approach; however, there is no

Table 41.4 Children's Oncology Group Wilms tumor staging system.

Stage I	Tumor limited to kidney, completely resected. The renal capsule is intact. The tumor was not ruptured or biopsied prior to removal. The vessels of the renal sinus are not involved. There is no evidence of tumor at or beyond the margins of resection.
Stage II	The tumor is completely resected and there is no evidence of tumor at or beyond the margins of resection. The tumor extends beyond the kidney, as is evidenced by any one of the following criteria: There is regional extension of the tumor (i.e., penetration of the renal capsule, or extensive invasion of the soft tissue of the renal sinus). Blood vessels within the nephrectomy specimen outside the renal parenchyma, including those of the renal sinus, contain tumor.
Stage III	Residual non-hematogeneous tumor present following surgery, and confined to abdomen. Any one of the following may occur: • Lymph nodes within the abdomen or pelvis are involved by tumor. • The tumor has penetrated through the peritoneal surface. • Tumor implants are found on the peritoneal surface. • Gross or microscopic tumor remains postoperatively. • The tumor is not completely resectable because of local infiltration into vital structures. • Tumor spillage occurring either before or during surgery. • The tumor is biopsied before removal. • The tumor is treated with preoperative chemotherapy before removal. • The tumor is removed in greater than one piece.
Stage IV	Hematogeneous metastases (lung, liver, bone, brain, etc.), or lymph node metastases outside the abdomino-pelvic region are present.
Stage V	Bilateral renal involvement by tumor is present at diagnosis.

upstaging to stage III based on biopsy. Each primary is staged separately to determine the need for radiotherapy. The current COG staging is listed in Table 41.4. The North American standard established by National Wilms Tumor Study (NWTS) and COG studies begins with initial surgery, followed by radiation if indicated, and then chemotherapy [178, 186]. Resectability is based on whether there is an extension of tumor thrombus above the hepatic veins, tumor extension to contiguous structures, if the child is at risk for pulmonary compromise secondary to metastatic disease, and the surgeon's discretion [185]. The rationale is to obtain an accurate pathologic diagnosis, prognostic information, and to surgically define the extent of disease in order to customize therapy. The International Society of Paediatric Oncology (SIOP) uses a different strategy of preoperative therapy, in an attempt to decrease intraoperative tumor spillage, assess response to therapy, with a goal of downstaging and reducing therapy [187]. Because previous studies have continued to lead to improved outcomes, COG radiation therapy treatment strategies are now risk-based, focusing on stage and pathology, while integrating age, tumor size and volume, response to chemotherapy, and loss of heterozygosity of chromosomes 1p and 16q [188, 189]. The details are listed in Table 41.5.

Patients diagnosed with stage I/II FH Wilms tumor do not require radiotherapy. Flank radiation is recommended for patients with stage III FH, stage I–III unfavorable histologies (FA and CCSK), and stage I–II DA. COG guidelines recommend that radiotherapy is commenced by postoperative day 9 if feasible, particularly for patients diagnosed with UH, and no later than postoperative day 14 for FH. Flank radiotherapy is indicated for residual/unresectable tumor following surgery, positive lymph nodes (LN), local spillage, transected tumor thrombus, or piecemeal resection. The standard dose for these patients is 10.8 Gy in fractions of 1.8 Gy, but higher doses are recommended for stage III DA and stage I–III RTK to a dose of 19.8 Gy at 1.8 Gy per fraction (limit of 10.8 Gy in infants aged ≤12 months). For flank radiotherapy, the GTV includes the involved kidney and associated tumor. A 1 cm margin, including below the level of ureteral disease extension, identifies the CTV. In the presence of a tumor thrombus that involves the inferior vena cava, the flank irradiation treatment volume should include the entire thrombus with a 1 cm margin. The PTV includes the CTV with an additional 0.5 cm margin to account for daily set-up error and patient movement. Flank radiotherapy is delivered to the anterior/posterior (AP/PA) fields or slightly oblique fields. A key point for flank radiotherapy is that the superior border of the treatment field is often below the dome of the diaphragm, unless there is tumor extension to that height. The medial border should cross the midline to include the vertebral body with an additional 1 cm; however, the medial border should not overlap with the contralateral kidney. Unresected LN metastases require an additional treatment to a total dose of 19.8 Gy. The entire para-aortic chain from L5 to the crus of the diaphragm should be included in the field.

An additional boost of 10.8 Gy is recommended for any gross residual disease present following resection, or 3.6 Gy for microscopically positive margins following surgery and chemotherapy. In patients with diffuse anaplasia treated to 19.8 Gy with residual tumor, a supplemental boost with 10.8 Gy for a total dose of 30.6 Gy is recommended. A boost GTV includes the postoperative residual tumor. A margin of 0.5 cm creates the CTV. A

Table 41.5 Children's Oncology Groups renal risk-based treatment.

Tumor risk classification	Multimodality treatment
Very Low-Risk FH WT	
<2 years, Stage I FH, <550 g	Surgery, NO therapy if central path review and LN sampling
Low-Risk FH WT	
≥2 years, Stage I FH, ≥550 g; OR	Surgery, No RT, Regimen EE4A
Stage II FH without LOH	
Standard-Risk FH WT	
Stage I and II FH with LOH; OR	Surgery, Regimen DD4A
Stage III FH without LOH	Surgery, RT, Regimen DD4A
High-Risk FH WT	
Stage III/IV FH w/ LOH;	Surgery, RT, Regimen M, WLI
Stage IV FH slow/incomplete response; OR	Surgery, RT, Regimen DD4A, No WLI
Stage IV FH: CR of lung mets at week 6/DD4A (rapid early responder)	
High-Risk UH WT	
Stage I–III FA	Surgery, RT, Regimen DD4A
Stage I DA	
High-Risk UH	
Stage IV FA; Stage II–IV DA Stage IV CCSK; Stage I–IV RTK	Surgery, RT, Regimen UH1
High-Risk UH	
Stage I–III CCSK	Surgery, RT, Regimen I

WT, Wilms tumor; LN, lymph nodes; RT, radiotherapy; FH, favorable histology; UH, unfavorable histology; LOH, loss of heterozygosity 1p and 16q; g, grams; mets, metastases; WLI, Whole-lung irradiation; FA, focal anaplasia; DA, diffuse anaplasia; CR, complete response; RTK, Rhabdoid tumor of the kidney; CCSK, clear-cell sarcoma of the kidney. EE4A, Vincristine/Dactinomycin.
DD4A, Vincristine/Dactinomycin/Doxorubicin.
Regimen M, Cyclophosphamide/Etoposide/Dactinomycin/Doxorubicin.
Regimen I, Vincristine/Doxorubicin/Cyclophosphamide.
Regimen UH1, Vincristine/Doxorubicin/Cyclophosphamide/Carboplatin/Etoposide.

0.5–1 cm PTV margin accounts for set-up error. Finally, a 1 cm block edge margin is recommended for the field design. 3DCRT or IMRT is the preferred planning technique for supplemental boost irradiation.

Whole-abdomen radiation therapy (WART) to a dose of 10.5 Gy at 1.5 Gy per fraction is recommended for positive cytology, preoperative tumor rupture, peritoneal metastases, diffuse spillage, prior biopsy, or peritoneal seeding. When the WART or liver dose exceeds 14.4 Gy the renal dose should be limited to <14.4 Gy by utilizing renal shielding. For example, a posterior partial transmission kidney block for the entire course of treatment could be incorporated, with the thickness determined based on treatment planning. The dimensions of the block should be 0.5 cm wider than the projection of the kidney on the posterior (PA) digitally reconstructed radiograph (DRR). For WART, the CTV is the entire peritoneal cavity. For field design, the superior border is 1 cm above the diaphragm. The inferior border is the bottom of the obturator foramen. Laterally, the field extends 1 cm beyond the abdominal wall. The femoral heads and heart should be shielded using cerrobend blocks or multileaf collimator. AP/PA fields should be used to deliver the treatment, with 3DCRT or IMRT for a boost. Radiation therapy field design is described in Figure 41.5.

Brain, liver, and bone irradiation is indicated when metastases are present. In the setting of pulmonary lesions, evaluation for resection should be considered at diagnosis for the confirmation of metastatic disease, incomplete response of pulmonary lesions with chemotherapy, and prior to additional treatment [190–192]. Whole-lung irradiation (WLI) to 10.5 Gy is recommended for patients with pulmonary metastases seen by chest X-radiography, but the treatment of CT-only pulmonary metastases that respond to chemotherapy has remained controversial. In the most recent AREN0533

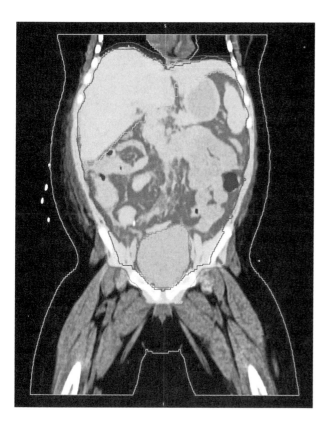

Figure 41.5 Whole-abdomen radiation therapy (WART) field for a patient with Wilms tumor. The field encompasses the entire peritoneal cavity with shielding of the femoral heads and heart. For a color version of this figure, see the color plate section.

protocol, patients with stage IV favorable histology Wilms tumor and lung metastasis only (no LOH 1p and 16q deletion) were treated using the DD4A regimen [193]. A central review of imaging at six weeks determined that patients with a complete response to chemotherapy would continue DD4A and omit WLI, while those with incomplete response would transition to Regimen M and receive WLI. Patients with incomplete response maintained excellent three-year EFS and OS at 88% and 92%, respectively. Omitting WLI did not compromise outcomes in patients who achieved a complete response, with three-year EFS and OS of 78% and 95%, respectively. For children aged ≥18 months, the bilateral lungs should be treated to a total dose of 12 Gy in eight fractions. For children aged <18 months, radiotherapy is indicated if there was no response to chemotherapy, and WLI should be delivered to a total dose of 9 Gy in six fractions [193]. For WLI, the target volume includes the entire lung volume, mediastinum, and pleural recesses. The superior, inferior and lateral borders should be 1 cm beyond the defined borders. The lateral borders should be placed 1 cm beyond the CTV, while the inferior border is often located at the level of L1. The key point here is to shield the humeral heads.

Bilateral Wilms tumor is present in approximately 5–6% of cases, and about 12% of these children are at risk of developing end-stage renal failure. AREN0534 was designed to improve the EFS and prevent the complete removal of at least one kidney. This study has implemented the SIOP histological classification system for guiding subsequent chemotherapy [194]. Radiotherapy is indicated in stage III completely necrotic, intermediate-risk tumors, blastemal predominant tumors, and stage I–III anaplastic tumors. In addition, it is indicated for metastases if present at diagnosis, and WLI is not allowed. In the setting of relapsed disease, the tumor volume and dose depend on involvement and age. If the patient requires flank or WART, infants aged ≤12 months would require 12.6–18 Gy, and older children 21.6 Gy to the involved region with a 9 Gy boost to gross residual disease.

Long-term survivors of Wilms tumor are at risk of significant morbidity and mortality, including – but not limited to – cardiac, renal failure, infertility, scoliosis, pneumonitis, soft tissue/bone hypoplasia, and secondary malignancies; however, there has been a trend over the past few years to reduce these risks [195–198]. Innovative approaches are being developed to further minimize normal tissue exposure to radiotherapy. This includes the use of IMRT for cardiac sparing during whole-lung radiotherapy, renal-sparing IMRT during whole-liver irradiation, and the introduction of proton beam therapy for flank irradiation [199–201]. The NWTS reported on 20-year congestive heart failure rates of 4.4% following initial treatment, and an increase to 17.4% following doxorubicin for the treatment of relapse. The recent cardiac-sparing whole-lung CS-IMRT prospective trial evaluated the feasibility of delivering the treatment in children and young adults diagnosed with lung metastases [200]. This approach was confirmed to be advantageous, demonstrating superior cardiac protection and dose coverage of four dimensional (4D) lung volumes [200]. There was no pulmonary toxicity during two years, with comparable tumor control and survival outcomes compared to historical outcomes. Future COG trials, and possibly also SIOP trials, will be utilizing CS-IMRT 4D lung volumes for treatment planning.

Rhabdomyosarcoma

Rhabdomyosarcoma (RMS) accounts for approximately 3.5% of malignancies in children aged <15 years, with two-thirds occurring under the age of seven years [202, 203]. RMS is the most common soft-tissue sarcoma of childhood and may occur in any location of the body, the most common sites being the genitourinary sites and the head and neck region [204]. Initial presenting symptoms are dependent on tumor location. Many children develop a mass causing pain or obstruction. In genitourinary sites, urinary obstruction is a common presenting symptom. Head and neck tumors may present with nasal obstruction or proptosis for orbital tumors. Parameningeal tumors may have cranial nerve findings due to invasion through the base of skull. The history and physical examination should focus on the extent of local disease and the possible occurrence of metastases. Less than 25% of patients have distant metastatic disease at presentation, involving lung, bone marrow, and bone. Lymph node involvement varies by site, most commonly seen in paratesticular and extremity primaries (20–30%), but is less likely for orbital primaries (<1%). CT and/or MRI of the primary site and regional lymph nodes are recommended. The metastatic work-up should include a CT scan of the chest, a bone scan, bone marrow biopsy, and evaluation of regional lymphatics [205]. Lumbar puncture for evaluation of cerebrospinal fluid (CSF) should be performed in patients with parameningeal tumors. A PET scan may be useful for the evaluation of metastases and lymphatic involvement [206]. If the primary is parameningeal, CSF cytology and MRI of the brain are indicated. Biopsy of the primary is required for diagnosis as well as to subtype RMS as embryonal (classic, spindle, and botryoid), alveolar, pleomorphic, and undifferentiated [207–209]. The histology is prognostic, with alveolar being least favorable, and is utilized for treatment recommendations along with the group and stage of disease [210]. Alveolar RMS is characterized by translocations involving the *FKHR* gene on chromosome 13, most commonly t(2; 13) (p35; q14), which fuses with the *PAX3*

gene, a transcription regulator. This is present in approximately 60–70% of children with alveolar RMS. A majority of alveolar RMSs are *PAX3-FOXO1* or *PAX7-FOXO1* translocation-positive; however, approximately 20–30% do not have translocations, and those without fusion genes behave like embryonal RMS, with more favorable prognoses [211, 212]. On the most current intermediate-risk protocol ARST 1431(260), *FOXO1* fusion status will be used to study eligibility because it is more predictive of outcomes compared to histology [213, 214].

The primary site is a strong determinant of outcome, with favorable sites including orbit, head and neck (excluding parameningeal), genitourinary (non-bladder, non-prostate), and biliary tract [215–218]. Parameningeal sites include mastoid, middle ear, nasal cavity, nasopharynx, infratemporal fossa, pterygopalatine fossa, paranasal sinuses, and parapharyngeal space. Stage and Group are also prognostic. Staging is dependent on site, size, nodal involvement, and metastases, with stage I tumors being favorable sites without metastases with or without nodal involvement, stage II representing small tumors ≤5 cm with negative lymph nodes in unfavorable sites (bladder/prostate, extremity, parameningeal, other), stage III tumors being those in unfavorable sites that are ≤5 cm with positive lymph nodes or >5 cm ± nodal involvement, and stage IV representing metastatic disease [219]. RMS is also categorized by the Intergroup Rhabdomyosarcoma Study Group (IRSG) post-surgical grouping, which represents the extent of resection and has been shown to be prognostic. Group I represents localized disease with complete resection, Group II signifies positive microscopic margins or resected regional disease, Group III represents gross residual disease, and Group IV distant metastatic disease [215, 216]. Staging and grouping are further described in Tables 41.6A–41.6C.

Treatment depends on risk and location. The achievement of local control with organ preservation and eradication of metastatic disease is the goal of combined-modality therapy. Surgery is performed initially for resectable tumors, and may be attempted following chemotherapy if tumors become resectable. If it is possible to achieve a complete resection initially with microscopic residual disease (Group II), then the process should proceed with surgery; otherwise, biopsy only is indicated. A nodal evaluation for extremity alveolar tumors or a paratesticular RMS for children aged >10 years, and a biopsy of any suspicious lymph nodes should always be performed prior to the initiation of therapy. Delayed surgery is often indicated for Group III.

Based on the most recent COG protocols, pediatric patients in North America with low-risk disease have been treated with four cycles of VAC (Vincristine, Dactinomycin, Cyclophosphamide) followed by Vincristine/ Dactinomycin for a total of six months to a year [217].

Table 41.6A Rhabdomyosarcoma pathologic pretreatment TNM staging system through the Intergroup Rhabdomyosarcoma Study Group.*

Classification	Description
Tumor	
T1	Confined to site of origin
• T1a	• Tumor size <5 cm
• T1b	• Tumor size ≥5 cm
T2	Extension to or infiltration of the surrounding tissue
• T2a	• Tumor size <5 cm
• T2b	• Tumor size ≥5 cm
Regional Lymph Nodes	
N0	Lymph nodes not clinically involved
N1	Lymph nodes clinically involved
NX	Clinical lymph node status is unknown
Metastasis	
M0	No distant metastasis
M1	Distant metastasis present

*This is not the TNM staging as seen for soft-tissue sarcomas described in the AJCC Cancer staging manual.

Table 41.6C Rhabdomyosarcoma clinical group based on Intergroup Rhabdomyosarcoma Clinical Grouping system surgical extent of disease.

Group	Extent of disease
Group I	**Excised localized disease**
• Ia	• Confined to the site of origin.
• Ib	• Infiltrative disease, beyond the site of origin. No lymph node involvement.
Group II	**Total gross resection with regional spread of disease**
• IIa	• Localized tumor with microscopic residual disease.
• IIb	• Regional disease with positive lymph nodes that are excised. No microscopic residual disease.
• IIc	• Regional disease with positive lymph nodes; grossly resected with microscopic residual disease.
Group III	**Gross residual disease**
• IIIa	• Biopsy only, with localized or regional disease.
• IIIb	• Resection of localized or regional disease (debulking of more than 50% tumor).
Group IV	**Distant metastasis**

The most recent intermediate risk COG RMS studies (IRS-IV, D9803, and ARST0531) were unable to demonstrate a significant improvement in outcome with the addition of one or more cytotoxic chemotherapeutic agents to the traditional VAC [211, 220, 221]. The current intermediate-risk protocol ARST1431 is a Phase III trial evaluating the benefit of biologically targeted agent Temsirolimus (TORI) in addition to the traditional VAC alternating with VI (Vincristine/Irinotecan) and impact on EFS and OS [222]. High-risk patients are treated on a single-arm COG protocol with VAC/IE (Irinotecan/Etoposide) every two weeks alternating with VI [222–224].

Currently, the COG protocols stratify patients into three risk groups (low, intermediate, and high) on the basis of site, stage, histology, and group; however, the definitions change over time depending on outcomes of

ongoing and future COG trials [225]. Historically, low risk included embryonal non-metastatic, any resected site (Group I/II) AND embryonal-favorable sites (Group III). Intermediate risk included embryonal incompletely excised (Group III) in unfavorable sites (stage II, III) and alveolar RMS non-metastatic (Group I–III) at any site (stage I–III). High-risk patients are those with metastatic disease (stage IV). However, based on the recent low-risk (ARST0331) and high-risk (ARST0431) RMS clinical trials, definitions have shifted so that patients aged <10 years with metastatic embryonal RMS will now be considered intermediate risk on the current ARST1431 protocol because of 60% EFS at three and four years on COG ARST0431 and COG D9803, respectively [220, 226, 227]. Furthermore, patients with embryonal

Table 41.6B Rhabdomyosarcoma clinical pretreatment TNM staging system through the Intergroup Rhabdomyosarcoma Study Group.

Stage	Site	T	Tumor size	N	M
Stage 1	Favorable*	T1 or T2	Any	N0, N1, NX	M0
Stage 2	Unfavorable#	T1 or T2	<5 cm	N0, NX	M0
Stage 3	Unfavorable	T1 or T2	<5 cm	N1	M0
	Unfavorable	T1 or T2	≥5 cm	N0, N1, NX	M0
Stage 4	Any	T1 or T2	Any	N0, N1	M1

*Favorable sites: Head and Neck (excluding parameningeal), biliary tract, orbit, genitourinary (excluding prostate and bladder).
#Unfavorable: Extremities, parameningeal, prostate and bladder, others, trunk.

RMS previously treated on protocols ARST0331 and D9502 for low risk disease (Stage 1 Group III, favorable sites/non-orbit), were found to have inferior three-year EFS and are now considered intermediate risk and eligible for the ongoing clinical trial [227–229].

The IRS studies have evaluated radiation dose and volume in combination with surgery and chemotherapy; this experience has improved outcomes tremendously and led to current recommendations for treatment [229]. Radiation plays an important role in local control for many tumors [230–232]. RMS is the most radiosensitive sarcoma. Contemporary treatment and the existing COG RMS trials require 3D/volumetric planning. Radiation is omitted only for patients with Group I favorable embryonal histology disease. Typically, 36 Gy is recommended for many patients with Group I and II disease, while nodal disease is treated to 41.4 Gy. The dose for Group III tumors, including orbital tumors, is now 50.4 Gy [233]. Based on the most recent intermediate-risk protocol ARST1431, patients with Group III tumors >5 cm can now be treated with an additional boost to a total of 59.4 Gy. Definitive stereotactic body radiotherapy (SBRT) is now being incorporated into the management of pediatric tumors, particularly for children and adolescents with bone metastases at presentation, as are being evaluated in ARST1431. SBRT is to be considered for patients with unresected/postoperative gross metastatic disease in bone <5 cm at diagnosis.

Definitive treatment doses may vary per patient, as the current intermediate-risk COG protocol ARST1431 recommends radiation dose according to *FOXO1* fusion status, clinical group, site, and treatment response to therapy [222]. The GTV1 includes the pre-chemotherapy volume and residual tumor volume, best delineated by registering pre-treatment and post-treatment CT, PET, and MRI with the planning scan. A margin of 1 cm around the GTV1 is recommended to define the clinical tumor volume (CTV1), confined by anatomic boundaries. When lymph nodes are involved, the nodal chains are also included within the CTV1. An additional margin of 0.3–0.5 cm added to the PTV to address set-up variation may depend on the location of the primary, institutional standards, and if IGRT is available. For patients scheduled to receive doses of 41.4–59.4 Gy, a cone-down should occur for patients with a decrease in tumor size following chemotherapy, which will be based on the post-chemotherapy volume (GTV2) [234]. CTV2 is defined as GTV2 with a 1 cm margin, modified to account for areas at risk and anatomic barriers. An additional 0.3–0.5 cm margin is delineated to create the PTV2 to balance set-up error and patient motion.

Special considerations include patients with bladder/prostate primaries. Although the amount of bladder involvement may vary from patient to patient, the preservation of organ function and growth must be considered during treatment planning. Placing a catheter daily can assist with bladder reproducibility. Growth plates (avoidance and/or symmetrical dosing of bony structures if unavoidable), bladder, anus/rectum, bowel, genitalia and bony structures should always be contoured in patients with pelvic or abdominal primaries. Young females diagnosed with vaginal tumors are at risk for late effects of surgery and radiotherapy, which can significantly impact on quality of life. ARST0331 and D9602 identified high local recurrence rates, especially in Group III vaginal primaries when radiotherapy was omitted [235]. Currently, radiotherapy to a dose of 36 Gy is recommended for young females diagnosed with Group II and III vaginal RMS, with goals to spare uterus, bladder, growth plates, and vagina. When treating extremity tumors, be sure to evaluate the need to treat regional nodes. Consider including scars/drains into the radiation treatment field. In addition, a strip of skin or portion of the joint/epiphysis should be spared. If proton beam therapy is used, a frog-leg set-up for the use of a perineal field is recommended in order to avoid organ and growth plate dose. Brachytherapy is also a useful modality to provide localized dosage, and minimize radiation to normal tissue. Despite the concern for late toxicities, radiotherapy should not be delayed or withheld in infants, because inferior outcomes have been reported as a result of decreased utilization of appropriate local therapy [236, 237]. Care should be taken to balance goals of care, including hope for cure, minimizing the risk of late toxicity, and maintaining quality of life. Advanced therapeutic modalities should be considered in order to decrease toxicities in these patients. For certain primary sites, proton beam therapy has demonstrated superior dose conformality compared to modern radiotherapeutic techniques, including IMRT, decreasing unnecessary dose to critical structures (including parotid and cochlea), which could have favorable implications on late morbidities and quality of life [231, 238, 239].

Non-Rhabdomyosarcoma Soft-Tissue Sarcoma (NRSTS)

Soft-tissue sarcomas represent approximately 7% of all childhood malignancies, with non-rhabdomyosarcoma soft-tissue sarcomas (NRSTS) comprising roughly half or approximately 500–550 of these pediatric diagnoses annually [240, 241]. Approach of management and indications for radiotherapy have differed vastly compared to adult studies, predominantly because of the concerns for the unique anatomy, late tissue toxicity, and risk for secondary malignancy. The goal of management has included limb-sparing surgery and adjuvant radiation as the standard for large, high-grade tumors. Negative margins is the goal of surgical resection, although when a tumor is in close proximity to neurovascular structures, either preoperative or postoperative radiotherapy should be considered. Pediatric Oncology Group (POG) 8653 recommended adjuvant radiotherapy following R1 surgical resection with initial field margins of 5 cm to target volumes prescribed to doses of 36–45 Gy, followed by a cone-down field with a margin of 2 cm to a total dose of 45–50.4 Gy. Local failure and grade 3/4 toxicity rates were reported at 12% and 15%, respectively [242]. However, with residual or unresectable disease dose escalation is required, as seen in both POG 8654 and POG 9553, potentially increasing the risk of some of these toxicities [243, 244]. In the Phase II RT-SARC prospective study initiated by St Jude Children's Research Hospital, the goal was to further limit target margin in this population. For treatment planning, MRI and CT-based imaging was used to delineate the postoperative bed and gross diseases, which generated the GTV. An additional 1.5–2 cm margin restricted along the fascial planes and adjacent bone shaped the CTV. The PTV was created afterwards, and a final margin of 0.4–1 cm was added to make up for patient and set-up errors. The overall five-year local and distal failure rates and Grade ≥3 were 14.8%, 31%, and 15%, respectively. Margin-positive patients continued to represent a high-risk group, and future trials should evaluate potential dose-escalation or radiosensitizers [245–247]. Based on the most recent protocols, ARST 0332 and 1321, the recommended CTV margin is 1.5 cm for children and up to 3.0 cm for adults diagnosed with NRSTS. The initial target volume is prescribed doses of 45–50 Gy, followed by a cone-down volume with a CTV margin of 1 cm anatomically constrained, prescribed to a final dose of 61.2–70 Gy.

Osteosarcoma

Osteosarcoma is the most common primary pediatric bone tumor, accounting for 3% of childhood malignancies and with approximately 400 cases diagnosed each year. For children, the peak incidence is seen in adolescent years as most patients present between the ages of 10 and 20 years, corresponding to growth spurts. A second peak occurs in patients aged >70 years, arising from Paget's disease. Males and females are equally affected, and the disease is 30% more common in African Americans. Osteosarcoma can occur in any bone, but is most commonly seen in the long bones of the lower extremities, with 80% of patients presenting with localized disease involving the metaphysis. Most commonly, the tumor occurs in the femur, followed by the tibia, and humerus. Risk factors include genetic predisposition (retinoblastoma/RB1 mutation, Li–Fraumeni/p53 mutation, Rothmund–Thomson syndrome), Paget's disease, primary RT. Classically at presentation, pain is the most

common symptom. If there is a palpable mass, it is tender, firm and fixed to the bone, but not inflamed. The adjacent joint is often restricted and the rest of the examination is normal. Levels of serum alkaline phosphatase and LDH may be elevated. Metastases are present in 10–20% of patients at diagnosis, with the most common site of metastases being the lung, followed by bone [248]. With local therapy alone, 80% of patients will develop metastatic disease, most commonly involving the lung, followed by the bone and bone marrow. Work-up includes laboratory studies (CBC, CMP, urinalysis, LDH, alkaline phosphatase). Initial X-ray evaluation often demonstrates both lytic (radiolucent) and blastic (radiodense) components. Osteosarcoma has an extraosseous component and periosteal reaction suggesting rapid growth, resulting in a Codman's triangle or sunburst pattern. MRI and/or CT (preferably both) help to define the primary lesion. The metastatic work-up should include chest CT and bone scan. A PET-CT scan may also be useful for initial staging and for follow-up [249]. The Enneking staging system incorporating grade (G1 or G2), whether or not the tumor is confined to the anatomic compartment of origin (T1 = confined, T2 = not confined), and whether or not metastases are present (M0 or M1), is the most common staging system used [250]. An initial core needle biopsy should be completed by the surgeon who will be performing the surgical resection. Measures should be taken to avoid hematoma formation. The most important prognostic factor for localized, completely resected disease is the degree of necrosis in response to neoadjuvant chemotherapy (>90% versus ≤90% necrosis) [251].

Treatment includes the use of multi-agent neoadjuvant chemotherapy with a regimen that includes methotrexate, cisplatin, and doxorubicin, among other agents [252, 253]. Local control should include wide-margin surgical resection, with the goal of preservation of function, followed by postoperative chemotherapy. Limb-sparing procedures are attempted for most patients, but some do still require amputation. For those patients with tumors in locations where a gross total resection is not feasible (base of skull, spine, and pelvis), in medically inoperable patients, inoperable metastatic disease, or palliation of metastatic disease, radiation is indicated. Several small series have reported a benefit of radiation, with most indicating that higher doses (50–76 Gy) are more likely to provide durable local control [254–259]. Key treatment planning points include an avoidance of circumferential irradiation, particularly in extremity primaries. Avoid the growth plate in pediatric patients and/or asymmetric coverage of vertebral bodies to minimize growth abnormalities and/or scoliosis. Proton radiation or brachytherapy may be required to deliver high doses of radiation while limiting a high dose to normal surrounding structures [258]. Of interest, osteosarcoma is the most common radiation-induced sarcoma, representing 50–80% of radiation-induced tumors of the bone. Higher radiation doses and chemotherapy with alkylating agents increase the risk of developing a secondary osteosarcoma [260, 261].

Ewing Sarcoma

Ewing sarcoma is the second most common pediatric sarcoma, with approximately 200–250 cases per year in the United States. Ewing's sarcoma is more common in adolescents and young adults, but less common in very young children. Males are more often affected than females. Pain is the most common presenting symptom, seen in more than 90% of cases. Patients may have a palpable mass. Almost one-fourth of patients present with metastatic disease, and most patients have micrometastatic disease at diagnosis. In advanced disease, there may be presentation of constitutional symptoms, elevation of LDH, and leukocytosis. Ewing sarcoma frequently originates in the diaphyseal region of the bone. Other tumors within the family of Ewing include Askin tumor (invading the chest wall), extraosseous Ewing sarcoma (8%), and peripheral primitive neuroectodermal tumor (PNET) (5%). Imaging reveals a mottled appearance, and a periosteal reaction is classic; this is commonly referred to as 'onion skin' because the tumor continues to grow through the reparative attempts of the bone. X-ray imaging may reveal a lytic destructive lesion with or without a soft-tissue mass. CT scanning is superior to define the bony abnormality, while MRI demonstrates a better definition of the soft-tissue component. It is preferable to obtain both studies at diagnosis. After a complete history and physical examination is completed, including laboratory studies (CBC, CMP, ESR, LDH), a metastatic evaluation should include bone scan, chest CT, and bone marrow biopsy. PET or PET-CT may also be very useful since many tumors are FDG-avid [262]. A biopsy of the lesion to evaluate for pathological diagnosis and cytogenetics is required, and will show a small round blue cell tumor [263]. Nearly all of these tumors contain a translocation between chromosomes (11:22) EWS/FLI fusion protein [264]. There is no recognized staging system for Ewing's sarcoma, but the prognosis is dependent on the presence of metastatic disease, age, location (with central tumors having a worse prognosis), cytogenetics, response to chemotherapy, and size of the tumor (diameter >8 cm or volume >200 ml) [265–268].

Treatment of Ewing's sarcoma includes chemotherapy and surgery and/or radiation. Survival is approximately 70% for localized disease. For tumors that are operable without substantial morbidity, surgery is indicated. Primary radiation is indicated for inoperable tumors for which surgical resection is either not feasible or would introduce unacceptable morbidity [269]. Some studies have shown superior outcomes for surgery as compared to radiation, but these results may be due to selection bias, as smaller tumors and those in more distal locations are more amenable to surgical resection [270, 271]. Radiation therapy is also indicated for either partially or inadequately resected tumors and tumors [272]. Several studies have helped to establish current radiation guidelines. The Pediatric Oncology Group showed that it is not necessary to treat the entire involved bone, and established the radiographic disease with an adequate margin as the target volume [273]. Several studies have shown a dose response to help define recommendations for a radiation dose in the range of 50–55.8 Gy [274, 275]. Most recently, the intensity of chemotherapy has resulted in superior outcomes, with shorter intervals on the most recent COG study AEWS0031; currently, patients are receiving vincristine/doxorubicin/cyclophosphamide alternating with ifosfamide/etoposide every two weeks [276].

Definitive radiation is recommended for unresectable tumors, and is to commence by weeks 12–14 of treatment. The initial tumor volume should be determined by CT, PET, and/or MRI prior to any surgical debulking and/or chemotherapy. It should include all areas of tumor involvement, including any soft tissue and/or bony abnormality identified at the time of diagnosis, and any enlarged but unresected lymph nodes. Adjustments should be made for tumors with 'pushing borders' that have regressed with chemotherapy (GTV1) (i.e., into thoracic or abdominal cavities), with a margin added for microscopic disease of approximately 1.0 cm in order to define to CTV1 (based on recent margin-reduction trials, St Jude institutional trials and AEWS 1031). An additional margin of approximately 0.3–0.5 cm, or based on various factors, is used to construct the PTV1, which should receive a dose of 45 Gy. Based on similar imaging following induction chemotherapy, the GTV2 is defined as any pre-treatment abnormalities of the bone and any residual visual or palpable tumor in the soft tissue, with a margin of approximately 1.0 cm (CTV2) accounting for anatomic boundaries. PTV2 is based on an added 0.3–0.5 cm margin for set-up error and patient day-to-day variability, ultimately receiving an additional dose of 10.8 Gy to a total of 55.8 Gy. Tumors arising in the vertebral body require dose de-escalation and receive a total 45 Gy due to spinal cord tolerance. Excellent treatment tolerance and outcomes have been demonstrated with the use of proton beam therapy for these patients, especially as a potential treatment option to reduce normal tissue exposure; however, longer follow-up is necessary [150]. Late toxicity includes skin discoloration, lymphedema, infertility in children who receive pelvic radiotherapy, secondary malignancies, muscular atrophy, permanent weakening of the affected bone (highest risk of fracture within 18 months of radiotherapy), and abnormal bone and soft-tissue growth. A limb length discrepancy of 2–6 cm can be addressed with a shoe lift; otherwise, surgical intervention should be considered. In patients who receive whole-lung radiotherapy, pneumonitis or pulmonary fibrosis remains a late toxicity [89, 168].

For refractory or recurrent Ewing's sarcoma, the prognosis remains poor, with long-term survival reported at 22–24%, and lower in patients with distant relapse [277]. No standard therapy has been described in this setting, and further research and randomized clinical trials are necessary. The implementation of multimodality therapeutic strategies will be necessary, as well as the development of new targeted agents in order to improve the outcomes of patients diagnosed and treated for Ewing's sarcoma [278, 279].

Retinoblastoma

Retinoblastoma (RB) accounts for 3% of childhood cancers, with approximately 250–300 new cases diagnosed in the United States annually. It is a disease of very young children, usually aged <3 years, with no predilection for gender, race, or eye. RB is well known for the discovery of tumor suppressor genes and Knudson's 'two-hit' hypothesis [280], and results from mutation in the tumor suppressor gene, *RB1* on the long arm of chromosome 13q14 [281]. To have the disease, both alleles must be affected. Some 40% of patients will have the hereditary form of RB, with one inherited mutation and one acquired mutation, and these children frequently have bilateral disease. Typically, 60% of patients have a non-hereditary form of RB, with disease involving only one eye that acquired two mutations in a retinal cell [282]. The tumors have a neuroepithelial origin, arising from the nucleated layers of the eye. Histologically, they are undifferentiated small anaplastic cells that may be round or polygonal, surrounded by scant cytoplasm. Calcifications are common in necrotic regions. Flexner–Wintersteiner rosettes are classic as they attempt to differentiate into photoreceptor cells. The tumors eventually display growth, either as endophytic, exophytic, diffuse plaque-like, or seeding throughout the vitreous. Spread of the tumor occurs by direct extension, or hematogeneously. Patients may develop lymph node involvement (through anterior extrascleral extension), local soft-tissue involvement, or metastatic (bone marrow, skull, long bones, or brain).

Children often present with leukocoria (white rather than red reflex due to white light reflected from tumor) on examination, or as noted in a photograph, or strabismus. Depending on the extent of disease, they may have symptoms of painful glaucoma, irritability, proptosis, or low-grade fever. The work-up includes an examination under anesthesia by a pediatric ophthalmologist for an ocular staging examination. MRI of the brain can show the primary ocular tumor and reveal extension into the extraocular space or involvement of the ocular nerve; it is useful if there are concerns of 'trilateral retinoblastoma' or a pineoblastoma that is rare but may occur in patients with hereditary disease [283, 284]. These patients can present with increased intracranial pressure, ataxia, or diabetes insipidus, and often have a grave prognosis without treatment [282].

A bone marrow biopsy, bone scan, and a lumbar puncture for CSF may be recommended if metastatic disease is suspected. All patients should have genetic counseling. Several classification systems exist, the most commonly used being the International Classification of Retinoblastoma (ICRB) grouping system, which was developed to better predict who is likely to be cured without the need for enucleation or external-beam radiotherapy (EBRT) [285]. Under this system, Group A is considered a small tumor away from the optic disc and fovea, Group B is a large tumor or tumor close to or involving the optic disc or fovea, Group C is a tumor with focal seeds, Group D is a tumor with diffuse seeds, and Group E is an extensive RB involving >50% of the globe, with glaucoma, or invasion of the optic nerve, choroid sclera, orbit, or anterior chamber. Treatment is dependent on the extent of involvement, whether the disease is unilateral or bilateral, whether or not it is hereditary, and sometimes by response to treatment and parental preference. For early disease, the goal is more often towards organ preservation. Systemic chemotherapy, cryotherapy and laser therapy are often preferred to avoid toxicities of radiation and enucleation for early cases [286]. Intra-arterial chemotherapy is being explored as another option for treatment [286, 287]. Radiation is generally recommended for disease refractory to systemic or intra-arterial chemotherapy and local consolidation, especially in an eye with useful vision [288]. Specifically, radiation is reserved for diffuse vitreous seeding, multifocal disease, or at the time of disease progression, particularly because of the toxicity risk and concern for second malignancies. For EBRT, the standard dose is 45 Gy at 1.8–2.0 Gy per fraction to the retina, using techniques that can spare the lens and cornea. Plaque brachytherapy may be an option for unifocal tumors of 0.2–1.6 cm base diameter and <1.0 cm thickness that are located in the peripheral retina [289]. Enucleation is recommended for advanced disease. For these rare advanced tumors, chemotherapy and often radiation are recommended. The most recent COG ARET0321 is utilizing multi-modality therapy, including chemotherapy, high-dose chemotherapy with stem cell rescue, and EBRT for the management of extra-ocular retinoblastoma to assess both response rate and toxicities [290].

Various radiation-related complications have been reported following previous local therapy or chemoreduction which include vitreous hemorrhage, nonproliferative retinopathy, bone hypoplasia, proliferative retinopathy, radiation maculopathy, cataracts, papillopathy, and secondary malignancies [89]. Although some toxicities cannot be avoided, continuous efforts are being made to reduce them in these patients. Most recently, proton beam therapy has been considered an excellent treatment modality in these children, demonstrating excellent tumor volume coverage while maximally avoiding non-target tissue compared to other radiotherapeutic techniques [291]. Radiation is often avoided in patients with germline mutations, because they are at significant risk of developing second malignancies within the treatment field, with cumulative incidence rates of up to 58.3% reported at 50 years after the initial diagnosis of hereditary retinoblastoma compared to those who did not receive radiotherapy [292]. It is important to bear in mind that the treatment fields used for these studies were very large. A recent study demonstrated markedly reduced risks of second malignancies for a proton cohort compared with a photon cohort [293]. Those patients with sporadic retinoblastoma are not at a significantly increased risk of developing secondary malignancies [289].

As children continue to have improved disease and survival outcomes, longevity puts them at risk for the toxicities from the therapies provided [1,2,169,294]. Strategies have been implemented to decrease radiotherapy-induced morbidity in children. In order to decrease the volume of tissue treated, a variety of techniques are utilized, including smaller margin expansions for treatment volume, the incorporation of adapted radiotherapy, advanced modern imaging to better define tumor margins, improved immobilization to treatment accuracy, and the application of innovative radiotherapeutic innovative technology (IGRT, IMRT, motion management, proton beam therapy).

Conclusions

A great deal of progress has been made during the past few decades, and as new treatments have emerged the role of radiation has evolved. For some pediatric malignancies, radiation was once the pivotal treatment and now plays an adjuvant role, or has been omitted entirely as a component of therapy. For other disease sites, new modalities allow for a more definitive treatment with decreased morbidity, thus facilitating improvement in survival [4]. As children continue to have improved disease and survival outcomes, they incur the risk of developing late toxicities inherent in the treatments provided [1, 2, 169, 294]. Imaging has enabled radiation oncologists to better target areas at high risk for recurrence, and to avoid or minimize dose to critical structures. Strategies have been implemented in order to decrease the volume of tissue treated. Various techniques are utilized, including smaller margin expansions for treatment volume, the incorporation of adapted radiotherapy, advanced modern imaging to better define tumor margins, improved immobilization for treatment accuracy, and the application of innovative radiotherapeutic technologies (IGRT, IMRT, motion management, proton beam therapy). Pediatric oncology is – and will continue to be – an evolving field, with new treatments and technologies emerging and being tested in the clinic. Physicians will continue to explore new therapies, with the goal of curing childhood malignancies while allowing children to grow into adults who can live a healthy life free from major late complications.

References

1 Oeffinger, K.C., Mertens, A.C., Sklar, C.A., *et al.* (2006) Chronic health conditions in adult survivors of childhood cancer. *N. Engl. J. Med.*, **355** (15), 1572–1582.

2 Armstrong, G.T., Kawashima, T., Leisenring, W., *et al.* (2014) Aging and risk of severe, disabling, life-threatening, and fatal events in the childhood cancer survivor study. *J. Clin. Oncol.*, **32** (12), 1218–1227.

3 American Cancer Society (2017) I. Cancer Facts & Figures 2017. Available at: http://www.cancer.org/content/dam/cancer-org/research/cancer-facts-and-statistics/annual-cancer-facts-and-figures/2017/cancer-facts-and-figures-2017.pdf.

4 Howlander, N., Noone, A.M., Krapcho, M., *et al.* (2016) SEER Cancer Statistics Review, 1975–2013, National Cancer Institute, Bethesda, Maryland. Available at: http://seer.cancer.gov/csr/1975_2013. Based on November 2015 SEER data submission, posted to the SEER web site. 04/2016.

5 Ostrom, Q.T., Gittleman, H., Fulop, J., *et al.* (2015) CBTRUS Statistical Report: Primary Brain and Central Nervous System Tumors Diagnosed in the United States in 2008–2012. *NeuroOncology*, **17** (Suppl. 4), iv1–iv62.

6 Merchant, T.E., Pollack, I.F., Loeffler, J.S. (2010) Brain tumors across the age spectrum: biology, therapy, and late effects. *Semin. Radiat. Oncol.*, **20** (1), 58–66.

7 Modak, S., Gardner, S., Dunkel, I.J., *et al.* (2004) Thiotepa-based high-dose chemotherapy with autologous stem-cell rescue in patients with recurrent or progressive CNS germ cell tumors. *J. Clin. Oncol.*, **22** (10), 1934–1943.

8 Gajjar, A., Chintagumpala, M., Ashley, D., *et al.* (2006) Risk-adapted craniospinal radiotherapy followed by high-dose chemotherapy and stem-cell rescue in children with newly diagnosed medulloblastoma (St Jude Medulloblastoma-96): long-term results from a prospective, multicentre trial. *Lancet Oncol.*, **7** (10), 813–820.

9 Polkinghorn, W.R., Tarbell, N.J. (2007) Medulloblastoma: tumorigenesis, current clinical paradigm, and efforts to improve risk stratification. *Nat. Clin. Pract. Oncol.*, **4** (5), 295–304.

10 Louis, D.N., Perry, A., Reifenberger, G., *et al.* (2016) The 2016 World Health Organization Classification of Tumors of the Central Nervous System: a summary. *Acta Neuropathol.*, **131** (6), 803–820.

11 Taylor, M.D., Northcott, P.A., Korshunov, A., *et al.* (2012) Molecular subgroups of medulloblastoma: the current consensus. *Acta Neuropathol.*, **123** (4), 465–472.

12 Northcott, P.A., Rutka, J.T., Taylor, M.D. (2010) Genomics of medulloblastoma: from Giemsa-banding to next-generation sequencing in 20 years. *Neurosurg. Focus*, **28** (1), E6.

13 Packer, R.J., Vezina, G. (2008) Management of and prognosis with medulloblastoma: therapy at a crossroads. *Arch. Neurol.*, **65** (11), 1419–1424.

14 Packer, R.J., Sutton, L.N., Elterman, R., *et al.* (1994) Outcome for children with medulloblastoma treated with radiation and cisplatin, CCNU, and vincristine chemotherapy. *J. Neurosurg.*, **81** (5), 690–698.

15 Packer, R.J., Goldwein, J., Nicholson, H.S., *et al.* (1999) Treatment of children with medulloblastomas with reduced-dose craniospinal radiation therapy and adjuvant chemotherapy: A Children's Cancer Group Study. *J. Clin. Oncol.*, **17** (7), 2127–2136.

16 Michalski, J.M., Janss, A., Vezina, G., *et al.* (2016) Results of COG ACNS0331: a phase III trial of involved-filed radiotherapy (IFRT) and low dose craniospinal irradiation (LDCSI) with chemotherapy in average-risk medulloblastoma: a report from the Children's Oncology Group. ASTRO Annual Meeting 2016, Boston Convention and Exhibition Center.

17 Albright, A.L., Wisoff, J.H., Zeltzer, P.M., Boyett, J.M., Rorke, L.B., Stanley, P. (1996) Effects of medulloblastoma resections on outcome in children: a report from the Children's Cancer Group. *Neurosurgery*, **38** (2), 265–271.

18 Zeltzer, P.M., Boyett, J.M., Finlay, J.L., *et al.* (1999) Metastasis stage, adjuvant treatment, and residual tumor are prognostic factors for medulloblastoma in children: conclusions from the Children's Cancer Group 921 randomized phase III study. *J. Clin. Oncol.*, **17** (3), 832–845.

19 Jakacki, R.I., Burger, P.C., Zhou, T., *et al.* (2012) Outcome of children with metastatic medulloblastoma treated with carboplatin during craniospinal radiotherapy: A Children's Oncology Group Phase I/II study. *J. Clin. Oncol.*, **30** (21), 2648–2653.

20 St Clair, W.H., Adams, J.A., Bues, M., *et al.* (2004) Advantage of protons compared to conventional X-ray or IMRT in the treatment of a pediatric patient with medulloblastoma. *Int. J. Radiat. Oncol. Biol. Phys.*, **58** (3), 727–734.

21 Eaton, B.R., Esiashvili, N., Kim, S., *et al.* (2016) Clinical outcomes among children with standard-risk medulloblastoma treated with proton and photon radiation therapy: a comparison of disease control and overall survival. *Int. J. Radiat. Oncol. Biol. Phys.*, **94** (1), 133–138.

22 Song, S., Park, H.J., Yoon, J.H., *et al.* (2014) Proton beam therapy reduces the incidence of acute haematological and gastrointestinal toxicities associated with craniospinal irradiation in pediatric brain tumors. *Acta Oncol.*, **53** (9), 1158–1164.

23 Yock, T.I., Bhat, S., Szymonifka, J., *et al.* (2014) Quality of life outcomes in proton and photon treated pediatric brain tumor survivors. *Radiother. Oncol.*, **113** (1), 89–94.

24 Goitein, M., Goitein, G. (2005) Swedish protons. *Acta Oncol.*, **44** (8), 793–797.

25 Engelsman, M., Schwarz, M., Dong, L. (2013) Physics controversies in proton therapy. *Semin. Radiat. Oncol.*, **23** (2), 88–96.

26 Seiler, G., De Vol, E., Khafaga, Y., *et al.* (2001) Evaluation of the safety and efficacy of repeated sedations for the radiotherapy of young children with cancer: a prospective study of 1033 consecutive sedations. *Int. J. Radiat. Oncol. Biol. Phys.*, **49** (3), 771–783.

27 Scott, M.T., Todd, K.E., Oakley, H., *et al.* (2016) Reducing anesthesia and health care cost through utilization of child life specialists in pediatric radiation oncology. *Int. J. Radiat. Oncol. Biol. Phys.*, **96** (2), 401–405.

28 Bindra, R.S., Wolden, S.L. (2016) Advances in radiation therapy in pediatric neuro-oncology. *J. Child. Neurol.*, **31** (4), 506–516.

29 ClinicalTrials.gov. A clinical and molecular risk-directed therapy for newly diagnosed medulloblastoma. St Jude Children's Research Hospital. Available at: https://clinicaltrials.gov/ct2/show/NCT01878617.

30 Gottardo, N.G., Hansford, J.R., McGlade, J.P., *et al.* (2014) Medulloblastoma Down Under 2013: a report

from the Third Annual Meeting of the International Medulloblastoma Working Group. *Acta Neuropathol.*, **127** (2), 189–201.

31 ClinicalTrials.gov. Reduced craniospinal radiation therapy and chemotherapy in treating younger patients with newly diagnosed WNT-driven medulloblastoma. Sponsored by National Cancer Institute. Available at: https://clinicaltrials.gov/ct2/show/NCT02724579.

32 ClinicalTrials.gov. Study assessing the feasibility of a surgery and chemotherapy-only in children with WNT positive medulloblastoma. Sponsored by Sidney Kimmel Comprehensive Cancer Center. Available at: https://clinicaltrials.gov/ct2/show/NCT02212574.

33 Rutkowski, S., von Hoff, K., Emser, A., *et al.* (2010) Survival and prognostic factors of early childhood medulloblastoma: an international meta-analysis. *J. Clin. Oncol.*, **28** (33), 4961–4968.

34 Duffner, P.K., Horowitz, M.E., Krischer, J.P., *et al.* (1999) The treatment of malignant brain tumors in infants and very young children: an update of the Pediatric Oncology Group experience. *NeuroOncology*, **1** (2), 152–161.

35 ClinicalTrials.gov. Combination chemotherapy followed by peripheral stem cell transplant in treating young patients with newly diagnosed supratentorial primitive neuroectodermal tumors or high-risk medulloblastoma. Sponsored by National Cancer Institute. Available at: https://clinicaltrials.gov/ct2/show/NCT00336024.

36 Dhall, G., Grodman, H., Ji, L., *et al.* (2008) Outcome of children less than three years old at diagnosis with non-metastatic medulloblastoma treated with chemotherapy on the 'Head Start' I and II protocols. *Pediatr. Blood Cancer*, **50** (6), 1169–1175.

37 PBTC.org. A feasibility study of SAHA combined with isotretinoin and chemotherapy in infants with embryonal tumors of the central nervous system. Sponsored by the National Cancer Institute. Available at: https://www.pbtc.org/public/PBTC-026%20Lay%20Summary.pdf.

38 ClinicalTrials.gov. Combination chemotherapy in treating younger patients with newly diagnosed, non-metastatic desmoplastic medulloblastoma. Sponsored by National Cancer Institute. Available at: https://clinicaltrials.gov/ct2/show/NCT02017964.

39 Fangusaro, J., Finlay, J., Sposto, R., *et al.* (2008) Intensive chemotherapy followed by consolidative myeloablative chemotherapy with autologous hematopoietic cell rescue (AuHCR) in young children with newly diagnosed supratentorial primitive neuroectodermal tumors (sPNETs): report of the Head Start I and II experience. *Pediatr. Blood Cancer*, **50** (2), 312–318.

40 Biegel, J.A., Fogelgren, B., Zhou, J.Y., *et al.* (2000) Mutations of the INI1 rhabdoid tumor suppressor gene in medulloblastomas and primitive neuroectodermal tumors of the central nervous system. *Clin. Cancer Res.*, **6** (7), 2759–2763.

41 Packer, R.J., Biegel, J.A., Blaney, S., *et al.* (2002) Atypical teratoid/rhabdoid tumor of the central nervous system: report on workshop. *J. Pediatr. Hematol. Oncol.*, **24** (5), 337–342.

42 Tekautz, T.M., Fuller, C.E., Blaney, S., *et al.* (2005) Atypical teratoid/rhabdoid tumors (ATRT): improved survival in children 3 years of age and older with radiation therapy and high-dose alkylator-based chemotherapy. *J. Clin. Oncol.*, **23** (7), 1491–1499.

43 ChildrensOncologyGroup.org. ACNS0333. Treatment of atypical teratoid/rhabdoid tumors (AT/RT) of the central nervous system with surgery, intensive chemotherapy, and 3-D conformal radiotherapy. Available at: https://www.childrensoncologygroup.org/index.php/acns0333.

44 Mahajan A. (2016) Radiotherapy for infant brain tumors. Panel 15: The changing role of radiotherapy of childhood cancer. ASTRO, Boston, September 27, 2016.

45 Merchant, T.E. (2002) Current management of childhood ependymoma. *Oncology (Williston Park)*, **16** (5), 629–642, 644; discussion 645–626, 648.

46 Greenlee, R.T., Murray, T., Bolden, S., Wingo, P.A. (2000) Cancer statistics, 2000. *CA Cancer J. Clin.*, **50** (1), 7–33.

47 Smyth, M.D., Horn, B.N., Russo, C., Berger, M.S. (2000) Intracranial ependymomas of childhood: current management strategies. *Pediatr. Neurosurg.*, **33** (3), 138–150.

48 van Veelen-Vincent, M.L., Pierre-Kahn, A., Kalifa, C., *et al.* (2002) Ependymoma in childhood: prognostic factors, extent of surgery, and adjuvant therapy. *J. Neurosurg.*, **97** (4), 827–835.

49 Hirano, A. (1988) *Color Atlas of Pathology of the Nervous system.* 2nd edition. Igaku-Shoin Ltd, Tokyo, New York.

50 Pajtler, K.W., Mack, S.C., Ramaswamy, V., *et al.* (2017) The current consensus on the clinical management of intracranial ependymoma and its distinct molecular variants. *Acta Neuropathol.*, **133** (1), 5–12.

51 Pajtler, K.W., Witt, H., Sill, M., *et al.* (2015) Molecular classification of ependymal tumors across all CNS compartments, histopathological grades, and age groups. *Cancer Cell*, **27** (5), 728–743.

52 Merchant, T.E., Fouladi, M. (2005) Ependymoma: new therapeutic approaches including radiation and chemotherapy. *J. Neurooncol.*, **75** (3), 287–299.

53 Merchant, T.E. (2009) Three-dimensional conformal radiation therapy for ependymoma. *Childs Nerv. Syst.*, **25** (10) 1261–1268.

54 MacDonald, S.M., Safai, S., Trofimov, A., *et al.* (2008) Proton radiotherapy for childhood ependymoma: initial clinical outcomes and dose comparisons. *Int. J. Radiat. Oncol. Biol. Phys.*, **71** (4), 979–986.

55 Zacharoulis, S., Levy, A., Chi, S.N., *et al.* (2007) Outcome for young children newly diagnosed with ependymoma, treated with intensive induction chemotherapy followed by myeloablative chemotherapy and autologous stem cell rescue. *Pediatr. Blood Cancer*, **49** (1), 34–40.

56 Foreman, N.K., Love, S., Gill, S.S., Coakham, H.B. (1997) Second-look surgery for incompletely resected fourth ventricle ependymomas: technical case report. *Neurosurgery*, **40** (4), 856–860; discussion 860.

57 ClinicalTrials.gov. Observation or radiation therapy and/or chemotherapy and second surgery in treating children who have undergone surgery for ependymoma. Sponsored by the National Cancer Institute. Available at: https://clinicaltrials.gov/ct2/show/NCT00027846.

58 Merchant, T.E., Li, C., Xiong, X., Kun, L.E., Boop, F.A., Sanford, R.A. (2009) Conformal radiotherapy after surgery for paediatric ependymoma: a prospective study. *Lancet Oncol.*, **10** (3), 258–266.

59 Merchant, T.E., Boop, F.A., Kun, L.E., Sanford, R.A. (2008) A retrospective study of surgery and reirradiation for recurrent ependymoma. *Int. J. Radiat. Oncol. Biol. Phys.*, **71** (1), 87–97.

60 Hoffman, L.M., Plimpton, S.R., Foreman, N.K., *et al.* (2014) Fractionated stereotactic radiosurgery for recurrent ependymoma in children. *J. Neurooncol.*, **116** (1), 107–111.

61 Gupta, N. (2004) *Pediatric CNS Tumors.* Springer-Verlag, Germany.

62 Rosser, T., Packer, R.J. (2002) Intracranial neoplasms in children with neurofibromatosis 1. *J. Child. Neurol.*, **17** (8), 630–637; discussion 646–651.

63 Pfister, S., Janzarik, W.G., Remke, M., *et al.* (2008) BRAF gene duplication constitutes a mechanism of MAPK pathway activation in low-grade astrocytomas. *J. Clin. Invest.*, **118** (5), 1739–1749.

64 Zapotocky, M., Lassaletta, A., Ryall, S., *et al.* (2016) The genetic characteristics of paediatric low-grade gliomas (O-020). Dublin, Ireland, October 20, 2016.

65 Fisher, P.G., Tihan, T., Goldthwaite, P.T., *et al.* (2008) Outcome analysis of childhood low-grade astrocytomas. *Pediatr. Blood Cancer*, **51** (2), 245–250.

66 Gajjar, A., Bhargava, R., Jenkins, J.J., *et al.* (1995) Low-grade astrocytoma with neuraxis dissemination at diagnosis. *J. Neurosurg.*, **83** (1), 67–71.

67 Mamelak, A.N., Prados, M.D., Obana, W.G., Cogen, P.H., Edwards, M.S. (1994) Treatment options and prognosis for multicentric juvenile pilocytic astrocytoma. *J. Neurosurg.*, **81** (1), 24–30.

68 Youland, R.S., Khwaja, S.S., Schomas, D.A., Keating, G.F., Wetjen, N.M., Laack, N.N. (2013) Prognostic factors and survival patterns in pediatric low-grade gliomas over 4 decades. *J. Pediatr. Hematol. Oncol.*, **35** (3), 197–205.

69 Merchant, T.E., Conklin, H.M., Wu, S., Lustig, R.H., Xiong, X. (2009) Late effects of conformal radiation therapy for pediatric patients with low-grade glioma: prospective evaluation of cognitive, endocrine, and hearing deficits. *J. Clin. Oncol.*, **27** (22), 3691–3697.

70 Packer, R.J., Ater, J., Allen, J., *et al.* (1997) Carboplatin and vincristine chemotherapy for children with newly diagnosed progressive low-grade gliomas. *J. Neurosurg.*, **86** (5), 747–754.

71 Merchant, T.E., Kun, L.E., Wu, S., Xiong, X., Sanford, R.A., Boop, F.A. (2009) Phase II trial of conformal radiation therapy for pediatric low-grade glioma. *J. Clin. Oncol.*, **27** (22), 3598–3604.

72 Marcus, K.J., Goumnerova, L., Billett, A.L., *et al.* (2005) Stereotactic radiotherapy for localized low-grade gliomas in children: final results of a prospective trial. *Int. J. Radiat. Oncol. Biol. Phys.*, **61** (2), 374–379.

73 Kuhlthau, K.A., Pulsifer, M.B., Yeap, B.Y., *et al.* (2012) Prospective study of health-related quality of life for children with brain tumors treated with proton radiotherapy. *J. Clin. Oncol.*, **30** (17), 2079–2086.

74 Merchant, T.E., Hua, C.H., Shukla, H., Ying, X., Nill, S., Oelfke, U. (2008) Proton versus photon radiotherapy for common pediatric brain tumors: comparison of models of dose characteristics and their relationship to cognitive function. *Pediatr. Blood Cancer*, **51** (1), 110–117.

75 Mayo, C., Martel, M.K., Marks, L.B., Flickinger, J., Nam, J., Kirkpatrick, J. (2010) Radiation dose-volume effects of optic nerves and chiasm. *Int. J. Radiat. Oncol. Biol. Phys.*, **76** (3 Suppl). S28–S35.

76 Wenkel, E., Thornton, A.F., Finkelstein, D., *et al.* (2000) Benign meningioma: partially resected, biopsied, and recurrent intracranial tumors treated with combined proton and photon radiotherapy. *Int. J. Radiat. Oncol. Biol. Phys.*, **48** (5), 1363–1370.

77 Gordon, K.B., Char, D.H., Sagerman, R.H. (1995) Late effects of radiation on the eye and ocular adnexa. *Int. J. Radiat. Oncol. Biol. Phys.*, **31** (5), 1123–1139.

78 Chapman, P.B., Hauschild, A., Robert, C., *et al.* (2011) Improved survival with vemurafenib in melanoma with BRAF V600E mutation. *N. Engl. J. Med.*, **364** (26), 2507–2516.

79 Reddy, A.T., Wellons, J.C, 3rd (2003) Pediatric high-grade gliomas. *Cancer J.*, **9** (2), 107–112.

80 Stupp, R., Mason, W.P., van den Bent, M.J., *et al.* (2005) Radiotherapy plus concomitant and adjuvant temozolomide for glioblastoma. *N. Engl. J. Med.*, **352** (10), 987–996.

81 Cohen, K.J., Pollack, I.F., Zhou, T., *et al.* (2011) Temozolomide in the treatment of high-grade gliomas in children: a report from the Children's Oncology Group. *NeuroOncology*, **13** (3), 317–323.

82 Gilbert, M.R., Dignam, J.J., Armstrong, T.S., *et al.* (2014) A randomized trial of bevacizumab for newly diagnosed glioblastoma. *N. Engl. J. Med.*, **370** (8), 699–708.

83 Jakacki, R.I., Cohen, K.J., Buxton, A., *et al.* (2016) Phase 2 study of concurrent radiotherapy and temozolomide followed by temozolomide and lomustine in the treatment of children with high-grade glioma: a report of the Children's Oncology Group ACNS0423 study. *NeuroOncology*, **18** (10), 1442–1450.

84 Espinoza, J.C., Haley, K., Patel, N., *et al.* (2016) Outcome of young children with high-grade glioma treated with irradiation-avoiding intensive chemotherapy regimens: Final report of the Head Start II and III trials. *Pediatr. Blood Cancer*, **63** (10), 1806–1813.

85 Wolff, J.E., Driever, P.H., Erdlenbruch, B., *et al.* (2010) Intensive chemotherapy improves survival in pediatric high-grade glioma after gross total resection: results of the HIT-GBM-C protocol. *Cancer*, **116** (3), 705–712.

86 NCI-CIRB.org. ACNS0423. A phase II study of concurrent radiation and temozolomide followed by temozolomide and lomustine (CCNU) in the treatment of children with high grade glioma. An intergroup study for participation by COG and the Dutch Childhood Oncology Group SKION (Stichting Kinderoncologie Nederland). Available at: https://ncicirb.org/cirb/protocols.action.

87 Gajjar, A., Bowers, D.C., Karajannis, M.A., Leary, S., Witt, H., Gottardo, N.G. (2015) Pediatric brain tumors: innovative genomic information is transforming the diagnostic and clinical landscape. *J. Clin. Oncol.*, **33** (27), 2986–2998.

88 Bunin, G.R., Surawicz, T.S., Witman, P.A., Preston-Martin, S., Davis, F., Bruner, J.M. (1998) The descriptive epidemiology of craniopharyngioma. *J. Neurosurg.*, **89** (4), 547–551.

89 Diller, L., Chow, E.J., Gurney, J.G., *et al.* (2009) Chronic disease in the Childhood Cancer Survivor Study cohort: a review of published findings. *J. Clin. Oncol.*, **27** (14), 2339–2355.

90 Stahnke, N., Grubel, G., Lagenstein, I., Willig, R.P. (1984) Long-term follow-up of children with craniopharyngioma. *Eur. J. Pediatr.*, **142** (3), 179–185.

91 Hopper, N., Albanese, A., Ghirardello, S., Maghnie, M. (2006) The pre-operative endocrine assessment of craniopharyngiomas. *J. Pediatr. Endocrinol. Metab.*, **19** (Suppl. 1), 325–327.

92 Desai, S.S., Paulino, A.C., Mai, W.Y., *et al.* (2006). Radiation-induced moyamoya syndrome. *Int. J.*

Radiat. Oncol. Biol. Phys., **65** (4), 1222–1227. Epub 2006 Apr 19. PMID:16626890. Doi: 10.1016/j.ijrobp.2006.01.038.

93 Mortini, P., Losa, M., Pozzobon, G., *et al.* (2011) Neurosurgical treatment of craniopharyngioma in adults and children: early and long-term results in a large case series. *J. Neurosurg.*, **114** (5), 1350–1359.

94 Hetelekidis, S., Barnes, P.D., Tao, M.L., *et al.* (1993) 20-year experience in childhood craniopharyngioma. *Int. J. Radiat. Oncol. Biol. Phys.*, **27** (2), 189–195.

95 Tomita, T., Bowman, R.M. (2005) Craniopharyngiomas in children: surgical experience at Children's Memorial Hospital. *Childs Nerv. Syst.*, **21** (8-9), 729–746.

96 Tomita, T., McLone, D.G. (1993) Radical resections of childhood craniopharyngiomas. *Pediatr. Neurosurg.*, **19** (1), 6–14.

97 Combs, S.E., Thilmann, C., Huber, P.E., Hoess, A., Debus, J., Schulz-Ertner, D. (2007) Achievement of long-term local control in patients with craniopharyngiomas using high precision stereotactic radiotherapy. *Cancer*, **109** (11), 2308–2314.

98 Kalapurakal, J.A. (2005) Radiation therapy in the management of pediatric craniopharyngiomas – a review. *Childs Nerv. Syst.*, **21** (8-9), 808–816.

99 Merchant TE, Kun LE, Hua CH, *et al.* (2013) Disease control after reduced volume conformal and intensity modulated radiation therapy for childhood craniopharyngioma. *Int. J. Radiat. Oncol. Biol Phys.*, **85** (4), e187–e192.

100 Merchant, T.E., Kiehna, E.N., Kun, L.E., *et al.* (2006) Phase II trial of conformal radiation therapy for pediatric patients with craniopharyngioma and correlation of surgical factors and radiation dosimetry with change in cognitive function. *J. Neurosurg.*, **104** (2 Suppl.), 94–102.

101 Fitzek, M.M., Linggood, R.M., Adams, J., Munzenrider, J.E. (2006) Combined proton and photon irradiation for craniopharyngioma: long-term results of the early cohort of patients treated at Harvard Cyclotron Laboratory and Massachusetts General Hospital. *Int. J. Radiat. Oncol. Biol. Phys.*, **64** (5), 1348–1354.

102 Winkfield, K.M., Linsenmeier, C., Yock, T.I., *et al.* (2009) Surveillance of craniopharyngioma cyst growth in children treated with proton radiotherapy. *Int. J. Radiat. Oncol. Biol. Phys.*, **73** (3), 716–721.

103 Beltran, C., Naik, M., Merchant, T.E. (2010) Dosimetric effect of target expansion and setup uncertainty during radiation therapy in pediatric craniopharyngioma. *Radiother. Oncol.*, **97** (3), 399–403.

104 Pereira, A.M., Schmid, E.M., Schutte, P.J., *et al.* (2005) High prevalence of long-term cardiovascular,

neurological and psychosocial morbidity after treatment for craniopharyngioma. *Clin. Endocrinol. (Oxford)*, **62** (2), 197–204.

105 Beltran, C., Roca, M., Merchant, T.E. (2012) On the benefits and risks of proton therapy in pediatric craniopharyngioma. *Int. J. Radiat. Oncol. Biol. Phys.*, **82** (2), e281–e287.

106 ClinicalTrials.gov. A phase II trial of limited surgery and proton therapy for craniopharyngioma or observation after radical resection. Sponsored by St. Jude Children's Research Hospital. Available at: https://clinicaltrials.gov/ct2/show/NCT01419067. First accessed: 08-16-2011; last update: 07-22-2016.

107 Merchant, T.E., Hua, C.H., Sabin, N.D., *et al.* (2016) Necrosis, vasculopathy, and neurological complications after proton therapy for childhood craniopharyngioma: results from a prospective trial and a photon cohort comparison (abstract 269). *Int. J. Radiat. Oncol. Biol. Phys.*, **96** (2 (Suppl.), S120–S121.

108 Jellinger, K. (1973) Primary intracranial germ cell tumours. *Acta Neuropathol. (Berl.)*, **25** (4), 291–306.

109 Jennings, M.T., Gelman, R., Hochberg, F. (1985) Intracranial germ-cell tumors: natural history and pathogenesis. *J. Neurosurg.*, **63** (2), 155–167.

110 Jubran, R.F., Finlay, J. (2005) Central nervous system germ cell tumors: controversies in diagnosis and treatment. *Oncology (Williston Park)*, **19** (6), 705–711; discussion 711–702, 715–707, 721.

111 Maity, A., Shu, H.K., Janss, A., *et al.* (2004) Craniospinal radiation in the treatment of biopsy-proven intracranial germinomas: twenty-five years' experience in a single center. *Int. J. Radiat. Oncol. Biol. Phys.*, **58** (4), 1165–1170.

112 Huh, S.J., Shin, K.H., Kim, I.H., Ahn, Y.C., Ha, S.W., Park, C.I. (1996) Radiotherapy of intracranial germinomas. *Radiother. Oncol.*, **38** (1), 19–23.

113 Ogawa, K., Shikama, N., Toita, T., *et al.* (2004) Long-term results of radiotherapy for intracranial germinoma: a multi-institutional retrospective review of 126 patients. *Int. J. Radiat. Oncol. Biol. Phys.*, **58** (3), 705–713.

114 MacDonald, S.M., Trofimov, A., Safai, S., *et al.* (2011) Proton radiotherapy for pediatric central nervous system germ cell tumors: early clinical outcomes. *Int. J. Radiat. Oncol. Biol. Phys.*, **79** (1), 121–129.

115 Alapetite, C., Brisse, H., Patte, C., *et al.* (2010) Pattern of relapse and outcome of non-metastatic germinoma patients treated with chemotherapy and limited field radiation: the SFOP experience. *NeuroOncology*, **12** (12), 1318–1325.

116 Goldman, S., Bouffet, E., Fisher, P.G., *et al.* (2015) Phase II trial assessing the ability of neoadjuvant chemotherapy with or without second-look surgery to eliminate measurable disease for nongerminomatous germ cell tumors: A Children's Oncology Group study. *J. Clin. Oncol.*, **33** (22), 2464–2471.

117 MacDonald, S., Murphy, E., Lavey, R., Morris, D., Merchant, T., Donahue, B. (2016) Whole ventricle target volume atlas for germ cell tumors. Available at: http://www.qarc.org/cog/ACNS1123_Atlas.pdf.

118 DeSousa, A.L., Kalsbeck, J.E., Mealey, J., Jr, Campbell, R.L., Hockey, A. (1979) Intraspinal tumors in children. A review of 81 cases. *J. Neurosurg.*, **51** (4), 437–445.

119 Tendulkar, R.D., Pai Panandiker, A.S., Wu, S., *et al.* (2010) Irradiation of pediatric high-grade spinal cord tumors. *Int. J. Radiat. Oncol. Biol. Phys.*, **78** (5), 1451–1456.

120 Rombi, B., Ares, C., Hug, E.B., *et al.* (2013) Spot-scanning proton radiation therapy for pediatric chordoma and chondrosarcoma: clinical outcome of 26 patients treated at Paul Scherrer Institute. *Int. J. Radiat. Oncol. Biol. Phys.*, **86** (3), 578–584.

121 Jemal, A., Siegel, R., Xu, J., Ward, E. (2010) Cancer statistics, 2010. *CA Cancer J. Clin.*, **60** (5), 277–300.

122 Hutchinson, R.J., Fryer, C.J., Davis, P.C., *et al.* (1998) MOPP or radiation in addition to ABVD in the treatment of pathologically staged advanced Hodgkin's disease in children: results of the Children's Cancer Group Phase III Trial. *J. Clin. Oncol.*, **16** (3), 897–906.

123 Smith, R.S., Chen, Q., Hudson, M.M., *et al.* (2003) Prognostic factors for children with Hodgkin's disease treated with combined-modality therapy. *J. Clin. Oncol.*, **21** (10), 2026–2033.

124 ChildrensOncologyGroup.org. AHOD1331. A randomized phase III study of brentuxima vedotin (SGN-35, IND #117117) for newly diagnosed high-risk classical Hodgkin lymphoma (cHL) in children and adolescents. Available at: https://childrensoncologygroup.org/index.php/ahod1331.

125 Peters, M.V. (1965) Current Concepts in Cancer. 2. Hodgkin's Disease. Radiation Therapy. *JAMA*, **191**, 28–29.

126 Friedman, D.L., Constine, L.S. (2006) Late effects of treatment for Hodgkin lymphoma. *J. Natl Compr. Cancer Network*, **4** (3), 249–257.

127 Hancock, S.L., Hoppe, R.T. (1996) Long-term complications of treatment and causes of mortality after Hodgkin's disease. *Semin. Radiat. Oncol.*, **6** (3), 225–242.

128 Mauch, P.M., Kalish, L.A., Marcus, K.C., *et al.* (1996) Second malignancies after treatment for laparotomy staged IA-IIIB Hodgkin's disease: long-term analysis of risk factors and outcome. *Blood*, **87** (9), 3625–3632.

129 Ng, A.K., Bernardo, M.V., Weller, E., *et al.* (2002) Second malignancy after Hodgkin disease treated with radiation therapy with or without chemotherapy: long-term risks and risk factors. *Blood*, **100** (6), 1989–1996.

130 Sklar, C. (2000) Paying the price for cure – treating cancer survivors with growth hormone. *J. Clin. Endocrinol. Metab.*, **85** (12), 4441–4443.

131 Willman, K.Y., Cox, R.S., Donaldson, S.S. (1994) Radiation induced height impairment in pediatric Hodgkin's disease. *Int. J. Radiat. Oncol. Biol. Phys.*, **28** (1), 85–92.

132 Donaldson, S.S., Link, M.P., Weinstein, H.J., *et al.* (2007) Final results of a prospective clinical trial with VAMP and low-dose involved-field radiation for children with low-risk Hodgkin's disease. *J. Clin. Oncol.*, **25** (3), 332–337.

133 Hudson, M.M., Krasin, M., Link, M.P., *et al.* (2004) Risk-adapted, combined-modality therapy with VAMP/COP and response-based, involved-field radiation for unfavorable pediatric Hodgkin's disease. *J. Clin. Oncol.*, **22** (22), 4541–4550.

134 Metzger, M.L., Weinstein, H.J., Hudson, M.M., *et al.* (2012) Association between radiotherapy vs no radiotherapy based on early response to VAMP chemotherapy and survival among children with favorable-risk Hodgkin lymphoma. *JAMA*, **307** (24), 2609–2616.

135 Mauz-Korholz, C., Metzger, M.L., Kelly, K.M., *et al.* (2015) Pediatric Hodgkin lymphoma. *J. Clin. Oncol.*, **33** (27), 2975–2985.

136 Keller, F.G., Nachman, J., Constine, L., *et al.* (2010) A phase III study for the treatment of children and adolescents with newly diagnosed low risk Hodgkin lymphoma (HL); (abstract 767). *Blood*, 116.

137 Friedman, D.L., Chen, L., Wolden, S., *et al.* (2014) Dose-intensive response-based chemotherapy and radiation therapy for children and adolescents with newly diagnosed intermediate-risk Hodgkin lymphoma: a report from the Children's Oncology Group Study AHOD0031. *J. Clin. Oncol.*, **32** (32), 3651–3658.

138 Charpentier, A.M., Friedman, D.L., Wolden, S., *et al.* (2016) Predictive factor analysis of response-adapted radiation therapy for chemotherapy-sensitive pediatric Hodgkin lymphoma: Analysis of the Children's Oncology Group AHOD 0031 Trial. *Int. J. Radiat. Oncol. Biol. Phys.*, **96** (5), 943–950.

139 Schwartz, C.L., Chen, L., McCarten, K., *et al.* (2016) Childhood Hodgkin International Prognostic Score (CHIPS) predicts event-free survival in Hodgkin lymphoma: A report from the Children's Oncology Group. *Pediatr. Blood Cancer*. Epub ahead of print-Oct 27. Doi: 10.1002/pbc.26278 [Epub ahead of print] PMID:27786406.

140 Kelly, K.M., Sposto, R., Hutchinson, R., *et al.* (2011) BEACOPP chemotherapy is a highly effective regimen in children and adolescents with high-risk Hodgkin lymphoma: a report from the Children's Oncology Group. *Blood*, **117** (9), 2596–2603.

141 Yahalom, J., Mauch, P. (2002) The involved field is back: issues in delineating the radiation field in Hodgkin's disease. *Ann. Oncol.*, **13** (Suppl. 1), 79–83.

142 Andolino, D.L., Hoene, T., Xiao, L., Buchsbaum, J., Chang, A.L. (2011) Dosimetric comparison of involved-field three-dimensional conformal photon radiotherapy and breast-sparing proton therapy for the treatment of Hodgkin's lymphoma in female pediatric patients. *Int. J. Radiat. Oncol. Biol. Phys.*, **81** (4), e667–e671.

143 Girinsky, T., Specht, L., Ghalibafian, M., *et al.* (2008) The conundrum of Hodgkin lymphoma nodes: to be or not to be included in the involved node radiation fields. The EORTC-GELA lymphoma group guidelines. *Radiother. Oncol.*, **88** (2), 202–210.

144 ILROG (2011) International Lymphoma Radiation Oncology Group. Available at: http://www.ilrog.com/.

145 Hodgson, D.C., Dieckmann, K., Terezakis, S., Constine, L, and the International Lymphoma Radiation Oncology Group (2015) Implementation of contemporary radiation therapy planning concepts for pediatric Hodgkin lymphoma: Guidelines from the International Lymphoma Radiation Oncology Group. *Pract. Radiat. Oncol.*, **5** (2), 85–92.

146 Campbell, B.A., Voss, N., Pickles, T., *et al.* (2008) Involved-nodal radiation therapy as a component of combination therapy for limited-stage Hodgkin's lymphoma: a question of field size. *J. Clin. Oncol.*, **26** (32), 5170–5174.

147 van der Pal, H.J., van Dalen, E.C., van Delden, E., *et al.* (2012) High risk of symptomatic cardiac events in childhood cancer survivors. *J. Clin. Oncol.*, **30** (13), 1429–1437.

148 van Nimwegen, F.A., Schaapveld, M., Cutter, D.J., *et al.* (2016) Radiation dose-response relationship for risk of coronary heart disease in survivors of Hodgkin lymphoma. *J. Clin. Oncol.*, **34** (3), 235–243.

149 Hancock, S.L., Tucker, M.A., Hoppe, R.T. (1993) Breast cancer after treatment of Hodgkin's disease. *J. Natl Cancer Inst.*, **85** (1), 25–31.

150 Wolden, S.L., Lamborn, K.R., Cleary, S.F., Tate, D.J., Donaldson, S.S. (1998) Second cancers following pediatric Hodgkin's disease. *J. Clin. Oncol.*, **16** (2), 536–544.

151 Murphy, S.B., Bleyer, W.A. (1987) Cranial irradiation is not necessary for central-nervous-system prophylaxis in pediatric non-Hodgkin's lymphoma. *Int. J. Radiat. Oncol. Biol. Phys.*, **13** (3), 467–468.

152 Loeffler, J.S., Leopold, K.A., Recht, A., Weinstein, H.J., Tarbell, N.J. (1986) Emergency prebiopsy radiation for mediastinal masses: impact on subsequent pathologic diagnosis and outcome. *J. Clin. Oncol.*, **4** (5), 716–721.

153 Chessels, J.M., Swansbury, G.J., Reeves, B., Bailey, C.C., Richards, S.M. (1997) Cytogenetics and prognosis in childhood lymphoblastic leukaemia: results of MRC UKALL X. Medical Research Council Working Party in Childhood Leukaemia. *Br. J. Haematol.*, **99** (1), 93–100.

154 Pui, C.H., Crist, W.M., Look, A.T. (1990) Biology and clinical significance of cytogenetic abnormalities in childhood acute lymphoblastic leukemia. *Blood*, **76** (8), 1449–1463.

155 Pui, C.H., Yang, J.J., Hunger, S.P., *et al.* (2015) Childhood acute lymphoblastic leukemia: progress through collaboration. *J. Clin. Oncol.*, **33** (27), 2938–2948.

156 Raimondi, S.C., Zhou, Y., Mathew, S., *et al.* (2003) Reassessment of the prognostic significance of hypodiploidy in pediatric patients with acute lymphoblastic leukemia. *Cancer*, **98** (12), 2715–2722.

157 Shuster, J.J., Wacker, P., Pullen, J., *et al.* (1998) Prognostic significance of sex in childhood B-precursor acute lymphoblastic leukemia: a Pediatric Oncology Group Study. *J. Clin. Oncol.*, **16** (8), 2854–2863.

158 Uckun, F.M., Nachman, J.B., Sather, H.N., *et al.* (1998) Clinical significance of Philadelphia chromosome positive pediatric acute lymphoblastic leukemia in the context of contemporary intensive therapies: a report from the Children's Cancer Group. *Cancer*, **83** (9), 2030–2039.

159 Gaynon, P.S., Angiolillo, A.L., Carroll, W.L., *et al.* (2010) Long-term results of the Children's Cancer Group studies for childhood acute lymphoblastic leukemia 1983–2002: A Children's Oncology Group Report. *Leukemia*, **24** (2), 285–297.

160 Nesbit, M.E., Jr, Sather, H.N., Robison, L.L., *et al.* (1981) Presymptomatic central nervous system therapy in previously untreated childhood acute lymphoblastic leukaemia: comparison of 1800 rad and 2400 rad. A report for Children's Cancer Study Group. *Lancet*, **1** (8218), 461–466.

161 Pui, C.H., Robison, L.L., Look, A.T. (2008) Acute lymphoblastic leukaemia. *Lancet*, **371** (9617), 1030–1043.

162 Salzer, W.L., Devidas, M., Carroll, W.L., *et al.* (2010) Long-term results of the Pediatric Oncology Group studies for childhood acute lymphoblastic leukemia 1984–2001: a report from the Children's Oncology Group. *Leukemia*, **24** (2), 355–370.

163 Schrappe, M., Reiter, A., Henze, G., *et al.* (1998) Prevention of CNS recurrence in childhood ALL: results with reduced radiotherapy combined with CNS-directed chemotherapy in four consecutive ALL-BFM trials. *Klin. Padiatr.*, **210** (4), 192–199.

164 Wofford, M.M., Smith, S.D., Shuster, J.J., *et al.* (1992) Treatment of occult or late overt testicular relapse in children with acute lymphoblastic leukemia: a Pediatric Oncology Group study. *J. Clin. Oncol.*, **10** (4), 624–630.

165 ChildrensOncologyGroup.org. AALL1331: risk-stratified randomized phase III testing of blinatumomab (IND# 117467, NSC#765986) in first relapse of childhood B-lymphoblastic leukemia (B-ALL) IND. Sponsor for blinatumomab: DCTD, NCI. A group wide phase III study participating countries: Australia, Canada, New Zealand and United States. Accessed at rpc.mdanderson.org/rpc/credentialing/files/AALL1331DOC.pdf, on December 28, 2016.

166 *Childhood Cancer Survivorship: Improving Care and Quality of Life*. National Academies Press, Washington, DC, 2003.

167 Halperin, E.C., Constine, L.S., Tarbell, N.J., Kun, L.E. (20110 *Pediatric Radiation Oncology*. 5th edition. Lippincott, Williams & Wilkins, alley Stream, New York.

168 Friedman, D.L., Whitton, J., Leisenring, W., *et al.* (2010) Subsequent neoplasms in 5-year survivors of childhood cancer: the Childhood Cancer Survivor Study. *J. Natl Cancer Inst.*, **102** (14), 1083–1095.

169 van Waas, M., Neggers, S.J., Pieters, R., van den Heuvel-Eibrink, M.M. (2010) Components of the metabolic syndrome in 500 adult long-term survivors of childhood cancer. *Ann. Oncol.*, **21** (5), 1121–1126.

170 Bhojwani, D., Sabin, N.D., Pei, D., *et al.* (2014) Methotrexate-induced neurotoxicity and leukoencephalopathy in childhood acute lymphoblastic leukemia. *J. Clin. Oncol.*, **32** (9), 949–959.

171 Diouf, B., Crews, K.R., Lew, G., *et al.* (2015) Association of an inherited genetic variant with vincristine-related peripheral neuropathy in children with acute lymphoblastic leukemia. *JAMA*, **313** (8), 815–823.

172 French, D., Hamilton, L.H., Mattano, L.A., Jr, *et al.* (2008) A PAI-1 (SERPINE1) polymorphism predicts osteonecrosis in children with acute lymphoblastic leukemia: a report from the Children's Oncology Group. *Blood*, **111** (9), 4496–4499.

173 Bhatia, S., Armenian, S.H., Armstrong, G.T., *et al.* (2015) Collaborative research in childhood cancer survivorship: the current landscape. *J. Clin. Oncol.*, **33** (27), 3055–3064.

174 Shimada, H., Ambros, I.M., Dehner, L.P., *et al.* (1999) The International Neuroblastoma Pathology Classification (the Shimada system). *Cancer*, **86** (2), 364–372.

175 Chen, Y., Takita, J., Choi, Y.L., *et al.* (2008) Oncogenic mutations of ALK kinase in neuroblastoma. *Nature*, **455** (7215), 971–974.

176 Cheung, N.K., Zhang, J., Lu, C., *et al.* (2012) Association of age at diagnosis and genetic mutations in patients with neuroblastoma. *JAMA*, **307** (10), 1062–1071.

177 Brisse, H.J., McCarville, M.B., Granata, C., *et al.* (2011) Guidelines for imaging and staging of neuroblastic tumors: consensus report from the International Neuroblastoma Risk Group Project. *Radiology*, **261** (1), 243–257.

178 Monclair, T., Brodeur, G.M., Ambros, P.F., *et al.* (2009) The International Neuroblastoma Risk Group (INRG) staging system: an INRG Task Force report. *J. Clin. Oncol.*, **27** (2), 298–303.

179 Hero, B., Simon, T., Spitz, R., *et al.* (2008) Localized infant neuroblastomas often show spontaneous regression: results of the prospective trials NB95-S and NB97. *J. Clin. Oncol.*, **26** (9), 1504–1510.

180 Yalcin, B., Kremer, L.C., Caron, H.N., van Dalen, E.C. (2015) High-dose chemotherapy and autologous haematopoietic stem cell rescue for children with high-risk neuroblastoma. *Cochrane Database Syst. Rev.* 2010(5):CD006301.

181 Yu, A.L., Gilman, A.L., Ozkaynak, M.F., *et al.* (2010) Anti-GD2 antibody with GM-CSF, interleukin-2, and isotretinoin for neuroblastoma. *N. Engl. J. Med.*, **363** (14), 1324–1334.

182 Paulino, A.C., Fowler, B.Z. (2005) Risk factors for scoliosis in children with neuroblastoma. *Int. J. Radiat. Oncol. Biol. Phys.*, **61** (3), 865–869.

183 Hill-Kayser, C., Tochner, Z., Both, S., *et al.* (2013) Proton versus photon radiation therapy for patients with high-risk neuroblastoma: the need for a customized approach. *Pediatr. Blood Cancer*, **60** (10), 1606–1611.

184 Ahmed, H.U., Arya, M., Levitt, G., Duffy, P.G., Mushtaq, I., Sebire, N.J. (2007) Part I: Primary malignant non-Wilms renal tumours in children. *Lancet Oncol.*, **8** (8), 730–737.

185 Irtan, S., Jitlal, M., Bate, J., *et al.* (2015) Risk factors for local recurrence in Wilms tumour and the potential influence of biopsy – the United Kingdom experience. *Eur. J. Cancer*, **51** (2), 225–232.

186 D'Angio, G.J. (2007) The National Wilms Tumor Study: a 40 year perspective. *Lifetime Data Anal.*, **13** (4), 463–470.

187 Bhatnagar, S. (2009) Management of Wilms' tumor: NWTS vs SIOP. *J. Indian Assoc. Pediatr. Surg.*, **14** (1), 6–14.

188 Dome, J.S., Fernandez, C.V., Mullen, E.A., *et al.* (2013) Children's Oncology Group's 2013 blueprint for research: renal tumors. *Pediatr. Blood Cancer*, **60** (6), 994–1000.

189 Dome, J.S., Perlman, E.J., Graf, N., *et al.* (2014) Risk stratification for Wilms tumor: current approach and future direction. American Society of Clinical Oncology Education. Available at: http://meeting library.asco.org/sites/meetinglibrary.asco.org/files/edbook_pdf/2014_E.

190 Cohen, M., Smith, W.L., Weetman, R., Provisor, A. (1981) Pulmonary pseudometastases in children with malignant tumors. *Radiology*, **141** (2), 371–374.

191 Green, D.M. (2016) Considerations in the diagnosis and management of pediatric patients with favorable histology Wilms tumor who present with only pulmonary nodules. *Pediatr. Blood Cancer*, **63** (4), 589–592.

192 McCarville, M.B., Lederman, H.M., Santana, V.M., *et al.* (2006) Distinguishing benign from malignant pulmonary nodules with helical chest CT in children with malignant solid tumors. *Radiology*, **239** (2), 514–520.

193 Dix, D.B., Gratias, E.J., Seibel, N., *et al.* (2015) Omission of lung radiation in patients with stage IV favorable histology Wilms tumor (FHWT) showing complete lung nodule response after chemotherapy: a report from Children's Oncology Group study AREN0533 (abstract 10011). *J. Clin. Oncol.*, 32:5s, 2014 (suppl; abstr 10001).

194 Breslow, N., Sharples, K., Beckwith, J.B., *et al.* (1991) Prognostic factors in nonmetastatic, favorable histology Wilms' tumor. Results of the Third National Wilms' Tumor Study. *Cancer*, **68** (11), 2345–2353.

195 Cotton, C.A., Peterson, S., Norkool, P.A., *et al.* (2009) Early and late mortality after diagnosis of Wilms tumor. *J. Clin. Oncol.*, **27** (8), 1304–1309.

196 Dorr, W., Kallfels, S., Herrmann, T. (2013) Late bone and soft tissue sequelae of childhood radiotherapy. Relevance of treatment age and radiation dose in 146 children treated between 1970 and 1997. *Strahlenther. Onkol.*, **189** (7), 529–534.

197 Green, D.M., Lange, J.M., Peabody, E.M., *et al.* (2010) Pregnancy outcome after treatment for Wilms tumor: a report from the national Wilms tumor long-term follow-up study. *J. Clin. Oncol.*, **28** (17), 2824–2830.

198 Termuhlen, A.M., Tersak, J.M., Liu, Q., *et al.* (2011) Twenty-five year follow-up of childhood Wilms tumor: a report from the Childhood Cancer Survivor Study. *Pediatr. Blood Cancer*, **57** (7), 1210–1216.

199 Kalapurakal, J.A., Pokhrel, D., Gopalakrishnan, M., Zhang, Y. (2013) Advantages of whole-liver intensity modulated radiation therapy in children with Wilms tumor and liver metastasis. *Int. J. Radiat. Oncol. Biol. Phys.*, **85** (3), 754–760.

200 Kalapurakal, J., Marcus, K., Mahajan, A., *et al.* (2016) Final report of a prospective clinical trial of cardiac sparing a whole lung IMRT in patients with metastatic pediatric tumors. ASTRO 2016. 28 September 2016, Boston Convention Center.

201 Vogel, J., Lin, H., Both, S., Tochner, Z., Balis, F., Hill-Kayser, C. (2017) Pencil beam scanning proton therapy for treatment of the retroperitoneum after nephrectomy for Wilms tumor: A dosimetric comparison study. *Pediatr. Blood Cancer*, **64** (1), 39–45.

202 Stat bite. (1999) Age-specific cancer incidence among children under 15. *J. Natl Cancer Inst.*, **91** (24), 2076.

203 Gurney, J.G., Severson, R.K., Davis, S., Robison, L.L. (1995) Incidence of cancer in children in the United

States. Sex-, race-, and 1-year age-specific rates by histologic type. *Cancer*, **75** (8), 2186–2195.

204 Wharam, M.D., Beltangady, M.S., Heyn, R.M., *et al.* (1987) Pediatric orofacial and laryngopharyngeal rhabdomyosarcoma. An Intergroup Rhabdomyosarcoma Study report. *Arch. Otolaryngol. Head Neck Surg.*, **113** (11), 1225–1227.

205 Breneman, J.C., Lyden, E., Pappo, A.S., *et al.* (2003) Prognostic factors and clinical outcomes in children and adolescents with metastatic rhabdomyosarcoma– a report from the Intergroup Rhabdomyosarcoma Study IV. *J. Clin. Oncol.*, **21** (1), 78–84.

206 Volker, T., Denecke, T., Steffen, I., *et al.* (2007) Positron emission tomography for staging of pediatric sarcoma patients: results of a prospective multicenter trial. *J. Clin. Oncol.*, **25** (34), 5435–5441.

207 Asmar, L., Gehan, E.A., Newton, W.A., *et al.* (1994) Agreement among and within groups of pathologists in the classification of rhabdomyosarcoma and related childhood sarcomas. Report of an international study of four pathology classifications. *Cancer*, **74** (9), 2579–2588.

208 Newton, W.A., Jr, Gehan, E.A., Webber, B.L., *et al.* (1995) Classification of rhabdomyosarcomas and related sarcomas. Pathologic aspects and proposal for a new classification – an Intergroup Rhabdomyosarcoma Study. *Cancer*, **76** (6), 1073–1085.

209 Parham DM. (2001) Pathologic classification of rhabdomyosarcomas and correlations with molecular studies. *Mod. Pathol.*, **14** (5), 506–514.

210 Parham, D.M., Ellison, D.A. (2006) Rhabdomyosarcomas in adults and children: an update. *Arch. Pathol. Lab. Med.*, **130** (10), 1454–1465.

211 Hawkins, D.S., Anderson, J.R., Mascarenhas, L., *et al.* (2014) Vincristine, dactinomycin, cyclophosphamide (VAC) versus VAC/V plus irinotecan (VI) for intermediate-risk rhabdomyosarcoma (IRRMS): a report from the Children's Oncology Group Soft Tissue Sarcoma Committee (abstract 10004). *J. Clin. Oncol.*, **32** (15_suppl):10004. http://meeting.ascopubs .org/cgi/content/abstract/32/15_suppl/10004.

212 Williamson, D., Missiaglia, E., de Reynies, A., *et al.* (2010) Fusion gene-negative alveolar rhabdomyosarcoma is clinically and molecularly indistinguishable from embryonal rhabdomyosarcoma. *J. Clin. Oncol.*, **28** (13), 2151–2158.

213 Missiaglia, E., Williamson, D., Chisholm, J., *et al.* (2012) PAX3/FOXO1 fusion gene status is the key prognostic molecular marker in rhabdomyosarcoma and significantly improves current risk stratification. *J. Clin. Oncol.*, **30** (14), 1670–1677.

214 Skapek, S.X., Anderson, J., Barr, F.G., *et al.* (2013) PAX-FOXO1 fusion status drives unfavorable

outcome for children with rhabdomyosarcoma: a Children's Oncology Group report. *Pediatr. Blood Cancer*, **60** (9), 1411–1417.

215 Crist, W., Gehan, E.A., Ragab, A.H., *et al.* (1995) The Third Intergroup Rhabdomyosarcoma Study. *J. Clin. Oncol.*, **13** (3), 610–630.

216 Crist, W.M., Garnsey, L., Beltangady, M.S., *et al.* (1990) Prognosis in children with rhabdomyosarcoma: a report of the intergroup rhabdomyosarcoma studies I and II. Intergroup Rhabdomyosarcoma Committee. *J. Clin. Oncol.*, **8** (3), 443–452.

217 Maurer, H.M., Beltangady, M., Gehan, E.A., *et al.* (1988) The Intergroup Rhabdomyosarcoma Study-I. A final report. *Cancer*, **61** (2), 209–220.

218 Maurer, H.M., Gehan, E.A., Beltangady, M., *et al.* (1993) The Intergroup Rhabdomyosarcoma Study-II. *Cancer*, **71** (5), 1904–1922.

219 Rodary, C., Gehan, E.A., Flamant, F., *et al.* (1991) Prognostic factors in 951 nonmetastatic rhabdomyosarcoma in children: a report from the International Rhabdomyosarcoma Workshop. *Med. Pediatr. Oncol.*, **19** (2), 89–95.

220 Arndt, C.A., Stoner, J.A., Hawkins, D.S., *et al.* (2009) Vincristine, actinomycin, and cyclophosphamide compared with vincristine, actinomycin, and cyclophosphamide alternating with vincristine, topotecan, and cyclophosphamide for intermediate-risk rhabdomyosarcoma: Children's Oncology Group study D9803. *J. Clin. Oncol.*, **27** (31), 5182–5188.

221 Crist, W.M., Anderson, J.R., Meza, J.L., *et al.* (2001) Intergroup rhabdomyosarcoma study-IV: results for patients with nonmetastatic disease. *J. Clin. Oncol.*, **19** (12), 3091–3102.

222 ClinicalTrials.gov. A randomized phase 3 study of vincristine, dactinomycin, cyclophosphamide (VAC) alternating with vincristine and irinotecan (VI) versus VAC/VI plus temsirolimus (TORI, Torisel, NSC# 683864, IND# 122782) in patients with intermediate risk (IR) rhabdomyosarcoma (RMS). NCI supplied agents: temsirolimus (NSC# 683864, INC# 122782). IND sponsor for temsirolimus: DCTD, NCI. An intergroup NCTN phase 3 study. ClinicalTrials.gov identified. NCT02567435. Available at: https:// clinicaltrials.gov/ct2/show/NCT02567435ARST1431.

223 Furman, W.L., Stewart, C.F., Poquette, C.A., *et al.* (1999) Direct translation of a protracted irinotecan schedule from a xenograft model to a phase I trial in children. *J. Clin. Oncol.*, **17** (6), 1815– 1824.

224 Rodriguez-Galindo, C., Crews, K.R., Stewart, C.F., *et al.* (2006) Phase I study of the combination of topotecan and irinotecan in children with refractory solid tumors. *Cancer Chemother. Pharmacol.*, **57** (1), 15–24.

225 Cosetti, M., Wexler, L.H., Calleja, E., *et al.* (2002) Irinotecan for pediatric solid tumors: the Memorial Sloan-Kettering experience. *J. Pediatr. Hematol. Oncol.*, **24** (2), 101–105.

226 Raney, R.B., Anderson, J.R., Barr, F.G., *et al.* (2001) Rhabdomyosarcoma and undifferentiated sarcoma in the first two decades of life: a selective review of intergroup rhabdomyosarcoma study group experience and rationale for Intergroup Rhabdomyosarcoma Study V. *J. Pediatr. Hematol. Oncol.*, **23** (4), 215–220.

227 Weigel, B., Lyden, E., Anderson, J.R., *et al.* (2010) Early results from Children's Oncology Group (COG) ARST0431: Intensive multidrug therapy for patients with metastatic rhabdomyosarcoma (RMS); (abstract 9503). *J. Clin. Oncol.*, **28**, 15s.

228 Walterhouse, D.O., Pappo, A.S., Meza, J.L., *et al.* (2014) Shorter-duration therapy using vincristine, dactinomycin, and lower-dose cyclophosphamide with or without radiotherapy for patients with newly diagnosed low-risk rhabdomyosarcoma: a report from the Soft Tissue Sarcoma Committee of the Children's Oncology Group. *J. Clin. Oncol.*, **32** (31), 3547–3552.

229 Raney, R.B., Walterhouse, D.O., Meza, J.L., *et al.* (2011) Results of the Intergroup Rhabdomyosarcoma Study Group D9602 protocol, using vincristine and dactinomycin with or without cyclophosphamide and radiation therapy, for newly diagnosed patients with low-risk embryonal rhabdomyosarcoma: a report from the Soft Tissue Sarcoma Committee of the Children's Oncology Group. *J. Clin. Oncol.*, **29** (10), 1312–1318.

230 Raney, R.B., Maurer, H.M., Anderson, J.R., *et al.* (2001) The Intergroup Rhabdomyosarcoma Study Group (IRSG): Major lessons from the IRS-I through IRS-IV studies as background for the current IRS-V treatment protocols. *Sarcoma*, **5** (1), 9–15.

231 Childs, S.K., Kozak, K.R., Friedmann, A.M., *et al.* (2012) Proton radiotherapy for parameningeal rhabdomyosarcoma: clinical outcomes and late effects. *Int. J. Radiat. Oncol. Biol. Phys.*, **82** (2), 635–642.

232 Cotter, S.E., Herrup, D.A., Friedmann, A., *et al.* (2011) Proton radiotherapy for pediatric bladder/prostate rhabdomyosarcoma: clinical outcomes and dosimetry compared to intensity-modulated radiation therapy. *Int. J. Radiat. Oncol. Biol. Phys.*, **81** (5), 1367–1373.

233 Yock, T., Schneider, R., Friedmann, A., Adams, J., Fullerton, B., Tarbell, N. (2005) Proton radiotherapy for orbital rhabdomyosarcoma: clinical outcome and a dosimetric comparison with photons. *Int. J. Radiat. Oncol. Biol. Phys.*, **63** (4), 1161–1168.

234 Eaton, B.R., McDonald, M.W., Kim, S., *et al.* (2013) Radiation therapy target volume reduction in pediatric rhabdomyosarcoma: implications for patterns of disease recurrence and overall survival. *Cancer*, **119** (8), 1578–1585.

235 Walterhouse, D.O., Meza, J.L., Breneman, J.C., *et al.* (2011) Local control and outcome in children with localized vaginal rhabdomyosarcoma: a report from the Soft Tissue Sarcoma committee of the Children's Oncology Group. *Pediatr. Blood Cancer*, **57** (1), 76–83.

236 Malempati, S., Rodeberg, D.A., Donaldson, S.S., *et al.* (2011) Rhabdomyosarcoma in infants younger than 1 year: a report from the Children's Oncology Group. *Cancer*, **117** (15), 3493–3501.

237 Bradley, J. (2016) Radiotherapy in infant sarcoma: patterns of failure for infants enrolled on ARST 0331/0531. COG/ASTRO. 27 September, Boston Convention Center.

238 Kozak, K.R., Adams, J., Krejcarek, S.J., Tarbell, N.J., Yock, T.I. (2009) A dosimetric comparison of proton and intensity-modulated photon radiotherapy for pediatric parameningeal rhabdomyosarcomas. *Int. J. Radiat. Oncol. Biol. Phys.*, **74** (1), 179–186.

239 Ladra, M.M., Edgington, S.K., Mahajan, A., *et al.* (2014) A dosimetric comparison of proton and intensity modulated radiation therapy in pediatric rhabdomyosarcoma patients enrolled on a prospective phase II proton study. *Radiother. Oncol.*, **113** (1), 77–83.

240 Ries, L.A., *et al.* (1999) Cancer incidence and survival among children and adolescents: United States SEER Program 1975–1995. National Cancer Institute, SEER Program. Bethesda, Maryland.

241 Ferrari, A., Miceli, R., Rey, A., *et al.* (2011) Non-metastatic unresected paediatric non-rhabdomyosarcoma soft tissue sarcomas: results of a pooled analysis from United States and European groups. *Eur. J. Cancer*, **47** (5), 724–731.

242 Pratt, C.B., Pappo, A.S., Gieser, P., *et al.* (1999) Role of adjuvant chemotherapy in the treatment of surgically resected pediatric nonrhabdomyosarcomatous soft tissue sarcomas: A Pediatric Oncology Group Study. *J. Clin. Oncol.*, **17** (4), 1219.

243 Pratt, C.B., Maurer, H.M., Gieser, P., *et al.* (1998) Treatment of unresectable or metastatic pediatric soft tissue sarcomas with surgery, irradiation, and chemotherapy: a Pediatric Oncology Group study. *Med. Pediatr. Oncol.*, **30** (4), 201–209.

244 Pappo, A.S., Devidas, M., Jenkins, J., *et al.* (2005) Phase II trial of neoadjuvant vincristine, ifosfamide, and doxorubicin with granulocyte colony-stimulating factor support in children and adolescents with advanced-stage nonrhabdomyosarcomatous soft tissue sarcomas: a Pediatric Oncology Group Study. *J. Clin. Oncol.*, **23** (18), 4031–4038.

245 Hua, C., Gray, J.M., Merchant, T.E., Kun, L.E., Krasin, M.J. (2008) Treatment planning and delivery of external beam radiotherapy for pediatric sarcoma: the

St. Jude Children's Research Hospital experience. *Int. J. Radiat. Oncol. Biol. Phys.*, **70** (5), 1598–1606.

246 Smith, K.B., Indelicato, D.J., Knapik, J.A., *et al.* (2011) Adjuvant radiotherapy for pediatric and young adult nonrhabdomyosarcoma soft-tissue sarcoma. *Int. J. Radiat. Oncol. Biol. Phys.*, **81** (1), 150–157.

247 Ferrari, A., Trama, A., De Paoli, A., *et al.* (2016) Access to clinical trials for adolescents with soft tissue sarcomas: Enrollment in European pediatric Soft tissue Sarcoma Study Group (EpSSG) protocols. *Pediatr. Blood Cancer.* Epub ahead of print- Pediatr Blood Cancer. 2016 Nov 24. doi: 10.1002/pbc.26348. [Epub ahead of print] PMID:27882658.

248 Kager, L., Zoubek, A., Potschger, U., *et al.* (2003) Primary metastatic osteosarcoma: presentation and outcome of patients treated on neoadjuvant Cooperative Osteosarcoma Study Group protocols. *J. Clin. Oncol.*, **21** (10), 2011–2018.

249 Brenner, W., Bohuslavizki, K.H., Eary, J.F. (2003) PET imaging of osteosarcoma. *J. Nucl. Med.*, **44** (6), 930–942.

250 Enneking, W.F. (1988) A system of staging musculoskeletal neoplasms. *Instr. Course Lect.*, **37**, 3–10.

251 Davis, A.M., Bell, R.S., Goodwin, P.J. (1994) Prognostic factors in osteosarcoma: a critical review. *J. Clin. Oncol.*, **12** (2), 423–431.

252 Meyers, P.A., Schwartz, C.L., Krailo, M., *et al.* (2005) Osteosarcoma: a randomized, prospective trial of the addition of ifosfamide and/or muramyl tripeptide to cisplatin, doxorubicin, and high-dose methotrexate. *J. Clin. Oncol.*, **23** (9), 2004–2011.

253 Goorin, A.M. (1988) Adjuvant chemotherapy for osteogenic sarcoma. *Eur. J. Cancer Clin. Oncol.*, **24** (2), 113–115.

254 DeLaney, T.F., Liebsch, N.J., Pedlow, F.X., *et al.* (2009) Phase II study of high-dose photon/proton radiotherapy in the management of spine sarcomas. *Int. J. Radiat. Oncol. Biol. Phys.*, **74** (3), 732–739.

255 DeLaney, T.F., Trofimov, A.V., Engelsman, M., Suit, H.D. (2005) Advanced-technology radiation therapy in the management of bone and soft tissue sarcomas. *Cancer Control*, **12** (1), 27–35.

256 DeLaney, T.F., Park, L., Goldberg, S.I., *et al.* (2005) Radiotherapy for local control of osteosarcoma. *Int. J. Radiat. Oncol. Biol. Phys.*, **61** (2), 492–498.

257 Wagner, T.D., Kobayashi, W., Dean, S., *et al.* (2009) Combination short-course preoperative irradiation, surgical resection, and reduced-field high-dose postoperative irradiation in the treatment of tumors involving the bone. *Int. J. Radiat. Oncol. Biol. Phys.*, **73** (1), 259–266.

258 Machak, G.N., Tkachev, S.I., Solovyev, Y.N., *et al.* (2003) Neoadjuvant chemotherapy and local

radiotherapy for high-grade osteosarcoma of the extremities. *Mayo Clin. Proc.*, **78** (2), 147–155.

259 Ciernik, I.F., Niemierko, A., Harmon, D.C., *et al.* (2011) Proton-based radiotherapy for unresectable or incompletely resected osteosarcoma. *Cancer*, **117** (19), 4522–4530.

260 Hawkins, M.M., Wilson, L.M., Burton, H.S., *et al.* (1996) Radiotherapy, alkylating agents, and risk of bone cancer after childhood cancer. *J. Natl Cancer Inst.*, **88** (5), 270–278.

261 Kuttesch, J.F., Jr, Wexler, L.H., Marcus, R.B., *et al.* (1996) Second malignancies after Ewing's sarcoma: radiation dose-dependency of secondary sarcomas. *J. Clin. Oncol.*, **14** (10), 2818–2825.

262 Charest, M., Hickeson, M., Lisbona, R., Novales-Diaz, J.A., Derbekyan, V., Turcotte, R.E. (2009) FDG PET/CT imaging in primary osseous and soft tissue sarcomas: a retrospective review of 212 cases. *Eur. J. Nucl. Med. Mol. Imaging*, **36** (12), 1944–1951.

263 Kovar, H. (2005) Context matters: the hen or egg problem in Ewing's sarcoma. *Semin. Cancer Biol.*, **15** (3), 189–196.

264 Douglass, E.C., Valentine, M., Green, A.A., Hayes, F.A., Thompson, E.I. (1986) t(11;22) and other chromosomal rearrangements in Ewing's sarcoma. *J. Natl Cancer Inst.*, **77** (6), 1211–1215.

265 Wilkins, R.M., Pritchard, D.J., Burgert, E.O., Jr, Unni, K.K. (1986) Ewing's sarcoma of bone. Experience with 140 patients. *Cancer*, **58** (11), 2551–2555.

266 Leavey, P.J., Mascarenhas, L., Marina, N., *et al.* (2008) Prognostic factors for patients with Ewing sarcoma (EWS) at first recurrence following multi-modality therapy: A report from the Children's Oncology Group. *Pediatr. Blood Cancer*, **51** (3), 334–338.

267 Krasin, M.J., Rodriguez-Galindo, C., Davidoff, A.M., *et al.* (2004) Efficacy of combined surgery and irradiation for localized Ewings sarcoma family of tumors. *Pediatr. Blood Cancer*, **43** (3), 229–236.

268 Gobel, V., Jurgens, H., Etspuler, G., *et al.* (1987) Prognostic significance of tumor volume in localized Ewing's sarcoma of bone in children and adolescents. *J. Cancer Res. Clin. Oncol.*, **113** (2), 187–191.

269 Rombi, B., DeLaney, T.F., MacDonald, S.M., *et al.* (2012) Proton radiotherapy for pediatric Ewing's sarcoma: initial clinical outcomes. *Int. J. Radiat. Oncol. Biol. Phys.*, **82** (3), 1142–1148.

270 Barbieri, E., Emiliani, E., Zini, G., *et al.* (1990) Combined therapy of localized Ewing's sarcoma of bone: analysis of results in 100 patients. *Int. J. Radiat. Oncol. Biol. Phys.*, **19** (5), 1165–1170.

271 Yock, T.I., Krailo, M., Fryer, C.J., *et al.* (2006) Local control in pelvic Ewing sarcoma: analysis from

INT-0091 – a report from the Children's Oncology Group. *J. Clin. Oncol.*, **24** (24), 3838–3843.

272 Schuck, A., Ahrens, S., Paulussen, M., *et al.* (2003) Local therapy in localized Ewing tumors: results of 1058 patients treated in the CESS 81, CESS 86, and EICESS 92 trials. *Int. J. Radiat. Oncol. Biol. Phys.*, **55** (1), 168–177.

273 Donaldson, S.S., Torrey, M., Link, M.P., *et al.* (1998) A multidisciplinary study investigating radiotherapy in Ewing's sarcoma: end results of POG #8346. Pediatric Oncology Group. *Int. J. Radiat. Oncol. Biol. Phys.*, **42** (1), 125–135.

274 La, T.H., Meyers, P.A., Wexler, L.H., *et al.* (2006) Radiation therapy for Ewing's sarcoma: results from Memorial Sloan-Kettering in the modern era. *Int. J. Radiat. Oncol. Biol. Phys.*, **64** (2), 544–550.

275 Krasin, M.J., Rodriguez-Galindo, C., Billups, C.A., *et al.* (2004) Definitive irradiation in multidisciplinary management of localized Ewing sarcoma family of tumors in pediatric patients: outcome and prognostic factors. *Int. J. Radiat. Oncol. Biol. Phys.*, **60** (3), 830–838.

276 Womer, R.B., West, D.C., Krailo, M.D., *et al.* (2012) Randomized controlled trial of interval-compressed chemotherapy for the treatment of localized Ewing sarcoma: a report from the Children's Oncology Group. *J. Clin. Oncol.*, **30** (33), 4148–4154.

277 Rodriguez-Galindo, C., Navid, F., Liu, T., Billups, C.A., Rao, B.N., Krasin, M.J. (2008) Prognostic factors for local and distant control in Ewing sarcoma family of tumors. *Ann. Oncol.*, **19** (4), 814–820.

278 Erkizan, H.V., Scher, L.J., Gamble, S.E., *et al.* (2011) Novel peptide binds EWS-FLI1 and reduces the oncogenic potential in Ewing tumors. *Cell Cycle*, **10** (19), 3397–3408.

279 Boro, A., Pretre, K., Rechfeld, F., *et al.* (2012) Small-molecule screen identifies modulators of EWS/FLI1 target gene expression and cell survival in Ewing's sarcoma. *Int. J. Cancer*, **131** (9), 2153–2164.

280 Knudson, A.G., Jr (1971) Mutation and cancer: statistical study of retinoblastoma. *Proc. Natl Acad. Sci. USA*, **68** (4), 820–823.

281 Lee, W.H., Bookstein, R., Hong, F., Young, L.J., Shew, J.Y., Lee, E.Y. (1987) Human retinoblastoma susceptibility gene: cloning, identification, and sequence. *Science*, **235** (4794), 1394–1399.

282 Abramson, D.H., Servodidio, C.A. (1993) Retinoblastoma. *Optom. Clin.*, **3** (3), 49–61.

283 Blach, L.E., McCormick, B., Abramson, D.H., Ellsworth, R.M. (1994) Trilateral retinoblastoma – incidence and outcome: a decade of experience. *Int. J. Radiat. Oncol. Biol. Phys.*, **29** (4), 729–733.

284 Paulino, A.C. (1999) Trilateral retinoblastoma: is the location of the intracranial tumor important? *Cancer*, **86** (1), 135–141.

285 Chantada, G.L., Doz, F., Orjuela, M., *et al.* (2008) World disparities in risk definition and management of retinoblastoma: a report from the International Retinoblastoma Staging Working Group. *Pediatr. Blood Cancer*, **50** (3), 692–694.

286 Kim, J.W., Abramson, D.H., Dunkel, I.J. (2007) Current management strategies for intraocular retinoblastoma. *Drugs*, **67** (15), 2173–2185.

287 Klufas, M.A., Gobin, Y.P., Marr, B., Brodie, S.E., Dunkel, I.J., Abramson, D.H. (2012) Intra-arterial chemotherapy as a treatment for intraocular retinoblastoma: alternatives to direct ophthalmic artery catheterization. *Am. J. Neuroradiol.*, **33** (8), 1608–1614.

288 Orman, A., Koru-Sengul, T., Miao, F., Markoe, A., Panoff, J.E. (2014) The modern role of radiation therapy in treating advanced-stage retinoblastoma: long-term outcomes and racial differences. *Int. J. Radiat. Oncol. Biol. Phys.*, **90** (5), 1037–1043.

289 Hernandez, J.C., Brady, L.W., Shields, C.L., Shields, J.A., DePotter, P. (1993) Conservative treatment of retinoblastoma. The use of plaque brachytherapy. *Am. J. Clin. Oncol.*, **16** (5), 397–401.

290 ChildrensOncologyGroup.org. ARET0321. A trial of intensive multi-modality therapy for extra-ocular retinoblastoma. A group-wide phase III study. GALOP - Groupo America Latina de Oncologia Pediatrea (coordinating centers include Hospital de Pediatria Juan P. Garrahan, Buenos Aires, Argentina; Instituto de Oncologia Pediatrica/GRAAC Sao Paulo, Brazil) and Children's Cancer Hospital, El Saida Zenab, Egypt 57357. Activated 02-04-2008.

291 Lee, C.T., Bilton, S.D., Famiglietti, R.M., *et al.* (2005) Treatment planning with protons for pediatric retinoblastoma, medulloblastoma, and pelvic sarcoma: how do protons compare with other conformal techniques? *Int. J. Radiat. Oncol. Biol. Phys.*, **63** (2), 362–372.

292 Wong, F.L., Boice, J.D, Jr, Abramson, D.H., *et al.* (1997) Cancer incidence after retinoblastoma. Radiation dose and sarcoma risk. *JAMA*, **278** (15), 1262–1267.

293 Sethi, R.V., Shih, H.A., Yeap, B.Y., *et al.* (2014) Second nonocular tumors among survivors of retinoblastoma treated with contemporary photon and proton radiotherapy. *Cancer*, **120** (1), 126–133.

294 Geenen, M.M., Cardous-Ubbink, M.C., Kremer, L.C., *et al.* (2007) Medical assessment of adverse health outcomes in long-term survivors of childhood cancer. *JAMA*, **297** (24), 2705–2715.

Index